AF705439

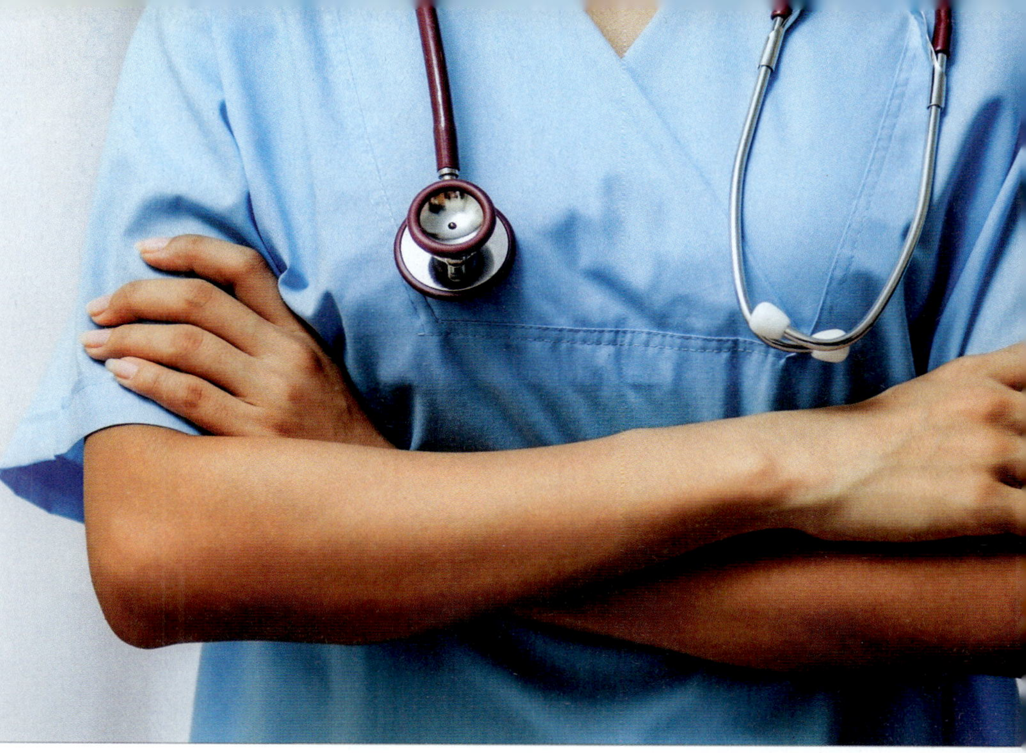

94%

of students said Davis Advantage improved their test scores

Personalized Learning

Unlock your personalized path to success with a custom learning plan based on your strengths and weaknesses. Dynamic interactive exercises bring concepts to life to help you master key topics.

Clinical Judgment

Strengthen your clinical reasoning skills with Next Gen NCLEX®-style case studies featuring complex patient situations that challenge you to apply your knowledge, make informed decisions, and evaluate outcomes.

Quizzing

Assess your understanding of course content with NCLEX®-style questions and detailed rationales. Complete assignments or create your own practice quizzes to further test your knowledge.

Simulations

Practice clinical judgment in a safe space while also earning clinical hours. Realistic video-based simulations challenge you to make clinical decisions and know the proper technique for any intervention.

eBook

Reference your text anywhere, anytime to complete readings and study for exams. Add notes, highlights, and bookmarks.

READY TO GET STARTED?

Scan the code below for step-by-step instructions

FOR INSTRUCTORS

Health Assessment & Physical Examination

SIXTH EDITION

Mary Ellen Zator Estes, MSN, APRN, FNP-BC, FNP-C, FAANP
Family Nurse Practitioner in Internal Medicine,
Fairfax, Virginia *and* Nurse Consultant
Vienna, Virginia

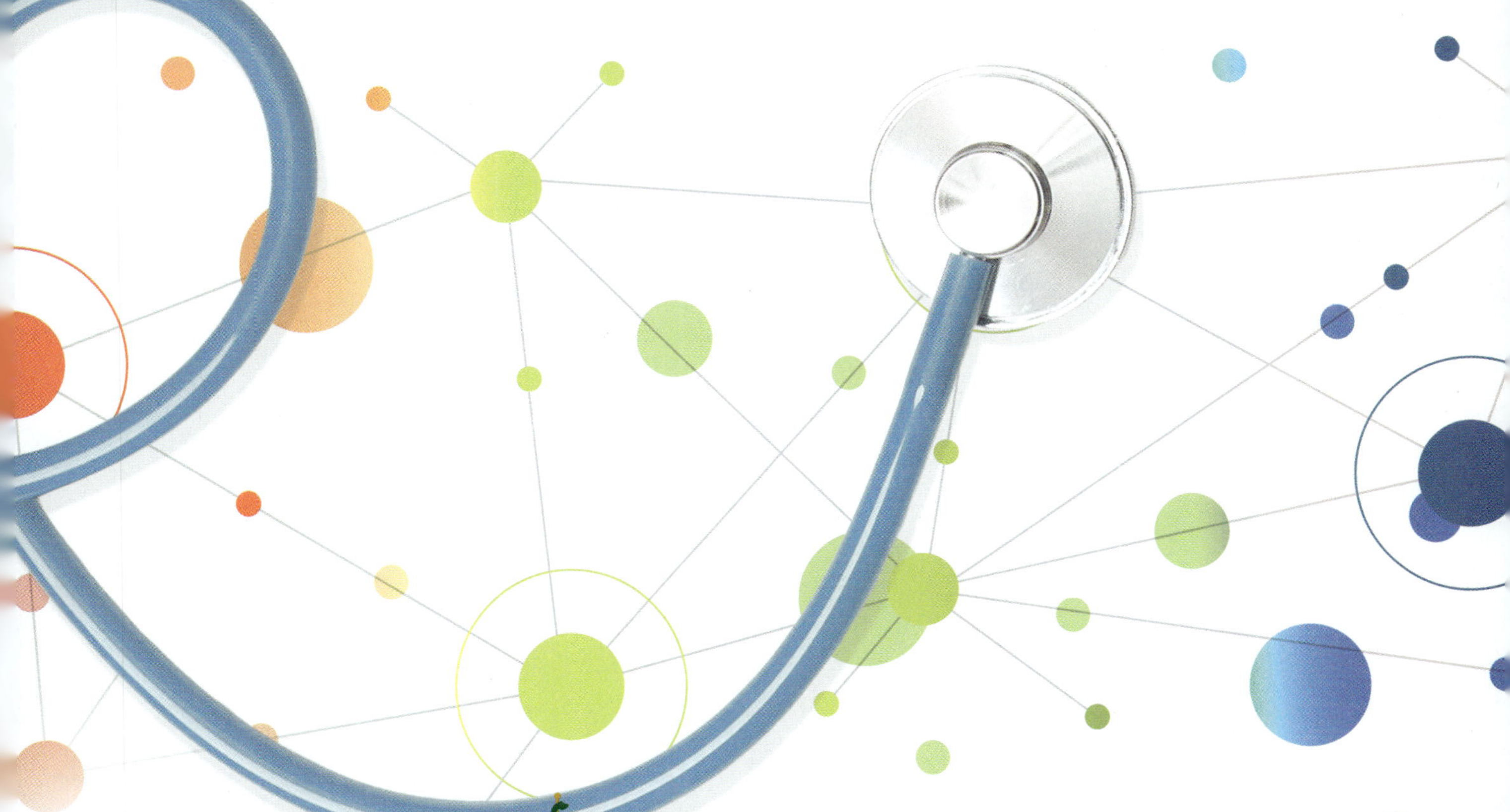

F.A. DAVIS
Philadelphia

F. A. Davis Company
1915 Arch Street
Philadelphia, PA 19103
www.fadavis.com

Copyright © 2027 by F. A. Davis Company

Copyright © 2027 by F. A. Davis Company. All rights reserved. This book is protected by copyright. No part of it may be reproduced, stored in a retrieval system, or transmitted in any form or by any means, electronic, mechanical, photocopying, recording, or otherwise, without written permission from the publisher.

Printed in the United States of America

Last digit indicates print number: 10 9 8 7 6 5 4 3 2 1

Acquisitions Editor: Haleahy Craven
Director of Project Management: Catherine Carroll
Content Project Manager 2: Sean West
Digital Asset and eBook Manager: Alison Enright
Senior Manager of Art and Design: Carolyn O'Brien

As new scientific information becomes available through basic and clinical research, recommended treatments and drug therapies undergo changes. The author(s) and publisher have done everything possible to make this book accurate, up to date, and in accord with accepted standards at the time of publication. The author(s), editors, and publisher are not responsible for errors or omissions or for consequences from application of the book, and make no warranty, expressed or implied, in regard to the contents of the book. Any practice described in this book should be applied by the reader in accordance with professional standards of care used in regard to the unique circumstances that may apply in each situation. The reader is advised always to check product information (package inserts) for changes and new information regarding dose and contraindications before administering any drug. Caution is especially urged when using new or infrequently ordered drugs.

Library of Congress Cataloging-in-Publication Data is available upon request.

Authorization to photocopy items for internal or personal use, or the internal or personal use of specific clients, is granted by F. A. Davis Company for users registered with the Copyright Clearance Center (CCC) Transactional Reporting Service, provided that the fee of $.25 per copy is paid directly to CCC, 222 Rosewood Drive, Danvers, MA 01923. For those organizations that have been granted a photocopy license by CCC, a separate system of payment has been arranged. The fee code for users of the Transactional Reporting Service is: 978-1-7196-5314-5/27 0 +$.25

Health Assessment & Physical Examination, sixth edition, is dedicated to my family for their continued love and support, most especially my husband of 41 years, Matthew.

And to...

The next generation of nurses who will navigate an evolving and challenging health care environment with the proliferation of artificial intelligence and scientific advances.

Yesterday is gone. Tomorrow has not yet come. We have only today. Let us begin.
-Mother Teresa

Brief Table of Contents

Contributors xvii

Reviewers xviii

Preface xix

Acknowledgments xxv

About the Author xxvii

Unit 1 Laying the Foundation 1

CHAPTER 1 **Critical Thinking and Clinical Reasoning in Nursing 2**

CHAPTER 2 **Communication Techniques and the Client Interview 20**

CHAPTER 3 **The Complete Health History Including Documentation 46**

Unit 2 Special Assessments 91

CHAPTER 4 **Developmental Assessment 92**

CHAPTER 5 **Cultural Assessment 121**

CHAPTER 6 **Spiritual Assessment 140**

CHAPTER 7 **Nutritional Assessment 157**

Unit 3 Physical Examination 197

CHAPTER 8 **Physical Examination Techniques 198**

CHAPTER 9 **General Survey, Vital Signs, and Pain 219**

CHAPTER 10 **Skin, Hair, and Nails 252**

CHAPTER 11 **Head, Neck, and Regional Lymph Nodes 298**

CHAPTER 12 **Eyes 319**

CHAPTER 13 **Ears, Nose, Mouth, and Throat 354**

CHAPTER 14 **Breasts and Regional Lymph Nodes 392**

CHAPTER 15 **Thorax and Lungs 417**

CHAPTER 16 **Heart 463**

CHAPTER 17 **Peripheral Vasculature System and Lymphatic System 502**

CHAPTER 18 **Abdomen 533**

CHAPTER 19 **Musculoskeletal System 573**

CHAPTER 20 **Mental Status and Neurological System 637**

CHAPTER 21 **Female Genitalia 695**

CHAPTER 22 **Male Genitalia 735**

CHAPTER 23 **Anus, Rectum, and Prostate 763**

Unit 4 Special Populations 783

CHAPTER 24 **The Pregnant Client 784**

CHAPTER 25 **The Pediatric Client 823**

CHAPTER 26 **The Older Adult Client 889**

Unit 5 Putting It All Together 927

CHAPTER 27 **The Complete Health History and Physical Examination 928**

APPENDIX A: Functional Assessments 954

APPENDIX B: Abbreviations 956

GLOSSARY 962

INDEX 981

Contents

Contributors xvii

Reviewers xviii

Preface xix

Acknowledgments xxv

About the Author xxvii

Unit 1 Laying the Foundation 1

CHAPTER 1 **Critical Thinking and Clinical Reasoning in Nursing 2**

Critical Thinking, Clinical Reasoning, and Clinical Judgment 3
- Components of Critical Thinking 3
- Universal Intellectual Standards for Critical Thinking 4

Critical Thinking Frameworks: The Nursing Process and the NCJMM 5
- The Nursing Process 6
- The Nursing Clinical Judgment Measurement Model (NCJMM) 13

Standardized Verbal Communication or Hand-off 16
- SBAR 17

Written Documentation 18

Assessment in Brief 18

CHAPTER 2 **Communication Techniques and the Client Interview 20**

The Client Interview 20
- The Role of the Nurse 21
- The Role of the Client 21
- Motivational Interviewing 21

Factors Influencing the Interview 22
- Approach 22
- Environment 22
- Confidentiality 23
- HIPAA 23
- Note Taking 23
- Time, Length, Duration 24
- Self-Awareness 24

Stages of the Interview Process 24
- Stage I 24
- Stage II 24
- Stage III 24

Factors Affecting Communication 25
- Listening 25
- Nonverbal Cues 25
- Distance 25
- Personal Space 26

Effective Communication Techniques 26
- Using Open-Ended Questions 26
- Using Closed Questions 27
- Facilitating 27
- Using Silence 27
- Grouping Communication Techniques 27

Nontherapeutic Communication Techniques 32
- Requesting an Explanation 32
- Probing 33
- Offering False Reassurance 33
- Giving Approval or Disapproval 34
- Defending 34
- Advising 35
- Using Problematic Questioning Techniques 35

Sexual and Gender Minorities 37

Interviewing the Client with Differing Abilities 38
- The Client Who Is Deaf or Hard-of-Hearing 39
- The Client Who Is Visually Impaired 39
- The Client Who Has a Speech Impairment or Aphasia 39
- The Client Who Is Illiterate/Has a Low Literacy Level 40
- The Client Who Is Non-English-Speaking 40
- The Client Who Has a Low Level of Understanding 41
- The Client Who Is Crying 41
- The Client Who Is Anxious or Angry 41
- The Client Who Is Hostile 42
- The Client Who Is Sexually Aggressive 42
- The Client Who Is Under the Influence of Alcohol or Drugs 42
- The Client Who Is Very Ill 42

Telehealth and Telenursing 43

Assessment in Brief 43

CHAPTER 3 **The Complete Health History Including Documentation 46**
Types of Health History 47
Preparing for the Health History 47
Computerized Health History 47
Advance Medical Directive 48
The Complete Health History 48
Today's Date 48
Biographical Data 48
Source and Reliability of Information 49
Client Profile 49
Reason for Seeking Health Care and Chief Complaint 49
Present Health and History of the Present Illness 49
Past Health History 52
Family Health History 59
Social History 61
Health Maintenance Activities 71
Review of Systems 74
The System-Specific Health History 76
Assistive Devices 77
Concluding the Health History 77
Documentation 77
General Documentation Guidelines 77
Documentation Guidelines for Handwritten Client Records 78
Examination-Specific Documentation Guidelines 78
U.S. Preventive Services Task Force 79
ENAP Format 80
Case Study: Complete Health History: Well Client 80
Case Study: Complete Health History: Ill Client 84

Unit 2 Special Assessments 91

CHAPTER 4 **Developmental Assessment 92**
Developmental Theories 92
Ages and Stages Developmental Theories 93
Assessment in Brief 100
Developmental Stages, Tasks, and Life Events 101
Developmental Tasks of Infants (Birth to 1 Year) 102
Developmental Tasks of Toddlers (1 to 3 Years) 104
Developmental Tasks of Preschoolers (3 to 6 Years) 105
Developmental Tasks of School-Age Children (6 to 12 Years) 106
Developmental Tasks of Adolescents (12 to 18 Years) 107
Developmental Tasks of Young Adults (18 to 30 Years) 108
Developmental Tasks of Early Middle Adulthood (30 to 50 Years) 109
Developmental Tasks of Late Middle Adulthood (50 to 70 Years) 110
Developmental Tasks of Late Adulthood (70 Years to Death) 111
Stages of Family Development 112
Developmental Assessment Tools 112
SARS-CoV2 (COVID-19) Effects on Growth and Development 116
Case Study: Ineffective Coping After Divorce 116

CHAPTER 5 **Cultural Assessment 121**
Culture 121
Cultural Diversity in the United States 122
Assessment in Brief 123
Cultural Awareness 123
Cultural Congruence 123
Defining Cultural Identity 125
Subculture 125
The Core Elements of Culture 127
Racial Prejudice, Ethnic Discrimination, and Stereotyping 129
Value Orientations 129
Cultural Health Beliefs 130
Ethnic Customs and Cultural Rituals 133
Culturally Competent Assessment 134
Cultural Assessment 134
Case Study: A Vietnamese Au Pair With Dysmenorrhea 135

CHAPTER 6 **Spiritual Assessment 140**
Religion and Spirituality in the United States 140
Religion and Spirituality 141
The Health Effects of Religion and Spirituality 143
Role of the Nurse in Spiritual Care 144
Assessment in Brief 145
Spiritual Assessment 145
Nursing Interventions to Promote Spiritual Well-Being 147

Nursing Interventions to Avoid 151
Evaluation 152
COVID-19 Effects on Spirituality and Religiosity 152
Case Study: Parents Demand Treatment Changes for Their Transgender Child 153

CHAPTER 7 **Nutritional Assessment 157**
Dietary Guidelines 158
Nutrients 158
Carbohydrates 159
Proteins 160
Fats 160
Vitamins 161
Minerals 163
Water 166
Nutrition Through the Life Cycle 167
Children 167
Adolescents 170
Young and Middle-Aged Adults 171
Older Adults 173
Cultural Differences 174
Assessment in Brief 177
Equipment 177
Nutritional Assessment 177
The Nutritional History 177
Physical Examination 179
Anthropometric Measurements 179
Laboratory Data 185
Diagnostic Data 191
Case Study: The Underweight Client 192

Unit 3 Physical Examination 197

CHAPTER 8 **Physical Examination Techniques 198**
General Aspects of Physical Examination 198
Role of the Nurse 199
Standard Precautions 199
Transmission-Based Precautions 203
Equipment 203
Steps for Conducting a Physical Examination 205
Preparing for a Physical Examination 205
Conducting a Physical Examination 206
Ending the Visit 207
Physical Examination Techniques 207
Assessment in Brief 209
Inspection 209
Palpation 209
Percussion 212
Auscultation 215
Legal Considerations 216
Golden Rules for Physical Examination 216

CHAPTER 9 **General Survey, Vital Signs, and Pain 219**
General Survey 219
Assessment in Brief 220
Equipment 220
Physical Presence 220
Psychological Presence 223
Distress 224
Vital Signs 225
Respiration 225
Pulse 226
Temperature 230
Blood Pressure 234
Korotkoff Sounds 235
Measuring Blood Pressure 235
Measurement Sites 236
Equipment 236
Manual Blood Pressure Measurement 236
Automatic Blood Pressure Measurement 237
Pain 241
Types of Pain 242
Source of Pain 243
Duration of Pain 244
Perception of Pain 244
Variables Affecting Pain 244
Pain Health History 245
History of Present Illness 245
Past Health History 245
Family Health History 246
Social History 246
Health Maintenance Activities 247
Effects of Pain on the Body 247
Assessing Pain 247
Pain Management 248
The Opioid Crisis 249

CHAPTER 10 **Skin, Hair, and Nails 252**
Anatomy and Physiology 252
Skin 252
Hair 255
Nails 255
Function of Skin 256
Function of Hair and Nails 256

Assessment in Brief 261
Equipment 261
Examination of the Skin, Hair, and Nails 261
Inspection of the Skin 261
Palpation of the Skin 283
Inspection of the Hair 286
Palpation of the Hair 288
Inspection of the Nails 289
Palpation of the Nails 293
Case Study: The Client With a Lip Lesion 293

CHAPTER 11 **Head, Neck, and Regional Lymph Nodes 298**
Anatomy and Physiology 298
Skull 298
Face 298
Neck 299
Thyroid 299
Lymph Nodes 300
Blood Supply 300
Assessment in Brief 304
Equipment 304
Examination of the Head and Neck 304
Inspection of the Shape of the Head 304
Palpation of the Head 305
Inspection and Palpation of the Scalp 305
Inspection of the Face 306
Palpation and Auscultation of the Mandible 307
Inspection and Palpation of the Neck 308
Inspection of the Thyroid Gland 309
Palpation of the Thyroid Gland 310
Auscultation of the Thyroid Gland 312
Inspection of the Lymph Nodes 313
Palpation of the Lymph Nodes 313
Case Study: The Client With a Thyroid Nodule 315

CHAPTER 12 **Eyes 319**
Anatomy and Physiology 319
External Structures 319
Internal Structures 321
Visual Pathway 322
Assessment in Brief 326
Equipment 326
Examination of the Eye 326
Visual Acuity 326
Visual Fields 329
External Eye and Lacrimal Apparatus 330
Extraocular Muscle Function 334
Anterior Segment Structures 336
Posterior Segment Structures 343
Case Study: The Client With a Stye, Conjunctivitis, and Diabetic Retinopathy 349

CHAPTER 13 **Ears, Nose, Mouth, and Throat 354**
Anatomy and Physiology 354
Ear 354
Nose 356
Sinuses 357
Mouth and Throat 358
Assessment in Brief 364
Equipment 364
Examination of the Ear 364
Auditory Screening 364
External Ear 366
Otoscopic Examination 368
Examination of the Nose 373
External Inspection 373
Patency 373
Internal Inspection 373
Examination of the Sinuses 375
Inspection 375
Palpation and Percussion 375
Examination of the Mouth and Throat 376
Examination of the Mouth 377
Inspection of the Throat 385
Case Study: The Client With Streptococcal Pharyngitis 387

CHAPTER 14 **Breasts and Regional Lymph Nodes 392**
Anatomy and Physiology 393
Breasts 393
Regional Lymph Nodes 394
Breast Development Throughout the Life Span 395
Assessment in Brief 400
Equipment 400
Examination of the Female Breasts and Regional Lymph Nodes 401
Inspection 401
Palpation 405
Examination of the Client Who Has Undergone a Mastectomy and Breast-Augmentation 409

The Male Breasts 411
Anatomy 411
Breast Cancer Screening in Men 411
Examination of the Male Breasts 412
Case Study: The Client With a Breast Mass 412

CHAPTER 15 **Thorax and Lungs 417**
Anatomy 417
Thorax 417
Sternum 417
Ribs 418
Intercostal Spaces 419
Lungs 419
Pleura 421
Mediastinum 421
Bronchi 421
Alveoli 421
Muscles of Respiration 422
Physiology 422
Ventilation 422
External Respiration 423
Internal Respiration 423
Control of Breathing 423
Assessment in Brief 427
Equipment 428
Examination of the Thorax and Lungs 428
Inspection 428
Palpation 439
Percussion 444
Auscultation 446
Case Study: The Client With COVID-19 and Pneumonia 458

CHAPTER 16 **Heart 463**
Anatomy and Physiology 463
Heart 463
Coronary Circulation 465
Cardiac Cycle 467
Conduction System of the Heart 468
Assessment in Brief 483
Equipment 482
Examination of the Precordium 482
Inspection 484
Palpation 486
Auscultation 489
Case Study: The Client With Cardiac Tamponade 496

CHAPTER 17 **Peripheral Vasculature System and Lymphatic System 502**
Anatomy and Physiology 502
Peripheral Vascular System 502
Lymphatic System 503
Assessment in Brief 512
Equipment 512
Examination of the Peripheral Vasculature 513
Inspection of the Jugular Venous Pressure 513
Inspection of the Hepatojugular Reflux 515
Palpation and Auscultation of Arterial Pulses 516
Inspection and Palpation of Peripheral Perfusion 518
Inspection and Palpation of Lymph Nodes 525
Inspection and Palpation of Epitrochlear Lymph Nodes 525
Inspection and Palpation of Inguinal Lymph Nodes 526
Inspection and Palpation of Popliteal Lymph Nodes 526
Case Study: The Client With Leg Claudication 527

CHAPTER 18 **Abdomen 533**
Anatomy and Physiology 533
Abdominal Cavity 533
Abdominal Viscera (Organs) 535
Assessment in Brief 546
Equipment 546
Examination of the Abdomen 546
Inspection 546
Auscultation 550
Percussion 552
Palpation 558
Case Study: The Client With Pancreatitis 567

CHAPTER 19 **Musculoskeletal System 573**
Anatomy and Physiology 573
Bones 574
Muscles 574
Tendons 574
Cartilage 574
Ligaments 575
Bursae 575
Joints 576

Assessment in Brief 582
Equipment 583
Examination of the Musculoskeletal System 583
General Assessment 583
Inspection 587
Palpation 591
Range of Motion (ROM) 594
Muscle Strength 595
Examination of Joints 596
Case Study: The Client With Acute Shoulder Pain 632

CHAPTER 20 **Mental Status and Neurological System 637**
Anatomy and Physiology 637
Macrostructure 637
Meninges 637
Central Nervous System 638
Blood Supply 641
Peripheral Nervous System 643
Reflexes 645
Assessment in Brief 651
Equipment 651
Examination of the Neurological System 652
Mental Status 652
Sensory Examination 668
Cranial Nerves 672
Motor System 679
Cerebellar Function (Coordination, Station, and Gait) 679
Reflexes 682
Case Study: The Client With Numbness in the Hands and Feet 689

CHAPTER 21 **Female Genitalia 695**
Anatomy and Physiology 695
External Female Genitalia 695
Internal Female Genitalia 697
The Female Reproductive Cycle 699
Assessment in Brief 707
Equipment 707
Examination of the Female Genitalia 708
Inspection of the External Genitalia 708
Palpation of the External Genitalia 715
Speculum Examination of the Internal Genitalia 717
Collecting Specimens for Cytological Smears and Cultures 722
Inspection of the Vaginal Wall 726
Bimanual Examination 727
Rectovaginal Examination 729
Case Study: The Client With Atrophic Vaginitis 731

CHAPTER 22 **Male Genitalia 735**
Anatomy and Physiology 735
Essential Organs 735
Accessory Organs 736
Ducts 736
Supporting Structures 737
Sexual Development 737
Spermatogenesis 737
Male Sexual Function 738
Assessment in Brief 742
Equipment 742
Examination of the Male Genitalia 743
Inspection 743
Palpation 751
Auscultation 756
Case Study: The Client With a Penile Lump and Peyronie Disease 759

CHAPTER 23 **Anus, Rectum, and Prostate 763**
Anatomy and Physiology 763
Rectum 763
Anus 763
Prostate 765
Assessment in Brief 768
Equipment 768
Examination of the Anus, Rectum, and Prostate 769
Inspection 769
Palpation 773
Case Study: A Client With an Enlarged Prostate and Hemorrhoid 778

Unit 4 Special Populations 783

CHAPTER 24 **The Pregnant Client 784**
Anatomy and Physiology 784
Skin and Hair 785
Head and Neck 785
Eyes, Ears, Nose, Mouth, and Throat 785
Breasts 786
Thorax and Lungs 786
Heart 786
Peripheral Vasculature 787
Abdomen 788
Urinary System 788

Musculoskeletal System 788
Neurological System 789
Female Genitalia 789
Anus and Rectum 790
Hematological System 791
Endocrine System 791
Assessment in Brief 798
Equipment 798
Examination of the Pregnant Client 798
General Assessment, Vital Signs, Height, and Weight 798
Skin and Hair 803
Head and Neck 804
Eyes, Ears, Nose, Mouth, and Throat 804
Breasts 804
Thorax and Lungs 805
Heart 805
Peripheral Vasculature 805
Abdomen 805
Urinary System 806
Musculoskeletal System 807
Neurological System 807
Female Genitalia 807
Uterine Size 809
Fetal Heart Tone 809
Leopold Maneuver 811
Anus, Perineum, and Rectum 813
Hematological System 813
Endocrine System 813
Nutritional Assessment 813
Special Antepartum Tests and Evaluations 813
Psychosocial Assessment and Learning Needs 813
Subsequent or Return Prenatal Visits 816
Case Study: The Pregnant Client 818

CHAPTER 25 **The Pediatric Client 823**
Physical Growth 823
Anatomy and Physiology 830
Structural and Physiological Variations 830
Growth and Development 840
Developmental Assessment 840
Assessment in Brief 843
Equipment 843
Physical Examination 844
Vital Signs 844
Physical Growth 845
Apgar Scoring 847
Skin 848
Hair 851
Head 851
Eyes 853
Ears 858
Nose 859
Mouth and Throat 859
Neck 861
Breasts 862
Thorax and Lungs 862
Heart 864
Peripheral Vasculature 868
Abdomen 868
Musculoskeletal System 870
Neurological System 873
Female Genitalia 877
Male Genitalia 879
Anus 881
COVID-19 Effects on the Pediatric Client 882
Case Study: The Client With Ear Pain and a Hydrocele 883

CHAPTER 26 **The Older Adult Client 889**
Epidemiology 889
Variations in Presentation 890
Anatomy and Physiology 891
Structural and Physiological Variations 891
Interview of the Older Adult 898
Special Assessments 900
Developmental Assessment 900
Cultural Assessment 901
Spiritual Assessment 901
Geriatric Syndromes 901
Self-Determination Assessment 903
Palliative Care 904
Assessment in Brief 905
Equipment 905
Physical Examination 905
Functional Assessment 906
Cognitive Assessment 907
Vital Signs 907
Skin 910
Hair 911
Nails 911
Head and Neck 911
Eyes 912
Ears 913
Nose 914
Mouth and Throat 914
Breasts 914
Thorax and Lungs 915
Heart 915
Peripheral Vasculature 915

Abdomen 915
Musculoskeletal System 915
Mental Status and Neurological System 916
Female Genitalia 917
Male Genitalia 918
Anus, Rectum, and Prostate 918

Case Study: The Older Adult With Pneumonia and Altered Mental Status 920

Unit 5 Putting It All Together 927

CHAPTER 27 **The Complete Health History and Physical Examination 928**

Legal Considerations 929
Ethical Considerations 929
Electronic Health Records 930
Advances in Technology 930
Artificial Intelligence 931
Health History 932
Physical Examination 932
General Survey 933
Measurements 933
Neurological System 933
Skin 934
Head and Face 934
Eyes 934
Ears 935
Nose and Sinuses 935
Mouth and Throat 935
Neck 935
Upper Extremities 936
Back, Posterior and Lateral Thoraxes 936
Anterior Thorax 936
Heart 936
Female Breasts 936
Male Breasts 937
Jugular Veins 937
Female and Male Breasts 937
Heart 937
Abdomen 937
Inguinal Area 938
Lower Extremities 938
Neurological System 938
Musculoskeletal System 939
Neurological System 939
Female Genitalia, Anus, and Rectum 939
Male Genitalia 939
Male Anus, Rectum, and Prostate 939
Laboratory and Diagnostic Data 940
Problem List 940
Long COVID and Worldwide Pandemic 941
Preparticipation Athletic Evaluation 942
Healthy People 2030 943
The Future of Nursing 943
Conclusion 944
Case Study: The Client With Multisystem Problems 945

APPENDIX A: Functional Assessments: Instrumental Activities of Daily Living (IADLs) and Physical Self-Maintenance Activities 954

APPENDIX B: Abbreviations 956

GLOSSARY 962

INDEX 981

Contributors

Deirdre Carolan, PhD, ANP-BC, GNP-BC, CNS, FAANP, DEGN
VANAP Project Manager
Director of AGNP Program
Clinical Assistant Professor Conway School of Nursing
The Catholic University of America
Washington, DC
Nurse Practitioner, Geriatrics and Clinical Nurse Specialist, Geriatrics
Inova Fairfax Hospital
Falls Church, Virginia

Helen Crowe, AM. RN, BAppSci, GDip Epi Biostats, MNursSci
Urology Nurse Practitioner
Melbourne, Victoria,
Australia

Tammi L. Damas, PhD, MBA, WHNP-BC
Director of Education & Academic Affairs
Office of the Provost
Georgetown University
Washington, DC

Tracy Davidson, DNP, MPH, PMHNP-BC
Associate Professor
Accelerated BSN Program Director School of Nursing
George Mason University
Fairfax, Virginia

Barbara Springer Edwards, RN, BSN, MTS
Clinician, Sweeten Creek Mental Health and Wellness
Asheville, North Carolina
Former Director of Nursing Care
Cardiac Surgical Unit
INOVA Alexandria Hospital
Alexandria, Virginia

Nicole Goitia, MSN, AGPCNP-BC
Nurse Practitioner, Gastroenterology
Denver, Colorado

Constance C. Kozachek, PhD, MSN, NPD-BC, CCRN
Associate Dean
RWJBarnabas Health
Trinitas School of Nursing
Elizabeth Campus
Elizabeth, New Jersey

Robbie McCauley, DNP, APRN, FNP-BC, NEA-BC, CNE
Associate Dean of Graduate Programs
Assistant Professor
Eleanor Wade Custer School of Nursing
Shenandoah University
Leesburg, Virginia

Jessica Olsen, DNP, CNM, WHNP-BC, FACNM
Certified Nurse-Midwife, Women's Health Nurse Practitioner
Obstetrics and Gynecology
Orlando, Florida

Susanne Quallich, PhD, ANP-BC, NP-C, CUNP, CMHE, FAUNA, FAANP
Assistant Professor of Urology
Andrology Nurse Practitioner
Division of Men's Health and Reconstruction
Department of Urology, Michigan Medicine
University of Michigan
Ann Arbor, Michigan

Whitney Hodges Shanley, DNP, MSN-Ed, APRN, FNP-BC
Assistant Professor
School of Nursing
The George Washington University
Ashburn, Virginia

Sharon R. Simon, DNP, APRN, FNP-C, PMHNP-C, CNE
Director, Family Nurse Practitioner Program
Associate Professor
Eleanor Wade Custer School of Nursing
Shenandoah University
Leesburg, Virginia

Catherine C. Tierney, RN, DNP, ACNP-BC
Associate Professor
Director, AG-ACNP Program
School of Nursing
Georgetown University
Washington, DC

Jennifer M. Walsh, DNP, CPNP-PC, CNE
Pediatric Nurse Practitioner, Primary Care
Clinical Assistant Professor
School of Nursing
The George Washington University
Washington, DC

Michael E. Zychowicz, DNP, ANP, ONP, FAAN, FAANP, FNAON
Clinical Professor of Nursing
Director, Orthopedic NP Specialty
Director, Veterans' Health Care Specialty
School of Nursing
Duke University
Durhan, North Carolina

REVIEWERS

Deirdre Conroy, DNP, APN, NP-C
Assistant Teaching Professor
Rutgers University, Camden, School of Nursing
Camden, New Jersey

Karen Diane Groller, PhD, RN, CV-BC, CMSRN
Associate Professor of Nursing and Public Health
Moravian University
Bethlehem, Pennsylvania

Taryn Hill, PhD, MPH, MSN, RN
Senior Director of Curriculum and Learning
Arizona College of Nursing
Phoenix, Arizona

Patricia Newton, DNP, RN, APN, FNP-BC, RNC-OB
Assistant Professor II
Rowan College of South Jersey
Vineland, New Jersey

Tasha Pfenning, MSN, RN
Assistant Professor Undergraduate Nursing/Skills Lab Coordinator
Bryan College of Health Sciences
Lincoln, Nebraska

Jennifer Rice, DNP, APRN, AGNP-C, ACHPN
Assistant Clinical Professor
University of Memphis, Lambuth
Jackson, Tennessee

Camden Seal, PhD, MSN-Ed, RN
Director of Curriculum and Instruction
Arizona College of Nursing
Gahanna, Ohio

Chasya Wiseman, DNP, MSN-Ed, RN
Curriculum and Instruction Specialist
Arizona College of Nursing
Phoenix, Arizona

Preface

Health assessment and physical examination comprise the foundation of all nursing care. Assessment is an ongoing process that evaluates the whole person as a physical, psychosocial, and functional being, whether the client is young or old, well or ill. ***Health Assessment & Physical Examination,*** sixth edition, provides an extensive illustrated approach to the process of holistic assessment, including health assessment, physical examination skills, advanced techniques, disease risk assessments, assistive device assessments, and client teaching guidelines.

Nursing students will welcome the text's clear presentation as they learn comprehensive health assessment and physical examination skills. Practicing and experienced nurses will find the book valuable as a review of the pathophysiological basis for abnormal findings and a quick reference to polish up on forgotten or seldom used examination techniques.

Nurses are privileged and challenged to care for individuals of all races, ethnicities, cultural backgrounds, religions, beliefs, and nationalities. Many times, nurses interface with individuals when they are most vulnerable due to their health status. The sixth edition of this text recognizes the evolution of the American society and provides inclusive language that is respectful to all, wherever the client may be on the health/illness continuum. Nurses are challenged to be self-aware of any personal biases or misconceptions so that holistic, caring, and evidence-based care is delivered. In other words, respect and dignity for all human life is modeled in the following pages.

Conceptual Approach

This text presents comprehensive content to educate the reader on how to assess a client in a holistic manner by incorporating physical, psychological, social, emotional, developmental, cultural, spiritual, nutritional, and functional elements. The skills of interviewing, inspection, palpation, percussion, auscultation, and documentation are thoroughly presented to guide readers on making clinical assessments and judgments to promote positive client outcomes.

The need for ***Health Assessment & Physical Examination***, sixth edition, arises from the necessity to present a comprehensive, straightforward, well-organized examination textbook that can be easily read and assimilated. The goals that form the foundation of this text are empowering readers as educated decision makers, developing their skills of analysis, critical thinking, and clinical reasoning while conducting a health assessment and physical examination on clients of all ages.

Health Assessment & Physical Examination, sixth edition, embraces a dual focus based on nursing as the art and science of caring. Strong emphasis on science encompasses all the technical aspects of anatomy and physiology, and examination, while highlighting clinically relevant information. Emphasis on the art of nursing and caring is displayed through themes of assessment of the whole person; developmental, cultural, spiritual, familial, and environmental considerations; client dignity; and health promotion. This approach encourages nursing students and practicing nurses to conduct a self-evaluation that leads to appropriate health care in a client-centered environment.

Health Assessment & Physical Examination, sixth edition, offers a user-friendly approach that delivers a wealth of information. The consistent, easy-to-follow format with recurring pedagogical features is based on two frameworks:

1. The **IPPA** method of examination (**I**nspection, **P**alpation, **P**ercussion, **A**uscultation) is consistently applied to body systems for a complete, detailed physical examination.
2. The **ENAP** format (**E**xamination, **N**ormal Findings, **A**bnormal Findings, **P**athophysiology) is followed for every IPPA technique, providing a useful and valuable collection of information. Pathophysiology is included for each abnormal finding, acknowledging that nurses' clinical decisions must be based on scientific rationale.

Readers of ***Health Assessment & Physical Examination***, sixth edition, need an understanding of anatomy and physiology, as well as a familiarity with basic nursing skills.

Organization

Health Assessment & Physical Examination, sixth edition, consists of 27 chapters organized into five units. **Unit 1** lays the foundation for the entire assessment process by guiding the reader through critical thinking and clinical reasoning using both the nursing process, the nursing clinical judgment measurement model (NCJMM), and communication techniques for the client interview and the health history. Specific tips on professionalism, approaching clients, and discussing sensitive topics help the reader understand the importance of the nurse-client partnership in the assessment process. A template for eliciting a comprehensive health history completes this unit.

Unit 2 highlights developmental, cultural, spiritual, and nutritional areas of assessment, emphasizing the holistic nature of the assessment process. These chapters are key in encouraging the reader to be aware of personal feelings and biases and how they may impact interactions with clients and colleagues.

Unit 3 opens with a description of fundamental examination techniques, including measuring vital signs and assessing pain, and then details examination procedures and findings for specific body systems. The format used for all applicable physical examination chapters in this unit includes:

1. Anatomy and physiology
2. Health history
3. Assessment in Brief
4. Equipment
5. Physical examination
   a. Inspection
   b. Palpation
   c. Percussion
   d. Auscultation
6. U.S. Preventive Services Task Force Recommendations
7. Case study
8. Clinical Judgment in Action
9. Review Questions

The examination techniques presented are described for adult clients. Because examination techniques and findings may differ in pregnant clients, children, and the older adult, these populations are discussed in separate chapters in **Unit 4.** The chapter on the pregnant client includes variations in examination techniques and special techniques used only on pregnant clients, as well as normal and abnormal findings related to pregnancy. The chapter on the pediatric client presents physical differences in the examination and explains special techniques used only with children. The chapter on older adults highlights the functional, developmental, cognitive, and self-determination assessments, geriatric syndromes, and physical examination skills that are appropriate for this population.

Unit 5 helps the reader assimilate and synthesize the wealth of information presented in the text in order to perform a thorough, accurate, and efficient health assessment and physical examination. Specific guidelines and reminders on gaining clients' cooperation, being sensitive to legal and ethical considerations, and documenting accurately make this unit a complete health assessment and physical examination resource tool.

NEW TO THIS EDITION

- The word "patient" was changed to "client" throughout. This action more closely aligns with the language used in the NCLEX/Next Gen NCLEX Exam and helps readers familiarize themselves with this change in terminology.
- All-new multicultural case studies humanize the material and help readers apply the critical thinking concepts that are learned in the chapters.
- More than 1,000 photographs and illustrations, of which 800 are new to this edition.
- The theme of "respect and dignity for all" permeates all aspects of this text.
- The effect that SARS-CoV2 (COVID-19) has had on client's health and body systems has been added to relevant chapters.
- Current U.S. Preventive Services Task Force recommendations are presented in each chapter where they apply.
- Each Case Study is followed by Clinical Judgment in Action which allows the reader to critically analyze the Case Study and apply nursing theory to each scenario.
- New review questions have been added at the end of each chapter.
- Updated bibliographies and Websites allow readers to broaden their knowledge base regarding the material presented in each chapter. (Note: These can be found on FADavis.com).

Chapter-specific enhancements and new and current content included in the sixth edition include:

- **Chapter 1, *Critical Thinking and Clinical Reasoning in Nursing***
  - Introduces the Nursing Clinical Judgment Measurement Model (NCJMM) as well as the Nursing Process. It is imperative that the student nurse possesses this knowledge as the Next Generation NCLEX (NEXT GEN) licensing examination will incorporate questions based on the NCJMM.
  - The SBAR Communication tool is discussed with an interactive example shown.
- **Chapter 2, *Communication Techniques and the Client Interview***
  - Includes an expanded section on sexual and gender minorities (LGBTQIA+).
  - Discusses communication with telenursing and telehealth.
- **Chapter 3, *The Complete Health History Including Documentation***
  - New content on human trafficking and an expanded section on Advance Medical Directive
  - Updates CDC/ACIP Immunization schedule
  - AUDIT-C and SASQ alcohol screening tools
  - HARK intimate partner violence screening tool
  - Addresses current trend of increased use of psychedelics and cannabis

- **Chapter 4, *Developmental Assessment***
  - Expanded list of Developmental Assessment tools
  - Addresses Social Determinants of Health
- **Chapter 5, *Cultural Assessment,***
  - The ANA Scope and Standards of Practice, Standard Eight addresses: What Every Nurse Should Know About Culturally Congruent Practice. This chapter describes the elements of cultural assessment to promote the development of culturally competent practice.
  - An adaptation of the well-known Cultural Assessment tool (2017) by Rachel Spector is used in the Case Study.
- **Chapter 6, *Spiritual Assessment***
  - Revised spirituality in America section
  - Revised health effects of religion and spirituality
  - Updates FICA Spiritual Assessment tool
  - Effect of COVID-19 on religion and spirituality
- **Chapter 7, *Nutritional Assessment***
  - Introduces *Dietary Guidelines for Americans, 2025–2030*
  - Addresses pediatric obesity epidemic
  - Provides content on GLP-1 medications and continuous glucose monitors
- **Chapter 8, *Physical Examination Techniques***
  - Updates Standard Precautions section based on current CDC guidelines
  - Introduces Smart stethoscope content
- **Chapter 9, *General Survey, Vital Signs, and Pain***
  - 2025 ACC/AHA Blood Pressure guidelines for adults
  - Use of noncontact infrared thermometer
  - Expanded pain section includes nociplastic pain
  - Addresses opioid crisis
- **Chapter 10, *Skin, Hair, and Nails***
  - Introduces the Monk Skin Tone system
  - Updates skin cancer Risk Factors
- **Chapter 11, *Head, Neck, and Regional Lymph Nodes***
  - Updated for currency
  - Updates headache Risk Factors
  - Updates thyroid cancer Risk Factors
- **Chapter 12, *Eyes***
  - Updated for currency
  - Updates Risk Factors for ophthalmological eye pathology
- **Chapter 13, *Ears, Nose, Mouth, and Throat***
  - Addition of assistive devices checklist for hearing aids, oral appliances, and nasal rinse devices
  - Updates Risk Factors for oral cancers
  - Updates Risk Factors for ear conditions
- **Chapter 14, *Breasts and Regional Lymph Nodes***
  - Expanded content on male breast cancer and screening
  - Transitional breast development in a transgender man
  - Breast examination in the pregnant and breastfeeding client
  - Breast self-awareness
  - Updates breast cancer Risk Factors
- **Chapter 15, *Thorax and Lungs***
  - Describes the 6-minute walk test
  - Addresses smoking cannabis, vaping, and e-cigarette use
  - Alerts readers to pertussis trends
  - Updates lung cancer Risk Factors
  - Updates Risk Factors for lung pathology
- **Chapter 16, *Heart***
  - New content on Mechanical Circulatory Assistive Devices
  - New content on dextrocardia
  - Introduces the Duke Activity Status Index
  - Updates Risk Factors for cardiac disease
- **Chapter 17, *Peripheral Vasculature System and Lymphatic System***
  - Additional content on TIA
  - Assistive devices now include compression garments for lymphedema and intermittent pneumatic compression pump for lymphedema
  - Updates Risk Factors for peripheral vasculature pathology
  - Updates Risk Factors for lymphatic system pathology
- **Chapter 18, *Abdomen***
  - Updates Risk Factors for gastrointestinal cancers
  - Updates Risk Factors for gastrointestinal pathology
  - Updates Risk Factors for urinary cancer
  - Updates Risk Factors for urinary pathology
  - New American Cancer Society Guidelines for the early detection of colorectal cancer and polyps
- **Chapter 19, *Musculoskeletal System***
  - Expanded assistive devices section including motorized scooters and wheelchairs
  - Introduces the Relative Energy Deficiency in Sports (RED-S) condition
  - Updated Risk Factors for musculoskeletal pathology
  - Updates Risk Factors for sports injuries
- **Chapter 20, *Mental Status and Neurological System***
  - Addition of the new 988 Suicide Hotline
  - FAST and BE FAST pneumonics for stroke recognition/prompt treatment

- Discusses traumatic brain injury
- Updates Risk Factors for neurologic pathology
- Updates Risk Factors for suicide

- **Chapter 21, *Female Genitalia***
  - Updates Risk Factors for female genitalia cancers
  - Updates Risk Factors for female genitalia pathology
  - Updates cervical cancer screening guidelines including the American Cancer Society 2025 recommendations
  - Gynecological examination after a hysterectomy
  - Hernias in females
  - Transgender practices
  - Addresses self-collection of samples for HPV, STI, and Pap testing
- **Chapter 22, *Male Genitalia***
  - Updates Risk Factors for HIV
  - Updates Risk Factors for male genitalia cancers
  - New content on men's unique health issues, male sexual health disparities, and transgender practices
- **Chapter 23, *Anus, Rectum, and Prostate***
  - Guidelines for early detection of prostate cancer
  - Helpful hint on palpating the prostate gland
  - Updates Risk Factors for anorectal and prostate cancer
- **Chapter 24, *The Pregnant Client***
  - Drug safety in pregnancy
  - Revised 2025 hypertensive disorders of pregnancy content
  - Updates Risk Factors for high-risk pregnancy
- **Chapter 25, *The Pediatric Client***
  - Updates CDC/ACIP immunization chart
  - HEADSSS 3.0 assessment tool
  - Neonatal abstinence syndrome
  - Accidental marijuana poisoning in children
  - Updates Risk Factors for adolescent suicide
  - Includes BMI chart for children that extends to 60 kg/m^2
- **Chapter 26, *The Older Adult Client***
  - Additional screening tools for the older adult
  - Expanded content on abuse and neglect of the older adult
  - STIs in older adults
  - Content on the complex issue of older adults and driving
- **Chapter 27, *The Complete Health History and Physical Examination***
  - Additional content on personal health record and electronic health record
  - Advances in technology and artificial intelligence and their impact on nursing practice
  - Long COVID and worldwide pandemic
  - Updates Speak Up™ initiatives
  - Healthy People 2030 update
  - Merging Health History and public health issues
  - The Future of Nursing, 2020–2030

Special Features

Many successful features from the previous editions of *Health Assessment & Physical Examination* have been retained in this new edition. These features stimulate critical thinking and self-reflection, develop technical expertise, and encourage readers to synthesize and apply the information presented in the text.

- **Nursing Checklists** offer an organizing framework for the examination of each body system or for approaching a given task. Nursing Checklists are also included in the Special Assessments and Special Populations Units.
- **Assistive Devices** present a brief checklist of items to verify when a client is using an assistive device. If the Assistive Device is not programmed or functioning correctly, it can adversely affect a client's health.
- **Nursing Tips** help the reader to apply basic knowledge to real-life situations for both new and experienced nurses.
- **Risk Factor** boxes highlight risk factors for many types of cancer and clinical conditions and pathology.
- The **ENAP** format (examination, normal findings, abnormal findings, pathophysiology) allows the reader to study the content that is specifically relevant to personal practice. The **IPPA** format (inspection, palpation, percussion, and auscultation) is applied consistently to each examination skill.
- **Health Histories** outline all areas of history taking related to each body system. The standard format used throughout the text teaches the importance of consistency and organization when discussing topics with clients during the health history interview.
- **U.S. Preventive Services Task Force Recommendations** provide guidelines for clinical practice that highlight actions to be taken to place the client in an optimal state of health.
- **Case Studies** humanize the material and help readers apply critical thinking concepts. The Case Studies present realistic scenarios and offer readers an opportunity to apply the chapter material, thereby encouraging extrapolation and intuitive thinking. These case studies list normal and abnormal examination findings in the context of a clinical scenario. Each case

study includes a sample client health history, physical examination findings, and (when appropriate) laboratory data and diagnostic studies. Case studies exemplify objective documentation to serve as models for accurate charting. The case studies deliberately use different charting styles to reflect the wide variety of norms in actual clinical practice. The case study scenarios are based on an amalgamation of real-life individuals, thus making the scenario realistic.

Pedagogical Features

Health Assessment & Physical Examination, sixth edition, also includes many pedagogical features that promote learning and accessibility of information. This text guides the novice as well as the experienced nurse in the art and science of conducting a comprehensive health history, health assessment, and physical examination.

- **Learning Objectives** open each chapter and introduce the main areas targeted for mastery in each chapter. They also provide a checkpoint for study and crucial physical examination skills.
- **Outstanding, high-quality photographs and illustrations** depict anatomy and physiology, examination techniques, normal clinical findings and abnormal clinical findings. There are more than 1,000 photos and illustrations in *Health Assessment & Physical Examination, sixth edition,* of which 80% are new to this edition.
- **Key Terms** are highlighted and defined in the text the first time they are used. These terms are also found and defined in the Glossary.
- **Assessment in Brief** provides a conceptual framework for the chapter, highlighting main points of the system-specific assessment/ physical examination.
- **Advanced Techniques** provide content on how to address specific abnormal clinical findings in order to accurately determine their etiology. Advanced Techniques also describe how to evaluate specific conditions for diagnostic purposes.
- **Clinical Judgment in Action** allows the reader to synthesize the assessment/ examination findings in the context of what is occurring in the client's physical and psychological environment presented in the case study.
- **Review Questions** offer readers an opportunity to assess their understanding of the content and better define areas where additional study is needed. All chapters include self-quizzes, written in an NCLEX/Next Gen NCLEX-style, on key information to test knowledge.
- A list of **Abbreviations** includes common abbreviations used in charting for quick reference.
- The **Glossary** at the end of the book defines all key terms used in the text and serves as a comprehensive resource for study and review.
- The **Index** facilitates access to material and includes special entries for tables and illustrations.

Acknowledgments

It is with great pride that I announce that *Health Assessment & Physical Examination* has found a new home with F. A. Davis for its sixth edition! F. A. Davis is an independent, family-owned publisher of educational solutions for Nursing and the Health Sciences. Since 1879 F.A. Davis has been committed to serving the needs of students with innovative products powered by the technology that is changing how learning occurs and nurses are practicing. It has been my privilege to join the F. A. Davis family! Specifically, I would like to thank the F. A. Davis staff who guided me through another successful textbook revision:

Haleahy Craven, Nursing Acquisitions Editor
Sean West, Content Project Manager 2
Liz Schaeffer, Manager of Development Editing
Catherine Carroll, Director of Project Management
Megan Schindele, Senior Project Editor, Content Solutions
Carolyn O'Brien, Senior Manager of Art and Design
Maria Everitt, Project Manager
Kate Margeson, Senior Illustration Coordinator
Alison Enright, Digital Asset and eBook Manager
Jaclyn White, Senior Marketing Manager

Many individuals have assisted me in my journey to see this sixth edition to market. I especially want to thank the following individuals:

- Contributors, old and new, who are experts in their respective fields. They are actively practicing advanced practice nurses who hail from various locations both within the United States as well as Australia! Twelve contributors are Nurse Practitioners and three are Fellows in the American Association of Nurse Practitioners. The collective expertise of these clinicians is unparalleled in other assessment texts. The geographical distribution of the contributors is always a plus as we learn that there is more than one way to accomplish the same goal. The contributors thoughtfully revised their chapters to ensure that timely research and national guidelines are current. I appreciate their candid use of actual clients in their case studies, which provide a wealth of knowledge and diversity. Truth can be stranger than fiction!
- Many thanks to the folks at N.Y. Vintage Camera Works, LTD, who produced a first-class photo package for this edition. Thank you, Chris, and especially to Jason. I enjoyed our time together for the photo shoot!
- Jacque Ginn and the team at GW Inc. who guided the assembly of the text.
- The colleagues who shared photographs of clinical conditions: Dr. Salim I. Butrus, Dr. Mark Dougherty, Dr. Joseph Konzelman, Dr. Jessica L. Olsen, Dr. Laura Pickford, Dr. Daniel D. Rooney, Dr. Andrew B. Silva, Dr. Robert A. Silverman, and Dr. Catherine C. Tierney. In addition, thank you to friends Mary Hitcho and the Ballard Family who shared photos.
- The many people who graciously agreed to pose for photos for the sixth edition and the patients/clients who graciously allowed me to take photos of their clinical abnormalities.
- The various individuals and organizations who granted permission to use copyrighted material.
- My family and friends, who are always there to encourage me. Most especially, my husband, Matt, who helped me through the ever-changing world of technology. You helped preserve my sanity many times!

Mary Ellen Zator Estes

About the Author

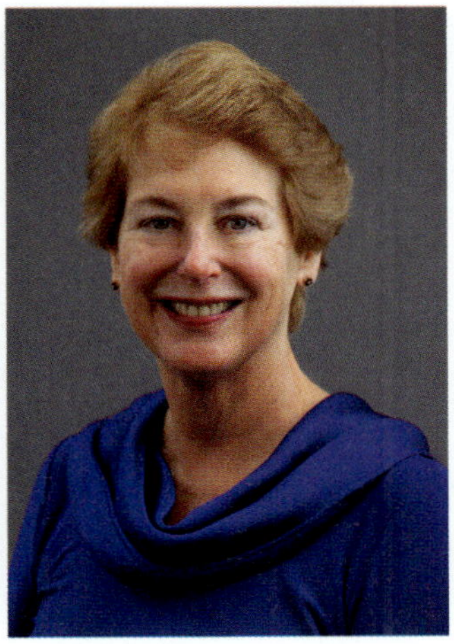

Mary Ellen Zator Estes obtained her Baccalaureate and Master's degrees and her Family Nurse Practitioner certificate from the University of Virginia School of Nursing. As an academician she has been on the faculty at the University of Virginia, Marymount University, and Northern Virginia Community College. Ms. Estes was the former Critical Care Nursing Education Coordinator at The George Washington University Medical Center in Washington, DC.

As a Nurse Practitioner Ms. Estes served as a clinical preceptor for numerous institutions of higher learning (The George Washington University, University of Virginia, James Madison University, Virginia Commonwealth University, George Mason University, Chamberlain University, Samford University, University of Cincinnati, and University of Southern Indiana) where she guided students' mastery of history taking and physical examination skills. Ms. Estes has also functioned as Clinical Faculty for Ball State University.

With more than 45 years' experience as a clinician and academician, Ms. Estes has taught health assessment and physical examination courses to nurses and nursing students from a variety of backgrounds. Her hands-on approach in the classroom, clinical laboratory, and health-care setting has consistently led to positive learning experiences for her students and colleagues.

Ms. Estes's professional expertise is well demonstrated at the local, regional, and national levels. In 2016 Ms. Estes was inducted as a Fellow into the American Association of Nurse Practitioners (FAANP). As a Fellow she engages in various national committees. In addition, Ms. Estes has served on the Virginia Council of Nurse Practitioners–Northern Virginia Region Board for many years as well as the Virginia Council of Nurse Practitioners State Nominations and Awards Committee. She has been an active member of the Virginia Council of Nurse Practitioners and the AANP for over 25 years. Prior to becoming a Nurse Practitioner Ms. Estes was active in the regional chapters of Sigma Theta Tau (Beta Kappa and Eta Alpha), American Association of Critical-Care Nurses (at the local and national levels), the American Nurses Association, and the Virginia Nurses Association (local and state levels). In addition, Ms. Estes has authored numerous articles in peer reviewed periodicals and served as a reviewer for numerous publishing houses and professional journals. She has delivered numerous presentations at local, state, and national levels.

Ms. Estes is passionate about protecting the health of her community. For almost 20 years she has led the automated external defibrillator (AED) programs in numerous counties in Northern and Central Virginia. She is the volunteer AED Coordinator for the Office of Risk Management for the Catholic Diocese of Arlington where she leads the AED program to help safeguard the health of over 430,000 Virginians. Ms. Estes currently works as a nurse practitioner at an Internal Medicine practice in Fairfax, Virginia, and as a Nurse Consultant.

UNIT

I Laying the Foundation

Chapter 1 Critical Thinking and Clinical Reasoning in Nursing, 2

Chapter 2 Communication Techniques and the Client Interview, 20

Chapter 3 The Complete Health History Including Documentation, 46

Critical Thinking and Clinical Reasoning in Nursing

CHAPTER 1

It is often thought that medicine is the curative process. It is no such thing; medicine is the surgery of functions, as surgery proper is that of limbs and organs. Neither can do anything but remove obstructions; neither can cure; nature alone cures. Surgery removes the bullet out of the limb, which is an obstruction to cure, but nature heals the wound. So it is with medicine; the function of an organ becomes obstructed; medicine so far as we know, assists nature to remove the obstruction, but does nothing more. And what nursing has to do in either case, is to put the patient in the best condition for nature to act upon him.

Florence Nightingale

Learning Outcomes

1. Discuss the components of critical thinking, clinical reasoning, and clinical judgment.
2. Define the American Nurses Association (ANA) Standards of Professional Nursing Practice.
3. Describe the steps of the Nursing Process.
4. Describe the components of the National Council of State Boards of Nursing (NCSBN) Nursing Clinical Judgment Measurement Model (NCJMM).
5. Describe verbal and written tools used to communicate client status and care.

"Nursing is a learned profession built on a core body of knowledge that reflects multiple ways of knowing, integrating both art and science" (ANA, 2021). The art of nursing allows nurses to incorporate aspects of caring and sharing into their practice. Over time, nurses build repertoires of professional experiences that serve as a clinical portfolio of responses to various client situations (Fig. 1-1). Experienced nurses make intuitive links that are not made by novice nurses because experienced nurses can delve into their professional portfolio of experiences and select strategies that have been successful in the past. Professional intuition develops over time as nurses begin to link certain patterns or events to specific outcomes. Experienced nurses seem to do this with little conscious effort. The novice, in contrast, may need guidance to perceive links that are intuitively recognized by the experienced nurse.

For example, a critical care nurse may feel that a client is declining even though the client's vital signs are stable. The experienced nurse has a "feel" for the client and the situation. A few hours later, the client goes into cardiopulmonary arrest. How did the experienced nurse know this might happen? That is part of the art of nursing.

The science of nursing involves using analytical thinking and nursing interventions and should be based on evidence-based research and rigorous scientific inquiry (Vega & Hayes, 2019). According to the Academy of Medical-Surgical Nurses, evidence-based practice (EBP) is "a method that allows the practitioner to assess research, clinical guidelines, and other information resources based on high quality findings and apply the results to practice" (2018). In analytical thinking, the nature of information is studied, the information is broken into its constituent parts, and relationships and patterns are identified. Causation, key factors, and possible outcomes of situations may all be identified. The science of nursing is based on evidence-based research. For example, with knowledge of lung physiology, the pathophysiology of asthma, and environmental triggers, a nurse can analyze why an asthmatic client is having an acute attack in a room filled with cigarette smokers and a wood-burning fire. Analytical thinking skills can be learned and are developed as clinical experience is gained. In 1992 Martha Rogers identified the art of nursing as the creative use of the science of nursing for human betterment (Butcher, 2021). Critical thinking, clinical reasoning, and clinical judgment are essential elements of this process.

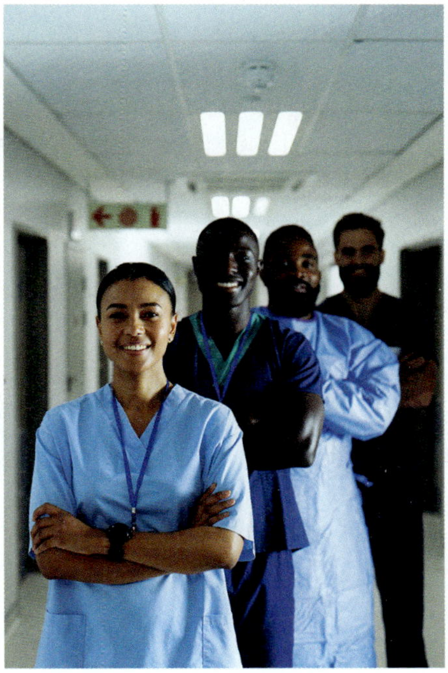

Figure 1-1 Nurses possess a wide variety of experiences that they take into each client encounter.

Critical Thinking, Clinical Reasoning, and Clinical Judgment

Critical thinking, clinical reasoning, and clinical judgment are related concepts that are often used interchangeably but are not the same. The American Association of Colleges of Nursing (AACN) (2021) defines critical thinking as "the skill of using logic and reasoning to identify the strengths and weaknesses of alternative health-care solutions, conclusions, or approaches to clinical or practice problems" (p. 56). Critical thinking is one of the key factors in the cognitive processes of clinical reasoning (Simpson & Courtney, 2002). Clinical reasoning in practice-based disciplines is the application of critical thinking to a clinical situation. It is the ability to understand the relevance of evidence and scientific knowledge as it applies to a client. In 2006 Tanner defined clinical judgment as "an interpretation or conclusion about a client's needs, concerns, or health problems, and/or the decision to act (or not), use or modify standard approaches, or improvise new ones as deemed appropriate by the client's response." In 2019 the National Council of State Boards of Nursing (NCSBN) defined clinical judgment "as the observed outcome of critical thinking and decision making. It is an iterative process that uses nursing knowledge to observe and assess presenting situations, identify a prioritized client concern, and generate the best possible evidence-based solutions to deliver safe client care." Critical thinking, clinical reasoning, and clinical judgment skills are essential to every nurse's clinical practice. For example, a client in the cardiac care unit complains of chest pain after eating dinner and immediately lies down for a nap. Your critical thinking skills lead you to assess all aspects of the client's condition to determine the etiology of the pain and treat it accordingly. You recognize that in addition to the client's diagnosis of angina, the client also has a history of gastroesophageal reflux disease (GERD) and a hiatal hernia. The client takes omeprazole 40 mg every morning. You pursue a line of questioning that teases out more information about the client's pain. You use clinical reasoning skills to determine that the client's pain is most likely gastrointestinal in nature because the pain is in the epigastric area, whereas recent chest pain was in the substernal region. In addition, the client had no EKG (electrocardiogram) changes with the pain, and the pain was relieved when the client sat up. You use clinical judgment to educate the client to remain sitting up for half an hour after eating to prevent pain.

Components of Critical Thinking

According to Pesut and Herman (1999), critical thinking encompasses many skills, including interpretation, analysis, inference, explanation, evaluation, and self-regulation. These skills will be discussed to show their relationship with health assessment and physical examination.

Interpretation of situations requires the nurse to decode hidden messages, clarify the meaning of the information, and categorize the information. For example, a client may claim to be seeking health care for a bad cough and

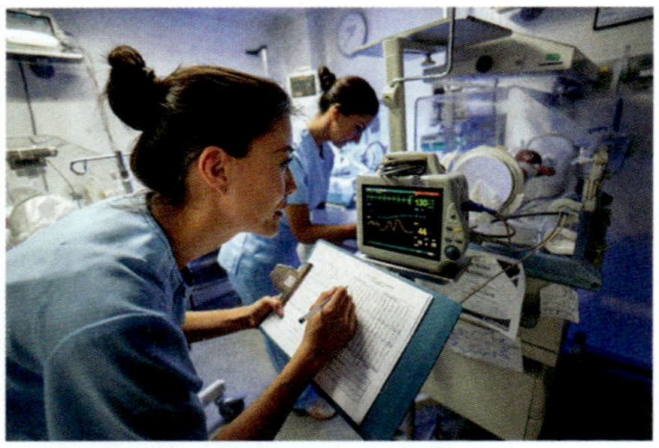

Figure 1-2 Critical thinking involves analysis, in which the nurse examines client data available from a variety of sources.

cold but may actually be concerned about whether the cough is a sign of lung cancer. Accurate interpretation implies that the nurse is clinically competent and professionally capable of obtaining information.

During analysis, the nurse examines the ideas and data that were presented, identifies any discrepancies, and reflects on the reason for the discrepancies. The nurse can then begin to frame the main points of the client's story (Fig. 1-2). For instance, a client complains of insomnia but, upon questioning, reveals that they sleep 6 hours at night and take a 2-hour nap each afternoon. Often discrepancies lead to a clearer picture of the client's overall situation.

Inference speculates, derives, or reasons a specific premise based on information and assumptions obtained from the client. Inference can be a challenging skill for the novice nurse because one must possess a certain level of knowledge and experience to draw conclusions and provide alternatives in any given scenario. If a client complains of an exacerbation of asthma every morning, the nurse can inquire about a history of heartburn or GERD. An experienced nurse would make the association between these causative factors.

Explanation requires that the conclusions drawn from the inferences be correct and justifiable. The use of scientific and nursing literature constitutes the basis for clinical justification. To continue with the example in the preceding paragraph, GERD as a contributing factor of asthma is well documented in the literature; that is, there is a documented scientific link between GERD and asthma.

The evaluation process examines the validity of the information and hypothesis. This leads to a conclusion that can be implemented. For example, the nurse assesses a 5-year-old child with cystic fibrosis who is experiencing labored breathing and wheezing. Based on the findings, the nurse implements a nebulizer treatment, postural drainage, and chest physiotherapy. The nurse reassesses the client after treatment and finds that there is no wheezing, and the respiratory rate is within normal limits.

Self-regulation is a key component of the critical thinking process. During this process, the nurse reflects on the critical thinking skills that were used and then determines which techniques were effective and which were problematic. After interviewing a client, for example, the nurse reflects on whether the questions posed to the client were leading, biased, or judgmental. The nurse might also reflect on the use of open-ended questions and the effectiveness of an interpreter. The recognition of both positive and negative outcomes is crucial to developing higher-level thinking skills and professional expertise. The nurse must also consider the client's health literacy level to ensure that the client understands what is being asked.

Universal Intellectual Standards for Critical Thinking

The quality of critical thinking can be evaluated by applying the nine Universal Intellectual Standards (UIS) proposed by Paul and Elder (2013). These standards are clarity, accuracy, precision, relevance, depth, breadth, logic, significance, and fairness.

Clarity, simply stated, asks whether the message or information is clear. For example, a client who drinks excessively may report a substance abuse problem. The nurse, using critical thinking skills, would need to clarify the substance abuse specifically as an alcohol use disorder versus abuse with another substance.

The second key element of the UIS is accuracy. Have the thinking process and information been accurate? For example, thinking that a client drinks to excess every day may be inaccurate. The client may be more of a binge drinker, consuming large amounts of alcohol only on certain occasions. The nurse would need to ask questions to ensure accurate understanding of information.

Precision is the third UIS. To state that a client "drinks excessively" is judgmental and not precise. How much is excessive? Precision in thinking and data collection is essential. The statement "The client reports drinking a fifth of whiskey every day" is precise.

Has the thinking been relevant? If the client with an alcohol use disorder presents with the need for rehabilitation secondary to alcohol withdrawal and delirium tremens, then the information that the client's grandfather died at age 82 of renal failure is not relevant at this time. This latter information may be true, but it does not connect to the central issue of alcohol use disorder rehabilitation.

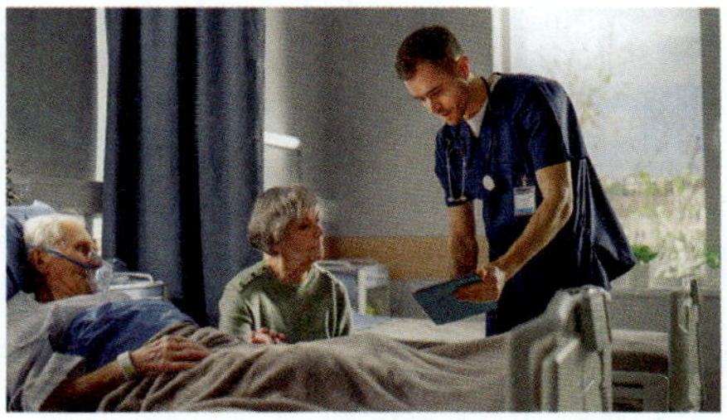

Figure 1-3 The nurse can speak with the spouse, relative, friend, or significant other to gain additional information about the client in order to make sound clinical decisions.

The UIS of depth can be a challenging standard for novice nurses to apply because they may not possess the appropriate knowledge base to prompt them to delve deeper into a given problem for related data. For instance, perhaps the nurse did not ascertain that the client has four relatives who also have alcohol use disorder, or that the client recently experienced the death of a child and was fired from their job, which led to an exacerbation of the drinking.

The sixth UIS is breadth. Does the client's (with an alcohol use disorder) story have more to it than was relayed to the nurse? Is there a need to consider the views of another person, such as a spouse, relative, friend, or significant other (Fig. 1-3)? Are there additional data that should be obtained to gain an accurate impression of the client's situation?

The UIS of logic must be applied to clinical reasoning. Does the client's or significant other's story seem logical? If the client stated that their only child recently died and that caused them to drink heavily, and then later this child comes to visit the client, what does this imply? Another way to think logically is attributing signs and symptoms to disease entities. The client experiences tremors: Is this due to alcohol withdrawal or Parkinson disease? Logical thinking would seem to point to the former etiology.

The eighth UIS is significance. The client's alcohol use, misuse, or abuse are important factors to consider for a healthy lifestyle, but if the client is admitted to the hospital with a stroke, then addressing alcohol use can be addressed at a later time. Likewise, if a client is admitted to the hospital with acute alcohol poisoning, immediate care is needed to prevent adverse outcomes.

Finally, the UIS of fairness should be considered. According to Paul and Elder (2013), human thinking is skewed toward our personal needs and thought processes. Thus, the nurse needs to reflect how the encounter was conducted with the person with an alcohol use disorder and determine whether an accurate representation of the client was made.

Consistent application of these standards to critical thinking leads to development and refinement of clinically useful skills.

Critical Thinking Frameworks: The Nursing Process and the NCJMM

There are many frameworks for critical thinking and clinical judgment in health-care professions. The nursing profession has developed its own unique tools to frame critical thinking: the Nursing Process and the NCSBN Nursing Clinical Judgment Measurement Model (NCJMM). Each of these frameworks will be discussed.

The Nursing Process is the framework on which the American Nurses Association developed the Scope and Standards of Practice (ANA, 2021). Refer to Table 1-1. These standards give the profession broad guidelines to which nurses can be held accountable in their practice. These nursing standards are the tenets on which the entire health assessment and

Table 1-1 ANA Standards of Professional Nursing Practice

Standard Number	Standard
1. Assessment	The registered nurse collects pertinent data and information relative to the health-care consumer's health or the situation.
2. Diagnosis	The registered nurse analyzes assessment data to determine actual or potential diagnoses, problems, and issues.
3. Outcomes Identification	The registered nurse identifies expected outcomes for a plan individualized to the health-care consumer or the situation.
4. Planning	The registered nurse develops a collaborative plan encompassing strategies to achieve expected outcomes.
5. Implementation	The registered nurse implements the identified plan. Standard 5A: Coordination of Care The registered nurse coordinates care delivery. Standard 5B: Health Teaching and Health Promotion The registered nurse employs strategies to teach and promote health and wellness.
6. Evaluation	The registered nurse evaluates progress toward attainment of goals and outcomes.

American Nurses Association (2021). Nursing Scope and Standards of Practice (4th ed.). Silver Spring, MD.

physical examination of the client are conducted. According to the NCSBN, clinical judgment is the observed outcome of critical thinking and decision making (2018). The NCJMM is a process that allows the nurse to combine knowledge and assessment to prioritize and deliver safe client care (NCSBN, n.d.).

The Nursing Process includes six steps: assessment, diagnosis, outcomes identification, planning, implementation, and evaluation. It is a dynamic process that uses information in a meaningful way through problem-solving strategies to place the client, family, or community in an optimal health state. The primary focus of this text is assessment. The physical, emotional, social, psychological, developmental, cultural, spiritual, nutritional, and functional assessments provide the foundation for the other steps of the Nursing Process.

The NCJMM is an expansion of the Nursing Process and is an evidence-based model that identifies six cognitive skills that are needed to make appropriate clinical judgments. These skills include recognize cues, analyze cues, prioritize hypotheses, generate solutions, take action, and evaluate outcomes. The idea of a clinical judgment model is not new. Tanner's Clinical Judgment Model (2006) and the National League for Nursing have suggested clinical judgment is a better problem-solving approach than the Nursing Process.

Table 1-2 illustrates how NCJMM cognitive skills can be aligned with the Nursing Process. The Nursing Process and clinical judgment using the NCJMM will be discussed to demonstrate how they provide a framework for critical thinking and clinical judgment to provide safe care to clients. It is imperative that the student nurse possess this knowledge as the Next Generation NCLEX (NEXT GEN) licensing examination will incorporate questions based on the NCJMM. *(https://www.ncsbn.org/news/ncsbn-launches-next-generation-nclex-exam).*

The Nursing Process

ANA Standard 1: Assessment

The registered nurse collects pertinent data and information relative to the healthcare consumer's health or the situation (ANA, 2021).

Table 1-2 Comparison of the Nursing Process and NCJMM

Nursing Process	NCJMM
Assessment	Recognize cues
Diagnosis	Analyze cues
Outcomes Identification	Prioritize hypotheses
Planning	Generate solutions
Implementation	Take action
Evaluation	Evaluate Outcomes

Assessment is the first step of the Nursing Process. It consists of the orderly collection of information concerning the client's health status. The assessment process aims to identify the client's current health status, actual and potential health problems, and areas for health promotion. The sources of information for the assessment include health history, physical examination, and diagnostic and laboratory data. Collectively, these data constitute the nursing database from which the nurse will develop a plan of care for the client, and they serve as a baseline against which future comparisons can be made (Fig. 1-4).

Health History

The health history interview is a means of gathering **subjective data**, usually from the client. These data are subjective in that they cannot always be verified by an independent observer. Subjective data include what the client says and what the client thinks, including the client's attitudes and beliefs. In some instances, however, this information can be validated during the physical examination; for instance, the existence of a client-reported breast lump can be evaluated with palpation.

The health history can also be obtained from sources other than the client. Relatives, neighbors, and friends of the client can provide insightful data for the health history (Fig. 1-5). In some instances, total strangers may be the only source of information, as in the case of a severe accident in which the client is rendered unconscious. The client's old charts or medical records are additional sources of information, as are healthcare colleagues. The nurse can and should use every available medium to gather as much information about the client as possible. The health history is further discussed in Chapter 3.

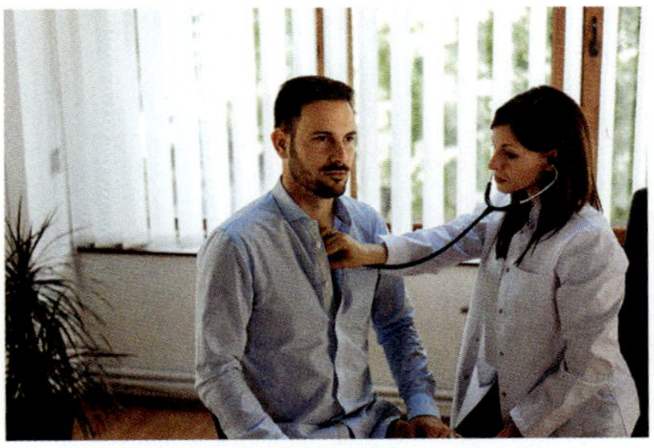

Figure 1-4 Physical examination is one component of the nursing database.

Physical Examination Findings

Physical examination findings are a second source of information that is used in the assessment step of the Nursing Process. Physical examination findings constitute **objective data**, or information that is observable and measurable and can be verified by more than one person. These data are obtained using the senses of smell, touch, vision, and hearing. This text describes the systematic and comprehensive physical examination techniques that will elicit these data (see Chapters 7–26).

The physical examination data can be obtained using a head-to-toe approach, grouping body systems in an organized manner. While physical examination data can be collected and grouped in various ways, this text uses the head-to-toe approach for physical examination. The body systems that will be assessed are:

- General survey, vital signs, and pain
- Skin, hair, and nails
- Head, neck, and regional lymph nodes
- Eyes

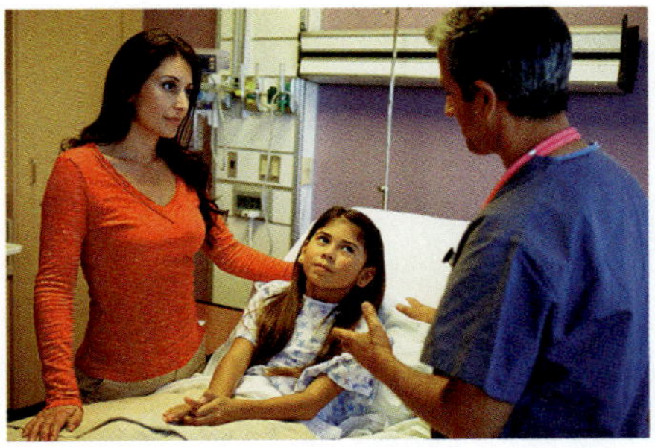

Figure 1-5 The health history can be gathered from many sources. In the case of a child, the health history is usually provided by a parent or caregiver.

- Ears, nose, mouth, and throat
- Breasts and regional lymph nodes
- Thorax and lungs
- Heart
- Peripheral vasculature system and lymphatic system
- Abdomen
- Musculoskeletal system
- Mental status and neurological system
- Female genitalia
- Male genitalia
- Anus, rectum, and prostate

Diagnostic and Laboratory Data

The final element that contributes to information gathering in the assessment step of the Nursing Process is diagnostic and laboratory data. Results of blood and urine studies, cultures, X-rays, CT scans, MRI scans, and diagnostic procedures constitute objective data about the client's status.

It is imperative that the nurse document all examination findings. The written record is a legal tool used to chart the client's current health status. Chapter 27 discusses documentation and covers the legal issues of the written client record. The documented client examination also serves as a means of communicating information to other healthcare colleagues.

Remember that the assessment step of the Nursing Process is dynamic. The nurse is continuously adding information to the database, validating the data, and interpreting the data. With these data the nurse is ready to progress to the second step of the Nursing Process, the nursing diagnosis.

ANA Standard 2: Diagnosis

The registered nurse analyzes assessment data to determine actual or potential diagnoses, problems, and issues (ANA, 2021).

The National Conference Group for Classification of Nursing Diagnoses convened in 1973 to establish a nomenclature to describe conditions treated by nurses. In 1982 the organization changed its name to the North American Nursing Diagnosis Association (NANDA). Later, in 2002, NANDA expanded globally and was renamed NANDA-I, or NANDA International. NANDA-I is the recognized leader in the formulation, classification, and testing of nursing diagnoses. NANDA-I defines a nursing diagnosis as "a clinical judgment concerning a human response to health conditions/life processes, or a vulnerability for that response, by an individual, family, group, or community. A nursing diagnosis provides the basis for selection of nursing interventions to achieve outcomes for which the nurse has accountability" (NANDA-I, 2019). There are currently 333 NANDA-I nursing diagnoses. Nursing diagnoses are holistic. Nurses identify "actual or potential risks to the health care consumer's health and safety or barriers to health, which may include but are not limited to interpersonal, systematic, cultural, socioeconomic, or environmental circumstances" (ANA, 2021, pp. 77–78). Nurses are licensed to treat clients based on nursing diagnoses by virtue of their educational and clinical preparation. The purpose of a nursing diagnosis is to create a standardization of language that identifies possible interventions for clients, families, and communities (Gaines, 2022). However, Rivera et al found that nurses think nursing diagnoses are "academic" in nature, time consuming, and ineffective (2013). The terminology of nursing diagnoses do not reflect the language nurses use when talking about client care and do not accurately reflect a client's changing symptoms (Ros et al, 2015). Additionally, NANDA-I nursing diagnoses are not universally used in health care. It is important that nurses learn and use the language used by the interprofessional healthcare team.

Diagnosis Formulation

The nursing diagnosis is formulated after the assessment data are analyzed. The process involves four steps as identified by Gordon (2016): collecting information, interpreting information, clustering information, and naming a cluster or problem formulation. The first step, collecting information, refers to the data collected in the assessment step of the Nursing Process. This process is used continuously to gain as much information about the client as possible.

In the second step, the nurse interprets the data. The nurse collects data for the purpose of positively impacting the client's health status, not merely to fill in blanks on a chart. The diagnostic importance of the information becomes relevant through the interpretation of it. The data, or cues, are evaluated against the standards for a client population. Using inferential reasoning, the nurse begins to see patterns or clusters of data.

Clustering of information is performed in the third step of nursing diagnosis development. The data are sorted into meaningful groups, such as NANDA-I's domains. There are thirteen NANDA-I domains: health promotion, nutrition, elimination and exchange, activity/rest, perception/cognition, self-perception, role relationship, sexuality, coping/stress tolerance, life principles, safety/protection, comfort, and growth/development.

Naming the cluster is the final step in the formulation of the nursing diagnosis. This is the step in which the NANDA-I nursing diagnosis is applied. Patterns can surface that lead to the development of more than one nursing diagnosis. Conversely, the data may seem unrelated, and no nursing diagnosis can be formulated from the data. In this case, the nurse needs to review the data to ensure it is comprehensive and accurate.

Types of Nursing Diagnoses

There are three types of nursing diagnoses: problem-focused, health promotion, and risk. A problem-focused diagnosis is "a clinical judgment concerning an undesirable human response to health condition/life processes that exists in an individual, family, group or community" (NANDA International, 2024). A health promotion diagnosis is a "clinical judgment concerning motivation and desire to increase well-being and to actualize human health potential. These responses are expressed by a readiness to enhance specific health behaviors, and can be used in any health state. Health promotion responses may exist in an individual, family, group, or community" (NANDA International, 2024). A risk nursing diagnosis is a "clinical judgment concerning the vulnerability of an individual, family, group, or community for developing an undesirable human response to health conditions/life processes" (NANDA International, 2024). None of these types of nursing diagnoses carries more weight than any other. Each client is a unique individual, and the importance of any one diagnosis can be different in different clients.

NANDA-I also includes syndrome in its taxonomy. A syndrome is "a clinical judgment concerning a specific cluster of nursing diagnoses that occur together, and are best addressed together and through similar interventions" (NANDA International, 2024). Some client problems are not completely within the domain of the nurse's scope of practice and require the nurse to look beyond the nursing diagnosis. For instance, the client experiencing cardiac tamponade (medical diagnosis) needs immediate nursing and medical attention. The nurse is not ethically or legally permitted to do all that the situation requires to alleviate the tamponade; the nurse, physician, and health-care team will work collaboratively to treat the problem. Thus, a collaborative problem is a client problem that requires the nurse to work jointly with the physician and other health-care workers in monitoring, planning, and implementing a client's care (Fig. 1-6).

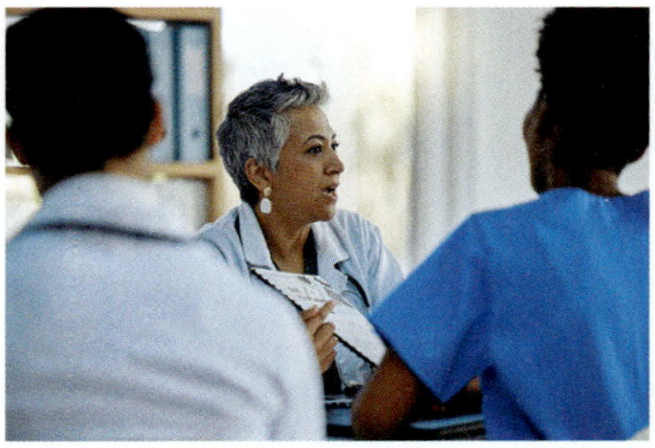

Figure 1-6 Nurses may collaborate with social workers, physicians, and other members of the health-care team to maximize client care.

ANA Standard 3: Outcomes Identification

The registered nurse identifies expected outcomes for a plan individualized to the healthcare consumer or the situation (ANA, 2021).

Outcomes identification represents the third step in the Nursing Process. After the nursing diagnoses have been formulated, client goals are established. The client goal is directed toward the removal of adverse conditions or client response to an adverse condition. Goals are broad statements that are not measurable. For example, if a nursing diagnosis is *Anxiety related to change in health status,* the client goal might be *The client will experience a reduction in anxiety.*

A client outcome is a statement of the expected change in client behavior denoting progress toward resolution of the altered human response over a specific period. These are written after the client goals. Client outcomes indicate the progression toward goal achievement. The nurse writes realistic and measurable client outcomes to ensure continuity in a client's care. Adjectives such as *more, less, increased,* and *decreased* and verbs such as *know* and *understand* are avoided because they are subjective and not measurable. Quantitative phrases such as "walk 15 feet" and "lose 8 pounds" are used as appropriate objective outcomes. Measurable verbs such as *state, identify,* and *list* are used.

Every client outcome must include a time frame that designates the time by which the client outcome should be met. The time frame can be short or long term. Short-term outcomes denote a time frame over a relatively short period of time, such as 1 hour, 1 day, or 1 week. Long-term outcomes usually extend over weeks or months. Each nursing diagnosis can have more than one client outcome. The complexity of the client's problem and the type of problem dictate the number of client outcomes required to develop a comprehensive plan of care.

Client outcomes should be evaluated consistently to determine the effect of the nursing care. The Nursing Outcomes Classification (NOC) taxonomy has developed 612 client outcomes (Moorhead et al, 2023). The nurse can define client outcomes using standardized language and refer to a set of indicators with a measurement scale to evaluate these outcomes. The NOC outcomes were developed to complement NANDA-I nursing diagnoses and are used in nursing practice, nursing education, and nursing research.

ANA Standard 4: Planning

The registered nurse develops a collaborative plan encompassing strategies to achieve expected outcomes (ANA, 2021).

Planning is the fourth step in the Nursing Process. It involves the prioritization of nursing diagnoses and care and the selection of nursing interventions.

Prioritization

The nurse formulates all the nursing diagnoses that are derived from the clustering of data. When there is more than one nursing diagnosis, the nurse must determine which problem or problems are the most vital to the client's well-being at that time. It is necessary to prioritize, or rank, the importance of each nursing diagnosis. When possible, the client should assist the nurse with the prioritization of needs. Clients who are actively involved in the decision-making process are more likely to be amenable to nursing care, to assist with their own care, and to be agreeable to the plan of care.

A theoretical framework that can be used to prioritize nursing diagnoses is Maslow's Hierarchy of Needs (Fig. 1-7). According to Maslow, basic needs such as food and oxygen take priority over all other issues. For example, the client experiencing a myocardial infarction must have their physiological needs met before safety needs are attended to. In some instances, however,

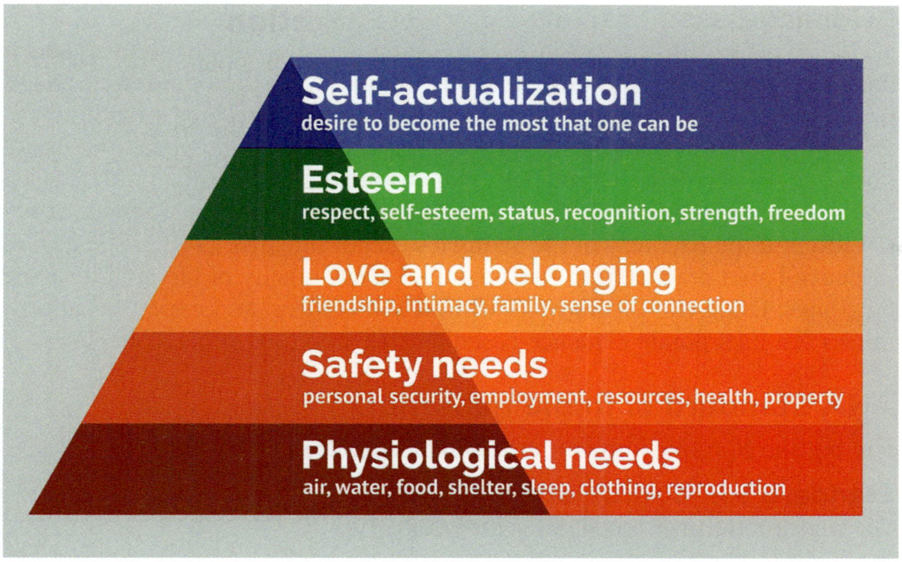
Self-actualization
desire to become the most that one can be
Esteem
respect, self-esteem, status, recognition, strength, freedom
Love and belonging
friendship, intimacy, family, sense of connection
Safety needs
personal security, employment, resources, health, property
Physiological needs
air, water, food, shelter, sleep, clothing, reproduction

Figure 1-7 Maslow's Hierarchy of Needs. *Adaptation based on* Maslow's Hierarchy of Needs.

clients' needs may not follow Maslow's hierarchy, or they may change over time, requiring reprioritization of nursing diagnoses. A client with terminal breast cancer may be more concerned with playing with their children than staying well hydrated. Some nursing diagnoses are equally important and can be prioritized together at the same level. The nurse, in conjunction with the client and family, continually reevaluates and revises the priority of the nursing diagnoses.

Intervention Selection

Interventions are planned strategies, based on scientific rationale, devised by the nurse to assist the client in meeting the client outcomes. When appropriate, the client, family, and significant others can assist in planning the interventions. As with nursing diagnosis prioritization, clients are more likely to be motivated and follow the interventions if they have been involved in the decision-making process.

Every client outcome has its own nursing interventions. When appropriate, a frequency is included in each intervention, such as "turn every 2 hours." The number of interventions per client outcome varies. What is essential is that the plan of care is comprehensive, to ensure that the client can meet the outcome. The interventions can be independent or collaborative nursing actions. Independent nursing interventions are those that the nurse is legally capable of implementing based on education and experience. Collaborative interventions are physician-prescribed and nurse-implemented. With all interventions, sound nursing judgment is required. The critically ill hypertensive client in an intensive care unit on a sodium nitroprusside infusion, with a blood pressure of 74/49, needs immediate nursing action. The nurse, using sound judgment, turns the infusion off and consults with the physician about a new plan of care. The nurse may also have standing orders indicating the parameters of treatment that lead to discontinuance of the infusion.

The Nursing Interventions Classification (NIC) complements the taxonomies of NANDA-I and NOC by devising research-based nursing interventions (Wagner et al, 2023). Currently 614 independent and collaborative interventions for nursing care delivered to individual clients, families, and communities have been identified. These interventions encompass both physiological and psychological realms.

Evidence-Based Practice

No longer are health-care practices being done "because they have always been done that way," nor are they being done intuitively. Rather, **evidence-based practice** uses the outcomes of well-designed and well-executed scientific studies to guide clinical decision making and clinical care. For example, the use of hormone replacement therapy (HRT) for postmenopausal women has changed dramatically because of the Heart and Estrogen/Progestin Replacement Study (HERS) and the HRT arm of the Women's Health Initiative (WHI). The goal of evidence-based practice is to enhance the client's quality of life by improving outcomes. Using clinical research, clinical conferences, and expert testimony, nurses can incorporate evidence-based practice into their professional lives.

ANA Standard 5: Implementation

The registered nurse implements the identified plan (ANA, 2021).

Standard 5A: Coordination of Care

The registered nurse coordinates care delivery.

Standard 5B: Health Teaching and Health Promotion

The registered nurse employs strategies to teach and promote health and wellness.

Implementation

The fifth step in the Nursing Process is implementation. In this step, the nurse executes the interventions that were devised during the planning stage to help the client meet predetermined outcomes. The time frame of the implementation step varies from client to client and from nursing diagnosis to nursing diagnosis. Remember that the nurse usually simultaneously implements interventions from multiple nursing diagnoses for a client at any given time. The client may achieve the outcome for one nursing diagnosis while progressing toward the outcome for another.

Implementation is a dynamic process. The nurse is continually interacting with the client, the family, and other health care colleagues, obtaining new data and making new judgments (Fig. 1-8). Plans of care can be changed or eliminated altogether based on the continuous flow of information.

ANA Standard 6: Evaluation

The registered nurse evaluates progress toward attainment of goals and outcomes (ANA, 2021).

Evaluation is the final step of the Nursing Process. During evaluation, the client's progress in achieving the outcomes is determined. Even before the time frame for assessing outcomes is reached, the nurse is continually assessing the client's progress toward the outcomes. This makes evaluation a continual and dynamic process.

The nurse, in conjunction with the client and the family, evaluates the status of the plan of care. One of two of the following conclusions can be made about the client outcome: It was met, or it was not met. When the client outcome has been met, the nurse documents this information and then periodically reevaluates the client's need for knowledge on the health matter. When evaluating a client's progress toward targeted outcomes, remember to also ask about the client's perception of whether goals were met or not, and to what degree.

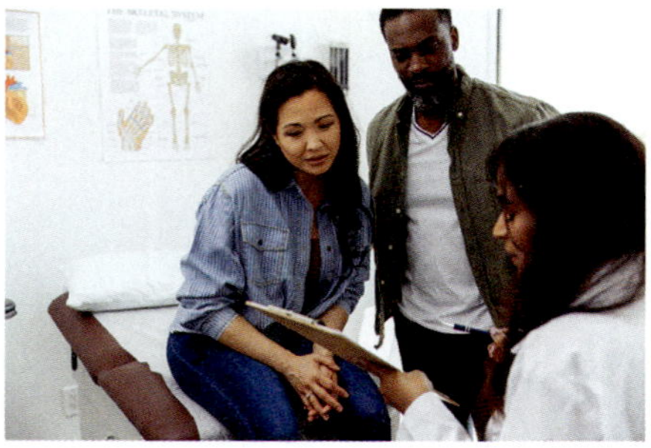

Figure 1-8 The client and family meet with the nurse to discuss progress on the client care plan.

If the outcome was not met, this too should be documented. Some factors to consider are: Was the diagnosis appropriate? Was the time frame adequate? Were the interventions accurate and comprehensive? Was the client outcome accurate? Had the client's condition changed sufficiently that the outcome was no longer appropriate? Did the client understand their role in the process? After considering these factors, the nurse and the client can decide to revise the client outcome and nursing interventions or to eliminate them. Based on the ongoing assessment and evaluation, new nursing diagnoses may be formulated that warrant other nursing interventions. These will be added to the client's plan of care.

Each outcome is evaluated separately. A frequent mistake is the practice of evaluating the interventions rather than the outcomes; the outcome should be evaluated, not the mechanics of achieving it.

The Nursing Clinical Judgment Measurement Model (NCJMM)

NCJMM: Recognize Cues

The NCJMM expands on the Nursing Process step of assessment with recognizing cues by identifying relevant and important information from different sources, such as the client's medical history and vital signs.

The nurse needs to consider the following:

- What information is relevant/irrelevant?
- What information is most important?
- What is of immediate concern?

The following client scenario demonstrates how the NCJMM is used in clinical practice:

Client Scenario

Adella Gul is a 68-year-old client who presents to the emergency department with a productive cough for 1 week, chest pain on the right side when taking a deep breath, fatigue, and chills. The client has a history of hypertension and coronary artery disease. The assessment findings are:

- Temperature of 100°F (37.8°C)
- Heart rate 112 beats per minute
- Productive cough
- Capillary refill less than 2 seconds
- Oxygen saturation 93% on room air
- Crackles in right lower lung
- Blood pressure 145/82 mm Hg
- Respiratory rate 20 breaths per minute

The nurse analyzes the client's condition and identifies clinical findings that require immediate care and treatment:

- Temperature of 100°F (37.8°C)
- Oxygen saturation 93% on room air
- Productive cough
- Crackles in right lower lung

The nurse recognizes these cues represent a serious illness and anticipates the client will need further evaluation, assessment, and treatment for this illness.

NCJMM: Analyze Cues

The NCJMM expands on the Nursing Process step of diagnosis with organizing and linking the recognized cues to the client's clinical presentation. The nurse needs to consider the following:

- What client conditions are consistent with the cues?
- Are there cues that support or contraindicate a particular condition?
- Why is a particular cue or subset of cues of concern?
- What other information would help establish the significance of a cue or set of cues?

Client Scenario continued

Adella Gul's physical examination is significant for crackles in the right lower lung. A chest X-ray shows a right lower lobe infiltrate. A complete blood cell count (CBC) results show a white blood cell count (WBC) of 14,000 µ/L (the normal range is 4000–11,000 µ/L). The client is admitted to the hospital's medical floor for observation and antibiotic therapy.

The nurse analyzes the cues and formulates potential complications from the client's clinical presentation:

- Diarrhea
- Nausea and vomiting
- Respiratory failure
- Sepsis
- Allergic reaction to medications
- Methicillin-resistant *Staphylococcus aureus* infection (MRSA)
- Venous thromboembolism
- Dehydration

After analyzing the cues, the nurse can take preemptive actions such as using standard precautions and proper hand hygiene, having the client ambulate regularly, and observing for signs and symptoms of adverse reaction to the antibiotics.

NCJMM: Prioritize Hypotheses

The NCJMM expands on the Nursing Process step of outcomes identification with evaluating and ranking hypotheses according to priority (e.g., urgency, likelihood, risk, difficulty, time). The nurse needs to consider the following:

- Which explanations are most and least likely?
- Which possible explanations are the most serious?

Client Scenario continued

On day 3 of hospitalization, Adella Gul continues to have a productive cough and pain on inspiration. The client refuses to ambulate because of fatigue.

The nurse creates a list of actual or potential problems that the client may experience:

Actual or Potential Problems	Reasons for Actual or Potential Problems
Diarrhea	Side effect to antibiotic therapy
Nausea and vomiting	Side effect to antibiotic therapy
Respiratory failure	Inappropriate treatment or progression of illness
Sepsis	Inappropriate treatment or progression of illness
Allergic reaction to medications	Adverse reaction to antibiotic therapy
MRSA infection	Prolonged hospital stay; increased risk of nosocomial infection
Venous thromboembolism	Reluctance to ambulate due to fatigue
Dehydration	Inability to drink fluids due to frequent cough

The nurse then prioritizes actual or potential problems. When prioritizing hypotheses, the nurse needs to rank in order of priority actual or potential client problems based on the cues that pose the greatest danger to the client.

The top four analyzing cues that have the highest priority for the nurse (listed in order of priority) are:

1. The client is at risk for a venous thromboembolism because of the reluctance to ambulate due to fatigue.
2. The client is at risk for an allergic reaction from the antibiotic.

3. The client is at risk for diarrhea as a side effect from the antibiotic therapy.
4. The client is at risk for a MRSA infection due to prolonged hospital stay.

Prioritizing the cues, the nurse recognizes that the client is at the highest risk for developing venous thromboembolism due to the client's fatigue and reluctance to ambulate. The nurse plans to ambulate the client at least three times a day to help prevent this adverse outcome.

NCJMM: Generate Solutions

The NCJMM expands on the Nursing Process step of planning by identifying expected outcomes and using hypotheses to generate solutions, or interventions, to achieve the expected outcomes. The nurse needs to consider the following:

- What are the desirable outcomes?
- What interventions can achieve those outcomes?
- What should be avoided?

The nurse must be able to identify interventions that are indicated to guide client care while also recognizing interventions that are contraindicated and to be avoided. Conceptually the nurse designs a grid similar to the one shown below to identify these actions. Nursing interventions that are appropriate to assist the client in attaining desirable outcomes are identified as "indicated." Recognizing that the nurse has limited time to spend with a single client, it becomes imperative that the prioritized essential elements of care are done and interventions that are safe, but "nonessential" are omitted.

Client Scenario continued

Health Teaching	Indicated	Contraindicated	Nonessential
"Use abdominal muscles for more forceful cough."	X		
"Ambulate three times a day."	X		
"Lie in supine position when sleeping."		X	
"Change position every 10 minutes."			X
"Perform deep breathing and coughing exercises every hour."	X		

NCJMM: Take Action

The NCJMM expands on the Nursing Process step of implementation by taking action(s) that addresses the highest priorities. The nurse needs to consider the following:

- Which intervention or combination of interventions is most appropriate?
- How should the intervention(s) be accomplished (performed, requested, administered, communicated, taught, documented, etc.)?

Client Scenario continued

The physician writes a list of orders for the client:

- Oxygen by nasal canula at 2 liters per minute (LPM)
- Levofloxacin 750 mg IV every 24 hours
- Acetaminophen 500 mg orally every 4 to 6 hours for fever >100°F (37.8°C)
- 0.9% sodium chloride (normal saline) 75 mL/hour, IV
- Laboratory tests: blood culture and sensitivity (C&S), complete blood cell count (CBC), arterial blood gas (ABG)

- Activity: bedrest with bathroom privileges
- Diet: low sodium

The nurse recognizes that all the physician's orders will be implemented but prioritizes them by importance. The nurse identifies the three orders that should be performed immediately:

- Oxygen by nasal canula at 2 LPM
- Laboratory tests: blood culture and sensitivity (C&S), complete blood cell count (CBC), arterial blood gas (ABG)
- Levofloxacin 750 mg IV every 24 hours

The priority for Adella Gul is oxygenation, laboratory work, and antibiotics. The nurse recognizes that the blood work needs to be drawn before starting the antibiotics to prevent interference with the results.

NCJMM: Evaluate Outcomes

The NCJMM expands on the Nursing Process step of evaluation by comparing observed outcomes against expected outcomes. The nurse needs to consider the following:

- What signs point to improving/declining unchanged status?
- Were the interventions effective?
- Would other interventions have been more effective?

As in the step of generate solutions, the nurse in the NCJMM conceptualizes a grid to evaluate various aspects of a client's care, determining whether the client's status has improved, not changed, or declined.

Client Scenario continued

Applying this step to Adella Gul's case, the nurse evaluates the client's condition and mentally notes the impact of care on various parameters:

Assessment Finding	Improved	No Change	Declined
Crackles in right lower lobe		X	
WBC 8,000 μ/L	X		
Temperature 101ºF (38.3°C)			X
Pulse oximetry reading 98%	X		
No chest pain when coughing	X		

After the nurse reviews the above data, their evaluation reveals the client's need for additional interventions for the rising temperature and persistent crackles in the right lower lobe of the lungs.

Standardized Verbal Communication or Hand-off

A hand-off is a transfer and acceptance of client care responsibility achieved through effective communication (The Joint Commission, 2014). It is a real-time process of passing client-specific information from one caregiver to another or from one team of caregivers to another for the purpose of ensuring the continuity and safety of the client's care (The Joint Commission, 2014). The hand-off requires a sender and a receiver. Senders are responsible for sending or transmitting client data and releasing the care of the client to receivers, who have been identified as those who will receive client data and accept care of the client. It is reported that differences in communication styles between nurses and physicians are contributing factors in communication errors (Greenfield, 1999). Nurse-physician communication is subject to differences in training and reporting expectations (Shahid & Thomas, 2018). According to a 2015 study by The Joint Commission, communication failures were partly responsible for 30% of all malpractice claims, resulting in 1,744 deaths and $1.7 billion in malpractice costs (CRICO Strategies, 2015), and responsible for 70% of adverse events (Dingley et al, n.d.). In 2006, The Joint Commission established a National Patient Safety Goal that addressed hand-off communication. In 2010, the requirement became a standard. Provision of Care Standard PC.02.02.01, element of performance (EP) 2, requires the following: The organization's process for hand-off communication provides for the opportunity for discussion between the giver and receiver of client information. Note: Such information may include the client's condition, care, treatment, medications, services, and any recent or anticipated changes to any of these (The Joint Commission, 2015).

SBAR

Within the multiple health-care settings and interdisciplinary health-care teams, there are many standardized communication tools. The gold standard communication tool is SBAR (situation, background, assessment, recommendation).

The SBAR protocol was introduced at Kaiser Permanente in 2003 as a framework for structuring conversations between physicians and nurses about situations requiring immediate attention (Doucette, 2006). SBAR was originally implemented in health-care settings with the intent of improving nurse-physician communication in acute care situations; however, it has also been shown to increase communication satisfaction among health-care providers and their perceptions that communication is more precise (Woodhall et al, 2008; Shahid & Thomas, 2018). In Table 1-3 the left-hand column shows the information needed for SBAR communication, and the right-hand column shows how SBAR is used in the clinical setting using the client Adella Gul.

Table 1-3 Example of Effective SBAR Communication

S	**Situation**: What is the situation you are calling about? • Identify self, unit, client, room number. • Briefly state the problem, what is it, when it happened or started, and how severe.	"Hello, Dr. Davidson, this is Mohammad from 8 west, the RN caring for Adella Gul who was admitted for right lower lobe pneumonia."
B	**Background**: Pertinent background information related to the situation could include the following: • The admitting diagnosis and date of admission • List of current medications, allergies, IV fluids, and laboratory results • Most recent vital signs • Laboratory results: provide the date and time test was done and results of previous tests for comparison • Other clinical information • Code status	"Adella Gul was admitted this afternoon to treat right lower lobe pneumonia and was started on levofloxacin 750 mg IV."
A	**Assessment**: What is the nurse's assessment of the situation?	"Adella Gul is complaining of itching. A physical assessment reveals a red papular rash on the chest. IV levofloxacin was discontinued."
R	**Recommendation**: What is the nurse's recommendation or what does he/she want? Examples: • Notification that client has been admitted • Client needs to be seen now • Order change	"I believe Adella Gul needs IV diphenhydramine and a different antibiotic."

Institute for Healthcare Improvement (ihi.org). This SBAR tool was developed by Kaiser Permanente. Please feel free to use and reproduce these materials in the spirit of client safety, and please retain this footer in the spirit of appropriate recognition.

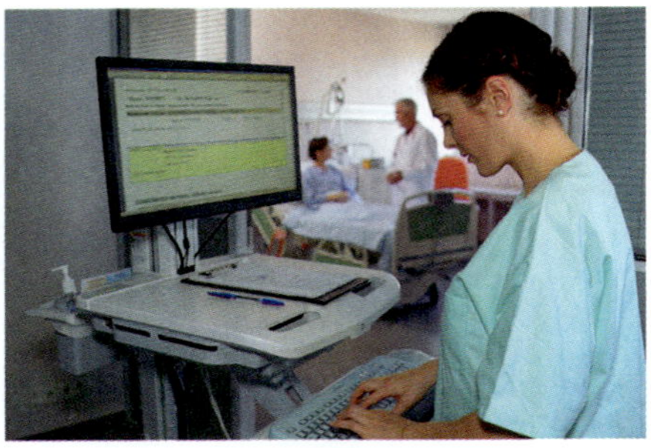

Figure 1-9 Documenting a client's clinical condition accurately is a vital component of client care.

Written Documentation

There are many documentation methods nurses use to document client care (Fig. 1-9). A progress note documents the client's progress toward achieving stated goals and outcomes. Frequently used documentation methods are:

CBE: Charting by exception
DAR: Data, action, response/revision
Focus charting
PIE: Problem/diagnosis, intervention, evaluation
PIO: Problem/diagnosis, intervention, outcome
SOAP: Subjective data, objective data, analysis of data stated as a nursing diagnosis, plan
SOAPIER: Subjective data, objective data, analysis of data stated as a nursing diagnosis, plan, intervention/implementation, evaluation, revision

Of the above documentation methods, SOAP notes are still routinely used. SOAP notes are used frequently in both academic and clinical settings. An example of a SOAP note for the client Adella Gul is:

S: "I have an itchy rash on my chest that started about 15 minutes ago."
O: Scattered red papules on client's chest that started 15 minutes after IV levofloxacin was infused, respiratory rate 18 breaths per minute without use of accessory muscles; breath sounds with crackles in right lower lobe that do not clear with coughing, no wheezing, blood pressure 145/85 mm Hg, heart rate 108 bpm; oxygen saturation 93%
A: Probable adverse/allergic reaction to antibiotic, levofloxacin
P: Stop levofloxacin; contact physician on call to report adverse reaction and get new client care orders for treatment

Institutions may have their own method for charting. Each charting method has advantages and disadvantages. With electronic charting the structure of the selected electronic health record system dictates the documentation format.

Assessment in Brief

Critical Thinking and Clinical Reasoning in Nursing

1. Critical thinking, clinical reasoning, and clinical judgment are incorporated into all aspects of client care.
2. The quality of critical thinking can be evaluated by applying the Universal Intellectual Standards.
3. Nurses frame their critical thinking by using the Nursing Process and Nursing Clinical Judgment Measurement Model.
4. Client status and response to treatment is communicated in both verbal and written forms using standardized formats or tools.

Review Questions

1. All of these are steps of the Nursing Process except which of the following?
   a. Evaluation
   b. Assessment
   c. Recognize cues
   d. Planning
2. On midshift assessment, the nurse notes the client has an acute mental status change. The nurse anticipates the client will need IV fluids. This is an example of what part of the Nursing Process?
   a. Take action
   b. Evaluation
   c. Planning
   d. Nursing diagnosis
3. Which of the following are included in SBAR communication?
   a. Subjective information, background, assessment, and revisions needed
   b. Situation, background, assessment, and recommendation
   c. Scientific findings, background, all vitals, requests
   d. Summary, backdrop, analysis, recommendation
4. The nurse uses logic and reasoning to identify the strengths and weaknesses of a solution. What skill is the nurse using?
   a. Critical thinking
   b. Clinical judgment
   c. Critical reasoning
   d. Clinical experience
5. The NCSBN Clinical Judgment Measurement Model consists of which of the following components? Select all that apply.
   a. Take action
   b. Diagnosis
   c. Analyze cues
   d. Prioritize hypotheses
   e. Recognize cues
6. Physical examination by the nurse is considered which of the following?
   a. Subjective data
   b. Health history
   c. Functional health pattern
   d. Objective data
7. A nurse on a medical-surgical unit calls a health-care provider to give SBAR communication. The nurse reports, "Rafqa Hadid is complaining of severe abdominal pain despite taking the prescribed pain medication. The client states the pain is so severe that getting out of bed to ambulate as prescribed is not possible." Which element of SBAR communication does this information represent?
   a. Situation
   b. Background
   c. Assessment
   d. Recommendation
8. The nurse is writing a SOAP note regarding the client's recent episode of hematuria. The documentation "My urine is bright red!" is best placed in which section of the SOAP note?
   a. Subjective data
   b. Objective data
   c. Analysis of data
   d. Plan
9. Which of the following is the correct order of Maslow's Hierarchy of Needs?
   a. Self-actualization, love and belonging, safety and security needs, self-esteem, physiological needs
   b. Physiological needs, safety and security needs, love and belonging, self-esteem, self-actualization
   c. Self-actualization, safety and security needs, self-esteem, love and belonging, physiological needs
   d. Physiological needs, self-esteem, safety and security needs, love and belonging, self-actualization
10. Which of the following are some of the Universal Intellectual Standards proposed by Paul and Elder? Select all that apply.
   a. Clarity
   b. Analysis
   c. Precision
   d. Explanation
   e. Fairness

CHAPTER

2 Communication Techniques and the Client Interview

Learning Outcomes

1. Discuss the role of the nurse and the client in a health-care interview.
2. Describe the role of motivational interviewing in the client interview.
3. Recognize factors that facilitate or hinder the communication and interview processes.
4. Describe effective communication techniques.
5. Describe the communication techniques of listening responses.
6. Describe the communication techniques of action responses.
7. Describe nontherapeutic communication techniques.
8. Describe problematic questioning techniques and interviewing behaviors and how they can be transformed into more appropriate responses.
9. Describe the opportunities and challenges in communicating with sexual and gender minorities.
10. Identify how to facilitate the communication and interview process for the client with a differing ability.

The nursing health assessment interview is a purposeful, time-limited verbal interaction between the nurse and the client. It is initiated to collect specific information regarding the client and the client's health status. Other purposes include validating appropriate health and illness information provided by the client or found in the client's record and identifying the client's knowledge of personal health and illness status. Accurate and complete information about the client serves as a foundation for subsequent nurse-client interactions and for medical and nursing interventions. The nurse-client interaction requires skill in communication and interviewing techniques that the nurse can learn and refine.

The Client Interview

The nursing assessment interview can be differentiated from the traditional medical interview. The medical interview typically focuses on the client's physical or emotional state, whereas the nursing interview is holistic and includes comprehensive information about the whole client. The nursing interview includes an assessment of the client's physical, mental, emotional, developmental, social, cultural, and spiritual health. Data are collected concerning the client's present and past states of health, including the client's family status and relationships, cultural background, lifestyle preferences, and developmental level. Other factors considered in data collection are the client's self-concept, religious affiliation, social supports, burden of care, sexuality, and reproductive processes. Remember, the health assessment interview is a goal-directed interview. It is not a social interaction.

The Role of the Nurse

The nurse is often the first person on the health-care team to interact with the client. The nurse frequently assumes the role of intermediary between the client and the larger health-care system. A critical role of the nurse is to assist the client in effectively using the system. The climate and tone of the initial client interview can influence all future interactions the client has in the health-care setting (Fig. 2-1). The nurse's attitude and expectations, both positive and negative, set the stage for the interview and can affect its outcome.

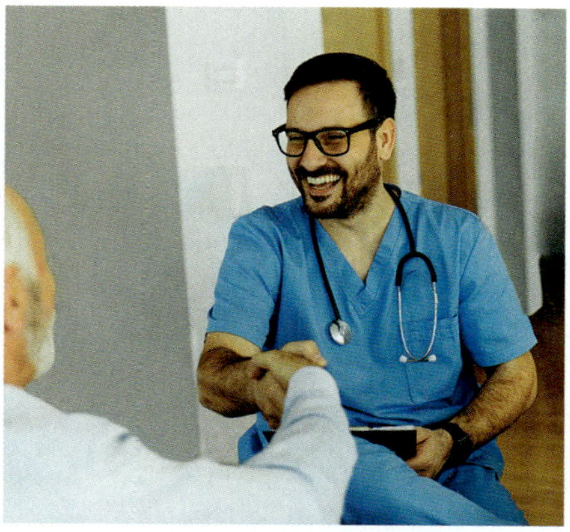

Figure 2-1 The tone of the nurse-client introduction sets the stage for the client interview and client care.

First impressions of individuals are important and can imprint long-lasting thoughts and feelings. The personal appearances of both the client and the nurse contribute significantly to the formation of first impressions. In U.S. culture, it is expected that health-care providers present a professional appearance by wearing clean and appropriate clothing for the particular setting in which they work. Hair should be pulled back from the face, nails should be neatly trimmed, and perfumes or other odor enhancers should be avoided. Jewelry should be kept to a minimum to avoid being distracting. Likewise, the manner in which the client physically presents to the nurse may influence the nurse's perceptions of the client.

The nurse is the facilitator of the interview and thus collaborates with clients in establishing a mutually respectful dialogue. Encouraging clients to speak freely and expressing concern for the clients are essential in this process. For example, if clients think that no one in the health-care setting listens to their concerns and feelings, then they may speak very little. Because accurate data collection is the primary purpose of the interview, clients must feel comfortable and safe to provide information, ask questions, and express fears or concerns. The nurse can foster an atmosphere of safety and comfort by approaching all clients with an accepting, respectful, and nonjudgmental attitude.

The nurse is also in the position of assessing the client as a unique, holistic being. As many aspects of the client's life experiences are discussed, the nurse may recognize "teachable moments" that promote health during the course of the interaction.

The Role of the Client

The client is an active and equal participant in the interview process and should feel free to openly communicate thoughts, feelings, perceptions, and factual information. Most clients possess previous knowledge of or experience with the health-care system that influences their current perceptions and behavior. Understanding how clients see their role in this system is vital to the successful completion of any health interview.

In today's health-care arena, clients are taking a more active role in both their own health care and in health-care decisions (Fig. 2-2). Clients are much more apt to question health-care providers, research their personal health needs, perform self-treatment, and demand a role in decision making. Frequently, clients actively seek health-care providers who possess clinical competence as well as a willingness to provide individualized attention in a genuine, caring relationship.

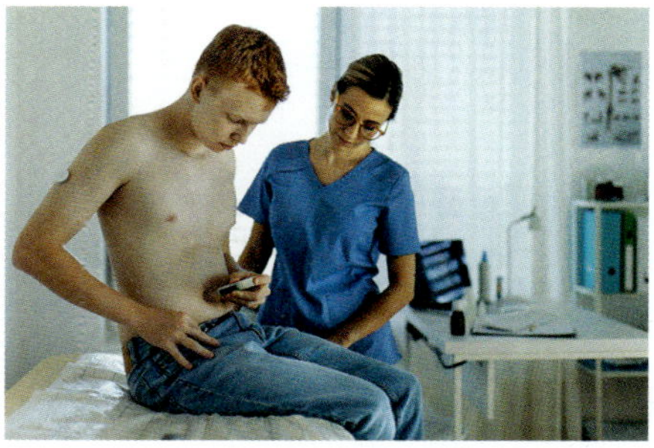

Figure 2-2 Clients are encouraged to take an active role in their health care. This adolescent is learning to administer his own insulin shots.

Motivational Interviewing

When interviewing clients, the nurse can also assume the role of motivational interviewer. This technique was originally developed to work with

NURSING CHECKLIST

Preparing for the Interview

1. Gather all available client information.
2. Seek out an appropriate setting for the interview.
3. Set aside a block of time for the interview.
4. Assess yourself for possible problematic thoughts or feelings.
5. Stay focused on the client. Avoid multitasking and being occupied with other clients and their needs (or your own).
6. If possible, sit at an appropriate distance from the client and make frequent eye contact throughout the interaction. Sometimes the client interaction will be conducted while the nurse is standing. This can possibly intimidate the client if the nurse is perceived as looming over them in a position of superiority. When a nurse stands during an interview, it can also send a message to the client that the nurse is in a hurry to complete the interview.
7. Begin the interview with a friendly introduction.
   - Introduce yourself by name and title.
   - Ask how the client wants to be addressed or which name the client wants to be called. Address clients using their preferred name(s).
8. Be cognizant of the allotted time for the interview and try to avoid rushing the client through the interview process.

clients who use addictive substances. Motivational interviewing can also be used to positively affect clients' lives by changing long-term behavior that is deleterious to their health (e.g., smoking, unhealthy diets). Through empathy, the nurse can gain clients' trust when using this technique. First, clients must be able to identify that a situation exists that needs to be changed in their lives. In addition, clients must be willing to acknowledge that a change in behavior is needed to reach a better health state, and clients must be ready to accept assistance. In other words, clients must assume ownership of the deleterious behavior before the process can move forward.

The nurse, in conjunction with clients, must jointly set realistic healthcare goals. It is the nurse's responsibility to motivate clients to become independent and self-motivated as the behavior-change process begins. Verbal encouragement and review of behavior diaries at visits; phone calls; e-mails; and providing appropriate reading material, resources, and location of community self-help groups (if indicated) are all ways that the nurse can help clients sustain motivation to change the deleterious behavior. Thus, to have the highest chance of success, the nurse should meet with clients on a regular basis (the interval depends on the clients' situation and can vary from daily to weekly). The nurse must also recognize that clients may backslide during the intervention period; this, too, can be a normal part of the motivational process.

Factors Influencing the Interview

Factors that can affect the client's comfort level and, therefore, the effectiveness of the interview are discussed in the following sections.

Approach

Before approaching the client, gather all available client information; admission data and past medical records are often available and may significantly reduce the time needed for the interview.

Begin the interview with an introduction that includes your name and title. Address the client by the previously established preferred name. Communication using appropriate names is respectful and helps identify clients as unique individuals at a time when they may be feeling quite anxious. Giving recognition helps lower client anxiety.

Examples of approaches you can use:

"Good morning, Ms. Ahmed."

"Hello, Mr. Coffey. It's nice to see you again."

Providing the client with an explanation of what is to follow and an approximate time frame for the interview helps establish trust. This information also helps to increase the client's feeling of control. The more effective you are in establishing trust, the easier it will be to obtain information from the client, for example: "Good morning, Colonel Vasquez; my name is Gracia Pereira. I'm a registered nurse. I'd like to ask you some questions about what brought you here today."

Environment

The setting for the interview has a direct influence on the amount and quality of information gathered. Time and effort spent in seeking out an appropriate setting for the interview indicate concern for the client and for the quality and quantity of information collected. Whenever possible, the interview should be conducted in a private room with controlled lighting and temperature. Televisions, cell phones, iPads, and computers should be silenced. When a private setting is impossible, control the environment to minimize distractions and interruptions and to increase the client's comfort level. Use any physical barriers available in the room to provide as much privacy as possible. When all efforts to ensure even minimal privacy fail, conduct a shortened interview to gather only immediately pertinent information. Defer the complete interview until a later time when privacy can be ensured.

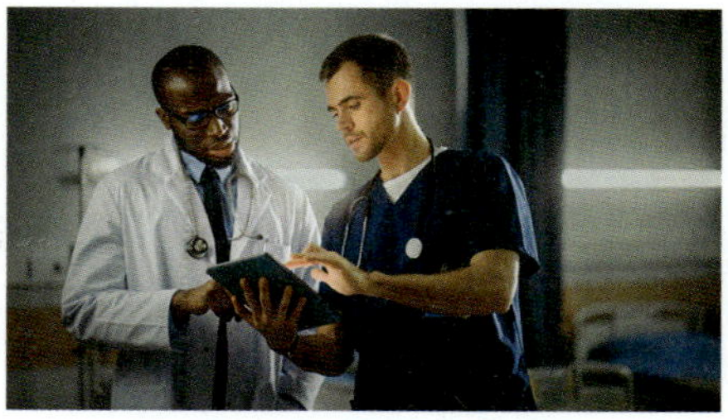

Figure 2-3 Sharing client information with colleagues is an important nursing role. Confidentiality must be observed at all times.

Confidentiality

Confidentiality is essential in developing trust between the nurse and the client. The client's willingness to communicate private and personal information is predicated on the assumption that this information will be used with discretion and for the benefit of the client (Fig. 2-3). Your verbal assurance of confidentiality often eases the client's concerns and fosters trust in the relationship.

In practice, there are certain exceptions to absolute confidentiality. For example, in a teaching institution where a team approach is used, information must be shared. Another important reason for sharing confidential information is when the client is a danger to self or others. Nurses need to be familiar with institutional policy and legal statutes on client confidentiality as well as the consequences of not adhering to them. It is essential to inform the client, before the interview, under what circumstances their information will be shared with others. Frequently, clients will have friends or family members with them. To ensure client comfort and confidentiality, ask the client whether these people should remain in the room for the interview.

HIPAA

Compliance with the privacy rule of the Health Insurance Portability and Accountability Act (HIPAA) became mandatory on April 14, 2003. This regulation affects all health-care providers, health care institutions, as well as service organizations, information system vendors, and universities. The goal of HIPAA is to safeguard the confidentiality of all client information, as well as to provide security for this information, whether it is in electronic or other form. In addition, HIPAA states that individuals have a right to access their medical records and to be informed of who else has been granted permission to view those records. Inappropriate use and release of confidential client information is punishable by law.

Note Taking

Although it is advisable to note information during the interview, the simple act of writing down or keyboarding what the client says may cause some client discomfort (Fig. 2-4). Early in the interview, explain the necessity of documenting pertinent information and, if possible, show the client the form or computerized program you will be using. You will become adept in skills that expedite charting information. Frequently, the client will lead the interview or discuss sensitive issues. When this occurs, give full attention to the client and defer formal recording of information. Key or jot down short phrases, words, and dates that can be used to complete formal data recording following the interview.

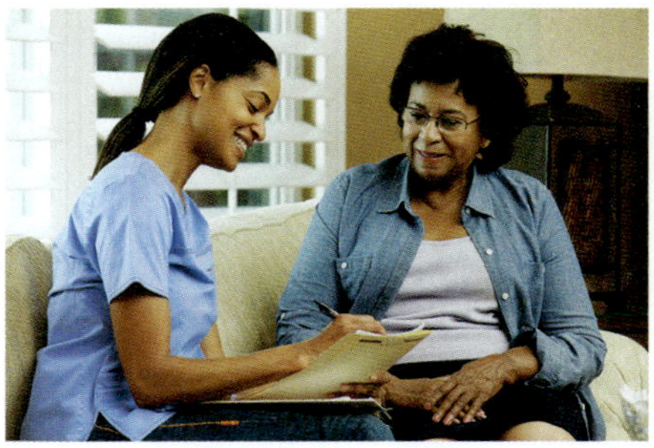

Figure 2-4 The client interview often requires note taking. Maintain rapport and eye contact as much as possible while taking notes.

Most health-care settings use computer-based charting for the client record. Input specific information, such as medications, allergies, and so forth, as you review this information with the client. If you are skilled at keyboarding, it is best to key information as the client relays it. For the less accomplished typist, it is advisable to key in main topics as they are discussed with the client. After the client interview, you can return to the electronic health record (EHR) and complete the documentation ensuring the information is complete and accurate.

Time, Length, Duration

To become fully involved with the client, enough time must be set aside for the interview. When scheduling an interview for the hospitalized client, look at the client's daily activities, then select a block of time for the interview that does not conflict with the client's mealtime or other planned activities. Do not hesitate to ask the client what interview times would be least disruptive to their daily routine and try to accommodate the client's request. For health-care visits outside the hospital setting, try to see the client at a time that does not conflict with a physical therapy session or other service.

Self-Awareness

Nurses' personal beliefs and value systems, attitudes, biases, and preconceptions can influence the sending and receiving of messages. Nurses need to possess self-awareness to avoid faulty assumptions, biases, and preconceptions. The nurse must continually validate information through the use of careful data gathering and effective interviewing techniques. Strive to treat all clients fairly, respectfully, and with dignity.

Generally, the nurse's subjective feelings during the interview are an indication of the climate of the interview and can be used to provide additional assessment information. For example, the nurse's feelings of anxiety during an interview may be an indication or a reflection of the client's feelings of fear, anxiety, or anger. Careful attention to these feelings may direct you to change the interview format (to lower client anxiety) or to refocus the questions (to gather specific data).

Stages of the Interview Process

The interview process has three stages: the introduction or the joining stage, the working stage, and the termination stage.

Stage I

The **joining stage** is the introduction or first stage of the interview process, during which the nurse and the client establish trust and get to know one another. During this stage, work with the client to define the relationship and establish goals for this and any subsequent interactions.

Stage II

The **working stage** of the interview process is the time during which the bulk of the client data is collected. It is a nursing responsibility to keep the interview goal directed, including refocusing the client and redefining the goals established in the joining stage.

Stage III

The **termination stage** is the last stage of the interview process, during which information is summarized and validated. During this stage, give the client an indication of the amount of time left in the interview and allow the client the opportunity to give additional information and make comments or statements. For example, "We have about five more minutes, Mr. Nguyen; is there anything else you would like to add or mention?" Other important steps in the termination stage are summarizing and validating information and planning for future interviews.

Factors Affecting Communication

Elements that can affect the sending and receiving of messages are discussed in the following sections.

Listening

Active listening, or the act of perceiving what is said both verbally and nonverbally, is a critical factor in the success of the health assessment interview. The primary goal of active listening is to decode client messages in order to understand the situation or problem as the other person perceives it. Pay careful attention to all sensory data to better understand the client's message and formulate an appropriate response. Be aware of how personal characteristics, choice of communication techniques, and the manner and timing of their use can affect communication.

Nonverbal Cues

Nonverbal communication is communicating a message without words. Nonverbal behaviors effectively supplement the spoken word and provide information about both nurse and client. These behaviors can provide insight into the client's cultural expectations, current physical and emotional states, and perceived self-image. Nonverbal cues, such as body position, nervous repetitive movements of the hands or legs, rapid blinking, lack of eye contact, yawning, fidgeting, excessive smiling or frowning, and repetitive clearing of the throat, may be indications both of the client's health and of feelings that the client may not be comfortable expressing verbally.

Health-care settings often evoke a great deal of anxiety, uncertainty, or fear in clients. Loss of personal control is a major obstacle confronting clients in health-care settings, regardless of whether they are seriously ill. In an attempt to maintain some control in unfamiliar circumstances and to decrease anxiety, clients frequently look to nurses for cues on how to behave or how to respond to questions. Nonverbal behaviors by the nurse can indicate empathy and attention or indifference and inattention. Such behaviors powerfully influence client comfort levels, feelings of control, and willingness to share information. Because of this, nurses need to continuously monitor their own nonverbal behaviors (Fig. 2-5).

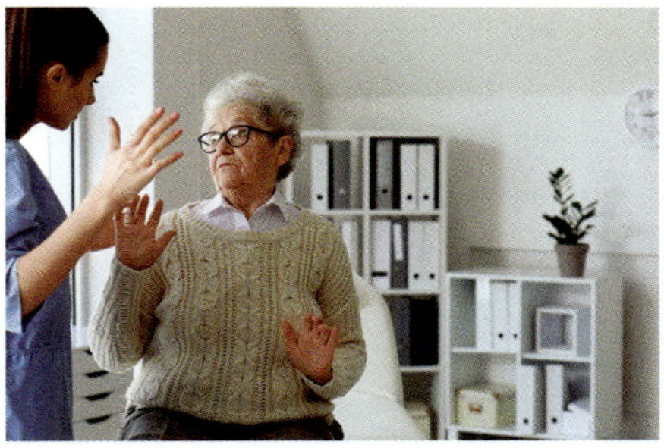

Figure 2-5 The nurse's nonverbal communication in this interaction may negatively impact the nurse/client interview.

Distance

The amount of space a person considers appropriate for interaction is a significant factor in the interview process and is determined in part by cultural influences. In the United States, distances are generally categorized as follows:

- Intimate distance is from the client to approximately 1.5 feet.
- Personal distance is approximately 1.5 to 4 feet.
- Social distance is approximately 4 to 12 feet.
- Public distance is approximately 12 feet or more.

Intimate distance is the closest and involves some touching or physical contact. Personal distance may also involve some touching or physical contact, and it may ease communication in some instances, such as for clients who are hearing impaired. In other instances, personal distance may be threatening or invasive to the client. Social distance is considered appropriate for the interview process because it allows for good eye contact and for ease in hearing and in seeing the client's nonverbal cues. Public distance is usually used in formal settings, such as in a classroom where the teacher stands in front of the class. It is not considered appropriate for an interview.

Personal Space

Personal space can be defined as the space over which a person claims ownership. In a health-care facility, the client's hospital room, bed, and bathroom are considered the client's personal space. The client may be very protective of this space and consider unauthorized use of it an invasion of privacy.

Effective Communication Techniques

Effective communication techniques facilitate or support interactions between the nurse and the client and foster their continuation. These techniques encompass both verbal and nonverbal approaches. The more skilled you can become in understanding the communication process, the more effectively you can use it in a purposeful, goal-directed manner to meet your needs for information and the client's need for attention to health concerns or problems. Because individuals who come to a health-care provider are frequently anxious, effectively communicating your interest and concern greatly enhances the effectiveness of the interview and interaction.

Certain specific verbal communication techniques are available to help you facilitate this interaction. The effectiveness of these techniques will vary from individual to individual. At first, these techniques may feel awkward, stilted, or forced; keep in mind that communicating effectively is a learned skill (similar to other nursing skills) and, as such, improves with practice.

> **NURSING TIP**
>
> **The Use of Touch in the Client Interview**
>
> You must be mindful of the use of touch during the client interview. Although a caring touch, a pat on the hand, or other gesture may send a message of empathy to a crying individual, it may not be appropriate in all situations. The client's cultural background may dictate what is or is not appropriate (see Chapter 5). Also, if a client has a history of physical abuse or neglect or is recovering from a skin disorder such as a burn, a well-meaning touch may be interpreted in a hostile manner.

Using Open-Ended Questions

Open-ended questions encourage the client to provide general rather than more focused information (Fig. 2-6). Beginning the health assessment interview with open-ended questions provides the client with a sense of control, leaving the choice of what to say, how much to say, and how to say it up to the client. These questions indicate respect for the client's ability to articulate important or pressing health concerns, and thus to help set priorities.

Examples of open-ended questions:

Nurse: *What are some of your concerns about caring for your terminally ill father at home?*

OR

Nurse: *How do you typically deal with a sore throat?*

Open-ended questions that begin with the words *how, what, where, when,* and *who* are usually more effective in eliciting the maximum amount of information than those that begin with the word *why. Why* questions can cause clients to become defensive and can trigger their need to explain or defend their ideas and behaviors, thus setting up an adversarial relationship between nurse and client. Although open-ended questions are quite helpful in the health assessment interview, they can be time consuming and may not be appropriate in situations requiring rapid access to information and rapid response by health-care providers. Overuse of open-ended questions, especially with clients who are confused, vague in their responses, or extremely talkative, can cause the nurse to miss important information and face time constraints.

In certain situations, perhaps because of anxiety or unfamiliarity with the health-care system, clients may attempt to ascertain what answers the nurse wants or expects and what areas the nurse seems to feel are important. The client will then focus on those rather than on areas that are most important to the client. With open-ended questions, you can encourage the client to define what is important. When eliciting health history, it is usually best to let the client speak uninterrupted. After the client completes an answer, you can proceed with further questions or clarification.

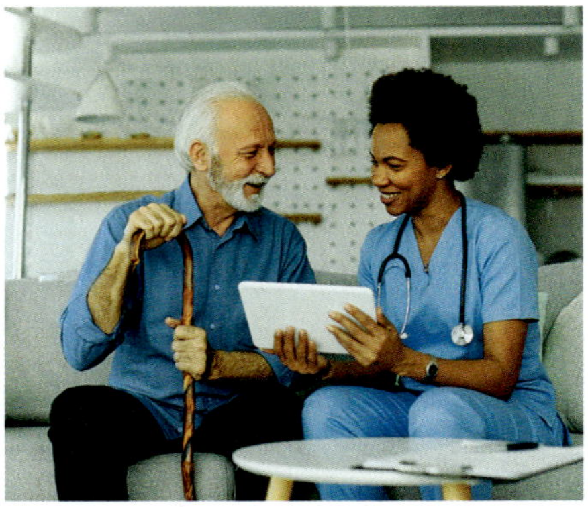

Figure 2-6 The nurse uses open-ended questions to gather general information in the client interview.

Using Closed Questions

Closed questions are those that regulate or restrict client response. They can frequently be answered with a "yes" or a "no." Closed questions can be used to focus the interview, pinpoint specific areas of concern, and elicit valuable information quickly and efficiently.

Examples of effective closed questions:
Nurse: *Do you have a plan to end your life?*
OR
Nurse: *Has this type of allergic reaction ever happened to you before?*

However, if used too frequently, closed questions can disrupt communication because they limit client responses and interaction. Even well-directed closed questions may take the initiative away from clients, giving them the impression that the nurse is in charge of the interview, already knows the answer to the question being asked, and is directing the client's responses.

Examples of ineffective closed questions:
Nurse: *Do you still feel sad and depressed?*
OR
Nurse: *Are you afraid to tell your parents that you are sexually active?*

Facilitating

Once the health assessment interview has started, there may be periods when clients stop talking because of anxiety, uncertainty, or embarrassment. You can use a variety of both verbal and nonverbal means to encourage clients to continue talking. Phrases such as "go on" or "uh-huh," the simple repetition of key words the client has spoken, or even head nods prompt the client to resume speaking and also indicate your continued interest and attention.

Using Silence

Silence, too, has its place in the assessment interview. When understood and used effectively by the nurse, periods of silence can help structure and pace the interview; convey respect and acceptance; and, in many cases, elicit additional client data. Silence on the part of the client may indicate feelings of anxiety, confusion, or embarrassment or simply a lack of understanding about the question asked or an inability to speak English. Nonverbal data such as these are often lost if the nurse is a persistent talker (Fig. 2-7). Conversely, if overused, silence can contribute to an awkward, disjointed interview providing minimal structure or direction for the client and little helpful data for the nurse.

Using silence effectively may seem like a difficult skill to master. Frequently, silences seem longer than they actually are. When silences occur, you may feel discomfort and pressure to speak in order to be actually "doing" something therapeutic; instead, handle silences by being quiet and observing the client's behavior for what is not being said verbally.

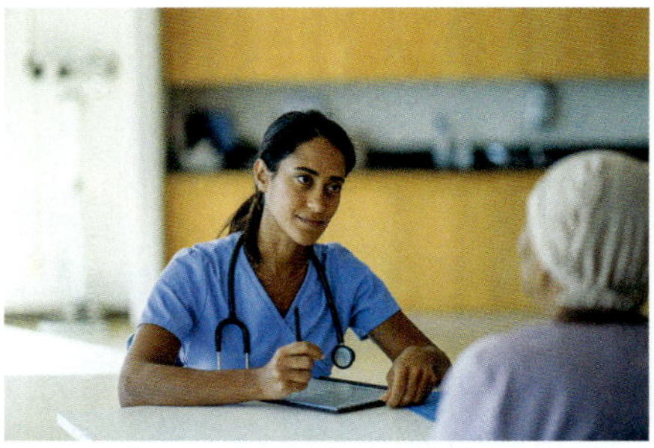

Figure 2-7 The nurse is using the communication technique of silence with this client who has cancer. She is observing the client's nonverbal communication to prompt additional dialogue.

Grouping Communication Techniques

Communication techniques often seem mechanical and artificial to the beginning nurse; one way to make them less so is to group or cluster them according to their primary purposes. One simple way to group interview techniques is to divide them into two groups: listening responses and action responses.

Listening Responses

Listening responses are attempts to accurately receive, process, and then respond to client messages. They provide a way for the nurse to communicate empathy, concern, and attentiveness. To truly listen to what the client says, the nurse must not only process the words spoken by the client but also understand the context of the client's experience.

Listening responses provide the nurse with a vehicle for understanding the client's perspective. Clients will realize that they are heard and that the nurse is an advocate for them. Listening responses include making observations, restating, reflecting, clarifying, interpreting, sequencing, encouraging comparisons, and summarizing.

Making Observations.

When making observations, the nurse verbalizes perceptions about the client's behavior, then shares them with the client. Calling to attention behavior about which the client might be unaware may prove insightful and help increase the client's conscious awareness of this behavior. Sharing observations is also a way to validate client competency and sense of control in an environment or situation where a client often feels out of control, uncertain, or overwhelmed.

Examples of making observations:

Nurse: *Speaking about these symptoms seems to make you tense. I notice that you are clenching your fists and grimacing.*

OR

Nurse: *I notice that each time you've been confronted with that problem, you've known how to handle it appropriately.*

Restating

Restating involves repeating or rephrasing the main idea expressed by the client and lets the client know you are paying attention. It promotes further dialogue and provides the client with an opportunity to explain or elaborate on an issue or concern.

Example of restating:

Client: *I don't sleep well anymore. I find myself waking up frequently at night.*

Nurse: *You're having difficulty sleeping?*

Reflecting

Reflecting is another listening response; it focuses on the content of the client's message as well as the client's feelings. In reflecting, the nurse directs the client's own questions, feelings, and ideas back to the client and provides an opportunity for the client to reconsider or expand on what was just said (Fig. 2-8). The client's point of view is given value, and the nurse, although indicating an interest in what the client has to say, refrains from giving advice, passing judgment, or assuming responsibility for the client's thoughts or feelings.

Examples of reflecting:

Client: *Do you think I should tell the doctor I stopped taking my medication?*

Nurse: *What do you think about that?*

Client: *Well, yes, I think that I probably should. Not taking my medication could be one of the reasons I'm feeling so run down. But that medication just makes me so teary and agitated.*

Nurse: *You sound a bit agitated. It seems as if you've been thinking about this a lot.*

Client: *I told that young doctor that I had problems with this medication, and he just didn't listen.*

Nurse: *Sounds as if you are pretty angry.*

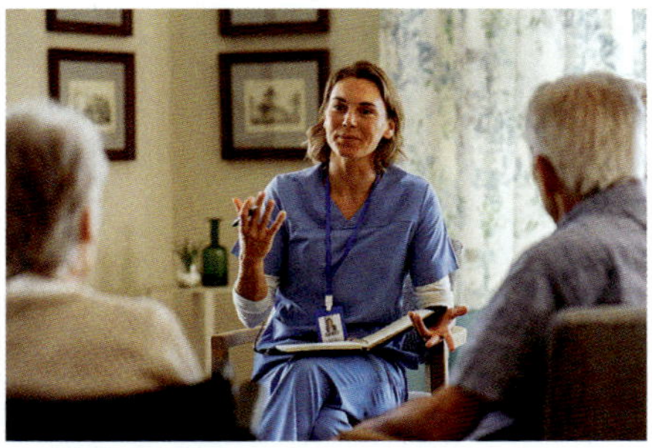

Figure 2-8 The nurse assists the client and family in reflecting on their feelings.

Clarifying

Clarifying is a communication technique the nurse can use to make clear something the client says or to pinpoint the message when the client's words and nonverbal behavior do not agree. Be sure you understand exactly what the client means before continuing, because communication may stop if the client feels misunderstood or not heard (Fig. 2-9). Distortions or misunderstandings about client data can occur if the nurse interprets client statements using only personal experiences and perceptions. Even more crucial is that making assumptions may cause the interviewer to proceed from a faulty database.

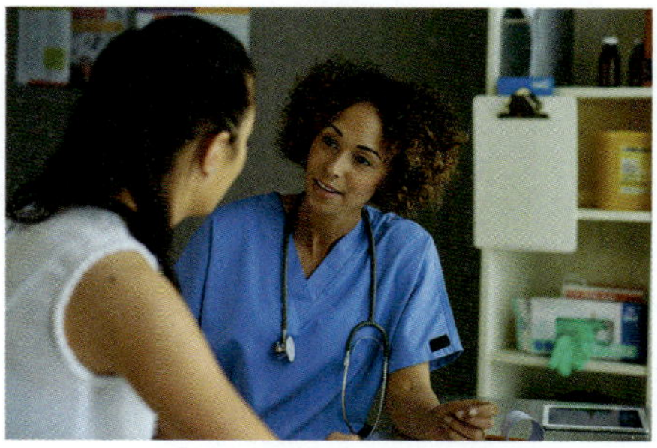

Figure 2-9 The nurse is clarifying the client's statements in order to understand what the client is saying.

Example of a clarifying response:

Client: *During yoga class, I get the most awful pain in my back.*

Nurse: *Please describe the back pain that you experience in yoga class.*

Interpreting

With interpreting, you have the opportunity to share your inferences or conclusions gathered from the client's interview. Although there is always the risk that your interpretation of the facts is incorrect, you are well poised to link events that perhaps the client was not able to piece together.

Examples of interpreting:

Nurse: *Your headaches seem to occur every time you eat nuts and chocolate.*

OR

Client: *My stomach pains occur only from late summer to midspring.*

Nurse: *From what you have just told me, could the stress of your teaching job [client works from September to May] be causing your pain?*

Sequencing

To effectively assess client needs, the nurse often requires knowledge of a time frame within which symptoms or problems developed or occurred. One way of getting at this information involves asking the client to place a symptom, a problem, or an event in its proper sequence. Sequencing also helps both client and nurse become aware of any patterns in the client's behavior that might indicate recurring themes. They can relate to feelings (depression or anxiety), behavior (refusal to take appropriate medications, consistently putting self in risky situations), or experiences (being beaten, being hurt, being misunderstood by health-care providers). Pattern identification provides the nurse with clues for further focus.

Examples of sequencing:

Nurse: *Did this sharp pain occur each time you had sexual intercourse or only when you didn't empty your bladder first?*

OR

Nurse: *What specific events led you to feel overwhelmed and suicidal?*

Encouraging Comparisons

Encouraging comparisons is a technique that enables both participants in the health assessment interview to become more aware of patterns, themes, or specific symptomatology in the client's life. It also helps the client to deal more effectively with unfamiliar situations by placing the symptoms or problems in the context of something else that is familiar and therefore more comfortable to the client. Often an awareness of successful prior dealings with similar situations increases client confidence levels.

Examples of encouraging comparisons:

Nurse: *Have you had similar experiences? What occurred?*

OR

Nurse: *In what way was this asthma attack different from or the same as your previous ones?*

OR

Nurse: *In what way was your reaction to this medication similar to or different from your reaction to other antibiotics you've taken?*

> **NURSING TIP**
> **The Use of Humor in the Client Interview**
> Humor can be an effective communication technique in the client interview. It can make an anxious client more at ease, defuse tension, and make it easier for a client to discuss sensitive issues. However, ill-timed humor or the use of inappropriate humor can offend individuals and make them distrustful of you.

Summarizing

Summarizing is a communication technique that helps clients to organize their thinking. Because of this, summarizing is especially useful at the end of the health assessment interview. A brief, concise review of the important points covered helps the client identify anything that has been left out and helps the nurse confirm understanding of what the client said. In addition, summarizing indicates interest and concern that the client feels heard as well as finished.

Example of summarizing:

Nurse: *During this past hour, you have shared with me several health concerns, of which the most vexing to you is your difficulty in losing weight. Is that correct?*

Summarizing also provides a means of smoothly transitioning to a new topic or section of the health assessment.

Example of transitioning:

Nurse: *You talked about your past experience with diabetes and what happened to you yesterday; now let's talk about what brought you in today.*

Action Responses

Action responses are the second group of effective interviewing techniques. These responses stimulate clients to make some change in their thinking and behavior. Action responses include such communication techniques as focusing, exploring, presenting reality, confronting, informing, collaborating, limit setting, and normalizing.

Focusing

Focusing allows the nurse to concentrate on or "track" a specific point the client has made. This technique is particularly useful with clients whose heightened anxiety level causes increased confusion, altered concentration, or jumping from topic to topic. With the nurse's assistance in focusing, the client is able to proceed with the health history in a clearer, more organized, thoughtful, thorough manner.

Examples of focusing:

Nurse: *Tell me more about the chest pain you experience when you begin to exercise.*

OR

Nurse: *You've mentioned several times that your partner is concerned about your smoking. Let's go back to that.*

Exploring

In exploring, the nurse is attempting to develop, in more detail, a specific area of content or client concern. The purpose of exploring is to identify patterns or themes in symptom presentation or in the way clients handle problems or health concerns.

Examples of exploring:

Nurse: *Tell me more about how you feel when you do not take your medication.*

OR

Nurse: *Please describe how you handle those periods in your life when you feel out of control?*

Presenting Reality

This technique, while typically used with clients who have mental health issues or clients who are confused, is also useful in the health assessment interview when the nurse is confronted with a client who exaggerates or makes grandiose statements. Presenting reality, when done in a nonargumentative way, encourages the client to rethink a statement and perhaps modify it.

Example of presenting reality:

Client: *I can never get an appointment at this clinic.*

Nurse: *But, Mr. Zsilavetz, I've seen you several times in the past 4 months.*

Client: *Well, yes, but I can never get an appointment at a time that is convenient for me.*

Confronting

Confronting is a verbal response that the nurse makes to some perceived discrepancy or incongruency in the client's thoughts, feelings, or behaviors. Gently challenging an incongruency can help the client reframe a situation and begin to see things differently. Confrontation can be used to help direct the client's focus on a behavior, which can lead to improved health or functioning. When confronting is used in a caring, empathetic manner rather than in a critical or accusatory one, clients feel encouraged to see themselves as competent and effective individuals.

Example of confronting:

Client: *I have been working on lowering my risk for a heart attack. I take my atorvastatin daily and have been watching my diet.*

Nurse: *You say that you are working on reducing your cardiovascular risk, yet you continue to smoke two packs of cigarettes every day and your cholesterol level has doubled in the past 9 months. Let's review your heart-healthy care plan and discuss risk factor reduction.*

Informing

Providing the client with needed information, such as explaining the nature of or the reasons for any necessary tests or procedures, is a nursing action that can help build trust and decrease client anxiety. In addition to providing clients with needed facts or details, information giving is appropriate when trying to help clients become aware of possible choices and then evaluate those choices correctly (Fig. 2-10).

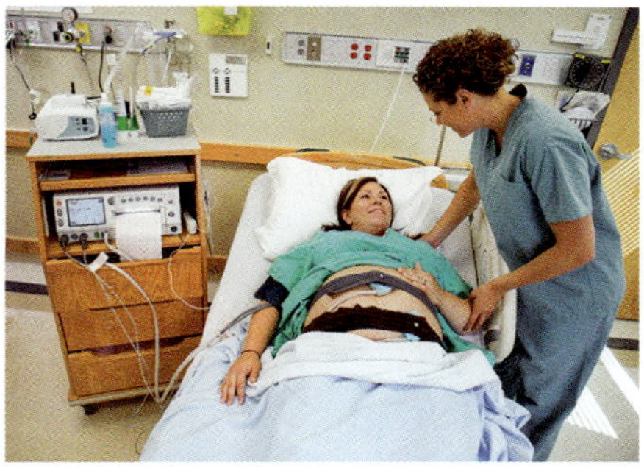

Figure 2-10 The nurse is using the action response of informing to provide the client with pertinent information.

Example of informing:

Client: *Dr. Sahib told me that I need to have my gallbladder taken out.*

Nurse: *Did you understand what she told you about your gallbladder surgery?*

Client: *No, I didn't understand what she said about the surgery. She said something about a tube.*

Nurse: *There is a technique where the surgeon inserts a tube in your abdomen to remove the gallbladder rather than making a large incision.*

Client: *Yes, that was it; please tell me more about that.*

Collaborating

In collaborating, the client is offered a relationship in which both nurse and client work together rather than one in which the nurse is in total control of the interaction. Use of this technique conveys the message that the client has important personal knowledge and information to share (Fig. 2-11). Collaborating provides a respectful way for the nurse to encourage clients' active involvement in their own health care, in setting goals, in gathering information, and in problem-solving.

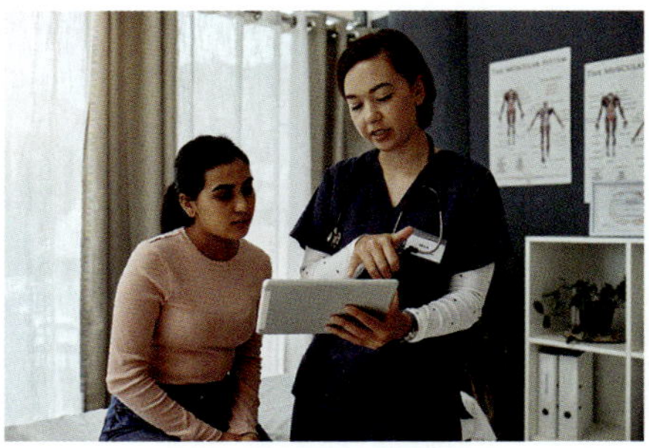

Figure 2-11 In the communication technique of collaborating, the nurse sends the message that the client and nurse can work together to achieve health goals.

Example of collaborating:

Nurse: *Let's talk more about your heartburn and discuss your diet and other lifestyle modifications.*

Limit Setting

During the interview with a hostile or talkative client, the nurse may find it necessary to set specific limits on client behavior. If, for example, the client persists in asking the nurse personal questions or rambles despite frequent attempts by the nurse to focus, it will be difficult to obtain the information needed for task completion. This client behavior may be a manifestation of stress produced by the interview situation itself or simply a characteristic specific to that particular client. In such situations, clients may require some direction as to how to behave; provide guidance by calmly, clearly, and respectfully telling the client what behavior is expected. Limit only the behavior that is problematic or detrimental to the purpose of the interview and avoid making a big issue of whatever it is that the client is doing. When limit setting, do not argue or use empty threats or promises, but rather offer the client alternatives.

Example of ineffective limit setting:

Nurse: *If you don't start answering my questions, we'll never finish, and you'll never get to see the nurse practitioner.*

Example of appropriate limit setting:

Nurse: *You know, it seems that you are feeling pretty unsure of how to behave now.*

Client: *What do you mean?*

Nurse: *Well, you're asking me a lot of personal questions and making it difficult for me to find out what is bothering you. The reason you are here is because you have some health concerns. How can I help you more clearly tell me what brought you to the clinic?*

> **NURSING TIP**
>
> **Answering Personal Questions**
>
> You bring a lifetime of experiences and emotions to each client encounter. Your client is in a similar position. It is only natural for the client to be curious about you as the health-care provider. Sharing personal experiences makes you a real person to the client and helps to develop a respectful nurse-client interaction. You need to be certain, however, that the information you divulge to the client remains generic so that you do not cross the professional boundary to a more social interaction. Also, remember that the client may ask personal questions in order to divert the interview to avoid uncomfortable or sensitive issues.

Normalizing

Very often, individuals faced with unexpected or life-threatening illnesses or possible surgeries respond in ways that seem extreme or out of the ordinary (e.g., becoming depressed or overly tearful). Normalizing allows the nurse to offer appropriate reassurance that the client's response may be quite common for this situation. This helps to decrease clients' anxiety and encourages clients to share thoughts and feelings they might otherwise keep to themselves for fear of being judged or misunderstood. However, if used inappropriately or out of context, normalizing may give false reassurance.

Example of normalizing:

Nurse: *It is no wonder you've been feeling shocked and overwhelmed since you first found that lump in your breast. Most women who have that experience react in a similar way.*

Nontherapeutic Communication Techniques

Just as there are certain communication techniques that facilitate communication between nurse and client, there are also some techniques that change, distort, or block communication and should be avoided. Verbal and nonverbal behaviors that involve inattentiveness, imposition of values, judgment, lack of interest, or an "I know what's best for you" attitude hinder communication by creating distance rather than connection. Clients on the receiving end of these behaviors may feel angry, defensive, or incompetent and may refuse to actively participate. Such ineffective techniques include requesting an explanation, probing, offering false reassurance, giving approval or disapproval, defending, and advising.

Requesting an Explanation

Clients often perceive questions that begin with "why" as challenging or threatening. Such questions ask the client to provide a reason or justification for personal beliefs, feelings, thoughts, and behaviors, and they imply criticism. If clients are unable to answer, either from lack of sufficient knowledge or because the answer is not known, clients can feel inadequate, defensive, or angry; some such questions are really unanswerable, in that individuals are frequently unaware of why they do things. Asking the client to describe the beliefs, feelings, or behaviors is preferable to asking why. Providing a description about what happened often helps the client elaborate. Enlarging the context provides opportunities for the client to increase self-awareness and for the nurse to learn relevant information.

Examples of requesting an explanation:

Client: *I guess I drink two or three six-packs of beer a weekend.*

Nurse: *Why do you drink that much?*

Client: *That's not very much; every one of my friends drinks the same amount.*

A more appropriate response in the preceding example might be:

Nurse: *It sounds as if you might be concerned about the amount of beer you are drinking. (reflecting)*

OR

Client: *I'm not sure why I came to the clinic today; I just feel miserable. I don't want to see anyone. I just want to stay in bed with the covers pulled over my head.*

Nurse: *Why do you feel that way?*

Client: *I don't know.*

A more effective response would be:

Nurse: *What happened that caused you to feel so miserable? (clarifying)*

OR

It sounds as if you are feeling rather overwhelmed today. (reflecting)

Probing

Repeated or persistent questioning of the client about a statement or a behavior increases client anxiety and can cause confusion, hostility, and a tendency to withdraw from the interaction. This client withdrawal and the increasing periods of silence resulting from it can escalate the nurse's anxiety. Anxious nurses tend to become more active and more directive in the interview. The client's unwillingness or hesitance to discuss a certain event or health concern may indicate client misunderstanding, misinformation, or a major problem area that requires further clarification or exploration.

A helpful rule of thumb for nurses to use in identifying probing is to pay particular attention to their own behavior and feelings. If in attempting to gather information, nurses feel frustrated or irritated, feel that they are pursuing the client, or have become involved in a verbal tug of war with the client, then they are most likely probing. More useful responses may include going on to the next part of the health assessment interview, asking the client's permission to return to this subject later if it seems likely that more information will be needed, or just sitting quietly until the client begins to speak.

Examples of probing:

Nurse: *What makes you drink a six-pack of beer after dinner each night?*

Client: *I'm not sure.*

Nurse: *Well, are there things going on in your life right now that would cause you to drink that much?*

OR

Nurse: *What made you try cocaine in college? What were you thinking?*

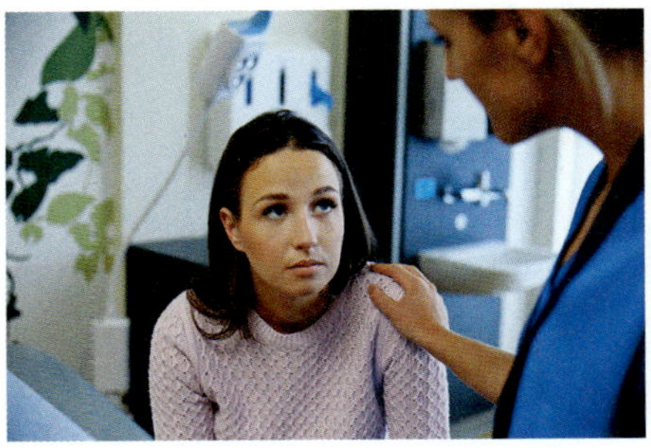

Figure 2-12 Giving false reassurance to a client or their family members does not help to build a trusting, therapeutic relationship.

Offering False Reassurance

False reassurances are vague and simplistic responses that question the client's judgment, devalue and block client feelings, and communicate a lack of understanding and sensitivity on the part of the nurse (Fig. 2-12). The impulse to provide false reassurance typically originates in the nurse's own feelings of helplessness. Giving false reassurance is an attempt by the nurse to take care of themself rather than the client and to relieve personal feelings of anxiety. This behavior often increases client anxiety. A more valuable nursing response is first to acknowledge personal feelings of anxiety and then to acknowledge the client's feelings.

Examples of false reassurance:
Nurse: *Everything will be fine.*
OR
Nurse: *I wouldn't worry about that.*

Example of an appropriate response:
Nurse: *It must be frightening to think about the possibility of surgery.*

Giving Approval or Disapproval

During the health assessment interview, nurses can feel pressured to comment judgmentally on a client's statements, feelings, or behaviors, especially if these contradict the nurse's personal beliefs or feelings. Telling a client what's right or wrong is moralizing. This may limit the client's freedom to verbalize or behave in certain ways that might not please the nurse. Comments such as "What a good idea," "You shouldn't feel that way," or "That is bad" hinder the nurse's attempts to establish rapport, support client competence, and facilitate communication. When there is concern that the client's expressed beliefs or personal behaviors are ill-informed, harmful, or destructive, the nurse might more effectively explore the source of the belief or the impact of the client's behavior on others.

Examples of effective responses:
Nurse: *What led you to that conclusion?*
OR
Nurse: *What do you think the consequences will be if you continue to keep your illness from your wife?*

Defending

Occasionally, clients who have had previous stressful or unpleasant experiences with the health-care system will engage in criticism or verbal attack. It is not helpful for the nurse to defend the object of the attack. Defending implies that the client has neither the right to hold such opinions or feelings nor the right to express them, especially if they are hostile or angry. The nurse will not be able to change the client's opinions or feelings by defending the individual or the object attacked. Rather, deflection or criticism of client feelings more often either blocks expression of these feelings or reinforces them. Defending is not therapeutic because it requires the nurse to speak not just for themselves, but also for others, something that nurses truthfully and realistically are not able to do.

Examples of defending:
Nurse: *This hospital has an excellent reputation. I'm sure that if you were kept waiting as long as you say, there was a good reason.*
OR
Nurse: *No one here would lie to you.*

It is more respectful and more useful to accept and support clients' rights to feel as they do and to express those feelings. The nurse can do this without agreeing with the expressed feelings. This empathetic behavior defuses any antagonism and minimizes client resistance to the continued interaction.

Examples of appropriate responses:
Nurse: *You sound pretty angry about your previous experiences in this hospital.*

Client: *Of course I am. Wouldn't you be upset if no one ever told you what was going on and no one answered your call bell?*

Nurse: *I guess I'd be pretty upset if I thought people were not treating me respectfully.*

Advising

Consistently telling a client what to do does not foster competence. Advising encourages clients to look to others for answers, deprives them of the opportunity to learn from past mistakes, and discourages independent judgment. Because some clients may resort to dependent, passive behavior when faced with illness, it is important that the nurse not reinforce such dependence but rather support the client's healthy functioning as much as possible.

Example of advising:

Client: *Do you think that I should start a glucagon-like peptide-1 agonist (GLP-1) to lose weight?*

Nurse: *You absolutely should! You have not lost any weight in the past 3 years, and your body mass index has increased from 35 to 40.*

A more helpful response would be for the nurse to support the client's own problem-solving ability through the use of therapeutic communication techniques such as exploring.

Examples of exploring:

Nurse: *What weight loss methods have you tried? Tell me what happened when you followed each weight loss method.*

OR

Nurse: *What weight loss methods have you considered but not yet tried?*

Using Problematic Questioning Techniques

Both experienced nurses and neophyte interviewers will occasionally find themselves feeling nervous and perhaps unsure of how to proceed during the health assessment interview. This anxiety can lead to the use of questioning techniques and interviewing responses that, although not specifically identified as nontherapeutic, are potentially problematic. Such techniques increase client anxiety, decrease the flow of needed information, and have the potential to provide the nurse with irrelevant data. The following are several examples of problematic interviewing techniques.

Posing Leading Questions

Leading questions may indicate to the client that the nurse already has a certain answer in mind. Their use can be intimidating to the client and curtail further communication. This is especially true if these leading questions concern topics that the client perceives as sensitive or possible sources of anxiety.

Examples of leading questions:

Nurse: *You've never had any type of sexually transmitted infection, have you, Mr. Barboza?*

OR

Nurse: *Of course, you've told your daughter that her smoking really bothers you, Mrs. Fayazi. Isn't that correct?*

Interrupting the Client

Changing the subject or interrupting the client prevents completion of a thought or idea and introduces a new focus. Such behavior may ease the nurse's discomfort, but it shows a lack of respect and often confuses or irritates the client. Questions should focus on one particular topic until all relevant data have been collected and the client feels finished. Changing the subject or interrupting cuts off the flow of ideas and communicates the message that whatever the client was addressing is not as important as what the nurse wants to discuss next.

Neglecting to Ask Pertinent Questions

Neglecting to ask pertinent questions can lead to faulty client data. For instance, if a married client is seen for a malodorous discharge in their genitals, remember to ask them if they are sexually active with more than one person. It is easy to become complacent when conducting client interviews. Do not let clients' outward physical appearances, personalities, or social standing distract you from ascertaining pertinent information.

Engaging in Talkativeness

Extreme talkativeness may indicate nervousness and uncertainty on the part of the nurse. Attempts to maintain control of the interview and ease personal anxiety can cause the nurse to talk more than necessary. Increased verbal activity minimizes client spontaneity and can increase client passivity, causing the nurse to work even harder at obtaining necessary information. The message to the client is that what the nurse thinks is more important than what the client thinks and feels.

Using Multiple Questions

Nurses may confuse their clients by asking several questions at once. Too many questions may put clients on the defensive, minimizing client participation and impeding the flow of necessary information.

Example of using multiple questions:

Nurse: *Is your headache dull? Severe? Causing nausea and vomiting? (no break in between questions)*

Example of more effective questioning:

Nurse: *Please tell me where your headache is located? (client responds)*
What makes your headache better? (client responds)
What makes your headache worse? (client responds)

Using Medical Jargon

The use of medical terms can make a client quite anxious or confused. Nurses who belong to the larger health-care system, which has its own culture and language, frequently use medical jargon; clients who may feel frightened and powerless in this unfamiliar environment are further disadvantaged by their lack of comprehension and any perceived language barrier. The use of medical jargon can be seen by the client as unwillingness to share or attempts to hide information, or it can give the impression that the nurse feels superior to the client and is unwilling to engage in collaboration or mutual problem-solving. Conduct the health assessment interview in a language that is common to both participants and check periodically with the client as to clarity; this will indicate an interest in the client's perspective and a desire to work collaboratively.

Example of using medical jargon:

Nurse: *Do you have dyspnea or diaphoresis when the angina occurs?*

Example of avoiding the use of medical jargon:

Nurse: *Do you have any shortness of breath with your chest pain? Do you have any sweating with the chest pain?*

Being Authoritative

The use of authority as a health-care professional can be a problematic technique. It reinforces an imbalance of power in the nurse-client relationship and can in effect discourage client cooperation.

Example of negative use of authority:

Nurse: *Mr. Haddad, I've been a nurse for over 10 years, and I think I know what's best for you.*

In a few situations, though, the use of authority can be an effective communication technique.

Example of positive use of authority:

Nurse: *As your health-care provider, knowing about your previous heart attack, history of high blood pressure, and family history of stroke, I would suggest you consider stopping smoking.*

Having Hidden Agendas

Frequently, clients seek health care for one problem but actually are concerned about other problems. The client may believe that the overriding concern is embarrassing, private, or insignificant. Once in the presence of a health-care provider, the client may open up and discuss concerns. For example, a client may seek care for a sore throat and then ask for a prescription for attention-deficit/hyperactivity disorder medication. The nurse should deal with the client's concerns in the best way possible and then follow up when indicated.

Sexual and Gender Minorities

Sexual and gender minorities are a subgroup of the American population. Sexual and gender minorities encompass all races, ethnicities, religions, and socioeconomic groups. These individuals often experience societal marginalization, bullying, and verbal and physical abuse, even in the health-care system. For these reasons, and for fear of bias and discrimination, they may have reservations about accessing the health-care system. Consider a person who has an office visit for a health-care concern. One of the first actions done at the visit is the completion of paperwork. Some insurance and demographic forms do not provide options for sexual and gender identities. Even this basic step of completing paperwork ignores or dismisses this population. Hence, sexual and gender minorities may identify a barrier even before they enter the health-care system. They may distrust the health-care arena since the system is not understanding of where they are coming from. Sexual and gender minorities want what everyone desires from the health-care system—to be treated in a nonjudgmental manner where they can be themselves without fear of bias or ridicule.

Clinical research demonstrates sexual and gender minorities have unique needs about which health-care providers need to be cognizant. Research data shows that sexual and gender minorities have an increased risk of mental health disorders such as anxiety and depression. The CDC (2021) reported that lesbian, gay, or bisexual teens in high school attempted suicide at a rate five times higher than heterosexual high school students. In 2021 Hatchel, Polanin, and Espelage's meta-analyses found that suicide was the second leading cause of death in sexual and gender minorities ages 15 to 24. In addition, sexual and gender minorities have a disproportionally elevated rate of substance abuse (Medina-Martinez, Saus-Ortega, Sanchez-Lorente, Dosa-Palanca, Garcia-Martinez, & Marmol-Lopez, 2021) and eating disorders (Drabish & Theeke, 2022; Yesildemir & Akbulut, 2023). Sexual and gender minorities expect their health-care providers to be educated on their unique needs as well as to be advocates so that they receive clinically competent care in a system where they feel valued as a person.

The acronym LGBTQIA+ has become part of everyday vernacular. Different people, groups, and organizations may define these terms differently, and it's important to recognize that a client may offer a correction on how to use a term during the health-care interaction; in this case it's important to defer to the term(s) the client uses. As the acronym, terms, and definitions are evolving in real time, it is a good idea to refer to reputable online resources for the most up-to-date definitions and additional terms. Two example sites are the National LGBTQIA+ Health Education Center (*https://lgbtqiahealtheducation.org*) and the APA style guide (*https://apastyle.apa.org/*).

For the purposes of this text the following terms and definitions will be used and are provided as a guide and starting point in understanding:

- ***Lesbian:*** A sexual orientation that describes a woman or a non-binary person who is primarily emotionally and physically attracted to other women.
- ***Gay:*** A sexual orientation describing people who are primarily emotionally and physically attracted to people of the same sex and/or gender as themselves. Commonly used to describe men who are primarily attracted to men but can also describe women attracted to women.
- ***Bisexual:*** A sexual orientation that describes a person who is emotionally and physically attracted to women and men. Some people define bisexuality as attraction to all genders.
- ***Transgender:*** Describes a person whose gender identity and assigned sex do not correspond based on traditional expectations; for example, a person assigned female sex at birth who identifies as a man; or a person assigned male sex at birth who identifies as a woman. Transgender can also include people with gender identities outside the girl/woman and boy/man gender binary structure—for example, people who are gender fluid or nonbinary.
- ***Queer:*** An umbrella term describing people who think of their sexual orientation or gender identity as outside of societal norms. Some people view the term *queer* as more fluid and inclusive than traditional categories for sexual orientation and gender identity. Although *queer* was historically used as a slur, it has been reclaimed by many as a term of empowerment. Nonetheless, some still find the term offensive.
- ***Questioning:*** Describes a person who is unsure about or is exploring their sexual orientation and/or gender identity.
- ***Intersex:*** Describes a group of congenital conditions in which the reproductive organs, genitals, and/or other sexual anatomy do not develop according to traditional expectations for females or males. Intersex can also be used as an identity term for someone with one of these conditions. The medical community sometimes uses the term *differences of sex development* (DSD) to describe intersex conditions; however, the term *intersex* is recommended by several intersex community members and groups.
- ***Asexual:*** Describes a person who experiences little or no sexual attraction to others and has little or no interest in having sexual relationships. Asexual people may still engage in sexual activity.
- ***Ally:*** A person who actively supports the rights of a marginalized community even though that person is not a member of that community—for example, a heterosexual person who campaigns for the rights of gay people.
- +: The + sign refers to people who feel that none of the above categories correctly identifies their sexual or gender identity.

Source: National LGBTQIA + Health Education Center. *https://www.lgbtqiahealtheducation.org*

Interviewing the Client with Differing Abilities

Clients with differing abilities can sometimes present a challenge to the nurse during the interview. Although the goal of the interview and specific interviewing techniques remain the same, the process can change according to the client's differing ability. Conducting a successful assessment interview with the client who has a differing ability may require more time than usual and often requires the help of an intermediary, such as a family member or a friend of the client. Remember that HIPAA laws require client consent when an interpreter or other assistive individual is used.

The Client Who Is Deaf or Hard-of-Hearing

Often, clients who are Deaf or hard-of-hearing will read lips, so it is important to remain within sight of the client and face the client when talking. When working with such a client, ensure that any hearing aid is in working order and turned on. Background noise should be at a minimum level because noise can be very distracting to the client who uses a hearing aid. Even if an **intermediary**, or an individual who is a liaison between the client and a member of the health-care team, is with the client to assist in communication, always face the client and direct all communication to the client (Fig. 2-13). It is common for those speaking to a client who is hard-of-hearing to speak loudly or slowly; though well intentioned, such actions detract from the client's ability to read lips. Tone and inflection of voice are lost on the client who is hard-of-hearing. However, other nonverbal cues, such as facial expression and body movements, can be used to convey the meaning of what is said. The U.S. government stipulates in the Americans with Disabilities Act (ADA) that a client who is Deaf or hard of hearing is entitled to assistance via an American Sign Language interpreter when using the health care system *(https://www.ada.gov/resources/effective-communication/)*.

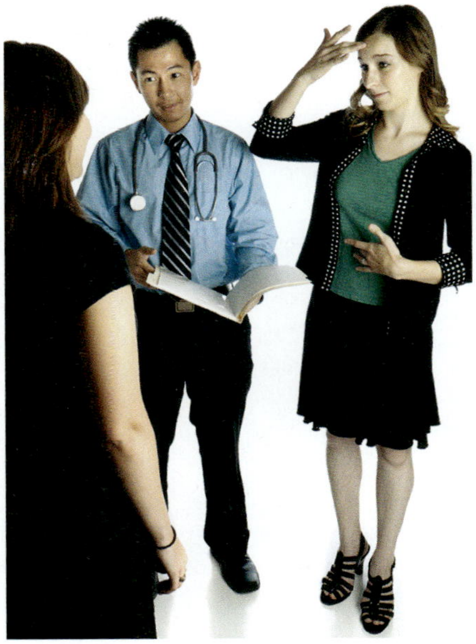

Figure 2-13 When working with a client who is Deaf, the interviewer should direct questions to the client, not the interpreter.

Clients who have never had the ability to hear and those who have not heard for a long time may have speech that is difficult to understand. Often, the best approach to interviewing these clients is to allow additional time with them and to use a written form for gathering data. When communicating through writing, always remain with the client to clarify questions and answers. Information can be reinforced with written instructions. Keep in mind that if masks are being worn by the nurse, the client, or both, the mask material may mute phonation. In addition, the client who reads lips will be unable to use this skill when the nurse wears a mask.

The Client Who Is Visually Impaired

When interviewing a client who is visually impaired, always look directly at the client as if the client were sighted. Because the client cannot rely on visual cues, voice intonation, volume, and inflection are important to the client who is visually impaired. It is common for those speaking to a client who is visually impaired to speak loudly; this is insulting and can hinder communication.

Touch is especially important to the client who is visually impaired; however, an unanticipated touch can be frightening. Before touching the client, be certain to inform the client and ask permission to touch (Fig. 2-14). Advise the client when you are entering or leaving the room and orient the client to the immediate environment. Use clock hours to indicate position of items in relation to the client. Those clients who are partially sighted may prefer to rely on the independence that their limited vision allows; offer assistance to the partially sighted and follow their cues or responses.

According to the ADA, clients who have a visual impairment are entitled to have a qualified reader or other services to facilitate their health-care needs with appropriate communication (e.g., Braille material, large print information, and audio assistance) *(https://www.ada.gov/resources/effective-communication/)*.

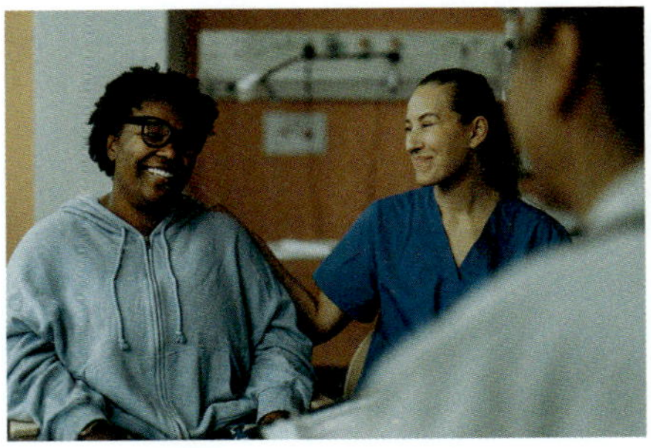

Figure 2-14 The nurse needs to inform a client who is visually impaired when a touch is to occur and ask permission.

The Client Who Has a Speech Impairment or Aphasia

When interviewing the client who has a speech impairment, ask simple questions that require only "yes" and "no" answers and allow additional time for client responses. Using this technique, it is often necessary to convert open-ended questions such as "How are you today?" to closed questions such as "Are you feeling well today?" You may need to repeat or rephrase the question if the client did not understand. If you are unable to understand the client's responses, use a written interview format, communication board, letter board, or "yes" or "no" cards. Some institutions have computers with adaptive mechanisms that can aid communication. Also, pay close attention to the client's nonverbal cues, such as blinking, clicking, or other gestures.

Even when all questions in the interview are asked and answered using closed questions, allow the client the opportunity to contribute to the information gathering; for example, "I have asked all the questions I have for you. Would you like to tell me anything related to any of the questions I have asked?" Then continue with, "Would you like to say anything else before we conclude the interview?"

When someone else is speaking for the client, the nurse should speak and direct questions to the client, not to the intermediary. If you ask the client with aphasia to complete a written format of the interview, remain with the client to clarify questions and to explain data requirements.

The ADA guidelines state that a client with a speech impairment must have the assistance of a person trained to intervene and clarify the client's speech in a health-care setting if necessary *(https://www.ada.gov/resources/effective-communication/)*.

The Client Who Is Illiterate/Has a Low Literacy Level

The client who is illiterate or has a low level of literacy may be unable to complete or verify written data. This must be done verbally or with the assistance of a trusted friend or family member. In addition, use alternative strategies to ensure that appropriate treatment and follow-up are clear. Illustrated charts can be used to describe procedures and treatments. A picture of a clock can be used to illustrate time for procedures such as blood glucose finger sticks. Medications can be color-coded for simplicity of administration. Clients should be able to repeat all instructions to verify accuracy. Home health care clinicians can follow a client who has a low level of literacy in the client's home environment to assess treatment adherence and accuracy.

The Client Who Is Non-English-Speaking

The Joint Commission estimates that over 300 languages are spoken in the United States. For this reason, it is critical to determine the client's language capabilities at the outset of the interaction. According to The Joint Commission (2015), failure to adequately communicate with the client can have adverse physical outcomes: increased infections, falls, pressure ulcers, and an increased risk of hospital readmission.

Interviewing clients who do not speak English requires the assistance of an interpreter. Federal law mandates that recipients of government aid cannot be discriminated against based on their race, color, or national origin. These persons must be provided a qualified interpreter if they have limited English proficiency *(https://www.hhs.gov/sites/default/files/yourrightsundertitleviofthecivilrightsactfactsheet.pdf)*.

Many health-care agencies have a register of interpreters who can assist with translations. Additional ways to assist with translation include the use of a telephone interpreter, the use of staff members, or the use of Internet resources. Sometimes the client will bring a translator to the interview; often this translator is a friend or family member. The nurse should not assume that the translator can answer questions for the client. It is important to direct interview questions to the client and not to the interpreter.

Remember that pure translation from one language to another does not take into account dialects or **colloquialisms** (words and phrases particular to a community), which have the potential to offend someone. For example, the question "Are you pregnant?" when translated without taking into account colloquialisms, may mean "Do you have intercourse outside of marriage?"

Pay special attention to nonverbal cues, especially facial expressions and body movements. Often, information that is lost in the translation to English can be gained through nonverbal cues. The use of signs, such as communication boards, can be helpful in an emergency situation; however, a more complete interview should be deferred until an interpreter is present.

> **NURSING TIP**
>
> **How to Use an Interpreter**
>
> 1. Use a trained medical interpreter whenever possible.
> 2. When possible, allow the interpreter and client a few minutes to converse before initiating the interview.
> 3. Instruct the interpreter to translate the client's replies sentence by sentence, thus avoiding summarization. This will ensure that important information is not omitted.
> 4. Keep your questions brief. Inform the interpreter what information you are trying to obtain.
> 5. Maintain eye contact with the client, not the interpreter, during the questioning and translating.
> 6. Observe the client's nonverbal communication, being sensitive to cultural influences.
> 7. Be patient. Extra time must be allotted for this interview exchange.
> 8. When available, use preprinted questions and health care instructions in the client's native language.

The Client Who Has a Low Level of Understanding

Interviewing the client with a low level of understanding requires time and patience because the client may require more time than usual to process questions and formulate answers and may need clarification of the meaning or intent of questions. Rushing the client may cause them to become confused, lose concentration, or refuse to answer (Fig. 2-15). It may be necessary to interview the client's family or caregiver for supplemental information. Request permission from the client to speak to someone else and respect the client's right to be present during all phases of the interview. Always direct interview questions to the client and allow the client to request assistance from family members or the caregiver. Observe the interaction between the client and the family or caregivers because nonverbal communication can provide valuable information about the client's present health or illness status as well as about the relationship between the client and the family member or primary caregiver.

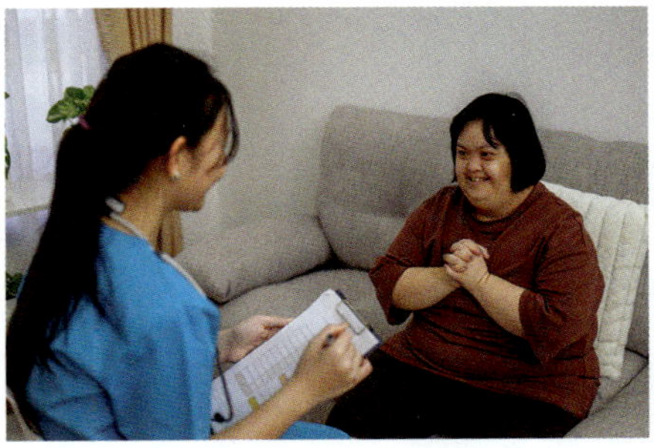

Figure 2-15 This client with Down syndrome may require more time to process and answer questions in the client interview.

The Client Who Is Crying

Clients may cry during the interview. On some occasions crying can be anticipated, such as when parents relate the events that led to their child's death. Other times a client may cry unexpectedly. The latter occurrence affords an opportunity for you to gain information about something of importance to the client by gently asking what is causing the emotional response. It is very important to show empathy and to allow the client to cry. Offering tissues indicates to the client that it is okay to cry and conveys a message of thoughtfulness. When the client has stopped crying, proceed with the interview.

The Client Who Is Anxious or Angry

Clients and those who are speaking for clients in health-care settings are frequently emotionally upset. For example, the parent of a sick child may be overwhelmed by events that led to the child's hospitalization. Emotional outbursts and crying are often the result of such stress. Allow the client, family member, or significant other to express emotions. If it is obvious that the person being interviewed is holding back tears, give permission to express emotion with a simple statement such as, "I can see that you are upset; it's okay to cry."

When interviewing an obviously angry person, recognize and acknowledge the emotion. A natural instinct is to personalize the anger and become angry in return; instead, recognize the emotion and bring it to the client's attention. "You appear very angry about something. Before we continue with the interview, please tell me about your feelings." Avoid statements such as "Take a moment to get hold of yourself," because this directive implies that the client's feelings are not appropriate and should not be expressed.

Acknowledging clients' emotions and giving them permission to express feelings will convey respect and enhance genuine communication (Fig. 2-16).

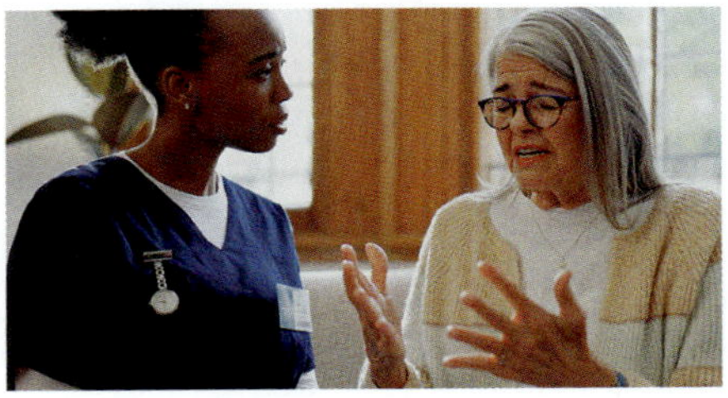

Figure 2-16 The nurse must recognize and acknowledge a client's anxiety in the client interview.

The Client Who Is Hostile

Before you begin the interview, review any documentation that might alert you to potential problems. Be especially cautious of those clients with a past history of violence or poor impulse control. Keep in mind that clients use hostile behavior because it gets them what they want. Hostility tends to be contagious. Do not reciprocate it.

You can minimize the risk of aggression through nonthreatening interventions such as limit setting and refocusing. Position yourself near an easily accessible exit. Do not turn your back on the client and never allow the client to walk behind you or come between you and the exit. Watch for signs of increasing tension in the client (e.g., clenched fists, loud voice, angry tone of voice, narrowed eyes). Consider leaving the door to the room open to some degree to deter a potentially hostile client.

Alert a colleague and security if the client makes you nervous or anxious. If feasible, have a colleague stand outside the door where you are located with the client. You may have a code word that alerts the second nurse to call for backup assistance if you feel threatened with the hostile client. Trust your instincts and remove yourself from potentially threatening and dangerous situations when necessary.

The Client Who Is Sexually Aggressive

A sexually aggressive client may act out during the interview. For example, the client may stand very close to the nurse and say, "You have been so nice to me, I would like the chance to be nice to you." The nurse may counter this behavior by defining appropriate boundaries, sharing personal reactions, and refocusing the client, for example, stating, "It makes me feel very uncomfortable when you stand this close to me. Let's get back to getting information to assist in your health-care needs." It is important to set limits and to focus on tasks when dealing with a client who is sexually aggressive.

The Client Who Is Under the Influence of Alcohol or Drugs

The client who is under the influence of alcohol or drugs presents a unique challenge to the nurse. Depending on the quantity of alcohol consumed and the type of drugs used, the client can have central nervous system (CNS) depression or can be very hyperactive and disruptive with CNS stimulation. The client's judgment may be impaired, which can lead to physical harm to those in the immediate environment. For this reason, when engaging with a violent or agitated client, security personnel should be alerted and stationed nearby.

Clients under the influence of some drugs have been known to exhibit extreme strength and are capable of inflicting serious physical harm on themselves and others. To care for this person, place yourself at a safe distance, remain calm, and provide care in a nonthreatening manner.

The Client Who Is Very Ill

Clients who are very ill may not have the strength or ability to go through a lengthy interview. Collect pertinent data from the client and defer the remainder of the interview until later (Fig. 2-17). If a client is very ill, it may be necessary to interview a family member or significant other. Show respect for the client by asking permission to do this and by allowing the client to be present during the interview. Allow the client to participate as much as possible in answering questions and giving information. A handheld dry-erase board can be provided to the client to write their answers to questions. Many institutions have a communication board that has letters which the client can point to and create words to express themselves. Other communication

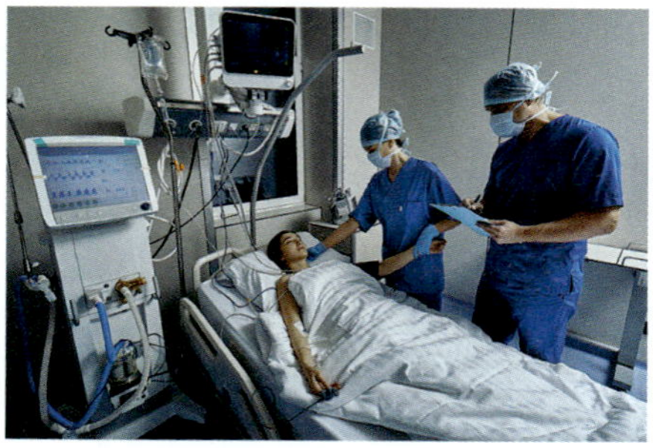

Figure 2-17 The nurse may need to defer components of the health history with a client who is very ill.

boards have pictures of items that the client may need, such as food, drinks, bathroom, adjustment of lights, adjustment to bed position, etc., that the client can point to when needed.

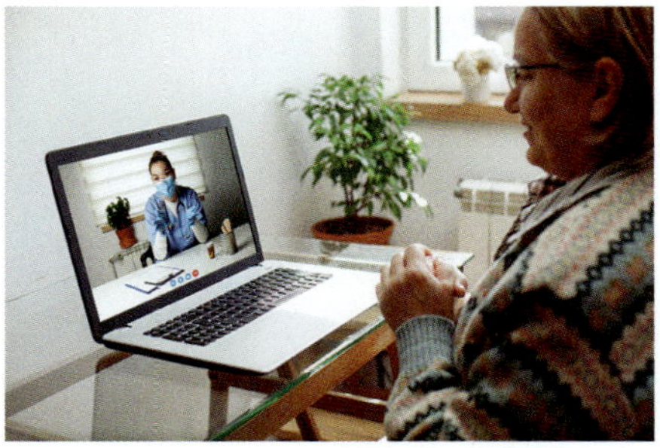

Figure 2-18 This nurse is conducting a preoperative history on a client via a telehealth visit.

Telehealth and Telenursing

Telehealth is the delivery of health care services remotely through the use of telecommunication technology. It can include both audio and audiovisual components. **Telenursing** is the use of telehealth to deliver health care. It can be conducted on a computer, iPad, or cell phone. The use of telehealth was greatly expanded in mid-2020 when the SARS-CoV2 (COVID-19) pandemic reached drastic proportions in the United States. This allowed nurses and other health care professionals to meet with their clients virtually to provide continuity of care. Telehealth is used by nurses of all educational backgrounds and clinical experiences. Though it can be used for research, administration, and education purposes, telehealth and telenursing as described here are limited to the practice arena. Many areas of clinical practice are represented in telenursing, as it encompasses clients with both acute and chronic illnesses. For example, the nurse may call a client to inquire about the client's health condition, such as blood pressure readings, serum glucose levels, or fetal movements. Telenursing can also include the nurse who calls a client before surgery to conduct a health history, as well as the nurse who calls after surgery to inquire about postoperative status (Fig. 2-18). In many rural areas, advanced practice nurses are using telenursing in very sophisticated ways to elicit clients' health histories and even conduct some select physical examination skills (e.g., the use of an electronic stethoscope to auscultate lung/cardiac/bowel sounds).

If the nurse is using only audio telenursing, all the communication and interviewing techniques discussed in this chapter can be employed to elicit information with which to formulate a client's plan of care. In these encounters the nurse's voice (tone, inflections, etc.) becomes paramount to conveying a respectful, active listener to the client on the other end of the phone line. Likewise, the nurse using audiovisual telenursing must remember that effective verbal and nonverbal communication techniques are essential to gain a client's trust and establish a therapeutic, working partnership. Thus, the goals of telenursing mirror those of face-to-face nursing: to deliver the best possible care to clients and empower them to make positive health choices.

Assessment in Brief

Effective Interviewing

- Be aware of personal beliefs. Avoid imposing your beliefs on those you interview.
- Remember that attitudes and feelings may be conveyed nonverbally.
- Consistently monitor your reactions to the client's verbal and nonverbal messages.
- Avoid being judgmental or critical.
- Listen and observe. Attend to verbal and affective demeanor as well as to nonverbal behavior.
- Keep your attention focused on the client. Do not listen with "half an ear." Do not think about other things while you are interviewing. Avoid multitasking.
- Maintain eye contact with the client as appropriate for the client's culture and comfort level.
- Notice the client's speech patterns and any recurring themes. Note any extra emphasis that the client places on certain words or topics.

- Do not assume that you understand the meaning of all client communications. Clarify frequently.
- Paraphrase and summarize occasionally to help clients organize their thinking, clarify issues, and begin to explore specific concerns more deeply.
- Allow for periods of silence.
- Avoid the use of nontherapeutic interviewing techniques.
- Use motivational interviewing techniques when appropriate.
- Reassure the client that the information obtained in the interview will be kept confidential. HIPAA regulations will be observed.

Review Questions

1. During which stage of the interview process does the nurse summarize and validate information?
   a. Joining stage
   b. Working stage
   c. Termination stage
   d. Refocusing stage
2. The nurse speaks to the client and is approximately 8 feet away. What term describes the distance of the nurse to the client?
   a. Intimate distance
   b. Personal distance
   c. Social distance
   d. Public distance
3. Which communication techniques are attempts made by the nurse to accurately receive, process, and respond to client messages?
   a. Action responses
   b. Presenting reality
   c. Listening responses
   d. Collaborating
4. Which of the following illustrates an example of an appropriate open-ended question? Select all that apply.
   a. Why are you vaping?
   b. How do you perform your breast self-examination?
   c. What are the over-the-counter medications that you take?
   d. Do you like your new blood pressure machine?
   e. Under what circumstances do you need to use your asthma rescue inhaler?
5. Which of the following is an appropriate situation for the nurse to use motivational interviewing?
   a. Teaching a client how to perform testicular self-examination
   b. Demonstrating to a client how to use a glucometer
   c. Assisting the client to explore different methods of weight loss
   d. Reviewing with the client possible side effects of a new medication
6. Which of the following actions by the nurse are appropriate when conducting a client interview? Select all that apply.
   a. Taking notes while interviewing the client
   b. Sitting on a client's bed and asking questions
   c. Avoiding eye contact with the client at all times
   d. Closing the door to the interview room
   e. Reaffirming that the client has a right to access personal medical records
7. The client begins to cry when she finds out that she will need a hysterectomy. The nurse hands the client a box of tissues and says to the client, "Many women who are told that they need a hysterectomy because of uterine cancer have a similar reaction." Which communication technique did the nurse use?
   a. Advising
   b. Collaborating
   c. Focusing
   d. Normalizing

8. A client was involved in a car accident and is in a coma. The client's spouse is crying outside the hospital room and asking why this happened. The nurse comforts the client's spouse and says, "Everything will be okay." What communication technique did the nurse use?
   a. Requesting an explanation
   b. Probing
   c. Giving disapproval
   d. Offering false reassurance

9. Which of the following is an appropriate use of telenursing? Select all that apply.
   a. Calling a client to discuss the blood pressure readings from the past week
   b. Having a cell phone audiovisual call to watch the client give a vitamin B_{12} injection
   c. Engaging a client on a Zoom call to assess postoperative status
   d. Speaking with a client in heart failure about their current weight compared with 3 days ago

10. Which of the following statements describes the appropriate use of an interpreter? Select all that apply.
    a. Use only legally bonded interpreters
    b. Use a trained medical interpreter
    c. Ask the interpreter to summarize what the client said
    d. Do not permit the interpreter and the client to be alone
    e. Inform the interpreter what information needs to be obtained

CHAPTER 3

The Complete Health History Including Documentation

Learning Outcomes

1. Provide the purpose of the four different types of health history and an example of when each is used.
2. Describe the client information that is documented in the Present Health and History of the Present Illness.
3. Identify the 10 characteristics of a chief complaint.
4. Describe the components of the Past Health History.
5. Construct a genogram based on the Family Health History.
6. Describe the components of Health Maintenance Activities.
7. Conduct a comprehensive Review of Systems.
8. Explain what constitutes legally advisable documentation.
9. Describe how the United States Preventive Services Task Force Recommendations direct client health care.
10. Document a Complete Health History on an ill and well client.

Conducting the health history is usually the first step of client assessment (Fig. 3-1). It is the collection of subjective information on the client's health status from the well or ill client and from other sources. The health history can provide information on a client's health status as well as social, emotional, mental, physical, cultural, developmental, and spiritual status. Client strengths and areas of health-care need can be identified. This information is combined with the physical examination findings to guide the nurse in formulating nursing diagnoses and devising the plan of care for the client.

The health history interview provides the mutual opportunity for the nurse and client to become more comfortable with each other. The client usually feels more at ease with the collection of health history data than with the physical contact necessary for the examination. For this reason, the health history is usually performed before the physical examination. The health history can be broadly or narrowly focused, depending on the client's needs and physical condition. The health history can also take different foci depending on whether it is conducted by a generalist or a specialist. Analysis of the information from the client in the health history provides the basis for planning the health-care education indicated by the client's condition and indicates areas requiring attention in the physical examination. The written health history also serves as part of the legal documentation of the client's health status and is a means of communicating information to other health-care team members. It also serves as a basis for acceptance or denial of insurance claims.

Refer to Chapter 2 for communication techniques and strategies for dealing with clients in various states of health.

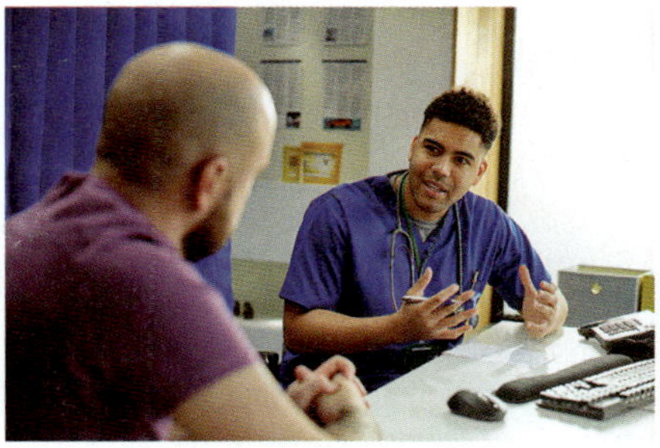

Figure 3-1 The client encounter usually starts with eliciting the health history.

Types of Health History

There are four types of health history: complete, episodic, interval or follow-up, and emergency. The **complete health history**, described in this text, is a comprehensive history of the client's past and present health status and covers many facets of a client's life. It is usually obtained during a client's initial visit to a health-care facility on a nonemergency basis and upon admission to the hospital. It establishes baseline information for future encounters. The **episodic health history** is shorter and is specific to the client's current reason for seeking health care. For example, the client who seeks care for a sore throat and fever would have an episodic health history taken. The episodic health history may center on just a single body system, or it can encompass more. The **interval** or **follow-up health history** builds on a preceding visit to a health-care facility. It documents the client's recovery/nonrecovery from illness, such as the sore throat and fever, or progress from a prior visit. Finally, the **emergency health history** is elicited from the client and other sources in an emergency situation. Only information that is required immediately to treat the client's emergent need is gathered; after the life-threatening condition is no longer present, the nurse may elicit a more comprehensive history from the client.

All four types of health history allow the nurse to identify specific health-care needs. The nurse can then devise a plan of care to promote wellness or a higher level of functioning.

Preparing for the Health History

Taking a complete health history with a client may require 30 to 60 minutes; inform the client before the interview starts of the amount of time that will be required. If the health history is not completed within the allotted time, it may be best to continue it at a later time to avoid fatiguing the client. If the client will be spending some time in the health-care facility, additional information can be obtained during routine nursing tasks such as bathing or assessing vital signs. Some health-care agencies request that the literate client complete detailed health history forms before the interview; in this instance, the nurse can validate the responses during the health history and save time. In addition, information can often be obtained from prior medical records and then updated during the interview.

Computerized Health History

Most health-care facilities use computerized electronic health records (EHRs). Various programs exist, but not all programs are compatible with each other, thus limiting their usefulness when many clinicians at various locations are involved in client care. The EHR establishes baseline client data that can be built on and modified in future client encounters. There are two types of computerized EHR for health histories: client-generated and health-care provider-generated. In client-generated health histories, the client responds via computer to various questions and then reviews information with the nurse for completeness. This type of computerized health history favors clients who may be embarrassed to verbally report specific information or those who freeze when asked for detailed information. When using a health-care provider-generated health history, the nurse completes the information on screen during or shortly after the client interview. These programs can be user friendly and time saving.

NURSING TIP

Eliciting Birthplace Information From Reluctant Clients

Some clients may seem reluctant to answer your questions regarding birthplace. Undocumented immigrants may fear deportation if they are identified in the health-care system, especially if they are seriously ill. Remind these clients that you are there to assist them with their health-care needs and encourage them to provide accurate information to assist you in appropriate diagnosis and treatment because some diseases are specific to geographic locations.

NURSING TIP

Ensuring an Accurate Chronological Age

Some Asian cultures calculate age from conception, not from the actual birth date. For example, a newborn infant is considered to be 1 year old. As the child ages, their age may be related to their horoscope at birth or a predetermined day such as January 1 of each year. You should clarify the actual chronological age with the client or caregiver. This is particularly important for pediatric clients because of the link between age and developmental milestones. Refer to Chapter 25 for the method to calculate the adjustment for premature infants.

NURSING CHECKLIST

General Approach to the Health History

1. Present with a professional appearance. Avoid extremes in dress so that your appearance does not become a hindrance to information gathering. Avoid wearing perfume or other odor-producing substances.
2. Ensure an appropriate environment: for example, good lighting, comfortable temperature, lack of noise and distractions, and adequate privacy. Refer to Chapter 2 for additional information.
3. Sit facing the client at eye level, with the client in a chair or on a bed. Ensure that the client is as comfortable as possible, because obtaining the health history can be a lengthy process.
4. Ask if the client has any questions about the interview before you start.
5. Avoid the use of medical jargon. Use terms the client can understand.
6. Wait to ask intimate and personal questions until rapport has been established.
7. Remain flexible in obtaining the health history. It does not have to be obtained in the exact order it is presented in this chapter or on institutional forms.
8. Remind the client that all information will be treated confidentially.

Advance Medical Directive

When admitting a client to a hospital or delivering care to a client outside the hospital, most health-care facilities document whether the client has an Advance Medical Directive. An **Advance Medical Directive** is a legal document that a client completes expressing what care should be provided if the client is unable to communicate these wishes due to illness or incapacity. When a client provides a copy of the Advance Medical Directive to the nurse, the document becomes a component of the client's chart or EHR. An Advance Medical Directive should be sought from every adult client.

The Complete Health History

All elements of a complete health history are outlined in the following pages. Two examples of the complete health history are given, one for the well client and one for the ill client, at the end of the chapter.

Today's Date

If using a paper chart, record the month, day, year, and time that the health history is recorded. An EHR will automatically document this information. If the health history is not written immediately, document both the time that the health history was taken and the time when it is recorded.

Biographical Data

The client usually completes the biographical identifying information before the actual physical examination. The following biographical data are usually requested from the client:

Client name	Occupation
Home address	Employer
Home phone number	Work address
Cell phone number	Work phone number
Date of birth	Insurance information
Birthplace	Usual source of health care
Social security number or other identifying number	Source of referral
Preferred language	Emergency contact name(s), relationship, and phone number(s)

Source and Reliability of Information

Usually the adult client is the historian (Fig. 3-2). However, in some instances, such as trauma, the historian may be someone other than the client. Note the name of the historian as well as the relationship between the historian and the client.

In addition, assess the reliability of the historian. Consider the historian's mental state, because emotions and certain medical conditions can influence the retelling of events. For example, the information provided by a client who has advanced Alzheimer disease may not be accurate. Note whether an interpreter is used.

Client Profile

The **client profile** provides demographics that may be linked to health status. Note the client's age, sex (for the purposes of this text the term *sex* will refer to the client's biological sex, the sex the client was assigned at birth), gender identity, preferred name, sexual orientation, race, and marital status. Many disease processes can be linked to a client's age, sex, and race. Documenting the client's gender identity, preferred name, and sexual orientation demonstrates respect for every client's uniqueness. Also note the client's marital status, as this may provide clues to support systems.

Reason for Seeking Health Care and Chief Complaint

The **reason for seeking health care** is the reason for the client's visit and is usually focused on health promotion. The **chief complaint** (CC) is the **sign** (objective finding) or **symptom** (subjective finding) that causes the client to seek health care. The client may present with multiple chief complaints for a single visit. The reason for seeking health care and the CC should be recorded as direct quotes from the client. The nurse can pose questions such as these:

"What concern(s) bring(s) you here today?"
OR
"What caused you to seek health care today?"

Present Health and History of the Present Illness

If the client is seeking health promotion, the present health states the client's current health status.

The **history of the present illness** (HPI) is a chronological account of the client's CC and the events surrounding it. The chronology can be taken

NURSING TIP

Nontraditional Health-care Sources

As a nurse, you can appreciate the need to base your clinical decisions and nursing care on evidence-based practice. However, not all clients hold similar views of health-care practices. You need to be sensitive to clients' nontraditional sources of health care, such as curandero, *yerbo, espiritualista,* voodoo, a shaman, or a medicine man. It is important to document these caregivers and their usual course of treatment. It may be possible—and desired in some instances—to allow the nontraditional healer to participate in the client's care.

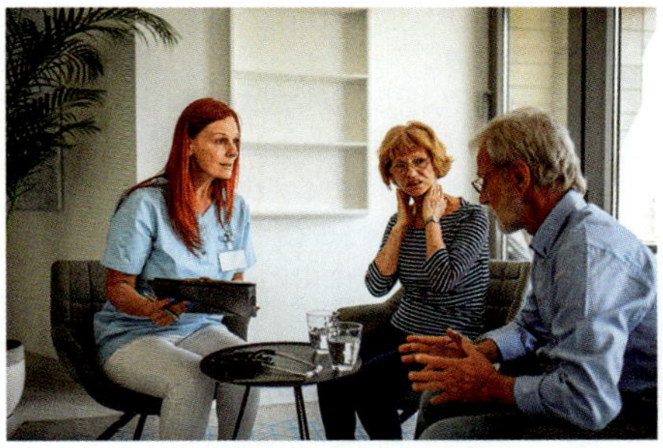

Figure 3-2 The nurse needs to note the source of the client health history. When working with adult clients, the client is usually the historian, although often a spouse will assist, especially during home health visits.

> **NURSING TIP**
>
> **Mnemonics to Remember Characteristics of a Chief Complaint**
>
> Another way to remember the characteristics of a chief complaint is to use the PQRSTU or OLD CARTS mnemonics.
>
> 1. PQRSTU
>   - **P** is for what Provokes the chief complaint (aggravating factors) and for Palliative measures (alleviating factors)
>   - **Q** is for the Quality
>   - **R** is for Region (location) and Radiation
>   - **S** is for Severity (quantity) and Setting
>   - **T** is for Timing
>   - **U** is for the Understanding of what the client's chief complaint means to the client (meaning and impact)
>
>   The PQRSTU mnemonic does not include associated manifestations, so remember to ask about these characteristics of a chief complaint.
> 2. OLD CARTS
>   - **O** is for the Onset
>   - **L** is for the Location
>   - **D** is for the Duration
>   - **C** is for the Character or quality
>   - **A** is for the Aggravating/ Alleviating factors and Associated manifestations
>   - **R** is for Radiation
>   - **T** is for the Timing
>   - **S** is for the Setting and Severity (quantity)
>
>   This mnemonic does not address meaning and impact, so remember to incorporate this factor into the description of the chief complaint.

in one of two ways: from the current state of the problem back to its origin (reverse chronology) or from the origin of the symptom leading to the current status (forward chronology). Either approach is acceptable as long as it is consistent with subsequent documentation of chronological events. Usually the client describes one or two signs or symptoms that are abnormal and their progression. Allow the client to give the detailed HPI without interruption, and then ask questions if the information is incomplete.

"Describe the condition that you are experiencing from the earliest time that it occurred to the present." (forward chronology)

Ten characteristics of each CC can be ascertained for a complete HPI:

1. Location
2. Radiation
3. Quality
4. Quantity
5. Associated manifestations
6. Aggravating factors
7. Alleviating factors
8. Setting
9. Timing
10. Meaning and impact

Note that some CCs may not involve all 10 qualifiers; hoarseness, for example, may not be objectively characterized by quantity. The CC of headache will be used to demonstrate the use of these 10 characteristics.

Location

Location refers to the primary area where the chief complaint or symptom occurs or originates.

"Where does your head hurt? Can you point to the location of the pain?"
"Is it in one location in your head or spread out (localized or diffuse)?"
"Have you ever experienced this type of headache in this location before? When?"
"Does this current headache differ from headaches you have had in the past?"

Radiation

Radiation is the spreading of the symptom or other CC from its original location to another part of the body. The areas of radiation can be diagnostic for specific pathologies.

"Does the headache move to another part of your head or body? If so, where?"
"Is the pain presently moving or radiating?"
"Describe how the pain feels in the area to which it radiated."

Quality

The quality of the CC describes the way it feels to the client. Use the client's own terms to describe the quality of the CC. If the client is having difficulty describing pain, for example, suggest some quality terms such as *gnawing, pounding, burning, stabbing, pinching, aching, throbbing,* and *crushing.*

"What does the headache feel like?"
"What word would you use to describe it?"
"Is the pain deep or closer to the skin (superficial)?"

Quantity

Quantity depicts the severity, volume, number, or extent of the CC. The client may refer to the CC with such terms as *minor, moderate,* or *severe* and *small, medium,* or *large.* Although this terminology is important to the HPI, this information is subjective and is therefore difficult to quantify. If the client consistently uses the same terms, a relative scale can be used to assess whether the CC is improving or becoming worse as reported by the client.

Another mechanism that can be used to assess the quantity of pain is a numerical scale, known as the **Numeric Rating Scale**, which rates pain from 0 (*no pain*) to 10 (*worst pain possible*). Refer to Chapter 9 for additional pain intensity scales.

"Using a scale of 0 to 10, where 0 represents no pain and 10 is the worst pain that you can imagine, rate the pain that you are having now."
"Has it been at this level before? When?"
"What level was the pain when it started?"
"When was the last time that your headache was at this level?"
"Has the severity of the headache changed? In what way?"
"Is this the worst headache of your life?"
"Has the headache interfered with your normal daily activities? How?"

Associated Manifestations

The signs and symptoms that accompany the CC are termed **associated manifestations**. Rarely does a CC occur without affecting other components of the involved system or another body system. Positive findings are those associated manifestations that the client has experienced along with the CC. Negative findings, also called **pertinent negatives**, are those manifestations expected in the client with a suspected pathology but which are denied by the client. If the client does not mention specific signs or symptoms that might be present with a given illness, ask whether they are present. Document both positive findings and pertinent negatives, because both give clues to the client's condition. For example, a client with headaches may have nausea, vomiting, and diaphoresis as positive associated manifestations. Photophobia and phonophobia are pertinent negatives because they might be present in a client with headaches but are absent in this client at this time; lack of these associated manifestations may lead to a different diagnosis.

"Beside your headache, are you experiencing any additional symptoms? What are they?"
"Have these symptoms occurred before? Do they always occur when you have a headache?"

Aggravating Factors

Those factors that worsen the severity of the CC are the **aggravating factors**.

"Have you done anything that makes your headache worse? What?"
"When you stopped this activity, did the pain lessen?"

Alleviating Factors

Alleviating factors are events that decrease the severity of the CC.

"Have you done anything that decreases the severity of the headache? What?"
"Has this worked in the past?"
"When you stopped this activity, did your headache become more severe?"

Setting

The setting in which the CC occurs can provide valuable information about the course of the HPI. The setting can be the actual physical environment in which the client is located, the client's mental state, or some activity in

> **NURSING TIP**
> **Variety of Alleviating Factors**
> Remember that alleviating factors encompass more than pharmacological interventions. You need to keep in mind the multitude of treatments that clients implement or seek out to relieve their discomfort. These include, but are not limited to, ice, heat, herbal supplements, exercise, animal-assisted therapy, magnet therapy, meditation, meridian therapy, yoga, massage, acupuncture, acupressure, homeopathy, heat wraps, and other alternative and complementary medicine interventions.

which the client was involved. The client may or may not be aware of any link between the setting and the occurrence of the CC. For instance, the odor of some chemicals, eating certain foods, or a drop in the barometric air pressure can induce headaches in some individuals.

"What were you doing when the headache started? Where were you?"
"Has this activity precipitated the headache on other occasions?"
"Has the headache occurred before in that setting? How many times?"
"What were you thinking about when the headache occurred?"
"Has the headache occurred before when you were feeling this way?"
"Does the headache occur at the same time each month during your menstrual cycle (for women)?"
"Does the headache occur after ejaculation (for men)?"

Timing

The timing used to describe a CC has three elements: onset, duration, and frequency. Onset refers to the time at which the CC begins and is usually described as gradual or sudden. Duration indicates the amount of time for which the CC is present. *Continuous* and *intermittent* are terms that can be used to describe the duration of a CC. When possible, the duration of the CC should be stated in specific time increments, such as minutes, hours, or days. Frequency describes the number of times the CC occurs and how often it develops (e.g., number of times per day, season of year).

"When did the headache first start? How long did the headache last?"
"Did the headache come on suddenly or gradually?"
"Is the pain continuous or intermittent? If intermittent, how much time elapsed between episodes?"
"When was the last time you experienced a headache? Is the pain different in any way from the first time that you experienced it?"
"How often does the headache occur in a week? In a month?"
"Have you detected a pattern to the headache's occurrence?"

Meaning and Impact

The last two pieces of information needed in the HPI are the meaning, or significance, of the CC to the client and the impact that the CC has on the client. For example, a client's father may have started having headaches at the client's age and been diagnosed with a malignant brain tumor, causing the client to be concerned about having headaches.

Second, you should investigate the impact that the CC has on the client's lifestyle. For example, consider the older adult client who complains of minor headache but admits to canceling routine activities because of it; in this case, the condition is presented as mild, but its effects are serious.

"What does it mean to you to have these headaches?"
"How do you see the headaches affecting your lifestyle?"
"Have you altered your daily activities because of the headache?"

Past Health History

The **past health history** (PHH) or past medical history (PMH) provides information on the client's health status from birth to the present. However, when you introduce this topic, the client may think you are ignoring the reason for seeking health care. The following statements can ease the transition:

"I will get back to the reason for your visit today in a few minutes. Now I would like to ask some questions related to your health in the past."
"Sometimes the reason for an illness is connected with your past health. For this reason, let's discuss your past health."

Medical History

The medical history comprises all medical problems that the client has experienced and their **sequelae**, or aftermath. Chronic illnesses as well as serious episodic illnesses are included. Forward or reverse chronology can be used to describe the medical history. It is best to be consistent and use the chronological format in the HPI. If the client denies medical illnesses, rephrase your questions. Some clients may discount "a little high blood pressure" as being insignificant.

"Are you presently under the supervision of a health-care provider for any medical illness?"
"Have you ever been diagnosed as having an illness or disease process? What was it?"
"When was the illness or disease process diagnosed?"
"Who diagnosed this illness or disease process?"
"What is the current treatment for this illness or disease process?"
"Do you follow the prescribed treatment? Do you have any difficulty following the prescribed treatment?"
"Have you ever been hospitalized for this illness or disease process? Where? When? For what period of time? What was the treatment? What was your condition after the treatment?"
"Have you ever experienced any complications (sequelae) from this illness or disease? What were they? How were they treated?"

> **NURSING TIP**
> **Expired Medications**
> Many clients keep unused medications past their expiration date. This presents a potential health hazard because some medications lose their potency after a period of time and others become toxic. Encourage clients to check their medicine cabinets at the same time every year so it becomes a routine practice. Encourage the client to discard any unused portion of medication by the stated date. Many communities have specific dates and locations when expired or unused medications can be dropped off and disposed of in a proper manner.

Surgical History

Record a complete account of each surgical procedure, both major and minor, including the year performed, hospital, surgeon, and sequelae, if known.

"Have you ever had surgery? What type?"
"When, where, and by whom was the surgery performed?"
"Were there any complications? How were they treated?"
"Were you hospitalized? For what period of time?"
"Tell me about your recovery period."
"Are you currently receiving any treatment related to this surgery?"
"Have you ever had an adverse effect from anesthesia?"

Allergies

Carefully explore all client allergies, which may include medications, foods, animals, latex, insect bites, beestings, and environmental allergens. Allergies are usually handwritten in a conspicuous location in red ink on a client's paper chart in order to stand out. In an EHR system, client allergies are prominently placed so as to be very visible. Many EHR systems alert the nurse via visual and/or audio warnings if a medication appears to which the client has a documented allergy.

"Are you allergic to any medications? Foods? Animals? Latex? Insect bites? Beestings?"
"Are you allergic to anything in the environment?"
"Are you allergic to anything that you touch?"
"What symptoms do you get when you are exposed to this substance?"
"What treatment do you use? Is it effective?"
"Have you experienced any complications from the allergies? Which?"
"Have you ever seen an allergist for this problem? What happened?"
"Do you carry an epinephrine autoinjector/nasal spray with you? What is its expiration date?" (for clients with life-threatening allergies, such as beestings or food allergies)
"Have you ever had an allergic or anaphylactic reaction with a known cause? What happened? Have you ever had an allergic or anaphylactic reaction, and no cause was identified? Tell me what happened."

> **NURSING TIP**
> **Allergies versus Side Effects**
> Many clients report that they are allergic to specific medications. When questioned further on the specific reaction to a medication, clients frequently report signs/symptoms such as headache, nausea, vomiting, and diarrhea. Though you must not discount such client experiences, it is vital to keep in mind that these examples are not drug allergies but adverse reactions to the medication. True drug allergies usually manifest as urticaria, breathing difficulties, or anaphylaxis.

> **NURSING TIP**
> **Prescription Drug Abuse**
> Prescription drug abuse is the consumption of a prescribed medication for a purpose for which it was not originally intended. Usually the abused drugs are controlled substances. Prescription narcotics (e.g., oxycodone, hydrocodone), sedatives/tranquilizers (e.g., diazepam, alprazolam), and stimulants (e.g., methylphenidate, lisdexamfetamine) are the classes of medications that are most often abused. Continued drug abuse can lead to addiction, problems in school or on the job, emotional and social difficulties, and serious health problems, including death. For these reasons, the nurse must be vigilant in obtaining a thorough medication history, especially the use of controlled substances.

> **NURSING TIP**
> **Obtaining an Accurate Medication History**
> Frequently, the client discounts OTC medications such as aspirin, acetaminophen, ibuprofen, vitamins, herbal or other supplements, cathartics, enemas, douches, cold remedies, and antacids. Ask the client whether such products are used, because they can adversely interact with prescribed medications and with one another. Also, women frequently overlook contraceptive devices (e.g., oral contraceptives, intrauterine device (IUD), vaginal ring, injection, implants); keep this in mind when interviewing women of childbearing age.
>
> The information gathered during the medication history may point to a need for client education. If contact is made with the client before the health-care visit, ask the client to bring in all medications (prescription and OTC) currently being taken. A review of all medications should be conducted at every client encounter (see Fig. 3-3).

Medications

Past and present consumption of medications, both prescription and over-the-counter (OTC), can affect the client's current health status.

Prescription Medication

"What prescription medications are you currently taking? For what reason are you taking these medications? Who prescribed them?"

"What prescription medications have you taken in the past? Who prescribed them?"

"What is the dose? How often do you take this medication?"

"How do you take this medication (e.g., pills, liquid, dissolvable tablet, patch, suppository, drops, inhaled, nasal sprays, topical, IV, injection)?"

For medications that require injection:

"Do you self-administer the medication, or do you have someone else administer the medication? Please describe how the injection is given."

"How do you dispose of the needle?"

"How long have you been taking this medication?"

"Have you ever experienced any side effects with this medication?"

"Have you ever had an allergic reaction to this medication? What happened?"

"Do you ever share your medications with others? Who? Which substances?"

Over-the-Counter Medication

"Do you currently take any over-the-counter medications? Which ones?"

"For what reason do you take this medication?"

"Do you take any home remedies? Which ones? For what purpose?"

Repeat all but the first and last questions from the "Prescription Medication" section.

"Do you ever take aspirin, acetaminophen, ibuprofen, antacids, calcium supplements, nutritional or herbal supplements, vitamins, probiotics, or laxatives? Do you douche? Administer enemas? Do you take allergy pills or cold medications?" (If yes, repeat all but the first and last questions of the previous section).

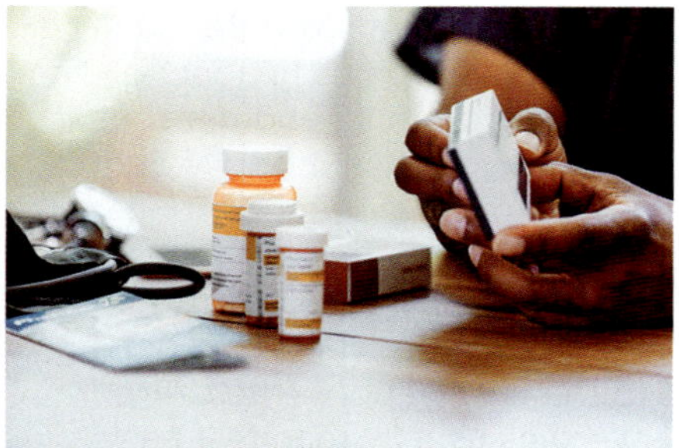

Figure 3-3 A review of all medications at every client encounter is essential to client safety.

General Medication Questions

"How often do you check the expiration date of your prescription and over the counter medications?"
"How long do you save unused medications?"
"How do you dispose of unused medications?"
"Where do you keep or store your medications?"
"Do you ever share needles with another person? Who?"
"Do you have any questions concerning your medications?"
"Do you ever take more than the prescribed or recommended amount of prescription or OTC medication?"
"Can you afford your medications? What do you do if you can't afford your medications?"
"Do you receive any of your medications through a special savings program? Which ones? How does it work?"

Communicable Diseases

Communicable diseases can have a grave impact on the individual as well as on society. Some communicable diseases generate enough concern to the community that they are reportable to the public health department. Consult your state's department of health to determine which communicable diseases must be reported. In recent years, there has also been a major focus on measles, pertussis, and hepatitis C outbreaks. In addition, human immunodeficiency virus (HIV) is a major concern throughout the world. There is substantial value in asking the client about possible exposure to communicable diseases, because pathology may not manifest itself until many years after exposure.

"Have you ever been diagnosed with an infectious or communicable disease? Which one(s)?"
"What were your symptoms?"
"How were you treated?"
"Did you have any complications? What were they? Were there any permanent consequences?"
"Have you ever had any of the following illnesses: varicella (chickenpox), diphtheria, pertussis (whooping cough), measles, mumps, rubella, polio, rheumatic fever, or scarlet fever?" (If yes, repeat the second, third, and fourth questions in this list).
"Have you ever had gonorrhea, chlamydia, syphilis, herpes, or any other sexually transmitted infection?" (If yes, repeat the second, third, and fourth questions in this list).
"Have you ever had tuberculosis?" (If yes, repeat the second, third, and fourth questions in this list).
"Have you ever been diagnosed with MRSA (methicillin-resistant staphylococcus aureus) or VRE (vancomycin-resistant enterococcus)?"
"Have you ever had hepatitis? Which type?" (If yes, repeat the second, third, and fourth questions). If other than hepatitis A, ask these follow-up questions:
"Do you have any tattoos? Where were they done?"
"Do you have any body piercings? Where were they done?"
"Have you ever been told that you are HIV positive? (If yes, repeat the second, third, and fourth questions.) Ask if the client has any tattoos or body piercings.
"Did you ever test positive for COVID-19? Did you have any complications?"
"Have you ever been diagnosed with respiratory syncytial virus (RSV)?"
"Have you ever been diagnosed with Mpox?"
"Have you ever been exposed to someone who had a communicable disease? Which disease(s)?"

NURSING TIP
Herbal Products

Herbal products are consumed by more of the U.S. population than ever before. Whether to improve health or combat illness and pain, this branch of complementary and alternative medicine deserves the nurse's attention. Glucosamine chondroitin, turmeric, ephedra, black cohosh, and St. John's wort are just a few of the many herbal products that clients ingest. Because these products are considered dietary supplements in the United States, they are not held to the same level of purity as prescription medications. Different brands of the same herbal product can have varying levels of potency and purity. Because many people consider these products to be natural (and therefore safe), clients rarely consider the possibility of herbal products interacting adversely with one another or with prescription medications. For this reason, clients need to be asked at every encounter which OTC herbal products they are consuming. Remember, just because a product is natural does not necessarily mean that it is healthful and safe. For example, arsenic is a naturally occurring substance, but when consumed, it can cause illness and death. Also, herbal products such as St. John's wort can adversely affect prescription medications such as antibiotics and antidepressants.

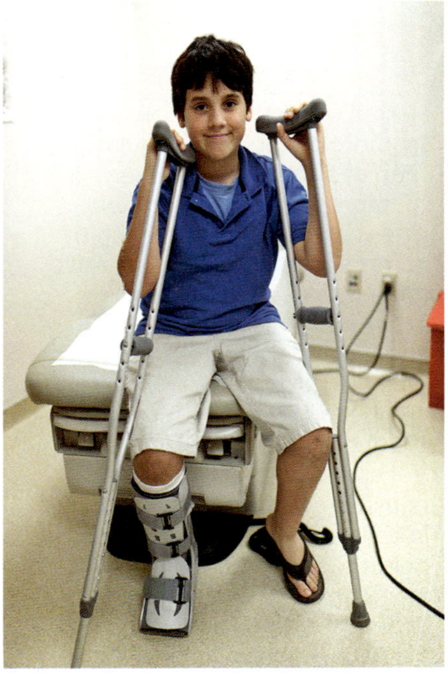

Figure 3-4 Seeing a client with injuries, sutures, or a cast prompts the nurse to inquire about the events that led to the incident, as well as past accidents.

Injuries and Accidents

A client's injury and accident history can reveal a pattern that is amenable to health promotion (Fig. 3-4). For example, an older adult female who sustains an injury from slipping on throw rugs in the home would be a candidate for health teaching on maintaining a safe home environment.

"Have you ever been involved in an accident?"
"Have you ever been injured in any way?"
"What occurred? Did you lose consciousness?"
"Did you take any precautionary measures? What were they?"
"Were you hospitalized? For how long?"
"Were there any complications? What were they?"
"Were there any long-term effects from this injury/accident?"
"Have you ever sustained an injury in a car accident? Describe."
"Have you ever had a broken bone? Stitches? Burns?"
"Have you ever been assaulted? Raped? Shot? Stabbed?"
"Have you ever been bitten by an animal or insect (e.g., dog, cat, brown recluse spider, tick)?"

Differing Abilities

The awareness of any cognitive, physical (Fig. 3-5), or psychosocial disability/differing ability is essential to providing individualized health care to a client. A client with Down syndrome, a client with paraplegia, and a client with autism all have unique needs. These clients may receive less than optimal health care if their particular limitations are not identified and considered when planning treatment. Sometimes additional time will be required to complete the health history and physical examination with a client with a disability.

"Do you have any disabilities/differing abilities? Describe."
"Does this disability/differing ability limit you in any way? If yes, how?"
"What strategies do you use to limit the effect the disability/differing ability has on your lifestyle?"
"What support systems help you cope with this disability/differing ability?"
"Does your disability/differing ability place an extra financial burden on you? How do you handle that?"

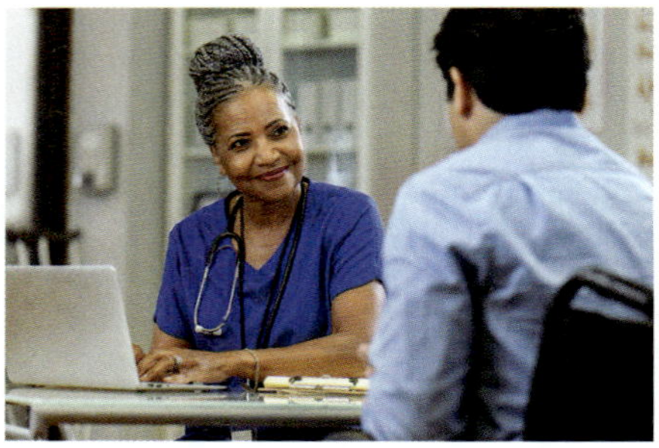

Figure 3-5 Clients' physical needs, such as use of a wheelchair, should be documented in their health histories.

Blood Transfusions

The chance of contracting an infectious disease from a blood transfusion is greatest in clients who receive a large number of transfusions, such as clients with hemophilia, clients with cancer, and clients who experience trauma (Fig. 3-6). The American Red Cross and other organizations are continuously updating their screening tools and history-taking procedures to protect the nation's blood supply. Still, the recipient assumes some risk with every transfusion. Tests are available to screen blood-borne diseases such as hepatitis and HIV.

"Have you ever received a blood transfusion (whole blood or any of its components)? When?"
"Why did you receive this blood product?"
"What quantity did you receive?"
"Did you experience any reaction to this blood product? What was it?"

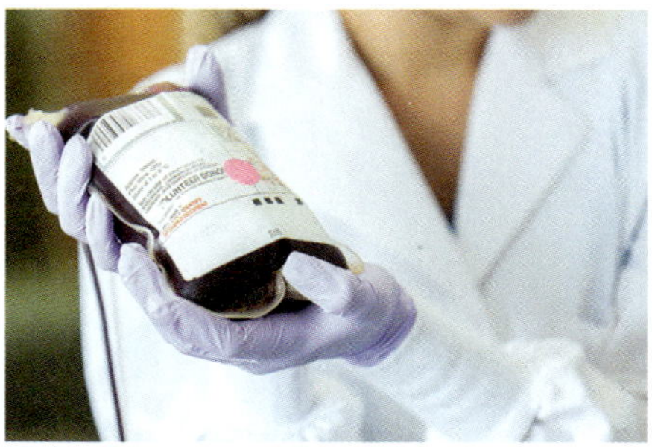

Figure 3-6 Inquiring about a client's past blood transfusions is a vital component of the health history.

Childhood Illnesses

Rarely are adults familiar with a complete history of their childhood illnesses. Ask the client about specific childhood diseases by name.

"Have you ever had any of the following illnesses: varicella (chickenpox), diphtheria, pertussis (whooping cough), measles, mumps, rubella, polio, rheumatic fever, scarlet fever, COVID-19, RSV, or rotavirus?" (This question is eliminated if previously asked during the communicable diseases section).
"How old were you when the illness occurred?"

"Was the diagnosis confirmed by a laboratory test, or was it based on clinical findings? By whom?"
"Were there any complications? What were they?"

Immunizations

The history of immunizations is closely tied to childhood illnesses. The majority of immunizations are received in childhood (Fig. 3-7), though many are given in adulthood. The adult client may not recall the exact dates when the immunizations were given, as with childhood illnesses, but will be aware that "I received everything that I should have." Routine immunizations are also associated with different groups. Health-care workers and laboratory workers are administered the hepatitis B vaccine if not previously inoculated. Every fall and winter most people 6 months and older are eligible for the influenza vaccine. In addition, travelers to underdeveloped areas of the world may receive additional vaccines before visiting specific countries or regions.

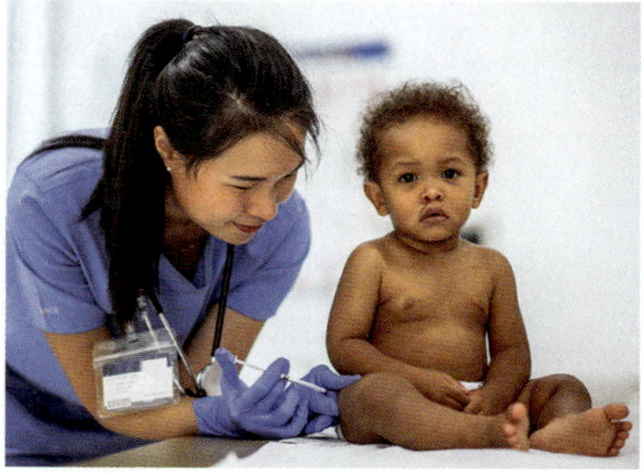

Figure 3-7 Initial immunizations are given as injections starting in infancy, with boosters administered throughout childhood and adulthood.

"As a child, did you receive the following immunizations: measles-mumps-rubella (MMR), polio, smallpox, diphtheria-pertussis-tetanus (DPT), *Haemophilus influenzae* type b (Hib), hepatitis A, hepatitis B, rotavirus, pneumococcal, varicella, meningococcal, human papillomavirus (HPV), COVID-19, dengue, or RSV?"
"Did you experience any reactions to the immunizations? What were they? Were there any complications?"
"What immunizations did you receive as an adult: varicella zoster, hepatitis A, hepatitis B, influenza, diphtheria, tetanus, pertussis, pneumococcal, meningococcal, HPV, Hib, MMR, COVID-19, RSV, Mpox?"
"When was your last TB test, and what was the result?"
"If born outside the United States, have you received the Bacillus Calmette-Guérin (BCG) vaccine?"
"Have you ever received any other immunizations, perhaps before visiting a specific geographical region (e.g., cholera, typhoid fever, yellow fever, Japanese encephalitis, rabies)?"

NURSING TIP

Immunization Schedules

Routine vaccinations can vary among different age-groups as well as in different geographic regions. Some immunizations have been eliminated, whereas others have been added to the vaccination schedule as recommended by the American Academy of Pediatrics (AAP) and the Centers for Disease Control and Prevention (CDC). For example, the smallpox vaccination was discontinued in 1977. In the 1990s, the AAP added the Hib and hepatitis B vaccines to its recommended immunization schedule. In some areas where there is a known increased risk for hepatitis A, this immunization is routinely administered. In December 2020 the CDC granted Emergency Use Authorization (EUA) for the SARS-CoV2 (COVID-19) vaccine. First administered to health-care workers and first responders, the COVID-19 vaccine is now included in the CDC's recommended annual immunizations. In addition, the 2024 immunization guidelines added the RSV and Mpox vaccines for eligible clients. Immunization guidelines are revised early each calendar year, so be alert to these changes in immunization schedules when interviewing clients, to ensure that they have received what is or was appropriate for them. The CDC can also issue revisions and/or additions of vaccines depending on current health conditions. Also, be sensitive to the prospect that clients from other countries may present with a significantly different immunization history than clients brought up in the U.S. health-care system. Table 3-1 shows the Recommended Adult Immunization Schedule, United States, 2025. Refer to the CDC Web site *(https://www.cdc.gov/vaccines/hcp/imz-schedules/index.html)* for the most recent immunization guidelines.

Table 3-1 Recommended Adult Immunization Schedule, United States, 2025

Article I. Adult Immunization Schedule by Age

Vaccine	19–26 years	27–49 years	50–64 years	≥65 years
COVID–19	1 or more doses of 2024–2025 vaccine (See Notes)			2 or more doses of 2024-2025 vaccine (See Notes)
Influenza inactivated (IIV3, ccIIV3) **Influenza recombinant** (RIV3)	1 dose annually			1 dose annually (HD–IIV3, RIV3, or aIIV3 preferred)
Influenza inactivated (aIIV3; HD–IIV3) **Influenza recombinant** (RIV3)	Solid organ transplant (See Notes)			
Influenza live, attenuated (LAIV3)	1 dose annually			
Respiratory syncytial virus (RSV)	Seasonal administration during pregnancy (See Notes)		60 through 74 years (See Notes)	≥75 years
Tetanus, diphtheria, pertussis (Tdap or Td)	1 dose Tdap each pregnancy; 1 dose Td/Tdap for wound management (See Notes) 1 dose Tdap, then Td or Tdap booster every 10 years			
Measles, mumps, rubella (MMR)	1 or 2 doses depending on indication (if born in 1957 or later)			For health care personnel (See Notes)
Varicella (VAR)	2 doses (if born in 1980 or later)		2 doses	
Zoster recombinant (RZV)	2 doses for immunocompromising conditions (See Notes)		2 doses	
Human papillomavirus (HPV)	2 or 3 doses depending on age at initial vaccination or condition	27 through 45 years		
Pneumococcal (PCV15, PCV20, PCV21, PPSV23)			See Notes	See Notes
Hepatitis A (HepA)	2, 3, or 4 doses depending on vaccine			
Hepatitis B (HepB)	2, 3, or 4 doses depending on vaccine or condition			
Meningococcal A, C, W, Y (MenACWY)	1 or 2 doses depending on indication (See Notes for booster recommendations)			
Meningococcal B (MenB)	19 through 23 years 2 or 3 doses depending on vaccine and indication (See Notes for booster recommendations)			
***Haemophilus influenzae* type b** (Hib)	1 or 3 doses depending on indication			
Mpox	2 doses			
Inactivated poliovirus (IPV)	Complete 3-dose series if incompletely vaccinated. Self–report of previous doses acceptable (See Notes)			

Recommended vaccination for adults who meet age requirement, lack documentation of vaccination, or lack evidence of immunity | Recommended vaccination for adults with an additional risk factor or another indication | Recommended vaccination based on shared clinical decision–making | No Guidance/Not Applicable

Adult Immunization Schedule by Medical Condition and Other Indication

Always use this table in conjunction with Article 1 and the Notes that follow. Medical conditions or indications are often not mutually exclusive. If multiple medical conditions or indications are present, refer to guidance in all relevant columns. See Notes for medical conditions or indications not listed.

VACCINE	Pregnancy	Immunocompromised (excluding HIV infection)	HIV infection CD4 percentage and count: <15% or <200mm³	HIV infection CD4 percentage and count: ≥15% and ≥200mm³	Men who have sex with men	Asplenia, complement deficiency	Heart or lung disease	Kidney failure, End–stage renal disease or on dialysis	Chronic liver disease; alcoholism[a]	Diabetes	Health care Personnel[b]
COVID–19		See Notes									
Influenza inactivated Influenza recombinant		Solid organ transplant (See Notes)	1 dose annually								
LAIV3					1 dose annually if age 19–49 years		1 dose annually if age 19–49 years				
RSV	Seasonal administration (See Notes)	See Notes				See Notes			Liver disease (See Notes)	See Notes	
Tdap or Td	Tdap: 1 dose each pregnancy	1 dose Tdap, then Td or Tdap booster every 10 years									
MMR	*										
VAR	*			See Notes							
RZV		See Notes									
HPV	*	3-dose series if indicated									
Pneumococcal											
HepA											
Hep B	See Notes									Age ≥ 60 years	
MenACWY											
MenB											
Hib		HSCT[c]: 3 doses				Asplenia: 1 dose					
Mpox	See Notes				See Notes						See Notes
IPV		Complete 3-dose series if incompletely vaccinated. Self–report of previous doses acceptable (See Notes)									

Recommended for all adults who lack documentation of vaccination, **OR** lack evidence of immunity | Not recommended for all adults, but recommended for some adults based on either age **OR** increased risk for or severe outcomes from disease | Recommended vaccination based on shared clinical decision–making | Recommended for all adults, and additional doses may be necessary based on medical condition or other indications. See Notes. | Precaution: Might be indicated if benefit of protection outweighs risk of adverse reaction | Contraindicated or not recommended *Vaccinate after pregnancy, if indicated | No Guidance/Not Applicable

a. Precaution for LAIV3 does not apply to alcoholism.
b. See Notes for influenza; hepatitis B; measles, mumps, and rubella; and varicella vaccinations.
c. Hematopoietic stem cell transplant.

The CDC Adult Immunization schedules list the recommended vaccines by age and medical condition. Access the CDC website for more specific information on vaccine contraindications, precautions, and updated guidelines. The website also provides additional information on the vaccines, frequency of administration, and considerations for special situations.

Family Health History

The **family health history** (FHH) records the health status of the client, as well as that of immediate blood relatives. It can help identify familial disease processes. When appropriate, the nurse can identify whether there are any screening tools for a condition that the client should undergo to determine whether the condition has been inherited (e.g., hemochromatosis, Factor V Leiden mutation). The FHH can alert the nurse of a need to refer clients for genetic counseling (e.g., cystic fibrosis, sickle cell disease). The FHH can also be a useful tool for providing anticipatory guidance to the client. For example, if there is a strong family history of diabetes, hypertension, and hyperlipidemia in an otherwise healthy adult who smokes, the nurse can use these familial conditions to help the client toward adopting therapeutic lifestyle changes before additional treatment is needed to avoid adverse events.

At a minimum, the FHH should contain the age and health status of the client, client's siblings, client's parents, and children. Ideally, the client's grandparents, aunts, and uncles should be incorporated into the history as well. Documentation of this information is done in two parts: the genogram, or family tree, and a list of familial diseases. A genogram is shown in Figure 3-8.

The second component of the family health history is the report of occurrences of familial or genetic diseases. Such information is crucial to the client and may not have been revealed previously because some familial illnesses do not occur in every generation. The pertinent negative findings are documented in the family health history beneath the genogram. Refer to the genogram illustration.

You may want to preface the FHH questions with the following statement:

> "Different diseases tend to run in families. I would like to ask you about your family and their health to gain a better understanding of your background."

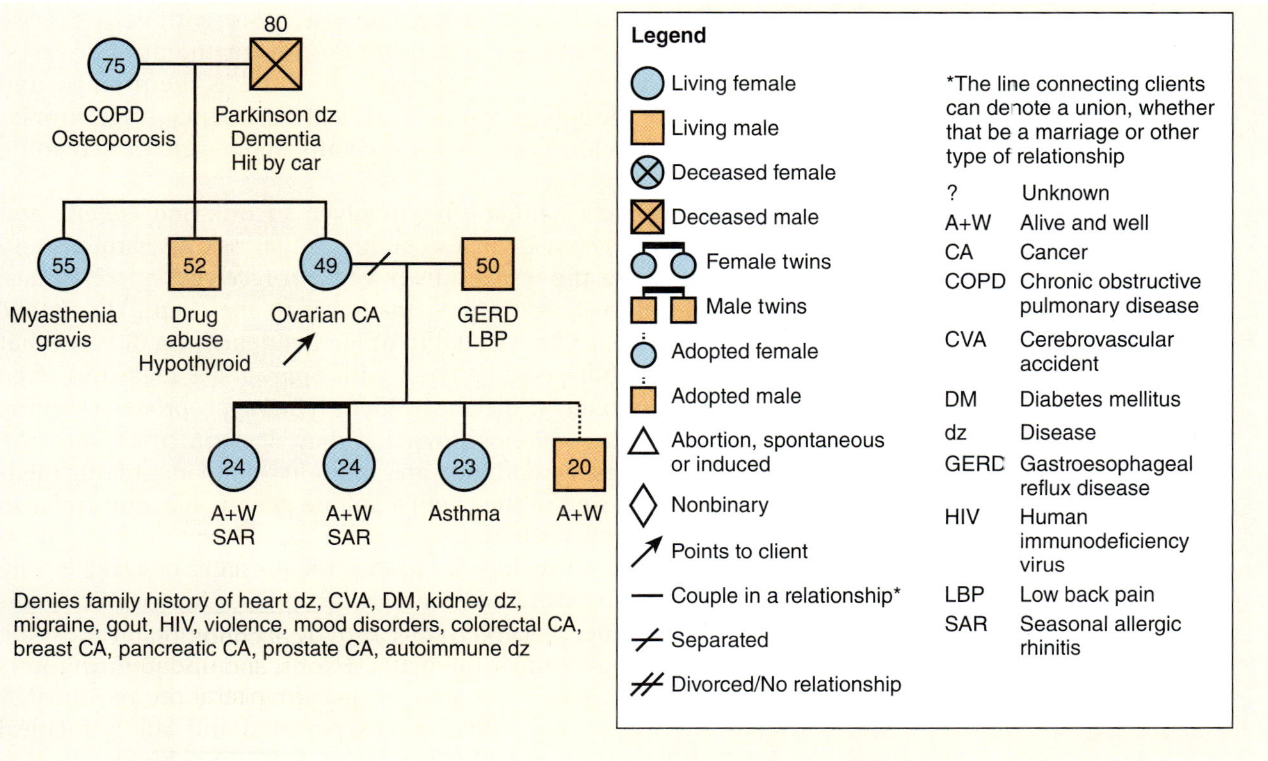

Figure 3-8 Genogram.

> **NURSING TIP**
>
> **Family Health History for a Client Who Was Adopted or Who Has Been in Foster Care**
>
> Clients who were adopted have varying degrees of information about their biological parents. Encourage adopted clients to be frank about their FHH. If the FHH of the biological parents is unknown, this is documented.
>
> Likewise, the FHH of adoptive parents can be equally important. Certain environmental factors (such as smoking, drug and alcohol use, and sanitation) may influence the health of the adopted child.
>
> Children who are in foster care may have been in many different environments during their lives. They are often placed in complex and difficult situations. The foster child's social worker may be a resource for obtaining needed information.

You can then continue with questions about the FHH:

"Tell me about the members of your family: children, siblings, and parents. How old are they?"

"Do any of these individuals have any medical illnesses or diseases? What are they?"

"Have there been any deaths in your immediate family? What was the cause of death? How old was this person at the time of death?"

"What is the current age of each of the following members of your family: maternal and paternal grandparents, aunts, uncles?"

Repeat questions 2 and 3.

"Has anyone in your family ever had any of the following illnesses: heart attack or heart disease, sudden cardiac death before age 50, high blood pressure, stroke, tuberculosis, diabetes, cancer (what kind?), kidney disease, blood disorders, sickle cell anemia, arthritis (what type?), seizure, migraine headaches, gout, thyroid disease, liver disease, asthma, allergic disorders, obesity, alcoholism, mental health disorders (e.g., anxiety, depression, bipolar depression, schizophrenia, suicide attempts or completions), learning disability, drug addiction, HIV, violent behavior? Who?"

Practice constructing the FHH genogram as the client describes the family's history to you. With time, the genogram can be completed much more quickly than narrative documentation.

Family Health History and Genomics

Genomics, or the study of the genetic makeup of the human cell, is increasingly becoming an area in which nurses need to be well versed. In 1990, the U.S. Department of Energy and the National Institutes of Health launched the U.S. Human Genome Project. The aim of this project was to identify the approximately 30,000 genes in human DNA and to determine the sequence of the roughly 3 billion chemical pairs that make up human DNA. This information is used to prevent disease, assist with early disease detection, develop a personalized and more precise treatment of diseases, and, ultimately, provide a cure for disease. All of this is the promise and future of genomics. Though genomics is still in its infancy stage, nurses must be prepared to field questions from clients about genetic screening and testing.

Many advanced practice nurses are involved in ordering genetic and genomic tests for their clients. Nurses conduct initial risk assessments and pretest counseling. After the test results have been received, a face-to-face meeting is conducted to share the information with the client. Ultimately, the goal is to improve the client's quality of life by identifying diseases that the client may inherit but possibly avoid with appropriate measures (e.g., familial hypercholesterolemia, diabetes), identifying appropriate screening tools (e.g., mammograms, colonoscopy) that may detect a condition early (with the hope of decreasing morbidity and mortality), and identifying medications that can be tailored to the client's unique genetic makeup (refer to the Nursing Tip on genetic testing).

Currently, health-care providers can test for the presence of a single gene as well as a gene panel (which looks for a group of genes for specific conditions, such as breast cancer). Larger scale genetics testing includes exome sequencing and whole genome sequencing. Exome gene sequencing tests for proteins in the DNA. Whole genome sequencing tests the entire DNA and is usually used in clients with complex personal and family medical histories (CDC, 2023). Some genetic tests can be performed by the client at home. These direct-to-consumer tests may or may not come with company support. The client frequently turns to the health-care provider to gain an understanding of the results. Thus, it is imperative that nurses who deal with genetics and genomics stay abreast of this ever-evolving clinical area through continuing education. The direct-to-consumer tests are informational but cannot be used to make diagnostic clinical decisions such as whether a client needs a mastectomy to prevent a high probability of developing breast cancer.

In 2008, the Genetics Information Nondiscrimination Act (GINA) was signed into law. GINA protects individuals who choose to have genetic and genomic testing from being discriminated against in their employment and with their health insurance company (National Human Genome Research Institute, 2022). Knowledge of GINA is crucial information to provide to clients when discussing genetic testing.

> **NURSING TIP**
> **Genetic Testing**
> In 2007, carbamazepine became the first mainstream drug to carry a recommendation that clients of Asian descent be tested for the HLA-B*1502 gene before starting drug therapy. Genetically, Asian clients are almost exclusively carriers of HLA-B*1502; if they are placed on carbamazepine, they are more likely to develop Stevens-Johnson syndrome or toxic epidermal necrolysis. This action by the Food and Drug Administration heralded the start of pharmacogenetic testing in which health care providers have the ability to make clinical decisions on appropriate medications based on a client's genetic profile.

Social History

The **social history** (SH) explores information about the client's lifestyle that can affect health. The information obtained in this section of the health history often leads the nurse to identifying educational areas to promote a healthier lifestyle. Introduce this area of questioning with statements similar to the following:

"Now I would like to ask you some questions about your lifestyle. This information is important because of the effects that different practices can have on your health."

Alcohol Use

The intermittent and prolonged use of alcohol can interfere with normal metabolism and normal body function. Chronic use of alcohol leads to many physiological changes that can lead to serious injury or death. In addition, alcohol abuse often leads to psychological, social, and emotional issues (Fig. 3-9). There are many alcohol assessment tools that can be used in the clinical setting (e.g., AUDIT-C, SASQ, AUDIT, TWEAK, MAST, CAGE, T-ACE). The U.S. Preventive Services Task Force recommends using the AUDIT-C or the SASQ alcohol screening tools. These screening tools are easily administered in the clinical setting and carry high sensitivity and specificity for unhealthy alcohol use (National Institutes of Health, National Library of Medicine, 2015; National Institute on Alcohol Abuse and Alcoholism, 2023). Additional questions can be posed to the client:

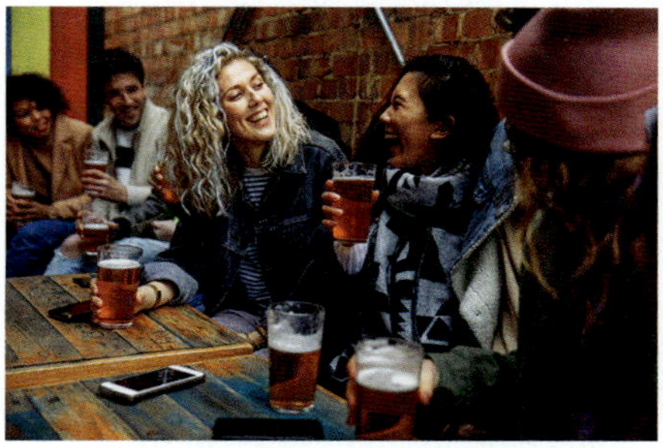

Figure 3-9 Alcohol consumption needs to be assessed to determine whether there are any health risks.

"How much alcohol do you drink per week?"
"How often do you drink?"
"What type of alcohol do you prefer (beer, wine, ale, hard cider, wine coolers, liquor, spirits, moonshine)?"
"Do you ever consume homemade alcoholic beverages?"
"What quantity do you usually consume at one time?"
"Has your drinking pattern changed? In what way?"
"When did you first start to drink?"
"How long have you been drinking the amount that you are currently consuming?"
"What time of the day do you drink?"
"Where do you obtain your drinks?"
"Do you have a special place to keep your alcohol?"
"Have you ever lost consciousness or blacked out after drinking?"
"Have you ever forgotten what happened when you were drinking?"
"Do you drink alone?"
"Do you drive after drinking?"
"Did you ever drink during pregnancy? How much?"
"Do you think you have a drinking problem?"

NURSING TIP

The AUDIT-C and SASQ Alcohol Screening Questionnaires

The AUDIT-C (Alcohol Use Disorders Identification Test-Concise) and the SASQ (Single Alcohol Screening Question) help identify clients who use excess alcohol or have hazardous alcohol consumption patterns.

AUDIT-C

How often did you have a drink containing alcohol in the past year?

	Points
Never	0
Monthly or less	1
Two to four times a month	2
Two to three times a week	3
Four or more times a week	4

How many drinks did you have on a typical day when you were drinking in the past year?

	Points
None, I do not drink	0
1 or 2	0
3 or 4	1
5 or 6	2
7 to 9	3
10 or more	4

How often did you have six or more drinks on one occasion in the past year?

	Points
Never	0
Less than monthly	1
Monthly	2
Weekly	3
Daily or almost daily	4

Each of the 5 responses to the above questions are scored from 0 to 4 points. A score of 4 or more is considered a positive screen in men while a score of 3 or more is positive for women. These elevated scores warrant additional investigation and possible intervention.

SASQ

For females:
"How many times in the past year have you had 4 or more drinks in a day?"
For males:
"How many times in the past year have you had 5 or more drinks in a day?"

A response of one or more days in the past year warrants further evaluation.

National Institutes of Health, National Library of Medicine (2015).
National Institute on Alcohol Abuse and Alcoholism (2023).

NURSING TIP

The Five As of Smoking Cessation

Ask: At every client encounter, the nurse *asks* the client about their smoking habits: type, amount, and duration.

Advise: The nurse strongly *advises* the client that quitting smoking is in their best health interest.

Assess: The nurse *assesses* the client's willingness to quit smoking.

Assist: The nurse *assists* the client in selecting an appropriate nicotine withdrawal method (e.g., cold turkey, patch, gum, nasal spray, prescription medication, acupuncture, hypnosis, or other method). Advantages and disadvantages of each method can be discussed to empower the client to make an informed decision.

Arrange: The nurse *arranges* for a close follow-up with the client once the smoking cessation is started. Studies demonstrate that clients who have a support mechanism (professional or nonprofessional) and encouragement have greater success in quitting smoking. The follow-up can be a scheduled appointment or successive phone calls during which the nurse inquires how the client is doing in meeting the smoking cessation goals and whether there are any questions about the chosen withdrawal method.

Tobacco Use

Because of the harmful nature of tobacco products, the client's use of tobacco should be ascertained at each visit. If tobacco is used, it is the role of the nurse to encourage the client to quit. Many resources are available to the nurse to assist the client in the smoking cessation process.

The quantity of cigarette smoking is usually described in **pack/year history**. To calculate the client's pack/year history, multiply the number of packs of cigarettes smoked on a daily basis by the number of years that the client has smoked. For example, to calculate the pack/year history for a client who has smoked 2½ packs a day for 30 years:

$$\text{pack/year history} = 2\tfrac{1}{2} \times 30 = 75$$

Some providers quantify tobacco use in the number of packs per day (PPD) for a specified number of years, for example, 2 PPD × 15 years.

"Do you use or have you ever used any tobacco product (cigarettes [filtered or nonfiltered], pipe, cigars, chewing tobacco, snuff)?"
"Do you use any electronic nicotine delivery system (ENDS) such as e-cigarette, vape pen, hookah?"
"Do you smoke/inhale any type of marijuana?"
"At what age did you start to use tobacco/marijuana?"
"What quantity do you use on a daily basis?"
"Has this amount changed? In what way?"
"Have you ever tried to quit? How many times? What method(s) did you use? What was the outcome?"
"How long ago did you quit?"
"Do you think you have a smoking (tobacco/marijuana) problem?"
"Do you live with someone who smokes?"

Recreational Drug Use

You may feel uncomfortable asking the client whether there has been recreational drug use; remind the client that the information will be kept confidential and that the withholding of information may delay necessary treatment. Keep in mind that recreational drugs can be called by various names. For instance, MDMA may be referred to as ecstasy.

"Do you use or have you ever used marijuana (keep in mind that it is legal to use marijuana in many states), amphetamines, MDMA (ecstasy), uppers, downers, cocaine, crack, heroin, PCP, inhalants, or other recreational or street drugs?"
"Do you use household products to get high (e.g., glue, aerosol substances, dextromethorphan)?"
"Do you do club drugs?"
"When did you first start to use recreational drugs?"
"What amount do you use?"
"How often do you use this drug?"
"Has this amount changed? In what way?"
"In what form do you use the drug (pill, needle, snort, other)?"
"Describe how you inject the drug."
"Do you share needles? Do you clean the needles between uses? How?"
"Have you experienced any health problems from the drug use?"
"Have you ever overdosed? What happened?"
"Have you ever been through a drug rehab program? What was the outcome?"
"Do you think you have a drug problem?"

NURSING TIP
Use of Psychedelics

A current trend exists in the use of psychedelic substances to affect cognitive and mental function. Substances such as lysergic acid diethylamide (LSD), psilocybin ("magic mushrooms"), MDMA (3,4-methylenedioxymethamphetamine), dimethyltryptamine, ibogaine, and mescaline are being used to treat mood disorders (such as depression, anxiety, PTSD), autoimmune disorders, chronic pain, substance use disorders, and palliative care. Psychedelics are also being used to enhance cognitive performance and creative thinking. Typically, small doses, or microdoses, of a psychedelic substance are administered over a period of time. Psychedelics act on brain receptors such as serotonin to alter perception and mood but at nonhallucinogenic doses. Ongoing clinical trials are investigating the efficacy of psychedelic substances, as they are being used more frequently. No current standards exist for their use in clinical practice.

NURSING TIP
Cannabis

Cannabis, or marijuana, is a psychoactive drug that has been used for centuries. Cannabis is a schedule 1 drug that is illegal under federal law, though it can be used legally for recreational and medicinal purposes in many states. The psychoactive ingredient that can cause a high is tetrahydrocannabinol (THC). Cannabidiol (CBD) is another active ingredient in cannabis that has no psychoactive properties. Cannabis can be ingested, smoked, and vaporized and is found in many forms: tablets, solution, oils, edibles, inhalants, topicals, and suppositories. Medicinally, cannabis and/or CBD may be used for seizures, chemotherapy-induced nausea and vomiting, pain, and multiple sclerosis spasticity relief. Ongoing research investigates the usefulness in various clinical conditions, and this body of knowledge is expanding. Though cannabis may help some people with serious health conditions, the negative side effects of cannabis cannot be ignored.

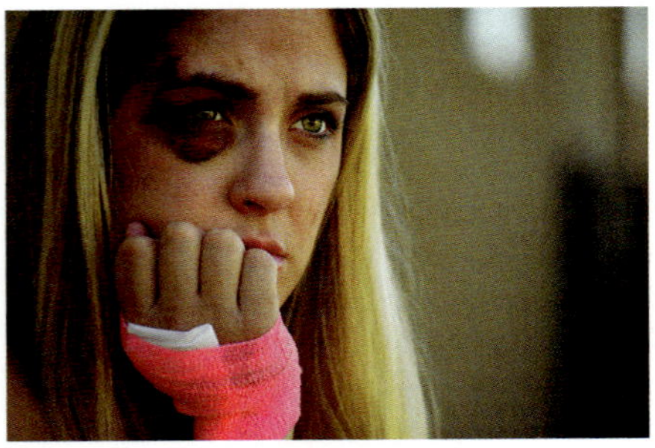

Figure 3-10 All people can be victims of domestic and intimate partner violence.

Intimate Partner Violence

The CDC (2022) defines Intimate Partner Violence (IPV) as "physical violence, sexual violence, stalking, and psychological aggression by a current or former intimate partner." IPV cuts across racial, cultural, geographic, and socioeconomic lines. Though men can be the victims of IPV, the majority of victims are women (Fig. 3-10). The CDC (2022) reports that about 33% of all women and 25% of men have experienced IPV in their lifetime. IPV also occurs in LGBTQ people and may even be increased in bisexual and transgender people compared with cisgender people (National LGBT Health Education Center, n.d.; Scott et al, 2023). It is vital to be familiar with your state's statutes regarding reporting actual and suspected violence and abuse. IPV involves more than physical abuse. It includes psychological, emotional, sexual, and financial abuse or coercion. Just as many health-care providers screen for tobacco and alcohol use at each health-care encounter, conducting routine screening for IPV at every health care is also imperative. The American Association of Colleges of Nursing published a White Paper in 1999 advocating for the incorporation of clinical content in nursing school curriculums on IPV as well as providing clinical experience in this area. In 2000 the American Nurses Association revised their 1991 position statement and recommended screening for IPV on a regular basis.

IPV can be an isolated incident or an ongoing condition. Some clues that might alert you to the possibility of domestic and intimate partner violence are:

- Frequent injuries, accidents, or burns
- Frequent urinary tract infections, frequent sexually transmitted infections
- Vaginal/rectal bleeding
- Multiple ecchymoses in various stages of healing
- Unexplained scars/skin disruptions
- Previous injuries for which the individual did not seek health care
- Injury that is inconsistent with the client's report of how it occurred
- Refusal of the client to discuss the injury
- Significant other accompanies the client to the emergency department (ED), answers questions for the client, and refuses to leave the client's side
- Significant other has a history of previous violent behavior or substance abuse
- Vague symptoms, such as chronic pain (e.g., headaches, back pain, pelvic pain) and fatigue

NURSING TIP
Dealing With Sensitive Topics

Alcohol use, drug use, and sexual practices are some of the most sensitive areas that are addressed in the health history. Some tips for dealing with these sensitive topics are:

- Ask these questions in the later stages of the interview after rapport has been established.
- Use direct eye contact; this demonstrates the importance of the topic to the client and your lack of embarrassment.
- Pose questions in a matter-of-fact tone.
- Adopt a nonjudgmental demeanor.
- Use the communication technique of normalizing when appropriate (e.g., "Many high school students drink alcohol or use drugs or engage in sexual relationships on a regular basis. Does this happen at your school? With you?").

NURSING TIP
The SANE Nurse

The sexual assault nurse examiner (SANE) is a nurse who has received extensive training in the handling of sexual assault victims. Intensive coursework combined with clinical training enables the nurse to take the SANE certification examination, which is administered by the International Association of Forensic Nurses (IAFN). The SANE nurse collects evidence with a physical evidence recovery kit (PERK) for legal proceedings and provides much-needed sensitivity during the collection of the physical evidence (e.g., mouth, vaginal, and anal swabs; head and pubic hair; blood samples). The SANE nurse is an expert in providing crisis intervention and support to the client, as well as guiding the client to community resources to help with the healing process. Finally, the SANE nurse is responsible for maintaining the chain of custody of the physical evidence so that it is admissible in a court of law. The SANE nurse may be called to testify at these legal proceedings.

Using the communication technique of normalizing, the nurse can screen for potential IPV. Some appropriate introductory comments might be:

"Many injured women who visit the Emergency Department (ED) have experienced some intimate partner violence. Is this what happened to you?"

"Intimate partner violence occurs very frequently in our community. Keeping this in mind, I would like to ask you some questions."

A single broad question can also be used to screen for domestic and intimate partner violence:

"In the past year, have you been hit, kicked, punched, or hurt in other ways by someone close to you?"

If the client answers "yes" to this question, you need to inquire whether the client feels safe in their current environment or situation. Most EDs have resources available to assist the client in moving to a climate where they can receive help and feel safe. In addition, there are many screening tools for IPV recommended by the U.S. Preventive Services Task Force (USPSTF) in primary care: Humiliation, Afraid, Rape, Kick (HARK); Hurt, Insult, Threaten, Scream (HITS); Extended–Hurt, Insult, Threaten, Scream (E-HITS); Partner Violence Screen (PVS); and Woman Abuse Screening Tool (WAST). These USPSTF screening tools are valid and reliable for IPV screening in women; unfortunately no tools exist in primary care that address IPV in men, older adults, and vulnerable adults who do not present with signs and symptoms of abuse (USPSTF, 2018).

It is imperative to document physical violence examination findings concisely and accurately. Incorporate drawings of injury locations or use printed anatomical maps on which injuries can be documented. Many EDs have cameras so that the staff can photograph injuries for the client's records.

Keep in mind that many victims of IPV experience anxiety, panic attacks, flashbacks, depression, sleep disorders, substance abuse, and post-traumatic stress disorder after the attack, and these conditions can last for years. Specific health-care procedures, such as a gynecological examination, may invoke memories of the IPV. The nurse must be sensitive to the client's needs at these times. For additional information, visit *https://www.ncbi.nlm.nih.gov/books/NBK533715/table/appf.tab1/.*

> **NURSING TIP**
> **Human Trafficking**
> Human trafficking is the exploitation and violation of a person by another where the oppressed person is made to engage in commercial labor or sex acts by the means of force, fraud, or coercion. Any person can be the victim of human trafficking—man or woman, boy or girl. According to the U.S. Department of State (2023), boys are the victims of the fastest-growing group of trafficked persons. Human trafficking is a crime if the exploited person is under the age of 18. Human trafficking is a human rights violation and occurs throughout the world (U.S. Equal Employment Opportunity Commission, n.d.). It is not unusual to see posters for reporting human trafficking in bathroom stalls at major interstate restrooms, airports, bus stations, etc. See Figure 3-11. To learn more about this critical issue and what you can do about it, visit the Web site of the National Human Trafficking Resource Center *https://www.eeoc.gov/national-human-trafficking-resource-center.*

Sexual Practice

Sexual practice histories focus on healthy sexual practices as well as the transmission of communicable diseases. Various medications can affect sexual function.

Questioning a client about sexual practices may be uncomfortable for both client and nurse. The client may notice your uneasiness with this topic and may feel embarrassed to answer the questions. Examine your personal feelings on human sexuality and attain a comfort level that will allow ease in questioning. The health histories in Chapters 21 and 22 provide additional information about female and male reproductive health.

"What term would you use to describe your sexual orientation?"

"Does your current sexual orientation represent your past sexual practice? If not, how has it changed?"

"At what age was your first sexual experience?"

"How many sexual partners have you had?"

"With how many partners are you currently involved? Has this changed?"

"What method of birth control do you use? Do you have any questions about it? Would you like additional information on other methods of birth control?"

"What measures do you use to prevent exchange of body fluids during sexual activity?"

"Do you engage in oral or anal intercourse?"

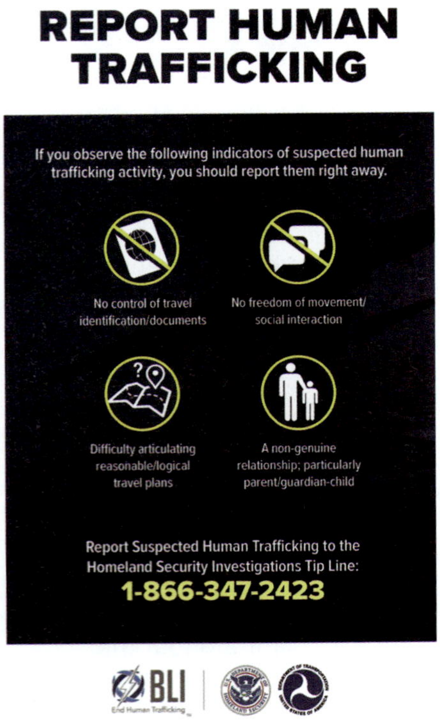
REPORT HUMAN TRAFFICKING
If you observe the following indicators of suspected human trafficking activity, you should report them right away.
No control of travel identification/documents
No freedom of movement/ social interaction
Difficulty articulating reasonable/logical travel plans
A non-genuine relationship; particularly parent/guardian-child
Report Suspected Human Trafficking to the Homeland Security Investigations Tip Line:
1-866-347-2423
BLI

Figure 3-11 Posters addressing Human Trafficking are often seen in heavily traveled areas.

NURSING TIP IPV SCREENING TOOLS

HITS Screening Tool

Sherin, Sinacore, Li, Zitter, and Shakil (1998) developed the HITS screening tool to assess for domestic and intimate partner violence. This is easily administered in a short period of time. The client is asked how many times in the past month or year each incident has occurred.

H—Have you been physically Hurt?
I—Have you been Insulted or did someone talk down to you?
T—Have you been Threatened with physical harm?
S—Has someone Screamed at you or cursed you?

HARK Screening Tool

H—Within the last year, have you been Humiliated or emotionally abused in other ways by your partner or ex-partner?
A—Within the last year, have you been Afraid of your partner or ex-partner?
R—Within the last year, have you been Raped or forced to have any kind of sexual activity by your partner or ex-partner?
K—Within the last year, have you been Kicked, hit, slapped, or otherwise physically hurt by your partner or ex-partner?

HARK score=
Each HARK question is equal to 1 point if the client answers "yes" with a total score range from 0 to 4. A HARK score of ≥1 indicates the client is affected by interpersonal violence (IPV). [PMID: 17727730]

From Sherin, K. M., Sinacore, J. M., Li, X. Q., Zitter, R. E., & Shakil, A. (1998). HITS: a short domestic violence screening tool for use in a family practice setting. *Family Medicine, 30*(7), 508–512. Reprinted with permission from the Society of Teachers of Family Medicine.
Feltner, C., Wallace, I., Berkman, N., Kistler, C., Middleton, J. C., Barclay, C., Higginbotham, L., Green, J. T., & Jonas, D. E. (2018). Screening for intimate partner violence, elder abuse, and abuse of vulnerable adults: an evidence review for the U.S. Preventive Services Task Force [Internet]. Retrieved July 29, 2025, from: https://www.ncbi.nlm.nih.gov/books/NBK533720/
For additional information on IPV screening tools, see
Retrieved October 8, 2025, from *https://www.ncbi.nlm.nih.gov/books/NBK533715/table/appf.tab1/*

NURSING TIP

Eliciting the Sexual History

Be aware that clients may refuse to answer questions pertaining to sexual history; try returning to these questions later. Ask the client whether a nurse of a different sex would make the client more comfortable in discussing sexual practice.

The adolescent client may refuse to answer these questions or may provide false answers if the parent or caregiver is in the room. It may be advisable to ask the caregiver to leave the room at the completion of the health history so that you can ask the client whether there is anything else that he or she would like to say.

Be alert for cues that demonstrate the client's desire for sexual education, such as questions or requests for written information. Answer the client's questions honestly.

"Have you ever had a sexual partner who had a sexually transmitted infection?"
"Are there other activities that satisfy your sexual needs?"
"Do you take any prescription or OTC medications to help your sexual performance?"
"Do you use any sexual aid devices?"
"Are you able to be aroused to orgasm?"
"Are you satisfied with your sexual performance?"
"Do you have any obstacles to achieving sexual satisfaction (e.g., sexually transmitted infection, children in the house)?"
"Do you have any infertility issues? How have you dealt with that?"
"Have you ever been sexually abused? What has transpired since?"
"Do you engage in sexual asphyxiation or similar practices?"

NURSING TIP

Dangerous Sexual Practices

Be alert for individuals who engage in potentially lethal sexual practices that involve near-strangulation. In adolescents, this practice is often referred to as the "choking game." Individuals literally choke one another with their hands, or they may use noose-like materials such as belts, scarves, and ropes. Adults usually use more sophisticated techniques to have this autoerotic experience. The premise of this "game" is to experience the euphoria that occurs when one is close to unconsciousness or becomes unconscious. In some instances, individuals have died during these activities.

Travel History

Endemic illnesses may be endogenous to specific regions in the world or to a single country (Fig. 3-12). Clients sometimes present with symptoms that cannot or may not be attributed to routine illnesses. For these reasons, a complete travel history is warranted when obtaining a health history.

"Where in the United States have you traveled? Is this a rural or an urban environment? When?"
"Have you ever traveled outside of the United States? Where? When?"
"For what period of time were you within this region?"
"Did you receive any immunizations before you visited that area?"
"Did you need to take any medications prophylactically before or while you were away (e.g., malaria, acetazolamide, dexamethasone)?"
"Were you ill when you were there?"
"Was a diagnosis made? By whom? What was it?"
"What treatment did you receive? Were there any complications?"
"Since returning from this area, have you been ill or not feeling normal?"
"If traveling for more than 2 to 4 hours, did you keep hydrated? How often did you get up and stretch or walk around?"
"Have you ever had a travel-related health issue (e.g., diarrhea, blood clot, altitude sickness)?"

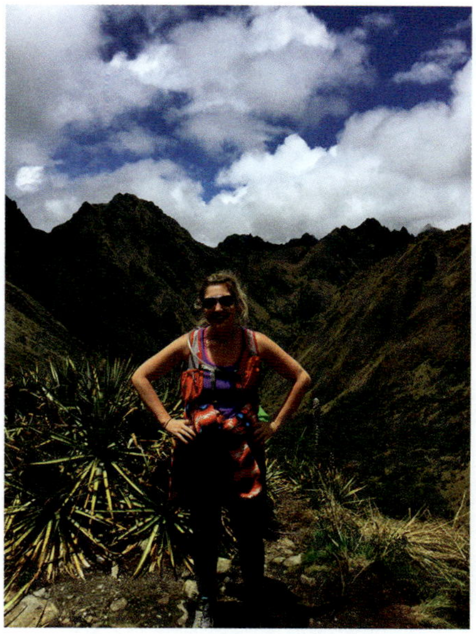

Figure 3-12 Travel to different parts of the world may require immunizations due to regional pathogens and illnesses.

Work Environment

The work environment can be hazardous. The nature of employment itself may present health hazards, regardless of whether safety measures are used. For example, carpenters may be prone to ischemia of their fingers from repeated exposure to handheld vibrating tools. Exposure to toxic substances in the work environment, such as asbestos and lead, is an additional factor to consider. Even traditional offices can be problematic due to noxious fumes, mold, asbestos, and other irritants (see Fig. 3-13).

"Describe the work that you do. Is it physically demanding? Is it mentally or emotionally demanding?"
"How many hours a day do you normally work? How long have you held this position?"
"Do the hours/shifts of your work change? How do you handle this?"
"Do you spend the majority of your workday sitting, standing, walking, running, lifting, or biking?"
"Do you work with any chemicals? Raw materials?"
"Are you exposed to radiation? Toxic fumes? Hazardous materials/conditions?"
"What safety measures do you practice at work?"
"Is there pollution near your place of employment?"
"What is the noise level at your place of employment?"
"Have you noticed that you are sick on the weekend or on your days off?"
"Have you had any work-related accidents or injuries?"
"Is there any construction at your work environment?"
"Do you enjoy your work?"
"What other jobs have you held in your lifetime?"

NURSING TIP

Travel Practices

As we become a society that travels more, both domestically and internationally, a new branch of health care has become a dominant force in helping to meet the needs of today's travelers. Travel medicine has boomed in the past decade for this reason. Travel medicine clinics assist the traveler in determining what immunizations are required for various parts of the world and then provide them for the client. In addition, the clinics teach travelers how to protect against illness while in particular regions. This information revolves around food, insect protection, and, in some cases, protection against potential violence. Effective travel clinics also educate the client on how to deal with jet lag and provide information on thrombosis prophylaxis.

Home Environment

When assessing the client's home environment, consider both the physical and the psychosocial aspects. The physical assessment of the home encompasses a broad spectrum of topics: physical condition of the house, safety

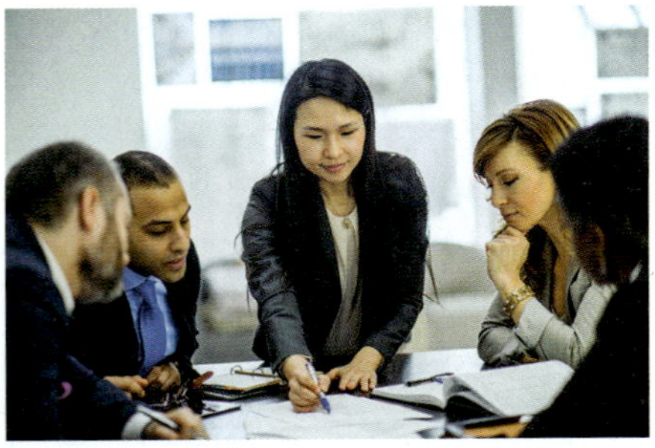

Figure 3-13 Assessment of the client's work environment is a component of the health history.

> **NURSING TIP**
> **Guidelines for Assessing the Home Environment**
> Not all of the questions for the home environment assessment have to be asked of every client. However, you need to be attentive to clues that signal the necessity of performing an in-depth home environment assessment. Some clues include, but are not limited to, poor hygiene, frequent infections, smoke inhalation, burns, malnutrition, and falls (especially among older adults).

from toxic substances, and the presence of modern conveniences such as a refrigerator, furnace, and electricity. Older houses may have been painted with lead-based paint, which poses a health threat to a young child who eats the paint chips. The presence of radon gas in the home is also a health concern.

Physical Environment

"How old is your residence/home (i.e., house, condo, trailer, or apartment building)?"
"In what condition is your residence/home?"
"Is your residence/home cleaned regularly?"
"Do you have heat, air conditioning, and electricity? What type of heat do you have? Do you use space heaters?"
"Do you have running water?"
"From what source does your water originate (e.g., well, reservoir, municipality)?"
"What is the temperature on your hot water heater?"
"Do you have a toilet, tub, or shower? Do you have a grab bar in the shower or bathtub?"
"What type of stove do you use (e.g., gas, electric, induction, wood, coil, radiant, pellet, propane, solar)?"
"Do you have any mold or wet/damp areas in your house?"
"Do you have a rodent or infestation problem?"
"Do you have a working telephone (landline, cell phone)?"
"Do you have smoke detectors? Do you have carbon monoxide detectors? Where? Do you inspect the batteries on a regular basis?"
"How many steps separate each floor? Is there a railing?"
"Do you have any throw rugs? Are they taped to the floor?"
"Do you use a nightlight when it is dark?"
"Do you have grab bars in the bathroom by the toilet"?
"Have you adapted your residence/home for any reason?"
"Do you think your living space is adequate for the number of people who live with you?"
"Have you ever had your residence/home tested for the presence of radon? What was the result?"
"How often do you have your fireplace cleaned?"
"How often do you replace the filter in your ventilation system?"
"What pets do you have? Do they live inside or outside?"
"What type of transportation do you use?"
"Who does your shopping?"
"Do you have easy access to a grocery store? Drug store? Health-care facility?"
"Where do you store your medications, cleaning supplies, and other toxic substances? How are they secured?" (if children live in the living quarters)
"Do you have a gun in the residence/home? Where is it stored? How is it stored? Where are the bullets stored? Is the gun loaded?"
"Where do you store gasoline and automotive supplies?"
"Is there a problem with pollution near your residence/home?"

Clients who are unhoused or have no fixed address pose unique challenges. The nurse needs to ascertain additional information and assist the client in accessing appropriate social services.

"What is your current living situation?"
"Do you reside in a specific location? Is this outdoors? Indoors? A shelter?"
"Do you feel safe with your current living condition?"
"Where do you eat? How do you get your food?"

The psychosocial component of the home environment assessment identifies the relative safety of the neighborhood.

Psychosocial Environment

"With whom do you live?"
"Do you feel safe in your neighborhood?"
"Do you know your neighbors?"
"Does your neighborhood have a crime prevention program?"
"What measures have you taken to ensure home safety?"
"Do you have some type of home security system?"

Hobbies and Leisure Activities

Acquiring information on clients' hobbies and leisure activities is necessary because some activities can pose health risks (Fig. 3-14). For example, repeated exposure to glue used in constructing model cars and planes can lead to respiratory ailments. People with asthma who do woodworking or pottery are at risk for attacks due to small particle exposure. People who work with sheep or wool from sheep can be at risk for contracting anthrax.

"What hobbies do you have?"
"What do you like to do in your spare time?"
"During or after this activity, have you ever felt sick? What happened?"
"Have you ever given up some leisure activity because of the effect it had on your health? What happened?"
"Have you ever had an injury from your hobby?"
"Are the hobbies and leisure activities relaxing?"
"Do you take any precautions (e.g., eye protection, mask) with your hobby?"

NURSING TIP
Technology Addiction

Computers are a vital component of our lives, and they have radically changed how business is conducted. In addition, computers and access to the Internet have altered the way many people now spend their free time. As a consequence, Internet addiction has become a health concern as individuals spend more time in front of computers. Whether the computer user frequents shopping sites, gambling sites, pornography sites, or multiplayer online role-playing games or engages in cybersex, the outcome can be the same—loss of control, social isolation, difficulties at home and/or work. In addition, other technology such as cell phone use, which engages people in texting, e-mailing, instant messaging, and sexting, poses similar concerns. Social networking sites have grown exponentially around the globe and engross millions in online interactions on a regular basis. The American Psychiatric Association added Internet Gaming Disorder to the Diagnostic and Statistical Manual of Mental Disorders (DSM-5-TR) as a clinical condition that requires further research.

Stress

Stress is a physiologically defined response to changes that disrupt the resting equilibrium of an individual. **Distress** is negative stress, or stress that is harmful and unpleasant (Fig. 3-15). **Eustress** is positive stress: stress that challenges the individual, provides motivation, and prevents stagnation.

"What are the current stressors in your life?"
"What do you feel is your greatest stress at the present time?"
"Are there recurring themes with the stress that you experience?"

NURSING TIP
Tracking Care Provided to People Who Are Unhoused

People who do not have permanent housing may reside at shelter facilities. The shelter staff follows their health needs, when possible, and ensures appropriate care. If a person experiencing homelessness does not reside at a shelter but lives on the street, it may be difficult to ensure appropriate follow-up care. If follow-up is essential, as in a client with tuberculosis, you may need to initiate actions to locate the person. Law enforcement officials or social service workers may be called upon to help locate seriously ill people who are unhoused so that their illnesses do not pose public health risks.

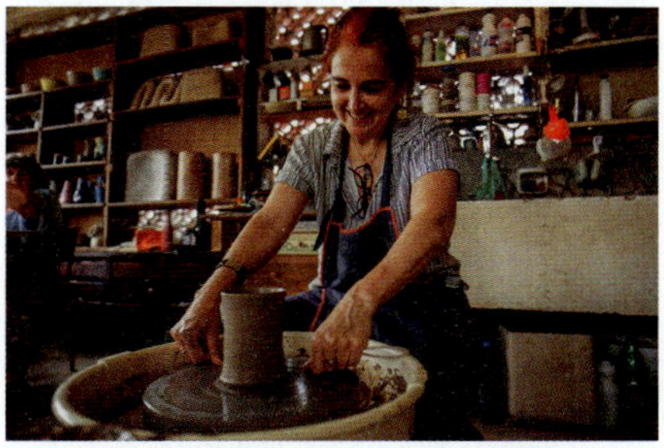

Figure 3-14 A client's hobbies can impact their health. This potter is exposed to small dust particles that can affect respiratory health.

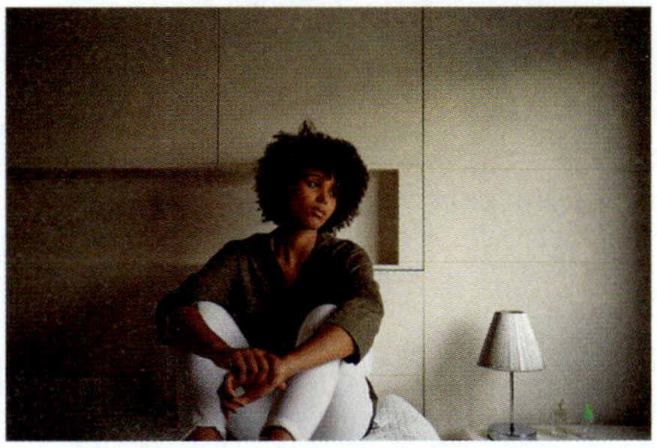

Figure 3-15 Distress can negatively impact health status.

"Have you ever progressed from the point of being stressed to panic? What were the circumstances? How did you handle it?"
"Are you able to recognize when you become stressed? What happens?"
"When you are stressed, do you experience palpitations, shortness of breath, light-headedness, sweating, or other symptoms?"

Education

Elicit information about the client's ability to read and write, and tailor your questions and information to this level.

"What was the highest grade level that you completed?"
"Describe the type of student you were."

Economic Status

Clients and nurses may be equally uncomfortable discussing financial status. The essence of the information needed is how the client lives on their income. Clients who lack adequate financial resources may be referred to social services for assistance in meeting their health-care needs.

"What are the sources of your income?"
"How would you describe your economic status?"
"Are you able to meet food, medication, housing, clothing, and personal expenses for you and your family?"
"Are you able to save any money?"
"Do you hesitate to seek health care because of the cost? Do you have health-care insurance?"
"Are you satisfied with your current economic status?"

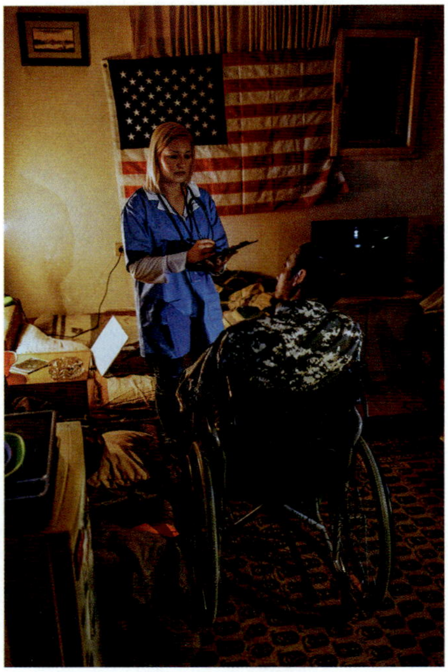

Figure 3-16 Knowledge of a client's military experience can provide information concerning geographic illnesses as well as exposure to toxic substances.

Military Service

Knowledge of overseas tours of duty may provide a vital link to current health status (Fig. 3-16); a client may not reveal this information during the travel history because it was work rather than leisure travel. For instance, many military personnel who served in Operation Desert Storm in 1990–1991 have multisystem health conditions collectively called Gulf War Illness (Cruz-Hernandez, Roney, Goswami, Tewari-Singh, & Brown, 2022). Knowledge of deployment to a specific geographical location, particularly in a hostile environment, can provide clues to the client's health condition.

"Are you or have you ever been in the military? What branch?"
"How long have you been in the military? Are you on active duty or reserve?"
"In what regions have you been assigned? How long were you there? When? Did you have any illnesses when you were abroad?"
"Have you ever been in combat? What were your experiences? Do you have flashbacks?"
"Have you ever been diagnosed with post-traumatic stress disorder (PTSD)?"
"Were you exposed to any chemical/biological agents? Radiation?"

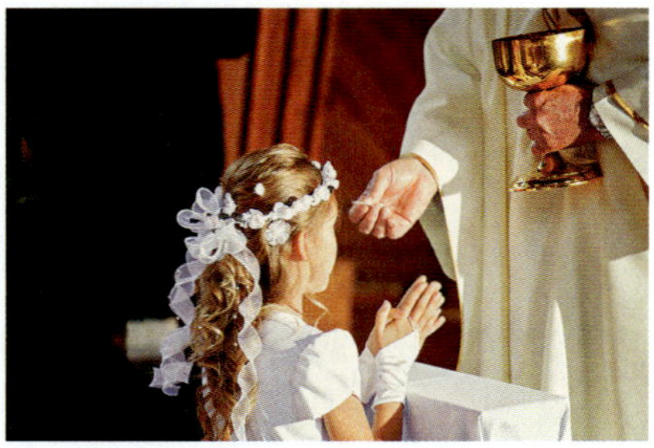

Figure 3-17 Assessing a person's religious and spiritual beliefs is an important aspect of nursing care. For example, the young girl in this photo is receiving First Holy Communion in the Roman Catholic Church. She has been required to complete an educational program, fulfill various religious requirements, and fast for a period of time to reach this special occasion in her faith.

Religion

Religion and spirituality can be powerful forces in a client's life. You need to be aware of and sensitive to implications of spirituality or religious beliefs on the client's health status and health-care practices (Fig. 3-17). Chapter 6 goes into greater depth on assessing religious and spiritual practices.

"Are you affiliated with a specific religion?"
"Do you currently practice your faith?"
"Do your religious beliefs affect your health status? In what way?"
"Are there any beliefs that you feel are compromised by seeking health care?"
"Are there any religious practices that you may need assistance with?"

Ethnic Background

Closely associated with religious practices is the client's culture or ethnic background, which can penetrate all facets of a client's life. Integrate familiarity with various cultures into your knowledge base so you will be sensitive to and more completely understanding of the client's ethnic heritage. Chapter 5 discusses the cultural assessment in greater detail.

"With what culture or ethnic group do you identify yourself?"
"What practices do you observe?"

Roles and Relationships

Family roles, work roles, and interpersonal relationships provide clues about possible stressors, areas for health promotion, support systems, and sources of altered psychosocial patterns (Fig. 3-18).

"Who lives with you?"
"What type of relationship do you have with these individuals?"
"What is your role within your family (e.g., caregiver, breadwinner, child, student)?"
"What responsibilities go along with this role?"
"Who do you turn to for support?"
"Describe the relationship that you have with your friends and neighbors."

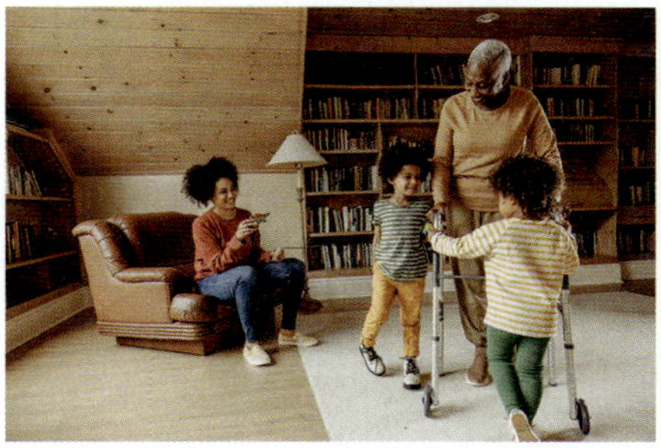

Figure 3-18 A person can assume many roles in life. The female on the left is a mother, full-time worker, and a caretaker for her own mother.

Characteristic Patterns of Daily Living and Functional Health Assessment

Questions about a client's usual lifestyle, or **characteristic patterns of daily living**, elicit information about the client's normal daily timetable: meals, work, sleep schedules, and social interactions (Fig. 3-19). If the client has a differing ability, a functional health assessment may need to be conducted (see Appendix B). The **Functional Health Assessment** documents a person's ability to perform instrumental activities of daily living (IADL) and physical self-maintenance activities. These data serve as baseline information upon which the effectiveness of nursing interventions can be evaluated.

"Describe a typical day for you, starting from the time you wake up to the time you go to bed."
"Do you need assistance with any activities of daily living? (If yes) Is assistance readily available?"
"Do you socialize, meet, or talk with people outside your house on a daily basis?"
"Does your schedule change on certain days or on the weekend? Describe."

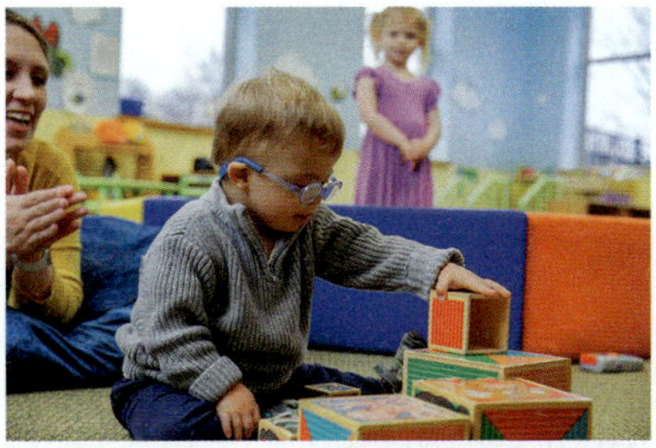

Figure 3-19 Part of this child's pattern of daily living is attending childcare during the workday.

Health Maintenance Activities

Health maintenance activities (HMA) are practices people incorporate into their lifestyle to promote healthy living. You can make the transition from the social history to HMAs with the following statements:

"Now I would like to discuss things that you do that promote health."
"There are many things you can do to promote healthy living. I would like us to discuss some of those practices."

Sleep

Many illnesses and diseases can lead to sleep disturbances. Increased or decreased sleep patterns can both occur. For this reason, you need to learn about the client's current and usual sleep habits (Fig. 3-20).

A standardized sleep tool can also be used to assess sleep and wakefulness patterns. One example of this is the Epworth Sleepiness Scale (Johns, 1991).

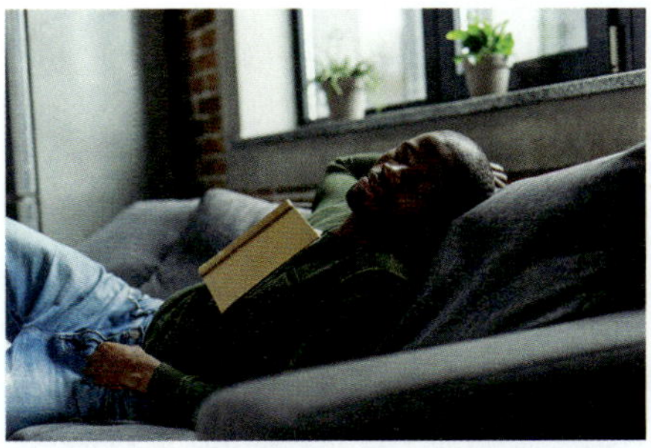

Figure 3-20 The nurse must inquire about a client's sleeping patterns and remember to ask about any napping in the daytime.

"At what time do you usually go to bed? What time do you usually awake?"
"Is this an adequate amount of sleep for you? How do you feel when you awaken?"
"How long does it take you to fall asleep?"
"Is the sleep undisturbed? Do you have difficulty staying asleep? If you awaken, is it easy for you to fall back to sleep?"
"Do you have any discomfort in your legs when you are in bed trying to sleep? Have you ever been diagnosed with restless legs syndrome?"
"Describe the environment in which you sleep (noise level, amount of light, temperature of the room, sleeping arrangement)."
"Are there any bedtime rituals that you practice?"
"What strategies do you use to fall asleep if you are having difficulty (medication, warm milk, other)? How many times per week do you do this?"
"What is your usual emotional state or mental condition when you go to bed? When you awaken?"
"Do you ever have difficulty falling asleep? How often does this occur? Have you ever been told that you have insomnia?"
"Have you ever been told that you snore loudly or excessively?"
"Do you ever have difficulty staying awake? Have you ever been told that you gasp while sleeping, stop breathing while sleeping, or that you have sleep apnea or narcolepsy?"
"Does the usual time of your sleep-awake cycle change (working rotating shifts)?"
"Do you have a job that requires rotating shifts or varies the time of work by a number of hours?"
"Do you take a nap during the day? For how long?"
"Do you fall asleep unintentionally at times other than nighttime?"
"Do you have nightmares? How frequent are they?"
"Do you walk in your sleep or do other activities such as driving? Eating?"
"Do you experience bedwetting?"
"Do you often wake up with dark circles under your eyes? Puffy eyelids? Bloodshot eyes?"
"Do you ever wake in the night because of pain, shortness of breath, or the need to urinate?"
"Do you have alcohol, nicotine, or caffeine within 2 hours of bedtime?"
"Do you take any prescription medications to help you sleep?"
"Have you been diagnosed with obstructive sleep apnea (OSA)? Do you use a continuous positive airway pressure (CPAP) machine? Have you ever had surgery for OSA?"

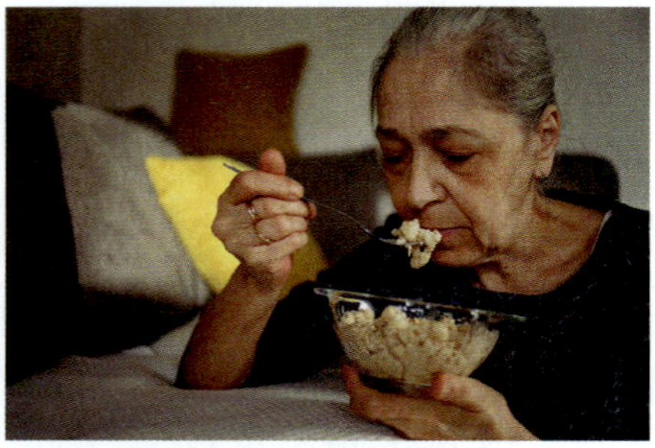

Figure 3-21 This woman requires a soft-food-only diet.

Diet

Refer to Chapter 7 for a more thorough discussion of nutrition and diet history.

"Are you on any special therapeutic diet (soft foods, low salt, low cholesterol, low fat, etc.)?" (Fig. 3-21).
"Do you follow any particular diet plan (vegetarian, liquid, paleo, commercially available diet food, rice diet, Mediterranean, DASH, Atkins diet, South Beach diet, etc.)?"
"How many meals a day do you eat? At what times do you eat? Do you snack? When? Do you practice intermittent fasting?"
"Has your weight fluctuated in the past year? Explain."

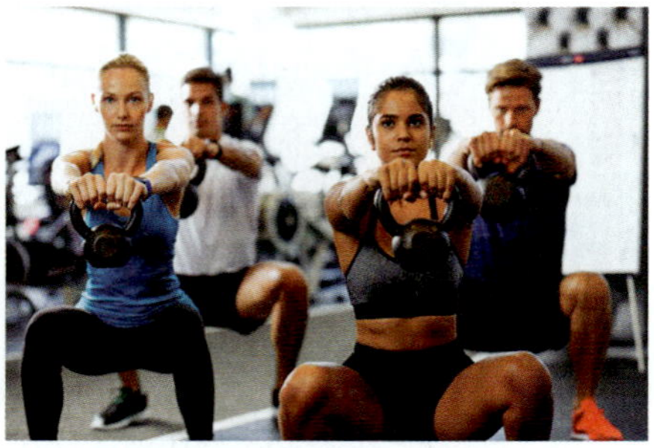

Figure 3-22 In this fitness class kettle bells are used for strength training.

Exercise

Aerobic exercise appropriate to the client's age and physical condition leads to cardiovascular, respiratory, and musculoskeletal fitness as well as mental alertness (Fig. 3-22). The American Heart Association (2021) guidelines for exercise call for 150 minutes of moderate-intensity exercise every week or 75 minutes of vigorous exercise per week, or a combination of both regimens. In addition, shorter 10- to 15-minute segments of exercise 2 to 3 times per day are encouraged if the individual is unable to be active for a longer period of time. Walking is always encouraged, but to be more heart healthy, aerobic activities such as running, biking, and swimming are recommended. Combining aerobic exercise with resistance training or weightlifting (which increases muscle strength) and calisthenics (which enhance flexibility) establishes a complete physical fitness regimen.

"Do you participate in a formal or informal exercise program?"
"What type of exercise do you do?"
"How many times per week do you exercise?"
"How long do you exercise (in minutes)?"
"What type of warm-up and cool-down exercises do you do?"
"What is your resting heart rate?"
"What is your heart rate at the most intense time of your exercise?"
"For what period of time do you maintain this elevated heart rate?"
"Have you ever experienced any injuries from your exercise regimen? What type?"
"How long have you been involved with this exercise program?"
"Does your health pose any restrictions on your ability to exercise?"

> **NURSING TIP**
> **"FIT" Acronym**
> An easy way to remember what questions to ask a client regarding an exercise regimen is to use the "FIT" acronym:
> **F**—is for the Frequency of the activity
> **I**—is for the Intensity of the activity
> **T**—is for the Timing, or duration, of the activity

Stress Management

The assessment of stress management practices is vital. Some commonly used stress management techniques are exercise, eating, biofeedback, yoga, progressive muscle relaxation, aromatherapy, imagery, massages, therapeutic touch (Fig. 3-23), verbalization, prayer, humor, pet therapy, music therapy, magnet therapy, reflexology, journaling, storytelling, support groups, and transcendental meditation. For others, stress management techniques include smoking, drinking, drugs, and violence. Many stress management apps are available (e.g., Calm, Happify, Breathe2Relax, Headspace, BetterSleep, the Mindfulness App, MindShift CBT, Sanvello, Smiling Mind, PTSD Coach, Panic Relief).

"When you become stressed, what do you do to help alleviate the stress?"
"When do you use this skill? Is it effective for you?"
"How do you evaluate the effectiveness of this technique?"
"How long do you need to perform this technique before your stress is reduced?"
"How many times per day do you use this technique? Per week?"
"Have you tried other stress management skills? How did they work?"

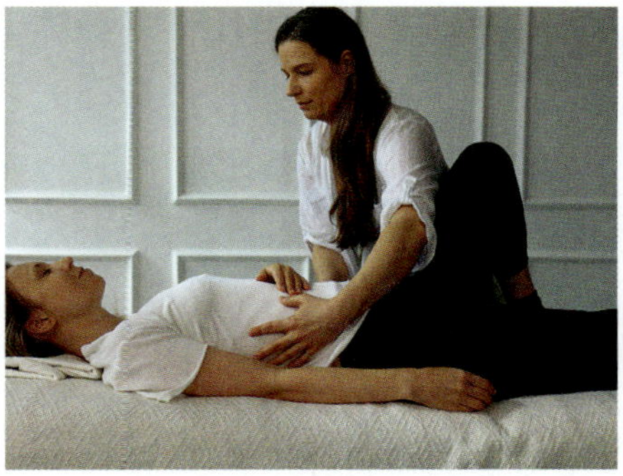

Figure 3-23 Somatic therapist using therapeutic touch is one of the many stress management techniques available to clients.

Use of Safety Devices

The client's use or lack of use of safety devices on the job, in the home, and in the environment provides an opportunity to teach health promotion skills (Fig. 3-24).

"Do you wear a seat belt when you are in an automobile?"
"Do you wear a helmet when riding a motorcycle/bicycle?"
"Do your hobbies and leisure activities require the use of safety devices? Do you use them?"
"Do you wear ear protection if you are engaged in an activity that produces loud noises?"
"What precautions do you take when using pesticides/fertilizers or other potentially harmful substances?"
"Do you wear sturdy shoes and goggles when you mow the lawn or do yard work?"
"Do you use mosquito repellent when outside?"

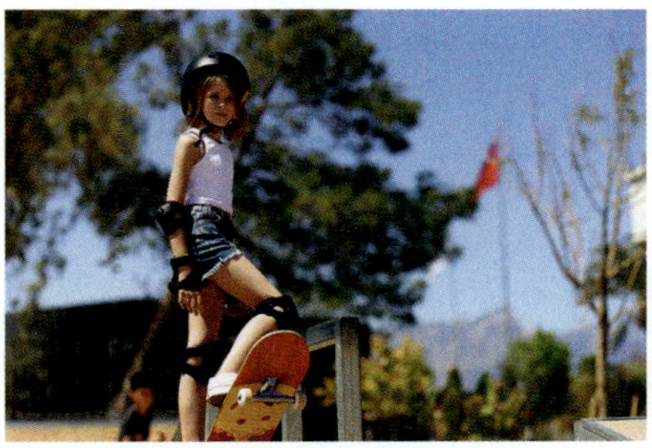

Figure 3-24 The proper use of safety equipment can help prevent or minimize injury.

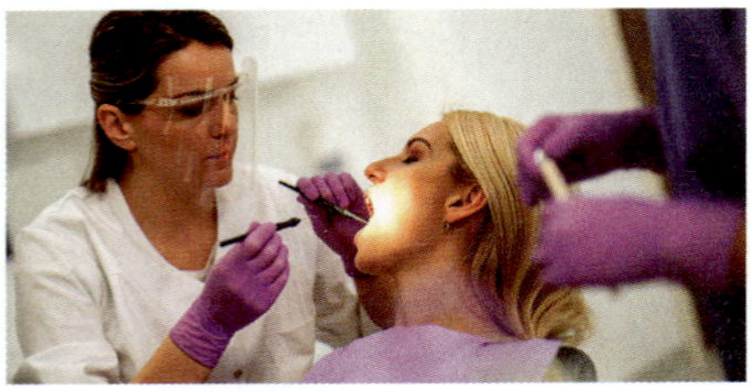

Figure 3-25 It is important to ask clients what other health-care providers they are seeing, such as a dentist.

Health CheckUps

Health checkup information demonstrates patterns of health-care practices by the client during illness and health, and reveals potential areas for health education.

"When was the last time you had the following performed: heart rate and blood pressure checks, complete physical examination, chest X-ray, TB test, EKG, urinalysis, complete blood cell count, blood chemistry, blood sugar, cholesterol? What were the results?"

"How often do you see a dentist (Fig. 3-25)? For what reason?"

"How often do you see an eye doctor? For what reason? Have you been checked for glaucoma?"

"How often do you have a gynecological checkup? By whom? What was the date and result of your last Pap smear?" (for women)

"Do you know how to perform a breast self-examination? How often do you perform it? Do you have any questions about it?" (for women)

"What was the date and the result of your last mammogram?" (for women)

"Do you know how to perform a testicular self-examination? How often do you perform it? Do you have any questions about it?" (for men)

"How often do you have a prostate examination? What was the date and result of your last PSA blood test and examination?" (for men)

"Have you had any screening for colon cancer? What test or procedure was done? What were the results?"

"Have you ever had a bone density or DEXA to screen for osteoporosis? What were the results?"

"Have you had any DNA testing? For what reason? If yes, what were the results?"

"Do you have any other health-care providers (e.g., cardiologist, pulmonologist, neurologist, gastroenterologist, ophthalmologist/optometrist, orthopedist, urologist, gynecologist, otolaryngologist, dermatologist, psychiatrist, psychologist, gerontologist, infectious disease, podiatrist, occupational, speech, or physical therapist, chiropractor, nutritionist)? For what reason? How often do you see them?"

Review of Systems

The **review of systems** (ROS) is the client's subjective response to a series of body system–related questions and serves as a double-check that vital information is not overlooked. The ROS covers a broad base of clinical states, but it is by no means exhaustive. The ROS follows a head-to-toe, or **cephalocaudal**, approach and includes two types of questions: sign or symptom related and disease related. The signs or symptoms and diseases are grouped according to physiological body parts and systems. Some of the diseases may have been discussed earlier in the interview.

Both positive and pertinent negative findings are documented in the ROS. When a response is positive, ask the client to describe it as completely as possible. Refer to the 10 characteristics of a chief complaint when gathering more information about positive responses. Table 3-2 lists the signs, symptoms, clinical conditions, and diseases that can be ascertained during the ROS. Many institutions have preprinted ROS sheets. These are convenient to use because positive findings can be circled and noted. Negative responses are not circled. In addition, computerized EHRs usually have ROS screens where the nurse can "check off" the pertinent information for the client. As you become more experienced, you can combine the ROS with the physical examination of the client. This technique often shortens the interview time with the client.

Table 3-2 Review of Systems

System	Signs/Symptoms/Clinical Conditions/Diseases/Tests
General	Client's perception of general state of health at the present, difference from usual state, vitality and energy levels, body odors, fever, chills, night sweats, metal or foreign objects in body (e.g., shrapnel), mechanical devices in the body (e.g., pacemaker, insulin pump)
Skin	Rash, itching, changes in skin pigmentation, lesions, ecchymoses, change in color or size of mole, sores that don't heal, lumps, dry or moist skin, pruritus, change in skin texture, odors, excessive sweating, acne, hives, warts, eczema, psoriasis, piercings, amount of time spent in the sun, use of sunscreen, skin cancer, skin self-examination
Hair	Alopecia, balding, excessive growth of hair or growth of hair in unusual locations (hirsutism), use of chemicals on hair, dandruff, pediculosis, scalp lesions, scalp conditions
Nails	Change in nails: color, splitting, breaking, thickening, texture change; onychomycosis, use of chemicals, use of false nails
Eyes	Visual acuity, blurred vision, visual field defect, use of glasses, use of contact lenses, sunglass use, photophobia, excessive tearing, difficulty seeing at night, diplopia, drainage, bloodshot eyes, infections, pain, itching, blind spots, flashing lights, halos around objects, floaters, glaucoma, cataracts, use of sunglasses, eye injury, use of protective eyewear, LASIK
Ears	Cleaning method, hearing deficits, hearing aid, pain, phonophobia, discharge, ringing in the ears (tinnitus), usual noise level, chronic exposure to loud noises, earaches, infection, ear discharge, itching, piercings, use of ear protection, amount of cerumen
Nose and Sinuses	Number of colds per year, nasal discharge, itching, hay fever, postnasal drip, stuffiness, sinus pain/pressure, chronic sinusitis, nasal polyps, itching, obstruction, epistaxis, change in sense of smell, environmental/seasonal allergies
Mouth	Dental habits (brushing, flossing, mouth rinses), bleeding or swollen gums, gingival hyperplasia, difficulty chewing, sore tongue, change in taste, palate itching, oral lesions, change in salivation, halitosis, tooth pain, tooth abscess, dentures, dental caries, teeth extractions, teeth implants, mouth appliances, orthodontics, dentures, dental checks
Throat and Neck	Hoarseness, change in voice, frequent sore throats, dysphagia, neck pain or stiffness, enlarged thyroid (goiter), lymphadenopathy, tonsillectomy, adenoidectomy, thyroidectomy
Breasts and Axilla	Pain, tenderness, discharge, lumps, change in breast size, dimpling, rash, benign breast disease, breast cancer, breast self-examination, results of recent mammogram
Respiratory	Dyspnea on exertion, shortness of breath, sputum, cough, sneezing, wheezing, hemoptysis, orthopnea, frequent upper respiratory tract infections, snoring, pneumonia, emphysema, asthma, chronic bronchitis, pulmonary emboli, tuberculosis, tuberculosis exposure, oxygen use, nebulizer treatments, obstructive sleep apnea/CPAP use, result of last chest X-ray or PPD
Cardiac	Paroxysmal nocturnal dyspnea, chest pain, heart murmur, congestive heart failure, coronary artery disease, palpitations, syncope, orthopnea (state number of pillows used), myocardial infarction, dysrhythmia, rheumatic fever, valvular disease, pacemaker, result of last EKG or other cardiac tests
Peripheral Vasculature	Hypertension, cyanosis, edema, cold or discolored hands or feet, leg cramps, peripheral vascular disease, peripheral artery disease, intermittent claudication, varicose veins, thrombophlebitis, deep vein thrombosis, use of support hose
Gastrointestinal	Change in appetite, nausea, vomiting, diarrhea, constipation, usual bowel habits, change in bowel habits, melena, rectal bleeding, hematemesis, change in stool color, flatulence, belching, heartburn, dysphagia, abdominal pain, bloating, jaundice, ascites, hemorrhoids, hepatitis, *Helicobacter pylori* infection, peptic ulcers, gallstones, gastroesophageal reflux disease, appendicitis, ulcerative colitis, Crohn disease, celiac disease, diverticulosis/diverticulitis, colostomy, ileostomy, umbilical/ventral hernia, result of last colonoscopy or other gastrointestinal tests

Continued

Table 3-2 Review of Systems—cont'd

System	Signs/Symptoms/Clinical Conditions/Diseases/Tests
Urinary	Change in urine color, voiding habits, dysuria, hesitancy, urgency, frequency, nocturia, polyuria, dribbling, difficulty starting/stopping urine stream, loss in force of stream, overactive bladder, bedwetting, change in urine volume, incontinence, urinary retention, suprapubic pain, flank pain, kidney stones, frequent urinary tract infections, pessary use, ileal conduit
Musculoskeletal	Joint stiffness, muscle pain, cramps, back pain, limitation of movement, redness, swelling, weakness, bony deformity, bone fractures, dislocations, sprains, crepitus, gout, arthritis, osteoporosis/osteopenia, herniated disc, muscle spasm
Neurological	Headache/migraine, change in balance, incoordination, loss of movement, change in sensory perception or feeling in an extremity, paresthesia, change in speech, change in smell, syncope, loss of memory, tremors, involuntary movement, loss of consciousness, concussions/head injury, seizures, limb weakness, head injury, vertigo, tremor, tic, paralysis, stroke, spasm
Psychological	Irritability, nervousness, tension, increased stress, difficulty concentrating, mood changes, suicidal thoughts, suicide attempts, depression, anxiety, other mental health condition, sleep disturbances, eating disorders, claustrophobia, memory loss, learning difficulty, attention-deficit/hyperactivity disorder (ADHD)
Female Reproductive	Vaginal discharge, change in libido, infertility, sterility, past history of STIs, pelvic pain, pain during intercourse, postcoital bleeding; menses: last menstrual period, menarche, regularity, duration, amount of bleeding, premenstrual symptoms, intermenstrual bleeding, dysmenorrhea, menorrhagia, fibroids; menopause: age of onset, duration, symptoms, bleeding; obstetrical: number of pregnancies, number of miscarriages, number of abortions, number of children, type of delivery, complications; type of birth control, hormone replacement therapy
Male Reproductive	Change in libido, infertility, sterility, impotence (erectile dysfunction), past history of STIs, pain during intercourse, age at onset of puberty, testicular or penile pain, penile discharge, erections, emissions, hernias, enlarged prostate, type of birth control, scrotal abnormalities, testicular cancer, testicular self-examination
Nutrition	Present weight, usual weight, desired weight, unintentional weight loss, unintentional weight gain, food intolerances, loss of appetite, food likes and dislikes, where meals are eaten, caffeine intake
Endocrine	Exophthalmos; fatigue; change in size of head, hands, or feet; weight change; heat and cold intolerances; excessive sweating; polydipsia, polyphagia, polyuria; increased hunger; change in body hair distribution; goiter; diabetes mellitus
Lymph Nodes	Enlargement, tenderness
Hematological	Easy bruising or bleeding, anemia, sickle cell anemia, other blood disorders, blood type, blood product infusions, exposure to radiation

Remember to ask the questions in terms that the client can understand. An appropriate statement for making the transition from the HMA to the ROS would be:

> "Now I would like to ask you if you have experienced a variety of conditions. Most of the questions can be answered with 'yes' or 'no.'"

Pose the same question for each item in the ROS:

> "Have you ever had . . . ?"

The System-Specific Health History

This text uses a system-specific health history in each body system chapter (refer to Chapters 10–23). The system-specific health history provides detailed information that guides questioning and provides clues of related pathology. Not every item in the complete health history is addressed in every body-system history. Only those sections relevant to the body system being assessed are addressed, and this can differ from chapter to chapter due to the nature of the material.

Assistive Devices

Some chapters in this text contain a section on assistive devices for that body system. These assistive devices are important to assess, as they are health extenders for the client. Whether the assistive device is supplemental oxygen, a walker, or a feeding tube, ask the client about their use/functioning in the health history and evaluate them as you examine the client. Correct use and functioning of these devices will help the client maintain a current level of health, whereas incorrect use can harm the client.

Concluding the Health History

After completing the ROS, ask the client whether there is any additional information to discuss. At the conclusion of the interview, thank the client for the time spent in gathering the health history. Inform the client what the next step will be (for example, physical examination, diagnostic tests, laboratory tests, treatment) and when to expect it.

Documentation

The documentation of the health assessment and physical examination is the legal record of the client encounter (Fig. 3-26). It also serves as the medium for communicating the client's condition among health professionals. The client record represents a description of the client's status and the care delivered to the client. The documentation may be read by a multitude of professionals: nurses; physicians; dietitians; respiratory, physical, speech, and occupational therapists; risk managers; utilization reviewers; quality assurance personnel; accreditation organizations; lawyers; insurance companies; and, ultimately, the client! Because all of these people may have access to the client's chart, you must document everything in a professional and legally acceptable manner. Each institution also has its own documentation system. If you perform computerized charting in your workplace, always safeguard your access code to protect yourself.

Many health-care facilities have preprinted health history forms that are checklists and require few narrative notes. Other facilities require the nurse to document the health history in its entirety. The health histories at the end of the chapter illustrate how to document the complete health history of an ill client and a well client.

General Documentation Guidelines

These general guidelines outline principles to guide your documentation:

- Ensure that you are documenting in the correct client record whether in the computer, on paper, or other system (e.g., oral dictation).
- Document as soon as the client encounter is concluded to ensure accurate recall of data (follow the institution's guidelines on frequency of charting).
- Avoid distractions while documenting. This is frequently when errors are made.
- If interrupted while documenting, reread what you wrote to ensure accuracy.
- Use quotation marks to indicate direct client responses (e.g., "I feel lousy").

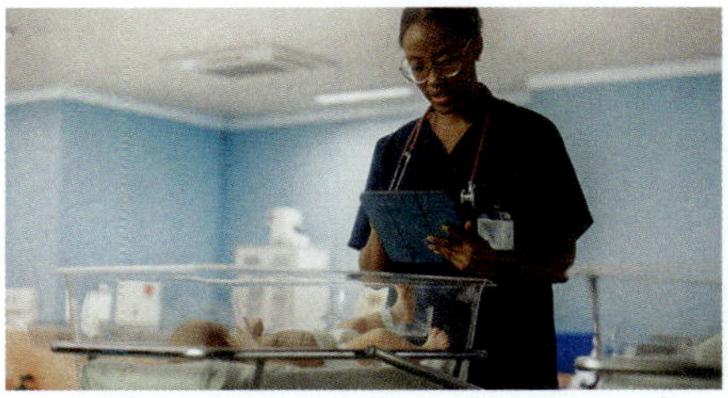

Figure 3-26 Documenting the health history is a crucial step in providing client care.

- Document in chronological order (forward or reverse).
- Document in a complete but concise manner by using phrases and abbreviations as appropriate. Avoid using dangerous abbreviations, acronyms, and symbols as specified by the Joint Commission (formerly the Joint Commission on Accreditation of Health Care Organizations [JCAHO]) and the Institute for Safe Medication Practices.
- When documenting numbers less than 1, write a zero to the left of the decimal point; this avoids confusion as to the placement of a decimal point.
- Document telephone calls that relate to the client's case.
- Always reread your notes for accuracy.
- Identify the name of an interpreter if one is used or other mediator.
- Avoid using words that have more than one meaning.
- If using electronic health records, protect your access code and electronic signature.
- Remember: From a legal standpoint, if you didn't document it, it wasn't done.

Documentation Guidelines for Handwritten Client Records

These guidelines outline principles to guide your handwritten documentation:

- Ensure that the client's name and identifying information are on every page of the record.
- Record the date and time of each entry.
- Sign each entry with your full legal name and your professional credentials, or per your institution's policy.
- Do not sign a note that you did not write.
- Do not leave space between entries.
- Do not insert information between lines.
- If an error is made while documenting, use a single line to cross out the error, then date, time, and sign the correction (check institutional policy); avoid erasing, crossing out, or using correction fluid.
- Never change another person's entry, even if it is incorrect.
- Use legible writing.
- Use a permanent ink pen. (Black is usually preferred because of its ability to photocopy well.)

Examination-Specific Documentation Guidelines

These examination-specific guidelines provide examination-oriented do's and don'ts for documentation:

- Record all data that contribute directly to the examination (i.e., positive examination findings and pertinent negatives).
- Document any parts of the examination that are omitted or refused by the client.
- Avoid using judgmental language such as "good," "poor," "bad," "normal," "abnormal," "decreased," "appears to be," and "seems."
- Avoid evaluative statements (e.g., "Client is uncooperative," "Client is lazy"); cite instead specific statements or actions that you observe (e.g., "Client said, 'I hate this place' and kicked trash can").
- State time intervals precisely (e.g., "every 4 hours," "daily," instead of "seldom," "occasionally").
- Do not make relative statements about findings (e.g., "mass the size of an egg"); use specific measurements (e.g., "mass 3 cm × 5 cm").

- Draw pictures when appropriate (e.g., location of scar, masses, skin lesion, decubitus, deep tendon reflex, etc.).
- Refer to findings using anatomical landmarks (e.g., left upper quadrant [of abdomen], left lower lobe [of lung], midclavicular line, etc.).
- Use the face of the clock to describe findings that are in a circular pattern (e.g., breast, tympanic membrane, rectum, vagina).
- Incorporate appropriate photos into the client's record if this feature is available in the EHR (e.g., wound, mass).
- Document any change in the client's condition during a visit or from previous visits.
- Describe what you observed, not what you did.

U.S. Preventive Services Task Force

Since its inception in 1984, the U.S. Preventive Services Task Force (USPSTF) has been charged with reviewing evidence-based research to formulate preventive service guidelines for primary care clinicians. Preventive services are recommended for adults in the following areas: cancer (prevention, screening, chemoprevention, counseling, and genetic risk assessment); heart, vascular, and respiratory diseases; infectious diseases; injury and violence; mental health conditions and substance abuse; metabolic, nutritional, and endocrine conditions; musculoskeletal conditions; obstetric and gynecological conditions; and vision disorders. Separate recommendations are made for pregnant females in Chapter 24 and for children and adolescents in Chapter 25.

The USPSTF has devised a system with five letter grades to convey the strength of the recommendation based on the review of literature. These are:

- **Grade A:** The USPSTF recommends the service. There is high certainty that the net benefit is substantial. *Suggestions for Practice:* Offer or provide this service.
- **Grade B:** The USPSTF recommends the service. There is high certainty that the net benefit is moderate, or there is moderate certainty that the net benefit is moderate to substantial. *Suggestions for Practice:* Offer or provide this service.
- **Grade C:** The USPSTF recommends selectively offering or providing this service to individual patients based on professional judgment and patient preferences. There is at least moderate certainty that the net benefit is small. *Suggestions for Practice:* Offer or provide this service for selected patients depending on individual circumstances.
- **Grade D:** The USPSTF recommends against the service. There is moderate or high certainty that the service has no net benefit or that the harms outweigh the benefits. *Suggestions for Practice:* Discourage the use of this service.
- **I Statement:** The USPSTF concludes that the current evidence is insufficient to assess the balance of benefits and harms of the service. Evidence is lacking, of poor quality, or conflicting, and the balance of benefits and harms cannot be determined. *Suggestions for Practice:* Read the clinical considerations section of USPSTF Recommendation Statement. If the service is offered, patients should understand the uncertainty about the balance of benefits and harms (USPSTF, 2018).

In this text, recommendations that carry a Grade A or Grade B Recommendation will be included at the end of each chapter for the appropriate content area. In addition, realize that because the Patient Protection and Affordable Care Act was enacted, Grade A and B recommendations that are performed will be covered in health insurance plans.

U.S. Preventive Services Task Force (USPSTF)

Grade A Recommendations

- The USPSTF recommends that clinicians ask all adults about tobacco use, advise them to stop using tobacco, and provide behavioral interventions and US Food and Drug Administration (FDA)-approved pharmacotherapy for cessation to nonpregnant adults who use tobacco.
- The USPSTF recommends that clinicians screen for HIV infection in adolescents and adults aged 15 to 65 years. Younger adolescents and older adults who are at increased risk of infection should also be screened.
- The USPSTF recommends that clinicians prescribe preexposure prophylaxis using effective antiretroviral therapy to persons who are at increased risk of HIV acquisition to decrease the risk of acquiring HIV.

Grade B Recommendations

- The USPSTF recommends that clinicians screen for intimate partner violence (IPV) in women of reproductive age, including those who are pregnant and postpartum. See the "Practice Considerations" section for information on evidence-based multicomponent interventions for information on IPV in men.
- The USPSTF recommends screening for unhealthy alcohol use in primary care settings in adults 18 years or older, including pregnant women, and providing persons engaged in risky or hazardous drinking with brief behavioral counseling interventions to reduce unhealthy alcohol use.
- The USPSTF recommends screening by asking questions about unhealthy drug use in adults age 18 years or older. Screening should be implemented when services for accurate diagnosis, effective treatment, and appropriate care can be offered or referred. (Screening refers to asking questions about unhealthy drug use, not testing biological specimens.)

Retrieved October 8, 2025, from *https://USPreventiveServicesTaskForce.org uspstf/recommendation-topics/uspstf-and-b-recommendations*

ENAP Format

The physical examination chapters in this text use the ENAP format. The "E" represents the examination component, a step-by-step procedure on how to perform each physical examination skill. The "N" states the normal examination finding for that skill. "A" lists many common abnormal findings for each physical examination skill. Finally, the "P" explains the pathophysiology of the abnormal finding. There is a key at the bottom of each examination page spread to remind the reader what these initials mean.

CASE STUDY

Complete Health History: Well Client

This case study illustrates documentation of a complete health history of a well client. Agapito is an 18-year-old male who will graduate from high school in 2 months. He will be traveling from his home in Virginia to work as a counselor-in-training at a summer camp in Brevard, NC. He presents today for a well check. His camp employer requires a physical examination attesting to his good health for working at a 6-week sleepover camp. He could not get an appointment at his usual pediatric practice, so he made an appointment at the urgent care clinic.

HEALTH HISTORY

TODAY'S Date April 20, 2026; 2PM

BIOGRAPHICAL DATA

Client Name Agapito Nido
Home Address 1414 W. Jefferson Street, Arlington, VA 22209
Home Phone Number (703) 244-1111
Cell Phone Number (703) 244-1112
Date of Birth March 1, 2008
Birthplace Arlington, VA
Social Security Number xxx-xx-1234
Occupation Student
Insurance Information United Health
Usual Source of Health Care Arlington Pediatric Associates since birth
Source of Referral Father
Emergency Contact Adonis Nido, father, same home phone number as above
Preferred Language English
Source and Reliability of Information Self; reliable historian
Advance Medical Directive Client does not have one

CLIENT PROFILE

Age 18 years old
Sex Male
Gender Identity Identifies as a male
Preferred Name Nido (client states all his friends call each other by their last names)
Sexual Orientation Heterosexual
Race Brown
Marital Status Single

REASON FOR SEEKING HEALTH CARE

"I am working at a sleepover camp this summer, and I need to get this form completed stating that my health is OK to do this job. I feel great!"

PRESENT HEALTH

Describes self as a healthy high school student.

PAST HEALTH HISTORY

Medical History

- Bee sting reaction age 4 requiring emergency room visit due to facial swelling
- Seasonal allergies in spring/fall, controlled with OTC meds; never had allergy testing
- Facial acne, pediatric nurse practitioner prescribes topical medication for past 2 years, acne has improved

Surgical History Wisdom teeth extractions × 4 in 2021 without sequelae; outpatient surgery; no anesthesia complications

Allergies No medication allergies; bee sting reaction of facial swelling

Medications

Prescription

- Adapalene and benzoyl peroxide 0.3%/2.5% gel to face once daily
- Epinephrine autoinjector 0.3 mg; has never used but carries with him spring/summer/fall

OTC

- Multivitamin one every morning
- Loratadine 10 mg orally daily in spring/fall
- Triamcinolone acetonide nasal spray: one spray each nostril twice daily in spring/fall
- Ibuprofen 200 mg: 1–2 orally prn

Communicable Diseases

- Denies hepatitis and STIs

Injuries and Accidents Concussion in 2022 after he hit his head while skiing, no loss of consciousness; evaluated at ED, had to refrain from strenuous activity for 2 weeks, no sequelae

Differing Abilities Denies

Blood Transfusions Denies

Childhood Illnesses Chickenpox age 4 without sequelae; denies MMR, diphtheria, polio, scarlet fever

Immunizations "My dad told me I had everything I needed—even that HPV vaccine."

FAMILY HEALTH HISTORY

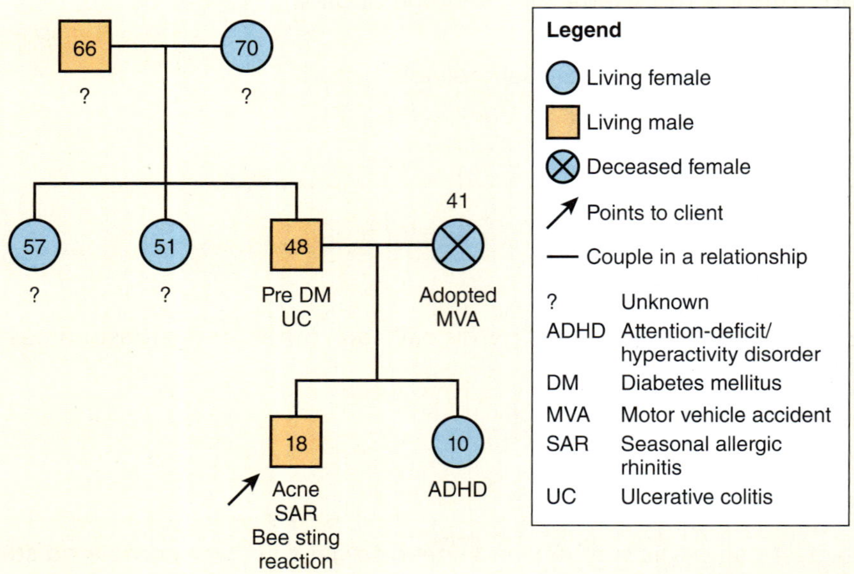

Denies family history of mental health disorders, kidney disease, heart disease, pulmonary disease, strokes, cancers, tuberculosis, blood disorders, drug addiction

SOCIAL HISTORY

Alcohol Use 1–2 beers every weekend with my friends; my dad gives me a beer on occasion at home when we watch a football game together

Tobacco Use Denies

Recreational Drug Use Denies

Intimate Partner Violence Denies

Sexual Practice Denies any previous/current sexual activity

Travel History Parents are from the Philippines. He traveled there last summer with his dad to meet some relatives. Completed hepatitis A series 3 months before he traveled. No other immunizations were received. All other travel on the East Coast.

Work Environment Lifeguards a few shifts every month at the local recreation center

Home Environment

Physical Environment Lives at home with father and sister. His mother died 5 years ago. Comfortable suburban neighborhood. House has all modern appliances. Not sure if smoke detectors or carbon monoxide detectors are checked. No guns in the house. Has a golden retriever that he cares for.

Psychosocial Environment Feels safe in house/neighborhood

Hobbies and Leisure Activities Ran cross-country every fall in high school. Plays basketball in the city league. Enjoys playing frisbee with his dog. Socializes with friends from school and neighborhood. Helps out at soup kitchen once a month.

Stress Keeping up his grades before graduation. Was accepted "early decision" to a VA college.

Education High school senior. Taking 2 Honors and 2 Advanced Placement courses, 3.5 GPA.

Economic Status "My dad takes care of that. He will take out loans for my college education."

Military Service Denies

Religion Does not follow any particular faith tradition.

Ethnic Background Parents emigrated from the Philippines before he was born. When mother was alive, she made some traditional dishes like *kare-kare* and cassava cake. On occasion the family goes to a Filipino restaurant.

Roles and Relationships Lives with father and sister. Feels he has a better relationship with his dad since his mother died. Tolerates his little sister.

Characteristic Patterns of Daily Living "I go to school. I do homework. Get a little exercise. Hang out a little. Work a little."

HEALTH MAINTENANCE ACTIVITIES

Sleep Sleeps 6–7 hours on school nights. Likes to sleep 10 hours on the weekend. Denies any difficulties in falling/staying asleep.

Diet "I try to eat healthy."

Exercise Cross-country practice every day in the fall (running 5–6 miles at least 5 days/week); basketball games and practice 2 days/week now. Swims 45 minutes once a week to keep in shape for his lifeguarding job.

Stress Management Plays computer games.

Use of Safety Devices Wears seat belt, wears helmet for skiing since his concussion.

Health Checkups Last physical was 1 yr ago, needed it to participate in high school sports; denies any problems. Sees dentist twice a year. Saw eye doctor last month—no problems.

REVIEW OF SYSTEMS

General High energy levels, healthy, denies recent illness, denies night sweats

Skin Uses sunscreen at the beach only; facial acne controlled with Rx medication. Denies: rashes, itching, change in skin pigmentation, ecchymoses, pruritus, hives, change in moles, sores, lumps, change in skin texture, body odors

Hair Denies: alopecia, hirsutism, dandruff, pediculosis, scalp lesions

Nails Denies: change in nails, splitting, breaking, onychomycosis

Eyes Does not require glasses/contacts. Recent eye examination showed 20/20 vision. Wears sunglasses on bright days. Denies: blurry vision, photophobia, increased tearing, diplopia, eye drainage, bloodshot eyes, eye pain, blind spots, floaters, flashing lights, halos around objects

Ears Denies: hearing deficits, hearing aid, pain, discharge, vertigo, tinnitus, earaches, infection

Nose and Sinuses Allergies per PHH, averages 1–2 colds/yr; Denies: nasal discharge, itching, postnasal drip, sinus pain, polyps, obstruction, epistaxis; no change in sense of smell

Mouth Brushes teeth in the morning and before bed, flosses at bedtime; no orthodontics used. Denies: toothache, tooth abscess, caries, bleeding/swollen gums, sore tongue, lesions, halitosis, difficulty chewing; no change in taste or salivation

Throat and Neck Denies: hoarseness, frequent sore throats, dysphagia, pain/stiffness, goiter

Breasts and Axilla Denies: change in size, pain, tenderness, lumps, nipple discharge

Respiratory Denies: sputum, sneezing, wheezing, hemoptysis, pneumonia, exercise-induced asthma, asthma

Cardiac Denies: paroxysmal nocturnal dyspnea, heart murmur, palpitations, dysrhythmia, chest pain, syncope, anemia, rheumatic heart disease

Peripheral Vasculature Denies: edema, cold hands/feet, leg cramps, intermittent claudication, varicose veins, thrombophlebitis

Gastrointestinal Regular bowel habit: stool every morning, soft and brown; Denies: nausea/vomiting, diarrhea, constipation, melena, change in stool color, hematemesis, flatulence, belching, heartburn, bloating, regurgitation; dysphagia, abdominal pain, jaundice, peptic ulcers, hemorrhoids, hepatitis, gallstones, umbilical hernia

Urinary Denies: change in urine color, voiding habits, hesitancy, urgency, frequency, nocturia, polyuria, suprapubic pain, kidney stones, incontinence, UTIs

Musculoskeletal Denies: bony deformity, weakness, decreased ROM, swelling, sprains, dislocations, arthritis, herniated disc, back pain

Neurological Concussion as per PHH. Denies: change in balance, incoordination, loss of movement, change in sensory perception, change in speech, anosmia, tremors, syncope, loss of memory, involuntary movement, loss of consciousness, seizure, weakness, vertigo, tremors, tics

Psychological

Anxious about starting college.

Denies: nervousness, difficulty concentrating, mood changes, depression, suicidal thoughts

Male Reproductive Denies: testicular/penile pain, penile discharge, STIs, ED, hernia

Nutrition

Usual and present weight 176 lbs (80 kg)

Food preferences: burgers, fruit

Food dislikes: brussels sprouts, peas

Denies: food intolerances/allergies

Endocrine Denies: exophthalmos; heat/cold intolerance, polyuria, polydipsia, polyphagia

Lymph Nodes Denies: enlargement or tenderness

Hematological Blood type: B negative (he found out when he donated blood at a school drive last year); Denies: easy bruising/bleeding, anemia

CLINICAL JUDGMENT IN ACTION

1. What medical conditions require counseling prior to the client working at the summer camp and attending college?
2. What cues indicate the need for health prevention before the client attends summer camp and college?

CASE STUDY

Complete Health History: Ill Client

This case study illustrates documentation of a complete health history of an ill client. Angela Tabatabai is a 66-year-old female who woke today with hematuria and dysuria. She recently retired from her job. She and her husband are scheduled to fly tomorrow to Honolulu for vacation. She is very anxious because she has planned this retirement vacation for many years, and she does not want to miss it. Angela presents for evaluation of her symptoms.

HEALTH HISTORY

Today's Date April 23, 2026; 10 AM

BIOGRAPHICAL DATA

Client Name Angela Tabatabai
Home Address 200 Larimer Street Denver, CO 80205
Home Phone Number (303) 405-2222
Cell Phone Number (303) 515-3434
Date of Birth January 28, 1960
Birthplace Colorado Springs, CO
Social Security Number xxx-xx-2348
Occupation Retired hairdresser
Insurance information Medicare
Usual Source of Health Care Urgent Care
Source of Referral Friend
Emergency Contact Husband, Ali (same home phone # as above)
Preferred Language English
Source and Reliability of Information Client is reliable historian
Advance Medical Directive Client does not have one but would like information on this

CLIENT PROFILE

Age 66
Sex Female
Gender Identity Female
Preferred Name Angel
Sexual Orientation Identifies as a heterosexual
Race White
Marital Status Married

CHIEF COMPLAINT

"I'm peeing blood. My side hurts."

HISTORY OF THE PRESENT ILLNESS

Client was in her usual state of health until this morning when she woke at 6 AM with blood-tinged reddish-pink urine and right-sided flank pain. She never had this occur in the past. She is urinating every 30 minutes. She denies doing any recent heavy lifting/strenuous activity. She describes the pain as "stabbing" without radiation. Her pain level is currently 3/10, but about an hour ago she said the pain was 7/10. She took ibuprofen 800 mg, and that brought the pain level down to its current level. The pain is continuous. Moving around makes the pain worse, so she was reclining in a chair until she came into the clinic. Her temperature was 99ºF (37.2C) orally this morning. Denies: urinary incontinence, suprapubic pain, frequent UTIs, STIs, kidney stones, nausea, vomiting, change in bowel habits, dysphagia, loss of appetite, heartburn, bloating, hernias, weight loss, gastrointestinal conditions, and trauma. Client does not want to miss her flight for her Hawaiian vacation tomorrow morning.

PAST HEALTH HISTORY

Medical History

- Anemia diagnosed age 55, takes daily iron, no labs in past year
- Asthma diagnosed age 18, takes medication only as needed
- Hypothyroidism diagnosed age 62, never filled prescription for medication
- Pneumonia age 58, finished antibiotics and recovered without additional treatment

Surgical History
- C-sections ages 22 and 25, no complications
- Appendectomy age 10, no complications

Allergies No known medication allergies. No insect/bee sting/food/latex/environmental allergies

Medications

Prescription Albuterol sulfate HFA: 1–2 inhalations every 4–6 hours as needed; she can't recall the last time she used it

OTC Ferrous sulfate 325 mg once daily

Communicable Diseases Hepatitis A age 45, drank a smoothie from a smoothie shop that had a local hepatitis A outbreak; was out of work for 4 weeks due to fatigue, no sequelae other than she can never donate blood

Injuries and Accidents "I occasionally cut myself on the scissors at work."

Differing Abilities Denies

Blood Transfusions Denies

Childhood Illnesses Chickenpox age 3, denies other diseases

Immunizations "I need to look at my records. I may have missed a few. I did receive the hepatitis B vaccine after I recovered from my other hepatitis."

FAMILY HEALTH HISTORY

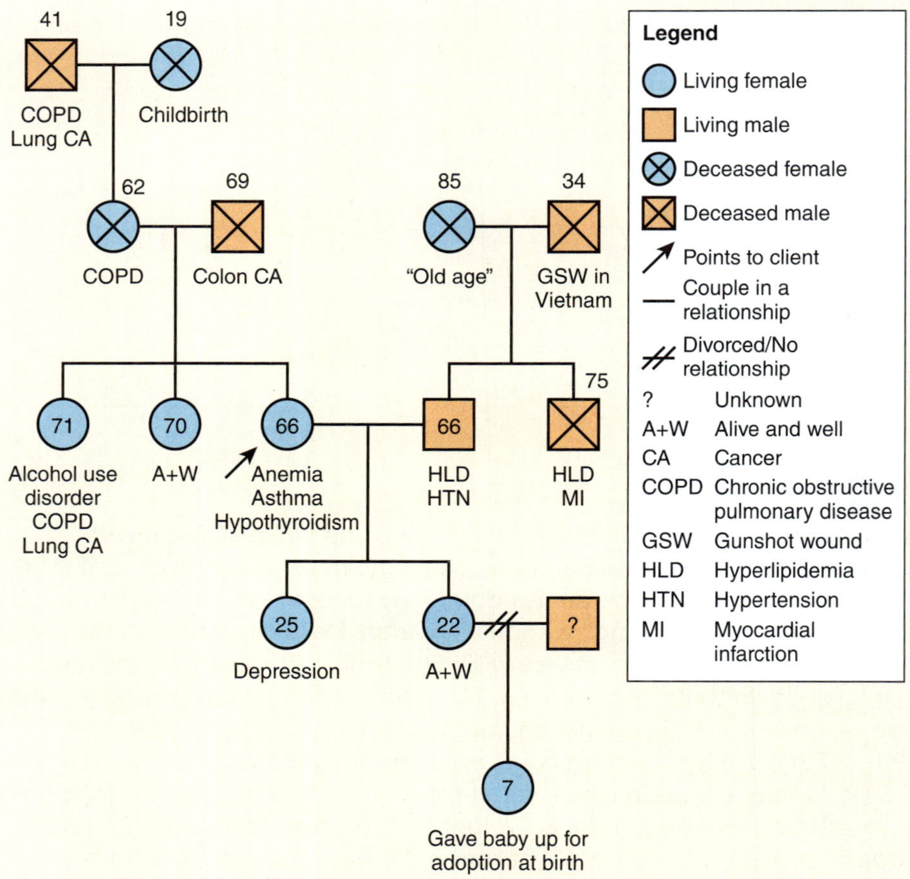

Denies family history of kidney disease, blood disorders, rheumatoid arthritis, migraines, gout, allergies, sudden cardiac death, stroke, diabetes, breast cancer, colorectal cancer

SOCIAL HISTORY

Alcohol Use Does not drink alcohol since she had hepatitis A.

Tobacco Use Started smoking cigarettes at age 18, 1 PPD × 40 years. Quit 8 years ago when she had pneumonia.

Recreational Drug Use Denies

Intimate Partner Violence Denies

Sexual Practice Monogamous relationship with husband

Travel History No travel outside the U.S.; all travel within 4 hours of her home

Work Environment Retired hairdresser

Home Environment

Physical Environment Has lived in the same 2-bedroom apartment for 20 years; has all modern appliances. Has air conditioning. She thinks husband checks smoke/carbon monoxide detectors.

Psychosocial Environment Feels safe but is fearful that her apartment complex will be sold and she will be priced out of the neighborhood.

Hobbies and Leisure Activities Needlepointing; wants to learn how to play pickle ball.

Stress "I really don't have any...I'm retired!"

Education Graduated high school

Economic Status "Things are tight!"

Military Service Denies

Religion Denies any church affiliation/practices but believes in a "higher power."

Ethnic Background "I grew up in CO when it was not very diverse. I met my husband at a bar. He's Iranian. Sometimes we eat his type of food."

Roles and Relationships Has 2 daughters who live out of state. They call on a regular basis and visit once a year. Married for 43 years. "We have our ups and downs."

Characteristic Patterns of Daily Living "I need to get into a routine now that I'm retired. After my trip."

HEALTH MAINTENANCE ACTIVITIES

Sleep Sleeps 9 hours every night, has no difficulty falling or staying asleep.

Diet Not too healthy now. "I gained a lot of weight since I retired."

Exercise None

Stress Management "I watch TV."

Use of Safety Devices Wears seat belt. Wore gloves when worked with chemicals when she worked as a hairdresser.

Health Checkups "I'll start taking care of myself when I get back from Hawaii."

REVIEW OF SYSTEMS

General "I feel terrible!"

Skin Uses sunscreen with SPF 30 when outside. Denies: rashes, itching, change in skin pigmentation, ecchymoses, warts, eczema, psoriasis, pruritus, change in moles, sores, lumps, change in skin texture, body odors, acne

Hair Dyes her hair every 6 weeks; Denies: alopecia, hirsutism, dandruff, pediculosis

Nails Denies: change in nails, splitting, breaking, onychomycosis

Eyes Cannot recall when she had her last eye examination; wears reading glasses from the drug store. Denies: blurry vision, photophobia, tearing, diplopia, eye drainage, bloodshot eyes, pain, blind spots, floaters, flashing lights, halos around objects, glaucoma, cataracts.

Ears Denies: hearing deficits, hearing aid, pain, discharge, vertigo, tinnitus, earaches, infection

Nose and Sinuses Denies: frequent colds/sinus infections, sinus pain, nasal discharge, itching, snoring, polyps, obstruction, epistaxis, change in sense of smell

Mouth Currently has bad taste in mouth. Brushes teeth 2–3 times daily, flosses at bedtime; has not seen a dentist in 3 years. Denies: toothache, tooth abscess, dentures, bleeding/swollen gums, sore tongue, lesions, change in salivation, bad breath, difficulty chewing

Throat and Neck Denies: sore throat, hoarseness, change in voice, pain/stiffness, goiter

Breasts and Axilla Does not do breast self-examination; last mammogram was at least 5 years ago. Denies: change in size, pain, tenderness, nipple discharge, lumps, dimpling, rash

Respiratory Cannot recall the last time she used her albuterol rescue inhaler. No URIs since she quit smoking. Denies: sputum, sneezing, wheezing, dyspnea, hemoptysis, recent pneumonia, emphysema, TB exposure

Cardiac Denies: paroxysmal nocturnal dyspnea, palpitations, dysrhythmia, chest pain, heart failure, heart disease, syncope, orthopnea, rheumatic heart disease

Peripheral Vasculature Had some bilateral lower leg edema when she worked—she was on her feet all day. Never wore compression hose. Has varicose veins. Has varicose veins since her early 30s and was told to see a vein specialist—did not make appointment. Denies: current edema, leg cramps, intermittent claudication, thrombophlebitis

Gastrointestinal Right flank pain per HPI. Never had colonoscopy.

Regular bowel habit: stool every morning soft and brown. Denies: nausea/vomiting, diarrhea, constipation, melena, change in stool color, hematemesis, increased flatulence, belching, peptic ulcers, hemorrhoids, gallstones

Urinary Hematuria per HPI. Denies: change in voiding habits, urinary hesitancy, urgency, frequency, polyuria, dribbling, UTIs, suprapubic pain, kidney stones, incontinence

Musculoskeletal Hand joints are sore in the morning. She thinks they are a little swollen. Denies: joint erythema, muscle cramps, weakness, fractures, sprains, dislocations, gout, arthritis, herniated disc, low back pain

Neurological Denies: change in balance, incoordination, loss of movement, change in sensory perception, change in speech, change in smell, tremors, syncope, loss of memory, involuntary movement, loss of consciousness, seizures, vertigo, spasm, tics

Psychological Currently anxious about leaving for her trip tomorrow. Denies: irritability, nervousness, difficulty concentrating, mood changes, suicidal thoughts, depression, anxiety

Female Reproductive Menopause age 48. Cannot remember when her last Pap smear was. Not sexually active. Denies: vaginal discharge, pelvic pain

Nutrition Present weight: 175 lbs (79.5 kg), was around 160 lbs (73 kg) until she retired, admits to binge eating and junk food sprees. Denies: food intolerances/allergies

Endocrine Diagnosed with hypothyroidism but never started medications. Does not recall laboratory values. Gets cold even in the summer. Denies: polyuria, polydipsia, polyphagia

Lymph Nodes Denies any enlargement

Hematological Blood type A+. Denies easy bruising/bleeding

CLINICAL JUDGMENT IN ACTION

1. What cues indicate that the client is having urinary distress?
2. What interventions have the highest priority?
3. What assessment findings indicate clinical improvement or decline in this client?

Review Questions

1. Ms. Kunkle was seen 3 days ago for an itchy rash on her arms and legs that erupted the day after she worked in the yard. She presents again today for a visit to document the response she has had from the treatment. What type of health history is most appropriate for the nurse to conduct on this visit?
   a. Complete health history
   b. Emergency health history
   c. Episodic health history
   d. Interval health history
2. The nurse documents the following characteristics of a client's back pain: stabbing pain in the sacral area that moves down the right leg; no loss of bowel or bladder control or paresthesia. Which characteristics of a chief complaint are described in this scenario? Select all that apply.
   a. Quality
   b. Location
   c. Quantity
   d. Setting
   e. Radiation
   f. Associated manifestations
3. The nurse assesses Mr. Satz's alcohol use using the AUDIT-C screening tool. The client states he has three beers daily after work and six beers on the weekends. What does the nurse conclude about Mr. Satz's alcohol consumption?
   a. The client has an AUDIT-C score of 27.
   b. The client needs immediate detoxication.
   c. The client is a social drinker.
   d. The client most likely is abusing alcohol.
4. The USPSTF recommends selectively offering or providing this service to individual clients based on professional judgment and client preferences. There is at least moderate certainty that the net benefit is small. Which Grade recommendation is this statement?
   a. Grade A
   b. Grade B
   c. Grade C
   d. Grade D
5. Mrs. Garcia tells the nurse that she has smoked cigarettes for 24 years. Most days she smokes a total of one and one-half packs. Which of the following statements best describes Mrs. Garcia's smoking habit?
   a. Mrs. Garcia has a 36 pack/year history.
   b. Mrs. Garcia smoked unfiltered cigarettes for 5 out of the 24 years; thus she has a 41 pack/year history.
   c. Mrs. Garcia has used CBD oil for the past 3 years, thus giving her a 39 pack/year history.
   d. Mrs. Garcia's pack/year history cannot be calculated based on the information provided.
6. Ava tells the nurse that she handles stress by walking, doing yoga, and meditation. In which section of the health history is this information documented?
   a. Medical History
   b. Psychosocial Environment
   c. Characteristic Patterns of Daily Living
   d. Health Maintenance Activities
7. Which of the following statements reflect(s) objective documentation? Select all that apply.
   a. The client reports being tired when waking in the morning.
   b. The client is wearing bilateral hearing aids.
   c. The client is uninterested in getting a colonoscopy.
   d. The client has a 1-cm lump in her right breast at the 11 o'clock position.
   e. The client reports that she gets moody around her menstrual cycle.
   f. The client is vomiting bright red blood.
8. The client denies having any limb cyanosis, limb edema, intermittent claudication, varicose veins, or deep vein thrombosis. In which section of the Review of Systems will this information be documented?
   a. Musculoskeletal
   b. Cardiac
   c. Neurological
   d. Peripheral vasculature

9. Which of the following situations warrants further investigation for possible intimate partner violence? Select all that apply.
   a. An 8-year-old client who has frequent urinary tract infections
   b. A 4 mm brown nevus on a 99-year-old client
   c. A 25-year-old female who refuses to tell you how her arm became broken in two places
   d. A 45-year-old male who has had two emergency room visits in the past 6 months for multiple cigarette burns on his back and buttocks
   e. The client's 65-year-old spouse refuses to allow the client to answer any question on the presenting injury

10. According to the American Heart Association, what is the optimal exercise regimen recommended for heart health?
    a. 10- to 15-minute segments of exercise 2 to 3 times per day
    b. 70 minutes of vigorous exercise per week
    c. 20 to 30 minutes of resistance training or weight lifting daily
    d. 150 minutes of moderate-intensity exercise every week

UNIT

II Special Assessments

Chapter 4 Developmental Assessment, 92

Chapter 5 Cultural Assessment, 121

Chapter 6 Spiritual Assessment, 140

Chapter 7 Nutritional Assessment, 157

CHAPTER

Developmental Assessment

4

Let us never consider ourselves finished nurses.... we must be learning all of our lives.

Florence Nightingale

Learning Outcomes

1. Identify the defining concepts and principles of major developmental theories.
2. Apply the developmental tasks and life events from each major theory of development to age-related developmental tasks and life events throughout the life span.
3. Describe developmental screening tools that can be used in clients from birth to older adult life.
4. Identify the effects of the SARS-CoV2 (COVID-19) lock down on normal development of clients of all ages.

All individuals, from birth to death, pass through identifiable, cyclical stages of growth and development that determine who and what they are and can become. **Growth** refers to an increase in body size and function to the point of optimum maturity. **Development** refers to patterned and predictable increases in the physical, cognitive, socioemotional, and moral capacities of individuals that enable them to successfully adapt to their environments.

Assessing the growth and development status of clients, adults, as well as children, is an integral part of client assessment. It must be noted, however, that although most development is patterned and predictable, you should not impose these expected patterns on a particular client; assess instead the individual client's unique development compared with these general guidelines.

Developmental Theories

A variety of theories have been developed that depict and predict growth and development. The theories most widely used for the clinical assessment of clients are the "ages and stages" theories of Piaget (1952), Freud (1946), Erikson (1974), and Kohlberg (1981). The **ages and stages developmental theories** are based on the premise that individuals experience similar sequential physical, cognitive, socioemotional, and moral changes during the same age periods, each of which is termed a **developmental stage**. During each developmental stage, there are specific physical and psychosocial skills, known as **developmental tasks**, that must be achieved. An individual's readiness for each new developmental task is dependent on success in achieving prior developmental tasks and on the presence of environmental opportunities to develop new skills. If prior developmental tasks have been insufficiently achieved or appropriate environments in which the tasks can be achieved are not available, mastery of subsequent developmental skills may not occur, may be delayed, or may occur in a defective way, thereby decreasing the individual's capacity to successfully adapt to the environment during their life span. A key nursing role in assessment is to help identify areas of deficiency and then develop a plan of care designed to address the client's needs.

A second group of theories includes the life events or transitional theories of development. **Life-event** or **transitional developmental theories** are based on the premise that development occurs in response to specific events, such as new roles (e.g., parenthood) and life transitions (e.g., career changes). Life events and transitions require an adaptive, coping behavior as well as often-significant changes in an individual's life patterns. Each of these events, which can occur singly or together and may be positively or negatively stressful, is not tied to a specific time or stage in the life span. Each event, however, does have certain tasks associated with it that must be achieved. For example, getting married is associated with specific developmental tasks that must be achieved regardless of the age of the individual at the time of marriage. The degree of success or failure with these tasks influences the individual's potential for success with concurrent and subsequent developmental tasks that occur in response to any other life events.

A variety of factors have been found to affect how an individual responds to life events: biological status, personality, cultural orientation, socioeconomic status, interpersonal support systems, number, timing, and intensity of life events, adverse childhood experiences, new roles (e.g., marriage, parenthood), life transitions (e.g., entering the workforce, learning a new job, losing a job), emotional malleability, and orientation to life (Kettlewell et al, 2020; Oh et al, 2018; Trinidad, 2021). Although the stress associated with each life event or transition can serve as an impetus for growth, excessive stress can disrupt the individual's equilibrium and lead to a variety of physical and psychological health problems (Shonkoff et al, 2021; Wykle, Kahana, & Kowal, 1992). In identifying life events and stressors, nurses can play a critical role in helping clients maintain health and control stress.

Ages and Stages Developmental Theories

The major tenets of Piaget, Freud, Erikson, and Kohlberg are discussed next; these are summarized in Table 4-1.

Piaget's Theory of Cognitive Development

Jean Piaget's (b. 1896–d. 1980) theory of cognitive development (1952) depicts age-related, sequential stages through which all developing children must progress to learn to think, reason, and exercise judgment and to learn the cognitive life skills (e.g., language development, problem-solving, decision making, critical thinking, and oral and written communication) needed to successfully adapt to their environments. The individual's cognitive development is influenced by innate intellectual capacity, maturation of the nervous and endocrine systems, and varied environmental interactions during which sensory and motor input is experienced and processed. Piaget's theory is based on the theory that cognitive development occurs by making discoveries, and it divides cognitive development into four periods: sensorimotor stage, preoperational stage, concrete operational stage, and formal operational stage (Bonham, 2019).

Table 4-1 Summary of Ages and Stages Developmental Theories

Stage/Age	Piaget's Cognitive Stages	Freud's Psychosexual Stages	Erikson's Psychosocial Stages	Kohlberg's Moral Judgment Stages
Infancy Birth to 1 yr	**Sensorimotor** (birth to 2 yr): Begins to acquire language Task: Object permanence	**Oral:** Pleasure from exploration with mouth and through sucking Task: Weaning	**Trust vs. Mistrust** Task: Trust Socializing agent: Mothering person Central process: Mutuality Ego quality: Hope	
Toddler 1–3 yr	**Sensorimotor** continues **Preoperational** (2–7 yr): Begins use of representational thought Task: Use language and mental images to think and communicate	**Anal:** Control of elimination Task: Toilet training	**Autonomy vs. Shame and Doubt** Task: Autonomy Socializing agent: Parents/caregivers Central process: Imitation Ego quality: Self-control and willpower	**Preconventional Level:** • **Morality Stage:** Avoid punishment by not breaking rules of authority figures
Preschool 3–6 yr	**Preoperational** continues	**Phallic:** Attracted to opposite-sex parent Task: Resolve Oedipus/Electra complex	**Initiative vs. Guilt** Task: Initiative and moral responsibility Socializing agent: Parents/caregivers Central process: Identification Ego quality: Direction, purpose, and conscience	• **Individualism, Instrumental Purpose, and Exchange Stage:** "Right" is relative; follow rules when in own interest
School Age 6–12 yr	**Preoperational** continues **Concrete Operational** (7 to 12 yr): Begins to engage in inductive reasoning and concrete problem-solving Task: Learn concepts of conservation and reversibility	**Latency:** Identification with same-sex parent Task: Identify with same-sex parent and test and compare own capabilities with peer norms	**Industry vs. Inferiority** Task: Industry, self-assurance, self-esteem Socializing agent: Teachers and peers Central process: Education Ego quality: Competence	**Conventional Level:** • **Mutual Expectations, Relationships, and Conformity to Moral Norms Stage:** Need to be "good" in own and others' eyes, believe in rules and regulations
Adolescence 12–18 yr	**Formal Operational** (12 yr to adulthood): Begins to engage in abstract reasoning and analytical problem-solving Task: Develop a workable philosophy of life	**Genital:** Develop sexual relationships Task: Establish meaningful relationship for lifelong pairing	**Identity vs. Role Confusion** Task: Self-identity and concept Socializing agent: Society of peers Central process: Role experimentation and peer pressure Ego quality: Fidelity and devotion to others, personal and sociocultural values	• **Social System and Conscience Stage:** Uphold laws because they are fixed social duties

Table 4-1 Summary of Ages and Stages Developmental Theories—cont'd

Stage/Age	Piaget's Cognitive Stages	Freud's Psychosexual Stages	Erikson's Psychosocial Stages	Kohlberg's Moral Judgment Stages
Young Adult 18–30 yr	**Formal Operational** continues		**Intimacy vs. Isolation** Task: Intimacy Socializing agent: Close friends, partners, lovers, spouse Central process: Mutuality among peers Ego quality: Intimate affiliation and love	**Postconventional Level:** • **Social Contract or Utility and Individual Rights Stage:** Uphold laws in the interest of the greatest good for the greatest number; uphold laws that protect universal rights
Early Middle Age 30–50 yr			**Generativity vs. Stagnation** (30–65 yr) Task: Generativity Socializing agent: Spouse, partner, children, sociocultural norms Central process: Creativity and person-environment fit Ego quality: Productivity, perseverance, charity, and consideration	
Late Middle Age 50–70 yr			**Generativity vs. Stagnation** continues	• **Universal Ethical Principles Stage:** Support universal moral principles regardless of the price of doing so
Late Adult 70 yr to death			**Ego Integrity vs. Despair** (65 yr to death) Task: Ego integrity Socializing agent: Significant others Central process: Introspection Ego quality: Wisdom	

Sensorimotor Stage

During the sensorimotor stage (birth to 2 years), the developing child perceives the world primarily through sensation and action response. The primary cognitive developmental task for this stage is to learn object permanence, that is, to form a mental image of an object and to recognize that although the object is removed from view, it still exists. Object permanence is usually achieved by the eighth month of life and facilitates the achievement of the second cognitive task, the development of a sense of self separate from one's environment. Beginning to use language and mental representations to think about events before and after they occur is an additional cognitive task that must be achieved during this stage.

Preoperational Stage

The second cognitive development period is the preoperational stage (2 to 7 years), which is characterized by **egocentrism**, that is, viewing the world in terms of self only and interpreting actions and all other events in terms of the consequences they have for self. Learning during this stage usually occurs through imitation of others, physical and cognitive exploration of the environment, and asking numerous questions. Thinking is concrete, and oftentimes magical in nature, and reasoning is intuitive and based on the observable; that is, what is directly seen, heard, or personally experienced. The major cognitive developmental task for this stage is to use language and mental representations to think and communicate about objects and events in the environment. Core behaviors seen during this stage include imitation, symbolic play, drawing, associating names with mental images, and using language to imitate and explain events (Scott, 2022).

Concrete Operational Stage

During the third cognitive development period, the concrete operational stage (7 to 12 years), thinking becomes socialized in that thought becomes less self-oriented and others' points of view are given consideration. Thinking becomes increasingly logical and coherent; facts are organized through sorting, ordering, and classifying; the concept of time evolves; different aspects of situations are dealt with simultaneously; reasoning is inductive; problems are solved concretely and systematically; and communication is enhanced through expanding oral skills and learning to read and write. The major developmental tasks are mastering the concept of **conservation** (understanding that altering the physical state of an object does not change the basic properties of the object) and **reversibility** (understanding that an action need not be experienced or performed before one can anticipate the results or consequences of the action).

Formal Operational Stage

The fourth cognitive development period is the formal operational stage (12 years to adulthood), in which thinking becomes increasingly abstract, logical, analytical, and creative. Ideas are combined to form concepts, and concepts are combined to form constructs and hypotheses. Theories are developed and beginning to be tested, and alternative solutions for problems are generated and examined. The antecedents, moderators, and outcomes of ideas, concepts, situations, and actions are recognized and incorporated into the individual's worldview. The primary cognitive developmental task for this stage is to develop a workable philosophy of life.

Freud's Psychoanalytic Theory of Personality Development

Sigmund Freud (b. 1856–d. 1939) contended that human behavior is motivated by psychodynamic forces within an individual's unconscious mind (1946). Driven to act by these internal forces, individuals repeatedly interact with the external environment. The individual's personality and psychosexual identity are developed through the accumulation of these interactional experiences.

Personality

Personality, according to Freud, consists of three components with distinctly separate functions: id, ego, and superego. The id, evident at birth, is inborn and unconscious and is driven by biological instincts and urges to seek immediate gratification of needs such as hunger, thirst, and physical comfort. The **ego** is conscious and rational and emerges during the first year of life as infants begin to test the limits of the world around them. The ego seeks realistic and acceptable ways to meet needs. The **superego**, appearing in early childhood, is the internalization of the moral values formed as children interact with their parents/caregivers and significant others. The superego acts as a moral arbitrator by blocking unacceptable behavior generated by the id that could threaten the social order, creating feelings of guilt when the internalized moral code is compromised, and generating feelings of pride when the moral code is upheld.

Freud believed that individuals experience an ongoing struggle among their id, ego, and superego. Achieving a balance among the three, however, is a prerequisite to the development of socially acceptable behavior and an integrated personality. To assist the personality to achieve this balance and to protect itself from excess anxiety created by the ongoing struggle, the ego uses unconscious defense mechanisms such as repression, denial, projection, and rationalization.

Psychosexual Stages

Freud perceived the desire to satisfy biological needs, primarily sexual, as the major drive governing human behavior. At different psychosexual developmental stages, individuals experience tension associated with a specific body region that prompts them to seek the gratification of the needs and conflicts thereby engendered. Each developmental stage is centered on a specific body region and the associated conflicts. If an individual's needs are met during a given stage and conflicts are resolved, development will proceed normally to the next stage, and the developing personality will be integrated in a healthy way. If resolution of the conflict does not occur, however, the individual will become fixated at that stage, and personality and psychosexual identity will be arrested or impaired. Freud identified five psychosexual stages of development: oral, anal, phallic, latency, and genital.

Oral Stage. The oral psychosexual stage (birth to 1 year) is focused on the sensory area of the mouth, lips, and tongue. Sucking, biting, chewing, swallowing, and vocalizing provide pleasure and reduce tension. The major conflict during this stage centers around weaning. Oral personality traits that begin to emerge are optimism versus pessimism, cockiness versus self-belittlement, admiration versus envy, determinism versus submission, and gullibility versus suspiciousness.

Anal Stage. In the anal psychosexual stage (1 to 3 years), the focus is on the anal and urethral sensory areas. Expulsion and retention of body wastes provide pleasure and reduce tension. The major conflict centers around toilet training. Anal personality traits that begin to emerge during this period are orderliness versus messiness, acquiescence versus stubbornness, overgenerosity versus stinginess, rigid punctuality versus tardiness, and expansiveness versus constrictedness.

Phallic Stage. The phallic psychosexual stage (3 to 6 years) is focused on the sensory areas of the genitals. Pleasure is provided and tension is reduced through penile and clitoral exploration and stimulation. The major conflicts center around the controversial **Oedipus** (young boys' sexual attraction toward their mothers and feelings of rivalry toward their fathers) and **Electra** (young girls' sexual attraction toward their fathers and rivalry with their mothers for their fathers' attention) **complexes**, **castration anxiety** (young boys' fear of having the penis cut off or mutilated), and **penis envy** (young girls' desire to have a penis). Phallic personality traits that begin to emerge are gaiety versus sadness, gregariousness versus isolationism, stylishness versus plainness, blind courage versus timidity, and brashness versus bashfulness.

Latency Stage. During the latency psychosexual stage (6 to 12 years), the focus is on the exploration and discovery of the total body's relatedness, coordination, and uses rather than on a specific body region. Channeling generalized psychic and physical activity into knowledge acquisition and vigorous play provides pleasure and reduces tension. The major conflict during this stage centers around identifying with the same-sex parent, learning and testing mental and physical capabilities, and comparing one's capabilities with peer norms.

Genital Stage. The genital psychosexual stage (12 years to adulthood) is focused on full sexual maturity and function. Self- and mutual sexual stimulation and the formation of friendships and sexual relationships provide pleasure and reduce tension. The major conflicts during this period center around becoming sexually desirable to others and establishing meaningful relationships in preparation for lifelong pairing.

Erikson's Epigenetic Theory of Personality

The most frequently used theory of personality development is Erikson's (b. 1902–d. 1994) epigenetic theory (1974), which is based on the biological concept that all growing organisms have an inherent plan of growth for all parts of the entity. Each part of a growing entity has a designated time of ascendancy and forms the basis for the growth of the next part until the functional whole is fully developed. Erikson's theory was built on Freud's theory of personality but goes beyond it by depicting personality development as a passage through eight sequential stages of ego development from birth through old age.

According to Erikson, developing individuals must master and resolve, to some extent, a core conflict/crisis during each stage by integrating their personal needs and skills with the social and cultural demands and expectations of their environment. Passage to each developmental stage is dependent on the resolution of the core conflict of the preceding stage. No core conflict is ever completely mastered, however. Rather, in each new life situation, the conflict may present in a new form that can then be resolved more readily if the conflict was initially resolved favorably. If the conflict was initially resolved unfavorably, subsequent encounters with new forms of the core conflict can provide opportunities to try again to resolve it favorably. Thus, the potential for further development and refinement always exists. For each of the eight core conflicts/crises, there is a key socializing agent, an associated central process for resolving the conflict, and an ego quality that results from a favorable resolution of the core conflict.

Trust versus Mistrust Stage

The core conflict/crisis for the first developmental stage (birth to 1 year) is trust versus mistrust. When developing infants' basic needs are met by prompt, consistent, predictable, loving parent figures, basic, relative trust evolves. If infants' needs are intermittently, inadequately, or perfunctorily met, then mistrust results (Fig. 4-1).

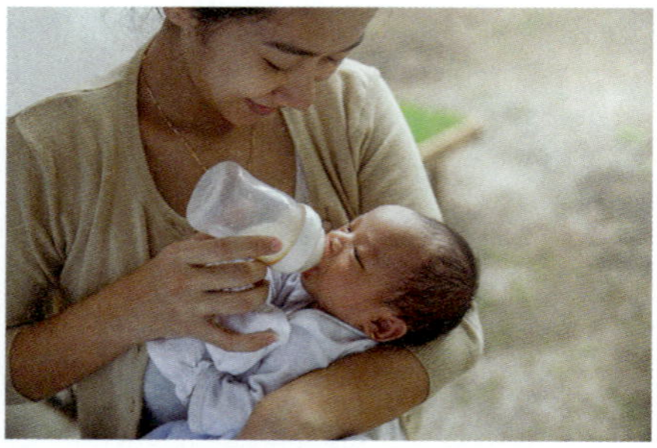

Figure 4-1 Trust develops in a baby when needs are met, such as with feeding.

Autonomy versus Shame and Doubt Stage

The second developmental stage (1 to 3 years) is focused on autonomy versus shame and doubt core conflict/crisis. If parental figures overprotect their children and overly criticize and punish their attempts to explore and control their environments and body activities, as well as their attempts to make independent decisions, then shame, doubt, and uncertainty about their abilities and themselves will result.

Initiative versus Guilt Stage

During the third developmental stage (3 to 6 years), the core conflict/crisis is initiative versus guilt. When children are encouraged to explore their environments and to plan and work toward goals that do not infringe on the rights of others, they develop initiative and moral responsibility (Fig. 4-2). In contrast, if children are restricted from exploring their environments or are made to feel that their enterprise and active imaginations are bad, they will experience guilt and lose the courage to conceive of and pursue valued goals.

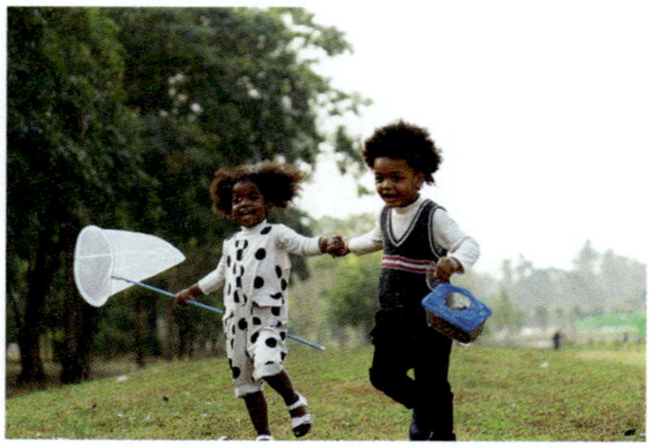

Figure 4-2 These young children are exploring their environment as they try to catch a butterfly.

Industry versus Inferiority Stage

The central conflict/crisis for the fourth developmental stage (6 to 12 years) is industry versus inferiority. Competence is the favorable result of being encouraged to, and successfully engage in achievable tasks and activities, competing and cooperating with others, and learning the rules and norms of a widening social and cultural environment. If children are not given sufficient opportunities or encouragement to develop their abilities or are pushed to achieve beyond their present abilities and thus repeatedly fail, feelings of inadequacy and inferiority result, and new learning activities will be increasingly avoided.

Identity versus Role Confusion Stage

The fifth stage of development (12 to 18 years) is focused on the identity versus role confusion core conflict/crisis. Adolescents must make the transition from childhood to adulthood, redefine themselves in terms of the roles they hope to play in society, explore life-work possibilities, and integrate self-concept and values with those of their peers and society (Fig. 4-3). Supportive, understanding interactions with peers and adult role models help clarify self-identity and lead to the ego quality of fidelity and devotion to others as well as personal and sociocultural values and ideologies. Unfavorable interactions or overidentification with popular teen fads and peer culture heroes can result in role confusion and difficulty in clarifying personal identity.

Intimacy versus Isolation Stage

Intimacy versus isolation is the core conflict/crisis associated with the sixth developmental stage (18 to 30 years). The capacity for intimate affiliation with and the love of significant others is what results from the favorable resolution of this core conflict. Feelings of aloneness and social isolation are the result of an unsuccessful resolution.

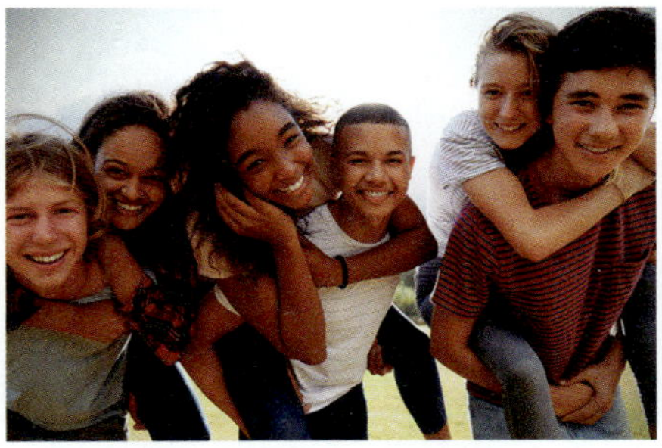

Figure 4-3 Peers become more important during the teen years.

Generativity versus Stagnation Stage

The seventh developmental stage (30 to 65 years) is focused on the core conflict of generativity versus stagnation. Generativity is when one's focus on meeting the needs of others is of equal concern to that of providing for oneself (Fig. 4-4). Qualities of productivity, perseverance, charity, and consideration result from the development of generativity. Generative young and middle-aged adults nourish and nurture the products of their creativity at home, at work, and in their communities. Individuals who are unsuccessful in resolving the core conflict during this stage of development become self-absorbed and feel chronically unfulfilled.

Ego Integrity versus Despair Stage

During the eighth and last stage of development (65 years to death), the core conflict/crisis is ego integrity versus despair. After reviewing one's life in its entirety, acceptance of what has passed and satisfaction with the present result in a sense of integrity. In contrast, remorse for the past and what might have been results in despair.

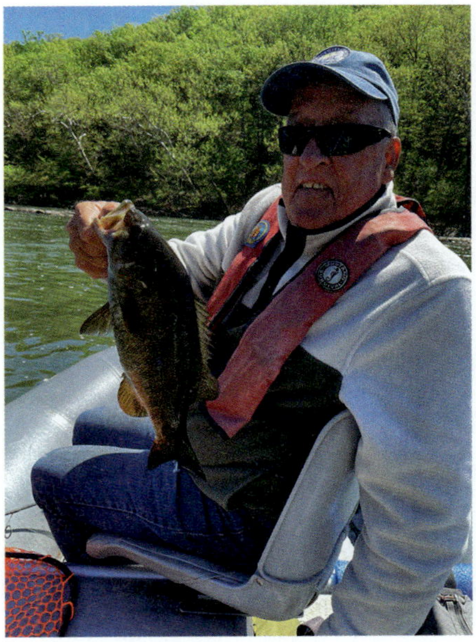

Figure 4-4 This male is exploring fishing as a new avenue of enjoyment to avoid stagnation in later years.

Kohlberg's Theory of Moral Development

The basic premise of Kohlberg's (b. 1927–d. 1987) theory of moral development (1981) is that when a conflict occurs among any of several universal values (e.g., punishment, affection, authority, truth, law, life, liberty, and justice), the moral choice that must be made and justified requires cognitive capabilities, including systematic problem-solving, which constitute moral reasoning. Thus, the development of the individual's moral reasoning and associated behaviors primarily parallels the development of cognitive behavior. According to Kohlberg, moral development is contingent upon children's ability to learn and internalize parental and societal rules and standards, develop the ability to empathize with others' responses, and form their own standards of conduct. Moral development progresses through three levels, with two distinct stages per level, for a total of six stages. Keep in mind that Kohlberg's theory of moral development has fallen under heavy criticism because it was based on studies of an all-male population.

Preconventional Level

The first level of moral development, the Preconventional Level, is divided into two stages. In stage 1, the Morality Stage, individuals have an egocentric point of view and avoid breaking rules and damaging persons and property to avoid being punished by authority figures with superior power. In stage 2, the Individualism, Instrumental Purpose, and Exchange Stage, individuals have a concrete individualistic perspective and follow rules only when doing so is primarily in their own (or sometimes in someone else's) immediate interest, and because "right" is relative and what is "fair" represents an equal exchange.

Conventional Level

The second level of moral development is the Conventional Level. This level is divided into two stages. The first stage at this level, stage 3, is Mutual Expectations, Relationships, and Conformity to Moral Norms Stage, in which individuals can envision the perspective of another and try to live up to the expectations of self and others through conformity to moral norms; have "good" motives; are concerned about others; believe in rules and regulations; and maintain relationships by being trustworthy, loyal, respectful, and appropriately grateful. In stage 4, the Social System and Conscience Stage, individuals can differentiate societal points of view from interpersonal agreements and motives and avoid the breakdown of the social system by recognizing and supporting how the system defines roles and rules, by fulfilling the duties to which they have agreed, and by upholding laws because they are fixed social duties. According to Kohlberg, most adults in the United States have not progressed beyond this stage of moral judgment.

Postconventional Level

The third level of moral development, the Postconventional Level, is divided into two stages: stage 5, Social Contract or Utility, and Individual Rights, in which adult individuals recognize that there are moral and legal points of view that may sometimes be in conflict and that although most rules are relative to the group that makes them, they warrant being upheld in the interest of the greatest good for the greatest number. Individuals in this stage recognize that as people's needs change, laws may have to be changed by working through the system to do so. Nonetheless, laws that protect some universal rights (such as life and liberty) must be upheld regardless of people's changing opinions or desires. Stage 6, Universal Ethical Principles, occurs when some middle-aged or older adults develop a rational, universal moral perspective and a commitment to laws and social agreements based on universal moral principles of justice, equal rights, and respect for human dignity. When laws violate these moral principles, it is the principle, rather than the law, that must be followed, regardless of the price that must be paid for doing so. Kohlberg contends that few people attain and even fewer maintain this state of moral development.

Assessment in Brief

Developmental Assessment

1. Note the client's stated chronological age.
2. Tailor your questions to the client's expected level of ability according to developmental parameters until you can accurately assess the actual developmental level.
3. When assessing small children, verify information with the parent/caregiver.
4. If a third party is assisting in the interview (for an older adult or client with differing abilities), address all questions to the client, not the intermediary.

Developmental Stages, Tasks, and Life Events

As is evident from a review of the preceding theories of development, there is no complete agreement about the age associated with each developmental stage. In addition, improved nutrition, medical advances (in particular, immunizations), and healthier lifestyles have contributed to greater longevity in the United States and other Western countries. Indeed, in 1900, approximately 1 in 25 U.S. citizens was 65 years of age or older; this statistic has nearly quadrupled—there are now more than 1 in every 6, and by 2030 it is estimated that 1 in every 5 will be over the age of 65 (Vespa, Armstrong, & Medina, 2018). As a result, what was once considered to be the beginning of late adulthood (55 to 70 years) is now a part of middle adulthood, and what was considered to be the latter part of late adulthood (70+ years) is now recognized as the beginning rather than the end of this period. The developmental assessment process presented in this text, therefore, uses the following stages:

Stage 1: Infancy (birth–1 year)
Stage 2: Toddler (1–3 years)
Stage 3: Preschooler (3–6 years)
Stage 4: School-age child (6–12 years)
Stage 5: Adolescence (12–18 years)
Stage 6: Young adulthood (18–30 years)
Stage 7: Early middle adulthood (30–50 years)
Stage 8: Late middle adulthood (50–70 years)
Stage 9: Late adulthood (70 years–death)

The following section combines the developmental tasks and life events and transitions from each major theory of development, thereby giving a composite of the developmental tasks and possible life events that characterize each developmental stage. The lists of tasks for each stage are not exhaustive, nor do they reflect all the tasks facing the full range of normal human conditions and circumstances. Generally, ask yourself whether the individual's overall development seems consistent with the tasks usually associated with the person's chronological age. In addition, the life events included in each stage are not restricted to that stage, but may occur or reoccur during several developmental stages. Failure to meet tasks in one area does not always indicate abnormal development. It is expected that the following will form a general framework on which you can base your assessment of a client's growth and development. Remember to consider each individual as a whole entity, not just a collection of tasks met or not met.

Adverse childhood experiences (ACE), social determinants of health (SDOH), structural racism, and health care bias can impact the development of clients. ACE refer to childhood traumatic or adverse events (e.g., abuse, neglect, parental mental illness, exposure to violence, food insecurity, etc.). It is well known that ACE play a significant role in negative health outcomes throughout the life span, in physical as well as psychological and mental health outcomes. SDOH are the conditions in which people are born, learn, work, and play (WHO, 2022). "Structural racism refers to the totality of ways in which societies foster racial discrimination through mutually reinforcing systems of housing, education, employment, earnings, benefits, credit, media, health care, and criminal justice. These patterns and practices in turn reinforce discriminatory beliefs, values, and distribution of resources (Bailey et al, 2017). Structural racism is entrenched within social, political, and economic systems, including our health care systems. Structural racism can exert a cumulative effect, resulting in changes in brain structure and function. Furthermore, internalized racism is associated with lower self-esteem, psychological well-being, life satisfaction, quality of life, and higher levels of alcohol use, depression, and anxiety (Shonkoff, Slopen, & Williams, 2021). Assessing for potential inequities due to ACE, SDOH, and structural racism is key to improving health outcomes across the life span (Phillips et al, 2020; Shonkoff, 2021).

Developmental Tasks of Infants (Birth to 1 Year)

Infancy is a period of dramatic and rapid physical, motor, cognitive, emotional, and social growth, which marks it as one of the most critical periods of growth and development. During the first year of life, infants change from totally helpless, dependent newborns to unique individuals who actively interact with their environments and form meaningful relationships with significant others. A list of key gross and fine motor, language, and sensory milestones associated with this period can be found in Table 4-2.

One of the major tasks of infancy is weaning, which requires children to give up the breast or bottle, which has been a major source of gratification, and learn to use a cup. Readiness for weaning usually occurs between the ages of 6 months and 12 to 14 months, when the child has learned that good things also come from a spoon, when more motor control has been developed so a cup can be grasped and brought to the mouth, and when the desire for freedom of movement begins to lessen the desire to be held while eating.

Conducting a comprehensive assessment of an infant requires an evaluation of the degree to which the infant has achieved the developmental tasks of infancy. It is important to remember that although individuals experience similar sequential physical, cognitive, socioemotional, and moral changes during the same age periods, there is still a degree of normal variability from one child to another. Furthermore, when evaluating the development of a child, one must take prematurity into account and age-adjust expectations accordingly. A 4-month-old infant who was born prematurely at 26-weeks gestation would not be expected to have the developmental skills

Table 4-2 Growth and Development During Infancy

Age	Gross Motor	Fine Motor	Language	Sensory
Birth to 1 month	• Assumes tonic neck posture • When prone, lifts and turns head	• Holds hands in fists and progresses to slightly opening fists when at rest • Draws arms and legs to body • Begins to bring hand to mouth to self-soothe	• Cries • Begins to make cooing (vowel) sounds	• Comforts with holding and touching • Looks at faces • Follows objects when in line of vision • Alert to high-pitched voices • Smiles
2 months	• Can raise head and shoulders when prone to 45°–90° • Supports self on forearms • Keeps head steady when held in sitting position	• Hands mostly open • Looks at and plays with fingers • Begins to bring hands together • Grasps and tries to reach objects	• Vocalizes when talked to; coos	• Smiles responsively • Follows objects 180°

Table 4-2 Growth and Development During Infancy—cont'd

Age	Gross Motor	Fine Motor	Language	Sensory
4 months	• Rolls from stomach to back • When pulled to sitting, almost no head lag	• Can hold feet and put in mouth • Can hold bottle • Can grasp rattle and other small objects • Puts objects in mouth	• Laughs • Squeals • Turns head when hears voices or sounds	• Laughs out loud • Looks at you, moves, and makes sounds to get attention
6 months	• Can sit on floor with hands forward for support • Rolls back to stomach • Starts to put full weight on legs when held in standing position • Can sit briefly without support • Bounces when held in a standing position	• Transfers objects from one hand to the other • Can feed self a cookie • Can bang object on surface	• Babbles consonant-like sounds, "ga" or "ba" • Imitation of speech sounds beginning ("mama," "dada")	• Responds by looking and smiling • Recognizes own name
9 months	• Crawls on all fours or uses arms to pull body along floor • Can pull self to sitting position • Can pull self to standing position	• Beginning to use thumb-three finger grasp • Dominant hand use • Has good hand-mouth coordination • Lets go of object with intention • Bangs two objects together	• Uses dada/mama nonspecifically • Responds to verbal commands (i.e., looks for named object "Where's your bottle?") • Imitates speech sounds	• Recognizes sounds • Uses basic gestures (waves bye-bye, holds out arms to be picked up) • Plays peekaboo, looks for dropped objects
12 months	• Can sit down from standing • Cruises (walks around room holding onto objects) • Can stand alone • Takes first step	• Picks up and drops objects • Can put small objects into toys or containers through holes • Turns many pages in a book at one time • Picks up small objects with two-finger pincer grasp • Builds a tower of two cubes • Starts to feed self with cup and spoon	• Understands "no" and other simple commands • Uses dada/mama specifically • Learns one or two other words • Speaks gibberish	• Follows fast-moving objects • Indicates wants • Imitates new gestures • Develops binocular vision

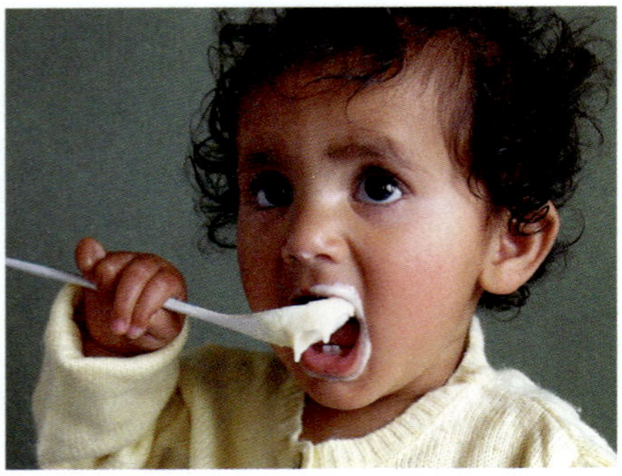

Figure 4-5 This infant is developing eye-hand coordination to feed herself.

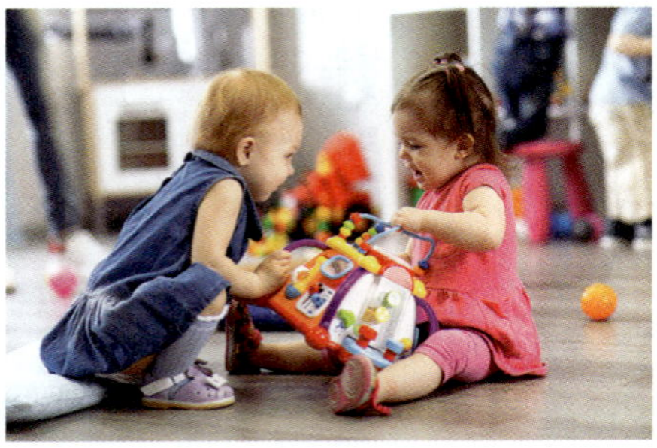

Figure 4-6 Refinement of skills and a growing sense of independence are most noted in toddlers.

of a full-term child of the same age. Developmental tasks that must be achieved during the infancy stage are to:

1. Develop a basic, relative sense of trust.
2. Develop a sense of self as dependent on but separate from others, particularly the mother.
3. Develop and desire affection for and response from others, particularly the mother.
4. Develop a preverbal communication system, including emotional expression, to communicate needs and desires.
5. Begin to develop conceptual abilities and a language system.
6. Begin to learn purposeful fine and gross motor skills, particularly eye-hand coordination and balance (Fig. 4-5).
7. Begin to explore and recognize the immediate environment.
8. Develop object permanence.

Developmental Tasks of Toddlers (1 to 3 Years)

The toddler period is one of steadily increasing motor development and control (Fig. 4-6), intense activity and discovery, rapid language development, increasingly independent behaviors, and marked personality development. Key gross and fine motor, language, and sensory milestones associated with the toddler period can be found in Table 4-3.

One of the major developmental tasks for toddlers is toilet training. Readiness for toilet training is usually evident in infants in the age-group of 18 to 24 months (girls tend to be ready to toilet-train earlier than boys) when the following are present: voluntary control of the anal and urethral sphincters; motor skills of sitting, walking, and squatting; fine motor skills needed to remove clothing; cognitive skills of recognizing the urge to defecate or urinate, and verbalizing the urge to do so; and willingness and ability to please the parents by sitting on the toilet for 5 to 10 minutes.

Table 4-3 Growth and Development During Toddlerhood

Age	Gross Motor	Fine Motor	Language	Sensory
15 months	• Squats to pick up objects • Can crawl up stairs • Begins to run	• May hold crayon or pencil and scribble • Able to put objects in and take objects out of container • Drinks from cup with little spilling	• Says three words other than names • Follows direction without a gesture included	• Looks around when asked "where's your toy" or "where's your blanket" • Points to ask for help/get attention
18 months	• Runs, falling often • Can jump in place • Can walk up stairs with two feet per step while holding on • Carries toy when walking • Plays with push-and-pull toys	• Can build a tower of three to four cubes • Scribbles spontaneously • Throws a ball	• Says 10 or more words • Points to at least five objects or two body parts when asked	• Visual acuity 20/40 • Engages with others for play • Helps dress and undress • Points to pictures in book/objects to gain attention • Looks to adult if sees something new happen

Table 4-3 Growth and Development During Toddlerhood—cont'd

Age	Gross Motor	Fine Motor	Language	Sensory
24 months	• Can walk up and down stairs • Can kick a ball • Jumps • Runs • Climbs up ladder	• Can draw a straight line • Uses spoon well • Tries to dress self • Stacks objects	• Talks a lot • Uses 50 words • Combines two words • Approximately 300-word receptive vocabulary • Understands commands • Names at least five body parts • Knows first name, refers to self • Verbalizes toilet needs • Language 50% understandable to strangers	• Plays alongside others (parallel play) • Removes clothing
30 months	• Throws a ball • Jumps with both feet • Can stand on one foot for a few seconds • Runs well without falling	• Can build a tower of eight blocks • Can use crayons with thumb and finger instead of fist • Learning to use scissors	• Knows first and last name • Knows the name of one color • Can sing • Expresses needs • Uses pronouns appropriately	• Increasingly engages in imaginary play

Parental recognition of the child's level of readiness and a willingness to invest the necessary time for toilet training are also essential for the toddler's successful mastery of this task.

A variety of life events and transitions may produce stress in the toddler. Among the most stressful are personal injury or illness, death of a parent, or loss through separation or divorce.

Children who have been successful in accomplishing the developmental tasks of infancy enter the toddler period with the basic relative trust needed for the achievement of the next tasks. The principal developmental tasks that must be mastered during the toddler stage are to:

1. Interact with others less egocentrically.
2. Acquire socially acceptable behaviors.
3. Differentiate self from others.
4. Tolerate separation from key socializing agents (parents or caregivers).
5. Develop increasing verbal communication skills.
6. Tolerate delayed gratification of wants and desires.
7. Control bodily functions (toilet training) and begin self-care (feed and dress self almost completely).

Developmental Tasks of Preschoolers (3 to 6 Years)

During the preschooler period, children are focused on developing initiative and purpose. Play provides the means for physical, mental, and social development and becomes the "work" of children as they use it to understand, adjust to, and work out experiences with their environment (Fig. 4-7). Preschoolers demonstrate an active imagination and an ability to invent and imitate. They constantly seek to discover the why, what, and how of objects

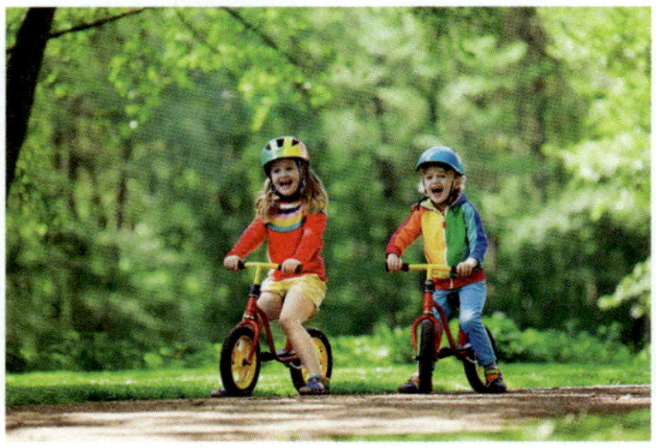

Figure 4-7 Play provides these preschoolers with the ability to interact with one another and develop their physical, mental, and social skills.

and events around them; are literal in their thinking; are increasingly sociable with other children and adults other than their parents; and are increasingly aware of their places and roles in their families. Key gross and fine motor, language, and sensory milestones associated with the preschooler period can be found in Table 4-4.

The preschooler stage of development is characterized by the refinement of many of the tasks that were achieved during the toddler stage and the development of the skills and abilities that prepare children for the significant lifestyle change of starting school. Readiness for school is demonstrated by increased attention span and memory, ability to interact cooperatively, ability to tolerate prolonged periods of separation from family, and independence in performing basic self-care activities. Unfortunately, recent studies estimate that only 40% of U.S. 3- to 5-year-olds are considered "healthy and ready to learn" (Campbell et al, 2014). Early identification of developmental and social concerns and prompt intervention continue to be our best hope at improving this statistic.

Among the principal developmental tasks that must be mastered during the preschooler stage are to:

1. Develop a sense of separateness as an individual.
2. Develop a sense of initiative.
3. Use language for increasing social interaction.
4. Interact in socially acceptable ways with others.
5. Develop a conscience.
6. Identify sex role and function.
7. Develop readiness for school.

Developmental Tasks of School-Age Children (6 to 12 Years)

With a well-developed sense of trust, autonomy, and initiative, school-age children increasingly reduce their dependency on the family as their primary socializing agents and move to the broader world of peers in their neighborhoods and schools, as well as to teachers and adult leaders of social, sports, and religious groups. They are increasingly exposed to others' views and seek approval from people outside the home. School-age children become industrious workers as they develop the significant physical, social,

Table 4-4 Growth and Development During Preschool Years

Age	Gross Motor	Fine Motor	Language (Expressive and Receptive)	Sensory
3–6 yr	• Pedals tricycle • Throws ball overhand • Skips and hops on one foot • Can climb well • Jumps forward	• Can draw a person with head and one other body part • Cuts with child scissors • Can draw circle • Likes art projects, likes to paste and string beads • Can brush teeth	• Uses three-word sentences • Speech is 75% understandable to strangers • Can retell a short story • Compares using adjectives like smaller, bigger, taller • Understands prepositions, such as under, over, on • Language skills are well developed, with the child able to understand and speak clearly • Vocabulary grows to more than 2,000 words • Talks endlessly and asks questions	• Visual acuity is well developed • Focused on learning letters and numbers • Knows colors

and intellectual skills needed to operate in the broader and more diverse environment (Fig. 4-8). They strive to be a part of a peer group and to achieve a variety of skills that are approved by others; in so doing, they become competent and confident in their own eyes. Key gross and fine motor, language, and sensory milestones associated with this period can be found in Table 4-5.

The principal developmental tasks that must be mastered during the school-age stage are to:

1. Become a more active, cooperative, and responsible family member.
2. Learn the rules and norms of a widening social, religious, and cultural environment.
3. Increase psychomotor and cognitive skills needed for participation in games and working with others.
4. Master concepts of time, conservation, and reversibility as well as oral and written communication skills.
5. Win approval from peers and adults.
6. Obtain a place in a peer group.
7. Build a sense of industry, accomplishment, self-assurance, and self-esteem.
8. Develop a positive self-concept.
9. Exchange affection with family and friends without seeking immediate payback.
10. Adopt moral standards for behavior.

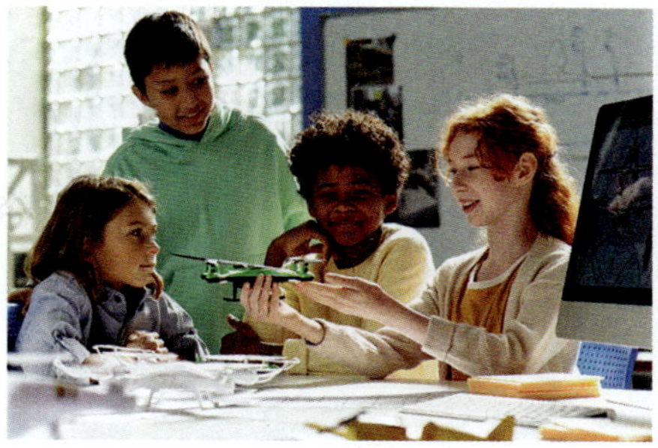

Figure 4-8 School-age children are often independent and industrious, with a developing sense of self-confidence.

Developmental Tasks of Adolescents (12 to 18 Years)

The adolescent period is one of struggle and sometimes turmoil as the adolescent strives to develop a personal identity and achieve a successful transition from childhood to adulthood. The biological, social, cognitive, and psychological changes associated with adolescence are the most complex and profound of any developmental period (Neinstein et al, 2016). For example, physical and sexual maturity are reached during adolescence, with girls tending to experience both puberty and a growth spurt roughly 2 years earlier than boys.

Furthermore, issues of gender and sexual identity may become more focused during adolescence and lead to potential conflict both for the individual and for the family unit. Gender dysphoria is defined as a conflict between the experienced or expressed gender and the gender assigned at birth (Kaltiala-Heino et al, 2018). The number of adolescents seeking gender identity services has risen significantly in recent years in the United States and Europe. Little is known to date, however, how gender dysphoria impacts the developmental attainment of identity. What is clear at the time is the increased risk for psychiatric disorders (including significant risk of suicide ideation in this population), bullying, violence, substance use, sexually transmitted infections (STIs), and health care bias. Nurses must create

Table 4-5 Growth and Development During School-Age Years

Age	Gross Motor	Fine Motor	Language	Sensory
6–12 yr	• Can use in-line skates or ice skates • Able to ride two-wheeler bicycle • Plays baseball	• Can put models together • Likes crafts • Enjoys board games, plays cards	• Vocabulary increases • Language abilities continue to develop	• Reading • Able to concentrate on activities for longer periods

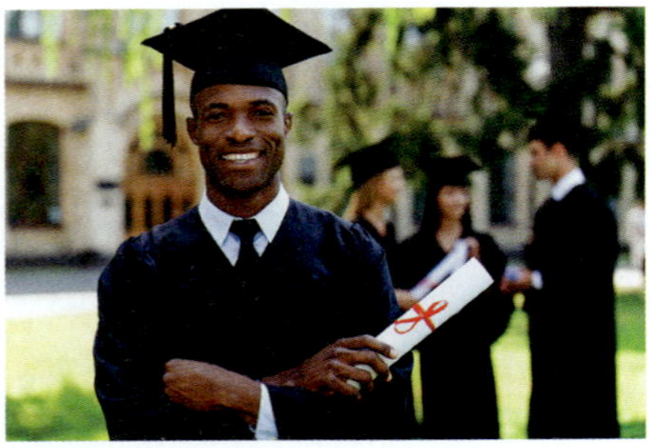

Figure 4-9 This high school graduate looks forward to the challenges of the future.

an inclusive and safe space for adolescents to have the confidence to express their concerns (Grimstad & Martinez, 2022).

Additionally, adolescents develop increasingly sophisticated cognitive and interpersonal skills, test out adult roles and behaviors, and begin to explore educational and occupational opportunities that will significantly influence future adult work life and socioeconomic status (Fig. 4-9). Key gross and fine motor, language, and sensory milestones associated with this period can be found in Table 4-6.

Adolescents who have the support and trust of their families as they tackle the developmental tasks of this period are more likely to have a smoother and successful transition from the dependency of childhood to the independence of adulthood. If their parents, however, are too controlling, too permissive, or too confrontational during this period, adolescents will experience difficulty in judging the appropriateness of their behavior and in forming self-identity as competent, worthwhile individuals. If adolescents can find sufficient acceptance in a desired peer group or receive more positive than negative responses from the objects of their growing sexual or friendship interests, they will be able to work through feelings of inadequacy and insecurity and become increasingly self-assured and competent in forming and maintaining adult relationships. The principal developmental tasks that must be mastered during the adolescent stage are to:

1. Develop self-identity and appreciate own achievements and worth.
2. Form close relationships with peers.
3. Gradually grow independent from parents.
4. Evolve own value system and integrate self-concept and values with those of peers and society.
5. Develop academic and vocational skills and related social, work, and civic sensitivities.
6. Develop analytic thinking.
7. Adjust to rapid physical and sexual changes.
8. Develop a sexual identity and role.
9. Develop skills in relating to people from different backgrounds.
10. Consider and possibly choose a career.

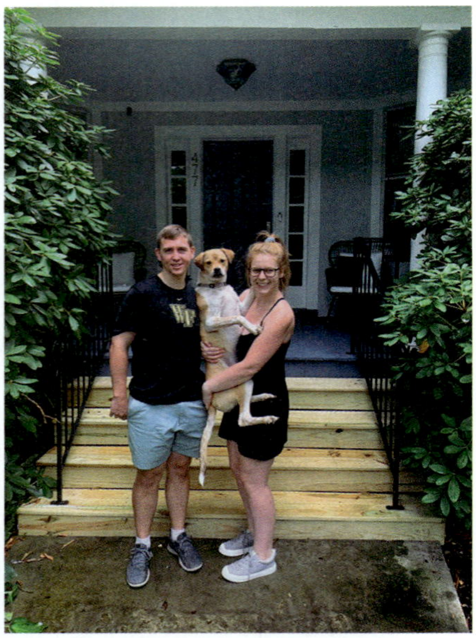

Figure 4-10 This couple moved into a home of their own to begin their married life.

Developmental Tasks of Young Adults (18 to 30 Years)

Young adulthood is a time of separation and independence from the family and of new commitments, responsibilities, and accountability in social, work, and home relationships and roles (Fig. 4-10). It is also a period when individuals are exposed to more diverse people, situations, and values and, in recent decades, to a more rapidly changing socioeconomic and technological environment than ever before. For example, the movement, particularly in the Western world, from an industrial to an information era has made extended education and a need to delay complete emancipation from the family, as well as to delay commitment to a lifelong partner, an increasing

Table 4-6 Growth and Development During Adolescence

Age	Gross Motor	Fine Motor	Language	Sensory
12–18 yr	• Muscles continue to develop • At times awkward, with some lack of coordination	• Well-developed skills	• Vocabulary is fully developed	• Development is complete

norm for young adults. More and more frequently, young adults are living with their parents after completing their education, while looking for a job in their area of academic specialization or getting a start in their career. Contrary to concern by some that this extended parental support and safety net will lead to young adults who are slackers, to the contrary, evidence indicates that it promotes definite growth in autonomy and self-reliance (Swartz et al, 2011). When parents and young adult offspring can resolve normal generational differences in philosophy and lifestyles, mastery of the young adult developmental tasks is greatly facilitated. Furthermore, trends resulting in disrupting, delaying, or avoiding cohabitative relationships have resulted in a change in the traditional structure and size of social relationships. Changes in marital and fertility rates have led to additional changes in family structure, with an increase in unmarried, remarried, or childless partnerships (Drewelies, Huxhold, & Gerstorf, 2019).

Among the developmental tasks that the young adult must achieve are to:

1. Establish friendships and a social group.
2. Grow independent of parental care and home.
3. Set up and manage one's own household.
4. Form an intimate affiliation with another and choose a mate.
5. Learn to love, cooperate with, and commit to a life partner.
6. Develop a personal style of living (e.g., shared or single) (Fig. 4-10).
7. Choose and begin to establish a career or vocation.
8. Assume social, work, and civic responsibility and roles in social, professional, political, religious, and civic organizations.
9. Learn to manage life stresses accompanying change.
10. Develop a realistic outlook and acceptance of cultural, religious, social, and political diversity.
11. Form a meaningful philosophy of life and implement it in home, employment, and community settings.
12. Begin a parental role for own or life partner's children or for young people in a broader social framework (e.g., teaching, health care, volunteer work).

Developmental Tasks of Early Middle Adulthood (30 to 50 Years)

Middle age, ranging from 30 to 70 years, is the longest stage of the life cycle and is now often divided into early and late middle adulthood. During early middle adulthood, individuals experience relatively good physical and mental health; settle into their chosen careers, socioeconomic lifestyles, patterns of relationships (married, parental, partnered, single), political, civic, social, professional, and religious affiliations and activities; and achieve maximum productivity in work and in influence over themselves and their environments. It is also a period when individuals experience a need to contribute to the next generation, that is, to raise children or produce something that will be socially useful to others. The generativity that characterizes this period consists of giving, sharing, facilitating the growth of others, and making a lasting contribution.

Many who choose to express their generativity through the parental role may, during this period, achieve both the successful launching of their children into responsible adult roles and the associated increase in leisure time and financial resources needed to pursue enjoyable, nonparental goals and activities. Others, following divorce and remarriage, may see a merging of offspring into new family groupings and the return to previous parental cycles. An increasing number of others, during or shortly after launching their young adult children into adult roles, may find themselves having to take on the responsibility of caring for chronically ill, aging parents. Each

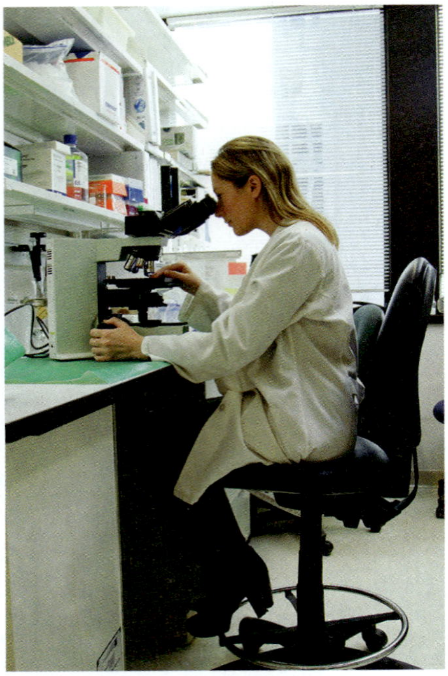

Figure 4-11 This young middle adult is establishing a career in the sciences.

such life event can generate stress and disruption in individuals' lives with which they must cope. Developing effective coping strategies to manage the stress of life events or role transitions is a developmental task facing individuals in all life stages.

Among the developmental tasks that must be achieved during early middle adulthood are to:

1. Attain a desired level of achievement and status in career (Fig. 4-11).
2. Review, evaluate, refine, and redirect career goals consistent with one's personal value system.
3. Continue to learn and refine competencies in areas of personal and career interests.
4. Manage life stresses accompanying change.
5. Continue developing mature relationships with life partner and significant others.
6. Participate in social, professional, political, religious, and civic activities.
7. Cope with an empty nest and possibly a refilled nest.
8. Adjust to aging parents and help plan for when they will need assistance.
9. Continue currently enjoyable hobbies and leisure activities and begin to develop ones for postretirement.
10. Begin to plan for personal, financial, and social aspects of retirement.

Developmental Tasks of Late Middle Adulthood (50 to 70 Years)

Many individuals during late middle adulthood may be diagnosed for the first time with a chronic health problem, such as arthritis, cardiovascular disease, cancer, diabetes, autoimmune conditions, or asthma. In addition, women generally experience a decrease in estrogen and progesterone production and undergo menopause during their late 40s or early 50s.

Changes also occur during late middle adulthood in work, family, social, and civic areas. For example, as the nuclear family contracts, parents rediscover being a couple and acquire new roles such as becoming grandparents. In addition, the gender developmental differences related to intimacy and autonomy seen in early adulthood begin to converge during late middle adulthood as men and women tend to take on similar life roles (Leidy & Darling-Fisher, 1995). Women generally become more involved and assume leadership roles in activities outside the home and work, such as politics and other civic activities, while men tend to become more aware and accepting of their nurturing and caring tendencies.

The well-known "midlife crisis" is rare in this age-group. Only 10% to 20% of individuals actually experience a midlife crisis (Infurna et al, 2020). Challenges during this time do exist as individuals may struggle to adapt to changing family dynamics. Of particular concern is the simultaneous balance that may be required when caring for an elderly parent with declining health and functioning, potentially relaunching adult children, maintaining one's career, and also planning for retirement during times of economic instability. Health disparities due to socioeconomic status, race, gender, sexuality, and SDOH continue to exist and influence middle age health outcomes, and in fact may even be magnified during this stage (Infurna et al, 2020).

A variety of development tasks must be achieved by individuals during late middle adulthood. Among these tasks are to:

1. Manage life stresses accompanying change.
2. Maintain interest in current political, cultural, and scientific advances, trends, and issues.

3. Maintain affiliation with selected social, religious, professional, civic, and political organizations.
4. Adapt to physical and mental changes and health status accompanying aging, including diagnosis of chronic health condition.
5. Continue current activities and develop new interests and leisure activities that can be pursued consistent with changing abilities.
6. Adjust to more interaction and time spent with life partner without the presence of children (Fig. 4-12).
7. Develop supportive, interdependent relationships with adult children and their significant others.
8. Help elderly parents and relatives cope with lifestyle changes (may include providing a home for them).
9. Adjust to possible or actual loss of parents, life partner, elder family members, and friends through death or their decreasing abilities to maintain independent living and self-care.
10. Prepare for and adjust to role changes, changing finances, and changing lifestyle resulting from retirement.

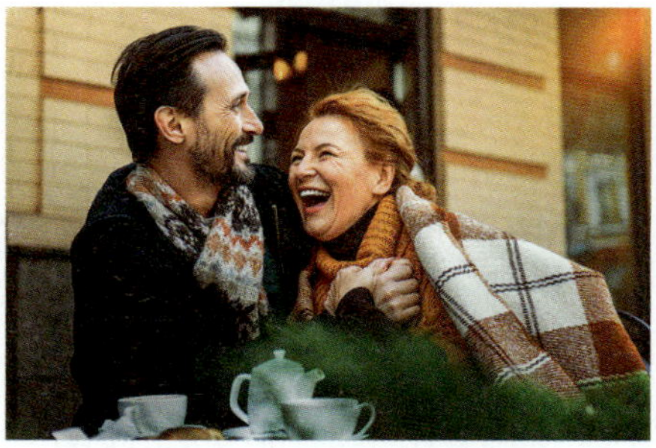

Figure 4-12 Adults in late middle adulthood frequently look forward to spending more time with their partner.

Developmental Tasks of Late Adulthood (70 Years to Death)

Individuals' health during late adulthood age (both physical and emotional) and how they confront and adjust to the changes associated with this stage are widely divergent. For those who have achieved the developmental tasks of middle adulthood and are comfortable with the life goals they have achieved, independence from the workplace and time to pursue more leisure activities are welcomed. Although a loss of work-related status and social outlets, reduced income, death of loved ones, decline in physical and some cognitive capabilities, decreased resistance to illness, and decreased recuperative powers are inevitable during late adulthood, they are often adjusted to with equanimity. Indeed, a high percentage of individuals will live out their lives managing their activities of daily living independently and in their own homes, enjoying new roles, giving requested advice and moral support to members of younger generations, and sharing leisure activities with new or old friends in their age-group.

Those that require residential care and are confronted with a loss of autonomy may struggle between finding ego-integrity or experiencing despair. Existential themes, such as isolation, hopelessness, meaninglessness, and fear and anxiety related to dying can cause an increase in depression and anxiety which can impact functioning. Performing a guided life review with the aid of a care professional is thought to be valuable, particularly for those struggling with transitions (Dezutter et al, 2020; Cavanaugh & Blanchard-Fields, 2015).

Among the developmental tasks that must be achieved during late adulthood are to:

1. Maintain and develop new activities that help retain functional capacities.
2. Accept and adjust to changes in mental and physical strength and agility and health status (Fig. 4-13).
3. Maintain and develop activities that contribute to a continuing sense of usefulness and self-worth and enhanced self-image.
4. Develop new roles in family as eldest member.
5. Establish affiliation with own age-group.
6. Accept and adjust to changing, possibly restricted circumstances—social, financial, and lifestyle.
7. Adapt to loss of life partner, family members, and friends.
8. Prepare for inevitability of own death.

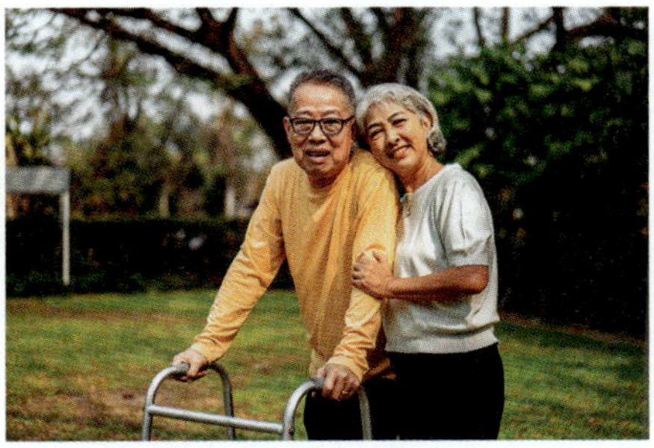

Figure 4-13 Adults in late adulthood may need to adapt to a new environment as they age and their health status changes.

NURSING CHECKLIST

General Approach to Developmental Assessment

1. Observe standard precautions and don personal protective equipment (PPE) such as gloves, gown, face shield, goggles, or N-95 respirator or face mask if the client's status warrants these protective measures.
2. If possible, choose a quiet, private room that will be free from interruptions. Position yourself at eye level with the client.
3. Greet the client, introduce yourself, and explain the purpose of the interview. Many aspects of a developmental assessment can be directly observed. Share with the client/caregiver any screening tools that will be used.

Stages of Family Development

A review of developmental stages, tasks, and life events is not complete without considering the family context of the child or adult being assessed. McGoldrick, Carter, and Garcia-Preto (2014) have described six stages in the life cycle of the average middle-class family and the emotional processes of transition and second-order changes in the family's status required for each developmental stage. Duvall, another family life-cycle theorist (Duvall & Miller, 1985), described the family in eight stages, starting with a childless married couple, progressing to a couple with children at various ages, and ending with aging family members and death.

Developmental Assessment Tools

A variety of developmental assessment tools are available for use by the nurse. Some of the most commonly used tools assess the mental, physical, emotional, and social functional status of individuals and families. It should be noted that use of some of these tools requires special training, cost and time varies, and none are diagnostic. Table 4-7 summarizes some of the tools that are frequently used.

Table 4-7 Developmental Assessment Tools

Tool	Target Population	Assessment Parameters	Special Considerations
Brazelton Neonatal Behavioral Assessment Scale (BNBAS)[1]	Newborns	Temperament characteristics: state of arousal, orienting responses to stimuli, ability to deal with disturbing stimuli, social behavior, motor skills	When results are shared with parents, increased and improved newborn-parent interactions have been noted
Ages and Stages Questionnaire[2]	1 month–5.5 yr	Developmental and social-emotional screening	Gender-specific questions can be omitted; translated into multiple languages
Denver II (DDST)[3]	1 month–6 yr old	Personal-social, fine motor-adaptive, language, gross motor skills	Standardized for minority populations
Revised Prescreening Developmental Questionnaire (R-PDQ)[4]	1 month–6 yr old	Personal-social, fine motor-adaptive, language, gross motor skills	Answered by parents to identify children who need more complete screening
Early Language Milestones Scale (ELM Scale-2)[5]	1 month–3 yr old	Early language development	Tests auditory visual, auditory receptive, expressive language in greater depth than Denver II
Parent Evaluation of Developmental Status (PEDS)[6]	Birth–8 yr	Global/cognitive, speech (expressive and receptive), behavioral, social-emotional, self-help, fine and gross motor	Appropriate to use with children from culturally and linguistically diverse backgrounds
Modified Checklist for Autism Toddlers (M-CHAT- R/F)[7]	16–30 months	Children at risk for autism	Currently available in over 57 languages and additional ones with pictures

Table 4-7 Developmental Assessment Tools—cont'd

Tool	Target Population	Assessment Parameters	Special Considerations
Pediatric Symptom Checklist (PSC)[8]	Ages 4 +	Checklist to identify social, emotional, and behavioral concerns	35-question parent form (shorter form also available, 17 questions) Y-PSC (youth self-report 11 yr +) Free Multiple languages Excellent sensitivity and specificity
Sense of Coherence (SOC) Scale[9]	School age through adults	Sense of coherence (comprehensibility, manageability, meaningfulness)	Gender, culturally, and socioeconomically neutral; results can be used for anticipatory guidance
Patient Health Questionnaire, 2 items (PHQ-2)[10]	Adolescents to middle-age adults	Functional Screening for depression	Can be self-administered or can be part of an interview. Two-questions client screen for depression. Should be followed by PHQ-9 if concerns; not appropriate for older adults.
Patient Health Questionnaire, 9 items (PHQ-9)[11]	Ages 12 yr and up	Functional screening for depression (includes perinatal depression)	Client self-administration <5 min; excellent sensitivity and specificity; available in over 49 languages (not all validated); free to use; preferred over PHQ-2 in older adults
HEEADSS 3.0 (Home, Education, Eating, Activities, Drugs, Sex, Suicide, and Safety) Adolescent Risk Profile[12]	Adolescents	Home, education, eating, activities, drugs, sex, suicide, and safety	Provider guidelines to identify high-risk adolescents, and provides a guide for anticipatory guidance
CRAFFT (car, relax, alone, forget, friends, trouble)[13]	Ages 12–21 yr	Screening for adolescent substance use disorder (SUD); use newest version (2.1 + N) includes questions related to tobacco, nicotine, marijuana, and vaping use	Clinician-administered; CRAFFT most widely used screen worldwide for substance use
Beck Depression Inventory (BDI)[14]	Ages 13–80	Mood, pessimism, sense of failure, dissatisfaction, guilt, sense of punishment, disappointment in oneself, self-accusations, self-punitive wishes, crying spells, irritability, social withdrawal, indecisiveness, body image, function at work, sleep disturbance, fatigue, appetite disturbance, weight loss, preoccupation with health, loss of libido	21 self-reported scale; Score indicating depression warrants referral to a mental health specialist

Continued

Table 4-7 Developmental Assessment Tools—cont'd

Tool	Target Population	Assessment Parameters	Special Considerations
Single Alcohol Screening Question (SASQ) (NIH, 2020)[15]	Adolescents and adults	Help identify clients who use excess alcohol	This single question can be self-administered or can be part of an interview. Refer to Chapter 3.
Alcohol Use Disorders Identification Test (AUDIT-C)[16]	Adolescents and adults	Screen for alcohol misuse from past year in 3 areas: current alcohol dependence; harmful drinking which has caused social, mental, or physical problems; and risks for future alcohol-related problems	Can be self-administered or can be part of an interview. Refer to Chapter 3.
CAGE* (Cut down, Annoyed, Guilty, and Eye-opener), 4 items[17] *The USPSTF recommends use of the AUDIT-C or SASQ alcohol screening tools as they are more sensitive and specific than the CAGE tool. CAGE is still used in practice by some clinicians.	Ages 16 yr and up	Screen for alcohol overuse	Self-administered; identifies clients for alcohol-related disorders
CAGE-AID** (Cut down, Annoyed, Guilty, and Eye-Opener adapted for alcohol and drug use)[18]	Ages 16 yr and up	Screen for alcohol and drug use	Clinician-administered
Beck Anxiety Inventory (BAI)[19]	Older adolescents and adults	Emotional, cognitive, and physiological symptoms of anxiety	Can be self-administered; distinguishes anxiety from depression
Edinburg Postnatal Depression Scale (EDPS)[20]	Birthing parents	Maternal ante- and postpartum depression	10-item scale
Transitional Impact Scale[21]	Adults	Measures both material and psychological change	12-item scale
Lives Daily Hassles Scale (LIVES- DHS)[22]	Adults	Everyday irritants that contribute to stress, and behaviors and feelings that promote well-being	Studies have suggested that day-to-day hassles are more strongly correlated with physical and psychosocial problems and outcomes than are life events; daily hassles negatively predict life satisfaction
Functional Activities Questionnaire (FAQ)[23]	Older adults	Level of independence demonstrated in the performance of activities of daily living	Can be completed by significant other or caregiver
Katz Index of Independence in Activities of Daily Living (Katz ADL)[24]	Older adults	Assesses functional status (as ability to perform six functions of bathing, dressing, toileting, transferring, continence, and feeding)	Assesses basic ADLs; often used in hospital discharge assessment; full geriatric assessment indicated with any concern

Table 4-7 Developmental Assessment Tools—cont'd

Tool	Target Population	Assessment Parameters	Special Considerations
Folstein Mini-Mental State Examination (MMSE)[25]	Older adults	Cognitive function	Can be easily administered in any clinical setting. A telephone version is also available. Assists in determining the need for a more definitive neurological examination
Functional Assessment Screening in the Elderly (FASE)[26]	Older adults	Functional disability	Suggests interventions when abnormal results are present
The Lawton Instrumental Activities of Daily Living Scale (IADL)[27]	Older adults	Functional disability	Assesses function at given time and improvement or deterioration of function over time; looks at items able to complete without assistance or unable to complete without assistance
Minimum Data Set (MDS 3.0) for Nursing Facility Resident Assessment and Care Screening[28]	Nursing home residents	Cognitive patterns, communication and hearing patterns, vision patterns, physical functioning and structural problems, psychosocial well-being, mood and behavior patterns, activity pursuit patterns, bowel and bladder status, disease diagnoses, health conditions, oral nutritional status, oral and dental status, skin condition, medication use, treatments and procedures, customary activities of daily living routines	Required by federal law for all clients residing in nursing homes
Geriatric Depression Scale-15 (GDS-15)[29]	Geriatric population	Functional screen for depression	Appropriate for those with mild to moderate dementia and physical illness
Calgary Family Assessment and Intervention Model (CFAM/CFIM)[30]	Families	Structural, developmental, and functional	Includes emphasis on diversity issues such as race, culture, ethnicity, gender, living environment, and sexual orientation; translated into over eight languages; focuses on assessment and both short and long-term interventions

Source: [1]Brazelton & Nugent, 2011; [2]Porter, Qureshi, Caldwell, Etchevarria et al, 2016; [3]Hagan et al, 2017, Frankenburg et al, 1996, Sansavini et al, 2021; [4]Marlow, Servili, & Tomlinson, 2019; [5]Lewis, 2013; [6]Porter et al, 2016, Liebzeit et al, 2018; [7]Zhang, 2022; [8]Weitzman et al, 2015; [9]Eriksson & Mittelmark, 2016; [10]Levis et al, 2020; [11]Costantini et al, 2021, Odone et al, 2021, Weitzman et al, 2015; [12]Levy et al, 2016, Klein et al, 2014; [13]Hadland et al, 2017, Levy et al, 2016, Weitzman et al, 2015; [14]Osman et al, 2004; [15]National Institute on Alcohol Abuse and Alcoholism, 2022; [16]Levy et al, 2016; [17]Mulvaney-Day et al, 2018; [18]Weitzman et al, 2015, Mulvaney-Day et al, 2018; [19]Beck & Steer, 1993, Beck et al, 1996; [20]Weitzman et al, 2015; [21]Svob et al, 2014, Uzer, 2020; [22]Udayar et al, 2021; [23]Marshall et al, 2015; [24]Wallace & Shelkey, 2007, Liebzeit et al, 2018; [25]Palsetia et al, 2018, Tsoi et al, 2015, Folstein et al, 1975; [26]Ward & Reuben, 2022; [27]Ward & Reuben, 2022, Graf, 2007, Lawton & Brody, 1969; [28]Centers for Medicaid and Medicare Services, 2019, Saliba & Bauchanan, 2008; [29]Krishnamoorthy et al, 2020; [30]Shajani & Snell, 2019, Leahey & Wright, 2016

SARS-CoV2 (COVID-19) Effects on Growth and Development

The COVID-19 pandemic affected everyone in the United States as well as around the world. The impact that this major life event has and will continue to exert on our lives is still largely unknown. The sense of isolation and social disconnect during the lockdowns, the shift to virtual learning and working, the anxiety and fear of the unknown, the public health threat, and the massive loss of life are anticipated to have ripple effects across the life span of all those who experienced the pandemic. Treglia et al (2023) estimated that as of mid-2022, over 216,000 children under the age of 18 lost a parent or other in-home caregiver to COVID-19 (COVID Collaborative, 2022- data updated in 2022). Mental health has been negatively impacted by increasing numbers of mental health diagnoses and suicide attempts continuing to rise in all age-groups. Time and long-term studies will likely bring to light new developmental crises and/or missed milestones. Nursing has the opportunity to play a pivotal role in assessing the impact COVID-19 has and will continue to have on our client's development and health outcomes (Heanoy et al, 2021).

U.S. Preventive Services Task Force (USPSTF)

There are no USPSTF recommendations, Grade A or B statements, for developmental assessment.

CASE STUDY
Ineffective Coping After Divorce

This case study illustrates a developmental assessment of a late middle-aged female. In addition, the application of the AUDIT-C questionnaire (refer to Chapter 3) is demonstrated. Ms. Alisha Miller is a 54-year-old accountant who is presenting to primary care for a renewal of her thyroid medication. Client currently lives with her two teen children, whom she shares custody of with her ex-husband. They have been divorced for 6 years. Ms. Miller is presenting at the Women's Health Center for renewal of her prescription medications.

HEALTH HISTORY

CLIENT PROFILE

54-year-old White divorced female

REASON FOR SEEKING HEALTH CARE

"I ran out of my thyroid medicine and need a refill."

PRESENT HEALTH

States her Irritable Bowel Syndrome (IBS), hypothyroidism, and hypertension (HTN) are under control with her current medications. Takes thyroid and blood pressure (BP) meds daily. Does not check her BP at home. States she does not have a lot of energy but has no trouble carrying out any activity she wishes to perform, such as housework, shopping, and traveling.

PAST HEALTH HISTORY

Medical History HTN 2018, hypothyroidism 2016; IBS, 2008

Surgical History Tonsillectomy and adenoidectomy, 1985 without complications

Allergies Allergy to amoxicillin (hives); some seasonal congestion and OTC use of antihistamines prn; denies food allergies, latex allergy, animal allergies

Medications Metoprolol succinate extended release 100 mg daily; levothyroxine 125 mcg daily; loratadine 10 mg daily prn for seasonal allergic rhinitis; loperamide HCl 2 mg capsules OTC prn for IBS symptoms, up to 8 capsules in 24 hr; multivitamin (MVI) daily; calcium 600 mg with vitamin D 400 International Units daily; omega-3 fish oil 1,200 mg daily

Communicable Diseases Denies

Injuries and Accidents Denies

Differing Abilities Denies

Blood Transfusions Denies

Childhood Illnesses Varicella age 5, no complications

Immunizations. Influenza vaccine last year.

COVID-19 vaccine mRNA x 2 doses 2021 and booster January 2022, declined other doses since then

Varicella zoster vaccine 2019—sore arm with erythema at the injection site for 1 week afterward, did not receive second dose

FAMILY HEALTH HISTORY

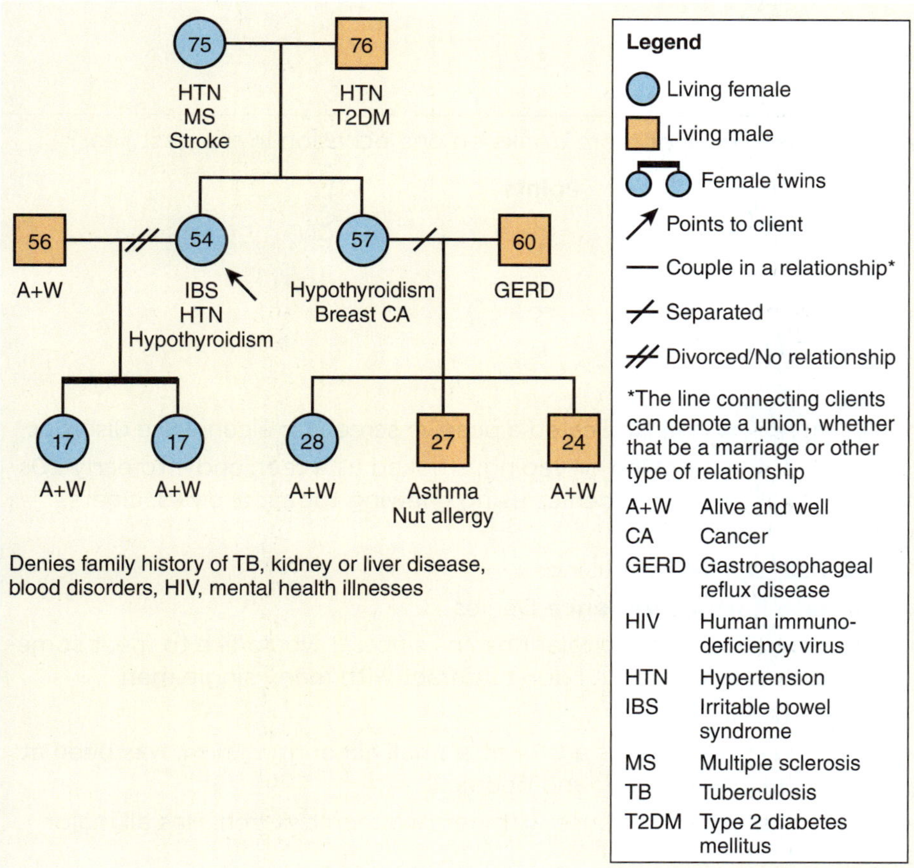

SOCIAL HISTORY

Alcohol Use Client stated, "I am probably drinking more than I should." Admits to drinking wine daily, sometimes five or more glasses per day (with dinner, any social activities, while watching TV, and an occasional nightcap). Has not tried to decrease her alcohol intake but believes she could stop now if she wanted to do so. Denies having blackouts with drinking. Has driven home after dinner with friends where she drank. Denies ever hurting herself or others while drinking. States "I'm not sure if I have a drinking problem." The AUDIT-C alcohol screening tool was administered:

AUDIT-C:

How often did you have a drink containing alcohol in the past year?

	Points
Never	0
Monthly or less	1
Two to four times a month	2
Two to three times a week	3
Four or more times a week	**4**

How many drinks did you have on a typical day when you were drinking in the past year?

	Points
None, I do not drink	0
1 or 2	0
3 or 4	**1**
5 or 6	2
7 to 9	3
10 or more	4

How often did you have six or more drinks on one occasion in the past year?

	Points
Never	0
Less than monthly	**1**
Monthly	2
Weekly	3
Daily or almost daily	4

AUDIT-C score = 6

A score of 3 or more in women indicated a positive screen for alcohol use disorder.

Tobacco Use Denies current smoking or vaping; smoked as a teen and into early 20s, 5 pack/year history, quit 28 yr ago; denies using chewing tobacco, pipes, cigars, snuff; does not smoke marijuana

Recreational Drug Use Denies ever using

Domestic and Intimate Partner Violence Denies

Sexual Practice Divorced 6 yr ago; no relationships since; "I would like to meet someone special, but I don't see how since I don't interact with many single men."

Travel History Enjoys traveling

Work Environment Works full-time as a CPA at a small accounting firm. Has been at this job for past 5 yr. Enjoys the work and people.

Home Environment Lives in a townhouse with her two teen children. Has all major appliances and air conditioning.

Hobbies and Leisure Activities Bunco group in neighborhood, visiting art museums and attending classical concerts, travel

Stress "I am very stressed about being an empty nester in the next year and affording my twins' college tuition. They are going to have to go to school in state, if I can even afford that!"

Education Master's degree in Accounting

Economic Status She can pay her bills each month but is concerned about retirement and paying for her children's college. She was a stay-at-home mom for most of her adult life until her divorce. Was able to make a sizable deposit on her current townhouse after her divorce settlement but doesn't have a lot of retirement money saved.

Military Status None

Religion Catholic but not currently active; stopped attending church when she divorced.

Ethnic Background English

Roles and Relationships Close relationship with teen twins, sister who lives in NYC, and neighborhood and work friends. Has monthly bunco group in neighborhood and several friends with whom she attends plays, visits museums, or travels. Contact with everyone has become a bit less since working full-time and raising two teens. Her parents live about 3 hr away and she visits them about every 2 months.

Characteristic Patterns of Daily Living No real pattern at present

HEALTH MAINTENANCE ACTIVITIES

Sleep 7 hr per night, does not feel rested in the morning

Diet Usually vegetables and fruit with some chicken or fish for dinner. Red meat maybe once a week. Has not had the energy to cook much lately. Usually has a protein shake for breakfast. Eats out 2 to 3 times a week. Regularly salts food. Caffeine intake: 4 cups of coffee daily. Does not consume energy drinks.

Exercise Dropped gym membership when realized she wasn't using it. Jogged a mile, then walked a mile around nearby park until last couple of months. Now walks around the neighborhood a couple times a week for 30 minutes.

Stress Management Listens to classical music, hot bath 3 to 5 times a week, wine

Use of Safety Devices Wears seatbelt

Health Checkups Annual physical and episodic visits prn; mammogram and Pap test 2 years ago; colonoscopy last year; last dentist visit was a year ago; cannot recall the last time she had her eyes checked.

DEVELOPMENTAL ASSESSMENT

Client has lived with IBS, hypothyroidism, and HTN for many years. As she has entered middle adulthood her medical conditions have not presented any change in her life or lifestyle. She has not experienced any complications from them.

Due to divorce, she has not been successfully managing her life stress, as evidenced by her heavy drinking.

She maintains her interest in her social activities, such as the bunco group and neighborhood/work friends.

Client has not had a life partner since her divorce.

Client would like to have partner in her life.

Relationship with teen children can be stressful at times. Anxious about having an empty nest next year.

Client visits her parents every couple of months. Is close with her sister, who lives about 4 hr away.

Concerned about her financial future.

CLINICAL JUDGMENT IN ACTION

1. What cues indicate that the client is having a developmental disorder?
2. What interventions have the highest priority?
3. What assessment findings indicate clinical improvement in this client?

Review Questions

1. An infant explores the environment using senses and starts to form mental images of objects. According to Piaget, which developmental stage characterizes these actions?
   a. Sensorimotor stage
   b. Preoperational stage
   c. Concrete Operational stage
   d. Formal Operational stage
2. A school-aged child states that the number 10 is greater than the number 4. According to Piaget, which developmental stage(s) characterizes this math concept?
   a. Sensorimotor stage
   b. Sensorimotor stage and Preoperational stage
   c. Preoperational stage and Concrete Operational stage
   d. Formal Operational stage
3. The nurse is assessing the fine motor skills of a 24-month-old child. Which skills will the child be expected to perform? Select all that apply.
   a. Cut using child scissors
   b. Draw a straight line
   c. Draw a circle
   d. Brush teeth
   e. Use a spoon well
   f. Stack 2 blocks
4. The adolescent is meeting with a guidance counselor to discuss post–high school plans. On which developmental task is the adolescent focused?
   a. Learning to trust
   b. Demonstrating ego integrity
   c. Being industrious
   d. Finding identity
5. The nurse is concerned about alcohol use in a 48-year-old client. Which tool would be most appropriate to use to assess potential alcohol overuse?
   a. HEEADSSS 3.0
   b. AUDIT-C
   c. CRAFFT
   d. PHQ-9
6. Which screening tool for depression is most appropriate for an older adult client with congestive heart failure and mild dementia?
   a. PHQ-2
   b. Beck's Depression Inventory
   c. Geriatric Depression Scale-15
   d. Edinburg Depression Scale
7. Which of the following gross motor movements are normal for a 9-month-old infant? Select all that apply.
   a. Takes a few independent steps
   b. Crawls using arms and legs
   c. Pulls self to sitting position
   d. Pulls self to standing position
   e. Stands alone
8. Which of the following describes Freud's Latency Stage of psychosexual theory?
   a. Pleasure from exploration with mouth and through sucking
   b. Compares own capabilities with peer norms
   c. Completes toilet training
   d. Develops sexual relationships
9. Which of the following is true about the Denver II developmental assessment tool? Select all that apply.
   a. It assesses fine motor-adaptive behaviors.
   b. It is used in children from birth to age 8.
   c. It is standardized for minority populations.
   d. It assesses gross motor skills.
   e. It assesses temperament characteristics.
10. According to Kohlberg, most adults do not reach or maintain which level?
    a. Preconventional Level
    b. Individualism, Instrumental Purpose, and Exchange Level
    c. Postconventional Level
    d. Social System and Conscience Level

CHAPTER

5 Cultural Assessment

Learning Outcomes

1. Explain the importance of cultural awareness and cultural humility in nursing practice.
2. Describe the American Nurses Association (ANA) competencies to promote culturally competent nursing care.
3. Describe the components of cultural identity.
4. Discuss the core elements of culture and the impact they can have on a client's health care.
5. Discuss how culturally driven folk illnesses and self-care practices can impact a person's health.
6. Conduct and document a cultural assessment of a client.

The racial, ethnic, and cultural diversification of the United States continues to shift at an unprecedented rate. According to the U.S. 2020 Census, an estimated 61.6% of the population identified themselves solely as White, 12.4% as Black, 18.7% Hispanic, 1.1% as American Indian and Alaska Native, 6% as Asian, and 0.2% as Native Hawaiian and Other Pacific Islander. The percentage of the population self-identified as "Some Other Race," is 8.4%, and 10.2% self-identified as being of two or more races/ethnicities (U.S. Census Bureau, 2021a). Between 2010 and 2020, the Hispanic population experienced the most growth in the U.S. (Fig. 5-1) compared with other racial/ethnic groups, increasing by 2.2 percentage points. Conversely, the White population decreased in growth by 4.1 percentage points (U.S. Census Bureau, 2021b).

According to the Pew Research Center, whereby, data is retrieved from the United Nations (UN) and analyzed, the projection in North America indicates migration from the rest of the world is expected to be the primary driver of persistent population growth. According to the UN projections, the immigrant population in the United States is expected to net an increase of 85 million people over the next 80 years (2020 to 2100) (Cilluffo & Ruiz, 2019). Given the increasing diversity in the U.S. population, it is critical for nurses to understand the impact these factors will have on their practice (National Academies of Sciences, Engineering, and Medicine, 2021; U.S. Census Bureau, 2021a).

Culture

Culture is a learned and socially transmitted orientation and way of life specific to a group of people with similar lifeways (Fig. 5-2). Culture

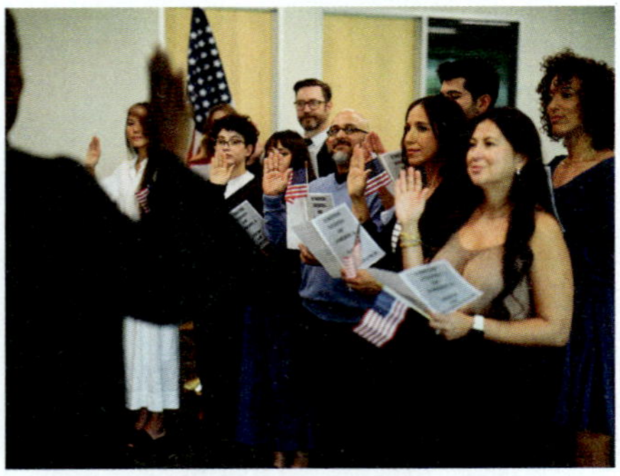

Figure 5-1 These new American citizens hale from various racial, ethnic, and cultural backgrounds.

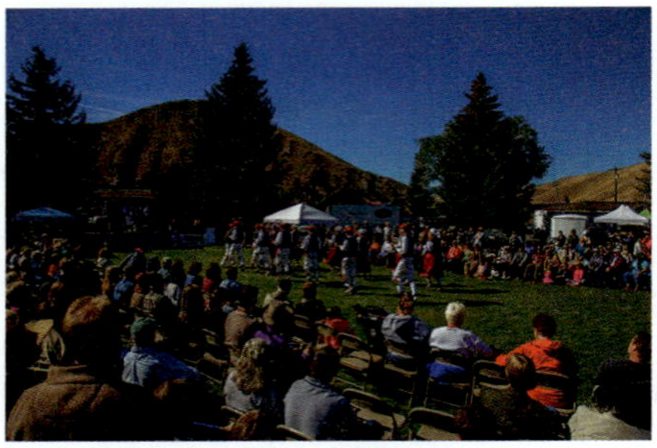

Figure 5-2 These dancers are preserving the sheepherding culture at the festival of the Trailing of the Sheep in Idaho.

enables members of large groups of people to find unity and survive in the world around them through the development of unique patterns of assumptions and shared meanings. Contrary to beliefs, cultures are not synonymous with countries. The cultural beliefs, values, customs, and norms that result from these assumptions and meanings shape how the group members think, act, and relate with others, as well as how they perceive aspects of life such as time, space, health, illness, family, work, and community-member roles.

The beliefs, values, and norms of a cultural group are passed informally from one generation of group members to the next. Family, cultural experiences, community, and the lived experience may have a profound impact on an individual's health, communication, and connection with those of different ethnic and cultural backgrounds.

Cultural Diversity in the United States

The population of the United States is shaped by centuries of migration, growth, and vast global origins. Thus, the American health-care system is one of **cultural diversity**, whereby, clients and health-care providers from diverse blends of ethnic (e.g., Hispanic), racial (e.g., Black), national (e.g., Turkey), religious (e.g., Hindu), generational (e.g., older adult), marital status (e.g., single), socioeconomic status (e.g., educational achievement and employment status), occupation (e.g., nurse), preference in life partner (e.g., heterosexual), health status (e.g., chronic illness), and cultural orientations coexist in a given location. For example, Chicago, Illinois is culturally and racially diverse. Its population is 44% White, 32% Black, 5% Asian, 28% Hispanic or Latino, and 2% two or more races. A few of the many languages other than English spoken in Chicago are Spanish, Chinese, German, French, and the African languages of Kru, Yoruba, and Ibo. The religiously diverse community includes Christians, Jews, Muslims, Buddhists, Hindus, and others (Population USA, 2022). Economically, Chicago neighborhoods are stratified by income; 21% live below the poverty line (earning less than $25,000 annually), medium household income is greater than $150,000, while 1% of the population earns greater than $600,000 annually (Crain's Chicago Business, n.d.).

Therefore the nurse needs to be able to communicate effectively with culturally diverse groups of individuals; make accurate cultural assessments; and plan, provide, and evaluate culturally competent care. Such care must be based on awareness of, and utilization of, knowledge and theories that explain client-specific situations and responses within the context of their cultural, ethnic, gender, and sexual orientation.

To further expand the concept of diversity, recent immigrants from countries such as Mexico, Columbia, Ecuador, the Dominican Republic, Haiti, El Salvador, the Philippines, China, Vietnam, Nigeria, Jamaica, Pakistan, India, Lebanon, Somalia, Russia, and Ukraine may have very different attitudes toward the health-care system, health behaviors, and perception of illness. These individuals grew up in their respective countries where they experienced **enculturation**, the informal process through which the beliefs, values, norms, and practices of a culture are learned by members born into that culture. Nurses must be mindful of the beliefs and attitudes of a client's heritage culture as they experience **acculturation,** the process of learning the beliefs, values, norms, and practices of the mainstream culture in their new homeland. Nurses must develop a perspective of **cultural relativity**, the belief that no culture is inferior or superior to another, and deliver culturally competent care that aligns with the values and beliefs of clients and their support system.

Assessment in Brief

Cultural Assessment

- The nurse must provide culturally competent care to all clients, being sensitive to the client's needs while providing nursing care with dignity and respect. The nurse needs to incorporate the American Nurses Association (ANA) competencies to promote culturally competent nursing care into their practice.
- The nurse needs to be self-aware of personal values and beliefs so that culturally sensitive approaches to care based on mutual respect can be provided.
- The nurse needs to recognize and understand the normal behaviors of different cultural groups and their unique behavioral responses to health and illness.
- The nurse needs to strive for an ethic of cultural relativism to provide nursing services. Personal behavior must be evaluated in relation to the cultural context in which it occurs, so that respect, equality, and justice are inherent in the nursing care provided to all clients.

Cultural Awareness

Cultural awareness is the process of critical self-reflection of one's own biases toward other cultures and exploration of one's cultural background. *The Future of Nursing 2020–2030: Charting a Path to Achieve Health Equity* (National Academies of Sciences, Engineering, and Medicine, 2021) emphasizes the concept of "cultural humility." According to Agner (2020), cultural humility is essential for the nurse. **Cultural humility** is defined by flexibility, awareness of bias, a life-long approach to working with diversity, and the recognition of the role of power in health-care interactions. Nurses cultivate cultural humility and dispose of stereotypical thinking and biases through self-reflection. Cultural humility enables nurses to develop respectful partnerships with clients to achieve equity in the delivery of health care (Agner, 2020). According to Foronda and colleagues (2016), cultural humility results in effective treatment, sound clinical decision making, communication, empathy, and improved care.

Biases are defined as social stereotypes that can be conscious or unconscious. Biases may lead nurses to generalize about clients based on appearance (e.g., tattoos, piercings, obesity), level of education, place of employment, and place of residence. These biases, which are socially constructed, are generalizations that may influence decisions in interactions and care. For example, in the aftermath of the 9/11 attacks on the United States, overt discrimination occurred toward persons of Muslim faith and Arab descent, as well as persons perceived to be members of these groups, in the United States (Campinha-Bacote, 2018; Foronda et al, 2016; Pacquiao & Douglas, 2019). The most serious barrier to cultural awareness and competence is not the lack of knowledge regarding a cultural group but the potential to generalize and stereotype individuals in the context of their culture (Campinha-Bacote, 2018).

Cultural Congruence

The American Nurses Association (ANA) advances the profession of nursing by fostering high standards of nursing practice, promoting a safe and ethical work environment, enhancing the health and wellness of nurses, and advocating on health-care issues that affect nurses and the public (ANA, 2021). *Nursing: Scope and Standards of Practice,* Standard Nine: Respectful and Equitable

Practice states, "the registered nurse practices with cultural humility and inclusiveness." Standard Nine outlines 13 competencies of the Registered Nurse to promote the development of culturally competent practice:

1. Demonstrates respect, equity, and empathy in actions and interactions with all health-care consumers.
2. Respects consumer decisions without bias.
3. Participates in life-long learning to understand cultural preferences, worldviews, choices, and decision-making processes of diverse consumers.
4. Reflects upon personal and cultural values, beliefs, biases, and heritage.
5. Applies knowledge of differences in health beliefs, practices, and communication patterns without assigning value to the differences.
6. Addresses the effects and impact of discrimination and oppression on practice within and among diverse groups.
7. Uses appropriate skills and tools for the culture, literacy, and language of the individuals and population served.
8. Communicates with appropriate language and behaviors, including the use of qualified health-care interpreters and translators in accordance with consumer needs and preferences.
9. Serves as a role model and educator for cultural humility and the recognition and appreciation of diversity and inclusivity.
10. Identifies the cultural-specific meaning of interactions, terms, and content.
11. Advocates for policies that promote health and prevent harm among diverse health-care consumers and groups.
12. Promotes equity in all aspects of health and health care.
13. Advances organizational policies, programs, services, and practices that reflect respect, equity, and values for diversity and inclusion. (ANA, 2021)

Culturally congruent care is the application of evidence-based nursing practice that aligns with the client/consumer's cultural values, beliefs, worldview, and practices, outlined above by the ANA (Fig. 5-3). Nurses provide culturally congruent care by applying the knowledge of how culture influences their own health beliefs, health practices, and communication patterns at each stage of the nursing process. Cultural assessment occurs in the first step of the nursing process: assessment (Marion et al, 2016).

Cultural Competence

Cultural competence represents the process by which the nurse demonstrates culturally congruent practice. The nurse provides culturally congruent care to diverse clients/consumers to improve access to care, enhance positive outcomes, and reduce disparities. Cultural competence aims to change the "one size fits all" approach to the care of individuals and groups.

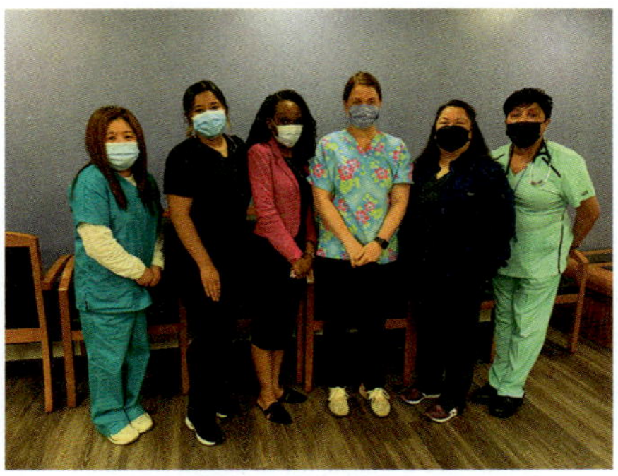

Figure 5-3 This diverse group of nurses works in an office setting and incorporates culturally competent care into their daily practice.

To provide culturally competent nursing care, the nurse first must be willing to confront personal cultural biases, or **ethnocentrism** (a condition that occurs when individuals or groups of people perceive their cultural group and cultural values, beliefs, norms, and customs to be superior to all others).

During the health assessment interview, the nurse needs to avoid stereotyping the client by depending too heavily on an "ideal" or normative racial, ethnic, or cultural characteristic or trait list. No one individual or family within a culture or subculture will display all the characteristics representative of that culture. Normative lists or summaries do not include all the diversity that may be part of a given culture. Nevertheless, an understanding of basic racial, ethnic, and cultural concepts associated with culturally competent health assessments can serve as a *guide* for the nurse. The nurse will benefit from experiences with a range of individuals and groups from any given cultural group to determine where, within the range, *this* client fits.

Assessing a client's cultural beliefs, values, and customs through observation and interview is an essential part of health assessment in the delivery of culturally competent nursing care. When assessing a client, the nurse must balance data related to the specific individual and data related to the client's support system. In addition, knowledge of the client's racial and ethnic group's physical and biological norms, as well as the risks to optimal health that are associated with the social determinants of health can be relevant to the assessment. The **Social Determinants of Health (SDOH)** are defined as economic and social conditions that influence the health status of individuals and groups, e.g., achieved education, immigration status, employment/ income, housing, and access to health care and the lived environment.

Cultural competence is built upon the values, trust, and respect for differences, and the ability to develop partnerships and collaboration to bridge diversity. The goal of cultural competence is to create a health-care system and workforce that are capable of delivering the highest quality care to every client regardless of race, ethnicity, culture, or language proficiency (Pacquiao & Douglas, 2019).

As the United States population becomes increasingly diverse, nurses will increasingly see clients with a broader range of perspectives regarding health, often influenced by their social or cultural backgrounds. Clients may have limited English proficiency, different thresholds for seeking care or expectations about their care, and unfamiliar beliefs that influence whether they adhere to their providers' treatment recommendations. Cultural competence among all members of the health-care team, of which nurses are the key stakeholders, can affect the delivery of care by minimizing racial and ethnic disparities.

Defining Cultural Identity

Subculture

Subculture is defined as a group of people whose values and experiences differ from those in the dominant culture with whom they identify. These smaller groups possess many of the values, beliefs, and customs of the larger culture, but also have unique characteristics that differentiate them from their heritage culture, such as race (Black, White), language (Hebrew, Yiddish), religion (Sikh, Christian), sexual orientation (bisexual, lesbian), country of origin (Black Caribbean, Arab American), preference in life partner, and generational status (Generation Z, baby boomers).

The nurse needs to recognize that all individuals have a combination of cultural influences, derived from membership in their heritage culture, as well as membership in one or more subcultures, which creates a **multicultural identity** (Fig. 5-4). An individual's unique multicultural identity makes it critical for the nurse to assess each client in the context of their culture(s) rather than simply as a normative member of a single culture, subculture, race, or ethnic group (Purnell & Fenkl, 2020).

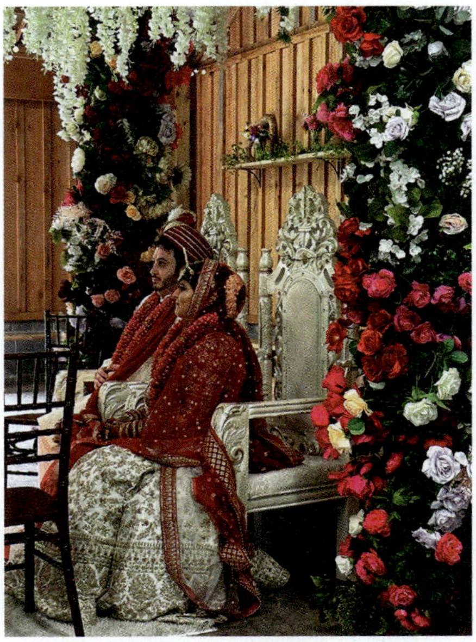

Figure 5-4 This Indian American couple celebrated their wedding by observing cultural and religious rituals in two ceremonies, one Hindu and the other Christian.

Race

Race is defined as the classification of individuals based on shared biological traits and physical characteristics such as skin color, physical features, and hair texture genetically inherited from biological ancestors, attributed to climate exposure and diet. Racial characteristics can have an impact on health status; for example, Asian and Native Americans have few apocrine glands and therefore perspire little and have mild or no body odor. Also, the incidence of skin cancer in dark-skinned individuals is much lower than in light-skinned individuals, due to a higher level of melanin in the pigmentation.

Racial identification must not be assumed by nurses. Therefore, nurses should ask clients to self-identify their race/ethnicity when performing a cultural assessment. The United States Office of Management and Budget (OMB) (Jensen et al, 2021) identifies the following six races in America:

- White
- Black
- American Indian or Alaska Native
- Asian
- Native Hawaiian or Other Pacific Islander
- Some other race (for people who do not identify with any of the OMB race categories)

Ethnicity

Ethnic group members share a unique national or regional origin and social, cultural, and linguistic heritage. Ethnic groups may exhibit distinguishing features, such as language, accent, physical features, family names, customs, and religion (Purnell, 2018). The following ethnic groups recognized by the OMB (U.S. Census Bureau, 2021a) are:

- Hispanic
- White alone, non-Hispanic
- Black alone, non-Hispanic
- American Indian and Alaska Native alone, non-Hispanic
- Asian alone, non-Hispanic
- Native Hawaiian and Other Pacific Islander alone, non-Hispanic
- Some other race alone, non-Hispanic
- Multiracial, non-Hispanic

Ethnic identity, or self-identification with an ethnic group, is subjective and not always obvious. Ethnic identity is affected by language acquisition, adaptation to culture and values, ancestry, biological attributes, values and beliefs, and the creation of social networks within the culture (Epstein & Heizler, 2015). For example, people may self-identify as Black; Asian or Filipino, European American, or White; Hispanic, Latino, or Columbian. They may identify with their country of origin (e.g., Egyptians may identify with Egypt) or their culture of origin. When a nurse conducts a culturally competent assessment, it is appropriate to determine the client's self-identified ethnic group, as well as the country of origin/ancestry.

Sexual Orientation and Gender Identity

Sexual orientation and gender identity are also components of an individual's culture and cultural identity. Based on data from the respondents in the "Household Pulse Survey," a national survey of adults in the United States, at least 20 million adults in the United States are estimated to be lesbian, gay, bisexual, or transgender. This equates to nearly 8% of the total U.S. adult population (U.S. Census Bureau, 2021b). The challenge in capturing the size and demographics of the LGBTQIA+ community in the United States is believed to be due to sampling and responder recall bias. Like other populations identified as at-risk, research has demonstrated that individuals who identify as LGBTQIA+ face disparities in care because of their sexual orientation. Gender and gender identity have complex effects on health; therefore a nurse must acquire a high level of cultural competence and sensitivity in their interactions and care of their clients. Culturally congruent nursing care aligns with each person's lifestyle, values, beliefs, and preferences (Fig. 5-5). This approach helps the nurse to understand the experiences of clients who identify as LGBTQIA+, to be aware of biases that are barriers to care, and to ensure that clients have access to the support person of their choice (Medina-Martínez et al, 2021).

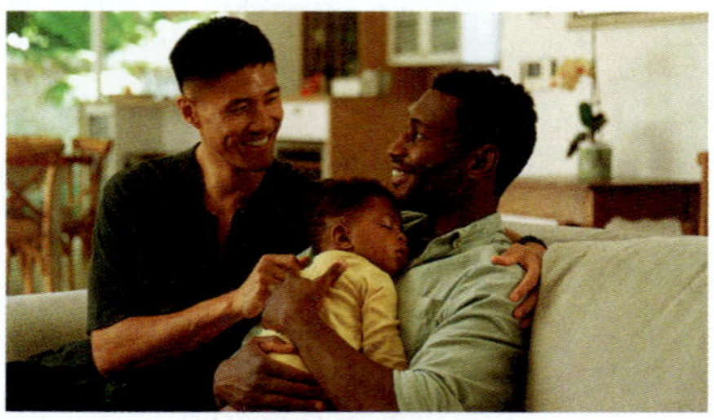

Figure 5-5 LGBTQIA+ individuals and families have unique health needs.

Nurses should not make gender assumptions based on name or appearance. Do not assume a person who has polished nails and makeup on their face self-identifies as a female. **Gender identity** refers to how a person manifests or expresses their gender, including male, female, or nonbinary. **Nonbinary individuals** do not identify with one specific gender; instead, they view themselves as somewhere on the spectrum. They may also identify as gender-fluid, whereby, their gender identity may change across their life span (Mendoza et al, 2020).

Affirmative care is defined as an approach to health-care delivery in which organizations and providers recognize, validate, and support the identity stated or expressed by the individuals served. Nurses should be mindful that people who belong to socially marginalized groups may present with mistrust and fear of the health-care system. Practicing culturally sensitive care while conducting comprehensive assessments and interviews will consist of eliciting information on gender identity as well as the individual's past interactions with the health-care system (Mendoza et al, 2020).

The Core Elements of Culture

The core elements of the client's culture should be known and understood to deliver culturally competent nursing care. The core elements of culture are language, communication variables, communication patterns, cultural norms, cultural values, symbols, and artifacts.

Language

Language is the principal method of human communication conveyed by speech, writing, or gestures. Health-care regulatory bodies such as The Centers for Medicare and Medicaid (CMS) and The Joint Commission (TJC) mandate health-care workers to assess and provide language assistance services to those with limited English proficiency to effectively communicate. Research shows that hospitalized clients with limited English proficiency are more likely to experience an adverse event that results in harm. Communication error is the most identified cause of adverse events. An exchange of information must ensure clients and providers are understood (Office of Disease Prevention and Health Promotion, 2019). Clear delivery and receipt of information and avoidance of ambiguous messages will enhance communication and facilitate the client's experience with admission assessment, management of care, end-of-life care, medication management, discharge, and transfer of care. Limited English proficiency in the United States is a barrier to accessing and navigating health care and health literacy, which is understanding health information. Title VI of the U.S. Civil Rights Act of 1964: Language Access for LEP Persons, ensures meaningful access for Limited English Proficient (LEP) individuals. Health-care organizations are mandated to provide interpreters who demonstrate proficiency in the ability to communicate information accurately in both English and other languages (The Joint Commission, 2016). In seeking clarification of the meaning that clients from other cultures attach to their illness experiences, it is important to accurately identify and then remove or overcome any language barriers that may exist. A variety of language barriers may exist even between two people for whom English is the first language, particularly if these individuals use different forms of English. Language barriers may be due to different connotative meanings of words, the use of clichés, a reliance on jargon specific to one individual's background, the complexity of the sentence structure, the different meanings attached to specific types of body language, and the use of value-laden terms. When English is the client's second language, a serious language barrier may arise (even for those proficient in their second language) if the client is anxious or ill and has limited energy to invest in speaking and understanding English (Fig. 5-6).

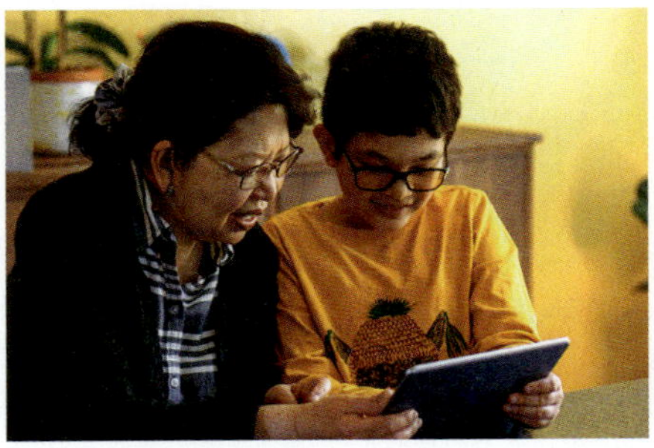

Figure 5-6 This boy is helping his non-English speaking grandmother complete a form in English.

Communication Variables

The process of communication is universal, however, the intonation, rhythm, speed, use of silence, facial expressions, eye contact, head movements, body posture, touch, social distancing, topics, and direct and indirect questioning—as well as other "rules" for communication—may be culturally unique.

In some cultures, movement of the head may mean the exact opposite of what it represents in Western cultures. For example, Bulgarians nod their head to indicate "no" and move their head back and forth to indicate "yes." In other cultures, a "yes" answer may be indicated in some other way, such as among the Tongans, from the Pacific Islands, who raise their eyebrows to answer "yes" to a question.

Communication Patterns

Communication patterns include both verbal and nonverbal means of expressing or concealing thoughts and feelings of joy, sorrow, grief, happiness, anger, acceptance, fear, love, and the full range of human experiences. Communication practices also reflect, determine, and ultimately mold the culture. Communication patterns include both verbal and nonverbal means of expressing or concealing thoughts and feelings of joy, sorrow, grief, happiness, anger, acceptance, fear, love, and the full range of human experiences.

Communicating distress associated with illness has cultural variability. Adults and children in some cultures are expected to endure pain stoically; in other cultures, individuals use expressive reactions to communicate distress. In some cultures, the expression of thoughts and feelings is open and dramatic, with frequent touching and sharing of territorial space. In other cultures, such open expressions are regarded as unacceptable. Some clients may consider it acceptable to avoid confrontation and unacceptable to overtly express annoyance or anger.

The nurse needs to listen to the client's description of symptoms, reflect on the meaning the client attaches to the symptoms (e.g., body language, grimaces, guarding), restate the inferred meaning, and allow the client time to determine whether the inferred-meaning statement accurately reflects the client's reality. In addition, the following may be helpful:

- Speak slowly and distinctly in a normal tone.
- Avoid clichés, jargon, and value-laden terms.
- Avoid defensive or offensive body language.
- Ask the client to restate information in their own words to confirm understanding.
- Provide reading material written in the appropriate language.
- Provide a language-proficient interpreter (remote access or in-person).
- Speak to the client, not to the interpreter.

Cultural Norms

Cultural norms are the often unwritten, but generally understood, actions for acceptable behavior in designated situations encountered by group members during their daily lives. Every group member is bound by these norms and may be criticized, punished, or ostracized by other group members when the norms are violated.

Cultural Values

Cultures and subcultures have a fundamental set of principles known as **values** that govern the behavior of all members of the group. These values prescribe how each member should think, act, and respond to their internal and external environments. **Cultural values** are a fundamental, often unshakable, and unwavering set of principles that serve as the foundation upon which an individual's beliefs, customs, goals, and aspirations are built.

Symbols

Symbols represent values and ideas that may be unique or may have shared meanings. Symbols are enduring identifiable behaviors (Fig. 5-7) or objects such as crosses, clothing, flags, colors, toasting with a glass in celebration, chants, and gestures. A symbol represents values, ideas, and traditions understood among members of the group. The nurse needs to understand that the meaning of cultural symbols/gestures is not universally understood/shared and may be perceived as offensive. For example, in some cultures "finger-pointing" is a sign of disrespect.

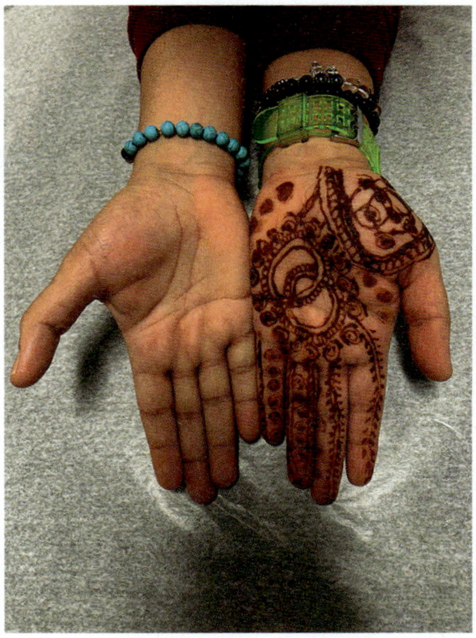

Figure 5-7 Henna-adorned hands are an important symbol for the Indian bride.

Artifacts

Artifacts are amulets/objects/trinkets used by individuals of different cultures to ensure health and luck or to ward off evil.

Racial Prejudice, Ethnic Discrimination, and Stereotyping

Individual or group experiences of racial prejudice, ethnic discrimination, and stereotyping, whether perceived or actual are harmful, hurtful experiences that can have both psychological and physiological impacts on the well-being and health conditions of the individual or group, often resulting in shame, fear, physical symptoms, and social isolation. **Prejudices** are negative, harmful, preconceived attitudes and beliefs directed toward an individual, group, culture, gender, or behavior that limit accurate perceptions. Examples of prejudice include homophobia, Islamophobia, and antisemitism. **Stereotyping** is classifying individuals and groups based on culture or race with rigid characteristics while failing to recognize individual and group variations (McFarland & Wehbe-Alamah, 2018). **Discrimination** is overt or covert actions that limit opportunities to access health care, housing, education, and employment based on cultural or racial biases. Discrimination can impact individuals or entire groups of people. An example of discrimination impacting a large group of people started with the SARS-CoV2 (COVID-19) pandemic.

The first coronavirus case was identified in Wuhan, China, in late December 2019. After the World Health Organization (WHO) officially declared the outbreak of the coronavirus to be a pandemic, almost two million excess deaths were reported globally within 6 months (WHO, 2021). The number of deaths caused by COVID-19 increased daily in the early pandemic, leading to shocking images of overcrowded hospitals and makeshift graveyards worldwide. In addition, prevention policies such as travel bans, closed schools, and complete lockdowns significantly altered people's daily lives. The fear of the virus as a physical threat tended to bring greater prejudice and racial intolerance toward the Chinese and mistrust related to theories regarding the circumstances surrounding the outbreak. The unprecedented course of events drew negative attention, by association, to those of Asian ethnicity/race. During the pandemic, emerging research indicates that people with an East Asian background, especially Chinese, experienced COVID-19-related acute racial-ethnic discrimination.

Most of the studies were conducted in the United States and collected data after the outbreak. The fact that this new virus was detected first in China led to racialized descriptions of the virus, such as it being labeled "the Chinese virus" in public discourse. Although discrimination experiences have negative mental health outcomes, they can also strengthen an individual's heritage-culture and ethnic identity and emphasize solidarity when dealing with negative attitudes regarding their ethnic group (Yang et al, 2022).

Value Orientations

All cultures have a fundamental set of values and concurrent **value orientations**, that is, patterned principles that provide order and give direction to individuals' thoughts and behaviors related to the solution of commonly occurring human problems (Weil, 2020). Three areas about which cultures have their own unique value orientations have major relevance for culturally competent assessments and care (Table 5-1). These value orientations are time, relational, and people to nature.

Cultural Health Beliefs

Cultural beliefs and preferences can influence the perception of health and illness and how individuals/groups make decisions related to their health. Asking clients to describe their cultural and ethnic beliefs can help the nurse to engage so that, together, they can create treatment plans that are consistent with the client's values.

Such beliefs influence the "meaning" individuals attach to health and illness, how clients prefer to treat illness (traditional/alternative), whom they prefer to be treated by (male/female/traditional/faith healer), and the health behaviors (preventative/curative/palliative/acceptance), in which they are willing to engage. Because health and illness are culturally determined, what may be health or illness in one culture may not be in another. In addition, many cultures distinguish between a **folk illness**, believed to be caused by disharmony or an imbalance or as punishment, and a **scientific illness**, in which the presence of pathology is the defining characteristic. In these cultures, a **folk practitioner** (a healer or other individual who is not part of the scientific health-care system but is believed to have special knowledge or power to prevent, treat, or provide resources needed to heal folk illnesses) is consulted for a folk illness, because health-care practitioners are not believed to be knowledgeable in recognizing or treating such illnesses.

Respectfully ask clients about their health beliefs and cultural preferences and note their responses in their clinical records. Address clients' cultural values specifically in the context of their health care. Understand that each person is an individual and may or may not adhere to certain cultural beliefs or practices common in their culture. Asking clients about their beliefs and preferences is the best way to be sure you know how their values may impact their care.

Nurses need to commit to life-long learning, which includes reading nursing professional and interdisciplinary journals, as well as valid, reliable, and secure Web sites to enhance skills and knowledge to gain cultural competency related to specific groups (Agency for Healthcare Research and Quality [AHRQ], 2015).

Table 5-1 Basic Cross-Cultural Values, Value Orientations, and Beliefs

Value	Value Orientation and Beliefs
Time What is the time orientation of human beings?	*Past* focus: Reverence for long-standing traditions. *Present* focus: Live in the "here and now," perceive time in a linear fashion. *Future* focus: Willing to defer gratification to ensure they can meet a future goal; tend to be disciplined in scheduling and using time.
Relational What is the purpose of human relations?	*Linear* relationships: Welfare and goals of the *hereditary and extended family* are emphasized. Goals of the family take precedence over the individuals. *Collateral* relationships: Welfare and goals of *social and family groups* are emphasized. Group goals take precedence. *Individual* relationships: *Individual* goals and accountability for own behavior emphasized.
People to Nature What is the relationship of human beings to nature?	Human beings *dominate nature* and have control over their environment. Human beings *live in harmony with nature* and must maintain that balance. Human beings are *subjugated to nature* and have no control over their environment.

Folk Illnesses

Two major types of folk illnesses are naturalistic and personalistic. **Naturalistic illnesses** are believed to be caused by an imbalance or disequilibrium between essentially impersonal factors. For example, the most common imbalance is between "hot" and "cold" (Table 5-2). Illnesses and treatments that are classified as either hot or cold are culturally determined and do not have any relationship to the actual temperature of the client or the substances used to treat the illness. In general, "hot" illnesses are treated with "cold" substances and vice versa to restore the balance between the two. These beliefs are held by many Hispanic, Middle Eastern, and Asian ethnic groups and cultures. Although most cultures that share these beliefs use the hot and cold terminology, among traditional Chinese, these forces are called *yin* (cold) and *yang* (hot).

Personalistic illnesses are believed to occur because an individual has committed some offense and is being punished, or the illness results from acts of aggression (sometimes unintentional) by other individuals. Witchcraft and the "evil eye" are two sources of personalistic illnesses (Fig. 5-8). Witchcraft is believed to be the cause of illness among some Haitians, Hispanics, and some Black Americans. Witchcraft may be used to punish individuals for an emotional or a physical injury, an illness, or a death they are thought to have caused, or occasionally because they possess something that is coveted by another.

The "evil eye" belief is shared by many Mediterranean (e.g., Italian, Sicilian, and Greek), African, and Hispanic cultures. The "evil eye" is often given unintentionally, for example, by complimenting a child who is unprotected by an amulet, gold cross, or other protective device, or by not touching the child while offering the compliment.

Table 5-2 Hot and Cold Conditions and Foods

Hot Conditions and Foods (Caliente/Yang)	
Hot Conditions	**Hot Foods**
Constipation	Beans
Diarrhea	Cheese
Fever	Chocolate
Hypertension	Eggs
Infections	Oils
Kidney problems	Onions
Liver problems	Vinegar
Pregnancy	Wine
	Peas
Cold Conditions and Foods (Frio/Yin)	
Cold Conditions	**Cold Foods**
Cancer	Avocado
Colds	Barley water
Depression	Bean curds
Earache	Cashew nuts
Headache	Dairy products
Infertility	Green vegetables
Joint pain	Tropical fruits
Teething	
Tuberculosis	

Compiled from data appearing in Ormsby, S. (2021). Hot and cold theory: Evidence in nutrition. *Advances in Experimental Medicine and Biology, 1343*, 87–107, doi: 10.1007/978-3-030-80983-6_6; and Yavari, M. (2021). *Hot and cold theory: The path toward personalized medicine* (Vol. 1343). Springer.

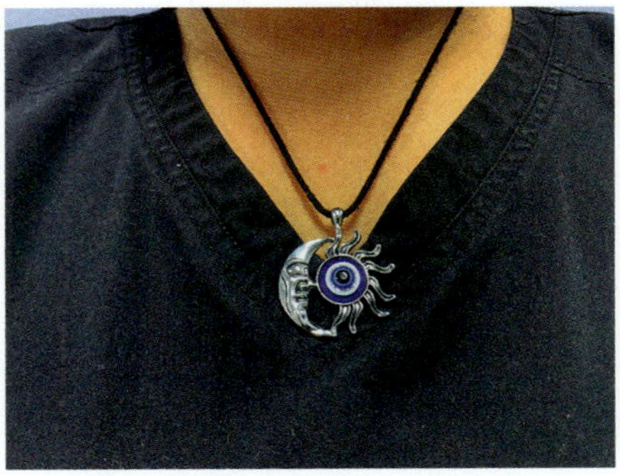

Figure 5-8 People who wear the evil eye believe it protects them against misfortune.

Preserving, Accommodating, and Repatterning Self-Care Practices

Cultural groups use a variety of self-care practices that may include the use of "folk medicine remedies." Self-care includes practices in which individuals/groups engage on their own behalf to aid in health promotion and maintenance, disease or injury prevention, or treatment. For example, a person of Vietnamese heritage may use *cao gio* (skin rubbing with a coin) to treat diseases they believe are caused by wind or cold air entering the body (e.g., upper respiratory infections). After applying oil or an ointment on the skin over the affected body area (chest, shoulders, upper back), the edge of a coin is moved along the skin until ecchymosis (bruised) stripes appear, demonstrating that the treatment is successful. *Cao gio* is rarely painful or injurious and often is perceived to be helpful by the recipient, whether coincidental or proof-positive that the treatment is therapeutic. Discovering these areas of ecchymosis may cause concern if nurses lack this knowledge regarding folk practices or fail to engage in discussion with the client/family support system regarding cultural healing practices.

According to pioneer nurse anthropologist and culture care nursing theorist Madeline Leininger, nurses must be able to make decisions and develop and implement plans of care for individuals/groups, regardless of culture by focusing on three principles: cultural care preservation or maintenance, cultural care accommodation or negotiation, and cultural care repatterning or restructuring. *Cultural care preservation or maintenance* is the principle of helping, facilitating, or focusing on cultural phenomena to enable individuals to determine their desired lifestyle and level of health. *Cultural care accommodation or negotiation* encompasses the principles of negotiation, support, assistance, or focus on cultural phenomena. It reflects ways to adapt and allow creative professional actions and decisions to assist clients from the culture designated to negotiate or consider health and lifestyle conditions. *Cultural care repatterning* or *restructuring* is the process of working with clients to reconstruct or change health behaviors to improve their health conditions and lifestyles. Cultural restructuring is carried out if the culture is detrimental to health status (Hidayat & Uliyah, 2019). For example, Hispanic clients may insist on being given penicillin, which is considered *caliente* (hot) treatment, for a viral upper respiratory infection (URI), which is considered a *frio* (cold) condition. Explanations about the lack of benefit in treating viral URIs with penicillin and the potential for building resistance to penicillin when used unnecessarily will rarely dissuade those who insist on its use. Alternatively, vitamins can be recommended by the prescriber, which are also considered a *caliente* (hot) treatment. This strategy demonstrates an acceptance of the client's beliefs and avoidance of harm. This exemplifies culture care accommodation, an effort to achieve the shared goal of an optimal health outcome for clients of a designated culture (McFarland & Wehbe-Alamah, 2018).

Assessing the Potential for Harm Associated With a Cultural Belief or Behavior

When assessing their own cultural values and beliefs and the behaviors that result from these values and beliefs, nurses are often faced with having to decide when it is appropriate for their cultural value orientation to take precedence over that of the client. In other words, how is a culturally competent nurse to evaluate and decide when a decision or procedure is adaptive, harmful, or neutral?

The nurse may be conflicted about participating in a procedure but be committed to ensuring quality client care. Each nurse must ultimately resolve their own cultural/ethical conflict with either reconciliation or refusal to participate on an individual client basis. The nurse is guided by the ANA Code of Ethics, which serves as a social contract with the public that it serves. The ANA Code of Ethics for nurses reflects the fundamental value, to do no harm (ANA, 2015).

Ethnic Customs and Cultural Rituals

Customs and rituals are culturally learned behaviors that are much easier to observe or learn about through interviewing than the values and beliefs on which the customs and rituals are based. **Customs** are frequent or common practices carried out by tradition and include communication patterns, family and kinship relations, work patterns, religious and dietary practices, and health behaviors and practices (Fig. 5-9). **Cultural rituals** are highly structured and prescribed patterns of behavior used by a cultural group to respond to or in anticipation of specific life events such as birth, death, illness, healing, marriage, worship, and other important events.

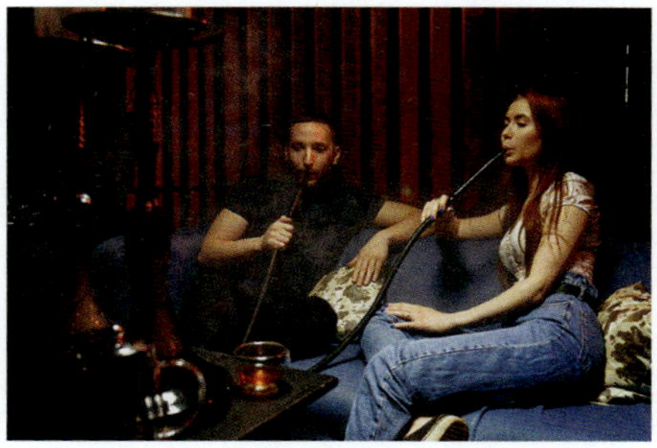

Figure 5-9 Young adults socializing while smoking shisha (hookah) and drinking Arabic tea.

Cultural Meaning of Symptoms

One of the most important techniques when performing a culturally competent health assessment is to make every effort to discover the cultural meaning of the client's perceptions and to encourage the client to communicate interpretations of health, illness, and symptoms. When people experience pain or other symptoms associated with sickness or illness, they interpret and react to the symptoms in ways that reflect their cultural norms. When attempting to discover the cultural meaning the client gives to symptoms, the nurse must be concerned with eliciting statements about symptoms the client considers to be significant, as well as symptoms the client believes to be an expected part of one's life.

In addition, each culture has its own system for communicating the distress associated with illness. For example, some cultures may endure pain stoically and expect this behavior from others. Others may use expressive reactions to communicate pain but hide pain from their families and closest friends.

The nurse should listen carefully to the client's description of symptoms, paying close attention to body language and gestures and reflecting on the meaning the client seems to attach to the symptoms. The nurse then can restate the inferred meaning and allow the client time to determine whether the reflected inferred-meaning statement accurately reflects the client's own reality. Then the nurse can restate and restructure the inferred meaning until the client validates its accuracy.

Family and Kinship Relations

Across cultures, family and kinship patterns have taken the form of linear, collateral, or individualistic, with the basic, traditional family unit being the nuclear family in all three patterns: parents living with children in one household. When the family has a linear pattern, that may consist of the nuclear family in addition to extended family members such as grandparents, aunts, uncles, and cousins. The collateral family structure consists of the individual's siblings and their children. Individualistic kinship patterns are independent of one another, and reliance is considered shameful and weak.

The linear family is usually patriarchal, led by the father figure, placing a strong emphasis on the decisions imposed on the family and respect for the elder family members. Asian, Middle Eastern, and some European American families tend to have linear family kinship patterns. The welfare, continuity, and goals of a linear family centered unit take precedence over those of the individual family member.

Families in which collateral patterns are the norm emphasize the welfare and goals of the lateral group members, such as the families of siblings and close peers, as well as of the nuclear family, and an individual's goals are subordinate to those of the social family group. These families tend to socialize primarily within their social family group, are generally open in their expressions of friendship, and highly value their children. Both parents, if present in the household, participate in decision-making, particularly in relation to child-rearing and caring. Examples of collateral family kinship

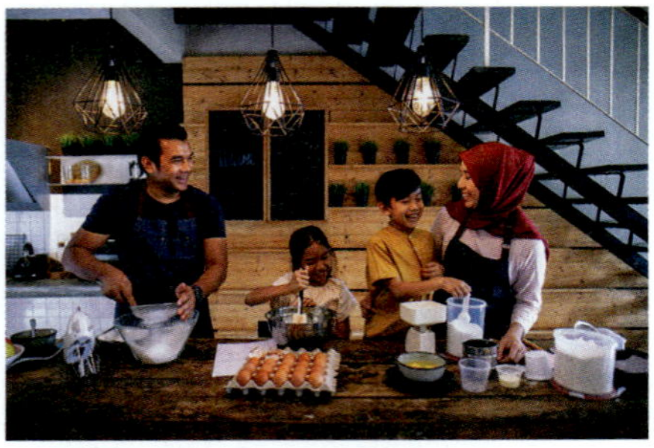

Figure 5-10 The number of traditional nuclear families is decreasing.

patterns are found among Hispanic American and American Indian families, and among many new immigrants to the United States, who tend to live in ethnically homogeneous neighborhoods and regions.

In cultures in which the individualistic, nuclear family pattern is prevalent, the individual family member's goals take precedence and self-responsibility and accountability for one's own behavior are the norm. Although there is less sense of responsibility for older adult family members, generosity in times of crises is characteristic. Sharing of parental responsibilities between parents is common.

Two-parent households are on the decline in the United States as divorce, remarriage, and cohabitation are on the rise. Families are smaller now, both due to the growth of single-parent households and the drop in fertility. Not only are Americans having fewer children, but the circumstances surrounding parenthood have changed. While in the early 1960s babies typically arrived within a marriage, today four-in-ten births occur to women who are single or living with a nonmarital partner. While family structures have transformed, so has the role of mothers in the workplace—and in the home. As more mothers have entered the labor force, more have become breadwinners—in many cases, *primary* breadwinners—in their families (Center, 2015).

As a result of these changes, there is no longer one dominant family configuration in the United States (Fig. 5-10). Parents today are raising their children against a backdrop of increasingly diverse and, for many, constantly evolving family forms. In 1960, the height of the post–World War II baby boom, the nuclear family was the dominant family form. At that time, 73% of all children were living in a family with two married parents in their first marriage. By 1980, 61% of children were living in this type of family, and today less than half (46%) are. The declining percentage of children living in what is often deemed a "traditional nuclear" family has decreased (Center, 2015).

Among these nontraditional families are blended families, single-parent families, intergenerational families, same-sex families, multiracial families, and foster families. Understanding the family characteristics and configuration is essential in determining who should be involved in health-care decisions and who should be taught about providing the health care needed by the family member who is ill.

When assessing the family, kinship, and work patterns, it is important to determine the family's actual structure. It may be helpful to draw a genogram (see Chapter 3) and an ecomap (refer to Case Study). An **ecomap** is a diagram depicting a person's relationship with their family, as well as with significant friends, peers, neighbors, and work associates, noting those with whom the client has the most frequent contact and their relative importance to the client.

> **NURSING CHECKLIST**
>
> **General Approach to Cultural Assessment**
>
> 1. Observe standard precautions and don personal protective equipment (PPE) such as gloves, gown, face shield, goggles, or N-95 respirator or face mask if the client's status warrants these protective measures.
> 2. If possible, choose a quiet, private room that will be free from interruptions.
>   Position yourself at eye level with the client.
> 3. Greet the client, introduce yourself, and explain that you will be discussing the client's culture and cultural background in order to provide culturally competent nursing care.
> 4. Portray an interested, nonjudgmental manner throughout the interview.

Culturally Competent Assessment

Assessing a client's cultural beliefs, values, and customs through observation during the client's health history and physical examination is an essential component of performing a culturally competent assessment and planning for culturally competent nursing care. The cultural health practices specific to the client's culture are critical to assessment, planning, and prescribing of nursing interventions.

Cultural Assessment

The cultural assessment should address those areas having a direct impact on the client's immediate health status. Many different cultural assessment tools can be used by the nurse in the clinical setting. This text illustrates an adaptation of the well-known tool by Rachel Spector (2017) (Fig. 5-11). Nurses need to be familiar with the culture of the client before conducting a cultural assessment.

Directions: The questions in bold print are recommended for use during the initial contact with the client. The remaining items can be used during the initial contact if time permits or if examples are needed to prompt the client's replies. If a long-term health-care relationship or prolonged hospitalization and/or home care is anticipated, it is advisable to complete all remaining questions during subsequent encounters (Spector, 2017).

Cultural Assessment Tool

- **Where were you born? Where were your parents born?**
- **What pronoun do you use (e.g., he/him, she/her, they/them)?**
- **In what language are you most comfortable speaking and reading?**
- **Did you grow up in a city, town, or rural setting?**
- **When you were growing up, who lived with you and your family?**
- Are your friends from the same cultural background as you?
- **What is your religious preference?**
- **Do you have any dietary preferences related to your religious or cultural beliefs?**
- In your culture, how do you celebrate the birth of a baby? A wedding?
- When a person is pregnant, are there any special customs they need to follow? Any special foods?
- **When someone in your family is ill, who cares for them? What foods are prepared? Is there anything the ill person should avoid or refrain from doing?**
- **What home remedies might be used if someone is ill?**
- As a family member is approaching death, what actions do you find comforting?
- After a loved one dies, what rituals are performed?
- **What do you think a nurse should know about your culture if a family member is hospitalized?**
- **Who makes the decisions in your family?**
- How are older adults viewed in your culture?
- **Are there any special beliefs regarding organ donation or blood transfusions that are held in your culture?**
- Is your culture known for any special customs (e.g., rites of passage, foods, holidays, etc.)?

Adapted from Spector, 2017.

Figure 5-11 Cultural Assessment Tool.

U.S. Preventive Services Task Force (USPSTF)

There are no USPSTF recommendations, Grade A or B Statements, for cultural assessment.

CASE STUDY

A Vietnamese Au Pair With Dysmenorrhea

Tran Le Mai, a 22-year-old female, has recently immigrated to the United States on a work/student visa from Vietnam. Mai has been sponsored by an American family, the Orems, to care for their two young children, as an au pair. Mai will also be able to enroll in remote classes offered at the city university to earn credits toward an accounting degree.

Before arriving in the United States, Mai began to experience severe pelvic cramping and passing of blood clots during her menses. She attributed these symptoms to the anxiety of leaving her family and beloved village, Duong Lam, in Hanoi. She has never traveled outside of her village. However, she knew her move to the United States would benefit her family.

One afternoon, Mrs. Kara Orem noticed Mai doubled over in pain as Mai was preparing to take the children to the park. Mai tried to dismiss the incident in fear she would be sent back to Vietnam and lose the opportunity to work, attend school, and leave this family she had grown to love.

Kara recognized Mai's fears and convinced Mai to make an appointment at the Women's Health Center. Kara assured Mai she would accompany her to the first appointment.

Initial Appointment at the Women's Health Center

Cultural Assessment

Introduction: *Hello, I am Judith Lepore, a Nurse Practitioner (NP).**

Please tell me your name and date of birth.

Response: Hello, Nurse Lepore, my name is Tran Le Mai, please call me, Mai.

My birthdate is: June 15, 2001.

** This question is added to provide additional client information and is not a part of the Spector tool.*

[The Nurse observes] Mai sits at the edge of the examination table, leans forward, and gently guards her pelvic area with her hands. In her right hand, she tightly clutches a small silk pouch, which she tells me has a piece of jade that her mother gave to her on her 21st birthday. She is quiet and shy and does not look directly at me when she speaks.* *This observation is added to provide additional client information and is not a part of the Spector tool.*

What has brought you to the Health Center today?*

"I do not think I am sick. I think I am out of balance. I think I am still experiencing some Lo ngại [anxiety] and homesickness being very far away from home. I have pain in my stomach [points to pelvis] and lose blood with clots during my kinh nguyệt [menses]."

** This question is added to provide additional client information and is not a part of the Spector tool.*

Where were you born? Where were your parents born?

"I am from a small village, Duong Lam, in Hanoi. I am Vietnamese. I am from Northern Vietnam. This my heritage and makes me feel close to my family even though I am in the United States. My family and our ways are all I know. My parents were born there, too."

What pronoun do you use (e.g., he, she, they)?

"I am a she."

In what language are you most comfortable speaking and reading?

"I speak and read Vietnamese, but I also learned to speak, read, and write English in school in Vietnam."

Did you grow up in a city, town, or rural setting?

"Duong Lam, in Hanoi, is in northern Vietnam, and it is a small village."

When you were growing up, who lived with you and your family?

"I lived with my mother, father, older sister, my father's parents, and my mother's sister."

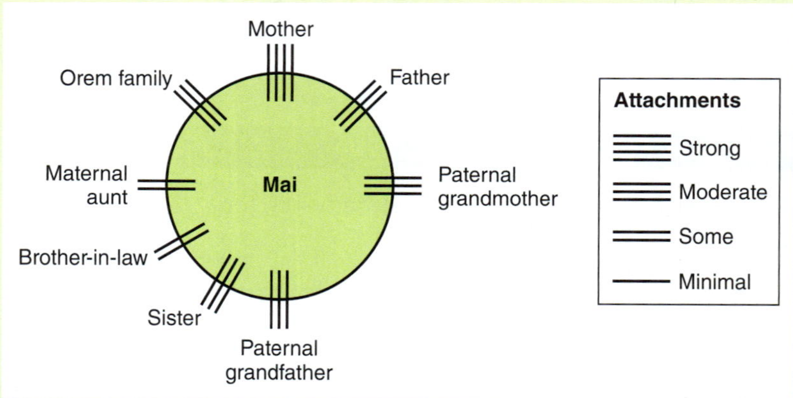

Ecomap

Are your friends from the same cultural background as you?

"Yes, back home in Vietnam. I have made few friends here. At school, I meet people from China and Korea."

What is your religious preference?

"We are Buddhist."

Do you have any dietary preferences related to your religious or cultural beliefs?

"Yes, I am vegetarian, as is my whole family. Kara always has fresh fruit and vegetables and noodles or rice for me. She make it easy for me. She like it too, she says, healthy."

In your culture, how do you celebrate the birth of a baby? A wedding?

"First, my sister's husband and his family ask my father for permission to get married. Then, "le an hoi," they announce engagement to whole family. Buddhist monk set their wedding date. On the wedding day, everyone brings small gifts to our house. There was an altar (small table) in my house, and my sister and husband pray for happiness and good luck in their marriage. Then a reception at her husband family house."

Initial Appointment at the Women's Health Center—cont'd

"When my sister gave birth, she could not shower for 1 month and had to rest indoors. We all help her. When baby was 1 month old, we have celebration."

When a person is pregnant, are there any special customs they need to follow? Any special foods?

"The first trimester of pregnancy is a 'cold' state. Women are recommended to eat 'hot' foods, including ginger and black pepper and to avoid 'cold' foods, including lemon, melon, pineapple, spinach, and green papaya. In the second trimester, which is 'neutral' state, women allowed to eat these foods. In the third trimester, which is a 'hot' state, women may decrease the amount of food they eat."

When someone in your family is ill, who cares for them? What foods are prepared? Is there anything the ill person should avoid or refrain from doing?

"I have not experienced bad sickness. Me [referring to her mother] takes care of us when we are sick."

"Me [my mother] would make sure we stay clean with sponge baths; this helps us to stay healthy. She would make me hot teas with ginger root, chamomile, and cinnamon, Yang [hot treatment] for my stomach cramps, this is Yin [cold condition]. She makes sure we are warm with woolen socks and hot water bottle on our bellies, even in summer. She also rubs Tiger balm over our bellies."

What home remedies might be used if someone is ill?

"Sometimes, Me would massage, scrape my skin with coin, make herb tea and soup."

As a family member is approaching death, what actions do you find comforting? After a loved one dies, what rituals are performed?

"We stay with our dying loved ones until they pass. Then we keep our loved one at home after their death for 3 days to a month. Family members dress their loved one in traditional white clothing, place rice and three coins in their mouth, and position a chopstick between their teeth."

What do you think a nurse should know about your culture if a family member is hospitalized?

"Please allow family or Vietnamese friend to stay with person. Please consider Yin and yang when assisting with meals. Arrange Buddhist priest to visit person. If family present, they may ask you to not discuss illness with person."

Have you ever been examined by a specialized doctor in Vietnam, called a gynecologist?*

No, my Me and Bố [father] *say only for my sister, Lin dahn, she is married. I am afraid, I am still a virgin, and a husband in my future would not accept me if I had this done." (*This question is added to provide additional client information and is not a part of the Spector tool.)*

Who makes the decisions in your family?

"My father makes decisions in our family, but my mother, in her quiet way, sometime influence my father. They have a special marriage. When I was younger, my grandfather made the decisions, but father says, his time to rest."

How are older adults viewed in your culture?

"Always respected."

Are there any special beliefs regarding organ donation or blood transfusions that are held in your culture?

"We accept blood transfusion. Buddha does not restrict us."

Is your culture known for any special customs (e.g., rites of passage, foods, holidays, etc.)?

"We love Tet, Vietnamese New Year! It lasts 7–9 days. This year it is February 17, year of the horse."

The NP returns to the examination room to discuss the plan of care:

Mai, with your permission, I would like to examine the area of your abdomen, where you feel discomfort. I will lightly touch your abdomen. Kara can remain in the room with you if you prefer. This will not be an internal pelvic examination. To do this, I will need to expose only your abdomen.

I would then like to perform an abdominal ultrasound, which means I will use a wand-like device that will scan externally over your abdomen. This will allow me to visualize the uterus and bladder in your pelvis. The device will have cool liquid jelly on it. It will not be painful. After this, I will prescribe a medication, which is a nonsteroidal anti-inflammatory medication, that you can begin 7 days before your next menstrual cycle until your menstrual flow is complete. I would like you to keep a journal of your menstrual cramping and bleeding for the next 6 weeks. Then I would like you to return in 6 weeks to have a follow-up appointment with me. The NP then asks Mai:

1. Are you comfortable with this plan?
2. Do you have questions/concerns for me?

Mai's response: "Thank you, Nurse Lepore, I am comfortable with this plan. I was afraid to come here. Afraid your clinic would not understand me. I am grateful to Kara for bringing me here today. I am no longer afraid."

CLINICAL JUDGMENT IN ACTION

1. What cues indicate that the client is experiencing a challenging medical appointment that can cause her anxiety?
2. What interventions have the highest priority?
3. What findings indicate a successful client encounter during which the nurse demonstrated cultural sensitivity and competence?

Review Questions

1. A client believes that treating their illness with *frio* (cold) foods will make them feel better. Which of the following foods are considered *frio*? Select all that apply.
   a. Cashew nuts
   b. Dairy products
   c. Onions
   d. Peas
   e. Cheese
   f. Barley water

2. Which of the following statements describes acculturation?
   a. Often unwritten, but generally understood, prescriptions for acceptable behavior by members of a cultural group.
   b. An informal process of adaptation through which the beliefs, values, norms, and practices of a dominant mainstream culture are learned by new members born into a different culture.
   c. Belief that no culture is either inferior or superior to another; that behavior must be evaluated in relation to the cultural context in which it occurs; and that respect, equality, and justice are basic rights for all racial, ethnic, subcultural, and cultural groups.
   d. Learned and socially transmitted orientation and way of life specific to a group of people with similar lifeways.

3. The nurse is educating a client newly diagnosed with diabetes and notices the client is looking away. This is the client's first health care visit in the United States since moving from another country. What action should the nurse take?
   a. Walk toward the client's gaze to ensure eye contact.
   b. Speak louder, as the client may be hearing impaired.
   c. Postpone the education, as the client appears disinterested.
   d. Confirm the client's understanding of the information after the teaching is completed.

4. The nurse admits a 14-year-old client, named Dylan, with the medical diagnosis of anxiety disorder. The medical record indicates the client's sex as male. The nurse notices that Dylan's fingernails are painted bright orange and facial makeup is worn. Which comment by the nurse indicates bias? Select all that apply.
   a. Dylan, why are you wearing nail polish? You're a boy.
   b. Dylan, you should have removed your nail polish before coming to the hospital. Only girls wear nail polish in public.
   c. Dylan, you are wearing eye makeup. Are you performing in a play at school?
   d. Dylan, no wonder you have anxiety. You have gender confusion!

5. A nurse whose background includes growing up in a linear family deeply committed to their faith is assigned to take care of a female client with pelvic pain. The client introduces her female visitor as her wife. The nurse proceeds to care for her client. Her care is thorough and her rapport with the client is professional and caring. Which term best describes the nurse's behavior?
   a. Cultural bias
   b. Ethnocentric
   c. Cultural indifference
   d. Cultural humility

6. The belief that illnesses occur because a person has committed some offense is called which of the following?
   a. *Cao gio* illness
   b. Personalistic illness
   c. Naturalistic illness
   d. Scientific illness

7. Which statement made by the nurse caring for an older adult client of Bolivian heritage with uncontrolled diabetes indicates a need for cultural competence training?
   a. Your high blood sugar levels are from all the rice, corn, and tortillas you eat.
   b. Would you like me to include your daughter in the conversation about meal preparation and your medications?
   c. Tell me how your diabetes medications make you feel.
   d. Show me how you use the glucometer.

8. Which of the following statements are components of the American Nurses Association standards for developing culturally competent nursing practice? Select all that apply.
   a. Demonstrates respect, equity, and empathy in actions and interactions with all health-care consumers
   b. Respects consumer decisions without bias
   c. Participates in life-long learning to understand cultural preferences, worldviews, choices, and decision-making processes of diverse consumers
   d. Reflects upon personal and cultural values, beliefs, biases, and heritage
   e. Applies knowledge of differences in health beliefs, practices, and communication patterns without assigning value to the differences

9. The nurse is caring for a client who is dying. The client's family practices a ritual of burning incense around a dying person. Which response by the nurse demonstrates cultural care accommodation/negotiation?
   a. Inform the family of fire codes in the hospital which prohibit the lighting of incense while suggesting the family bring fragrant potpourri from home.
   b. Tell the family that the door must be kept closed while burning incense.
   c. Inform the family that the scent will make the client nauseous.
   d. Inform the family that if they don't tell anyone, the incense can be burned for 1 hour.

10. Which of the following cultural groups do not typically incorporate *folk practices* as a routine course of treatment?
    a. Filipinos
    b. Haitians
    c. European Americans
    d. Vietnamese

CHAPTER

Spiritual Assessment

6

Learning Outcomes

1. Describe how different spiritual beliefs influence the client's health, growth and development, illness, and death.
2. Identify the role of the nurse in the spiritual care of a client.
3. Discuss how to conduct a client's spiritual assessment.
4. Identify signs and symptoms indicating that the client may be experiencing spiritual distress.
5. Describe nursing interventions that promote the client's spiritual well-being.
6. Identify the effects of COVID-19 on clients' spirituality and religiosity.
7. Conduct a spiritual assessment on a client.

Clients' spiritual and religious beliefs will influence whether or not they will take medication, agree to surgery, have an abortion, follow a special diet, vaccinate, or execute an advance directive (Fig. 6-1) because spiritual and religious beliefs provide a worldview that guides humans in their life journey. Research shows that spiritual and religious beliefs produce measurable improvements in healthy behaviors as well as decreased morbidity and mortality associated with illness (Koenig, 2018). The Spiritual Assessment is the key to understanding and engaging clients' inner thoughts and resources, which improves client care and the relationship between clients and nurses (Christensen, 2018). The Joint Commission requires a Spiritual Assessment of every hospitalized client (Joint Commission, 2020).

Religion and Spirituality in the United States

Americans are religious people (Fig. 6-2). The United States has the largest number of Christians of any country in the world (Fig. 6-3) (World Population Review, 2025). According to Pew Research, in 2023-2024 the majority of Americans were Christians (62%) (combining Protestants, Catholics, Orthodox, and members of the Church of Jesus Christ of Latter-Day Saints, commonly called "Mormons"), but their numbers dropped significantly in the past decades from 2007 when 75% of Americans identified as Christians (Pew Research Center, 2025). Jews, Muslims, Buddhists, Hindus, New Age, Native American religions, and others make up an additional 7% of the religious population (Pew Research Center, 2025). Among these religions, there are varieties of world views, rituals, diets, and beliefs about medical care (Taylor, 2019). Specific information can be accessed online for these groups. Consult the websites listed in the online resources for additional information.

Of note is the marked increase of the 29% of Americans who describe themselves as "unaffiliated" without any formal religion or spiritual practices (Pew Research Center, 2025). This group includes the 5% of Americans who identify as atheists. Atheists don't believe in any god (Fig. 6-4). The "unaffiliated" group also includes 6% of Americans who identify as agnostics; agnostics are unsure if there is a god(s). These percentages remain low but have increased (Pew Research Center, 2025). The largest "unaffiliated" group in the United States, however, is the 19% of American adults who describe themselves as "nothing in particular." This group includes a wide variety of beliefs and practices, from New Age spiritualities, atheists, and agnostics, to people who pray and believe in God but have drifted away from membership and participation in a church, synagogue, temple, or mosque. This group may "mix and match" religious and spiritual practices and includes almost 40% of American millennials (Burton, 2020). Americans over the age of 65 have the strongest proportion of identification with Christianity (Public Religion Research Institute, 2020).

It might be easy to conclude that religion is aging out and atheism will be the dominant force in the future, but the data do not bear that out. In the United States, the rise in the religiously unaffiliated has slowed, whereas the decline in Christian attendance has stabilized (PRRI, 2020). Births are low among the unaffiliated and are high among the religious. "Projections anticipate that a vast majority of the world's people will continue to identify with a religion, including six-in-ten who will be either Christian (31%) or Muslim (30%) in 2050. Just 13% are projected to have no religion" (Pew Research Center, 2022a).

Government persecution of religion globally has increased globally, involving 183 countries in 2021, "the largest number since the study began" (Pew Research Center, 2024a). The nurse should keep this in mind when discussing religion with clients. Some clients may be hesitant to open up about their religious or spiritual beliefs. In the United States, where religious and political tensions are high, many people believe that religion's role in life is important, but shrinking (Pew Research Center, 2024b).

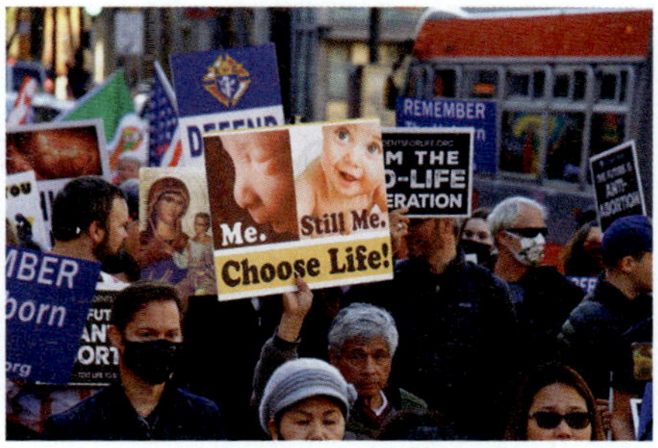

Figure 6-1 A client's religious beliefs can affect many aspects of health care.

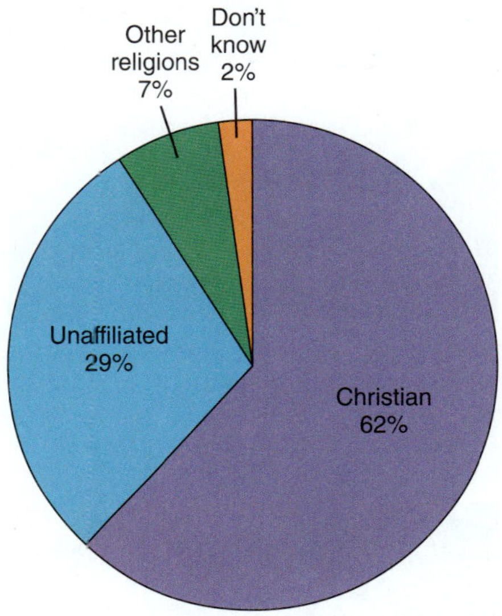

Figure 6-2 Most Americans identify themselves as Christians (62%), but this figure has dropped significantly over time. A sizable minority identify as "unaffiliated," and this percentage has increased over time (29%). The percentages have been rounded to the nearest whole number. *Pew Research Center, 2025.*

Religion and Spirituality

What is a religion? **Religion** is an organized system of beliefs usually centered around the worship of a sacred, supernatural force or being, which in turn defines the self and the self's purpose in life. Religion exists in group form over time and is a tradition of shared beliefs. Although many variances may exist among believers within any given religion, there will be common beliefs that unite the followers. A religious system of beliefs can be highly organized and include **rituals,** which are solemn, ceremonial acts that reinforce the faith. **Faith** is the assent to the truth of those beliefs and may also refer to the total orientation of the self's entire life to the belief structure. **Dogma** refers to the beliefs of a religion that are so essential to the identity of that religion that to deny them is to deny the religion itself. Religions also include **codes of ethics,** which are codified beliefs and lists of mandatory or prohibited acts that help define the self's relation to the object of worship.

An example of a religion is Judaism. Judaism has existed for thousands of years. Followers of the Jewish faith worship Yahweh (God) and define humans as the special creations of God who must in turn worship God. Judaism is highly organized. Who God is, why God should be worshipped, and how humans ought to act by virtue of being created by God are delineated in the Bible and a system of biblical commentary and teachings by the leaders of the religion. Judaism has different kinds of religious leaders

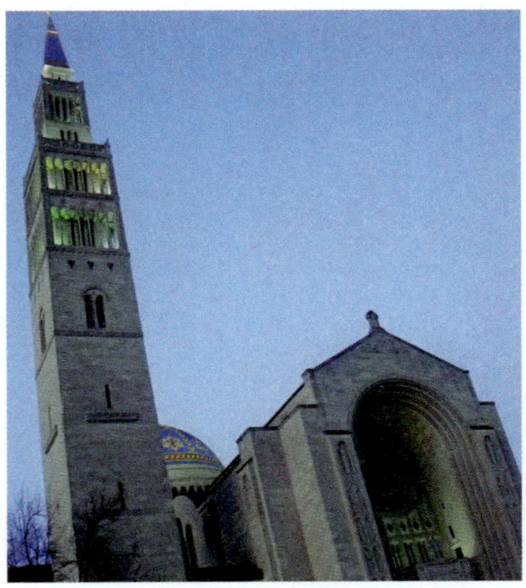

Figure 6-3 The United States has the largest Christian population in the world. They worship at churches such as this, the Basilica of the Shrine of the Immaculate Conception, a Roman Catholic church, in Washington, DC.

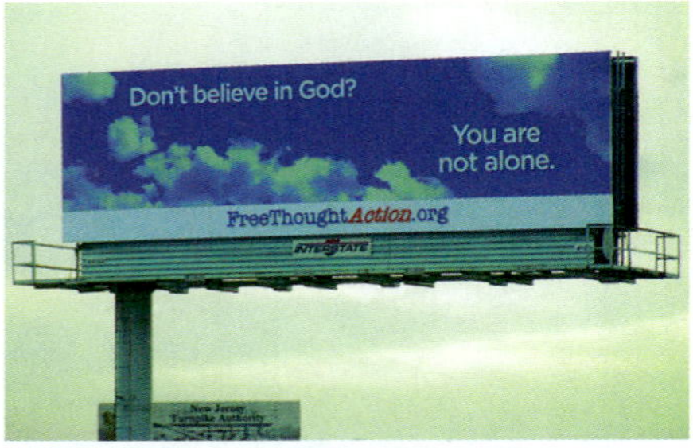
Don't believe in God?
You are not alone.
FreeThought.Action.org

Figure 6-4 This billboard reflects the growing prevalence of atheistic views.

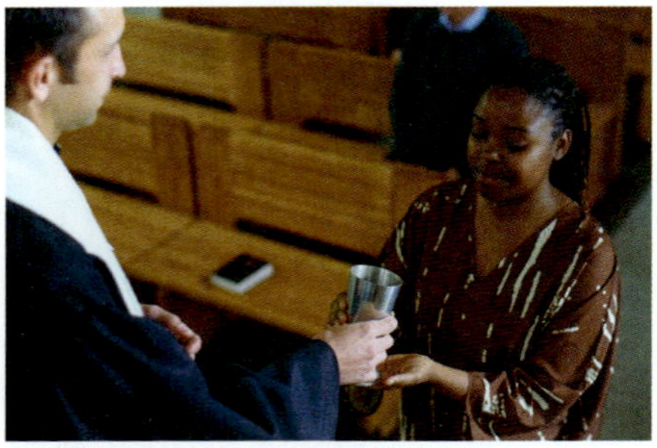

Figure 6-5 This woman is receiving wine during Communion at a Christian church.

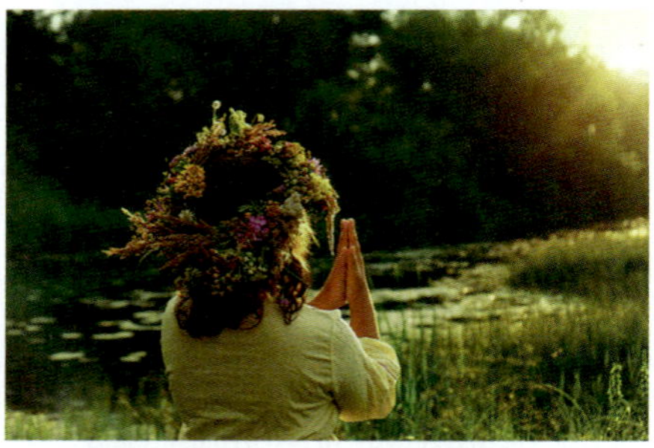

Figure 6-6 This woman is celebrating Wiccan Solstice Day.

(rabbis, cantors), codes of ethics (the biblical Ten Commandments is the best-known example), and rituals (circumcision, Bat Mitzvah). There are many forms of Judaism, but broadly speaking, implications for health care for a religious Jew could include a special diet (pork-free or kosher); men wearing a special prayer cap called a yarmulke and women keeping their heads covered; prayers on Fridays at sundown; rest on the Sabbath on Saturdays; and consultation with a rabbi before any complex bioethical decisions are made.

It is important to remember that religions are quite different. The concept of God may vary from a dispassionate, distant deity to a dynamic, personal, present being. "God" may be called by many names, such as Allah, Yahweh, Jehovah, or Shiva; one religion, Judaism, considers the name of God so sacred that believers are not supposed to pronounce the name at all (using "the Lord" instead). Orthodox Christians and Catholics believe that the prayers of a priest can transform bread and wine into the actual body and blood of Jesus Christ, whom they believe is God. When a priest or lay minister brings the consecrated wafer or wine to a client, Orthodox Christians and Catholics believe that God himself is being given to that client (Fig. 6-5).

Monotheistic (single-god) religions such as Judaism, Christianity, and Islam all believe in only one all-powerful, omnipresent, and omnipotent God (capital "G") who created the universe. **Polytheistic** (many-gods) religions such as Hinduism recognize many gods (lowercase "g") that may have different levels of power and status. The definition of a **cult** is controversial, but can best be described as a small, recently created religious organization often headed by a single charismatic leader and viewed as spiritually innovative or heretical in nature. Cults are thought to be fanatical and socially disapproved, but the difference between a cult and a religion may depend on the person making the definition.

The definition of *spirituality* is more complex. The term came into use in the 1960s when the rejection of authority became popular. The term "spiritual" came to be used in opposition to religion. An actual distinction between religion and spirituality is, however, difficult to make. A helpful distinction is that spirituality is a form of religion, but a private and personal form of religion, divorced from the rites, rituals, and codified beliefs of organized religion. Many New Age movements are examples of spiritualities. These movements often have no holy books, no formal organizations, no clergy, no dogma, and no creeds. New Age organizations often include elements of **animism,** that is, the belief that spirits inhabit natural objects and creatures, and **pantheism,** which is the belief that God is the world and the world is God. New Age movements may also embrace elements of **paganism.** "Paganism" is a term with multiple meanings. To members of the three monotheistic religions, a pagan is someone who is not monotheistic. Another definition of a pagan is someone who believes in an animistic, pantheistic, or polytheistic belief system (Fig. 6-6).

Medical studies of the effect of religion and spirituality on health struggle with how to measure religion and spirituality (Koenig, 2008). Some studies that claim to measure the effect of spirituality are actually measuring worship attendance as a measure of religion. Others rely on self-reporting descriptions of religion and spirituality—this creates difficulties in that the terms themselves are often used interchangeably. Because of the growth of those describing themselves as "unaffiliated," the nurse is likely to hear clients describe themselves as "spiritual but not religious." The vagueness of the term "spirituality" can be useful, however, when talking with clients, because religious clients usually believe themselves to be spiritual, and unaffiliated, atheistic, and agnostic clients are not put on the defensive by inquiries into "religion." In this chapter, the terms *spirituality* and *religion* are used interchangeably.

The Health Effects of Religion and Spirituality

Research shows that spiritual and religious beliefs produce measurable improvements in healthy behaviors. In a landmark analysis of hundreds of studies with a wide variety of researchers over decades, Dr. Harold Koenig showed that spiritual and religious beliefs and practices are associated with decreased rates of drug abuse, alcohol abuse, and smoking; decreased risky and criminal behavior; decreased numbers of sexual partners and decreased sexually transmitted infections; and an increase in altruism and volunteerism (Koenig, 2008, 2012). These are behaviors that nurses want to instill and foster in their clients. Koenig's research demonstrated that understanding and tapping into clients' religious and spiritual beliefs can assist in medical treatment. Further, research showed how spiritual and religious beliefs and practices are associated with decreased physical morbidity and mortality such as decreased rates of depression, anxiety, and suicide, decreased rates of hypertension and myocardial infarctions, improved coping with chronic illness, improved outcomes after cardiac surgery, and an increase in the immune factors that protect from infectious disease (Luchetti, 2021; Koenig, 2008, 2012). Research continues to show the benefits: Religious and spiritual beliefs and practices are associated with a decreased risk of heart disease (Hemmati, 2019), a significant decrease in smoking rates (Manzoor, 2019; Martinez 2021), an increased quality of life among stroke survivors and their caregivers (Pucciarelli 2020), improved response to SARS-CoV2 (COVID-19) threats and decreased infection rates (Ma, 2022), and a decreased suicide rate (Saiz, 2021). Religious-based interventions are effective in decreasing depression symptoms and should be considered (Marques, 2022). Spiritual well-being and meaning in life are protective factors against psychological stress at the end of life (Bernard, 2017).

However, not all effects of spirituality and religion are positively associated with health. Some specific religious and spiritual beliefs can forbid established medical care and have caused harm and even death. A landmark article in *Pediatrics* documented 172 children who died between 1975 and 1995 whose parents withheld medical care for religious reasons (Asser, 1998). Some examples of spiritual and religious beliefs and practices that may cause harmful outcomes are:

- Jehovah's Witnesses are a small Christian denomination with a unique biblical interpretation promulgated in 1961 that prohibits blood transfusions. One estimate is that 594 Jehovah's Witnesses die every year in the United States by refusing life-saving blood transfusions (Elder, 2017). About 1% of the population of the United States are Jehovah's Witnesses.
- The Church of Christ, Scientist ("Christian Science") is a Christian denomination that teaches that illness is "imaginary." Christian Scientists reject most forms of standard medical care in favor of prayer alone. Church members are allowed to have broken bones set, prenatal care, pain medication, eyeglasses, and hearing aids, but all other forms of standard medical care, including medicine, surgery, antibiotics, and vaccination, are rejected in favor of prayer alone. Members who receive standard medical care are excommunicated from the church and shunned. The refusal of needed medical care has led to the deaths of several minor children from such preventable causes as diabetes, meningitis, and tumors. In some cases, parents were prosecuted for neglect but their sentences after conviction were reduced or dismissed.
- Of the other religious groups in the United States that have opposed medical interventions, most are small, insular communities that are led by one charismatic leader who teaches a unique interpretation of the Bible.

- Additionally, individuals have caused the death of children through medical neglect based on their own personal spiritual views separate from a formal religious institution. One example is a New York parent whose 7-month-old son died of malnutrition after being fed only vegan food in accordance with following the Bible (Roberts, 2021).
- Many writers have accused religions of causing violence, especially after the 9/11 attacks in 2001 by Islamic terrorists (Dawkins, 2006; Hitchens, 2007). Their arguments are complex and will not be recounted here, but there are legitimate criticisms of their definitions of what is a religious or a nonreligious cause (Cavanaugh, 2007). On the contrary, a study of mass shooters showed that among the shooters, just 16% were religious (Pittaro, 2018; Crime Research, 2018).
- Parents who kill their children sometimes give religious reasons for doing so (getting rid of demons or preserving their eternal salvation, for example), but they are more likely to act because of a psychiatric illness (Lettieri, 2021). Half of the parents who murder their children have psychotic symptoms and have recently abused alcohol or illegal drugs; other motives may include a desire to spare a child from suffering, viewing the child as a hindrance to personal satisfaction, revenge against a spouse, or abuse that culminates in the child's death (Lettieri, 2021).

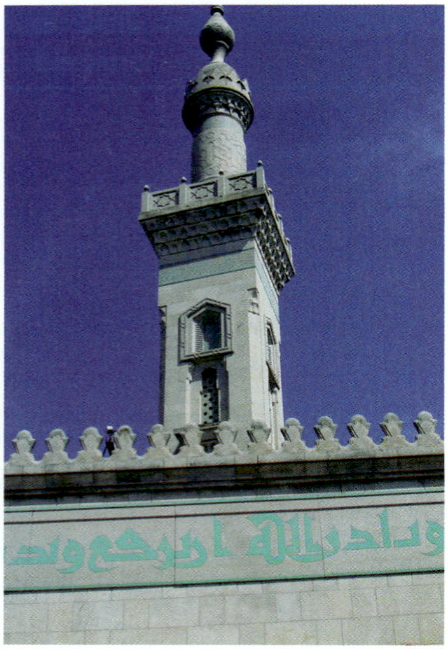

Figure 6-7 Muslims face east when praying, in order to face Mecca, Saudi Arabia, their holiest site. The facade of this mosque faces the street, but the minaret points toward Mecca.

Role of the Nurse in Spiritual Care

Nurses have a vital role to play in the spiritual care of clients. The nurse's role includes:

1. Becoming knowledgeable about different religions and spiritual practices so that you will recognize your client's particular beliefs.
2. Performing a spiritual assessment to learn more about your client's beliefs, which will assist in the understanding and treatment of the client.
3. Formulating a nursing care plan and clinical judgment based on the spiritual assessment.
4. Formulating nursing interventions to support clients' spiritual and religious practices.

Almost all religions attempt to explain why human beings suffer from illness and death and how higher powers can affect healing. It is important to realize that religion rarely, if ever, describes disease as resulting from a strictly biological cause that has a scientific solution. Instead, some religions explain that disease is sent by God, caused by sin or by the poor performance of a ritual act, or results from the malevolence of relatives, neighbors, or ancestors. Based on these explanations, the treatment or cure for disease is to be found in the confession of sin, purification rites, exorcism, or the transmission of power to the client by prayers or rituals. These acts of healing are not performed by physicians or nurses, but by priests, elders, mediums, and other specialists who have access to the higher powers that control disease. For example, it may be more important to the client to see a neighbor who has had experience with a disease and was successfully able to repel it with certain prayers than to take a prescribed medication.

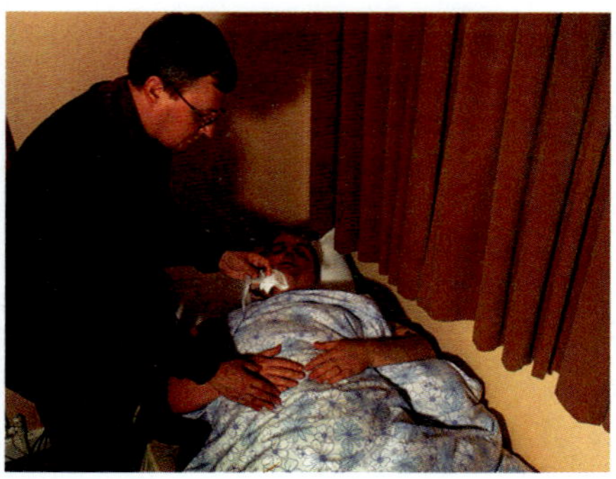

Figure 6-8 Rituals such as the sacrament of the Anointing of the Sick are important expressions of religious beliefs.

Become familiar with various religions and spiritual practices. Your understanding of religions and spiritualities will help you recognize and understand your client's religion or spiritual practice. A Muslim client may ask which direction is east, for example, in order to pray while facing Mecca (Fig. 6-7). A Catholic may refuse to enter the operating room even for life-saving surgery until the sacrament of Anointing of the Sick has been received (Fig. 6-8). A Buddhist may pace and pray. An Orthodox Christian client may wish to be able to see an icon from their bed.

Assessment in Brief

General Approach to Spiritual Assessment

1. If possible, choose a quiet, private room that will be free from interruptions.
2. Ensure that the room light is sufficiently bright to observe the client's verbal and nonverbal reactions.
3. Greet the client, introduce yourself, and explain that you will be taking a health history.
4. Position yourself at eye level with the client.
5. Portray an interested, nonjudgmental manner throughout the interview. Respect silence and diversity.
6. Use a spiritual assessment tool to engage the client.

Spiritual Assessment

The purpose of a spiritual assessment is to collect information in order to understand the client's religious or spiritual beliefs and practices. The Joint Commission requires that every client receive a spiritual assessment (Joint Commission, 2020).

The spiritual assessment is best done as part of the history taking but can also be performed conversationally during the client's physical examination or client care. It is performed in a supportive and nonjudgmental manner.

The spiritual assessment should be performed on every client for whom you do a screening assessment, but older clients, hospitalized clients, and clients with a terminal illness should be prioritized. Barriers to spiritual assessment include a lack of time, lack of experience, and difficulty in identifying clients who might want to discuss spiritual matters (Villagran, 2017). Nonreligious nurses and doctors are often reluctant to engage in spiritual assessment (Dein, 2018; Taylor, 2018). If this describes you, think about your own beliefs and why you might feel reluctant to engage in a spiritual assessment. Studies show that clients want to discuss spiritual and religious issues with the health-care team (Sajja, 2018). Engaging in a spiritual assessment can improve the relationship between nurses and clients (Tan, 2022).

NURSING TIP

Gaining Client Trust

Many people believe that spiritual issues are very private. Clients may fear that they will be ridiculed for their beliefs. It is important, therefore, to build an atmosphere of trust with the client before you delve into questions about the client's spiritual beliefs. Begin the health history interview with the expected questions concerning the client's physical history. As the client reveals personal or intimate details about their physical being, you will build trust with the client by remaining nonjudgmental and maintaining an attitude of respect, empathy, and understanding. The trusting client should gradually feel more comfortable discussing potentially personal issues in the psychological and spiritual portions of the interview.

Client History as a Source of Information about Religious and Spiritual Beliefs

Keep in mind that the client's history may raise spiritual and religious issues. For example, the client may reveal a requirement for a vegetarian diet (Hindu, New Age), or a history of circumcision (Jews). Similarly, a client may reveal that they are estranged from their family. This may be due to a conversion to a different, even conflicting, religious or spiritual belief, or a rejection of the religious or spiritual belief of the family of origin. The revelation of such facts serves as an invitation to perform the spiritual assessment.

Observe the Client Closely

Just as you observe the client for evidence of health and disease, observe the client for clues to their religious and spiritual beliefs. Beyond the obvious Bibles and religious jewelry, look for special clothing (members of the Church of Jesus Christ of Latter-day Saints, known as Mormons, Jews, Sikhs), religious objects draped or tied around the body (Catholics, Jews), uncut hair (Sikhs), prayer beads (Buddhists, Catholics, and Orthodox Christians), and even knives (Sikhs). Ask about any object with which you are unfamiliar. It may be fashion or it may be sacred (Fig. 6-9). In any case, your observations and questions will open the door to the spiritual assessment.

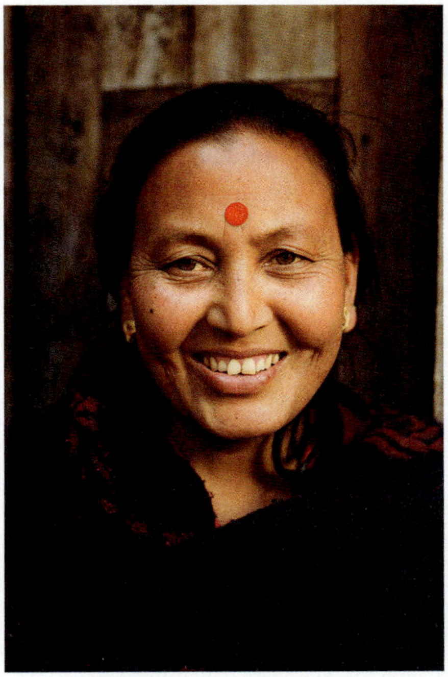

Figure 6-9 This Indian woman wears a red bindi to remind her to follow the tenets of the Hindu faith.

Non-Christian religions are growing, and it is now common to meet adherents of a much wider variety of religions and spiritualities than even 10 years

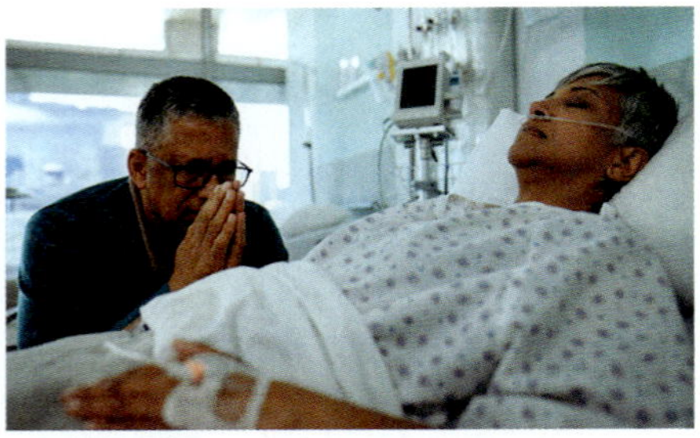

Figure 6-10 Prayer can be performed in both formal and informal ways.

NURSING CHECKLIST

General Approach to Spiritual Assessment

1. Observe standard precautions and don personal protective equipment (PPE) such as gloves, gown, face shield, goggles, or N-95 respirator or face mask if the client's status warrants these protective measures.
2. If possible, choose a quiet, private room that will be free from interruptions.
3. Ensure that the room's light is sufficiently bright to observe the client's verbal and nonverbal reactions.
4. Greet the client, introduce yourself, and explain that you will be taking a health history.
5. Position yourself at eye level with the client.
6. Portray an interested, nonjudgmental manner throughout the interview. Respect silence and diversity.

ago. If the nurse is expecting a client to pray by folding their hands and softly repeating a prayer, for example, that nurse might overlook expressions of prayer in other traditions. People at prayer may be sitting (Protestant; see Figure 6-10), kneeling (Islam, Catholic), standing (Protestant), rocking (some Jewish), or walking (Buddhist); silent (various religions) or chanting (Muslim, Jewish); with hands folded (Catholic) or arms raised (Protestant); holding a religious object (Catholic, Buddhist) or facing a specific direction (Muslim). An awareness of cultural and religious norms will help you deliver appropriate nursing care. It is important to know how different belief systems define acceptable behavior through the life cycle (Taylor, 2019).

Beware of stereotyping a client or jumping to conclusions. Don't assume that a holy book on the table means that the client is a devout believer. The book may have been left there by a family member or friend, distributed by a missionary group, or donated by a well-meaning volunteer. Additionally, the absence of a holy book does not mean the client is not spiritual or religious, as some religions (Native American, Unitarian, New Age) do not have holy books. Furthermore, many self-identified members of religious faiths do not follow the teachings of their religions. For example, a Jew may eat pork, a Jehovah's Witness may accept a blood transfusion, and a Catholic may request birth control. Some atheist clients may want to return to the religion of their youth in a time of crisis. Many clients may blend elements of one religion with those of another religion or spiritual belief. A good understanding of religious and spiritual practices is important, and an understanding of your client's specific beliefs is crucial.

Spiritual Assessment Tools

Many spiritual assessment tools exist such as the FICA (Puchalski & Romer, 2000, updated 2022), the HOPE tool (Kwok, 2022), and the Open Invite (Saguil, 2012). The information that is gathered in the spiritual assessment will assist the health-care team in planning respectful and appropriate client care. This text uses the FICA spiritual assessment tool. The FICA is a simple yet complete spiritual assessment that is brief and easy to use. This spiritual assessment tool has been clinically validated and provides a nonthreatening way to perform a spiritual assessment on everyone from the most adamant atheist to the most devoutly religious client.

FICA Spiritual Assessment Tool

F: Faith, Belief, Meaning. Ask: "Do you consider yourself to be spiritual?" "Is spirituality something important to you?" "Do you have spiritual beliefs, practices, or values that help you to cope with stress, difficult times, or what you are going through right now?" "What gives your life meaning?"

I: Importance and Influence. Ask: "What importance does spirituality have in your life?" "Has your spirituality influenced how you take care of yourself, particularly regarding your health?" "Does your spirituality affect your healthcare decision making?"

C: Community. Ask: "Are you part of a spiritual community?" "Is your community of support to you and how?" "Is there a group of people you really love or who are important to you?"

Communities such as churches, temples, and mosques; families; groups of like-minded friends; or yoga or similar groups can serve as strong support systems for some clients.

A: Address/Action in Care. "How would you like me, as your healthcare provider, to address spiritual issues in your healthcare?"

FICA tool used with permission of Christina M. Puchalski, MD, The George Washington Institute for Spirituality and Health (GWish), The George Washington University.

Record your assessment findings. Communicate them to the health-care team as appropriate. The information that is gathered in the spiritual assessment will assist the health-care team in planning respectful and appropriate client care.

Resistance to the Spiritual Assessment

If your client is resistant to the spiritual assessment, don't force the conversation. This may be an area more private to the client than bowel or sexual habits.

If the client is resentful or hostile to questions about religion and spirituality, focus on the client's support system only. Avoid a debate on the merits of religion and particularly avoid expressing your views or forcing them on the client. Be alert for an opportunity, an "open door," that makes it natural and permissible to ask questions or probe further into the client's religious and spiritual beliefs and support system. The client may even "open the door" for you and tacitly invite you to make inquiries in this area (Table 6-1).

The Importance of an Ongoing Assessment

Spiritual distress is the state in which a client feels that the belief system, or one's place within it, is threatened. Commonly, the circumstances in which nurses find themselves providing care—birth, accidents, illness, and the dying process—are the same events that provoke spiritual distress. Any threat to one's own life, any reminder of one's mortality, can serve to evoke both wonder about the meaning and purpose of life and disquiet about the answers that spirituality or religion provide.

Thus, in an ongoing therapeutic relationship with a client, it is vital to reevaluate the client's spiritual and religious beliefs continuously. A major life event or health crisis, or the long grind of a chronic illness, can put even long-held spiritual and religious beliefs to the test, and the client may welcome an intervention previously refused or consider an option previously ruled out. Spiritual distress may manifest itself as anxiety, withdrawal, distractedness, hopelessness, or crying behaviors. When caring for a dying or end-of-life client, it may help to ask if the client is at peace, as a brief means of conducting a spiritual assessment (Steinhauser, 2006).

Table 6-1 Some "Open Doors" for Discussing Religious and Spiritual Beliefs

- Use required queries regarding organ donation and advance directives to start a conversation.
- Discussions about difficult treatment options can lead to a conversation about beliefs.
- When bad news or a serious diagnosis is announced, encourage the client to discuss personal beliefs.
- When clients express hopelessness, ask, "Are you a praying person?"
- Ask the client how their spouse or family is "holding up."
- Respond to client's statement indicating spiritual distress with empathy and gentle queries about spiritual and religious beliefs.
- The client may ask you about your spiritual or religious beliefs, or those of another health-care team member, or make an observation about the hospital chaplain. Turn the conversation around to the client's beliefs.

NURSING TIP
Signs of Spiritual Distress

Signs of spiritual distress may be subtle or overt, but you should be alert to their deep meanings and not brush them off as the client is "having a bad day." Such signs may include:

- Crying, sighing, withdrawn behavior
- Verbalization of questions about spiritual beliefs, such as "What does it all mean?" or "An experience like this really makes you put things into perspective" or "I just don't understand why this is happening to me."
- Verbalizations about worthlessness, hopelessness, or death, such as "I'd be better off dead" or "I guess we've all got to go some time."
- Verbalizations about God and God's purposes, such as "I guess the gods have it in for me," or "It's payback time," or "I wonder what I did to deserve this," or "When God says it's your time to go, you go no matter what, I guess."
- Explicit requests to the nurse or others for spiritual assistance, such as requests for prayers or the special placement of religious artifacts.

NURSING TIP
Clues to a Client's Spirituality

When you are caring for a client in the home or an institution such as a hospital, a hospice, or a nursing home, use your access to the client to look for clues about the client's spirituality. Does the client pray before meals? Do the client's get-well cards contain religious or spiritual messages? Who visits the client—family and friends, or also members of the client's religious or spiritual organization?

Nursing Interventions to Promote Spiritual Well-Being

The following nursing interventions to promote spiritual well-being are appropriate for both religious and spiritual nursing care.

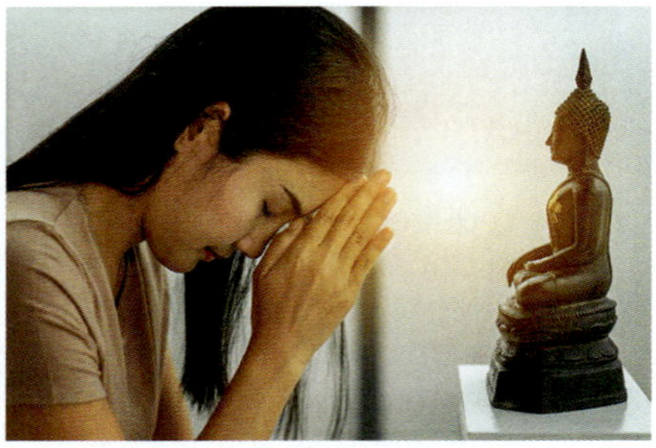

Figure 6-11 Some of the fastest-growing religions in America are non-Judeo-Christian religions. This woman is praying to Buddha.

Show Respect for the Client's Religious and Spiritual Beliefs

It is important to show respect for the client's religious and spiritual beliefs and practices, even those that are unusual and unfamiliar. Even clients who belong to more familiar mainstream religions may feel uneasy practicing their religions in unfamiliar institutional settings before strangers' eyes. A Buddhist in a Christian hospital, for example, may feel awkward displaying an icon of a guru or may be distressed if an arrangement of religious items is disturbed (Fig. 6-11). Muslims have been singled out for special scrutiny and criticism since the terrorist attacks of 9/11 and may be reluctant to call attention to their religion by praying five times a day in a hospital, where there is little privacy. Even mainstream Christians may find that their religious beliefs are thought of as amusing or quaint by the secular, scientific practitioners of health care. The health-care team needs to acknowledge the importance of spiritual and religious practices for the client and avoid verbal and nonverbal disrespect. Eye-rolling, disparaging comments, arguing with the client about religion, carelessness regarding religious and spiritual objects (such as placing used bandages or medical equipment on top of a holy book or object), or cursing using the name of the god worshipped by the client are some common instances of disrespect for the client's religious and spiritual practices. When the client has clearly pathological beliefs, such as a delusional belief that they are a god, it is advised to maintain a respectful but neutral stance. At some point, it may be necessary to gently challenge harmful spiritual and religious beliefs, but this is best left to trained people such as a psychiatrist or chaplain after a therapeutic alliance is established (Koenig, 2018). Compassion, active listening, and supportive actions show respect for clients' beliefs (Elk, 2017).

Allow Clients to Practice Their Religion and Spirituality

Nurses care for clients in distress: a client feeling the ill effects of chemotherapy or overwhelmed by a diagnosis; parents exhausted from labor and delivery; a person disfigured in an accident or undergoing painful débridement; clients who are frightened as they approach death. It is not sufficient to allow clients to lie and suffer quietly while the health-care team whirls busily around them, and it may not be sufficient to get a visitor to visit and hold the client's hand (sometimes visitors are not allowed and sometimes the client has no visitors). Spiritual and religious beliefs and practices help clients endure pain and misery, cope with a new reality, and deal with impending death. Thus, an effective nursing intervention is to allow clients to practice their religion and spirituality if they wish to do so. Clients may need your permission, because some reluctant clients may feel overwhelmed by unfamiliar institutional surroundings or by their medical treatment regimens and thus forego what might bring them profound relief in a time of crisis.

Allowing or assisting clients with religious practice may require some creativity. A Muslim client may require nursing assistance to maintain modest dress in a health-care setting. For example, a female client may need help keeping their head covered. This may require time and effort, but it is important for the client's well-being. Clients of many faiths may want religious objects or clothing worn, draped, tied, placed on top of, or wrapped around them. This may prove challenging when the client has a wound, incision, infection, or medical equipment attached to the body. Discuss the situation with the client or family member. An object that is supposed to be tied around the waist could perhaps be tied around a leg instead to avoid an abdominal incision. Do what you can to accommodate the client's desires and practices. Be creative: Battery-operated candles can substitute for real candles, and a towel or blanket may suffice for a prayer rug. The nurse can provide privacy for prayer or a special phone call. On a psychiatric unit where a long rosary might be prohibited for safety reasons, print out a picture of a rosary or see if the client could make a rosary by gluing beads or beans onto paper, or by making a "one-decade" rosary (a short rosary with only 10 beads instead of the normal 60 beads) in art therapy.

The client may want, additionally, to view or listen to a particular TV channel or podcast. It may be helpful to keep prayer beads or a favored crystal in a client's hand, even taping them to their bed or bedside table if the client is too ill to hold it. Holy cards or icons could be taped on IV poles or placed visibly on a bedside table where they can be seen. The client may appreciate reading or being read to from a holy book, spiritual book, or tract.

It is important to understand that the spiritual and religious beliefs of clients and families might be misperceived as behavior problems. A Muslim father, for example, may urgently want access to a distressed newborn to whisper, "There is no God but Allah and Mohammed is His Prophet" (the "Shahada") in the child's ear so that this sentence will be the first (and possibly last) thing the child hears. An Orthodox Christian family member may demand that a priest see a client during a resuscitation event. A malnourished client may refuse food if the food is not kosher, halal, vegan, or blessed. A brusque response during an emergency—"We can't do that now, we'll do that later" or "It's just food—food is food—just eat it, you need it"—may be seen as disrespectful or insulting to clients and their families. The nurse must understand these spiritual and religious requests and respect them even if fulfilling them is difficult. The nurse should clarify what is being requested, understand its importance, and accommodate the client's request on how this can be done given the circumstances. Be creative and persistent with the rest of the health-care team, who may be focused understandably elsewhere. Some requests can be accommodated. Clients in distress can be baptized by non-Christians as long as they say the correct words, "I baptize you in the Name of the Father, and of the Son, and of the Holy Spirit," while tracing a cross with water on the client's body (usually the forehead). The Muslim father may be able to be brought to his child's bedside to recite the Shahada even during a resuscitation attempt, or perhaps a Muslim staff person can do this. A priest or rabbi could be gowned and gloved and brought into a resuscitation area or even an operating room and safely positioned for prayers and rituals.

No health-care practitioner should be required to perform spiritual and religious rituals against their conscience. Understandably, an atheist may be reluctant to baptize, and a non-Muslim might be reluctant to recite the Shahada. The nurse should be persistent, however, in assisting clients to get their spiritual and religious needs met, even when it is challenging to meet the client's needs. See Table 6-2 for nursing solutions to difficult client spiritual problems.

Praying with Clients

Prayer is a means of speaking to God or a higher spiritual power. The practice can provide profound spiritual and religious relief, hope, and encouragement, and the nurse should provide the means and privacy necessary for the client to engage in prayer. But clients may ask the nurse to pray with them (Fig. 6-12). If so, what should you do? First, you might ask the clients what is required of them. When the nurse asks for more information and clarification, it implies respect and allows clients to be in control (Elk, 2017). Some clients may simply want the nurse to be present while the client prays aloud. Other clients prefer a joint silent prayer. Still others may want the nurse to lead them in prayer or want to be included in the nurse's private prayer. If the nurse shares the basic beliefs of the client or family, and the client or family asks or invites the nurse to join in prayer, and the nurse is

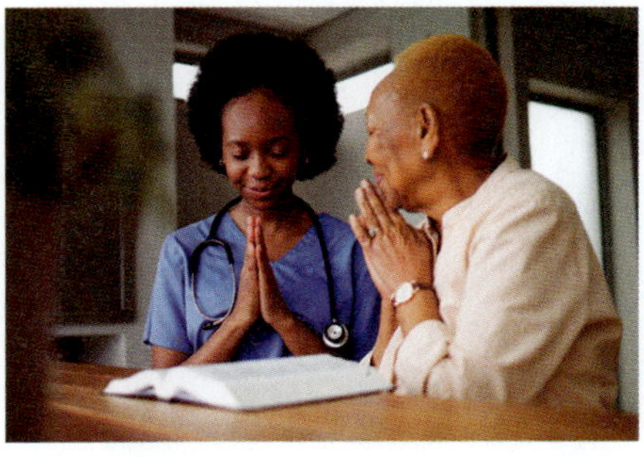

Figure 6-12 The nurse may join a client in prayer if they feel comfortable doing so.

Table 6-2 Overcoming Obstacles to a Client's Practice of Religion and Spirituality in the Health-Care Setting

Obstacles	Nursing Interventions
Secular health-care practitioners belittle or dismiss the client's spiritual or religious beliefs.	Show respect for the client's spiritual and religious beliefs. Educate self and health-care team members about the client's beliefs.
Client is of a faith different from the mainstream.	Same as above. Avoid the use of profanities with the name of religious deities. Encourage the client to engage in spiritual and religious practices that bring comfort and meaning.
Medical equipment/treatment interferes with client's practice of religion/spirituality.	Place spiritual/religious objects of importance within view of the client, on the client, or in the client's hand. For example, holy cards can be taped to an IV pump or ventilator tubing. Prayer beads can be placed in the client's hand. Put the TV on a religious channel of the client's choice. Read or encourage visitors to read religious/spiritual literature to the client. Mobilize the client's support system to visit. Consult your institution's chaplaincy service.
Client does not have proper religious/spiritual equipment (candles, rosary, holy book, prayer blanket, phylacteries, etc.) in the institution.	Contact friends, family, pastor, and so on to bring in necessary equipment. Consult the chaplaincy service. An institutional chaplaincy service is likely to have some of the proper equipment available for loan. If proper equipment cannot be used (e.g., candles cannot be used if the client requires oxygen therapy), suggest alternatives (e.g., battery-operated candles).
Lack of privacy to practice religion or spirituality.	Provide privacy as much as possible for spiritual and religious practices.
Religious/spiritual clothing or objects are taken off the client during the course of treatment.	Religious/spiritual clothing and objects can be draped over the client or placed on an extremity if the client's clinical condition allows.

comfortable and agrees, there should be no reason to prohibit such a powerful and reassuring intervention. But if the nurse is not comfortable praying with the client, there are several graceful responses (Christensen, 2018; Elk, 2017; Koenig, 2018; Taylor 2018):

- "I see that prayer is important to you. Can you tell me more?"
- "I'm not comfortable praying, but I'll stay here while you pray."
- "I personally do not pray, but I am sure I can find someone to pray with you."
- "I appreciate your trust in me in asking me to pray. I don't pray myself, but I will stand here quietly while you pray."
- "I don't pray with my clients directly, but I will promise to hold you in my thoughts and heart today."
- "Let's spend a few moments of silence together."

Contact and Mobilize the Client's Important Spiritual Resources

With the client's permission, it is important to mobilize the client's spiritual and religious resources. The client may be unable to do so, and due to HIPAA privacy laws, the client's spiritual community may be unable to find out whether one of their own is in a health-care institution. This may involve calling the client's worship community or religious leader, alerting an important group of friends, and so on. The ability to talk or visit with a spiritual or religious leader may prove very helpful in allaying fears, strengthening faith, and making difficult medical decisions. When policies prohibit visitation, prayer and support can be provided virtually.

Private prayer and virtual prayers with a spiritual or religious leader can be very helpful to clients. It is important to understand, however, that this is not religious practice as defined by many religions. Some religions require that rituals be performed in person by certain credentialed people. Catholic and Orthodox Christian teaching, for example, requires that the Sacrament of the Anointing of the Sick "Last Rites" and the Sacrament of Confession be performed only by a priest who must speak to the client in person (not on the phone) and who must also physically anoint the client with oil (an action that cannot be done by a nurse or family member).

Make Appropriate Referrals to the Hospital Chaplain

Hospital chaplains of any faith generally function as spiritual and religious resource people within a health-care institution. Do not fail to take advantage of their expertise just because the client is Buddhist and the chaplain is Jewish, for example. Research shows that faith affiliation is not as important as kindness, listening skills, and a nonjudgmental attitude (Advocat, 2023). The chaplain should feel comfortable visiting any client who is experiencing spiritual distress and discussing the client's spiritual and religious concerns without judging the client or trying to convert the client to the chaplain's own religion. Most institutional chaplains have received special training in **pastoral care,** which is the care and response needed when a person is in a spiritual crisis. In their practice of pastoral care, these chaplains can be valuable aids for the client. The nurse is in a unique position to act as a client's advocate and initiate a chaplaincy referral. The chaplain will provide a satisfying explanation for the visit, such as, "I normally visit with clients before surgery," and the client will not miss out on a valuable resource for alleviating spiritual or religious distress.

If the client has religious or spiritual beliefs that pose a risk, it is appropriate to notify the nursing supervisor and possibly obtain an ethics committee consultation to discuss the treatment plan.

Hospital chaplains may also be a source of holy books and spiritual and religious objects often requested by clients, and this in turn may trigger a visit to a client in need.

Hospital chaplains can also be useful in acting as a mediator between a client or family with spiritual and religious concerns and the health-care team in discussions about medical decisions (Weiner, 2017). Keep in mind that the chaplain is not acting to convince the client that the medical team is right, but to show respect and understanding of the client or family's spiritual and religious beliefs, explore those beliefs, speak their spiritual and religious language, and help them think about the decisions before them. In one example with a family that was resisting the withdrawal of life support, the chaplain, "through lengthy discussions about religious beliefs, ... helped them accept the idea that God was powerful enough to heal without extensive medical intervention. 'Then the family was able to have a conversation with the physician that they hadn't been able to have before.'" (Weiner, 2017). Clients want to be heard, understood, and respected. The nurse and hospital chaplain can help achieve these goals.

Nursing Interventions to Avoid

There are several nursing interventions to avoid when working with a client's spiritual condition, and these are listed in Table 6-3.

When Spiritual and Religious Beliefs May Pose a Risk to Client Care

When a client's spiritual and religious beliefs are harmful to client care, the health-care team needs to tread carefully. Showing respect for the client's right to a personal belief system is still appropriate. No one will make headway

Table 6-3 Nursing Actions to Avoid When Intervening in the Client's Spiritual Condition

It is important to show respect for your clients' religious and spiritual beliefs. These actions are considered disrespectful of such beliefs and should be avoided.

- Do not proselytize your own spiritual beliefs. You may share your beliefs if the issue comes up, but it is never appropriate to try to convert the client to another set of beliefs. In a worst-case scenario, you may instill fear in the client that you will not provide care unless the client espouses your own beliefs. You may also unwittingly undermine the client's support system at a time when the client needs support.
- Do not instruct the client in religious or spiritual doctrine. In a time of spiritual distress, a client needs support, not instruction. Let the religious or spiritual leader take the lead in any instruction that is required, and follow nursing interventions that will enhance spiritual well-being.
- Do not perform the function of a spiritual advisor for the client. You and the client may become confused about your role.
- Do not respond to the client with clichés. Well-known and overused clichés such as "no sense crying over spilled milk" or "there's always someone else who's worse off than you" are inappropriate because they tend to blame or diminish the importance of the client's anguish. Clichés about religion, such as "God helps those who help themselves" or "it was God's will," are just as inappropriate, because they are patronizing and tend to trivialize both the sufferer's problems and the sufferer's religion. Additionally, most well-known religious clichés are based on Western Judeo-Christian culture and have no bearing on those with other religions or spiritual beliefs. Respond instead with real, heartfelt words or, in some cases, with silence or with touch, if appropriate.
- Avoid taking on the role of spiritual advisor, spiritual healer, minister, priest, teacher, guru, and so on. Utilize instead the client's pastor, imam, priest, minister, or spiritual support system, family, or the health-care institutional chaplain to fill that role.

with a client by ridiculing—even subtly—the client's beliefs, or by trying to argue with the client about them. Clients should not be separated from visitors who support these difficult beliefs, although visitors, even families, may have to be separated and assigned to selected visiting times to decrease conflict. Nurses should avoid becoming angry with such religiously or spiritually difficult clients, or lecturing or instructing them. A hospital chaplain may be able to help mediate between the client and the health-care team.

When a child's health is harmed by the parents' religious and spiritual beliefs, it is appropriate to invoke your state's statutes on the required reporting of possible child abuse. Such reporting will ensure legal representation for the minor client and move the discussion to the legal realm.

> **NURSING TIP**
> **Answering the "Why Me?" Question**
>
> Don't answer. Listen instead.
>
> Nurses care for suffering clients who, in their spiritual distress, may pose the ancient question "Why me?" Different religions and spiritualities answer the question differently. Although you may offer some personal thoughts on the subject, it is a better and more helpful intervention to listen while clients talk about their struggles with the topic. Many times, surprisingly, listening and companionship alone are enough to bring comfort to a suffering client.

Evaluation

Evaluate the effectiveness of your nursing interventions by observing the client. Signs that the client's spiritual distress has decreased include:

1. Acceptance of spiritual support from the source with which the client feels most comfortable.
2. Decrease in crying, restlessness, and sleeplessness. There may even be a decrease in complaints of pain or the severity of pain.
3. Decrease in statements of worthlessness and hopelessness.
4. Verbalization of satisfaction with spiritual beliefs and the support and comfort they provide. The client may talk openly about spiritual beliefs and even offer spiritual insights to other clients, to you, or other health-care professionals. This is a healthy sign that the client is admitting acceptance of spiritual beliefs.

COVID-19 Effects on Spirituality and Religiosity

The COVID-19 pandemic posed challenges to every person in the United States as well as around the world. Just about every facet of life was affected. Due to the deleterious environment of COVID-19, "the incidence of mental disorders increased by 50% compared with prepandemic; alcohol and other substance abuse surged, and young adults were more than twice as likely to seriously consider suicide than they were in 2018. The only group to see *improvements* in mental health ... were those who attended religious services at least weekly" (Rosmarin, 2021, emphasis in original).

During the early days of the COVID-19 pandemic when little was known about the virus and people were hospitalized and dying, an understandable fear of contagion existed. Hospitalized clients were denied visits from their family, friends, and spiritual and religious leaders (Fussel, 2020; Morse, 2020). Hospital chaplains were not allowed to visit clients in the hospital even when they were dying (Barber, 2020). This was distressing to clients and clergy alike and led to a Health and Human Services ruling that guaranteed clients could see their spiritual and religious leaders (HHS, 2020).

U.S. Preventive Services Task Force (USPSTF)

There are no USPSTF recommendations, Grade A or B Statements, for spirituality or religion.

CASE STUDY

Parents Demand Treatment Changes for Their Transgender Child

This case study illustrates the application and objective documentation of the spiritual assessment. Fatima is a 13-year-old child, assigned female at birth, who was admitted to an inpatient psychiatric unit after attempting suicide by cutting both wrists. Once admitted to the unit, Fatima directs staff to use he/him pronouns and the name "Ali" because he identifies as a boy. Fatima's parents come to the hospital to visit their child. When the client's parents discover that their child is identifying as a boy, they demand the child's discharge because transgenderism is against their Islamic faith.

SPIRITUAL HISTORY

CLIENT PROFILE

13-year-old single person

HISTORY OF PRESENT ILLNESS

Fatima was brought to the Emergency Department (ED) by ambulance after being found in a school bathroom crying and bleeding from self-inflicted cuts to both forearms. In the ED the wounds were sutured, and Fatima was evaluated by a psychiatrist and admitted to the adolescent-locked psychiatric unit for further evaluation and treatment. Upon admission, the nurse performs an assessment. Fatima has a history of ADHD, depression, and anxiety. Fatima was taking escitalopram 10 mg daily, methylphenidate 18 mg every morning, and buspirone 7.5 mg twice daily before admission. Fatima has been in treatment with a private psychiatrist and therapist for 6 months. Fatima (client's legal name) immigrated to the U.S. 2 years ago, speaks English well, attends public school, and receives some services at school for ADHD. Fatima's parents are married. Fatima has three living siblings; a fourth older brother was killed in a shooting in Afghanistan. The family was separated from the father for 8 years after the father moved to the U.S. from Afghanistan 10 years ago for work and to obtain visas for the rest of the family. The client, mother, and siblings immigrated to the U.S. 2 years ago, reuniting with the father. The family is Muslim and attends a local mosque. Physical examination shows that the client's assigned sex is female. The sutures to both forearms are intact, and there is evidence of extensive prior cutting on both thighs, with both scabbed and scarred linear cuts. The client is otherwise physically healthy. During the initial assessment, directs staff to use he/him pronouns and the name "Ali" because he identifies as a boy. The staff accommodates this request. The psychiatrist adjusts the client's medications, and the client engages in the therapeutic milieu on the unit.

On the second hospital day, the client's parents visit for the first time. The parents are Mohammed, age 43, and Dimah, age 39, refugees from Afghanistan. Mohammed speaks English fluently and works as an engineer. He has lived in the U.S. for 10 years. Dimah speaks English haltingly and wears a hijab. She and the client and the client's three other siblings moved to the U.S. 2 years ago. Dimah does not have a work permit and stays home raising the children and caring for the home. Dimah is 6 months pregnant. Mohammed is surprised and outraged to find "Ali" written on his child's room door, and to hear the staff refer to his child as "he." He relates this in his native language to his wife, who also becomes irate. They have several loud and angry conversations with the nurse, the social worker, and a medical resident. They insist that their child is a girl named Fatima and want her treated so, otherwise, they "will take her home immediately and have her treated by their outpatient psychiatrist." They know that transgenderism is against their Islamic faith and that they have parental rights over their children. During these conversations, the client cries and yells, "This is so stupid! I hate my life!" and has to be removed to a calming room by the staff. After further discussion, the health-care team persuades the parents that the client is not yet stable enough for discharge that day.

SPIRITUAL ASSESSMENT: FICA TOOL

F: Faith, Belief, Meaning *"Do you consider yourself to be spiritual?" "Is spirituality something important to you?" "Do you have spiritual beliefs, practices, or values that help you to cope with stress, difficult times, or what you are going through right now?" "What gives your life meaning?"*

Parents: Islam means everything to them. Throughout their married lives, living in a war-torn country and then managing an 8-year separation while they immigrated to the U.S., they always felt like Allah helped and comforted them. Their current local mosque has provided them with companionship in their native language as well as a religious education for their children and financial and practical help with their relocation. They can't imagine going against Islamic teaching, which they are sure is against transgenderism.

Client: The client shrugs. Life in Afghanistan was chaotic; the religious restrictions there were irritating. When the father moved away to the U.S. and the older brother was shot and killed, the client became depressed. The client would pray to Allah, but nothing changed. The move to the U.S. was difficult, and the client does not feel comfortable in the new school, does not fit in, and does not want to wear the hijab the father requires. There is a lot of stress; cutting helped the stress a little but hiding it from the parents was stressful, as was the fear of getting caught. The client doesn't know what gives life meaning. "More friends?" When other students at a school suggested that perhaps Fatima was a boy, this seemed to fit. The client chose the name Ali in honor of an uncle killed in Afghanistan.

I: Importance and Influence *"What importance does spirituality have in your life?" "Has your spirituality influenced how you take care of yourself, particularly regarding your health?" "Does your spirituality affect your health-care decision making?"*

Parents: Islam means everything to them. They are trying to raise all their children as Muslims. They try to follow all Islamic teachings. They do not agree with transgenderism, which they think is anti-Islamic and a product of secular America.

Client: Again shrugs. The client is Muslim and believes it is the one true religion but does not believe the religion's rules need to be strictly followed. The client knew the parents would not like transgenderism and tried to hide it from them, but was surprised at the strength of their reactions. Uncle Ali, whose name is taken by the client, was a student at a Midrash (Islamic school) when he was killed by a bomb. The client feels that one can be a good Muslim and transgender.

C: Community *"Are you a part of a spiritual community?" "Is your community of support to you and how?" "Is there a group of people you really love or who are important to you?"*

Parents: They belong to the local mosque, which is the source of their friends, social life, and material support. It is the center of their life and faith.

Client: Again shrugs. The mosque is "OK." The Imam "talks too much," but can be nice sometimes. Head coverings are required at the mosque. Some of the adults there are "OK." The services are "boring." There is a friend there that the client likes, a girl, but she's been gone on a long trip to Pakistan, and they've been out of touch because the friend does not have a cell phone.

A: Address/Action in Care *"How would you like me, as your healthcare provider, to address spiritual issues in your healthcare?"*

Parents: They want the health-care team to respect their religious views and their authority as Fatima's parents, treat Fatima as a girl, and discharge Fatima home as soon as possible.

Client: "I want to be a boy Muslim. They have more freedom. I want to be an engineer like my dad. I don't want to get married and stay home raising children. That's boring."

FICA tool used with permission of Christina M. Puchalski, MD, The George Washington Institute for Spirituality and Health (GWish), The George Washington University.

CLINICAL JUDGMENT IN ACTION

1. What cues indicate that the client is experiencing spiritual distress?
2. What interventions have the highest priority?
3. What findings indicate resolution, improvement, or decline in this scenario?

Review Questions

1. A client is severely injured after a motor vehicle accident. The emergency department health-care team is working vigorously to stabilize the client. A medical assistant informs the nurse that a priest is in the waiting room and wants to see the client immediately. How should the nurse proceed?
   a. Bring the priest in immediately.
   b. Ask the medical assistant to tell the priest the visit will have to wait until later.
   c. Tell the client to say their prayers.
   d. Clarify with the client/family if the priest visit is wanted, and if it is desired, do what is feasible in this situation.

2. When assisting a client in disrobing for medical treatment, what attention should be paid by the nurse to the client's clothes and personal belongings?
   a. None; they are not important at this time.
   b. Little; they can be attended to later.
   c. Some; there may be valuables among them.
   d. They should be attended to with care as soon as possible because they may hold important spiritual or religious meaning and symbolism.

3. When is the best time to conduct a spiritual assessment?
   a. When the client is initially assessed as part of the health history
   b. When the client is about to undergo surgery
   c. When the client is near death
   d. When the client has been newly diagnosed with melanoma

4. A client describes to you a potentially harmful set of religious and spiritual beliefs. What is the best course of action?
   a. Listen respectfully while maintaining a neutral stance.
   b. Smirk and shake your head.
   c. Steer the conversation back to the medical history.
   d. Point out the obvious errors in the beliefs.

5. A Spanish-speaking client is 2 days postpartum and packing to go home. A nurse enters the room and begins teaching about the importance of birth control. The nurse hands over several pamphlets written in English and pressures the client to choose which kind to use. The client avoids eye contact, tosses the pamphlets into the suitcase, and says, "I'll look at home." What might the nurse have overlooked? Select all that apply.
   a. The nurse did not assess the client's need or desire for birth control.
   b. The nurse did not assess or know the client's religious or spiritual beliefs or social situation, which might impact the need for birth control information.
   c. The nurse did not know if the client had the desire for more children.
   d. The nurse did not assess the client's health literacy or written language preference.

6. A client goes to an urgent care center for fatigue, high fever, chest pain, and shortness of breath. A chest X-ray shows bilateral infiltrates indicative of pneumonia. The nurse informs the client that IV antibiotics have been prescribed by the nurse practitioner. As the nurse readies the antibiotic infusion, the client's partner bursts into the room and states the client requires intensive prayers to heal and nothing more. This belief aligns with which of the following religions?
   a. Jehovah's Witnesses
   b. Roman Catholic
   c. Hinduism
   d. Church of Christ, Scientist

7. The following clients are near death. For which client would you conduct a spiritual assessment and offer to help provide spiritual and religious support? Select all that apply.
   a. A 20-year-old client who is transgender
   b. An 80-year-old female client with a rosary wrapped around her wrist
   c. A 30-year-old 20-weeks-pregnant client who says she is "an avowed atheist"
   d. A 50-year-old client with substance use disorder who is homeless

8. The nurse wants to conduct a spiritual assessment on a client admitted to the oncology floor with a new diagnosis of pancreatic cancer. Which of the following assessment tools can be used? Select all that apply.
   a. FICA
   b. SASQ
   c. HOPE
   d. HITS
   e. OPEN INVITE

9. Which of the following is a true statement?
   a. A majority of Americans identify as following some kind of formal religion.
   b. A majority of Americans are unaffiliated.
   c. A majority of Americans are atheists or agnostics.
   d. A majority of Americans don't care about religion at all.

10. Which of the following statements best describes a dogma?
   a. The beliefs of a religion that are so essential to the identity of that religion that to deny them is to deny the religion itself
   b. Codified beliefs and lists of mandatory or prohibited acts that help define the self's relation to the object of worship
   c. An organized system of beliefs usually centered around the worship of a sacred, supernatural force or being, which in turn defines the self and the self's purpose in life
   d. The assent to the truth of those beliefs and may also refer to the total orientation of the self's entire life to the belief structure

CHAPTER

7 Nutritional Assessment

Learning Outcomes

1. Describe key recommendations of the *Dietary Guidelines for Americans*, 2025–2030.
2. Identify nutritional differences throughout the life cycle.
3. Conduct a nutritional health history.
4. Perform a nutrition-focused physical examination on a client including anthropometric measurements.
5. Describe laboratory results and their clinical significance to the nutritional assessment.
6. Identify the United States Preventive Services Task Force recommendations for nutritional health.
7. Document a complete health history and physical examination on a client with a nutritional disorder.

Nutrition, or the processes by which the body metabolizes and utilizes nutrients, affects every system in the body. We must have food and drink to sustain life—but what type, and how much? These are the questions that must be asked when assessing a person's nutritional health. Healthcare providers must also understand how the body digests and absorbs nutrients, the importance of meeting daily nutritional requirements, the causes and results of an imbalance of nutrients, and how to assess nutritional status. Social determinants of health (SDOH) including psychological, social, environmental, educational, financial, and cultural issues must also be considered during a nutritional assessment.

The U.S. Department of Health and Human Services' ***Healthy People 2030*** public health initiative identified two health behaviors focused specifically on nutrition and food: nutrition and healthy eating and safe food handling. The healthy eating objectives include increasing fruit, vegetable, and whole grain consumption, decreasing sugary drinks and sodium intake, reducing food insecurity, increasing intake of vitamins and minerals, increasing the number of infants breastfeeding, and reducing obesity. Safe food handling objectives include reducing foodborne infections and reducing allergen reactions requiring emergency department care. Proper nutrition greatly affects the development and course of many chronic conditions (e.g., coronary artery disease, diabetes mellitus, hypertension, osteoporosis, and some types of anemia). By promoting solid dietary practices, *Healthy People 2030* strives to increase each American's quality of life and the number of years of a healthy life and to eliminate health disparities.

Dietary Guidelines

The Dietary Guidelines Advisory Committee publishes its revision of the evidence-based **Dietary Guidelines for Americans** every 5 years. The committee aims to promote health and reduce the morbidity and mortality of chronic diseases by recommending foods and drinks that meet nutrient needs. The Dietary Guidelines also promote increased physical activity and less sedentary behavior. The U.S. Department of Agriculture (USDA) and the U.S. Department of Health and Human Services (HHS) use this information to formulate programs and policies for the American public. The Dietary Guidelines for Americans, 2025–2030 apply to healthy people from diverse racial and ethnic backgrounds. Refer to the website, *https://www.dietaryguidelines.gov,* for the complete report and recommendations.

Dietary guidelines are published by various government agencies to educate the general population regarding dietary needs. In 1997, the Food and Nutrition Board of the Institute of Medicine developed **Dietary Reference Intakes (DRIs)**. DRIs are used to assess an individual's diet and are the basis on which nutritious, balanced diets are devised. DRIs have four components: Adequate Intake (AI), Estimated Average Requirement (EAR), Tolerable Upper Intake Level (UL), and Recommended Dietary Allowances (RDA). AI is the specific intake value that is estimated to provide adequate nutrition for each sex and various age groups. EAR is the average daily nutrient level that should meet the needs of 50% of healthy men or women at a specific life stage. UL is the maximum level of daily nutrients that is unlikely to pose health risks for most of the general population. **Recommended Dietary Allowances (RDA)** are the recommended amounts of nutrients that should be eaten daily by healthy individuals. Recommendations differ based on sex, age, and whether the client is pregnant or lactating. These are recommendations, not requirements. Requirements are the amounts needed to prevent deficiencies. Recommendations exceed the required amounts to ensure that the entire population is considered.

Historically, a framework to guide dietary intake was the "Basic Four" food guide. The "Basic Four" food guide, first issued in 1956, divided foods into four groups: milk and dairy; meats; vegetables and fruits; and breads and cereals. The USDA published recommendations in 1992 using the Food Guide Pyramid, which expanded on the original basic four food groups to include guidelines on proportions and moderation.

In 2005, the USDA published a new food guidance system, the MyPyramid, to replace the original 1992 Food Guide Pyramid. This plan offered individuals a more personalized approach to nutrition that combined healthy eating with physical activity.

MyPlate debuted in 2011, replacing MyPyramid as the United States' guide for healthful eating. MyPlate incorporates the evidence-based data that are the basis of the *Dietary Guidelines for Americans.* MyPlate has five color-coded areas that represent the types of food one should eat daily. The size of each section correlates with the quantity of each food that should be consumed (see Figure 7-1). The website, *http://www.myplate.gov,* provides interactive tools that allow users to evaluate their current diet and structure a healthful daily food plan. Recommendations for how to eat healthy on a limited budget, healthy eating tips, information on food groups, and weight loss are available on the website. Information is also available in Spanish. Refer to the website periodically for updates.

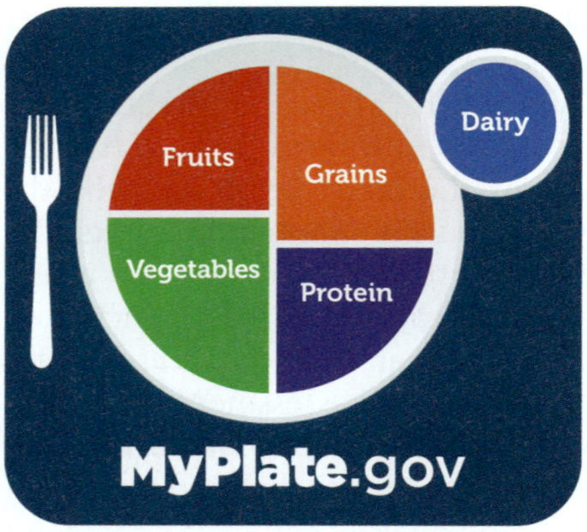

Figure 7-1 MyPlate Food Guide.

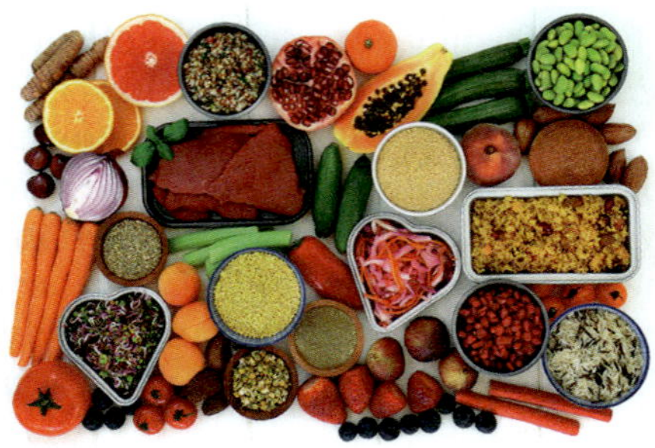

Figure 7-2 Accurate nutritional assessment necessitates knowledge of the nutrients within the food.

Nutrients

To perform a proper nutritional assessment, you must have a clear understanding of the various nutrients needed to provide an adequate diet, the reason they are needed, and the food sources that provide them (Fig. 7-2).

Nutrients are the substances found in food that are nourishing and useful to the body. Carbohydrates, proteins, fats, vitamins, minerals, and water are the nutrients essential for life.

Carbohydrates, proteins, and fats supply the body with energy, which is measured in units called **kilocalories (kcal)**. A kilocalorie (also called *calorie*) is the amount of heat required to raise 1 gram of water 1 degree centigrade. Table 7-1 lists the estimated calorie needs per day by age, gender, and physical activity level.

Carbohydrates

The major source of energy for the various functions of the body is **carbohydrates**. Each gram of carbohydrate contains four calories. Children older than age 1 and adults require 45% to 65% of their daily caloric intake in the form of carbohydrates to prevent ketosis and protein breakdown of muscles (Institute of Medicine, 2005).

Carbohydrates help form adenosine triphosphate (ATP), which is needed to transfer energy within the cells. Carbohydrates supply fiber and assist in

Table 7-1 Estimated Calorie Needs per Day by Age, Sex, and Physical Activity Level[a]

Estimated amounts of calories needed to maintain calorie balance for various sex and age groups at three different levels of physical activity. The estimates are rounded to the nearest 200 calories. An individual's calorie needs may be higher or lower than these average estimates.

		Physical Activity Level[b]		
Sex	**Age (Years)**	**Sedentary**	**Moderately Active**	**Active**
Child (female and male)	2-3	1,000-1,200[c]	1,000-1,400[c]	1,000-1,400[c]
Female[d]	4-8	1,200-1,400	1,400-1,600	1,400-1,800
	9-13	1,400-1,600	1,600-2,000	1,800-2,200
	14-18	1,800	2,000	2,400
	19-30	1,800-2,000	2,000-2,200	2,400
	31-50	1,800	2,000	2,200
	51 +	1,600	1,800	2,000-2,200
Male	4-8	1,200-1,400	1,400-1,600	1,600-2,000
	9-13	1,600-2,000	1,800-2,200	2,000-2,600
	14-18	2,000-2,400	2,400-2,800	2,800-3,200
	19-30	2,400-2,600	2,600-2,800	3,000
	31-50	2,200-2,400	2,400-2,600	2,800-3,000
	51 +	2,000-2,200	2,200-2,400	2,400-2,800

a. Based on Estimated Energy Requirements (EER) equations, using reference heights (average) and reference weights (healthy) for each age/gender group. For children and adolescents, reference height and weight vary. For adults, the reference man is 5 feet 10 inches tall and weighs 154 lb. The reference woman is 5 feet 4 inches tall and weighs 126 lb. EER equations are from the Institute of Medicine. *Dietary Reference Intakes for Energy, Carbohydrate, Fiber, Fat, Fatty Acids, Cholesterol, Protein, and Amino Acids.* National Academies Press, 2005.

b. *Sedentary* means a lifestyle that includes only the light physical activity associated with typical day-to-day life. *Moderately active* means a lifestyle that includes physical activity equivalent to walking about 1.5 to 3 miles per day at 3 to 4 miles per hour, in addition to the light physical activity associated with typical day-to-day life. *Active* means a lifestyle that includes physical activity equivalent to walking more than 3 miles per day at 3 to 4 miles per hour, in addition to the light physical activity associated with typical day-to-day life.

c. The calorie ranges shown are to accommodate the needs of different ages within the group. For children and adolescents, more calories are needed at older ages. For adults, fewer calories are needed at older ages.

d. Estimates for females do not include women who are pregnant or breastfeeding.

the utilization of fat. The primary sources of carbohydrates are bread, potatoes, pasta, corn, rice, dried beans, and fruits. Dietary deficiency of carbohydrates can result in electrolyte imbalance, fatigue, and depression. However, an excess of carbohydrates may produce obesity and tooth decay and may adversely affect those with diabetes mellitus.

Diets high in fiber have been shown to be beneficial in disease prevention. The possible benefits are decreased weight and a decrease in the risks of colorectal cancer, heart disease (through decreasing serum cholesterol levels), dental caries, constipation, and diverticulitis.

Proteins

There are four calories in every gram of protein, but foods usually are a combination of protein and fat (meats, milk) or protein and carbohydrates (legumes). Adults, 19 years and older, should have 10% to 35% of their daily caloric intake come from protein. Children ages 4 to 18 are advised to have protein constitute 10% to 30% of their diet. Children 1 to 3 years of age should consume 5% to 20% of their calories from protein sources (Institute of Medicine, 2005).

Protein is required to supply the body with the nine essential amino acids that the body is unable to synthesize. These amino acids form the basis of all cell structures in the body. Protein is needed to manufacture and repair body tissue; it helps to maintain osmotic pressure within the cells; it is a component of antibodies; and it is ultimately a source of energy.

A complete protein source contains all nine essential amino acids. The major sources of protein are meat, poultry, fish, eggs, cheese, and milk. Legumes (dried beans and peas) are a good source of protein when eaten with corn or wheat (e.g., a combination of beans and rice provides a good source of complete protein). This is helpful information for vegetarians and people whose incomes will not cover the purchase of meat and milk products.

Fats

Lipids, or fats, contain 9 calories per gram. The Institute of Medicine (2005) recommends that fats constitute 20% to 35% of the diet in adults 19 and older. Children ages 4–18 should have their diet consist of 25% to 35% fat, and for children 1 to 3 years this range increases to 30% to 40%. **Fats** supply the essential fatty acids, which form a part of the structure of all cells and must be supplied by the diet. They also help to lower the serum cholesterol level. Fats influence the texture and taste of food. The food sources of fat are animal fat (butter, shortening, and lard) and vegetable fat (vegetable oil, margarine, and nuts).

The types of fats consumed in the diet should be evaluated. **Saturated fats** come from animal sources (butter, lard, and fatty meats) and vegetable sources (coconut, palm, and the partially hydrogenated oils that are used in some processed foods). Saturated fats have been found to raise cholesterol levels. **Monounsaturated fats** (olive and canola oils) lower LDL cholesterol and do not lower HDL cholesterol. **Cholesterol** is a lipid found only in animal products. It is found in muscles, red blood cells, and cell membranes. Cholesterol is transported in the blood by **high-density lipoproteins** (HDLs) and **low-density lipoproteins** (LDLs). HDLs are useful in carrying cholesterol toward the liver. The LDLs carry the cholesterol toward the cells and then tissues, and deposit it there. There is a strong association between high levels of LDL and coronary artery disease (CAD). In contrast, high levels of HDLs protect against CAD.

Triglycerides account for most of the lipids stored in the body's tissues. In the bloodstream, triglycerides produce energy for the body. An elevated triglyceride level occurs in hyperlipidemia, a risk factor for CAD.

NURSING TIP
Omega-3 Fatty Acids

Both the medical literature and the public media publicize and promote omega-3 fatty acids. An omega-3 fatty acid is a polyunsaturated fat that is cardioprotective in nature. These fatty acids are found in salmon, sardines, nuts, avocados, mung beans, kidney beans, melons, broccoli, and spinach. The American Heart Association (Rimm et al., 2018) recommends eating one to two servings of fish per week to capitalize on the heart-healthy benefit of these fatty acids.

A deficiency of fat in the diet can cause a decrease in weight, a lack of satiety, and skin and hair changes. An excess of fat in the diet contributes to obesity and is linked to CAD. There has also been a correlation between high-fat diets and certain cancers (colorectal, breast, and prostate, in particular).

Vitamins

Vitamins are organic substances needed to maintain the function of the body. They are not supplied by the body in sufficient amounts and must be obtained from dietary sources. **Fat-soluble vitamins** are stored in dietary fat and absorbed in the fat portions of the body's cells; these are vitamins A, D, E, and K. **Water-soluble vitamins** include C, thiamine (B_1), riboflavin (B_2), niacin (B_3), pyridoxine (B_6), folacin (folate), cobalamin (B_{12}), pantothenic acid, and biotin. They are not stored in the body as they are excreted in the urine. Various disease conditions occur when a vitamin source is lacking. Table 7-2 discusses the signs and symptoms of vitamin deficiencies and excesses.

Table 7-2 Fat-Soluble Vitamins and Water-Soluble Vitamins

Name	Food and Other Sources	Functions	Deficiency/Toxicity
Vitamin A (retinol)	Animal: Kidney Liver Whole milk Butter Cream Cod liver oil Plants: Dark-green, leafy vegetables Deep yellow or orange fruit Fortified margarine	Dim-light vision Maintenance of mucous membranes Growth and development of bones	Deficiency: Night blindness Xerophthalmia Respiratory infections Bone growth cessation Toxicity: Cessation of menstruation Joint pain Stunted growth Enlargement of liver
Vitamin D (cholecalciferol)	Animal: Eggs Liver Fish liver oils Fortified milk Plants: Fortified cereals Other: Sunlight	Bone growth Tooth development	Deficiency: Rickets Osteomalacia Osteoporosis Poorly developed teeth Muscle spasms Toxicity: Nephrolithiasis Calcification of soft tissues
Vitamin E (alpha-tocopherol)	Animal: None Plants: Legumes Whole grains Dark-green, leafy vegetables Margarines Salad dressing	Antioxidant	Deficiency: Destruction of RBCs Toxicity: Hypertension

Continued

Table 7-2 Fat-Soluble Vitamins and Water-Soluble Vitamins—cont'd

Name	Food and Other Sources	Functions	Deficiency/Toxicity
Vitamin K	Animal: Egg yolk Liver Milk Plants: Green, leafy vegetables Cabbage	Blood clotting	Deficiency: Prolonged time for blood clotting Toxicity: Hemolytic anemia Jaundice
Thiamine (vitamin B_1)	Animal: Pork Beef Liver Eggs Fish Plants: Whole and enriched grains Legumes	Coenzyme in oxidation of glucose Normal appetite Healthy nervous system	Deficiency: Gastrointestinal tract, nervous, and cardiovascular system problems Toxicity: None
Riboflavin (vitamin B_2)	Animal: Liver Kidney Milk Plants: Green, leafy vegetables Cereals Enriched bread	Aids release of energy from food Healthy skin Healthy vision	Deficiency: Cheilosis Glossitis Photophobia Toxicity: None
Pyridoxine (vitamin B_6)	Animal: Fish Poultry Pork Milk Eggs Plants: Whole-grain cereals Legumes	Synthesis of nonessential amino acids Conversion of tryptophan to niacin Antibody production	Deficiency: Cheilosis Glossitis Toxicity: Liver disease
Vitamin B_{12} (cobalamin)	Animal: Seafood Meat Eggs Milk Plants: None	Synthesis of RBCs Maintenance of myelin sheaths	Deficiency: Degeneration of myelin sheaths Pernicious anemia Toxicity: None
Niacin B_3 (nicotinic acid)	Animal: Milk Eggs Fish Poultry Plants: None	Transfers hydrogen atoms for synthesis of ATP Healthy skin Healthy nervous system Healthy digestion	Deficiency: Pellagra Dermatitis Dementia Diarrhea Toxicity: Vasodilation of blood vessels

Table 7-2 Fat-Soluble Vitamins and Water-Soluble Vitamins—cont'd

Name	Food and Other Sources	Functions	Deficiency/Toxicity
Folacin (folic acid)	Animal: Liver Plants: Green, leafy vegetables Spinach Asparagus Broccoli Kidney beans	Synthesis of RBCs	Deficiency: Glossitis Macrocytic anemia Neural tube defects of fetus in pregnancy Toxicity: None
Biotin	Animal: Milk Liver Plants: Legumes Mushrooms	Coenzyme in carbohydrate and amino acid metabolism Niacin synthesis from tryptophan	Deficiency: Dermatitis Loss of hair Toxicity: None
Pantothenic acid	Animal: Eggs Liver Salmon Yeast Plants: Mushrooms Cauliflower Peanuts	Metabolism of carbohydrates, lipids, and proteins Synthesis of acetylcholine	Deficiency: Burning sensation in feet Toxicity: None
Vitamin C (ascorbic acid)	Animal: None Plants: All citrus Broccoli Tomatoes Brussels sprouts Potatoes	Prevention of scurvy Formation of collagen Healing of wounds Release of stress hormones Absorption of iron	Deficiency: Scurvy Easy bruising Muscle cramps Ulcerated gums Toxicity: Raised uric acid level Hemolytic anemia Kidney stones Rebound scurvy

ATP = adenosine triphosphate; RBC = red blood cell.

Minerals

Minerals are inorganic elements that build body tissue and regulate body processes. These processes include fluid balance; acid-base balance; nerve cell transmission; vitamin, enzyme, and hormonal activity; and muscle contraction. Minerals are divided into two classifications. **Macrominerals**, or major minerals, are needed by the body in large amounts (>100 mg/day) (Table 7-3). **Microminerals**, or trace minerals, are needed in smaller amounts by the body (<15 mg/day) (Table 7-4).

The most common nutrient deficiency in the world is iron deficiency. This is particularly prevalent among infants, adolescents, and pregnant and menstruating clients. It can result in iron-deficiency anemia.

Table 7-3 Major Minerals

Name	Food Sources	Functions	Deficiency/Toxicity
Calcium (Ca)	Milk Cheese Sardines Salmon Green vegetables	Development of bones and teeth Permeability of cell membranes Transmission of nerve impulses Blood clotting	Deficiency: Osteoporosis Osteomalacia Rickets Poor tooth formation Toxicity: Constipation Increased risk of nephrolithiasis when large amounts are taken in a short period
Phosphorus (P)	Milk Cheese Poultry Lean meat Fish Nuts Legumes	Development of bones and teeth Transfer of energy Component of phospholipids Buffer system	Same as calcium
Potassium (K)	Oranges Bananas Dried fruits Meat Cereals	Contraction of muscles Maintenance of water balance Transmission of nerve impulses Carbohydrate and protein metabolism	Deficiency: Hypokalemia Muscle cramps Irregular heart rhythm Toxicity: Hyperkalemia Irregular heart rhythm
Sodium (Na)	Table salt Beef Eggs Poultry Milk Cheese	Maintenance of fluid balance in blood Transmission of nerve impulses	Deficiency: Acid-base disturbance Seizures Toxicity: Increase in blood pressure Edema
Chloride (Cl)	Table salt Meat Eggs Seafood	Gastric acidity Regulation of osmotic pressure Activation of salivary amylase	Deficiency: Imbalance in gastric acidity Imbalance in blood pH Toxicity: None
Magnesium (Mg)	Green vegetables Milk Nuts Legumes Whole grains	Synthesis of ATP Transmission of nerve impulses Activation of metabolic enzymes Relaxation of skeletal muscles	Deficiency: CNS depression Seizures Toxicity: Diarrhea Hypersomnolence
Sulfur (S)	Eggs Poultry Fish	Protein structure maintenance Formation of high-energy compounds	Deficiency: None Toxicity: None

Table 7-4 Trace Minerals

Name	Food Sources	Functions	Deficiency/Toxicity
Iron (Fe)	Meat, organ meats, fish, poultry, dried fruits, beans, fortified cereals, dark-green, leafy vegetables	Transports oxygen and carbon dioxide	Deficiency: Iron deficiency anemia Toxicity: Hemochromatosis
Iodine (I)	Seafood, iodized salt	Regulates basal metabolic rate	Deficiency: Goiter Congenital hypothyroidism (cretinism) Myxedema Toxicity: Rare
Zinc (Zn)	Eggs, oysters, liver, legumes, milk	Formation of collagen Component of insulin Component of many vital enzymes Wound healing	Deficiency: Growth retardation Toxicity: Decreased copper and iron absorption
Selenium (Se)	Liver, seafood, grains	Antioxidant	Deficiency: Rare Toxicity: Rare
Copper (Cu)	Oysters, liver, nuts, legumes, whole grains	Oxidation of glucose	Deficiency: Rare Toxicity: Wilson disease
Manganese (Mn)	Nuts, peas, beans, fruits	Component of metabolic enzymes	Deficiency: Rare Toxicity: Rare
Fluoride (F)	Fluoridated drinking water, seafood	Reduces dental caries	Deficiency: Dental caries Toxicity: Mottled-looking teeth
Chromium (Cr)	Eggs, meats, whole grain cereals	Binds insulin to cell membranes	Deficiency: Impaired glucose intolerance (rare) Toxicity: Rare
Molybdenum (Mo)	Liver, legumes, whole grains, dark-green, leafy vegetables	Metabolism of nucleic acids to uric acid	Deficiency: Headache Tachycardia Toxicity: Rare

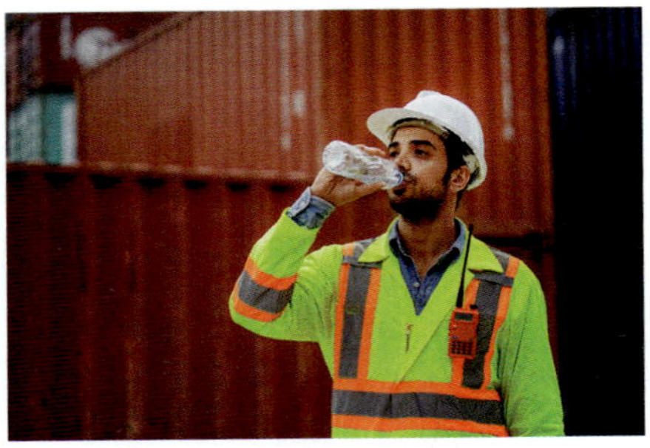

Figure 7-3 Hydration is essential to body function, especially when engaged in strenuous activities.

NURSING TIP

Signs and Symptoms of Dehydration

- Health history reveals inadequate intake of fluids
- Decrease in urine output
- Urine specific gravity >1.035
- Weight loss (% body weight): 3% to 5% for mild, 6% to 9% for moderate, and 10% to 15% for severe dehydration
- Eyes appear sunken; tongue has increased furrows and fissures
- Oral mucous membranes are dry
- Decreased skin turgor
- Sunken fontanels in infants
- Inability to produce tears
- Changes in neurological status (with moderate to severe dehydration)

NURSING TIP

Bottled Water

Many Americans drink bottled water exclusively, or are drinking a large quantity of bottled water. The reasons are many: belief that it is purer, safer, and healthier; social status (it is "cool"); transportability; storage; and concerns about the purity of tap water. However, most bottled water does not contain sufficient, if any, fluoride, so consumers are missing the trace mineral that helps prevent dental caries. Children may need fluoride supplements if they drink mostly bottled water. Also, the use of metal or hard plastic containers, to reduce the number of plastic water bottles that may not be recycled, is advocated by many communities.

Water

Water is essential to life; we cannot survive more than a few days without it. Water accounts for 50% to 60% of the body's weight. The daily amount needed depends on many factors, including gender, the climate, and the amount of activity. According to the *Dietary Guidelines for Americans*, 2025–2030, water should be the primary beverage in a healthy diet, along with beverages that contribute beneficial nutrients. Plain Water Intake (PWI) is the amount of water an individual drinks per day. Total Water Intake (TWI) is the combined total water obtained from drinking water, water in food consumed, and water in other beverages. Recent evidence indicates that 20 mL/kg of water daily may be the best recommendation for simultaneously meeting the hydration criteria and limiting chronic disease risk (Stookey, 2019). Athletes and those living in hot, dry climates require more. Thirst may not always be an adequate indicator of water intake needs, especially in infants or very ill individuals who may have a poor thirst mechanism. Those who engage in intense physical activity may have a decreased thirst sensation as well (Fig. 7-3).

In addition, it is important to determine the source of the water intake. Tap water is usually safe in most areas of this country. Since 1971, the CDC has monitored drinking water for contaminants, which include parasites, bacteria, viruses, chemicals, and soil deposits. Illnesses from tainted tap water range from gastroenteritis to cancer, hemolytic uremic syndrome, teratogenic effects, and even death. However, there is a trend of people consuming more bottled water than tap water (see Nursing Tip, Bottled Water). This may pose potential health problems. Also, people who live in less populated areas may have access to only well water, which must be carefully monitored for health risks. In some rural areas, rusty water pipes harboring unknown pathogens may be the only source of water. In other areas, local streams/rivers may be the only source of water (Fig. 7-4). Even regulated water systems can be contaminated, as occurred in Flint, Michigan. The alarm was sounded in 2014 when elevated levels of lead were found in the drinking water (Miracle, 2017). Regulated as well as unregulated water sources should be monitored by governments and individuals regularly to avoid the risk of illness.

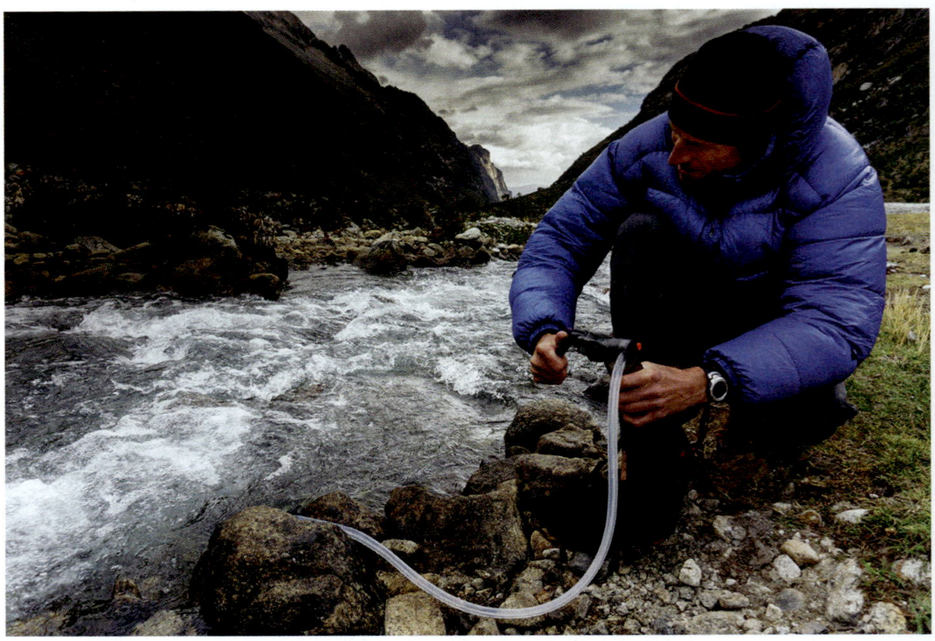

Figure 7-4 The source must be considered when evaluating the potability of water.

Nutrition Through the Life Cycle

Assessment of the client's developmental needs must always be included with a nutritional assessment. Nutritional needs change throughout the life cycle and are affected by both physical and developmental changes. A clear understanding of those changes, how they affect the client, and what anticipatory guidance is indicated is needed to conduct a nutritional assessment. **Anticipatory guidance** covers health promotion; informs at-risk individuals of physical, cognitive, psychological, and social changes that may occur; and explains their nutritional needs.

Children

Recommended daily requirements for children change with each age group. An understanding of development regarding physical, cognitive, and psychosocial changes is needed to properly assess the nutritional needs of children. This includes educating the caregiver about these changes before they occur. Families can then have more realistic expectations and an understanding of what is within the normal range and what should be cause for concern.

Infants

Infants grow more during the first 6 to 12 months of life than at any other time. This is also the time when there is rapid neurological development, which emphasizes the need for proper nutrients. The American Academy of Pediatrics recommends the exclusive use of breast milk for infants, instead of formula feeding, for the first 6 months and then recommends continued breastfeeding along with nutritious food for the first 2 years and beyond (Fig. 7-5) (Meek & Noble, 2022); if this is not possible, even a few weeks is beneficial, except in limited cases where the mother is HIV positive or has human T-cell lymphotropic virus type I or type II infection, untreated brucellosis, or suspected or confirmed Ebola virus because these infections can be transmitted via breast milk. Equity continues to be a challenge with breastfeeding; the rates of breastfeeding continue to be lower for non-Hispanic Black women, low-income women, younger women (<20 years old), and those with a high school education or less (Meek & Noble, 2022). Be prepared to educate clients on the benefits of breastfeeding, support the caregiver's feeding decision, and discuss schedules, habits, and warning signs of problems or inadequate intake (Fig. 7-6). Gender-diverse parents may prefer to use the term *chestfeeding* for milk from a human source (Meek & Noble, 2022). It is important even with infant feeding to consider personal preferences, cultural traditions, and budget factors.

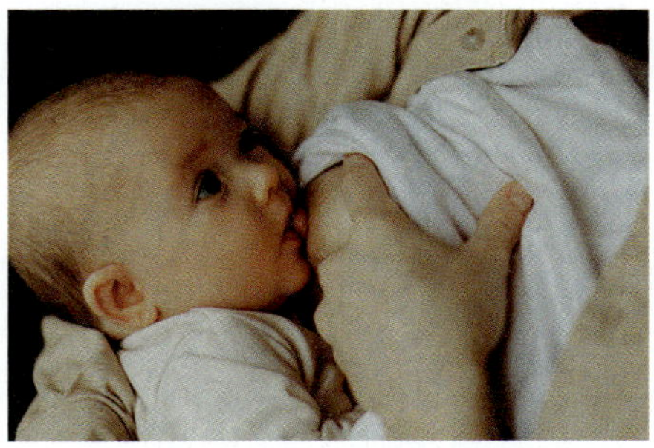

Figure 7-5 Breast milk is the preferred source of an infant's nutrition for the first 6 to 24 months.

Infants are born with several reflexes that should be assessed when evaluating their nutritional status: sucking, rooting, and swallowing. Infants can feel hunger and express the need to eat by crying. By 4 months old, infants can hold and bring teething rings or toys to their mouths. At 6 months old, infants can feed themselves a cracker. When infants are 8 to 12 months old, they may drink from a cup by themselves. The use of a developmental assessment tool helps monitor the infant's ability to achieve these milestones (see the Denver II, Chapter 25). Assessing the infant's physical development (such as head control and the ability to sit) is also helpful to determine readiness for solid food. Foods should be introduced one at a time to observe for possible allergic reactions. It is no longer advised for infants to delay the introduction of highly allergenic foods beyond 4 to 6 months to avoid atopic conditions; additionally, allergists now recommend peanut introduction as early as 4 to 6 months specifically in infants who have a higher risk for peanut allergies based on the existence of severe eczema and/or egg allergy (Greer et al., 2019). Also, infants under 12 months should not have honey, because of the possibility of botulism toxicity.

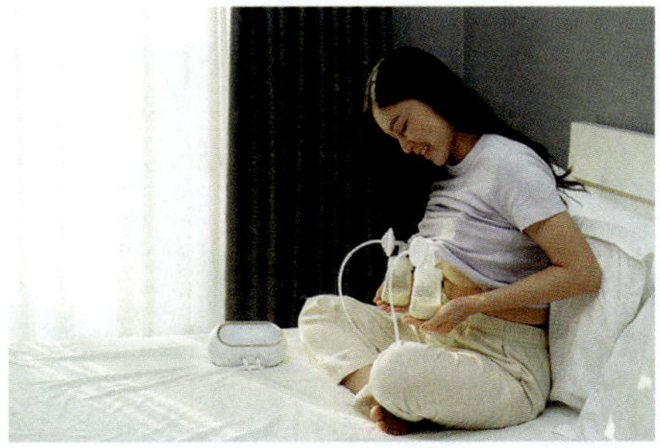

Figure 7-6 Many mothers pump their breast milk so that other people can be involved in infant feedings; fortified infant formulas are also a sound nutritional choice.

NURSING TIP
Preventing Choking

Instruct caregivers to:

- Avoid the use of foods that may cause choking in infants and small children (up to 3 years old), such as corn, nuts, raw peas and carrots, celery, small candies, hot dogs, popcorn, and any other small, hard food.
- Offer peanut butter only on bread or a cracker.
- Stress the importance of sitting up while eating; prohibit running with food or objects in the mouth.

NURSING CHECKLIST
Nutritional Assessment of Infants

- If the infant is breastfed, how often and for how long?
- How much formula does the infant take at each feeding, and how often does the infant eat? (Estimate how much is consumed in 24 hours.)
- How is the formula prepared? (It is important to make sure the formula is prepared correctly; this also helps establish how much the infant is eating). How is the prepared formula stored?
- How does the infant react to eating? Does the infant appear satisfied?
- Does the infant appear to have any respiratory distress or reflux while eating? Are there any problems with constipation or diarrhea, and if so, how are they treated? Have any allergies been diagnosed?
- Is the infant taking any supplemental food or vitamins?
- Is the infant ever put in bed with a bottle? If the answer is "yes", instruct the caregivers about infant bottle caries and the importance of not propping the bottle or placing it in the bed.

NURSING TIP
Lactose Intolerance

Lactose intolerance, which is caused by an insufficient amount of the enzyme lactase, is the inability of the body to digest foods containing the carbohydrate lactose. Lactose intolerance can affect people of all ages. Typically, people experience abdominal pain and cramping, bloating, flatulence, nausea, and diarrhea. Lactose-digesting enzymes and a lactose-free diet can limit the severity of the symptoms. If the client strictly follows these measures and symptoms persist, then another etiology should be explored.

Birth to 6 months: breast milk or infant formula only. Increases gradually to 28 to 32 oz per day by the third to fourth month of life and up to 40 ounces by 6 months.

6 to 8 months: iron-fortified cereals and other solid foods. Single-grain (rice or oat) cereals are usually introduced first. As the infant adjusts to eating a few solid foods, other food may be introduced. Help the infant adjust to spoon-feeding. Offer only one new food every 3 to 4 days to observe for signs of allergic reactions. Within a few months, the infant should have a variety of foods in the diet. Encourage parents to read the labels of all foods to determine what has been added. Fruit juices that are noncitrus may be introduced, but limited to 4 oz/day. It is helpful to use a cup. This prevents the infant from associating sweet fruit juices with a bottle and limits the amount ingested. Do not add sugar or seasoning to foods.

9 to 10 months: finger foods may be introduced. Small, bite-sized pieces that are cooked, mashed, and soft will allow the child independence and will provide increased texture, which requires chewing. Gradually increase foods with texture as the child's chewing skills improve and teeth emerge.

Toddlers

Toddlers have their own unique nutritional needs as their physical growth slows. Toddlers' development plays a very important role in their diet (Fig. 7-7) and in providing appropriate assessment and anticipatory guidance to caregivers. As children experience increased independence and control over their bodies, some of this independence is demonstrated in their eating patterns. There is an increased problem with food refusal or the desire for only certain foods. This is a normal response in this developmental stage and should not be a problem unless it is excessive. Toddlers may say "no" even to the food they desire to demonstrate that they are in charge.

Instruct parents to offer healthy foods that the toddler can self-feed in small portions and offer only one new food at a time. A serving size should be about 1 to 2 tablespoons of food for each year of age. Water and low-fat or fat-free milk are the best beverage choices for children over 2 years old. Toddlers are very good at imitating and often exhibit food dislikes that are shown at home (particularly if there is an older sibling). Encourage routine mealtimes that are enjoyed together to provide the toddler with role models for developing good eating habits (Jones, 2018).

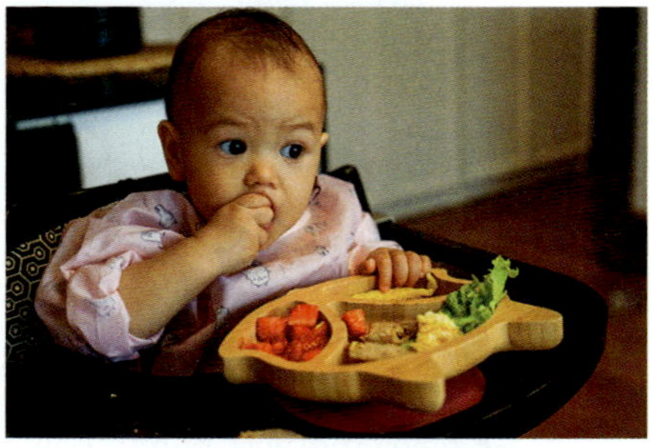

Figure 7-7 A toddler's developing motor skills allow the child to exert more independence and control with eating habits.

Preschoolers

Preschoolers continue to have food dislikes and may become picky eaters. They verbalize their likes and dislikes and show their independence by conflicting with their caregivers. Giving choices, serving small amounts of foods children can eat easily (finger foods), and providing a routine and enjoyable eating environment help to foster good eating habits by decreasing conflicts.

Preschoolers often have smaller appetites compared with toddlers. This may be caused by drinking too many liquids (milk, juice, and other beverages) and a slower increase in growth. They often are resistant to new foods and may eat only one food at a time. Encourage the caregivers to offer other foods. Discuss the need to provide healthy snacks and prevent the preschooler from eating foods that are too high in sugar. The preschooler benefits by helping to prepare food (Fig. 7-8), setting the table, and making some decisions. Providing preschoolers with acceptable options is an easy way to ensure an appropriate diet.

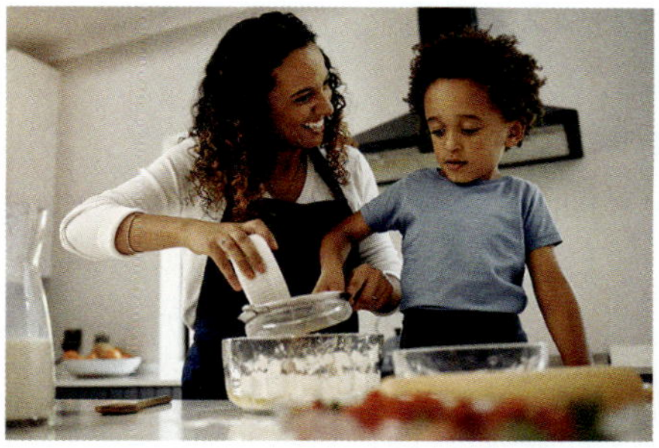

Figure 7-8 Preschoolers benefit from helping with meal preparation, especially with foods they like.

NURSING TIP

Obesity Epidemic in Children

A school-age child comes home from school; grabs a soda, chips, and cookies; and sits in front of the television. After some time, this child may move on to chat with friends on the Internet or play computer games (Fig. 7-9). This sedentary lifestyle and the child's dietary practices are some of the reasons for the alarming continuing increase in the rate of childhood obesity. Additional factors include gender, familial history of obesity, concurrent medical conditions, and Social Determinants of Health (SDOH) such as socioeconomic status, neighborhood environment, education, food security, and access to care. Racial and ethnic background disproportionately impact childhood obesity, namely, Hispanic and non-Hispanic Blacks (U.S. Department of Health and Human Services, 2022a). According to the CDC, 12.7% of children aged 2 to 5 years are obese, 20.7% of those aged 6 to 11 years are obese, and 22% of those aged 12 to 19 years are obese (Stierman et al., 2021). According to the U.S. Department of Health and Human Services (2022b), childhood obesity is associated with a higher risk for high blood pressure, high cholesterol, diabetes, asthma, anxiety, and depression. This obesity epidemic demands the attention of all nurses; those who are involved with children must be able to identify children at risk and intervene with those who are already overweight. The NHLBI's WE CAN! (Ways to Enhance Children's Activity and Nutrition available at: *https://www.nhlbi.nih.gov/health/educational/wecan/index.htm*) program in conjunction with health departments, universities, and community organizations, strives to reach children ages 8 to 13 with their educational programs. This science-based program's objectives are to improve food choices, increase physical activity, and decrease sedentary time spent at the computer or playing video games.

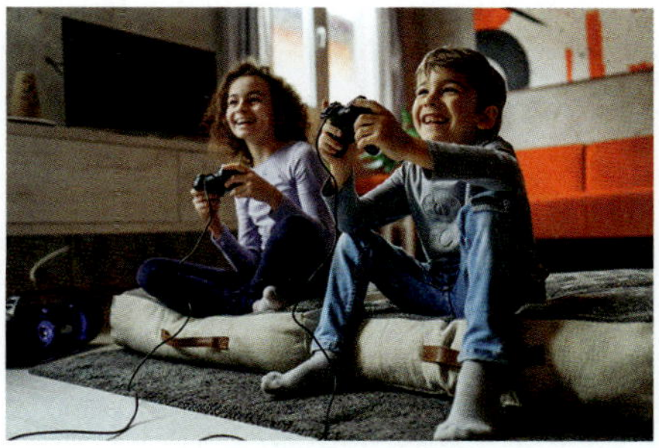

Figure 7-9 Playing sedentary games contributes to the childhood obesity epidemic.

School-Age Children

School-age children tend to have erratic growth patterns that are reflected in their equally erratic eating patterns. They also tend to continue having strong likes and dislikes. Encourage families to maintain a balanced diet and limit sweetened snacks and foods (Fig. 7-10). Caregivers should be advised to teach children proper nutrition and should be encouraged to show children how to read nutrition and ingredient labels. Advise caregivers and children that pubescent chubbiness—but not obesity—is a normal part of growth that often precedes a rapid increase in height.

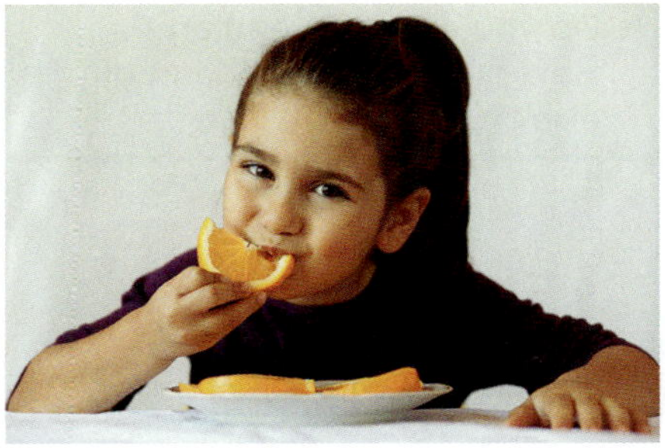

Figure 7-10 This school-age child is eating a healthy snack.

NURSING CHECKLIST

Nutritional Assessment of the Toddler, Preschooler, and School-Age Child

- Do you have any problem or concern with your child's eating?
- Is your child a picky eater, and how is this handled at home?
- Does your family eat together?
- What are your child's food likes or dislikes?
- What does your child eat for snacks?
- Is your child involved in sports or any other physical activity?
- What is your child's meal schedule? Where and when does your child eat?
- How much does your child eat during a meal?
- Does your child eat lunch at school?
- Does your child eat foods from all the groups in MyPlate?
- Does your child have any food allergies?
- Does your child drink beverages with added sugar (e.g., soda, fruit juices)? How much?

Adolescents

Adolescence is a period of rapid growth and change, and adolescents' nutritional needs fluctuate accordingly. Adolescents are concerned with body image and often compare their bodies to those of their peers and media images in an attempt to fit into an identity that is acceptable to them. A poor body image can lead to disordered eating (yo-yo dieting, preoccupation with food, or irregular eating habits) and progress to eating disorders such as anorexia nervosa, bulimia nervosa, and binge eating. Although eating disorders can occur at any age, they frequently begin in adolescence. Eating disorders are diagnosed through specific criteria set forth by the American Psychiatric Association (2022). Anorexia nervosa is characterized by severely low body weight, defined as being 85% or less of the client's ideal body weight; a distorted body image in which the individual perceives him-/herself to be fat; a fear of gaining weight; increased exercise patterns; and amenorrhea in women. Bulimia's hallmark is binge eating followed by purging. Purging can take many forms: self-induced vomiting and abuse of laxatives, diuretics, and enemas. These practices can lead to electrolyte imbalances. Clients with bulimia frequently complain of a sore throat and heartburn. They may also have tooth erosion, dental caries, and bleeding gums. In addition, the client with bulimia may be impulsive and have an addictive personality. A third eating disorder, Binge Eating, involves eating large amounts of food over short periods without regard for the sensations of hunger or fullness. This disorder does not involve purging as seen in bulimia. Individuals with eating disorders usually do not present for medical care unless physical symptoms manifest and they are hypotensive, have an acute electrolyte imbalance, or have abdominal complaints. Other more common, physical complaints include fatigue, dizziness, and low energy levels. Refer to the National Eating Disorder Association (NEDA) website (*https://www.nationaleatingdisorders.org/warning-signs-and-symptoms*) for common emotional and behavioral symptoms of eating disorders and additional information.

NURSING CHECKLIST

Nutritional Assessment of Adolescents

- Are you on any specific diet or meal plan?
- Do you skip any meals?
- Do you feel content with your weight? If not, how much do you feel you should weigh? What do you do to control your weight?
- How often do you weigh yourself?
- Are you involved in any sports? If so, are there any requirements regarding weight or food?
- Have you ever induced vomiting or used laxatives, diuretics, or diet pills to help with weight control?
- Do you eat snacks? What type of snacks? What are your between-meal eating habits?
- Do you exercise regularly? How often and what kind of exercise?

The level of physical activity must also be taken into account for a nutritional evaluation (Fig. 7-11). An understanding of the different sports and their requirements may help you screen for potential problems. In some sports (e.g., football), players are encouraged to be large and heavy; this puts them at risk for possible anabolic steroid use. Toxic effects of steroid use include possible cancer of the liver, short stature, behavioral changes, endocrine dysfunction (acne, impotence, testicular atrophy), and hypertension.

In sports where decreased weight is desirable (e.g., wrestling, gymnastics, dancing), athletes may try many methods to "make weight." Instruction about proper nutrition to help reduce body fat without compromising health is needed when working with all athletes.

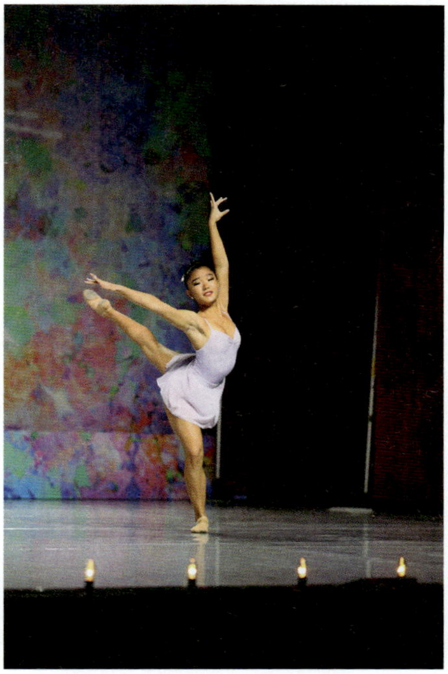

Figure 7-11 Female adolescents who participate in activities such as ballet are at risk for eating disorders.

Young and Middle-Aged Adults

Growth and caloric needs usually stabilize in young and middle-aged adults. Eating habits may be altered by changes in activity levels and by the effects of work and life stressors.

Obesity can be defined in several ways. **Obesity** is a weight greater than 120% of the ideal body weight (IBW). Obesity can also be defined as a body mass index (BMI) greater than 30 kg/m^2. Refer to the "Body Mass Index" section later in this chapter. Obesity occurs when the calories consumed exceed the calories expended. This can occur when there is an increase in food consumption, a decrease in activity level, or both. Obesity can occur at any age but is frequently seen in young and middle-aged adults. The CDC reports that 41.9% of adults aged 20 years and older are obese and 9.2% are extremely obese (Stierman et al., 2021). Many factors affect whether a person is prone to obesity: genetic, physiological, psychological, and environmental. Income and education also impact obesity with lower income and educational status increasing rates. Obesity unequally affects different races. Non-Hispanic Black adults have the highest prevalence of obesity (49.9%) at an almost 10% higher rate than non-Hispanic White adults; Hispanic adults are also more likely to be obese (45.6%) (Ogden et al., 2017). Obesity places a person at risk for hyperlipidemia, coronary artery disease (CAD), hypertension, diabetes mellitus, chronic disorders, and some cancers.

Clients who are overweight or obese frequently experience yo-yo dieting, or weight cycling. In weight cycling, clients diet for some time, achieve their goal weights, and cease dieting. The majority of people return to their usual eating habits and regain the lost weight and may add a few more pounds as well. Because many weight reduction programs do not address behavior modification or psychological factors associated with eating, nor do they include an exercise regimen, most diets fail. The use of fad diets (i.e., diets that promise results without effectively altering lifestyle) and fad exercise regimens (e.g., use of vibrating machines to lose fat, use of saunas to decrease weight) may be deleterious to a person's health. Some fad programs are relatively safe if followed for a short period with adequate professional supervision.

Noninsulin-dependent diabetes mellitus, or type 2 diabetes, can develop at any age but is usually diagnosed after age 40. It is associated with family history and obesity and is often undiagnosed until there are complications because, until then, the person often has few or only mild symptoms. The incidence of diabetes is increasing as the girth of Americans is increasing.

Coronary artery disease is one of the leading causes of death in the United States. The primary cause is **atherosclerosis**, which is the development of lipid plaques along the coronary arteries. The risk factors for atherosclerosis are discussed in Chapters 16 and 17.

Metabolic syndrome (MetS) is a cluster of conditions that, if present, cumulatively increases the risk of an adult developing cardiovascular disease and diabetes. The majority of the adults with MetS are overweight or obese. Lifestyle modification is the hallmark of treatment. Medications are used if the individual is unable to bring his or her risk factors to a normal level.

In the past, metabolic syndrome has been called syndrome X, insulin resistance syndrome, dysmetabolic syndrome, obesity syndrome, and

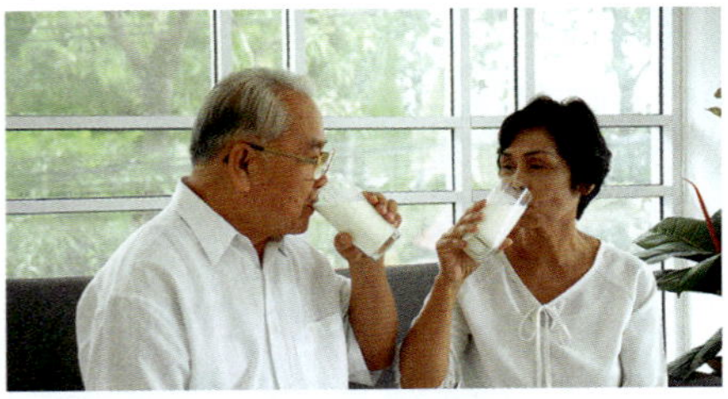

Figure 7-12 Calcium consumption is essential for all people. Both men and women can develop osteoporosis.

hypertriglyceridemic waist. The risk of developing MetS increases with age and is more prevalent in Blacks and Hispanics. Abdominal obesity, a family history of type 2 diabetes mellitus, and gestational diabetes also increase the risk of developing MetS. Other conditions that are associated with an increased risk of developing MetS are polycystic ovary syndrome and blood coagulopathies.

Under the most widely used diagnostic model, three of the following criteria must be present for a client to be diagnosed with MetS (Grundy et al., 2005):

- Waist circumference >35 in. (88 cm) in women
- Waist circumference >40 in. (102 cm) in men
- Fasting triglyceride level ≥ 150 mg/dL
- Fasting HDL cholesterol <50 mg/dL in women
- Fasting HDL cholesterol <40 mg/dL in men
- Blood pressure ≥ 130/ ≥ 85 mm Hg
- Fasting serum glucose ≥ 110 mg/dL

Osteoporosis is a disease that reduces bone mass. It is more common in women and often undiagnosed in men. (Fig. 7-12). Osteoporosis is often not detected until a person falls and fractures a bone. Suspect anorexia nervosa in a young, thin female with osteoporosis. See Chapter 19 for additional information.

Pregnant and Lactating Clients

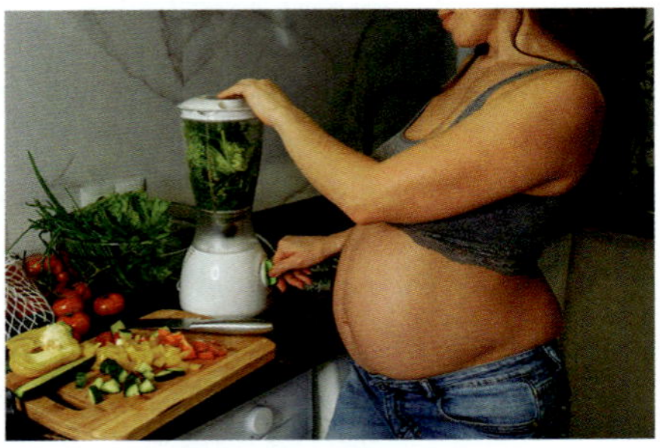

Figure 7-13 Optimal nutrition is essential in pregnancy.

It is important to assess and counsel a pregnant client regarding nutrition to promote a healthy pregnancy (Fig. 7-13). Proper nutrition for the client from the time of conception is required for the development of a healthy infant. The infant is at risk of being small for gestational age if the client does not gain adequate weight, and the client is at risk for gestational diabetes and hypertension if the weight gain is excessive. Target weight gain depends on the client's weight at conception. According to the Institute of Medicine (IOM) (2009), a client whose BMI is less than 18.5 kg/m^2 should gain 28 to 40 lb during pregnancy; a client with a preconception BMI of 18.5 to 24.9 kg/m^2 should gain 25 to 35 lb; a client with a BMI of 25 to 29.9 kg/m^2 should gain 15 to 25 lb; and a client with a BMI greater than 30 kg/m^2 should gain 11 to 20 lb. These recommended weight gains are for single fetuses. Guidelines for weight gain when carrying multiple fetuses can be viewed on the National Academy of Medicine (formerly IOM) website (*https://nam.edu/*). Assessment includes a general knowledge of physical changes during pregnancy and their relationships to nutrition. Some of the common complaints experienced during pregnancy (e.g., heartburn, constipation, nausea, hemorrhoids, and vomiting) can be alleviated by dietary changes such as small, frequent meals; increased fluid intake; and a well-balanced diet.

Iron supplements are routinely given during pregnancy because diet alone is not adequate to meet the body's requirements. Prenatal vitamins are also prescribed for all pregnant clients. There is evidence that folic acid helps to reduce the risk of neural tube defects, especially when the folic acid supplement is instituted three or more months before pregnancy.

In addition, the fluid requirements of a pregnant and lactating client are increased. Adequate fluid consumption helps to decrease the risk of premature labor. Lactating clients need additional fluid and may have to ingest 2 to 3 quarts of fluid daily.

Pica, or cravings for substances other than food, is a phenomenon documented primarily in pregnant clients. It is the practice of eating dirt, clay, starch, or even ice cubes, and may lead to nutritional difficulties, including an increased risk of anemia.

NURSING CHECKLIST

Nutritional Assessment of Pregnant Clients

- What was your prepregnancy weight?
- What is your activity level, and have there been any changes since you became pregnant?
- Do you take any supplemental vitamins?
- Do you have a history of problems during previous pregnancies? What were they? How were they resolved?
- How often do you use caffeine, artificial sweeteners, and alcohol?
- Do you experience constipation, nausea, vomiting, or heartburn?
- Do you have any food cravings?
- Do you have cravings for substances other than food?

NURSING TIP
Alternative Calcium Supplements

Most Americans consume calcium supplements in the form of calcium carbonate and calcium citrate. Calcium carbonate is best absorbed when taken with some food. Calcium citrate can be absorbed well with food or on an empty stomach. Many American men and women combine the food in their daily diet with one of these calcium supplements. Sometimes sufficient quantities of calcium are not consumed with these means to meet the recommended DRI. Additional treatment options are to consume calcium via calcium-fortified beverages (e.g., bottled water, orange juice, milk), calcium-fortified chocolate, calcium-fortified chewables, calcium-fortified aspirin, and calcium-fortified fiber. Corporations are developing new products to meet the tastes and lifestyles of today's diverse population.

Older Adults

Healthy eating habits and nutrition established early in life will benefit adults as they age, whereas unhealthy eating habits may contribute to disease processes (e.g., hypertension, diabetes mellitus, CAD, and obesity). Caloric needs decrease as a person ages, due to the reduction in basal metabolic rate, so health teaching should focus on modifications in portion size to coincide with reduced activity and decreased caloric requirements. Planning with the client to include acceptable modifications, and providing education and support, help to ensure compliance.

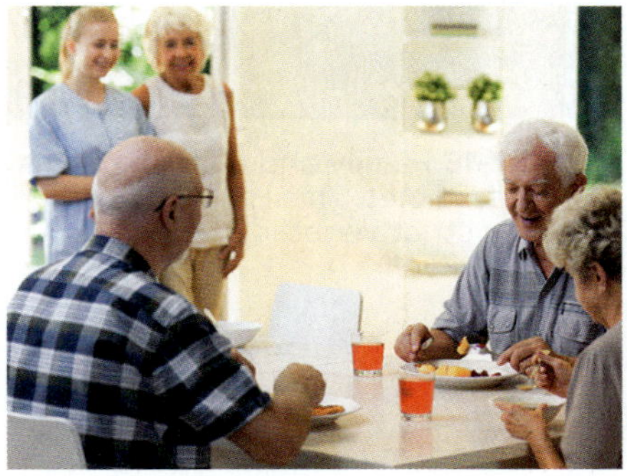

Figure 7-14 Eating is a nutritional as well as a social time. These people are enjoying camaraderie as well as a nutritional meal at their local senior center.

Possible problems that may be noted when assessing the older adult are difficulty chewing (oral problems), difficulty swallowing (possible stroke or Parkinson disease), decreased appetite, decreased ability to feed self (musculoskeletal diseases, such as osteoarthritis, and neurological diseases, such as stroke), and decreased taste and smell. There is also a decreased emptying time of the esophagus, making the older adult more susceptible to aspiration. The older adult should eat in a sitting position to avoid aspiration. Constipation, due to a decrease in gastrointestinal motility, is a common problem that can be alleviated through adequate fluid intake and foods high in fiber.

Numerous socioeconomic conditions can affect the nutrition of older adults: income, transportation, and social support are primary among them. First, many older adults do not work and therefore have no regular source of income, or they are on a fixed income. Their limited financial resources can adversely affect their food choices. Without adequate public or personal transportation, older adults may not have the means to obtain their food. Lastly, in the United States, eating is a social as well as a nutritional ritual (Fig. 7-14). Cooking responsibilities are often shared in a family, and eating is a bonding, congenial event. Many older adults live alone and may not "feel" like eating because of their solitary nature, depression, or both.

NURSING TIP
DASH Diet for Hypertension

The Dietary Approaches to Stop Hypertension (DASH) diet and reduced dietary sodium have been proven to help clients with hypertension eat a nutritionally sound diet while lowering their blood pressure. The DASH diet is low in total fat, cholesterol, saturated fats, red meats, sweets, and sugar-containing beverages, and is rich in vegetables, fruits, and low-fat dairy products. Refer to the website, *https://www.nhlbi.nih.gov/education/dash-eating-plan,* for additional information.

NURSING CHECKLIST
Nutritional Assessment of Older Adults

- Do you have any physical limitations that affect your eating?
- Do you have any difficulty swallowing (e.g., history of cerebrovascular accident, neuromuscular disorders)?
- Do you have any dental problems that interfere with eating?
- Who buys and prepares the food?
- Do you eat alone or with someone?
- How are your eating habits different from 10 years ago? 30 years ago?

NURSING TIP
Psychosocial Implications of Food

The psychosocial implications of food and eating cannot be stressed enough. Food elicits certain memories and feelings of when we were younger (e.g., the smell of our mom's pie baking or the taste of Aunt Edna's cookies). It is also important to take into account other aspects of the nutritional history. If an older adult lives alone, there may be a problem obtaining food or preparing it; loneliness at mealtimes may also be a factor.

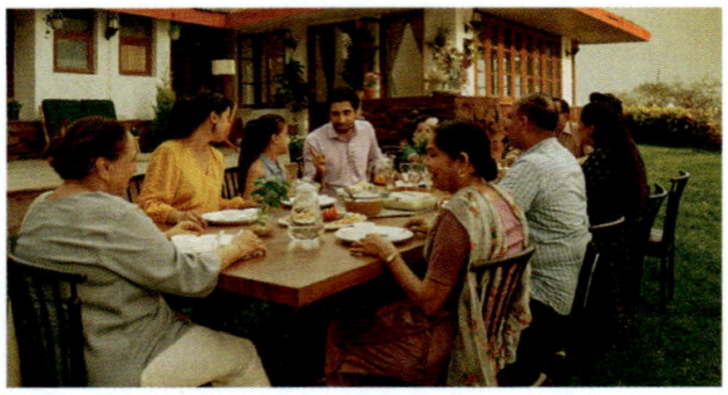

Figure 7-15 Family and cultural values often affect diet. This Hindu family follows a strict vegetarian diet.

Cultural Differences

It is not possible to know all cultural dietary differences, but an open and understanding attitude and acceptance of various religious and cultural beliefs is imperative. Certain foods may have special meanings and memories for individual clients or may be traditional among many with the same cultural backgrounds (e.g., turkey for Thanksgiving). There may also be regional considerations, food preferences, and religious beliefs that restrict the consumption or preparation of certain foods, times food is ingested, and periods of fasting (Fig. 7-15). An understanding of the food practices of various cultural groups is needed to provide appropriate nutritional assessment and education. This understanding is also helpful to establish rapport and individualize the nutritional plan. Be sure to inquire about various cultural and religious influences on dietary practices during the nutritional assessment; refer to Chapters 5 and 6.

HEALTH HISTORY

The nutritional history or subjective information gathered is one of the most significant aspects of the nutritional assessment. It gives an understanding of the client's dietary habits and practices. Nutrition information is gathered throughout the entire health history.

The nutritional health history provides insight into the link between a client's life/lifestyle and nutritional information and pathology.

CLIENT PROFILE

Disease that are age- and sex- specific for nutrition are listed.

Age Anorexia nervosa (adolescents)

Bulimia (adolescents)

Sex More than 90% of clients with anorexia nervosa are female. Pregnant clients and clients with heavy menses are more likely to develop iron deficiency anemia.

CHIEF COMPLAINT

Common chief complaints for nutrition are defined, and information on the characteristics of each sign or symptom is provided.

1. Anorexia Lost or decreased interest in and desire for food

Quantity Amount of food consumed in relation to client's normal intake

Associated Manifestations Physical weakness, fatigue, nausea, cramps, dietary intolerances, weight loss, abdominal distention, abdominal fullness, anxiety, depression

Aggravating Factors Smoking, sleeplessness, odors, pain, emotional status, cardiorespiratory distress

Timing Early morning, afternoon, bedtime, continuous, days, weeks, months, during pregnancy

2. Dysphagia Difficulty swallowing; associated with damage to the 9th or 10th cranial nerve, causing paralysis of the swallowing mechanism or disorders of the throat, neck, or esophagus

Associated Manifestations Weight loss, choking, or difficulty breathing when swallowing

Aggravating Factors Solid or liquid foods

Alleviating Factors Position, throat lozenges

Timing Associated with specific times and meals during the day

3. Weight Gain Number of pounds gained above usual weight

Associated Manifestations Use of medications (corticosteroids, insulin, oral contraceptives [OCPs], antidepressants), pregnancy, sedentary lifestyle, high-calorie diet, high-fat diet, increased appetite

Setting Stress, depression, negative body image

Timing Over what period

4. Weight Loss Number of pounds lost below usual weight

Associated Manifestations Nausea, vomiting, diarrhea, use of laxatives or diuretics, medication side effects, decreased appetite, increase in exercise, malabsorption diseases, diseases increasing demand of nutrients

Setting Stress, depression, negative body image, following a particular diet, participating in a structured weight-loss program (e.g., WeightWatchers)

Timing Over what period

PAST HEALTH HISTORY

The various components of the past health history are linked to nutrition pathology and nutrition-related information.

Medical History

Nutrition Specific Obesity, malnutrition, malabsorption diseases, anorexia nervosa, bulimia, binge eating, dysphagia, weight cycling, Metabolic Syndrome, iron deficiency anemia, pernicious anemia, food sensitivities

Nonnutrition Specific Diabetes mellitus, coronary artery disease, hyperlipidemia, cholesterol level, burns, trauma, cerebrovascular accident, hypertension, cancer, diverticulosis, muscular dystrophy, multiple sclerosis, Parkinson disease, Crohn disease, ulcerative colitis, gout, pancreatitis, cholelithiasis, dental disease, dialysis, current chemotherapy or radiation therapy, cystic fibrosis, Wilson disease, phenylketonuria

Surgical History Surgery for weight loss (e.g., gastric bypass such as Roux-en-Y, intragastric balloon, sleeve gastrectomy, gastric or lap banding, biliopancreatic diversion), jaw wiring to reduce intake of food in morbid obesity, any surgical procedure that would alter food intake from postsurgical complications, nausea, or normal recovery

Allergies Gastrointestinal disturbances may occur with medication, food, and environmental allergies; infants may manifest allergies as dietary disturbances (lactose intolerance)

Medications Review all medications for actual or potential side effects that may affect appetite or growth (antibiotics may cause gastrointestinal disturbances, methylphenidate may cause anorexia, and long-term steroid use may cause weight gain; in children, steroids can affect linear growth), some medications such as warfarin, when taken with green leafy vegetables, decrease the anticoagulant effect of the drug, prescription weight loss drugs (e.g., semaglutide, tirzepatide, liraglutide, phentermine, phentermine-topiramate, naltrexone-bupropion, orlistat), probiotics, vitamins, herbal supplements, protein supplements

Communicable Diseases Children with HIV: failure to thrive

Adults with HIV: wasting syndrome

Injuries and Accidents Affect eating or the ability to self-feed, such as facial or mouth trauma; need for nasogastric tube feeding; gastrostomy; severe burns

Differing Abilities Affect ability to cut, handle, chew, or swallow food

FAMILY HEALTH HISTORY

Familial nutritional diseases are listed.

Food allergies and intolerances, eating disorders, obesity, as well as any medical conditions that may contribute to nutritional problems (e.g., diabetes mellitus, hyperlipidemia, hypertension, CAD, celiac disease, cystic fibrosis, cancer, gout, osteoporosis, alcoholism)

SOCIAL HISTORY

The components of social history are linked to nutritional factors and pathology.

Alcohol Use Alcohol has very little nutritional value, and abuse may lead to nutritional deficiencies. These include an inadequate intake of food, decreased sense of taste and smell, altered metabolism of nutrients (by decreasing storage and increasing excretion of nutrients), and decreased absorption through intestinal mucosa. There is also an increased excretion of calcium with alcohol consumption, which increases the risk of osteoporosis. In a pregnant client, chronic alcohol consumption can lead to a baby with low birth weight and fetal alcohol syndrome in a newborn.

Tobacco Use Smoking is associated with decreased estrogen levels in women, which increases their risk of osteoporosis. Tobacco is an appetite suppressant that may stimulate weight gain when the person quits smoking. Tobacco may also alter the senses of taste and smell.

Recreational Drug Use Recreational drug abuse alters nutrition due to the client's increased dependence on the substance and decreased intake of proper nutrients. Many drugs alter food intake by causing anorexia (e.g., amphetamines) and decreasing sense of smell and taste (e.g., cocaine).

Travel History Recent travel may cause gastrointestinal disturbances. It may also temporarily change the normal dietary habits of the client.

Hobbies and Leisure Activities Food-related hobbies or food activities (gourmet cooking or eating out), amount of daily physical activity

Education Education level may not necessarily translate into an adequate knowledge of nutritional needs.

Economic Status Resources for purchase of adequate food and transportation to grocery store

Religion Refer to Chapter 6 for information on the impact of religion on diet.

Ethnic Background Refer to Chapter 5 for information on the impact of culture on diet.

HEALTH MAINTENANCE ACTIVITIES

This information provides a bridge between health maintenance activities and nutritional function.

Sleep Stress increases when a client is sleep deprived, which may contribute to nutritional problems.

Diet See Table 7-6 for questions to be asked during the diet history. This diet history is not intended for severely ill clients who may be receiving parenteral nutrition or for the client being fed exclusively via tube feedings/gastrostomy.

Exercise Clients with anorexia nervosa may exercise to excess

Stress Management Increasing or decreasing food consumption

Health Checkups Lipid panel results, fasting serum glucose, weight, height, waist circumference, anthropometric measurements, blood pressure, and any other laboratory or diagnostic results

Assessment in Brief

Nutritional Assessment

Nutritional History

Physical Examination

- General appearance
- Skin
- Hair
- Nails
- Eyes
- Mouth
- Head and neck
- Heart
- Peripheral vasculature
- Abdomen
- Musculoskeletal system
- Neurological system
- Female genitalia

Anthropometric Measurements

- Height
- Weight
- Body mass index
- Waist circumference and waist-to-hip ratio
- Midarm and midarm muscle circumference
- Skinfold thickness

Laboratory Data

- Hematocrit and hemoglobin
- Lipids
- Transferrin, total iron-binding capacity, and iron
- Total lymphocyte count
- Antigen skin testing
- Prealbumin
- Albumin
- Glucose
- HbA1c
- Creatinine height index
- Nitrogen balance
- Vitamin D
- Vitamin B_{12}
- Folic acid

Diagnostic Data

- X-rays
- DEXA scan

Equipment

- Appropriate PPE
- Wall-mounted unit (stadiometer), rod attached to the scale that has a right-angle headboard
- Tape measure
- Scale (preferably a balance-beam scale or electronic scale)
- Skinfold calipers (ideally one with a spring-loaded lever)

Nutritional Assessment

Table 7-5 illustrates a comprehensive nutritional assessment. It includes the nutritional history, physical examination, anthropometric measurements, laboratory data, and diagnostic data.

The Nutritional History

The first step in the nutritional assessment is the nutritional history. A comprehensive history is always warranted when the client has a chronic medical condition or unexplained weight loss or gain. Specific diet information is obtained via the Diet History (Table 7-6). The food intake history may be obtained in a variety of ways. The first is the 24-hr recall. In this approach, the client relates what has been consumed in the past day. Clients may also keep a food diary recording what foods and drinks were consumed over a specific 72-hr period. These histories can provide essential information; however, they may not truly represent a typical diet for the client. The client can change the usual dietary habits, omit foods that were eaten, or record incorrect entries, knowing that the information will be evaluated by the nurse. Such instances can lead to invalid information and incorrect diagnoses and treatment plans.

Direct observation of the food and drink consumed by the client and recorded by the nurse constitutes another method of recording food intake patterns. Caloric intake can then be calculated. This is most easily done with the client in a health care facility.

Table 7-5 Comprehensive Nutritional Assessment

Nutritional History (refer to Health History and Table 7-6)

Physical Examination General appearance Skin Hair Nails Eyes Mouth Head and neck Heart Peripheral vasculature Abdomen Musculoskeletal system Neurological system Female genitalia	
Anthropometric Measurements	
Height: _____ in or cm	Waist Circumference: _____ in or cm
Weight: _____ lb or kg	Waist/Hip Ratio: _____
	Mid-Arm Muscle Circumference: _____ cm
	Triceps Skinfold: _____ mm
	Mid-Arm Circumference: _____ cm
% Weight Change: _____	
Body Mass Index: _____ kg/m^2	
Laboratory Data	
Hematocrit (Hct): ____%	Hemoglobin (Hgb): _____ g/dL
Cholesterol: _____ mg/dL	HDL: _____ mg/dL
Triglycerides: _____ mg/dL	LDL: _____ mg/dL
Transferrin: _____ mg/dL	
TIBC: _____ mcg/dL	
Iron: _____ mcg/dL	
Total Lymphocyte Count: _____ $cells/mm^3$	
Antigen Skin Testing: _____	
Prealbumin: _____ mg/dL	Albumin: _____ g/dL
Glucose: _____ mg/dL	HbA1c: _____ %
CHI: _____%	Nitrogen Balance: _____ g
Vitamin D: _____ ng/mL	
Vitamin B_{12}: _____ pg/mL	Folic Acid: _____ ng/mL
Diagnostic Data	
X-rays: _____	DEXA Scan: _____

Table 7-6 Diet History

Part 1: General Diet Information
Do you follow a particular diet? What are your food likes and dislikes? Do you have any food allergies? Do you have any especially strong cravings? How often do you eat fast food? How often do you eat at restaurants? Do you have adequate financial resources to purchase your food? How do you obtain, store, and prepare your food? Do you eat alone or with a family member or another person? Do you observe any religious or cultural dietary practices? When do eat? Where do you eat? Do you consume any food supplements? What types of beverages do you drink? In the past 12 months, have you: • Experienced any weight change? • Had a change in your appetite? • Had a change in your diet? • Experienced nausea, vomiting, or diarrhea from your diet? • Changed your diet because of difficulty in feeding yourself, eating, chewing, or swallowing?

Part 2: Food Intake History (24-hr Recall, 3-Day Diary, Direct Observation)

Time	Food/Drink	Amount	Method of Preparation	Eating Location

Once the food intake history is recorded, the nurse evaluates the diet. Many frameworks can be used to evaluate food consumption. *The Dietary Guidelines for Americans,* MyPlate, the American Heart Association diets, and the American Dietetic Association diets are just a few standards against which a client's diet can be evaluated.

Physical Examination

Certain physical signs may indicate poor nutrition. See Table 7-7 for a list of signs and symptoms of poor nutritional status.

Anthropometric Measurements

Anthropometric measurements are the various measurements of the human body, including height, weight, and body proportions. They measure growth patterns in children and changes in nutritional status in adults. When an adult has had a severe illness, injury, or chronic disease, anthropometric measurements can be used to determine the client's response to enhanced nutrition therapy.

Measurements are easily obtained and can assist in an objective assessment that can be compared over time. Standardized charts should be used to compare the specific measurements with expected norms.

NURSING CHECKLIST

General Approach to Nutritional Assessment

1. Observe Standard Precautions and don PPE such as gloves, gown, face shield, goggles, N-95 respirator, or face mask if the client's status warrants these protective measures.
2. Explain all procedures to clients and family members.
3. Ask client to remove shoes before height measurement.
4. Have older children or adults remove heavy clothing (an adult may wear a hospital gown).
5. Explain and review results with client and family.

Table 7-7 Physical Signs and Symptoms of Poor Nutritional Status

	Subjective	Objective
General appearance	Fatigue, poor sleep, change in weight, frequent infections	Dull affect, apathetic, increased weight, decreased weight
Skin	Pruritus, swelling, delayed wound healing	Dry, rough, scaling, flaky, edema, lesions, decreased turgor, change in color (pallor, jaundice, acanthosis nigricans), petechiae, ecchymoses, xanthomas
Hair	Easily falls out, brittle	Less shiny, dry, change in color pigment, hair loss (patchy or complete)
Nails	Brittle	Dry, splinter hemorrhages, spoon-shaped, pale
Eyes	Vision changes, night blindness, eye discharge	Hardening and scaling of cornea, conjunctiva pale or red
Mouth	Mouth sores	Lips: cracked, dry, swollen, fissures around corners Gums: recessed, swollen, bleeding, spongy Tongue: smooth, beefy red, magenta, pale, fissures, sores, change in size, change in papillae Teeth: missing, caries
Head and neck	Headaches, decreased hearing	Xanthelasma, irritation and crusting of nares, swollen cheeks (parotid gland enlargement), goiter
Heart	Palpitations	Tachycardia, heart murmur, cardiomegaly
Peripheral vasculature	Swelling	Edema, changes in blood pressure
Abdomen	Tender, changes in appetite, nausea, changes in bowel habits	Edema, hepatosplenomegaly, vomiting, diarrhea
Musculoskeletal system	Weakness, pain, cramping, frequent fractures	Decreased muscle tone, flabby muscles, muscle wasting, bowing of lower extremities
Neurological system	Irritable, changes in mood, numbness, paresthesia	Slurred speech, unsteady gait, tremors, decreased deep tendon reflexes, loss of position and vibratory sense, paresthesia, decreased coordination
Female genitalia	Changes in menstrual pattern	None

Height

A standing height is obtained for clients 3 years and older (Fig. 7-16).

E 1. Have the client remove hats/braids/buns/headpieces from the top of the head.
2. Have the client stand erect with the feet together and weight evenly distributed.
3. The heels, buttocks, shoulder blades, and head should be against the wall or measuring device.
4. Place the headboard at a right angle to the wall and along the crown of the client's head.
5. Record height to the nearest 1/8 inch or 1 mm.

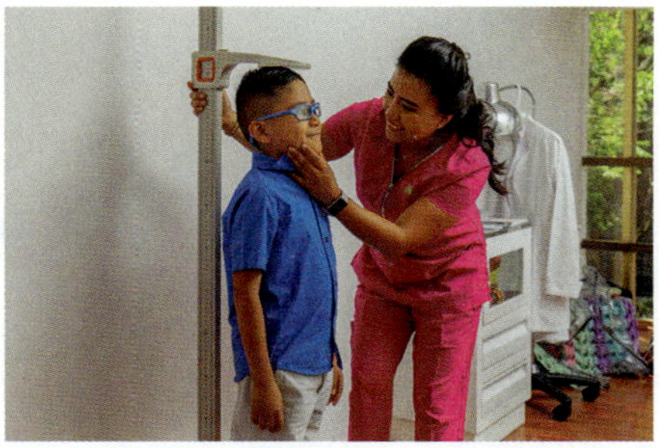

Figure 7-16 Measuring client height.

N **Compare height to standardized charts (refer to the tables of the National Health and Nutrition Examination Survey [NHANES] at *https://www.cdc.gov/nchs/data/series/sr_03/sr03-046-508.pdf*). Bear in mind that clients will reflect familial growth patterns. Also compare to the client's height and weight at the last visit.**

A Insufficient growth is abnormal.

P Chronic malnutrition may result in a decrease in height because the body does not have the nutrients necessary for proper growth.

P A client with osteoporosis may demonstrate a decrease in height due to thinning of the bones and possible vertebral compression fractures. A client with degenerative disc disease may also lose stature due to the nature of the musculoskeletal changes.

P Insufficient growth may also be due to an endocrinological cause such as pituitary gland dysfunction.

A Excessive growth is abnormal.

P Hormone abnormalities may cause excessive growth, as in acromegaly, giantism, and precocious puberty.

P Genetic and metabolic syndromes that affect growth are Marfan syndrome and Klinefelter syndrome.

Weight

E 1. Instruct the client to remove the shoes.
2. Have the client stand erect on the scale with hands at the side, facing the weights (Fig. 7-17).
3. Slide the weight until balanced.
4. Read and record to the nearest 100 g or 1/4 lb (10 g or 1/2 oz for infants).
5. If the current weight has changed from the client's usual weight, calculate the percentage of weight change using the formula:

$$\%\text{Weight Change} = \frac{\text{Usual Weight} - \text{Current Weight}}{\text{Usual Weight}} \times 100$$

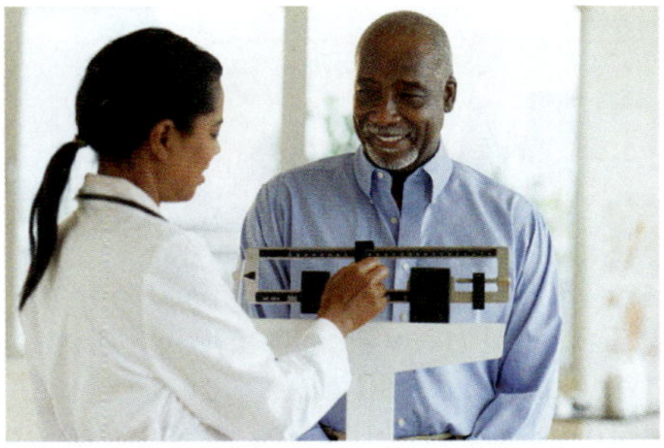

Figure 7-17 Measuring client weight.

N **Compare weight to standardized charts (refer to the tables from the National Health and Nutrition Examination Survey (NHANES) at *https://www.cdc.gov/nchs/data/series/sr_03/sr03-046-508.pdf*.**

A Obesity is abnormal. Obesity occurs when the client's BMI is 30 kg/m^2 or above. Morbid obesity occurs when a client has a BMI of 40 kg/m^2 or above or a BMI of 35 kg/m^2 or above with comorbid conditions such as diabetes or atherosclerotic heart disease.

P Obesity occurs when there is excess body fat because of increased food intake, decreased activity level, or both.

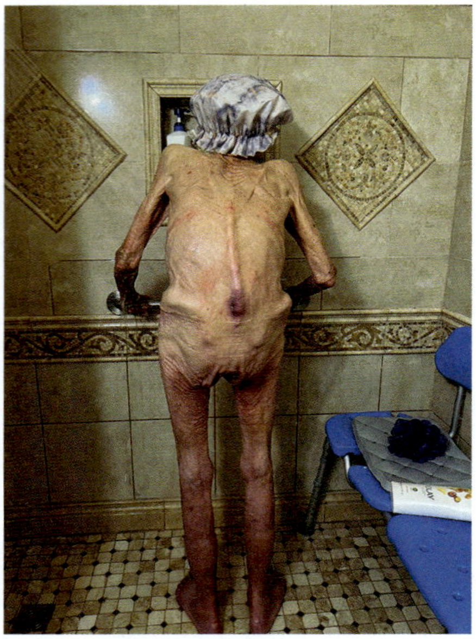

Figure 7-18 This 90-year-old woman with cachexia has a body mass index of 14 kg/m². Note the thin arms, legs, and bony structures.

P Some medications may contribute to weight gain (e.g., steroids).

P Some disease processes, such as hypothyroidism, may contribute to weight gain because of decreased metabolic rate.

P Genetics may influence weight gain.

A A BMI below 18.5 kg/m² is termed underweight.

P Decreased food intake may occur with dental problems, depression, medications, alcoholism, anorexia nervosa, and poverty.

P Inadequate nutrition may occur with impaired absorption, as present in malabsorption diseases (e.g., celiac disease), HIV, and small bowel disease.

P There may be a loss of nutrients with diarrhea, vomiting, and diabetes mellitus.

P Increased demand for nutrients may be present in malignancies, fever, burns, and hyperthyroidism. This increased demand may account for the weight loss that occurs early in cancer even when calories are not decreased. If this continues, the client will exhibit signs of extreme malnutrition and wasting, which is called **cachexia** (Fig. 7-18).

Body Mass Index

Body mass index (BMI) is a measurement that indicates body composition. The degree of overweight or obesity, as well as the degree of underweight, can be determined. The BMI can be associated with increased mortality at specific levels in both clients with known chronic diseases and those without.

The BMI takes into account a person's height as well as weight. Many electronic health record systems automatically calculate a client's BMI once the height and weight are entered. If this feature is not available on your system, the BMI can be manually calculated.

The formula to determine BMI is:

$$\text{BMI} = \frac{\text{Weight (in kg)}}{\text{Height (in m}^2\text{)}}$$

The BMI can be difficult to calculate because few people know their height in meters squared. Thus, the BMI can be determined by three different methods:

E
1. To determine the BMI measurement, enter the client's height and weight on the website *https://www.nhlbi.nih.gov/health/educational/lose_wt/BMI/bmicalc.htm*. This website automatically calculates the BMI. In addition, this site also offers the option of downloading an app to an iPhone or Android smartphone. OR
2. Multiply the weight in lb by 703.
3. Multiply the height in inches by the height in inches.
4. Divide the first number in step 2 by the second number in step 3.
5. The answer is the BMI.

For example: weight = 107 lb, height = 60 in.

$$107 \times 703 = 75221$$
$$60 \times 60 = 3600$$
$$75221 \div 3600 = 20.9 \text{ or } 21$$

N **A BMI of 18.5 to 24.9 kg/m² is considered a healthy weight and is within normal limits in adults. Weights in children and adolescents are plotted on growth charts. Refer to Chapter 25. A specialized BMI calculator which also provides percentiles based on**

> **NURSING TIP**
> **Interpreting Anthropometric Measurements**
> It is important to interpret anthropometric, laboratory, and diagnostic data collectively. One abnormal result does not provide sufficient evidence to diagnose malnutrition. Deficiencies and toxicities usually occur in more than one assessment area. Monitor the results of the nutritional assessment and observe trends.

the CDC growth charts is located at *https://www.cdc.gov/healthy weight/bmi/calculator.html.*

A A BMI of 25 to 29.9 kg/m^2 is considered overweight. A BMI of greater than 30 kg/m^2 is classified as obese.

P A BMI greater than 25 kg/m^2 is associated with increased morbidity and mortality from cardiovascular disease, cancer, and other diseases.

A A BMI less than 18.5 kg/m^2 is abnormal.

P A BMI less than 18.5 kg/m^2 is underweight and may be associated with malnutrition. The malnutrition can be self-induced (e.g., anorexia nervosa, bulimia), caused by illness (e.g., cancer, HIV), or result from a lack of available adequate nutrition.

Waist Circumference and Waist-to-Hip Ratio

Body fat distribution is linked to morbidity and mortality. This is frequently referred to as the "pears" and "apples" distribution. Women tend to deposit fat more in their hips and buttocks, giving them a pear-shaped appearance. Men, in contrast, tend to deposit fat around the abdominal midline, thus giving them an apple-shaped appearance. The latter is usually more closely connected with the adverse effects of obesity. The waist circumference and waist-to-hip ratio is a simple method of determining one's body fat distribution.

E

1. Have the client remove the shirt or gather the examination drape above the waist and cross the arms, placing them on the opposite shoulder. Ensure that no clothing is around the waist.
2. Measure the waist in inches around the narrowest point of the waist between the 12th rib and the iliac crest at end-expiration. This is the waist circumference.
3. Measure the hips at the widest point.
4. Divide the waist measurement by the hip measurement. This is the waist-to-hip ratio. For example:

$$\text{waist} = 25 \text{ inches, hips} = 35 \text{ inches}$$
$$25 \div 35 = 0.71$$

N **A waist circumference ≤ 35 in. (88 cm) in women and ≤ 40 in. (102 cm) in men is considered within normal limits. A waist-to-hip ratio less than 0.8 is normal in women. A waist-to-hip ratio less than 1.0 is normal in men.**

A A waist-to-hip ratio greater than 0.8 in women and 1.0 in men is abnormal.

A A waist circumference >35 in. (88 cm) in women and >40 in. (102 cm) in men is abnormal.

P Elevated waist circumference and waist-to-hip ratio measurements are associated with the adverse morbidity and mortality of obesity, cardiovascular disease, and diabetes.

Mid-Arm and Mid-Arm Muscle Circumferences

The **midarm circumference (MAC)** provides information on skeletal muscle mass. This measurement alone is not of great significance, but it is used to calculate the **midarm muscle circumference (MAMC)**.

E

1. Stand behind the client.
2. With the client standing, instruct the client to flex the right arm 90° at the elbow with the palm facing up.
3. Measure the distance from the uppermost edge of the posterior border of the acromion process to the tip of the olecranon process.

NURSING TIP

Health Benefits of GLP-1 Medications

Semaglutide and liraglutide are some of the medications in the class of glucagon-like peptide-1 (GLP-1) agonists. This class of medications is used in the treatment of type 2 diabetes. A GLP-1 stimulates the release of insulin from the pancreas and blocks glucagon secretion. Tirzepatide, is a glucose-dependent insulinotropic polypeptide (GIP)/GLP agonist with similar action. These medications are also known to slow gastric emptying and increase satiety, which leads to decreased food consumption. For these reasons the GLP-1 medications have in recent years been used extensively in treating overweight and obesity even in people who do not have type 2 diabetes. In addition, in March 2024, the U.S. Food and Drug Administration (FDA) approved semaglutide to be used in clients who are overweight or obese and have cardiovascular disease to decrease the risk of myocardial infarction, stroke, and death from cardiovascular disease.

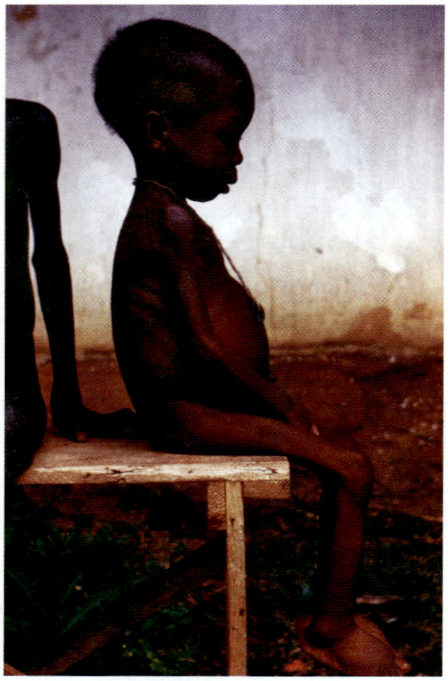

Figure 7-19 Clients with kwashiorkor may have a normal weight as well as TSF and MAC. Edema is common.

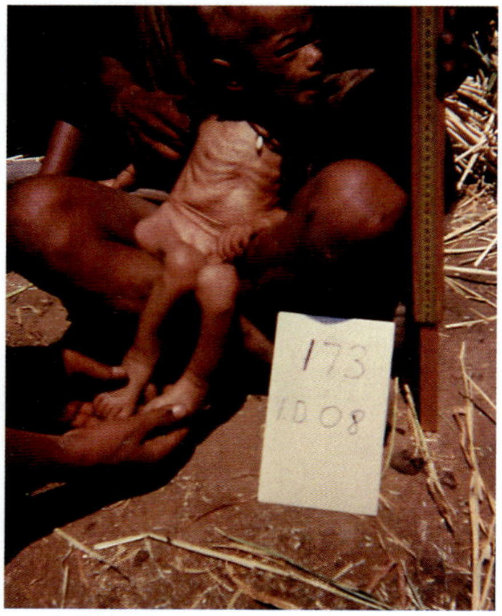

Figure 7-20 Marasmus is characterized by decreased weight, TSF, MAC, and muscle wasting.

4. Divide this distance in half and place a horizontal line on the client's arm at this location. This is the midarm landmark.
5. Measure the circumference of the arm (MAC) at this location.
6. Calculate MAMC using the formula:

$$\text{MAMC (cm)} = \text{MAC (cm)} - [3.14 \times \text{TSF* (cm)}]$$

*The TSF is measured in mm. You need to convert the TSF from mm to cm to calculate the MAMC.

N **Refer to the tables of the National Health and Nutrition Examination Survey (NHANES) at *https://www.cdc.gov/nchs/data/series/sr_03/sr03-046-508.pdf*. Normal measurements fall between the 5th and 95th percentiles.**

A Results less than the 5th percentile on the standard charts are abnormal.

P **Kwashiorkor**, or protein malnutrition, is a severe deficiency in good-quality protein. This can develop even if the client is consuming an adequate number of calories. Because of the decrease in visceral proteins (especially albumin), edema may develop, particularly in the abdomen. This can also lead to decreased immune function. The TSF, MAC, and weight can be within normal limits. Additional physical signs are scaly, flaky skin, depigmentation of the hair, enlarged liver, and mental apathy (Fig. 7-19). It can occur with the ingestion of liquid diets that are low in protein, malabsorption diseases, hypermetabolic states, cancer, and HIV.

P **Marasmus**, or protein-calorie malnutrition, is a severe nutritional disorder in which there is an inadequate intake of protein and calories. As a result, there is a wasting of skeletal muscle and subcutaneous fat. This disorder can also occur from poor absorption of proteins, such as with burns, anorexia nervosa, tuberculosis, cancer, HIV, and malabsorption diseases. Clients with marasmus have symptoms similar to kwashiorkor except that they appear more emaciated and do not have edema (Fig. 7-20). If the marasmus is severe enough, these clients may also develop impaired cell-mediated immunity.

P Marasmic kwashiorkor is a severe form of protein-calorie malnutrition. It is typically seen in clients who are in a severe hypermetabolic state (such as trauma or burns), as well as a near-starvation state. There is a reduction in subcutaneous tissue, visceral proteins, and somatic proteins.

A Results greater than the 95th percentile on the standard charts are abnormal.

P Obesity is suggested.

P If edema is present on the assessed body parts, the measurement may not be a reliable indicator of nutritional status.

NURSING TIP

Severe Malnutrition

Many nursing schools offer coursework abroad to expand the nursing student's global perspective of health care. In addition, many nursing schools sponsor trips to underserved areas of health care throughout the world. It is in instances of severe malnutrition, especially in third-world countries, where conditions such as marasmus and kwashiorkor are seen. Figures 7-19 and 7-20 depict these extreme states of malnourishment, which are rarely seen in the United States.

Skinfold Thickness

Skinfold thickness is used to determine body fat stores and nutritional status. It is a more reliable indicator of body fat than weight because more than half of the body's total fat is in the subcutaneous tissue. The most common measurement site is the **triceps skinfold** (TSF). Measurements can also be performed in subscapular and suprailiac skinfolds.

E
1. Place the client in a standing position with the arms hanging loosely at the side. Stand behind the client.
2. Take the measurements on the right arm, with the client in a relaxed position.
3. Locate the position of the MAC, and grasp a fold of skin and subcutaneous tissue 2 cm above or below this area.
4. Apply the caliper at this location and measure to the nearest 0.1 mm (Fig. 7-21).
5. Release the skin, wait 3 seconds, and repeat the measurement twice more.
6. Average the findings to determine the TSF.

N **NHANES stopped collecting this data in 2010. The TSF measurement is used to calculate the MAMC.**

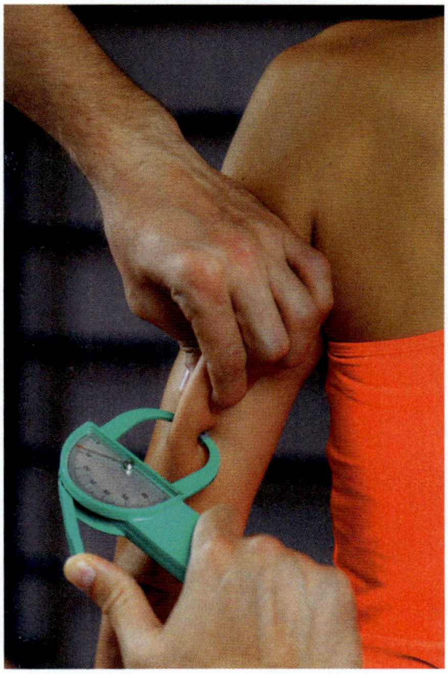

Figure 7-21 Measuring triceps skinfold.

Laboratory Data

Laboratory analysis is used when screening for potential nutritional problems and to assist with diagnosis when problems are suspected after a thorough history and a physical have been conducted. Caution must be exercised when interpreting laboratory values because many pathophysiological processes can affect the values. The laboratory data must be considered in context with the client's history, physical examination, and anthropometric measurements.

Hematocrit and Hemoglobin

Hematocrit determines the percentage of red blood cells to the volume of whole blood. It reflects the body's iron supply. **Hemoglobin** is the iron component of the blood that transports oxygen. Both values are obtained from a venous blood sample. Certified laboratories calibrate their equipment and determine the normal range of laboratory values with specified procedures to produce quantitative results for the client population. Refer to your laboratory for normal ranges.

N **Hemoglobin and hematocrit results should fall within expected values. Increased hematocrit and hemoglobin may normally occur in people living in high altitudes, due to the decrease in partial pressure of oxygen in those areas.**

A Decreased hematocrit and hemoglobin are abnormal.

P Moderate to severe anemia may indicate decreased iron intake, leukemia, cirrhosis, hyperthyroidism, hemorrhage, hemodilution, or hemolytic reactions.

A Increased hematocrit and hemoglobin are abnormal.

P Chronic hypoxia, such as cyanotic heart defects, can result in polycythemia. Severe dehydration may also result from hemoconcentration.

Lipids

The *Third Report of the National Cholesterol Education Program (NCEP) Expert Panel on Detection, Evaluation, and Treatment of High Blood Cholesterol in Adults (ATP III) (2002)* presented long-standing guidelines to assist health-care providers in assessing lipid levels. In 2018, following multiple clinical trials demonstrating the benefits of statins, the American College of Cardiology (ACC) released the 2018 Guideline on the Management of Blood Cholesterol to assist providers in managing hyperlipidemia, particularly regarding statin benefit groups. The ACC utilizes cholesterol laboratory values to calculate an Atherosclerotic Cardiovascular Disease (ASCVD) risk percentage (Grundy et al., 2019). Refer to the ASCVD Risk Calculator found at *https://tools.acc.org/ascvd-risk-estimator-plus/#!/calculate/estimate/*.

Keep in mind that cholesterol laboratory values are obtained from a fasting client. The following values are drawn from ATP III:

N **Total Cholesterol (in mg/dL)**

<200	**Desirable**
200–239	**Borderline high**
>240	**High**

HDL Cholesterol (in mg/dL)

<40	**Low**
>60	**High**

LDL Cholesterol (in mg/dL)

<100	**Optimal**
100–129	**Near optimal/above optimal**
130–159	**Borderline-high**
160–189	**High**
>190	**Very high**

Triglycerides (in mg/dL)

<150	**Normal**
150–199	**Borderline-high**
200–499	**High**
≥ 500	**Very high**

A Elevated cholesterol, LDL, and triglyceride levels above desirable range are abnormal. A HDL level less than 40 mg/dL is abnormal in adults.

A An ASCVD 10-year Risk >7.5% is abnormal in adults 40 to 79 years of age.

P Elevated cholesterol and/or triglycerides can be due to increased fat intake, genetics, and some medications (e.g., steroids, estrogens, cyclosporin). These lipid elevations can lead to an increased risk of cardiac disease. A low HDL level can also be due to genetics.

Transferrin, Total Iron-Binding Capacity (TIBC), and Iron

Transferrin is a protein that regulates iron absorption. Transferrin can be measured by the **total iron-binding capacity** (TIBC) (the amount of iron with which it can bind).

Serum iron is the amount of transferrin-bound iron. These data are obtained from a venous blood sample. Serum transferrin can be calculated using the following formula:

$$\text{Transferrin} = (0.8 \times \text{TIBC}) - 43$$

N **Normal adult levels are:**

Transferrin: 170–250 mg/dL
TIBC: 240–450 mcg/dL
Serum iron (women): 65–165 mcg/dL
Serum iron (men): 75–175 mcg/dL

A An increase in transferrin is abnormal.

P Increased levels of transferrin are found in inadequate dietary iron, iron deficiency anemia, hepatitis, and oral contraceptive use.

A Decreased levels of transferrin are abnormal.

P Decreased levels of transferrin are found in pernicious anemia, sickle cell anemia, anemia associated with infection or chronic diseases, cancer, and malnutrition.

A Increases in serum iron levels are abnormal.

P Increases in serum iron levels are found in hemolytic anemias, hemochromatosis, and lead poisoning.

A Decreases in serum iron levels are abnormal.

P Decreases in serum iron levels are found in iron deficiency, gastrointestinal bleeding, chronic diseases, third-trimester pregnancy, and severe physiological stress.

Total Lymphocyte Count

Total lymphocyte count (TLC) is measured in the complete blood count with differential; it measures immune function and visceral protein status. When the white blood cell count is abnormally elevated or decreased, such as in bacterial infections or HIV, respectively, the TLC is not always a reliable indicator of nutritional status.

N **Normal adult levels are 1500–1800 cells/mm^3.**

A A decrease in the total lymphocyte count of fewer than 1500 cells/mm^3 indicates moderate protein deficiency, whereas less than 900 cells/mm^3 indicates severe protein deficiency.

P Protein deficiency occurs when the body is malnourished, such as when a client is immunocompromised.

Antigen Skin Testing

Antigen skin testing is another test of immune function. Intradermal injections of various antigens can be used. Antigens commonly used are PPD tuberculin skin tests, mumps virus, *Candida albicans,* streptokinase, *Streptococcus, coccidioidin,* and *Trichophyton.* Results are read at 24 and 48 hr postinjection.

N **A negative skin reaction (no induration or erythema) after being tested with various antigens is normal. These are antigens to which most people have been exposed and have developed an antibody response.**

A A positive reaction to antigens placed intradermally is abnormal; a positive reaction is indicated by a red area or induration 5 mm or more around the test site 24 hr or more after the injection. A negative reaction to only one of the antigens tested or a delayed positive reaction may occur with malnutrition.

P Poor antibody response occurs in clients who are immunocompromised because they have a decreased ability to fight infection and build antibodies. Protein malnutrition has been shown to decrease immune function. This diminished reaction to antigens is called **anergy**. Antigen skin testing is often called anergy panels.

Prealbumin

Prealbumin (also called thyroxine-binding prealbumin) is the transport protein for thyroxine and retinol-binding protein. The half-life is 24–48 hr, so it is an excellent value with which to monitor the effects of recent nutritional support and changes in nutritional status.

N **The normal range for prealbumin is 10–40 mg/dL.**

A Liver diseases, such as cirrhosis and hepatitis, as well as severe stress from infection, burn injury, sepsis, prolonged surgery, hyperthyroidism, and cystic fibrosis, can all lead to decreased prealbumin levels.

P Severe acute conditions in which severe catabolism occurs tend to lower the prealbumin level. In the case of liver disease, the levels are lower because of decreased hepatic synthesis of proteins.

> **NURSING TIP**
> **Continuous Glucose Monitoring**
> A continuous glucose monitor (CGM) is a device attached to the client's upper arm or abdomen that continually measures in real time the client's blood glucose level (Fig. 7-22). The blood glucose reading assists the client and health care team in managing diabetes and prediabetes by measuring the body's blood sugar response to conditions such as food, exercise, stress, and illness. The CGM device is paired with a smartphone or smart watch and alerts the client when the blood glucose level is outside the preset ranges. If the blood glucose level drops to a dangerous level the client's phone or watch will alarm. The client will know to treat the hypoglycemia by consuming some type of glucose product. Conversely, if the blood glucose level elevates above the preset limit the client is alerted and appropriate action can be taken. In addition, the client can add contacts to the CGM network so that family/friends will also be notified in instances of hypoglycemia and hyperglycemia.

Albumin

Albumin is formed in the liver. It transports nutrients, blood, and hormones, and helps maintain osmotic pressure. The body must have functioning liver cells and an adequate amount of amino acids to synthesize albumin. It is an indicator of visceral protein status. Because albumin has a long half-life (about 20 days), it is not an indicator of subtle or early changes in nutritional status. It is measured from a venous blood sample.

N **The normal range for serum albumin is 3.5 to 5.0 g/dL.**

A Less than 3.5 g/dL is abnormal.

P Decreased levels of albumin may indicate malnutrition because of a decrease in visceral protein stores, or a decrease in the amount of protein stored in organs. The decrease may not be seen until the protein deficiency reaches a chronic stage.

P Decreased levels of albumin are also found in massive hemorrhages, burns, and kidney disease.

Glucose

Serum glucose tests the body's ability to metabolize glucose. It is best assessed after a fasting period and from a venous blood sample.

N **The normal fasting blood glucose levels in an adult are:**

Fasting serum:	**70–100 mg/dL**
Prediabetes:	**100–125 mg/dL**
Diabetes:	**≥ 125 mg/dL**

A An increase in glucose level is abnormal.

P **Hyperglycemia** occurs in **prediabetes** (a clinical state of hyperglycemia that places the individual at risk for developing diabetes and heart disease, but where the blood glucose levels are not yet high enough to be classified as diabetes), diabetes mellitus, vitamin B_1 deficiency, and convulsive states. This indicates that glucose is not being transported into the cells by insulin.

A A decrease in serum glucose level is abnormal.

P **Hypoglycemia** occurs in pancreatic disorders, liver disease, decreased food intake, and insulin overdose. This occurs when there is too much insulin and not enough glucose in the blood.

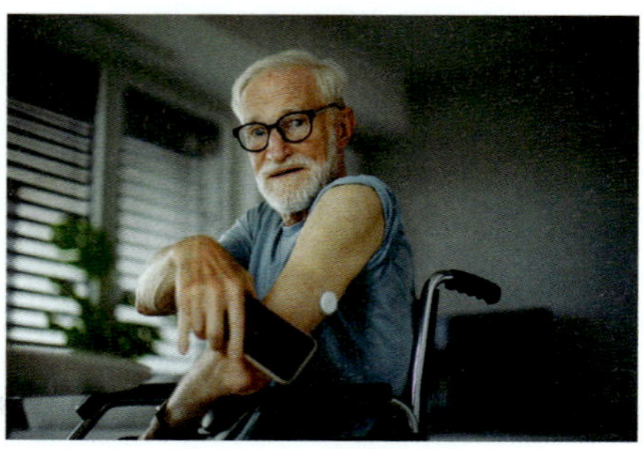

Figure 7-22 This male is checking his current blood sugar level via a continuous glucose monitor linked to his smartphone.

Glycosylated Hemoglobin (HbA1c)

Glycosylated hemoglobin (HbA1c) represents the amount of glucose that is permanently bound to hemoglobin. It is a long-term measure of blood sugar control, as it reflects the average serum glucose over a 2- to 3-month period. For this reason, it is usually not checked more than once every 3 months.

N **The normal HbA1c is less than 5.7%.**

A An HbA1c value of 5.7% and greater is abnormal.

P An HbA1c level between 5.7% to 6.4% is classified as prediabetes. An HbA1c greater than or equal to 6.5% is recognized as diabetes by the American Association of Clinical Endocrinologists and the American Diabetes Association. The higher the HbA1c value, the more uncontrolled the diabetes. Over a decade ago, the American Diabetes Association officially recognized HbA1c as the clinical test that should be used to monitor diabetes (American Diabetes Association, 2021).

Creatinine Height Index (CHI)

Creatinine is a substance normally excreted in the urine; it is dependent on the amount of skeletal muscle mass, and it measures the amount of protein reserves. Urine creatinine is tested after collecting a 24-hr urine sample. An ideal urine creatinine level by height table is used to establish the denominator in the equation used to calculate CHI. Use the following equation to calculate the creatinine height index:

$$\text{CHI} = \frac{\text{actual 24 hour creatinine excretion}}{\text{ideal 24 hour creatinine excretion}} \times 100$$

The CHI is not an accurate indicator of skeletal muscle mass in dehydrated clients or clients with renal dysfunction.

N **Normal CHI values are greater than 90%.**

A CHI between 80% and 90% indicates mild protein deficiency.

CHI between 70% and 80% indicates moderate protein deficiency.

CHI of less than 70% indicates severe protein deficiency.

P Protein malnutrition may be indicated by the loss of lean body mass, which can occur in severe trauma, prolonged fever, and stress.

Nitrogen Balance

Nitrogen is usually taken into the body in the form of food protein sources. It is one of the compounds of amino acids. Nitrogen is incorporated into protein and excreted in urine and feces. This balance of nitrogen intake to nitrogen output is compared, usually with a 24-hr urine sample. The nitrogen balance can be calculated using this formula:

$$\text{Nitrogen balance} = \frac{\text{grams of protein eaten}}{6.25} - (UUN^{*} + 4)$$

*UUN = 24-hour urine urea nitrogen (in grams)

N **A zero balance is normal. A positive balance indicates tissue formation, found in growing children and pregnant clients.**

A A negative nitrogen balance is abnormal and indicates a catabolic state (i.e., the body excretes more nitrogen than is consumed).

P More nitrogen is excreted than taken in, which means there is destruction or wasting of tissue. This can occur in malnutrition and catabolic states (e.g., burns, severe stress, trauma, surgery).

Vitamin D

Table 7-2 notes that vitamin D is essential for proper bone growth and teeth development. Vitamin D is unique because dietary consumption can help meet nutritional needs, but the body, with sufficient exposure to ultraviolet light radiation, can also produce vitamin D. Thus, vitamin D is actually a hormone and not a vitamin. A dietary deficiency of vitamin D levels can lead to vitamin D insufficiency, as can the lack of adequate sun exposure and/or the use of sunscreen agents. Extensive research is being conducted worldwide on the larger role that vitamin D may have in osteoporosis, decreased muscle strength, myopathy, and cancer. The laboratory marker used to evaluate vitamin D is the total 25-hydroxyvitamin, or vitamin D 25-OH, which is a combination of 25-hydroxyvitamin D_2 and D_3.

N **The normal vitamin D 25-OH is 32 to 100 ng/mL.**

A A serum vitamin D 25-OH less than 25 ng/mL is suboptimal. This results from a low consumption of food/beverages with vitamin D and/or decreased sun exposure (especially with the use of sunscreen).

P In adults, hypovitaminosis D, or vitamin D deficiency, can result in osteoporosis, osteomalacia, hepatobiliary disease, and calcium malabsorption; in children, it can result in rickets (see Figure 7-23).

P Low vitamin D levels can also lead to musculoskeletal pain, weakness, a sensation of heaviness in the legs, and fatigue.

Vitamin B_{12}

Vitamin B_{12} is a water-soluble vitamin that is needed for the synthesis of red blood cells and the maintenance of myelin sheaths. It is found in seafood, meat, eggs, and milk. It can take the body 2 years or more to deplete its store of vitamin B_{12}.

N **The normal vitamin B_{12} level is 211 to 911 pg/mL.**

A A vitamin B_{12} level below 211 pg/mL is abnormal. A high level of vitamin B_{12} should not pose any risks, as it is a water-soluble vitamin.

P An inadequate dietary intake of Vitamin B_{12} can lead to paresthesia of the fingers and toes, incoordination, delirium, depression, dementia, and pernicious anemia. This can occur in malnutrition, after prolonged or critical illness, and in HIV infection.

P Decreased absorption or utilization of vitamin B_{12} occurs in pernicious anemia, Crohn disease, celiac disease, gastrectomy, and with bariatric surgery.

P Some medications, such as methotrexate, metformin, vonoprazan, and proton pump inhibitors, can lead to a vitamin B_{12} deficiency.

Folic Acid

Folic acid is a water-soluble B vitamin that is needed for the synthesis of red blood cells. It is found in liver and plant sources such as spinach, asparagus, broccoli, kidney beans, and green, leafy vegetables. The body cannot store large quantities of folic acid.

N **The normal folic acid level is >5.4 ng/mL.**

A A folic acid level less than 5.4 ng/mL is abnormal. A high level of folic acid should not pose any risks, as it is a water-soluble vitamin.

P A deficiency of folic acid in pregnant clients increases the risk of a neural tube defect, such as spina bifida, in the fetus.

P Low folic acid levels lead to macrocytic anemia. Alcohol and substance abusers are prone to folic acid deficiency due to an inadequate diet.

P Some medications, such as methotrexate, metformin, phenytoin, and trimethoprim, can affect the utilization of folic acid.

P Celiac disease can lead to folic acid deficiency due to malabsorption.

Diagnostic Data

Radiographic studies are used to determine bone formation and to assess development. Rickets and scurvy are both examples of long-term nutritional deficiencies that have radiographic manifestations. Rickets is a deficiency of vitamin D (Fig. 7-23), and scurvy is a deficiency of vitamin C; both are characterized by softening and deformities of the bones. A bone density, or dual-energy x-ray absorptiometry (DEXA), scan is a low-radiation, noninvasive test that assesses the hip, lumbar spine, femoral neck, and wrist for osteoporosis. Though osteoporosis can result from many variables, nutritional deficiencies is one of the leading etiologies in various age groups.

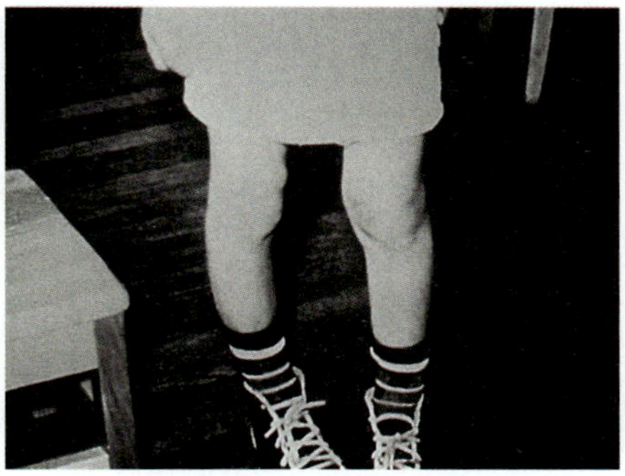

Figure 7-23 This child is suffering from malnutrition and rickets. Note the bowed legs.

U.S. Preventive Services Task Force (USPSTF)

Grade A Recommendation:

- The USPSTF recommends that all persons planning to or who could become pregnant take a daily supplement containing 0.4 to 0.8 mg (400 to 800 mcg) of folic acid.

Grade B Recommendations:

- The USPSTF recommends screening for gestational diabetes in asymptomatic pregnant persons at 24 weeks of gestation or after.
- The USPSTF recommends that clinicians offer pregnant persons effective behavioral counseling interventions aimed at promoting healthy weight gain and preventing excess gestational weight gain in pregnancy.
- The USPSTF recommends that clinicians provide or refer children and adolescents 6 years or older with a high body mass index (BMI) (≥95th percentile for age and sex) to comprehensive, intensive behavioral interventions.
- The USPSTF recommends offering or referring adults with cardiovascular disease risk factors to behavioral counseling interventions to promote a healthy diet and physical activity.
- The USPSTF recommends screening for osteoporosis with bone measurement testing to prevent osteoporotic fractures in postmenopausal women younger than 65 years who are at increased risk of osteoporosis, as determined by a formal clinical risk assessment tool.
- The USPSTF recommends screening for osteoporosis with bone measurement testing to prevent osteoporotic fractures in women 65 years and older.
- The USPSTF recommends screening for prediabetes and type 2 diabetes in adults aged 35 to 70 years who have overweight or obesity. Clinicians should offer or refer patients with prediabetes to effective preventive interventions.
- The USPSTF recommends that clinicians offer or refer adults with a body mass index (BMI) of 30 or higher (calculated as weight in kilograms divided by height in meters squared) to intensive, multicomponent behavioral interventions.

Retrieved September 23, 2025, from *https://preventiveservicestaskforce.org/uspstf/recommendation-topics/uspstf-a-and-b-recommendations*
https://www.uspreventiveservicestaskforce.org/uspstf/topic_search_results?topic_status

CASE STUDY
The Underweight Client

This case study illustrates the application and objective documentation of the nutritional assessment. Etsuko was widowed approximately 1 year ago. She has experienced weight loss to the degree that her clothes are much too large for her. The client presents for a clinical evaluation at the request of her adult daughter who is concerned about the weight loss.

HEALTH HISTORY

CLIENT PROFILE

68-year-old widowed Asian woman

REASON FOR SEEKING HEALTH CARE

"My daughter told me I had to be seen. She is worried that I'm not strong enough and I could get hurt."

PRESENT HEALTH

Etsuko is a retired schoolteacher whose husband died 1 year ago. Husband's death was unexpected and client struggled with "grief and lots of sadness" for 2 to 3 months after his passing but is now doing much better. Etsuko attended a few bereavement classes. Reports that she keeps busy with her friends, activities, and classes at the community center. "I miss my husband, but I am adjusting." Reports that her daughter is concerned because "when I was sad, I lost about 15 pounds. I wasn't eating well—I just wasn't hungry and I wasn't going to my classes at the community center." Etsuko reports that she is back to eating her normal diet and is not losing any more weight but has not been able to put back on the weight that she lost. Etsuko has been attending water aerobics classes 3 days a week at the community center for the past 3 weeks. Etsuko states that she needs to go shopping to buy some new clothes as her usual wardrobe is too big on her. Etsuko does not believe that there is any problem.

PAST HEALTH HISTORY

Medical History Hypothyroidism, managed with medication, postmenopausal age 53

Surgical History Cesarean section age 28.

Allergies Denies allergies to meds, food, insect bites, bee stings; denies seasonal and perennial allergies

Medications Multivitamin; levothyroxine 50 mcg every morning, 1 hr before breakfast.

Communicable Diseases Denies any recent illness or communicable disease.

Injuries and Accidents Denies any falls, accidents, or injuries.

Differing Abilities Denies special needs or diet.

Blood Transfusions Denies

Childhood Illnesses "Chicken pox as a child - maybe around age 8."

Immunizations COVID Vaccine (mRNA): completed two vaccines in March 2021 plus two boosters in 2022, and one a year since then. Current per CDC recommendation including annual flu vaccine, completed recombinant zoster vaccine in 2019, Pneumococcal 20-valent Conjugate vaccine in 2023 and Pneumococcal Vaccine Polyvalent 23 in 2017, Tdap 2024

FAMILY HEALTH HISTORY

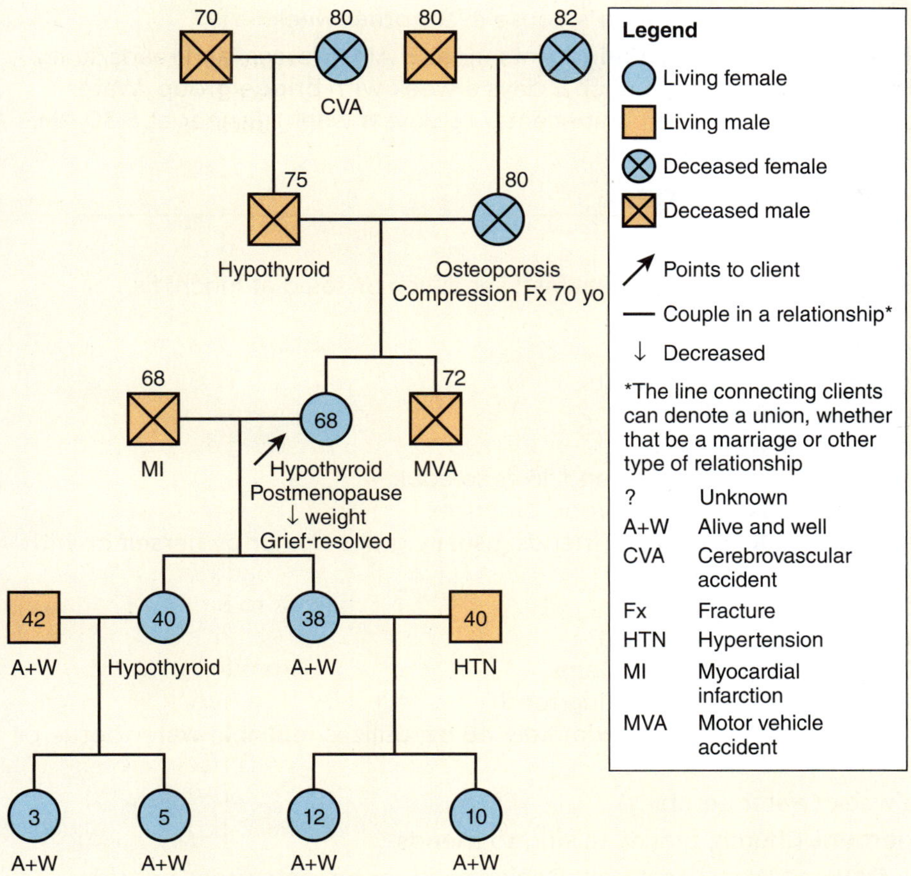

Denies family history of food allergies, eating disorders, obesity, celiac disease

SOCIAL HISTORY

Alcohol Use Denies

Tobacco Use Denies

Recreational Drug Use Denies

Domestic and Intimate Partner Violence Denies

Sexual Practice Denies any activity since husband's death.

Travel History Only local travel in past 12 months

Work Environment None—Retired.

Home Environment Feels safe in very upscale neighborhood in 3,500-square-foot house. Has not modified home décor and accessories to anchor/reduce throw rugs or to increase lighting. Has two flights of stairs in her home. Laundry room is in basement.

Hobbies and Leisure Activities Quilting, playing cards (bridge) with friends, going to the community center, and watching grandkids play sports.

Stress Husband's death

Education Master's Degree in Education

Economic Status "I am fine. My husband set up a very good retirement for us and the house is paid off. I have health insurance from my school retirement."

Military Status None.

Religion Protestant

Ethnic Background Korean

Roles and Relationships Widowed. Two grown daughters (one local and one 2 hr away), both married, each with two children. Enjoys visits with local grandchildren. Has Sunday dinner at local daughter's house every other week.

Characteristic Patterns of Daily Living Gets up at 6 AM, dresses, and reads/knits. Coffee with friend midmorning. Lunch 3 days a week with bridge group. Water aerobics from 3 to 4 PM at community center (3 days a week). Dinner at 5:30 PM. TV in the evening. Bedtime at 9 PM.

HEALTH MAINTENANCE ACTIVITIES

Sleep 9 hr every night

Diet "Regular"—1 egg and toast at breakfast; sandwich or salad at lunch; fish or chicken with veggies for dinner.

Diet History

- Eats a regular diet with few sweets
- Likes most foods; no dislikes
- Denies any food allergies
- Does her own grocery shopping and 'likes to cook'
- Observes no religious or cultural food practices
- Eats breakfast by self, lunch with friends, usually grabs dinner by herself or with family members (kids/grandkids)
- Denies food supplements
- Denies nausea, vomiting, diarrhea
- Denies chewing/swallowing problems
- Denies purging, binging, or avoiding food

Drinks water throughout the day. Approximately 48 oz; utilizes refillable water bottle or home filter.

Exercise 3x a week (water aerobics)

Stress Management Church, prayer, talking to friends

Use of Safety Devices Wears seat belt. Denies need for helmets (does not ride bike). Excellent swimmer. No firearms at home. Handrail in shower and on home stairs.

Health Checkups Dentist twice a year; annual physical with thyroid evaluation annually, last was 11 mos ago. Sick visits as needed.

NUTRITIONAL ASSESSMENT

	Subjective	Objective
General appearance	Recent change in weight	Thin, frail appearance
Skin	Dry skin throughout	Dry, normal turgor, pale
Hair	Thin	Dull, dry
Nails	Manicured, denies peeling	Pale, well-kept
Eyes	No complaints	Conjunctiva pale
Mouth	No complaints	Lips, gums, tongue, teeth within normal limits
Head and neck	Headache every few days	Thyroid without masses, nodules, or thyromegaly
Heart	Occasional racing heart	No heart murmur BP: 100/60 HR: 64

	Subjective	Objective
Peripheral vasculature	No complaints	No edema
Abdomen	Small, soft stools every other day	No hepatosplenomegaly, no edema
Musculoskeletal system	No complaints	Muscle tone within normal limits, height decreased by ½ inch since last measurement 12 months ago (64.5" down to 64"); m ld kyphosis/dowager's hump
Neurological system	Irritable, especially when tired	Within normal limits

PHYSICAL EXAMINATION

Height: 64 in
Current weight: 105 lb, Usual weight: 120 lb
Percent Weight Change: (120–105) / 120 = 0.125
0.125 × 100 = 12.5% ; percent weight change is 12.5%
BMI: 105 × 703 = 73,815
64 × 64 = 4096
73,815 / 4096 = 18.02 kg/m^2; BMI is 18.02 kg/m^2

Pt refused other anthropometric measurements. "Just not sure that it's necessary. This seems like a lot of fuss about nothing."

DIAGNOSTIC DATA

DEXA scan last year: no osteopenia or osteoporosis, within normal limits

CLINICAL JUDGMENT IN ACTION

1. What cues indicate that the client may be having a nutritional disorder?
2. What interventions have the highest priority?
3. What assessment findings indicate clinical improvement or decline in this client?

Review Questions

1. A school nurse is developing an education program designed to teach parents of high school athletes about common symptoms of eating disorders in adolescents. Which of the following information should the school nurse include in the teaching? Select all that apply.
   a. Skipping meals frequently
   b. Eating fast food once weekly
   c. Eating a vegan diet
   d. Preoccupation with food or weight loss
   e. Uncomfortable eating around others

2. A 70-year-old Asian female client is diagnosed with osteoporosis. Which of the following features can be associated with osteoporosis in an adult female?
   a. Rickets
   b. Sunscreen use
   c. Vitamin B_{12} level of 200 pg/mL
   d. Eating legumes, cabbage, and seafood

3. The pediatric nurse teaches parents that low-fat or skim milk is recommended beginning at what age?
   a. 6 months
   b. 1 year
   c. 2 years
   d. 5 years

4. A 48-year-old male with a history of hypertension provides a dietary recall that includes bacon and eggs for breakfast, fast food (hamburger with soda and fries) for lunch, and pepperoni pizza or fried chicken for dinner. What dietary modifications should be encouraged? Select all that apply.
   a. More soda intake
   b. Reducing fat
   c. Eating beef twice daily
   d. Limiting fruit
   e. Decreasing sodium

5. A 59-year-old postmenopausal female has been told that her vitamin D level is too low. Which of the following food selections can increase the vitamin D level? Select all that apply.
   a. Eggs
   b. Fortified milk
   c. Oranges
   d. Liver
   e. Tomatoes

6. A client is on medication for hypertension. Which of the following foods would you advise the client to eat if the serum potassium level decreases as a result of the diuretic medication? Select all that apply.
   a. Bananas
   b. Cereal
   c. Dried fruits
   d. Table salt
   e. Seafood

7. Which of the following physical findings make the nurse suspect that Metabolic Syndrome is present in a male client?
   a. Waist circumference of 45 inches, fasting triglyceride level of 175 mg/dL, fasting serum glucose level of 100 mg/dL
   b. Fasting HDL level of 41 mg/dL, blood pressure of 135/85 mm Hg, fasting serum glucose level of 180 mg/dL
   c. Fasting triglyceride level of 145 mg/dL fasting HDL level of 35 mg/dL, blood pressure of 110/75 mm Hg
   d. Waist circumference of 42 inches, fasting HDL level of 20 mg/dL, fasting serum glucose level of 128 mg/dL

8. A male client is 6′ 2″ tall and weighs 225 lb. What conclusion do you make about the client's body mass index (BMI)?
   a. The BMI cannot be calculated because the age is not provided.
   b. The BMI indicates that the client is overweight.
   c. The BMI indicates that the client is most likely anorexic.
   d. The BMI decreases the client's risk of developing cardiovascular disease.

9. A 67-year-old male takes metformin for diabetes, phenytoin for a seizure disorder, and methotrexate for rheumatoid arthritis. The nurse needs to assess this client for a deficiency of which substance impacted by all three medications?
   a. Biotin
   b. Thiamine
   c. Folic acid
   d. Vitamin K

10. A 27-year-old female with obesity has a HbA1c of 6.7%. What conclusion does the nurse make about this laboratory result?
    a. The client has diabetes mellitus.
    b. The client has prediabetes.
    c. The client has diabetes insipidus and diabetes mellitus.
    d. The client has a family history of diabetes.

UNIT

III Physical Examination

Chapter 8 Physical Examination Techniques, 198

Chapter 9 General Survey, Vital Signs, and Pain, 219

Chapter 10 Skin, Hair, and Nails, 252

Chapter 11 Head, Neck, and Regional Lymph Nodes, 298

Chapter 12 Eyes, 319

Chapter 13 Ears, Nose, Mouth, and Throat, 354

Chapter 14 Breasts and Regional Lymph Nodes, 392

Chapter 15 Thorax and Lungs, 417

Chapter 16 Heart, 463

Chapter 17 Peripheral Vasculature System and Lymphatic System, 502

Chapter 18 Abdomen, 533

Chapter 19 Musculoskeletal System, 573

Chapter 20 Mental Status and Neurological System, 637

Chapter 21 Female Genitalia, 695

Chapter 22 Male Genitalia, 735

Chapter 23 Anus, Rectum, and Prostate, 763

CHAPTER

Physical Examination Techniques

8

So never lose an opportunity of urging a practical beginning, however small, for it is wonderful how often in such matters the mustard-seed germinates and roots itself.

Florence Nightingale

Learning Outcomes

1. Discuss the purposes of the physical examination.
2. Describe how to follow Standard Precautions and Transmission-Based Precautions during the physical examination.
3. Establish an appropriate environment for conducting a physical examination.
4. Describe how to perform the physical examination technique of inspection and which areas of the body are assessed with this technique.
5. Describe how to perform the physical examination technique of palpation and which areas of the body are assessed with this technique.
6. Describe how to perform the physical examination technique of percussion and which areas of the body are assessed with this technique.
7. Describe how to perform the physical examination technique of auscultation and which areas of the body are assessed with this technique.
8. Discuss the legal considerations of conducting a physical examination.

Inspection, palpation, percussion, and auscultation are the techniques used by the nurse to assess the client during a physical examination. This chapter introduces the assessment techniques and equipment used to conduct physical examinations.

General Aspects of Physical Examination

Physical examination of a client serves many purposes:

1. Screening of general well-being. The findings will serve as baseline information for future examinations.
2. Linking physical examination findings to the symptoms that led the ill client to seek health care.
3. Monitoring health status and current health problems.
4. Formulating diagnoses and interventions based on the findings of the physical examination.
5. Recommending preventive health-care services to optimize client health.

How and when the physical examination is conducted depends on, among other factors, the client's health status and accessibility to healthcare. For example, a person with brittle diabetes, arthritis, and glaucoma who has access to health care is more likely to enter the health-care delivery system than a healthy college student. Similarly, a person who lives in a remote location may need health care, but access can be limited or nonexistent.

Role of the Nurse

The professional nurse plays a vital role in the assessment of client problems. Educational preparation and the clinical setting in part determine the extent to which the nurse participates in the assessment process. For example, a nurse in primary care may perform a comprehensive physical examination of clients, whereas a critical care nurse may conduct selected client assessments to monitor and evaluate current health problems. In either case, nurses are expected to be familiar with and comfortable using physical examination skills. Today's nurses are sophisticated professionals who require information to make clinical decisions based on scientific rationale and evidence-based research. The physical examination findings provide this information.

Standard Precautions

The transmission of hepatitis, SARS-CoV2 (COVID-19), human immunodeficiency virus (HIV), and other infectious diseases is a primary concern for the nurse and the client. **Standard Precautions**, formerly known as "universal precautions," were developed by the Centers for Disease Control and Prevention (CDC) to protect health-care professionals and clients (Fig. 8-1). The primary goal of Standard Precautions is to prevent the exchange of blood and body fluids. Standard Precautions should be practiced with every client throughout the entire encounter, whether or not the client has a known or suspected infectious process.

Standard Precautions are the minimum infection control practices that are practiced in *all* health-care settings; these recommendations recognize that more client care is being delivered in nonhospital settings. The CDC recommendations for Standard Precautions include:

1. Hand hygiene
2. Use of personal protective equipment
3. Respiratory hygiene/cough etiquette
4. Appropriate client placement
5. Proper handling of equipment and disinfecting the environment
6. Safe injection practices

Hand Hygiene

The most important infection control practice is hand washing. You must begin and end every physical examination with a thorough hand wash (Fig. 8-2A). Some nurses perform this in the examination area with the client present. It is a nonthreatening way to start the physical examination and allows the client time to ask questions.

The CDC's *Guideline for Hand Hygiene in Health-Care Settings* recommends the use of an alcohol-based hand rub for routine decontamination (Fig. 8-2B). Hand washing with soap and water is recommended when hands are visibly soiled or after working with clients with blood or body fluids. Complete guidelines can be found on the CDC Web site: *https://www.cdc.gov/mmwr/PDF/rr/rr5116.pdf.*

> **NURSING TIP**
> **Hand Hygiene Outside the Clinical Setting**
> COVID-19 impacted every facet of life when the virus became endemic in early 2020. Shortly thereafter disinfectant stations became commonplace in restaurants, gyms, public buildings ... just about everywhere (Fig. 8-3). Following CDC guidelines and recognizing the first line of defense as hand hygiene, these antibacterial stations provide convenient hand hygiene treatment when a person is outside the home.

Use of Personal Protective Equipment

Personal protective equipment (PPE) includes gloves, gowns, masks or respirators (such as N-95), and goggles/face shields (Fig. 8-4). The selection of personal protective equipment is related to the potential for exposure to body fluids and infectious processes when caring for a client. Properly donning and removing PPE protects the nurse from accidental exposure to infectious and communicable diseases. A thorough hand wash should be performed as soon as the PPE is removed. Additional information is available at the CDC Web site: *https://www.cdc.gov/infection-control/hcp/isolation-precautions.*

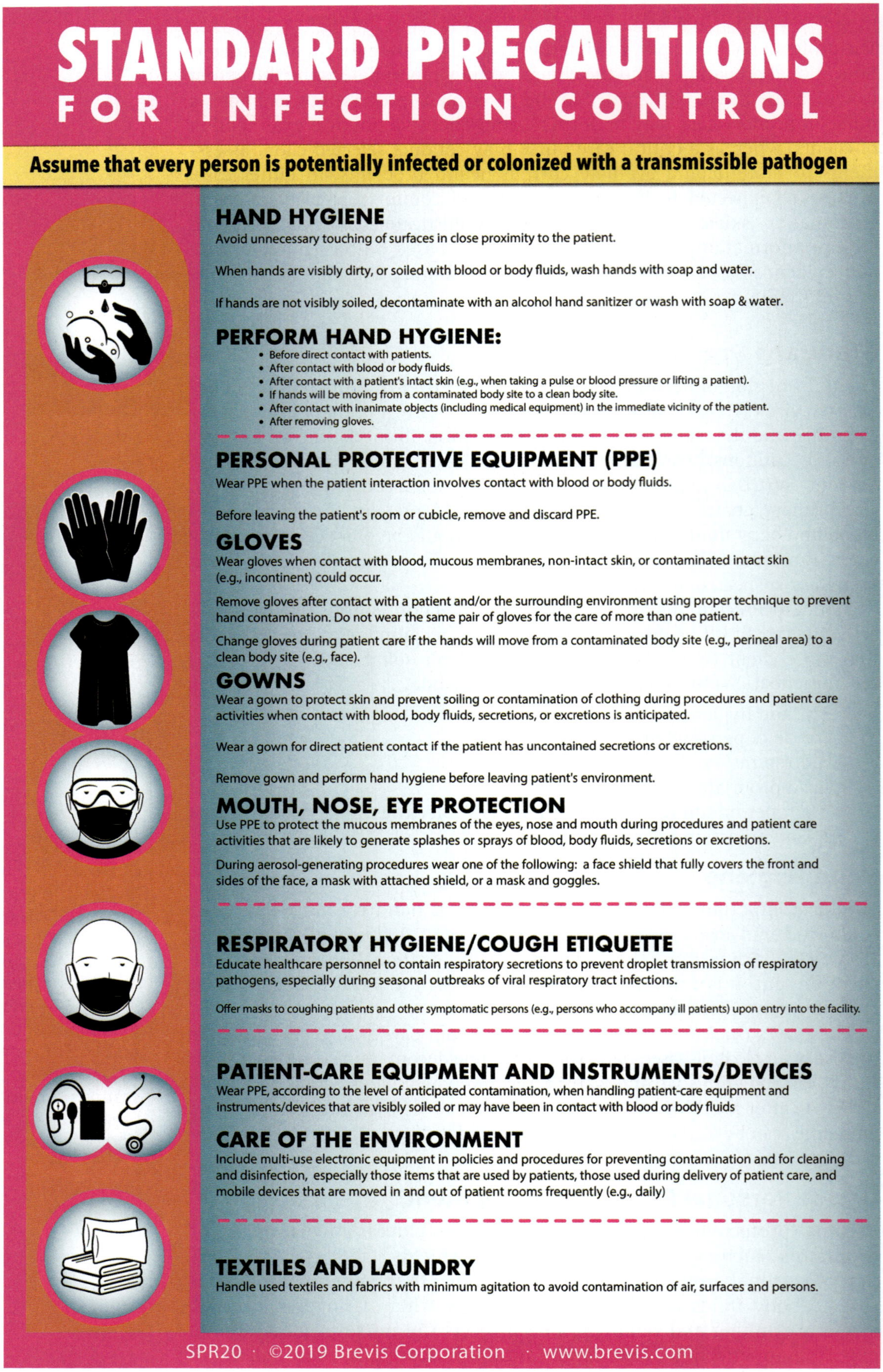

Figure 8-1 Standard Precautions.

NURSING TIP

Latex Allergies

In accordance with Standard Precautions, nurses frequently wear gloves when performing client care. Be alert to the possibility that you, as well as your client, may have a latex allergy. The possibility, as well as the severity, of a latex allergy increases with increased exposure to latex. In actuality, it is not the latex itself that causes an allergic reaction, but a protein found in the natural rubber from which latex is derived. This protein can bind to the powder that is found in latex gloves and can also become aerosolized. Thus direct contact is not always necessary to initiate an allergic reaction. The allergic reactions range from eczematous contact dermatitis to hives, wheezing, and even anaphylaxis. In addition, people with a latex allergy have an increased risk of reacting to foods such as bananas, kiwis, avocados, and European chestnuts. Be aware of any latex allergies in clients and use vinyl or nitrile gloves. Also, be aware that many medical products, such as blood pressure cuffs and tubing, wound drains, syringes, rubber-stopper medication vials, and tourniquets, contain latex; those individuals with latex allergies must use alternative products. Latex can also be found in everyday-use items such as baby pacifiers, rubber bands, erasers, balloons, and condoms. Clients need to be educated on items that should be avoided (AAAAI, 2023).

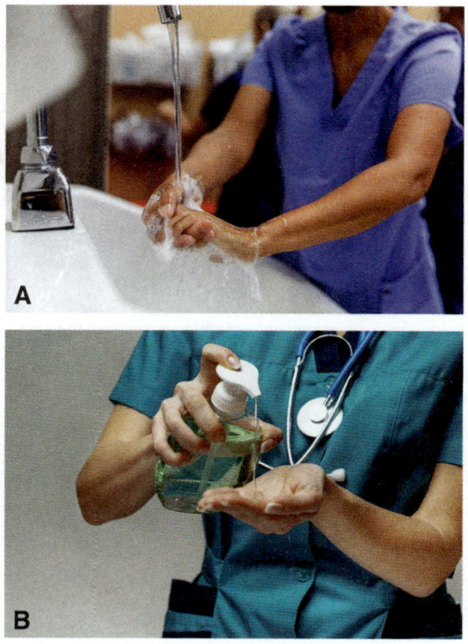

Figure 8-2 Hand hygiene practices. **A.** Hand washing using soap and water. **B.** Hand washing using an alcohol-based hand rub.

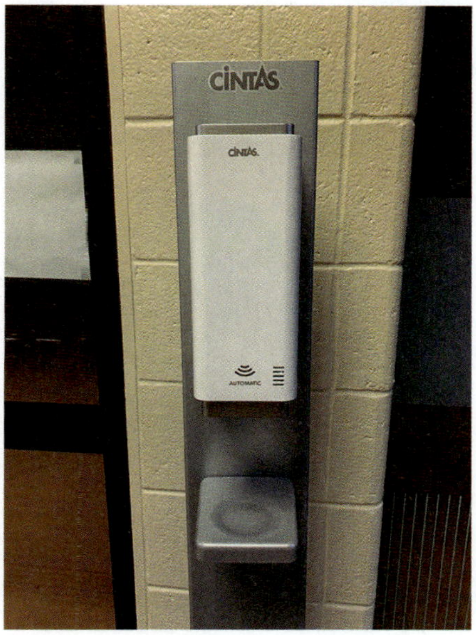

Figure 8-3 These antibacterial stations provide convenient hand hygiene treatment when outside the home.

Respiratory Hygiene/Cough Etiquette

Respiratory hygiene/cough etiquette measures were developed in response to the 2002–2004 outbreak of severe acute respiratory syndrome coronavirus (SARS-CoV1). They continued to be a vital component of Standard Precautions during the SARS-CoV2 (COVID-19) pandemic. From now on SARS-CoV2 will be referred to as COVID-19 in this text. Visual cues such as posted signs declaring "Cover Your Cough" serve as reminders that we are all responsible for containing our respiratory droplets whether in a health-care setting or the grocery store (Fig. 8-5). Outside the health-care setting many facilities posted signs reminding people to stay 6 feet away from others to help decrease contact with respiratory droplets. In the health-care setting, PPE is worn to protect the nurse from direct exposure to clients who present with suspected or confirmed respiratory illnesses and communicable or infectious diseases (Fig. 8-6). Refer to the CDC Web site: *https://www.cdc.gov/infection-control/hcp/basics/standard-precautions.html*

Appropriate Client Placement

The CDC identifies the need for appropriate client placement based on the client's presenting symptoms and pathology. Isolation guidelines based on clinical research help to prevent the transmission of infectious agents to health-care workers and other clients in health-care settings. The CDC describes the appropriate strategies to use in various settings: acute care hospital, ambulatory care center, long-term care facility, client transport, as well as in the client's home environment. For more information, refer to the CDC Web site: *https://www.cdc.gov/infection-control/hcp/basics/standard-precautions.html*

Proper Handling of Equipment and Disinfecting the Environment

Environmental infection control guidelines provide recommendations based on clinical research. Most of these guidelines do not fall within the domain of nursing practice. Extensive protocols describe how to minimize infections

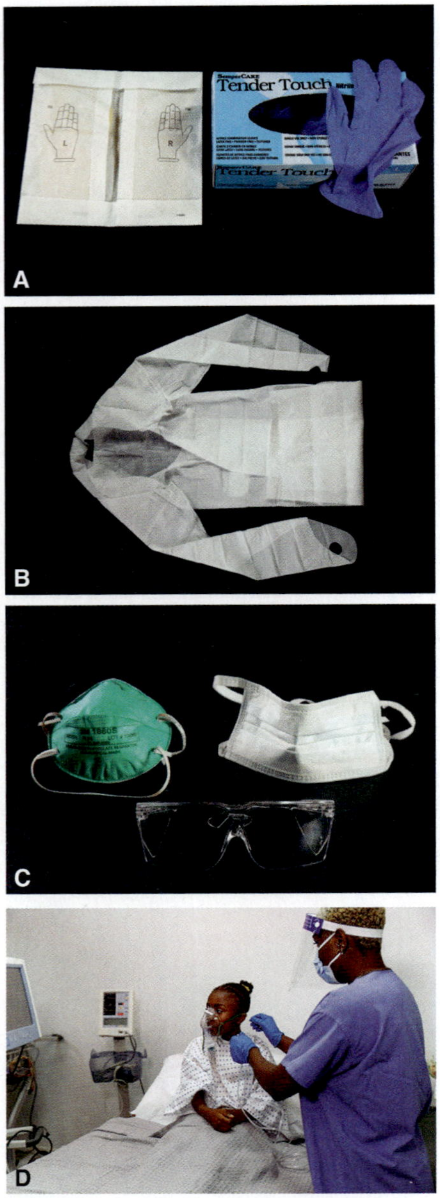

Figure 8-4 Types of personal protective equipment. **ABC.** The nurse must select the appropriate personal protective equipment for every client encounter. **D.** The nurse has donned appropriate personal protective equipment to provide care to this young child.

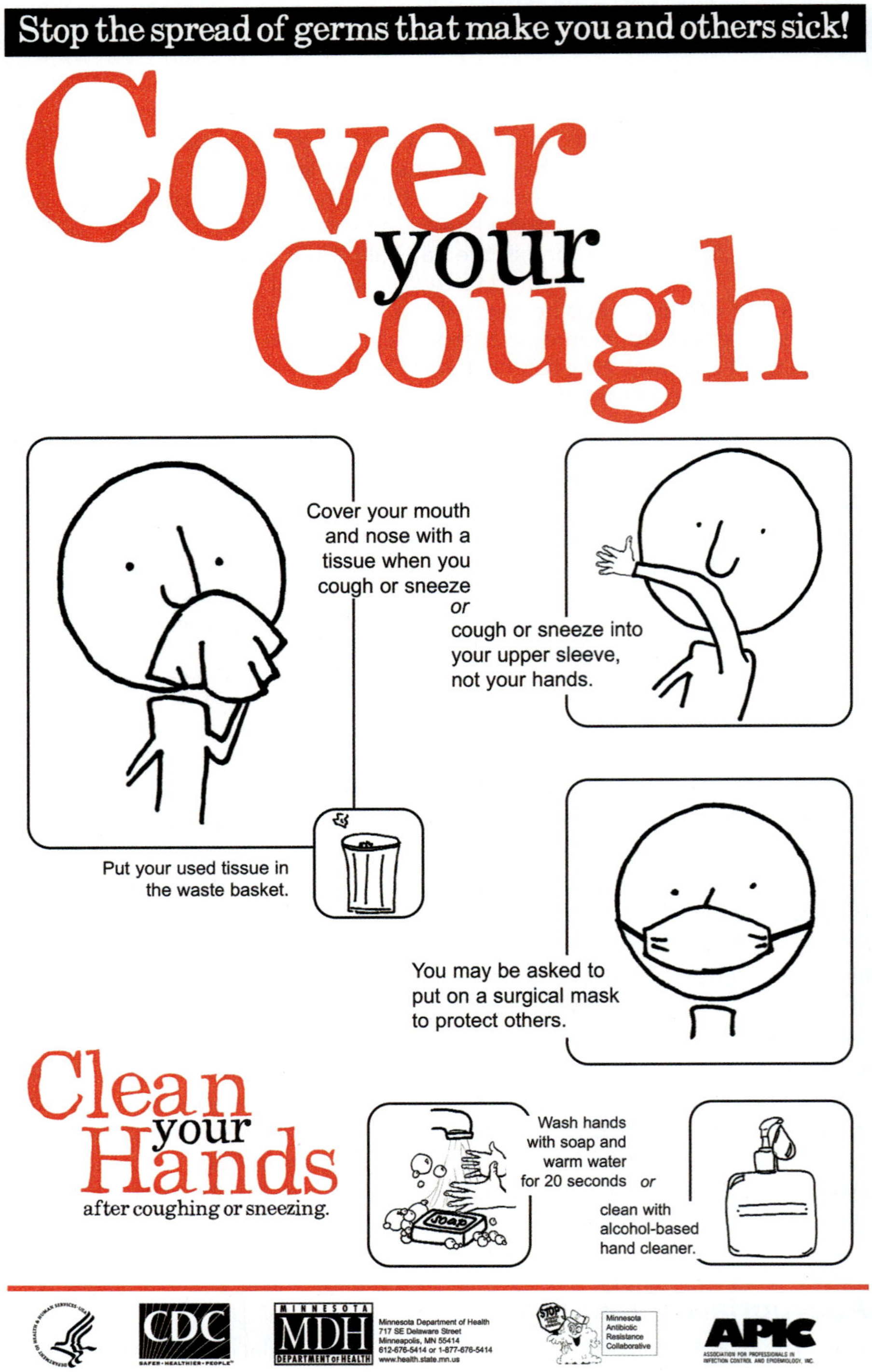

Figure 8-5 "Cover Your Cough" poster serves as a reminder that everyone needs to practice respiratory hygiene. Courtesy of the Centers for Disease Control and Prevention.

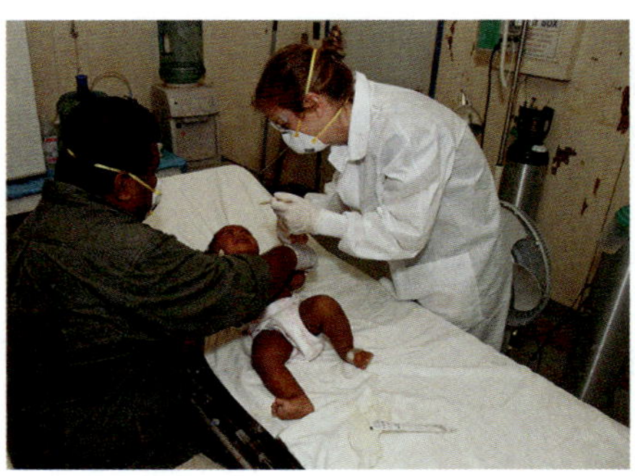

Figure 8-6 Note personal protective equipment worn by the nurse while delivering care to the small child with suspected measles. Courtesy of the Centers for Disease Control and Prevention.

in air handling systems, in a health-care setting construction, client room ventilation systems, water management systems, the cleaning of contact surfaces in client care areas, proper disinfection of laundry/bedding, and waste disposal. Guidelines also provide information on how animals can be safely incorporated into the health-care setting for animal-assisted therapy and other uses. The complete document is found on the CDC Web site: *https://www.cdc.gov/infection-control/hcp/basics/standard-precautions.html*

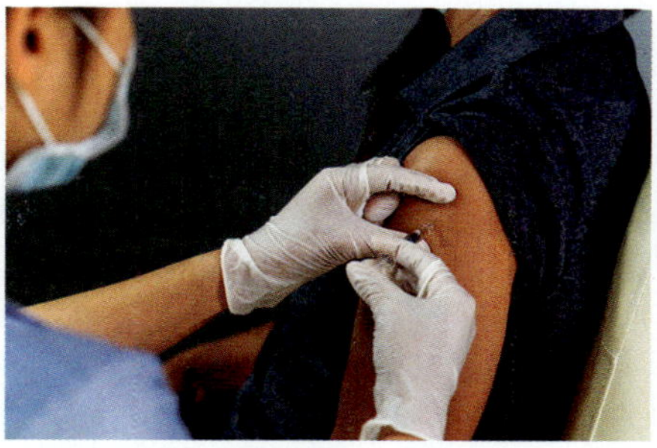

Figure 8-7 Safe injection practices are essential to preventing the spread of infections.

Safe Injection Practices

Safe injection practices specify how best to prevent the spread of infectious agents from client to client and from client to health-care providers from contaminated needles/sharps (Fig. 8-7). These practices are vital to the prevention of blood-borne diseases such as hepatitis B, hepatitis C, and HIV. In addition, the CDC recommends wearing a surgical mask when performing lumbar punctures to prevent bacterial meningitis. Safe injection practices also extend to the home environment. The frequent measuring of blood sugar in home glucose monitoring or the self-administration of insulin or other injectable medications are not uncommon practices. Refer to the CDC Web site for guidance on how best to conduct injections in a safe manner outside the health-care setting: *https://www.cdc.gov/infection-control/hcp/basics/standard-precautions.html*

Transmission-Based Precautions

The CDC has developed another level of precautions called **Transmission-Based Precautions** (Fig. 8-8). These precautions are to be used in conjunction with Standard Precautions. Contact, Droplet, and Airborne Precautions are employed to prevent the transmission of microorganisms that are known or suspected in a client. Contact transmission pathogens, such as in impetigo, scabies, varicella-zoster virus, and multidrug-resistant organisms (e.g., methicillin-resistant *Staphylococcus aureus*–MRSA), can be spread directly from person to person. Contact Precautions must also be implemented when the client has fecal incontinence, excessive wound drainage, or other body secretions, because of the risk of environmental contamination and subsequent transmission. Microorganisms can also be spread indirectly from a contaminated inanimate object to a person. Droplet transmission occurs when microorganisms are deposited on susceptible body parts via respiratory secretions (sneezing and coughing). Typically, the pathogens in the droplet remain infectious for only a short period. Suctioning a client's endotracheal tube or tracheostomy can also transmit droplets. *Bacillus pertussis, Haemophilus influenzae,* rhinovirus, adenovirus, group A *Streptococcus,* and *N. meningitidis* are examples of pathogens contracted through this mode of transmission. Airborne transmission spreads microorganisms by air currents and inhalation. These pathogens are infectious over long distances when they are airborne. They can also be passed through ventilation systems. Measles, the varicella virus, and *Mycobacterium tuberculosis* can spread in this mode. Additional information is available at: *https://www.cdc.gov/infection-control/hcp/basics/transmission-based-precautions.html*

Equipment

The physical examination will proceed efficiently if you have gathered all the necessary equipment beforehand. The equipment needed to perform a complete physical examination of the adult client includes:

- Personal protective equipment (PPE)
- Pen and paper
- Marking pen

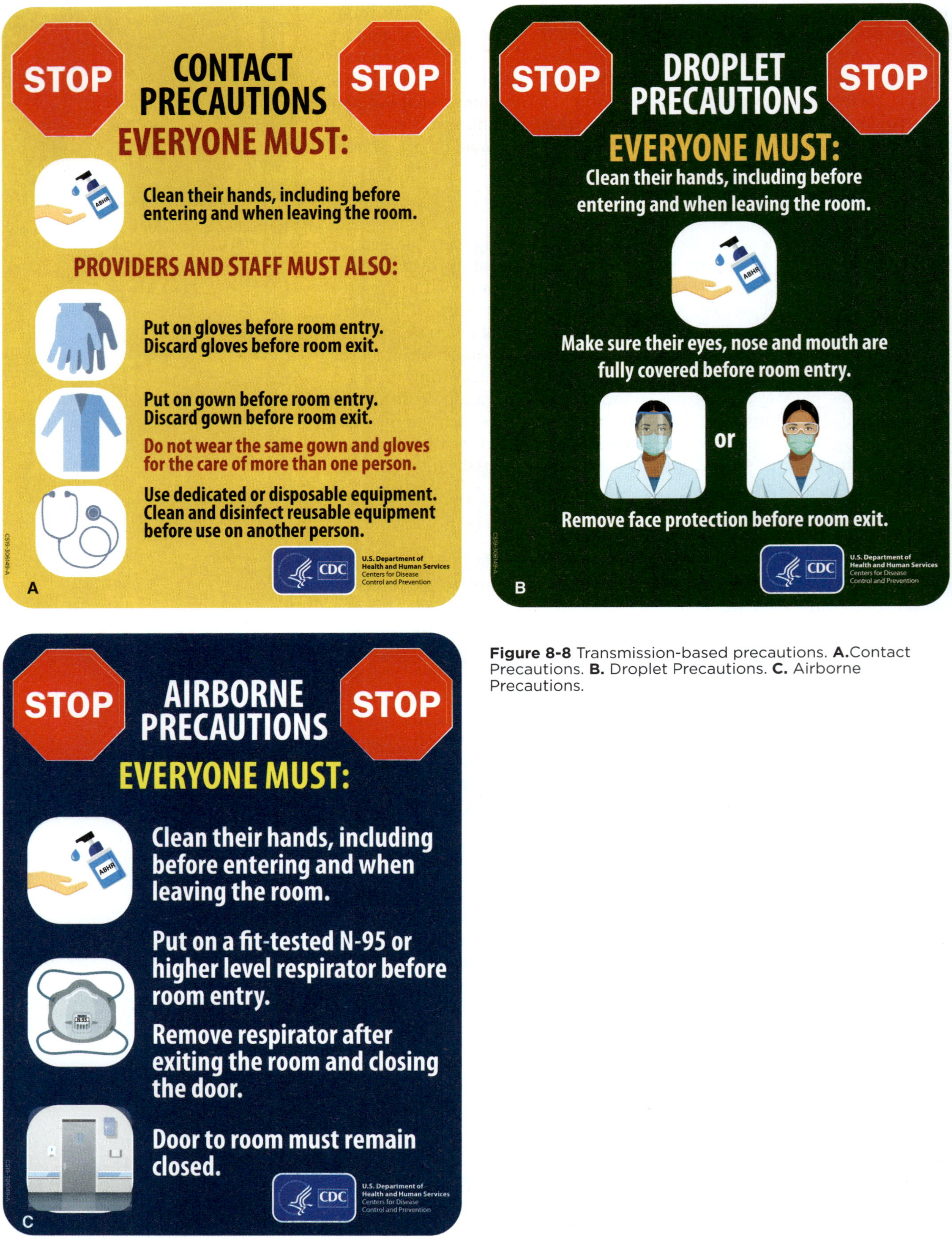

Figure 8-8 Transmission-based precautions. **A.**Contact Precautions. **B.** Droplet Precautions. **C.** Airborne Precautions.

- Tape measure
- Ruler
- Client gown/drape
- Penlight or flashlight
- Scale (you may need to walk the client to a central location if a scale cannot be brought to the client's room)
- Thermometer
- Sphygmomanometer
- Gooseneck lamp
- Tongue depressor
- Stethoscope
- Otoscope
- Nasal speculum
- Ophthalmoscope
- Transilluminator
- Visual acuity charts
- Visual occluder
- Tuning forks
- Reflex hammer
- Sterile needle
- Cotton balls; gauze pads
- Odors for cranial nerve assessment (coffee, lemon, flowers, etc.)
- Small objects for neurological assessment (paper clip, key, cotton ball, pen, etc.); single-fiber monofilament
- Water-soluble lubricant
- Various sizes of vaginal speculums
- Ayre spatula
- Cytobrush
- Cotton-tip swab, 6 inches
- Liquid-based cytology vial
- Guaiac material
- Specimen cup; culture tube
- Goniometer
- Scoliometer
- Gestation calculation wheel

The use of these items is discussed in the chapters describing the examinations for which they are used. Figure 8-9 illustrates some of the equipment used in the physical examination.

Steps for Conducting a Physical Examination

Preparing for a Physical Examination

- Always dress in a clean, professional manner; make sure your name pin or workplace identification is visible.
- Remove all bracelets, necklaces, or earrings that can interfere with the physical examination.
- Be sure that your fingernails are short and your hands are warm, for maximum client comfort.
- Be sure your hair will not fall forward and obstruct your vision or touch the client.
- Arrange for a well-lit, warm, and private room.
- Observe Standard Precautions and don personal protective equipment (PPE), such as gloves, gown, face shield, goggles, N-95 respirator, or face mask if the client's status warrants these protective measures.
- Ensure that all the necessary equipment is ready for use and within reach.

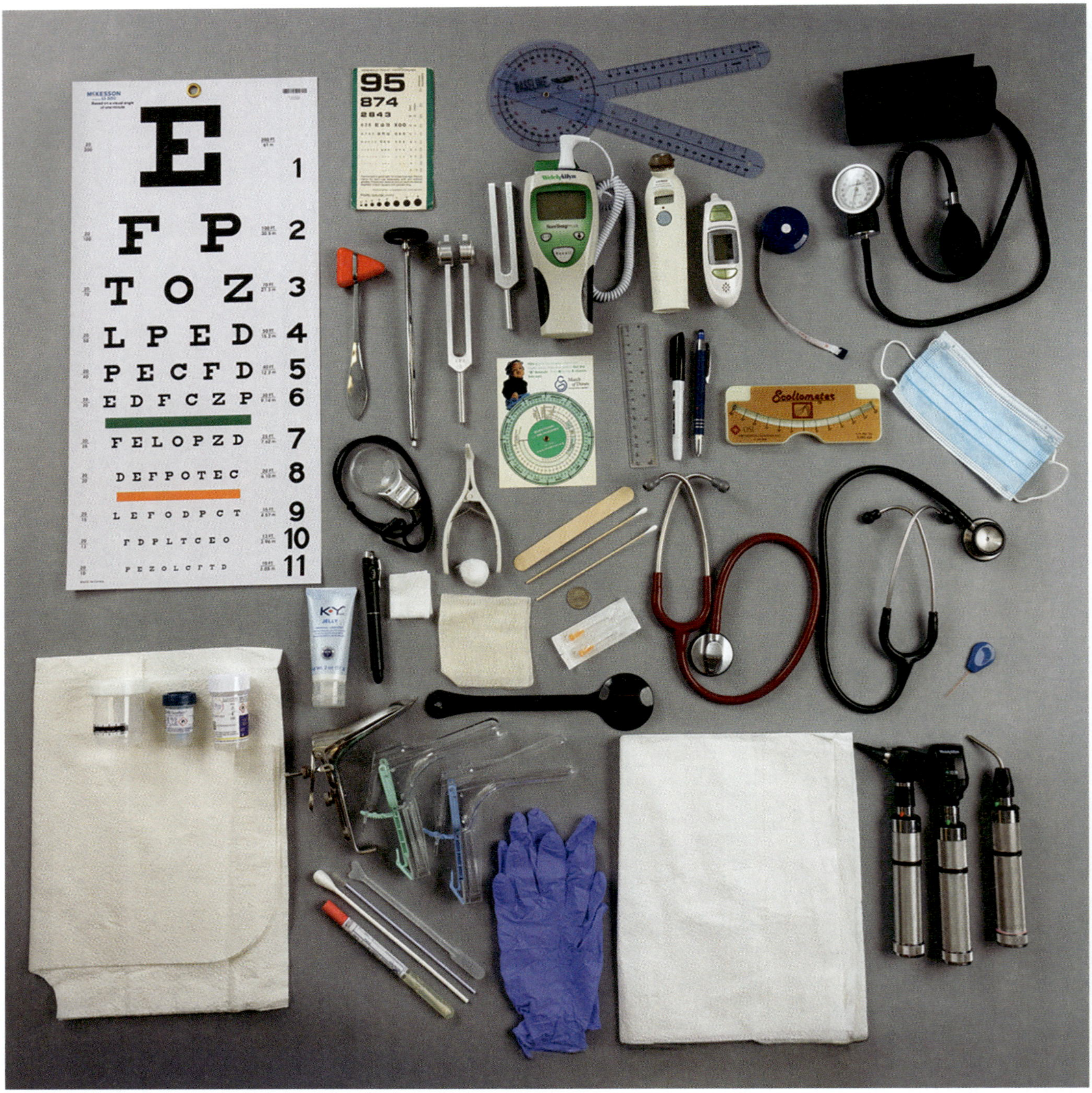

Figure 8-9 Equipment used in physical examination.

Conducting a Physical Examination

- Introduce yourself to the client: "My name is Mia Fernandez. I am the nurse taking care of you today."
- Clarify how the client wishes to be addressed: Miss Ahmed, José, Colonel Ballard, Reverend Grimes, etc.
- Explain what you plan to do and how long it will take; allow the client to ask questions.
- Have the client void before the examination.
- Instruct the client to undress; underwear can be left on until the end of the examination. Provide a gown and drape for the client and explain how to use them.

- Allow the client to undress privately; inform the client when you will return to start the examination.
- Wash your hands in front of the client to show your concern for cleanliness.
- Observe Standard Precautions and Transmission-Based Precautions.
- Ensure that the client is accessible from both sides of the examining bed or table.
- If a bed is used, raise the height so that you do not have to bend over to perform the examination.
- Position the client as dictated by the body system being examined. Figure 8-10 illustrates positioning and draping techniques.
- Enlist the client's cooperation by explaining what you are about to do, where it will be done, and how it may feel.
- Warm all instruments before using them.
- Examine the unaffected body part or side first if a client's complaint is unilateral.
- Explain to the client why you may be spending a long time performing one particular skill: "Listening to the heart requires concentration and time."
- If the client complains of fatigue, continue the examination later (if possible).
- Do not make crude or negative remarks; control your facial expression when dealing with clients who are malodorous or ones who have disturbing findings (infected wounds, disfigurement, etc.).
- Conduct the examination in a systematic fashion every time. (This decreases the likelihood of forgetting to perform a particular assessment.)

Ending the Visit

- Ask the client if they have any questions.
- Thank the client when the physical examination is concluded; inform the client what will happen next.
- Document examination findings in the appropriate section of the client record.

Physical Examination Techniques

Physical examination findings, or objective data, are obtained using four specific diagnostic techniques: inspection, palpation, percussion, and auscultation. Usually, these examination techniques are performed in this order when body systems are assessed. An exception is in the examination of the abdomen when auscultation is performed after inspection. Percussion and palpation can alter bowel motility, so they are performed after auscultation. These four techniques validate information provided by a client in the health history, or they can verify a suspected physical diagnosis.

Frequently inspection and auscultation skills are developed and used more by the novice nurse. Percussion and palpation may take more time and practice to perfect. With time and practice, the physical examination techniques become second nature, and you will develop your own rhythm and style. You may not perform all examination skills in the same order as they are presented in this text. This practice is acceptable if basic guidelines are observed.

<table>
<tr><td>Standing: Can be used to assess a client's skin; head and neck; eyes, ears, nose, mouth, and throat; breasts and axillae; thorax and lungs; heart and peripheral vasculature; abdomen; musculoskeletal system; neurological system; male genitalia</td><td>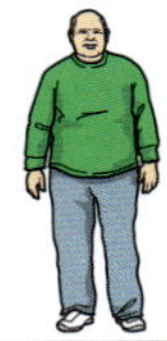</td></tr>
<tr><td>Semi-Fowler's: Can be used to assess a client's skin; head and neck; eyes, ears, nose, mouth, and throat; breasts and axillae; anterior thorax and lungs; heart and peripheral vasculature; abdomen; musculoskeletal system; neurological system</td><td>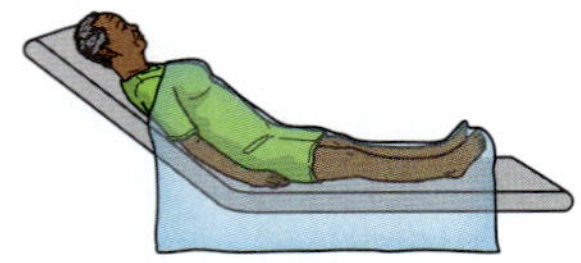</td></tr>
<tr><td>High-Fowler's/Sitting: Can be used to assess a client's skin; head and neck; eyes, ears, nose, mouth, and throat; breasts and axillae; thorax and lungs; heart and peripheral vasculature; abdomen; musculoskeletal system; neurological system</td><td>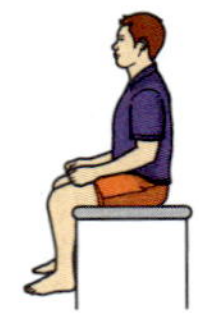</td></tr>
<tr><td>Supine/Horizontal Recumbent: Can be used to assess a client's skin; head and neck; eyes, ears, nose, mouth, and throat; breasts and axillae; anterior thorax and lungs; heart and peripheral vasculature; abdomen; musculoskeletal system; neurological system</td><td>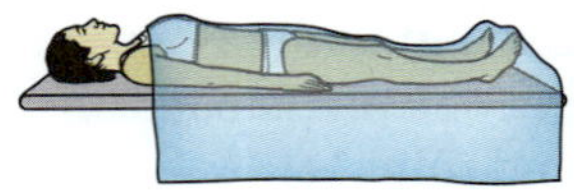</td></tr>
<tr><td>Dorsal Recumbent: Can be used to assess a client's skin; head and neck; eyes, ears, nose, mouth, and throat; breasts and axillae; anterior thorax and lungs; heart and peripheral vasculature; musculoskeletal system; neurological system; female genitalia</td><td>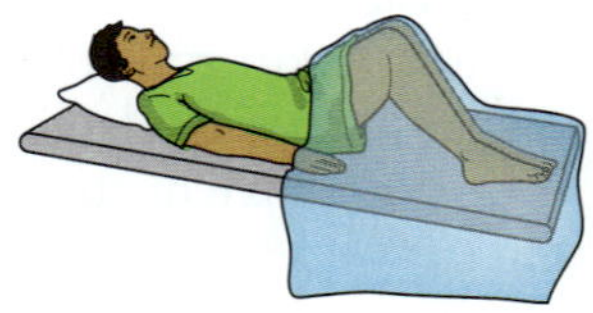</td></tr>
<tr><td>Side Lying: Can be used to assess a client's skin; thorax and lungs; heart and peripheral vasculature; musculoskeletal system; neurological system; prostate; rectum</td><td>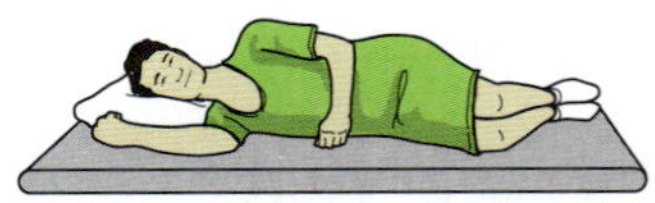</td></tr>
<tr><td>Lithotomy: Can be used to assess a female client's skin; genitalia; rectum</td><td>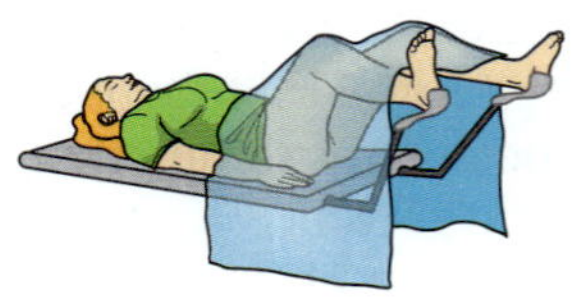</td></tr>
<tr><td>Knee-Chest: Can be used to assess a client's skin; musculoskeletal system; prostate; rectum</td><td>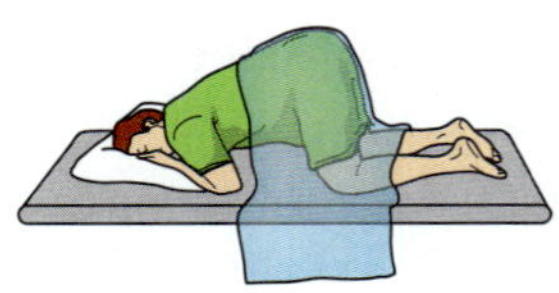</td></tr>
<tr><td>Sims': Can be used to assess a client's skin; musculoskeletal system; female genitalia; rectum</td><td>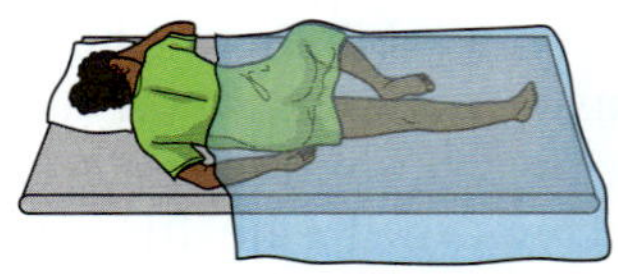</td></tr>
<tr><td>Prone: Can be used to assess a client's skin; posterior thorax and lungs; musculoskeletal system</td><td>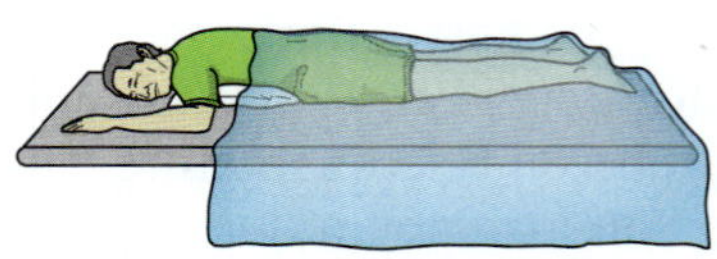</td></tr>
</table>

Figure 8-10 Positioning and draping techniques, including the body systems assessed while the client is in each position. Note that portions of many systems can be examined in various positions, even when not positioned ideally for a specific assessment.

Assessment in Brief

Inspection	Palpation	Percussion	Auscultation
• Vision • Smell	• Light palpation • Deep palpation	• Direct, or immediate percussion • Indirect, or mediate percussion • Direct fist percussion • Indirect fist percussion	• Direct, or immediate auscultation • Indirect, or mediate auscultation

Inspection

"A conscientious nurse is not necessarily an observing nurse; and life or death may lie with the good observer." This statement by Florence Nightingale provides inspiration and direction for inspection, which is usually the first examination technique used during the assessment process. **Inspection** is an ongoing process that you use throughout the entire physical examination and client encounter. Inspection is the use of one's senses of vision and smell to consciously observe the client.

> **NURSING TIP**
> **Practicing Physical Examination Techniques**
> Have a classmate use a cell phone to record you performing the physical examination techniques of inspection, percussion, palpation, and auscultation on another classmate. Evaluate your technique and ask for your classmate's feedback.

Vision

Use of sight can reveal many facts about a client. Visual inspection of a client's respiratory status, for example, might reveal a rate of 38 breaths per minute and cyanotic nailbeds. In this case, the client is tachypneic and possibly hypoxic and would need a more thorough respiratory examination. The process of visual inspection necessitates full exposure of the body part being inspected, adequate overhead lighting, and, when necessary, **tangential lighting** (light that is shone at an angle on the client to accentuate shadows and highlight subtle findings).

Smell

The nurse's olfactory sense provides vital information about a client's health status. The client may have a fruity breath odor characteristic of diabetic ketoacidosis. The classic, fruity, grape-like odor emitted by a *Pseudomonas* infection is another well-recognized smell to the experienced nurse.

Palpation

The second examination technique is **palpation**, which is the act of touching a client therapeutically to elicit specific information. Before palpating a client, you must observe some basic principles. You should have short fingernails to avoid hurting the client as well as yourself. Also, you should warm your hands before placing them on the client; cold hands can make a client's muscles tense, which can distort examination findings. Encourage the client to continue to breathe normally throughout the palpation. If pain is experienced during the palpation, discontinue the palpation immediately. Most significantly, inform the client where, when, and how the touch will occur, especially when the client cannot see what you are doing. In this way, the client is kept aware of what to expect in the examination process.

Your hands are the tools used to perform the palpation process. Different sections of the hands are best used for examining certain areas of the body.

The dorsum of the hand is most sensitive to temperature changes in the body. Thus it is more accurate to place the dorsum of the hand on a client's forehead to assess the body temperature than it is to use the palmar surface of the hand. The palmar surface of the fingers at the metacarpophalangeal joints, the ball of the hand, and the ulnar surface of the hand best discriminate vibrations, such as a cardiac thrill and tactile fremitus. The finger pads are the portion of the hand used most frequently in palpation. Because of their fine tactile discrimination, the finger pads are useful in assessing skin moisture and texture; the presence of masses, pulsations, edema, and crepitus; and the shape, size, position, mobility, and consistency of organs (Fig. 8-11).

Remember to observe Standard Precautions when you are performing palpation. Gloves *must* be worn when examining any open wounds, skin

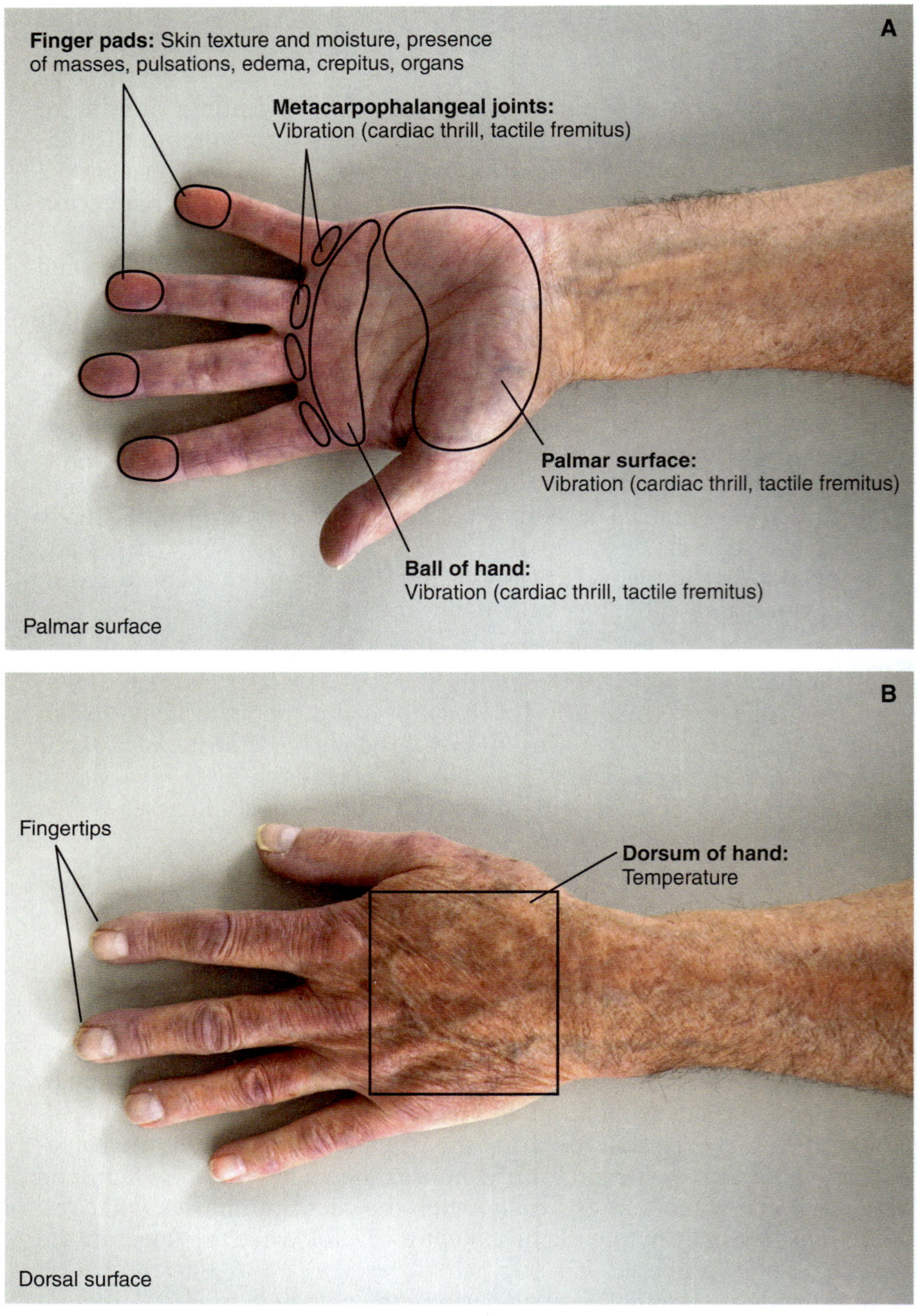

Figure 8-11 Parts of the hand used in palpation. **A.** Palmar surface. **B.** Dorsal surface.

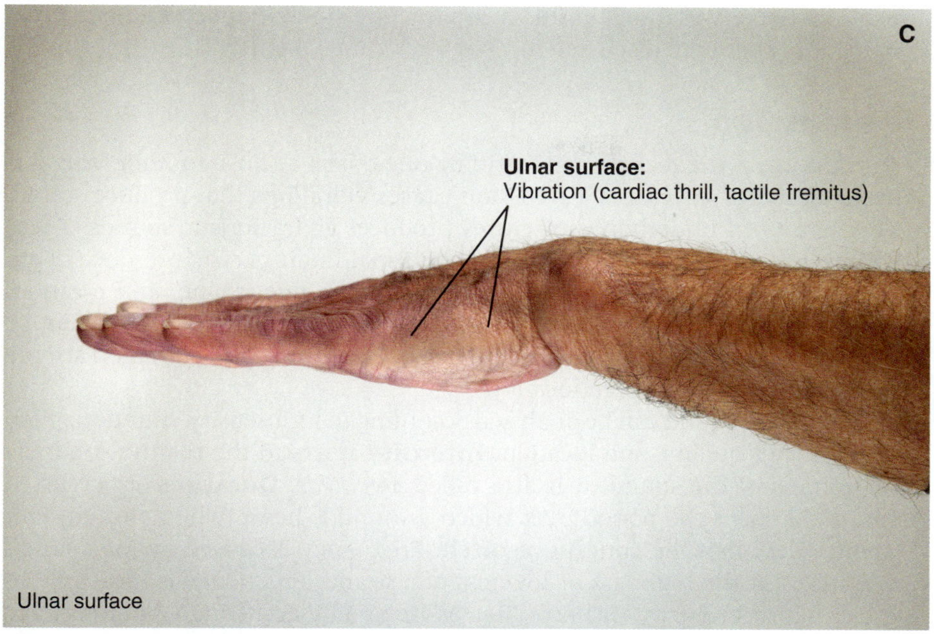

Figure 8-11—cont'd C. Ulnar surface.

lesions, or a body part with discharge, as well as internal body parts such as the mouth, vagina, and rectum.

There are two distinct types of palpation: light and deep palpation. Each of these techniques is described here and covered in greater detail in chapters describing body system examinations in which palpation is specifically used.

Light Palpation

Light palpation is done more frequently than deep palpation and is always performed before deep palpation. As the name implies, **light palpation** is superficial, delicate, and gentle. In light palpation, the finger pads are used to gain information from the client's skin surface to a depth of approximately 1 cm below the surface. Light palpation reveals information on skin texture and moisture; overt, large, or superficial masses; and fluid, muscle guarding, and superficial tenderness. To perform light palpation:

1. Keeping the fingers of your dominant hand together, place the finger pads lightly on the skin over the area that is to be palpated. The hand and forearm will be on a plane parallel to the area being examined.
2. Depress the skin 1 cm in light, gentle, circular motions.
3. Keeping the finger pads on the skin, let the depressed body surface rebound to its natural position.
4. If the client is ticklish, lift the hand off the skin before moving it to another area.
5. Using a systematic approach, move the fingers to an adjacent area and repeat the process.
6. Continue to move the finger pads until the entire area being examined has been palpated.
7. If the client has complained of tenderness in any area, palpate this area last. Figure 8-12 shows how light palpation is performed.

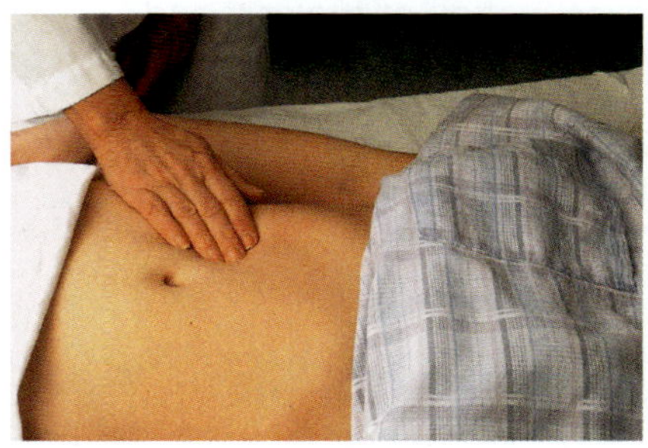

Figure 8-12 Technique of light palpation.

Deep Palpation

Deep palpation can reveal information about the position of organs and masses, as well as their size, shape, mobility, consistency, and areas of discomfort/pain. Deep palpation uses the hands to explore the body's internal structures to a depth of 4 to 5 cm or more (Fig. 8-13). This technique is most often used for abdominal, anal, rectal, and male and female genitalia

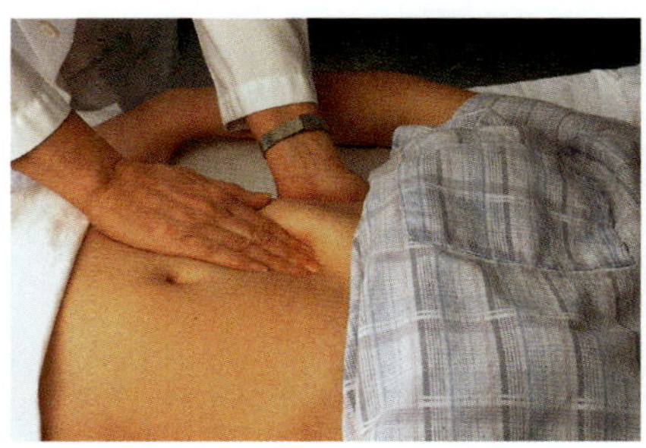

Figure 8-13 Technique of deep palpation.

examinations. Variations in this technique are single-handed and bimanual palpation; these are discussed in Chapter 18 and Chapter 21.

Percussion

Percussion is the technique of striking one object against another to evaluate underlying structures. Percussion causes vibrations that produce sound. The density of underlying structures produces characteristic sounds. These sounds are diagnostic of normal and abnormal findings. The presence of air, fluid, and solids can be confirmed, as can organ size, shape, and position. Any part of the body can be percussed, but only limited information can be obtained in specific areas such as the heart. The thorax and abdomen are the most frequently percussed locations.

Percussion sound can be analyzed according to its intensity, duration, pitch (frequency), quality, and location. **Intensity** refers to the relative loudness or softness of the sound. It is also called *amplitude*. **Duration** of percussed sound describes the period over which a sound is heard when elicited. Frequency describes the concept of **pitch**. Frequency is caused by the sound's vibrations or the highness or lowness of a sound. Frequency is measured in cycles per second (cps) or hertz (Hz). More rapidly occurring vibrations have a pitch that is higher than that of slower vibrations. Figure 8-14 illustrates this concept. The **quality** of a sound is its *timbre*, or how one perceives it musically. **Location** of sound refers to the area where the sound is produced and heard.

Percussion can produce five distinct sounds in the body: **flatness, dullness, resonance, hyperresonance,** and **tympany**. Specific parts of the body produce distinct sounds in response to percussion. Therefore, when an unexpected sound is heard in a particular part of the body, the cause must be further investigated.

Table 8-1 describes each of the five percussion sounds in relation to their respective intensity, duration, pitch, quality, location, and density. In addition, examples are provided of normal and abnormal locations of percussed sounds.

Sound waves are better conducted through a solid medium than through an air-filled medium because of the increased concentration of molecules. The basic premises underlying the sounds that are percussed are:

1. The more solid a structure, the higher its pitch, the softer its intensity, and the shorter its duration.
2. The more air-filled a structure, the lower its pitch, the louder its intensity, and the longer its duration.

NURSING TIP
Order of Examination Procedures

A good rule of thumb to follow when sequencing examination procedures is to progress from the least intrusive to the most intrusive. Examination techniques that may cause discomfort should be performed last whenever possible to prevent client anxiety, fear, and muscle guarding, which can affect the assessment process. For example, palpation of a tender area in the abdomen should be performed last. In the pediatric client, the examination of the ears and throat is usually performed last because these are usually the most uncomfortable for the child and may cause crying.

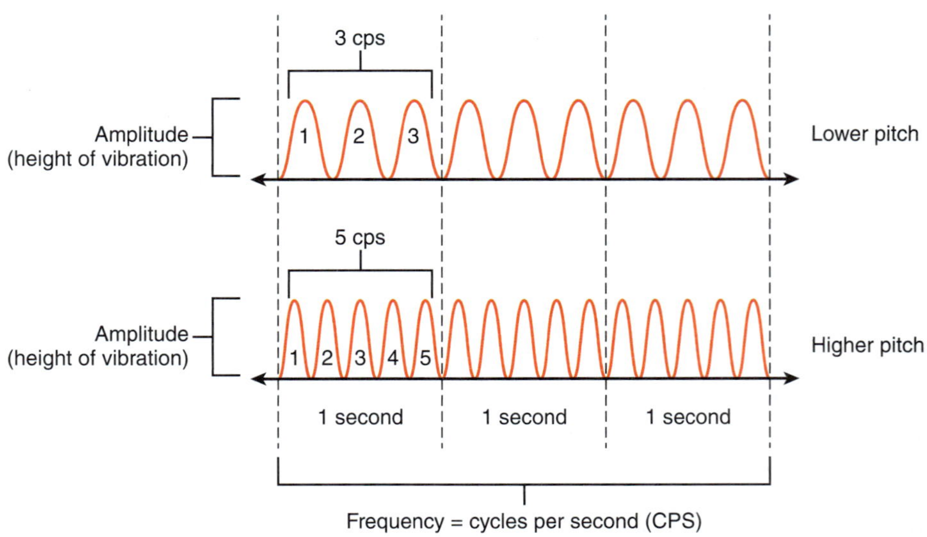

Figure 8-14 Percussion pitch.

Table 8-1 Characteristics of Percussion Sounds

Sound	Intensity	Duration	Pitch	Quality	Normal Location	Abnormal Location	Density
Flatness	Soft	Short	High	Flat	Muscle (thigh) or bone	Lungs (severe pneumonia)	Most dense
Dullness	Moderate	Moderate	High	Thud	Organs (liver)	Lungs (atelectasis)	↓
Resonance	Loud	Moderate-long	Low	Hollow	Normal lungs	No abnormal location	
Hyperresonance	Very loud	Long	Very low	Boom	No normal location in adults; normal lungs in children	Lungs (emphysema)	
Tympany	Loud	Long	High	Drum	Gastric air bubble	Lungs (large pneumothorax)	Least dense

There are four types of percussion techniques: direct (immediate), indirect (mediate), direct fist percussion, and indirect fist percussion. It is important to keep in mind that the sounds produced from percussion are generated from body tissue up to 5 cm below the surface of the skin. If the abdomen is to be percussed, the client should have the opportunity to void before the examination.

Direct Percussion

Direct percussion or **immediate percussion** is the striking of an area of the body directly. To perform direct percussion:

1. Spread the index or middle finger of the dominant hand slightly apart from the rest of the fingers.
2. Make a light tapping motion with the finger pad of the index finger against the body part being percussed.
3. Note what sound is produced.

Percussion of the sinuses (Fig. 8-15) illustrates the use of direct percussion in the physical examination.

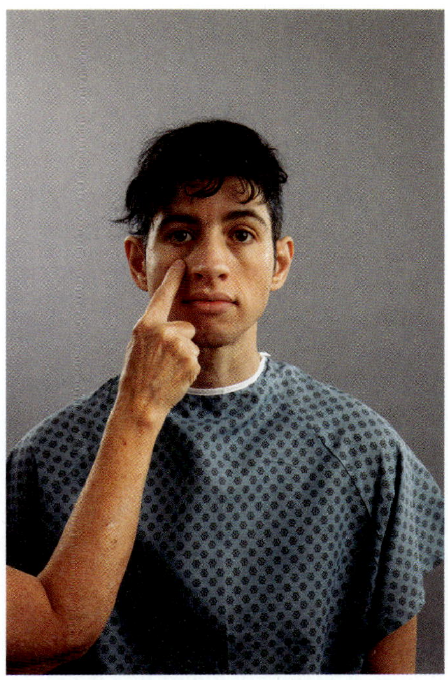

Figure 8-15 Technique of direct percussion.

Indirect Percussion

Indirect percussion is also referred to as **mediate percussion**. This is a skill that takes time and practice to develop and use effectively. Most sounds are produced using indirect percussion. Follow these steps to perform indirect percussion (Fig. 8-16):

1. Place the nondominant hand lightly on the surface to be percussed.
2. Extend the middle finger of this hand, known as the **pleximeter**, and press its distal phalanx and distal interphalangeal joint firmly on the location where percussion is to begin. The pleximeter will remain stationary while percussion is performed in this location.
3. Spread the other fingers of the nondominant hand apart and raise them slightly off the surface. This prevents interference, and thus dampening, of vibrations during the actual percussion.
4. Flex the middle finger of the dominant hand, called the **plexor**. The fingernail of the plexor finger should be very short to prevent

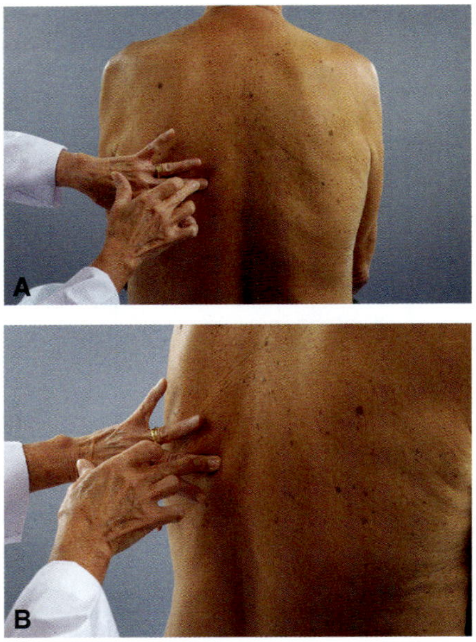

Figure 8-16 Technique of indirect percussion. A. Position of hands for posterior thorax percussion. B. Percussion strike.

undue discomfort and injury to the nurse. The other fingers on this hand should be fanned.

5. Flex the wrist of the dominant hand and place the hand directly over the pleximeter finger of the nondominant hand.
6. With a sharp, crisp, rapid movement from the wrist of the dominant hand, strike the pleximeter with the plexor. At this point, the plexor should be perpendicular to the pleximeter. The blow to the pleximeter should be between the distal interphalangeal joint and the fingernail. Use the finger pad rather than the fingertip of the plexor to deliver the blow. Concentrate on the movement to create the striking action from the dominant wrist only.
7. As soon as the plexor strikes the pleximeter, withdraw the plexor to avoid dampening the resulting vibrations. Do not move the pleximeter finger.
8. Note the sound produced by the percussion.
9. Repeat the percussion process one or two times in this location to confirm the sound.
10. Move the pleximeter to a second location, preferably the contralateral location from where the previous percussion was performed. Repeat the percussion process in this manner until the entire body surface area being assessed has been percussed.

> **NURSING TIP**
>
> **At-Home Practice of Percussion**
>
> - Percuss two glasses—one filled with water, the other empty. Compare the sounds.
> - Percuss the wall of a room and listen for the change in tones when a stud is reached.
> - Percuss your thigh. Puff your cheeks and percuss them. Compare the sounds.

Recognizing Percussion Sounds

When using direct and indirect percussion, the change from resonance to dullness is more easily recognized by the human ear than the change from dullness to resonance. To distinguish whether a change in sounds occurs, it is often helpful to close your eyes and concentrate on the sound. This concept has implications for patterns of percussion in areas of the body where known locations have distinct percussive sounds. For example, the techniques of diaphragmatic excursion (refer to Chapter 15) and liver border percussion (refer to Chapter 18) can proceed in a more defined pattern because percussion can be performed from an area of resonance to an area of dullness. Another helpful hint is to validate the change in sounds by percussing back and forth between the two areas where a change is noted to confirm this change.

As stated earlier, the percussion technique can take considerable time to develop and perfect. Practicing the technique in the home environment can be a helpful learning experience; see the Nursing Tip, At-Home Practice of Percussion.

Direct Fist Percussion

Direct fist percussion is used to assess the presence of tenderness and pain in internal organs such as the liver or the kidneys. Exercise caution when using direct fist percussion. Avoid hitting the client too hard, because this may cause injury.

To perform direct fist percussion (Fig. 8-17):

1. Explain the technique thoroughly so the client does not think you are hitting them.
2. Draw the dominant hand up into a fist.
3. With the ulnar aspect of the closed fist, directly hit the area where the organ is located. The strike should be of moderate force, and it may take some practice to achieve the right intensity.

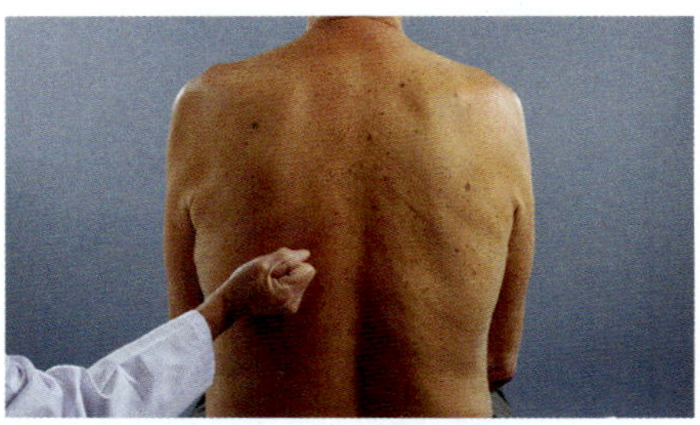

Figure 8-17 Technique of direct fist percussion: Left kidney.

The presence of pain in conjunction with direct fist percussion indicates inflammation of that organ or a strike that is too high in intensity.

Indirect Fist Percussion

The purpose of **indirect fist percussion** is the same as that of direct fist percussion. In fact, the indirect method is preferred over the direct method, but caution is still warranted to avoid client injury. It is performed in the following manner (Fig. 8-18):

1. Explain the technique thoroughly so the client does not think you are hitting them.
2. Place the palmar side of the nondominant hand on the skin's surface over the organ to be examined. Place the fingers adjacent to one another and in straight alignment with the palm.
3. Draw up the dominant hand into a closed fist.
4. With the ulnar aspect of the closed fist, use moderate intensity to hit the dorsum of the outstretched nondominant hand.

The nondominant hand absorbs some of the force of the striking hand. The resulting intensity should be of sufficient force to produce pain in the client if organ inflammation is present.

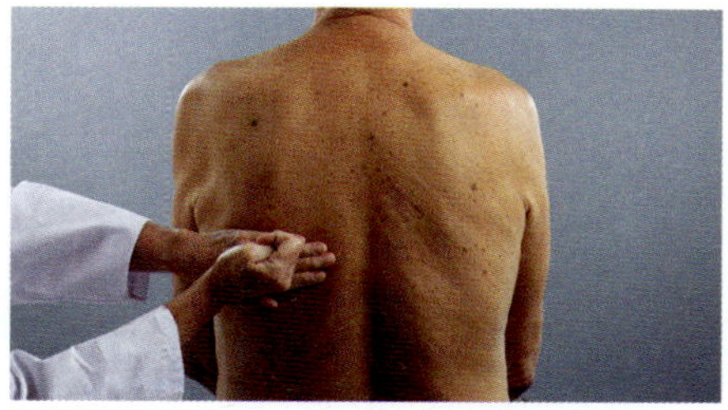

Figure 8-18 Technique of indirect fist percussion: Left kidney.

Auscultation

Auscultation is actively listening to body organs to gather information on a client's clinical status. Auscultation includes listening to sounds that are voluntarily and involuntarily produced by the body. A deep breath a client takes during lung auscultation is an example of a voluntary sound; heart sounds are an example of involuntary sounds. A quiet environment is necessary for auscultation. Auscultated sounds should be analyzed in relation to their relative intensity, pitch, duration, quality, and location. There are two types of auscultation: direct and indirect.

Direct Auscultation

Direct or **immediate auscultation** is the process of listening with the unaided ear. This can include listening to the client from some distance away or placing the ear directly on the client's skin surface. An example of direct auscultation is listening to the wheezing that is audible to the unassisted ear in a person having a severe asthmatic attack.

Indirect Auscultation

Indirect or **mediate auscultation** describes the process of listening with some amplification or mechanical device. The nurse most often performs indirect auscultation with an acoustic stethoscope, which does not amplify the body sounds, but instead blocks out environmental sounds.

Figure 8-19 shows two different acoustic or analog stethoscopes. The earpieces come in various sizes. Choose an earpiece that fits snugly in the ear canal without causing pain. The earpieces block out noises in the environment. The earpieces and binaurals should be angled toward the nose. This angle permits the natural direction of the ear canal to be accessed. In this manner, sounds will be directed toward the adult tympanic membrane. The rubber or plastic tubing should be between 30.5 and 40 cm (12 to 18 in.) long. Stethoscopes with longer tubing will diminish the body sounds that are auscultated.

> **NURSING TIP**
> **Headpiece Mnemonic**
> The word *bellow* can be used to remember which frequency is transmitted by the headpiece of the stethoscope. The "bell" transmits "low" sounds.

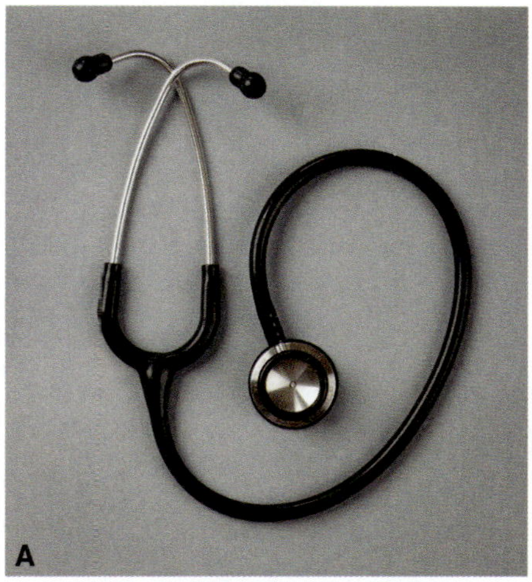

A

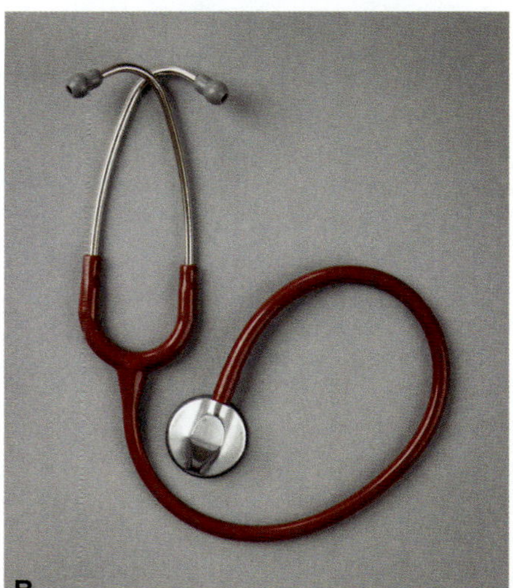

B

Figure 8-19 Types of acoustic stethoscopes. **A.** Acoustic stethoscope with the diaphragm and the bell. **B** Single-sided, dual-frequency acoustic stethoscope.

An acoustic stethoscope has two listening heads: the bell and the diaphragm (see Figure 8-19A). The diaphragm is flat, and the bell is a concave cup. The diaphragm transmits high-pitched sounds, and the bell transmits low-pitched sounds. Breath sounds and normal heart sounds are examples of high-pitched sounds. Bruits and some heart murmurs are examples of

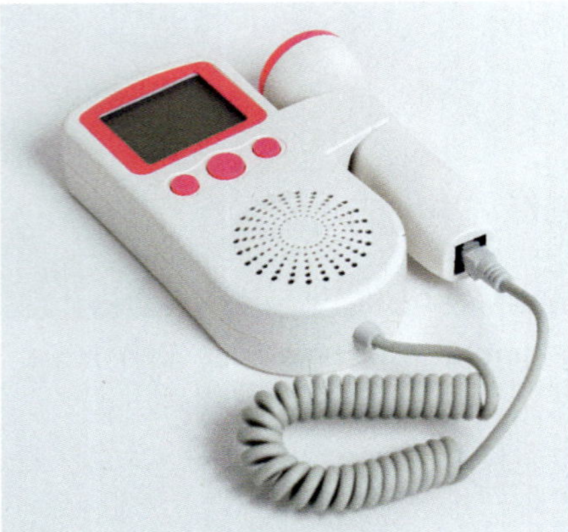

Figure 8-20 Doppler ultrasonic stethoscope.

> ## NURSING TIP
> ### Smart Stethoscopes
> For over 200 years the analog stethoscope has been the instrument used to assess heart and lung sounds. In a few years this type of stethoscope may become obsolete with the increased use of "smart stethoscopes." (Fig. 8-21). One type of "smart stethoscope" is the digital stethoscope. Digital stethoscopes, used initially in specialty areas, can now be found being used in primary care. Digital stethoscopes can amplify heart sounds up to 40 times. A mute feature to block the sound of background noise assists with the auscultation. Digital stethoscopes can detect a heart murmur as well as atrial fibrillation with a high rate of sensitivity and specificity. With the appropriate downloaded digital software package such as from Eko, a mobile phone can record a HIPAA compliant tracing of the auscultated sounds. These tracings can be added into the client's electronic health record for evaluation of disease status. Another type of smart stethoscope is the Stethophone from Sparrow BioAcoustics. Once the application is downloaded to a smartphone the phone acts as a medical grade stethoscope to analyze heart and lung sounds. Both digital and stethophone devices are portable and easy to use, and in a few years they may become the standard for auscultation.

low-pitched sounds. Another commonly used stethoscope has a single-sided, dual-frequency listening head (see Figure 8-19B). This stethoscope has a single chest piece. The nurse applies different pressures on the chest piece to auscultate high- and low-pitched sounds.

Another type of stethoscope is the stereophonic stethoscope. This type of stethoscope is a two-channel device that amplifies right- and left-sided auscultatory sounds. An adaptive tube allows two people to listen simultaneously.

Before auscultating, remove dangling necklaces or bracelets that could move during the examination and cause false noises. Warm the headpieces of the stethoscope in your hands before use, because shivering and movement can obscure examination findings. To use the diaphragm, place it firmly against the skin surface to be auscultated. If the client has a large quantity of hair in this area, it may be necessary to wet the hair to prevent it from interfering with the sound being auscultated. Otherwise, a grating sound may be heard. To use the bell, place it lightly on the skin surface that is to be auscultated. The bell will stretch the skin and act like a diaphragm and transmit high-pitched sounds if it is pressed too firmly on the skin. In both instances, auscultation requires a great deal of concentration. It may be helpful to close your eyes during the auscultation process to help you isolate the sound. Sometimes you can hear more than one sound in a given location. Try to listen to each sound and concentrate on each separately. It is important to clean your stethoscope after each client to prevent the transfer of pathogens. Remember, auscultation is a skill that requires practice and patience. Do not expect to become an expert overnight!

Amplification of body sounds can also be achieved with the use of an electronic stethoscope or a Doppler ultrasonic stethoscope (Fig. 8-20). An electronic stethoscope amplifies body sounds as it filters extraneous sounds. Both high and low frequencies can be auscultated with one headpiece. With the Doppler ultrasonic stethoscope, water-soluble gel is placed on the body part being assessed, and the stethoscope is placed directly on the client. The device amplifies the sounds in that region. Fetal heart tones and unpalpable peripheral pulses are frequently assessed via a Doppler ultrasonic stethoscope.

Legal Considerations

In today's litigious society, you must be ever vigilant when engaging in nursing practice. Documentation issues were discussed in Chapter 3. Equally important is how you execute the physical examination. Establishing a trusting and caring relationship is the primary element in avoiding malpractice claims. While performing each step in the physical examination process, you need to inform the client of what to expect, where to expect it, and how it will feel. Address protests by the client before continuing the examination. Otherwise, the client may claim insufficient informed consent, sexual abuse, or physical harm or harassment.

All examinations and procedures, including any injury that was caused during the physical examination, must be completely documented. The institutional policy regarding client injury in the workplace should be followed.

Golden Rules for Physical Examination

Now that you have been introduced to the physical examination techniques that will be used when conducting a head-to-toe or body system-focused examination, some general rules to observe are:

- Stand on the right side of the client; establishing a dominant side for examination will decrease your movement around the client.

- Perform the examination in a head-to-toe approach.
- Always compare the right- and left-hand sides of the body for symmetry.
- Proceed from the least invasive to the most invasive procedures for each body system.
- Always perform the physical examination using a systematic approach. If it is performed in the same order each time, you are less likely to omit a component of the examination.
- Minimize position changes of the bedridden/frail client as much as possible.
- Be flexible and adapt your examination to any unforeseen client situation.

Be patient with yourself as you learn the physical examination techniques in the following chapters. Repetition, attention to detail, and caring for a variety of clients in different settings will sharpen and refine your physical examination skills as you progress in your professional career.

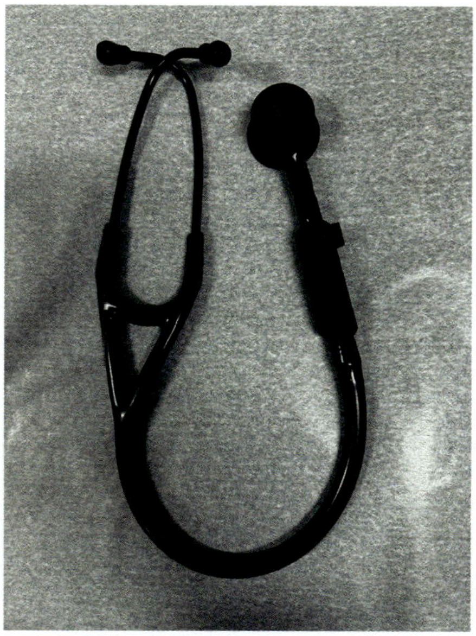

Figure 8-21 Digital stethoscope.

Review Questions

1. Which of the following characteristics describes the percussion sound of tympany in adults? Select all that apply.
   a. Loud in intensity
   b. Long in duration
   c. Very low in pitch
   d. Booming quality
   e. Normally heard over the gastric air bubble
   f. Can be found abnormally in a large pneumothorax

2. Which of the percussion sounds is usually located over the liver?
   a. Dullness
   b. Flatness
   c. Resonance
   d. Hyperresonance

3. Pain in the abdominal right upper quadrant can possibly elicit liver tenderness when using which of the following techniques?
   a. Direct percussion
   b. Immediate percussion
   c. Mediate percussion
   d. Indirect fist percussion

4. Which of the following is true about deep palpation? Select all that apply.
   a. It helps to reveal information about the position and shape of organs.
   b. Only a single-handed technique is used.
   c. The finger pads are depressed to a depth of approximately 5 cm.
   d. It should not be performed on ticklish clients.
   e. It is the technique of choice when examining female reproductive organs such as the uterus.
   f. It is used to examine the rectum and anus.

5. Which of the following statements describes an acoustic stethoscope and its use? Select all that apply.
   a. It allows the nurse to perform direct auscultation.
   b. To optimize sound, the earpieces and binaurals should be angled toward the nose.
   c. The rubber tubing should be 12–18 inches in length.
   d. The diaphragm of the stethoscope transmits high-pitched sounds.
   e. The bell is a convex-shaped cup.
   f. It amplifies auscultatory sounds.

6. Which of the following positions can be used to auscultate heart sounds? Select all that apply.
   a. Dorsal recumbent
   b. Sitting
   c. Knee-chest
   d. Semi-Fowler
   e. Prone
   f. Sims'

7. In what order would you conduct the physical examination of the abdomen?
   a. Inspection, palpation, percussion, auscultation
   b. Palpation, percussion, inspection, auscultation
   c. Inspection, auscultation, percussion, palpation
   d. Percussion, palpation, auscultation, inspection

8. A client asks you not to touch them with your gloved hands because they fear that they have a latex allergy. Which of the following statements are true regarding latex allergies? Select all that apply.
   a. Latex allergies are always manifested in childhood.
   b. Individuals with a latex allergy may also have allergies to bananas, kiwis, and avocados.
   c. Direct contact is necessary to develop an allergic reaction to latex.
   d. Manifestations of a latex allergy can include hives, wheezing, and dermatitis.
   e. A client with a latex allergy has an anaphylactic reaction with each exposure.

9. Which part of the hand should be used to assess for tactile fremitus or a cardiac thrill?
   a. Ulnar surface of the hand
   b. Dorsum of the hand
   c. Radial aspect of a closed-fisted hand
   d. Finger pads

10. Which statement represents the precautions the CDC outlines in Standard Precautions? Select all that apply.
    a. Visual cues such as posted signs declaring "Cover Your Cough"
    b. Hand washing with soap and water when hands are visibly soiled
    c. Personal protective equipment includes gloves, mask, goggles, and shoe covers
    d. Wearing a surgical mask when performing a lumbar puncture
    e. Procedures to follow when the client has fecal incontinence or excessive wound drainage

CHAPTER

9 General Survey, Vital Signs, and Pain

Learning Outcomes

1. Describe the assessment of a client's physical presence.
2. Describe the assessment of a client's psychological presence.
3. Describe how to assess for distress in a client.
4. Discuss factors affecting respiratory rate.
5. Identify the rate, rhythm, volume, and sites of pulse assessment.
6. Discuss factors influencing body temperature.
7. Discuss the advantages and disadvantages of body temperature measurement using different types of thermometers.
8. Identify factors influencing blood pressure and blood pressure measurement.
9. Define pain and the different types of pain.
10. Identify elements of a pain health history and tools that are used to assess pain.
11. Discuss the current opioid epidemic and the challenges it presents.
12. Identify the United States Preventive Services Task Force Recommendation for general survey, vital signs, and pain.

A complete physical examination is initiated by performing general observations of a client, obtaining the client's **vital signs**, and assessing the client for pain. These initial observations can provide data about the client's general state of health. Vital signs include the client's respiration, pulse, temperature, and blood pressure (BP). These measurements provide information about the client's basic physiological status. The presence of pain can affect a client's physical, emotional, and mental health; pain is thus often referred to as the "fifth vital sign."

General Survey

Initial observations include collecting information about the client's physical presence, psychological presence, and signs and symptoms of distress. The components of the general survey, vital signs, and assessment of pain are discussed later in the chapter.

Assessment in Brief

General Survey

- *Physical presence*
  - Stated age versus apparent age
  - General appearance
  - Body fat
  - Stature
  - Motor activity
  - Body and breath odors
- *Psychological presence*
  - Dress, grooming, and personal hygiene
  - Mood and manner
  - Speech
  - Facial expression
- *Distress*

Vital Signs

- Respiration
- Pulse
- Temperature
- Blood pressure

Pain

- Types of pain
- Source of pain
- Duration of pain
- Perception of pain
- Pain health history
- Effects of pain on the body
- Assessing pain
- Pain management

Equipment

- Appropriate personal protective equipment (PPE)
- Stethoscope
- Watch with a second hand
- Thermometer (gloves and lubricant if using a rectal thermometer)
- Sphygmomanometer
- Various pain scales (paper or digital)

Physical Presence

E Observe the client's:

1. Stated age versus apparent age
2. General appearance
3. Body fat
4. Stature
5. Motor activity
6. Body and breath odors

Stated Age Versus Apparent Age

N **The client's stated chronological age should be congruent with the apparent age.**

A It is significant for a client to appear older or younger than the stated chronological age.

P An endocrine deficiency of growth hormone (somatotropin) is associated with dwarfism and can manifest in a younger-than-chronological-age appearance in younger life and premature aging later in life.

P Children who have a genetic syndrome, such as Hutchinson-Gilford syndrome, age at an accelerated rate and appear much older than their actual age.

NURSING TIP

Environmental Cues

In addition to observing the client, look around the room for clues about the client's health status. For example, the smell of cigarettes, an asthma inhaler, hearing aid, or used tissues may all provide information about the client's health.

P Chronic illnesses/disease, alcoholism, drug abuse, severe illness (such as cancer and HIV), and prolonged sun exposure (that causes facial wrinkling) can all lead to a client looking older than their chronological age.

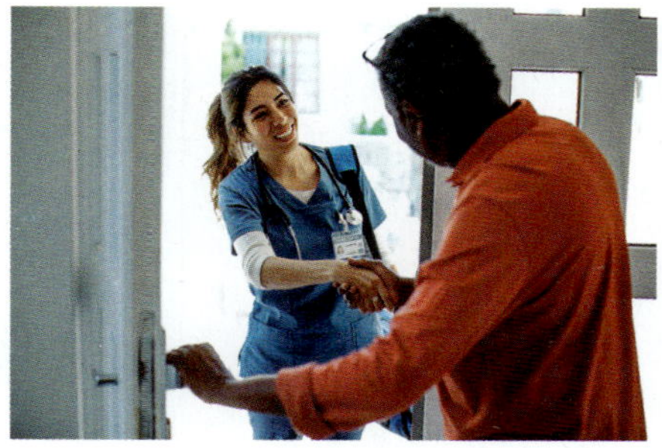

Figure 9-1 The nurse can make observations about the client's general appearance while talking with the client and preparing for the physical examination.

General Appearance

E Observe body symmetry, any obvious anomaly, and the client's apparent level of wellness (Fig. 9-1). In addition, note any gross observation, such as the use of a walker, assistance from a caregiver, or distinctive markings (e.g., burns, multiple piercings, tattoos).

N **The client should exhibit body symmetry, have no obvious deformity, and have the appearance of wellness. The level of gross normal observations varies.**

A Asymmetry is seen when a paired body part does not look the same on the contralateral side.

P The unilateral facial drooping of Bell palsy, a limb appearing at an abnormal angle (such as from a fracture), and unilateral paralysis are examples of body asymmetry.

A A missing limb, cleft lip, and burned skin are examples of obvious anomalies.

P The pathophysiology of each of these is varied and should be investigated further via history and physical examination.

A A fine white, crystal-like powder on the skin is abnormal.

P This is called uremic frost and is seen in clients with advanced chronic renal failure. Chapter 10 details many more examples of skin changes that may be detected during the general survey.

A The client who appears ill is an abnormal finding.

P A client who appears ill usually is ill and needs to be carefully assessed via the health history and physical examination.

Body Fat

N **Body fat should be evenly distributed. Body fat composition is difficult to estimate accurately without the use of immersion tanks or calipers. Research has indicated, however, that it is body fat content, not body weight, that is most closely linked to pathology. For example, a person can be within normal limits on height and weight charts but have a high proportion of body fat to lean body mass.**

A Obesity occurs when there are large amounts of body fat. This poses a serious health risk to the client and warrants comprehensive nutritional and metabolic assessments (refer to Chapter 7).

P Excess caloric intake and decreased energy expenditure are the most common causes of obesity.

P Some disease processes, such as hypothyroidism, which slows the basic metabolic rate, may result in obesity.

A Cushing syndrome manifests in a rounded, moonlike face, truncal obesity, fat pads on the neck, and relatively thin limbs (see Chapter 11).

P Excessive production of cortisol resulting from an anterior pituitary tumor or large doses of prolonged steroid use can lead to Cushing syndrome.

A A thin or frail appearance occurs when there are limited body fat stores. Severely limited fat stores can be a life-threatening condition.

P Energy expenditures that exceed caloric intake will result in decreased fat stores. This may be caused by several conditions, including:

- Eating disorders, which result in inadequate intake of calories from food, possible purging, and/or an overexpenditure of energy by means of exercise.
- Hyperkinetic states, in which the body's metabolic needs are greater than the ability to ingest calories. Adolescent growth spurts result in tall, thin teens because the increased metabolic demands for growing tissue exceed the calories teens can consume.
- Many chronic disease processes may be due to hyperkinetic states or a result of malabsorption diseases, such as celiac disease.
- Clients who have a malignant process can also result in a thin appearance with decreased fat stores due to the pathology of the cancer and probable decreased food consumption.

Stature

N **Limbs and trunk should appear proportional to body height; posture should be erect. A person's arm span (fingertip to fingertip) should be approximately equal to the person's height, and body length (crown to pubis) should be about equal to the length from the pubis to the feet.**

A A slumped or humpbacked appearance is abnormal.

P Osteoporosis, especially in postmenopausal women, may cause a slumped or humpbacked appearance.

P Clients experiencing depression may also present with a slumped posture.

A Long limbs relative to trunk length are abnormal.

P Marfan syndrome, an inherited disease that causes a defect in the elastic fibers of connective tissue, can result in the development of long limbs; long, thin fingers; a tall, thin appearance; and poorly developed muscles. A client with Marfan syndrome will have an arm span greater than their height.

Motor Activity

N **Gait, as well as other body movements, should be smooth and effortless. All body parts should have controlled, purposeful movement.**

A An unsteady gait or movements that are slow, absent, or require great effort are abnormal. Tremors or movements that the client seems unable to control are also abnormal.

P Arthritis can result in slow and difficult movement because joint movement is painful. See Chapter 19 for additional information on movement disorders.

P Neurological disturbances can result in tics, paralysis, or ataxia and can cause difficulty with the smoothness of movement. See Chapter 20 for additional information on neurological pathology.

Body and Breath Odors

N **Normally, there is no apparent odor from clients. It is normal for some people to have bad breath related to the types of foods ingested.**

A Severe body or breath odor is abnormal.

P Poor hygiene can cause body odors due to perspiration and bacteria left on the skin.

P An alcohol smell on the breath can result from alcohol ingestion or ketoacidosis in a diabetic client.

P Bad breath can result from poor oral hygiene, allergic rhinitis, gastroesophageal reflux disease, or from infections such as tonsillitis, rhinosinusitis, or pneumonia.

P Severe vaginal infections can result in an offensive body odor.

P Clients with a fecal odor may be experiencing fecal incontinence or intestinal obstruction. A leaking colostomy can also produce a fecal odor.

P In portal hypertension, liver encephalopathy, and liver failure, the strong musty-sweet fecal or sulfuric-smelling odor is called fetor hepaticus.

P An ammonia smell, or uremic fetor, is caused by the body breaking down urea to ammonia. This is seen in renal disease.

Psychological Presence

E Observe the client's:

1. Dress, grooming, and personal hygiene
2. Mood and manner
3. Speech
4. Facial expressions

Dress, Grooming, and Personal Hygiene

N **Normally, clients should appear clean and neatly dressed. Clothing choice should be appropriate for the weather. Norms and standards for dress and cleanliness may vary widely.**

A A disheveled, unkempt appearance or clothing that is inappropriate for the weather (such as a wool coat in hot weather) is abnormal.

P Psychological or psychiatric disorders such as depression, bipolar depression, schizophrenia, and dementia may be reflected in inappropriate appearance or clothing selection.

P People with poor self-esteem or people who are unhoused may present with a general neglect of personal hygiene, grooming, and dress.

P An unshaven, unclean appearance may reflect abuse or neglect of the client by the client's caregiver.

P Baggy clothes may indicate a recent weight loss from an acute illness, intentional weight reduction, or an eating disorder. Keep in mind that some people choose to dress in this fashion.

P Tight clothes may result from weight gain, whether intentional or unintentional.

P People who wear long-sleeved shirts in warm weather should be assessed for intravenous drug use and self-harm (e.g., "cutting," cigarette burns).

Mood and Manner

N **Generally, a client should be cooperative and pleasant.**

A An uncooperative, hostile, or tearful adult or an adult who seems unusually elated or who has a flat affect needs further assessment.

P Psychiatric conditions such as anxiety, depression, manic disorders, paranoid disorders, delusion disorders, and schizophrenia can manifest in a distortion in reality, with disorganized thinking and altered perceptions, which can result in abnormal behaviors. Dementia or confusion in older adults can also result in disturbances in mood and manner. Refer to Chapters 20 and 26 for a more complete discussion.

Speech

N **Assuming the nurse and client share a language they can converse in, the client should respond to questions and commands easily. Speech should be clear and understandable. Pitch, rate, and volume should be appropriate to the circumstances.**

A Speech that is slow, slurred, mumbled, very loud, or rapid needs to be assessed further.

P Hyperthyroidism can cause rapid speech because of an oversupply of stimulatory hormones that results in hypermetabolism and hyperactivity.

P Alcohol ingestion can cause slow, mumbled, or slurred speech because alcohol affects the central nervous system, causing transient brain dysfunction.

P Hearing difficulties may be associated with loud speech because individuals with decreased ability to hear may not be able to hear themselves at normal conversational decibels.

P A client who has experienced a stroke may have aphasia if the speech center in the brain is affected.

P A client with autism may speak in a monotone voice and have decreased eye contact in social interactions.

Facial Expressions

N **The client should appear awake and alert. Facial expressions should be appropriate for what is happening in the environment and should change naturally.**

A Unchanging or flat facial expressions, inappropriate facial expressions, tremors, or tics are abnormal.

P Apathy or depression may cause a lack of facial expression due to feelings of lethargy or sadness.

P Dementia may cause inappropriate facial expressions because the client's perception of reality is distorted.

P Bell palsy, a condition resulting in paralysis of the muscles in the face, may cause the mouth to droop and the affected side of the face to appear flaccid; it often makes the client unable to completely close the eyelid on the affected side.

Distress

E Observe for:

1. Labored breathing, wheezing or acute/chronic cough, and labored speech.
2. Painful facial expression, sweating, or physical protection of a painful area.
3. Serious or life-threatening occurrences such as seizure activity, active and severe bleeding, gaping wounds, and open fractures.
4. Signs of emotional distress or anxiety that may include, but are not limited to, tearfulness; nervous tics or laughter; avoidance of eye contact; cold, clammy hands; excessive nail biting; inability to pay attention; diaphoresis; or changes in breathing patterns.

N **Breathing should be effortless, without coughing or wheezing. Speech should not leave a client short of breath. The face should be relaxed, and the client should be willing to move all body parts**

freely. There should be no serious or life-threatening conditions. The client should not perspire excessively or show signs of emotional distress such as nail biting or avoidance of eye contact.

A The presence of shortness of breath with labored speech, wheezing, or cough is abnormal (Fig. 9-2).

P Pulmonary pathology may be present. Refer to Chapter 15 for additional information.

A Pain as evidenced by facial grimacing, crying, moaning, sweating, or protection of a body part is an abnormal finding.

P Tissue damage results in pain and requires further investigation into the character, location, intensity, and occurrence of the pain, as well as factors associated with increased and decreased pain.

A Excessive nail biting, avoidance of eye contact, nervous laughter, tearfulness, or lack of interest may be indicators of emotional distress or emotional pain.

P Nervous habits are often displayed when a person is in an uncomfortable or new situation. A tearful or sad affect can result from emotional pain related to situations the client may be experiencing or has experienced. Often, an attempt is made to disguise emotional distress.

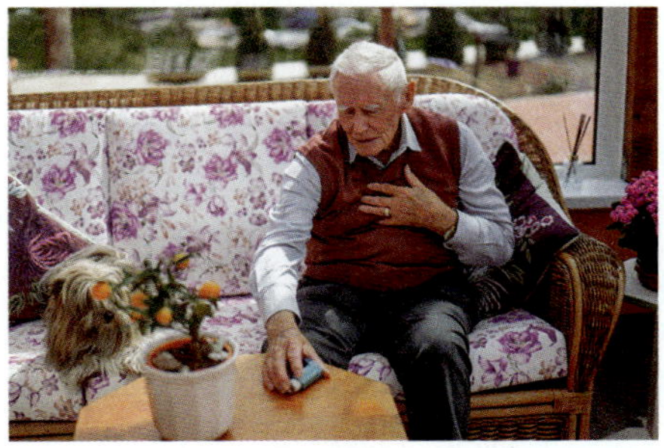

Figure 9-2 This man is experiencing respiratory distress and is reaching for his asthma rescue inhaler for relief.

Vital Signs

Vital signs should be assessed at the beginning of each visit. If the client is hospitalized, vital signs should be assessed as often as prescribed or as often as the client's condition requires. Vital sign measurements include respiration, pulse, temperature, and blood pressure.

Respiration

Respiration is the act of breathing. Breathing supplies oxygen to the body and occurs in response to changes in the concentration of oxygen (O_2), carbon dioxide (CO_2), and hydrogen (H+) in the arterial blood. Inhalation, or inspiration, occurs when air is taken into the lungs. Exhalation, or expiration, refers to the airflow out of the lungs.

Inspiration occurs when the diaphragm and the intercostal muscles contract. This can be observed by the movement of the abdomen outward and the movement of the chest upward and outward, resulting in the lungs filling with air. Expiration occurs when the external intercostal muscles and the diaphragm relax. The abdomen and the chest return to a resting position.

Respiratory rate is measured in breaths per minute. One respiratory cycle consists of one inhalation and one expiration. A complete discussion of respiratory assessment is found in Chapter 15.

To assess respiratory rate:

E
1. Stand in front of or to the side of the client.
2. Discretely observe the client's breathing (rise and fall of the chest). These observations are best done with the client unaware of what you are doing. If the client is aware that you are counting respirations, the breathing pattern may be altered.
3. Count the number of respiratory cycles that occurs in 1 minute.

N **Table 9-1 lists the normal respiratory rates for different ages. Respiratory rates decrease with age and may vary with excitement, anxiety, fever, exercise, medications, and altitude.**

NURSING CHECKLIST

General Approach to Vital Sign Assessment

1. Select equipment according to the client's age, size, and developmental level and the site selected for assessment. Specific decision-making criteria are discussed in each section.
2. Gather equipment.
3. Observe Standard Precautions and don personal protective equipment, such as gloves, gown, face shield, goggles, N-95 respirator or face mask if the client's status warrants these protective measures.
4. Explain the procedure to the client.
5. Always warm the stethoscope headpiece before placing it on the client. Clean the head/bell of the stethoscope before use with an alcohol swab or other cleaning solution.
6. Take the vital signs and record findings.

NURSING TIP

Respiration Assessment

Usually, respiration can be assessed while counting the radial or apical pulse. If respirations are shallow and the client is supine, place the client's arm across the chest while taking a radial pulse and feel the chest rise while observing for respiration.

Table 9-1 Respiratory Rate

Age	Resting Respiratory Rate (Breaths/Minute)	Average
Newborn	30–50	40
1 yr	20–40	30
3 yr	20–30	25
6 yr	16–22	19
10 yr	16–20	18
14 yr	14–20	17
Adult	12–20	18

A **Tachypnea** is a respiratory rate greater than 20 breaths per minute in an adult.

P Hypoxia and metabolic acidosis are common causes of tachypnea. The increased respiratory rate is a compensatory mechanism to provide the body with more oxygen and eliminate excess hydrogen ions when the body's metabolism is increased.

P Fever can cause tachypnea as the body reacts to a bacterial, viral, or fungal infection.

P Stress and anxiety cause the release of catecholamines, which can elevate the respiratory rate.

P Stimulants such as caffeine, cocaine, and amphetamines as well as medications such as albuterol and pseudoephedrine can cause tachypnea.

A **Bradypnea** is a respiratory rate of fewer than 12 breaths per minute in an adult at rest.

P Head injury resulting in increased intracranial pressure in the respiratory center of the brain can cause bradypnea.

P Medications such as narcotics and barbiturates as well as alcohol can depress the respiratory center of the brain and can cause bradypnea.

P A lower metabolic rate that occurs during normal sleep can result in bradypnea.

A **Apnea** is the absence of spontaneous breathing for 10 or more seconds.

P Central sleep apnea occurs with brain malfunction while obstructive sleep apnea occurs with some degree of blockage of the upper respiratory tract.

P Traumatic brain injury may lead to apnea from injury of the brainstem. Death ensues in the absence of respirations and pulse.

P Apnea can occur in newborns due to underdeveloped respiratory tracts, neurological impairment, structural obstruction, and other causes known and unknown.

Pulse

As the heart contracts, blood is ejected from the left ventricle (stroke volume) into the aorta. A pressure wave is created as the blood is carried to the peripheral vasculature. This palpable pressure is the **pulse**. Pulse assessment can determine heart rate, rhythm, and the estimated volume of blood being pumped by the heart.

Rate

Pulse rate is the number of pulse beats counted in 1 minute. Several factors influence heart rate or pulse rate. These include:

- The sinoatrial (S-A) node, which fires automatically at a rate of 60 to 100 times per minute and is the primary controller of pulse rate and heart rate.
- Parasympathetic or vagal stimulation of the autonomic nervous system, which can result in a decreased heart rate.
- Sympathetic stimulation of the autonomic nervous system, which results in an increased heart rate.
- Baroreceptor sensors, which can detect changes in blood pressure and influence heart rate. Elevated blood pressure can decrease heart rate as can occur in an arrhythmia, whereas decreased blood pressure can increase heart rate such as in shock.

Other factors influencing heart rate include:

- *Age:* The heart rate generally decreases with age.
- *Sex:* The average female's heart rate is higher than the average male's heart rate.
- *Activity:* The heart rate increases with activity and exercise. Athletes will have a lower resting heart rate than the average person because of their increased cardiac strength and efficiency.
- *Emotional status:* Heart rate increases with anxiety.
- *Pain:* Heart rate increases with pain.
- *Environmental factors:* Temperature and noise level can alter the heart rate.
- *Stimulants:* Caffeinated beverages and tobacco elevate the heart rate.
- *Medications:* Drugs such as digoxin and beta blockers decrease the heart rate, and drugs such as albuterol and amphetamines increase the heart rate.
- *Disease state:* Abnormal clinical conditions can affect the heart rate (e.g., increased heart rate in hyperthyroidism, fever, and hemorrhage).

Rhythm

Pulse rhythm refers to the pattern of pulses and the intervals between pulses. Pulses can be regular or irregular. A regular pulse occurs at regular intervals with even intervals between each beat. Normal sinus rhythm is an example of a regular pulse.

An irregular pulse can be regularly irregular or irregularly irregular. A regular irregular rhythm is one in which abnormal conduction occurs in the heart but at regular intervals. Ventricular bigeminy is an example of a regularly irregular rhythm. In ventricular bigeminy, irregular conduction, called a premature ventricular complex (PVC), occurs before the expected QRS complex. This PVC occurs in a regular rhythm (every other beat).

An irregularly irregular rhythm has no predictable pattern. Atrial fibrillation is an example of an irregularly irregular rhythm. Chapter 17 provides additional content on pulse rhythm alterations.

Volume

Pulse volume (also called pulse strength or amplitude) reflects the stroke volume and the **peripheral vasculature resistance** (afterload). It can range from absent to bounding. Table 9-2 displays the two most used scales: a 3-point and a 4-point scale. When reporting pulse volume, 2 +/4 + indicates a normal pulse (2 +) on a 4-point scale, whereas 2 +/3 + indicates a normal pulse (2 +) on a 3-point scale. Refer to the Nursing Tip, Documenting Pulses, for schematic representations. If a pulse is not palpable, then attempt to ascertain its presence with a Doppler ultrasonic stethoscope. The letter "D" in a pulse chart or stick figure represents the pulse that was detected by using this device.

Site

Peripheral pulses can be palpated where the large arteries are close to the skin surface. There are nine common sites for the assessment of pulse, as indicated in Figure 9-3. When routine vital signs are assessed, the pulse is generally measured at one of two sites: radial or apical.

Measuring the apical pulse is indicated for clients with irregular pulses or known cardiac or pulmonary disease. The assessment of apical pulse can be accomplished through palpation but is most commonly accomplished through auscultation.

Table 9-2 Scales for Measuring Pulse Volume

3-Point Scale

Scale	Description of Pulse
0	Absent
1 +	Thready/weak
2 +	Normal
3 +	Bounding

4-Point Scale

Scale	Description of Pulse
0	Absent
1 +	Thready/weak
2 +	Normal
3 +	Increased
4 +	Bounding

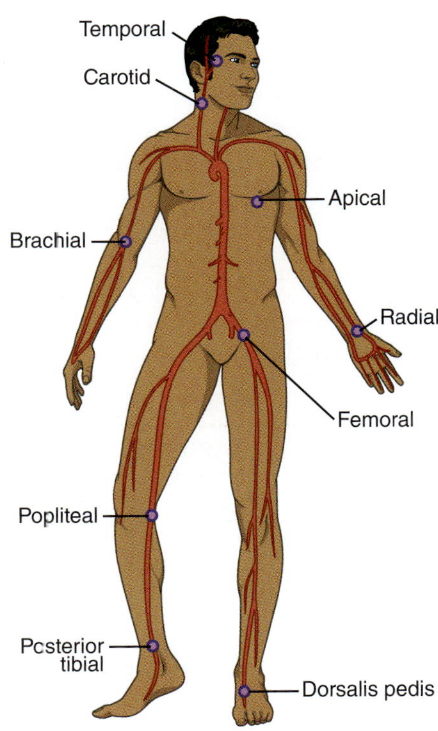

Figure 9-3 Peripheral pulse sites.

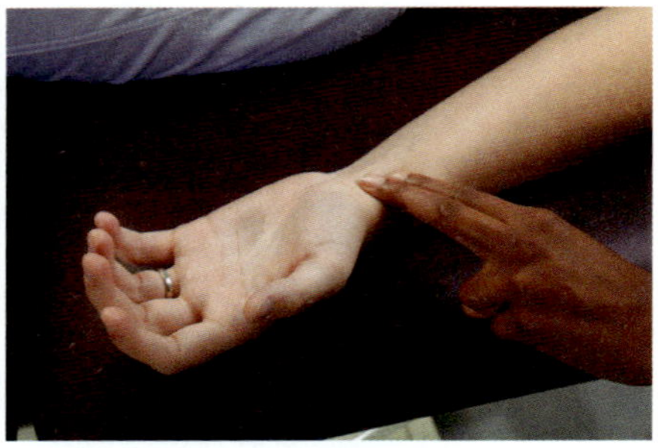

Figure 9-4 Palpation of the radial pulse.

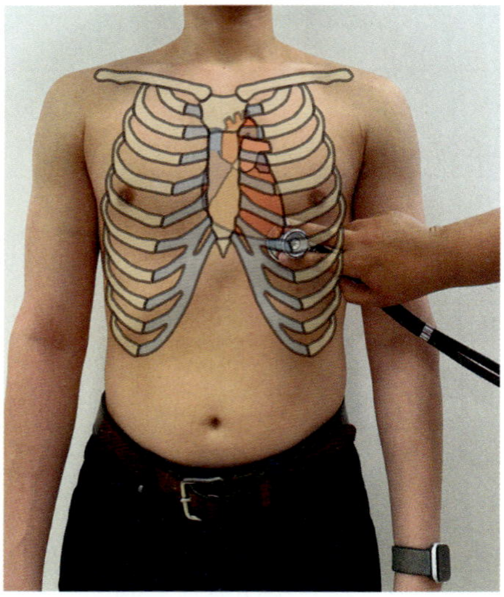

Figure 9-5 The apical pulse site is the best location to auscultate the heart rate of a client who has an irregular rhythm.

Table 9-3 Pulse Rate: Normal Range According to Age

Age	Resting Pulse Rate (Beats/Minute)	Average
Newborn	100–170	140
1 yr	80–160	120
3 yr	80–120	110
6 yr	70–115	100
10 yr	70–110	90
14 yr	60–110	85–90
Adult	60–100	72

Radial Pulse

To palpate the radial pulse:

E
1. Place the pad of your first, second, and/or third finger on the site of the radial pulse, along the radial bone on the thumb side of the inner wrist (Fig. 9-4).
2. Press your fingers gently against the artery with enough pressure so that you can feel the pulse. Pressing too hard will obliterate the pulse.
3. Count the pulse rate using the second hand of your watch. If the pulse is regular, count for 30 seconds and multiply by 2 to obtain the pulse rate per minute. If the pulse is irregular, count for 60 seconds.
4. Identify the pulse rhythm as you palpate (regular or irregular).
5. Identify the pulse volume as you palpate (using scales from Table 9-2).

N A P Refer to the following section on Rate.

Apical Pulse

To assess the apical pulse:

E
1. Place the diaphragm of the stethoscope on the apical pulse site (Fig. 9-5).
2. Count the pulse rate for 30 seconds if regular, and 60 seconds if irregular.
3. Identify the pulse rhythm.
4. Identify a **pulse deficit** (apical pulse rate greater than the radial pulse rate) by listening to the apical pulse and palpating the radial pulse simultaneously.

N A P Refer to the following section on Rate.

Rate

N **Normal pulse rates vary with age. Table 9-3 lists ranges for normal pulse rates by age. The heart rate normally increases during periods of exertion. Athletes commonly have resting heart rates below 60 beats per minute because of the increased strength and efficiency of the cardiac muscle.**

A **Tachycardia** refers to a pulse rate faster than 100 beats per minute in an adult.

P Psychophysiological stressors such as trauma, blood-volume losses, anemias, infection, fear, fever, pain, hyperthyroidism, shock, and anxiety can increase pulse rate because of increased metabolic demands placed on the body.

P Some tachycardia may not have clinical significance; however, in clients with myocardial disease, tachycardia can be a sign of decreased cardiac output, congestive heart failure, myocardial ischemia, or arrhythmias.

A **Bradycardia** refers to a slow pulse rate. Pulse rates that fall below 60 in adults are considered to be bradycardic.

P Medications such as cardiotonics (digoxin) and beta blockers decrease the heart rate.

P Bradycardia usually occurs with excessive vagal stimulation or decreased sympathetic tone. Conditions that may cause bradycardia are eye surgery, increased intracranial pressure, myocardial infarction, hypothyroidism, and prolonged vomiting.

A **Asystole** refers to the absence of a pulse.

P Cardiac arrest resulting from biological or clinical death can result in asystole.

P Pulseless electrical activity (electromechanical dissociation) caused by hypovolemia, pneumothorax, cardiac tamponade, or acidosis results in the absence of a pulse despite the presence of electrical activity in the heart muscle.

A A pulse deficit occurs when the apical pulse rate is greater than the radial pulse rate.

P Arrhythmias (such as atrial fibrillation, premature ventricular contractions, second-degree heart block, and third-degree heart block) and heart failure can cause pulse deficits because some cardiac contractions are too weak to produce a pulse pressure to the peripheral site. Severe vascular disease can also cause pulse deficits.

Rhythm

N **Normal pulse rhythm is regular, with equal intervals between each beat.**

A **Dysrhythmias**, or **arrhythmias**, refer to pulse rhythms that are not regular. They may consist of irregular beats that are random or irregular beats that present in a regular pattern.

P Cardiac dysrhythmias that are atrial and ventricular in origin cause abnormal rhythms, such as atrial flutter and ventricular fibrillation. Refer to Chapters 16 and 17 for additional information.

Volume

N **The pulse volume is normally the same with each beat. A normal pulse volume can be felt with a moderate amount of pressure of the fingers and obliterated with greater pressure.**

A Small, weak pulses are referred to as weak or thready pulses; these pulses are easily obliterated with light pressure.

P Decreased cardiac stroke volume caused by heart failure, hypovolemic shock, late septic shock, and cardiogenic shock can result in weak pulses.

P A low pulse amplitude occurs in states of increased peripheral vascular resistance, such as aortic stenosis and constrictive pericarditis.

P Weak pulses occur in conditions when ventricular filling time is decreased, such as in dysrhythmias.

A Bounding pulses are full, forceful pulses that are difficult to obliterate with pressure.

P Hyperkinetic states such as exercise, fever, anemia, anxiety, and hyperthyroidism can cause bounding pulses.

P Early stages of septic shock are characterized by bounding pulses because of decreased peripheral vascular resistance.

NURSING TIP
Documenting Pulses

You can document the amplitude of a client's pulses by recording the pulses in tabular format (Fig. 9-6A), or by drawing a small stick figure and labeling the pulses accordingly (Fig. 9-6B).

	Carotid	Brachial	Radial	Femoral	Popliteal	Posterior tibial (PT)	Dorsalis pedis (DP)
R	2+	2+	2+	1+	1+	D	D
L	2+	2+	2+	2+	1+	1+	1+

Scale = 4+; D = Doppler ultrasonic stethoscope; R = Right; L = Left

A

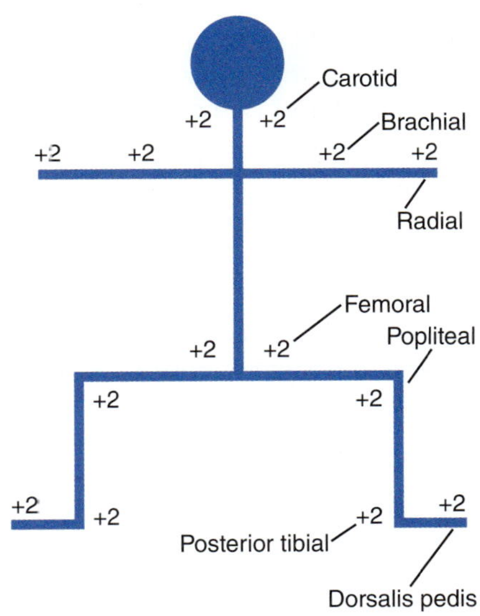

B Scale = 3+

Figure 9-6 Methods for charting peripheral pulses. **A.** Tabular peripheral pulse documentation **B.** Stick-figure peripheral pulse documentation.

E Examination **N** Normal Findings **A** Abnormal Findings **P** Pathophysiology

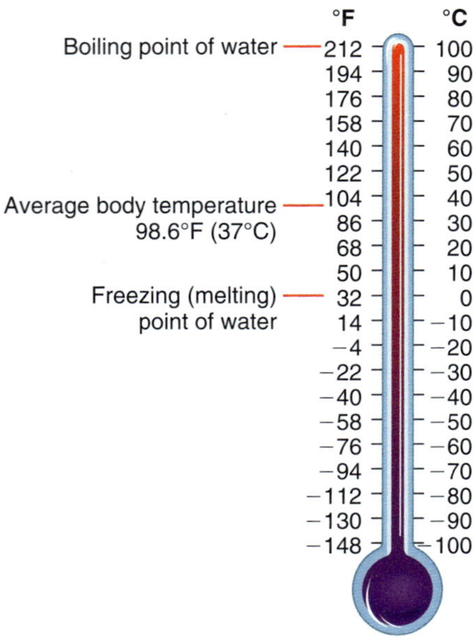

Figure 9-7 Correlation between Celsius and Fahrenheit scales.

Temperature

A client's temperature can provide objective information on general clinical status. Temperature scales, variables, routes, and measurement methods are discussed below.

Temperature Scales

Both the Celsius and the Fahrenheit scales are commonly used to measure **temperature**, which is the degree of core body heat. Clients are most often familiar with the Fahrenheit scale, whereas institutions often use the Celsius scale. Therefore it is important that you know temperature scale correlations. Figure 9-7 summarizes these correlations and provides the conversion formulas.

Variables Affecting Body Temperature

Core body temperature is established by the temperature of blood perfusing the area of the hypothalamus (the body's temperature control center), which triggers the body's physiological response to temperature. An ideal thermometer would accurately measure central brainstem temperature at the hypothalamus. Invasive procedures that provide temperatures of the arterial blood, esophagus, or bladder are reliable indicators of core temperature but are impractical. More practical methods for the measurement of body temperature are less reliable and can result in variations in body temperature readings. In addition, there are physiological variables that affect body temperature. These include:

- **Circadian rhythm** patterns: Normal body temperature (as well as pulse and blood pressure) fluctuates with a client's activity level and the time of day. Core body temperature is lower during sleep than during waking activities, being the lowest in the early morning just before awakening from sleep, and the highest in the afternoon or early evening. A 1°F to 2°F, or a 0.5°C to 1.0°C, fluctuation in body temperature throughout the day is considered within the normal range.
- Hormones: In women, increased production of progesterone at the time of ovulation raises the basal body temperature by about 0.5°F, or 0.35°C.
- Age: Infants and young children are affected by environmental temperature to a much greater extent than adults because their thermoregulatory mechanisms are not fully developed. Older adults are more sensitive to extremes of environmental temperature due to a decrease in thermoregulatory controls.
- Exercise: Body temperature rises due to increased metabolic activity.
- Stress: Stimulation of the sympathetic nervous system increases the production of epinephrine, resulting in increased metabolic activity and higher body temperature.
- Environmental extremes of hot or cold.
- Health status: Temperature deviations can occur in illnesses such as infections as well as in hypothalamus dysfunction.

> **NURSING TIP**
> **Using Oral and Rectal Thermometers**
> Do not use the same thermometer to take rectal and oral temperatures, because doing so may result in the transfer of pathogens.

> **NURSING TIP**
> **Limiting Mercury Exposure**
> The Joint Commission has mandated that mercury-containing products, such as thermometers and sphygmomanometers, be removed from U.S. health-care institutions. This action prevents possible mercury contamination in clients, health-care professionals, and the community. But some clients may still have mercury thermometers in their homes.
> If a mercury thermometer is broken, certain hazardous material precautions and client follow-up should be undertaken.

Measurement Routes

There are six frequently used routes by which temperature can be measured: oral, rectal, axillary, tympanic, temporal artery, and noncontact infrared. Each method has advantages and disadvantages. The advantages and disadvantages of each route are summarized in Table 9-4. Research is ongoing to determine "the best" route to evaluate a client's temperature throughout the life span.

Table 9-4 Advantages and Disadvantages of Routes for Body Temperature Measurement

Route	Normal Range	Advantages	Disadvantages
Oral Average 98.6°F (37.0°C)	96.8°–100.4°F (36.0°–38.0°C)	Convenient; accessible	**Safety:** Glass thermometers with mercury can be bitten and broken, causing client injury. Noncontained mercury poses a serious hazardous material risk requiring specific cleanup procedures. Glass thermometers are no longer used in health-care institutions in the United States. Clients need to be alert and cooperative and cognitively capable of following instructions for safe use. **Physical aspects:** Clients need to be able to breathe through the nose and be without oral pathology or recent oral surgery; this route is not appropriate for comatose or confused clients, infants, or toddlers. **Accuracy:** Oxygen therapy by mask, as well as ingestion of hot or cold beverages immediately before oral temperature measurement, affects the accuracy of the reading.
Rectal Average 0.7°F (0.4°C) higher than oral temperature	98.0°–100.4°F (36.7°–38.0°C)	Considered most accurate	**Safety:** Glass thermometers with mercury can break causing client injury. Noncontained mercury poses a serious hazardous material risk requiring specific cleanup procedures. Glass thermometers are no longer used in health-care institutions in the United States. **Physical aspects:** Contraindicated following rectal surgery, rectal abscess, or diarrhea. Should be avoided in clients with leukopenia. Risk of rectal perforation in children less than 2 yr of age. Risk of stimulating Valsalva reaction in cardiac clients. Invasive, uncomfortable, and possibly embarrassing.
Axillary Average 1°F (0.6°C) lower than oral temperature	95.8°–99.4°F (35.4°–37.4°C)	Safe; noninvasive	**Time frame:** Glass thermometer must be left in place for 5 minutes to obtain accurate measurement. **Safety:** Glass thermometers with mercury can break causing client injury. Noncontained mercury poses a serious hazardous material risk requiring specific cleanup procedures. Glass thermometers are no longer used in health-care institutions in the United States. **Accuracy:** Placement and position of thermometer tip affect reading.

Continued

Table 9-4 Advantages and Disadvantages of Routes for Body Temperature Measurement—cont'd

Route	Normal Range	Advantages	Disadvantages
Tympanic Calibrated to oral/rectal scales	See oral/rectal	Convenient, accessible, fast, safe, noninvasive. Does not require contact with any mucous membrane.	**Physical aspects:** Avoid in clients with ear pain or recent ear surgery. **Accuracy:** Research is inconclusive as to accuracy of readings and correlations with other body temperature measurements. Technique affects reading. Tympanic membrane is thought to reflect the core body temperature.
Temporal Artery Average 0.7°F (0.4°C) higher than oral temperature	98.0°-100.4°F (36.7°-38.0°C)	Convenient, accessible, fast, safe, accurate, noninvasive. Does not require contact with any mucous membrane.	**Physical aspects:** Cannot be used in clients with head injury/surgery/burns to the forehead. **Accuracy:** Possibly reduced accuracy with a diaphoretic forehead. Can show a low temperature reading if the scan button is released prematurely.
Noncontact Infrared Comparable to rectal values	Comparable to rectal values	Convenient, accessible, fast, safe, accurate, noninvasive. Does not require contact with any mucous membrane or any body part.	**Physical aspects:** Cannot be used in clients with head injury/surgery/burns to the forehead.

Oral Method

E

1. Place the thermometer (Fig. 9-8) at the base of the tongue and to the right or left of the frenulum. Instruct the client to close the lips and avoid biting the thermometer. Ensure that it has been at least 15 minutes since the client has consumed a hot or cold beverage or food.
2. Leave the thermometer in the mouth until the device has signaled that the maximum body temperature has been reached, or until the appropriate amount of time has passed according to the thermometer manufacturer's instructions.
3. Remove the thermometer from the client's mouth.

Rectal Method

E

1. Position the client with the buttocks exposed. Adults may be more comfortable lying on the side (with the knees slightly flexed), facing away from you, or prone.
2. Put on clean gloves.
3. Lubricate the tip of the thermometer with a water-soluble lubricant.
4. Ask the client to take a deep breath; insert the thermometer into the anus 0.5 to 1.5 inches, depending on the client's age and size.
5. Do not force the insertion of the thermometer or insert it into feces.
6. Leave the thermometer in the rectum until the device has signaled that the maximum body temperature has been reached, or until the appropriate amount of time has passed according to the thermometer manufacturer's instructions.

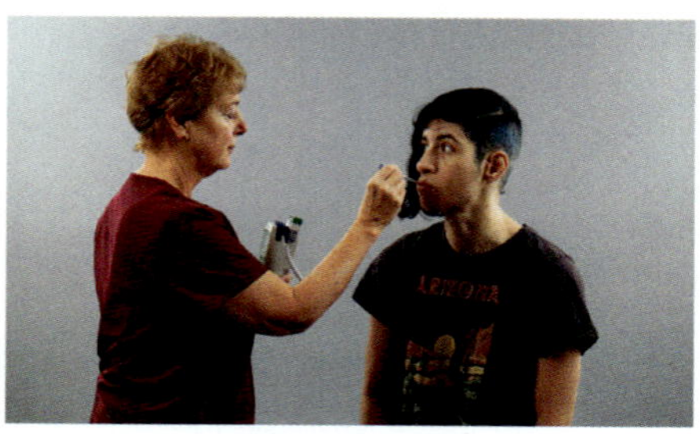

Figure 9-8 Taking a client's oral temperature with an electronic thermometer.

7. Remove the thermometer from the client's rectum.
8. Reposition the client.

Axillary Method

E
1. Place the thermometer into the middle of the axilla (Fig. 9-9) and have the client hold the arm close to the side to keep the thermometer in place.
2. Leave the thermometer in the axilla until the device has signaled that the maximum body temperature has been reached, or until the appropriate amount of time has passed according to the thermometer manufacturer's instructions.
3. Remove the thermometer from the client's axilla.

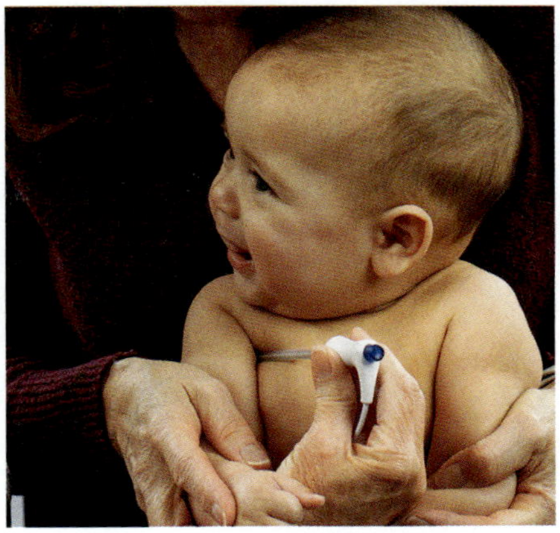

Figure 9-9 Taking a client's axillary temperature.

Electronic Thermometer Method

E
1. Remove the electronic thermometer from the charging unit.
2. Attach a disposable cover to the probe.
3. Using a method described (oral, rectal, or axillary), take the client's temperature.
4. Listen for the sound or look for the symbol indicating that maximum body temperature has been reached.
5. Observe and record the reading.
6. Remove and discard the probe cover.
7. Return the electronic thermometer to the charging unit.

Tympanic Method

E
1. Attach the probe cover to the nose of the thermometer.
2. Gently place the probe of the thermometer over the entrance to the ear canal. If the client is under 3 years old, pull the pinna down, aiming the probe toward the opposite eye (Fig. 9-10). If the client is over 3 years old, grasp the pinna and pull gently up and back, aiming the probe toward the opposite ear. Ensure there is a tight seal.
3. Press the start button on the thermometer handle.
4. Wait for the beep, remove the probe from the ear, and read the temperature.
5. Discard the probe cover.
6. Return the tympanic thermometer to the charging unit.

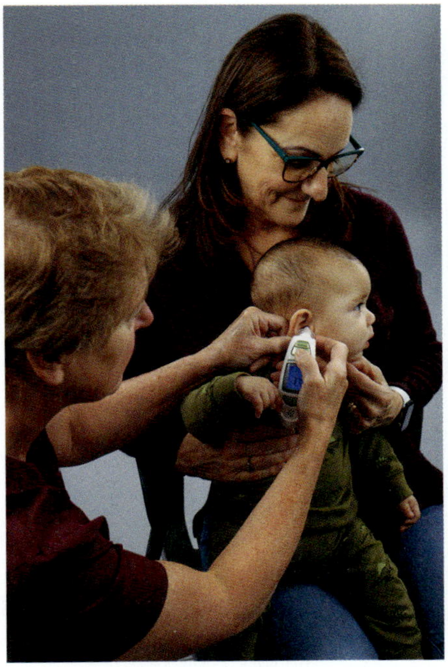

Figure 9-10 Taking a client's temperature with a tympanic thermometer.

Temporal Artery Method

The temporal artery thermometer is a battery-operated, noninvasive device that uses infrared technology to provide fast and accurate body temperature measurements that reflect core body temperature (Fig. 9-11). The device measures the body's temperature, but it can be affected by ambient temperature. For this reason, the temporal artery thermometer has to acclimatize to the air's temperature for at least 30 minutes before use. The probe head of the temporal artery thermometer is coated with a silver ion antimicrobial head that prevents bacterial and fungal growth. Thus it need not be cleaned after each use.

E
1. Remove the protective cap from the probe head.
2. Position the probe head on the center of the forehead, midway between the eyebrow and hairline. Avoid areas of the forehead that are covered by hair, wigs, hats, bandages, or scar tissue. Depress the scan button.
3. Gently move the thermometer across the forehead (in either direction), maintaining contact between the probe head and the client's forehead until the hairline is reached.

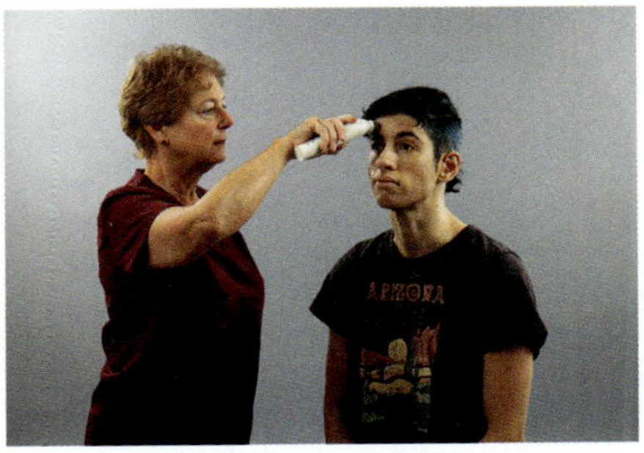

Figure 9-11 Measuring a client's body temperature with a temporal artery thermometer is noninvasive and accurate.

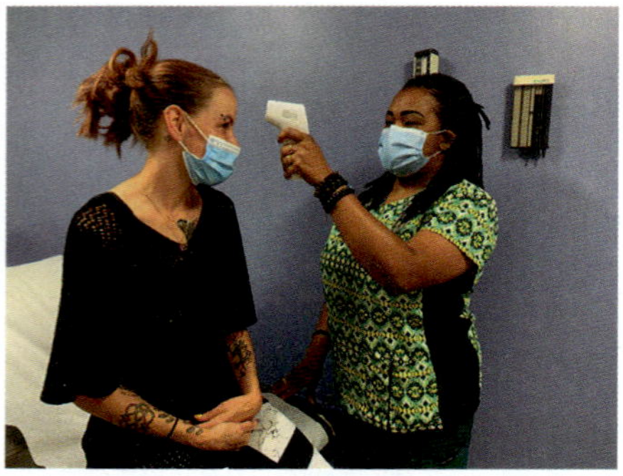

Figure 9-12 No direct client contact is required with the infrared thermometer.

4. A blinking light and/or beeping indicate that a measurement is being calculated.
5. Release the scan button and remove the thermometer from the client's forehead. Read the temperature on the display screen.
6. Replace the protective cap on the probe head.
7. If the client is diaphoretic, perform steps 1 through 3 as noted and, while continuing to depress the scan button, move the probe head to the mastoid process, just posterior to the lobule of the ear. Continue with steps 4 through 6 from above.
8. If additional measurements must be taken, wait 30 seconds to repeat the process.

Noncontact Infrared Method

The noncontact infrared thermometer is an easy-to-use battery-operated device that requires no direct contact with a client. This makes it an ideal device when obtaining the temperature in any clinical setting. Direct sunlight should be avoided when using the thermometer. Some devices have an audible alarm that sounds if the client has an elevated temperature. The forehead is frequently the location of choice for measurement though the wrist and behind the ear can be used.

1. Have the client remove any hat, scarf, or headband. Avoid any bandaged areas.
2. Ask the client to push any bangs to the side of the forehead.
3. Turn the thermometer on. Avoid being close to a source of radiant heat.
4. Aim the thermometer at the forehead at a distance that is specified by the manufacturer (Fig. 9-12) This can be as close as 2 inches and usually no farther away than 6 inches.
5. Depress the trigger button while keeping the device steady until the temperature reading appears.

N **Normal body temperatures are described in Table 9-4.**

A **Hyperthermia**, pyrexia, or fever are conditions in which body temperatures exceed 101.5°F, or 38.5°C. Clinical signs of hyperthermia include increased respiratory rate and pulse, shivering, pallor, and thirst.

P There are numerous causes of hyperthermia such as fungal, viral, and bacterial infections that result in an increased basal metabolic rate.

P Hyperthermia can also result from exposure to extremely high ambient temperatures and heating devices.

A **Hypothermia** occurs when the body temperature is below 95.2°F, or 35°C. Clinical signs of hypothermia include decreased body temperature and initial shivering that ceases as drowsiness and coma ensue. Hypotension, decreased urinary output, lack of muscle coordination, and disorientation also occur as hypothermia progresses.

P Hypothermia can be caused by prolonged exposure to cold, such as immersion in cold water or air, or by administration of large volumes of unwarmed blood products or IV fluids.

P Hypothermia may be clinically induced to decrease the tissues' need for oxygen, such as during cardiac surgery.

Blood Pressure

Blood pressure measures (in millimeters of mercury [mm Hg]) the force exerted by the flow of blood pumped into the large arteries. Arterial blood pressure is determined by blood flow and the resistance to blood flow as indicated in the following formula:

$$\text{MAP} = \text{CO} \times \text{TPR}$$

$$\text{mean arterial pressure (MAP)} = \text{cardiac output (CO)} \times \text{total peripheral resistance (TPR)}$$

Changes in blood pressure can be used to monitor changes in cardiac output. Ineffective pumping and decreased circulating volume, as well as changes in the characteristics of the blood vessels, can affect blood pressure. There is a normal diurnal variation in blood pressure, characterized by a high point in the early evening and a low point during the early deep stage of sleep.

Baroreceptors play a vital role in maintaining blood pressure. Baroreceptors are receptors located in the wall of the carotid sinus that sense hypotension and initiate reflex vasoconstriction and tachycardia to bring the blood pressure back to normal. They help a client to maintain normal blood pressure when changing from a supine to a sitting or a standing position.

Korotkoff Sounds

Korotkoff sounds are generated when the flow of blood through the artery is altered by inflating the blood pressure cuff that is wrapped around the extremity. Korotkoff sounds may be heard by listening over a pulse site that is distal to the blood pressure cuff. As the air is released from the bladder of the cuff, the pressure on the artery changes from that which completely occludes blood flow to that which allows free flow. As the pressure against the artery wall decreases, five distinct sounds occur. These are:

Phase I: The first audible sound heard as the cuff pressure is released. Sounds like clear tapping and correlates to systolic pressure (the force needed to pump the blood out of the heart).

Phase II: Sounds like swishing or a murmur. Created as the blood flows through blood vessels narrowed by the inflation of the blood pressure cuff.

Phase III: Sounds like clear, intense tapping. Created as blood flows through the artery, but cuff pressure is still great enough to occlude flow during diastole.

Phase IV: Sounds are muffled and are heard when cuff pressure is low enough to allow some blood flow during diastole. The change from the tap of Phase III to the muffled sound of phase IV is referred to as the first diastolic reading.

Phase V: No sounds are heard. Occurs when cuff pressure is released enough to allow normal blood flow. This is referred to as the second diastolic reading.

Measuring Blood Pressure

Systolic pressure represents the pressure exerted on the arterial wall during **systole** when the ventricles are contracting. Diastolic pressure represents the pressure in the arteries when the ventricles are relaxed and filling. Blood pressure is recorded as a fraction, with the top number representing the systole and the bottom number(s) representing the **diastole**. If the first and second diastolic sounds are recorded, the first diastolic sound is written over the second. For example, 120/90/80 indicates that 120 mm Hg is the systolic pressure, 90 mm Hg is the first diastolic sound, and 80 mm Hg is the second diastolic sound. **Pulse pressure** is the difference between diastolic and systolic blood pressure.

NURSING TIP

Home Blood Pressure Monitoring Devices

Many clients monitor their blood pressure at home to document their body's response to antihypertensive medications. Brachial artery-based monitors are the most accurate home monitoring devices. Periodically, clients should be instructed to bring their home devices to their appointments. You can observe how clients take their blood pressure and assess the process for accuracy. Reinforcing the correct technique can positively influence client compliance with the medical regimen.

It is also appropriate to compare the blood pressure reading on the home device with that obtained in the office. The measurements should correlate within 5 mm Hg of each other. This allows you to determine whether the readings from home parallel the client's blood pressure taken in a professional setting.

Technological advances in blood pressure monitoring that use artificial intelligence may soon be changing how blood pressure is obtained in the home environment. In July 2025, the U.S. Food and Drug Administration approved the first medical-grade cuffless blood pressure device. A specialized bracelet is worn that interfaces with a smartphone to provide continuous, accurate blood pressure readings in persons of different skin tones. This new blood pressure monitoring system can be used in a standing, sitting, or supine position. These devices are expected to be available in the U.S. sometime in 2026. However, the 2025 ACC/AHA blood pressure guidelines state that cuffless, including smartphone, blood pressure measurements cannot be used to diagnose and manage hypertension in adults at this time (Jones et. al, 2025).

Accessed October 11, 2025, from *https://www.fiercebiotech.com/medtech/fda-clears-over-counter-cuffless-blood-pressure-monitor-hilo-bracelet.*

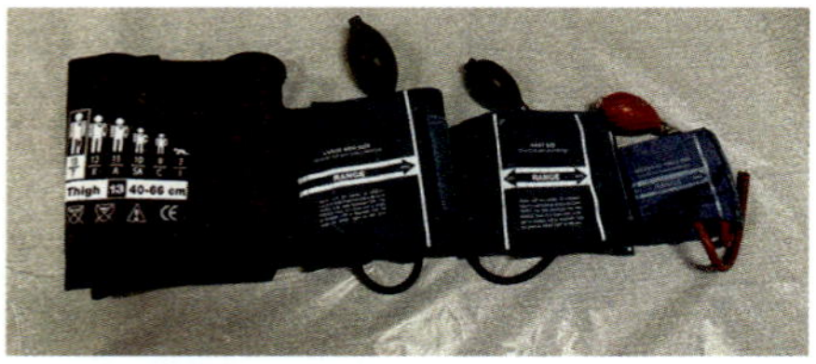

Figure 9-13 Blood pressure cuffs come in various sizes.

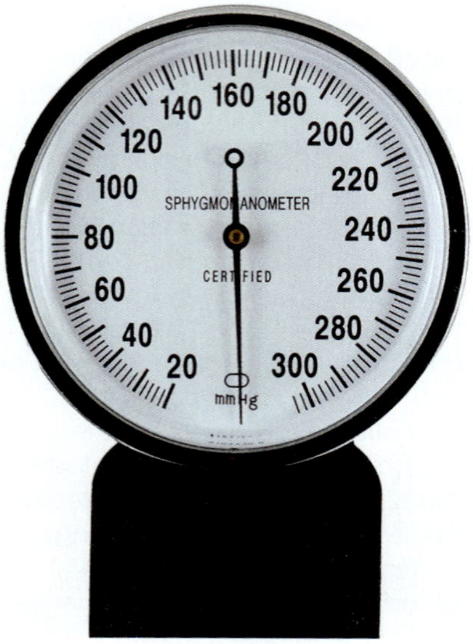

Figure 9-14 An aneroid sphygmomanometer dial.

Measurement Sites

There are several potential sites for blood pressure measurement. The preferred site is the brachial pulse site, where the brachial artery runs across the antecubital fossa. The posterior thigh, where the popliteal artery runs behind the knee joint, can also be used. A site should not be used if there is pain or injury around or near the site; for instance, a postmastectomy client should have blood pressure assessed on the unaffected side. Surgical incisions, intravenous, central venous, or arterial lines, or areas with poor perfusion should be avoided for blood pressure measurement. Clients with arteriovenous (AV) fistulas or AV shunts should not have blood pressure measured in those extremities.

Equipment

Blood pressure is measured indirectly with a stethoscope or Doppler and a **sphygmomanometer,** which consists of the blood pressure cuff, connecting tubes, air pump, and manometer. Blood pressure cuffs come in several sizes (Fig. 9-13). The inflatable bladder inside the cuff should be approximately 80% of the limb circumference. The cuff should completely encircle the limb. A manometer is attached to the cuff via a second tube.

The **aneroid manometer** is a calibrated dial with a needle that points to numbers representing the air pressure within the cuff (Fig. 9-14).

A Doppler ultrasonic stethoscope can also be used to obtain blood pressure. It is especially useful when blood pressure sounds are difficult to hear, such as with infants or very obese clients.

Manual Blood Pressure Measurement

E

1. Ensure that the client has not had any caffeine, tobacco products, or exercise in the past 30 minutes. The client should also have an empty bladder. Allow the client to rest for 5 minutes before the blood pressure is taken. Do not engage the client in conversation during this time or when the blood pressure is obtained. The room temperature should be at a comfortable level.
2. Select an appropriate size cuff.
3. Position the client. The client may be sitting, standing, or supine. At the first encounter, all three positions are recommended.
4. Position the arm or leg to be used so that the extremity is at a level equal to the heart to prevent a false reading (Fig. 9-15). At subsequent encounters, the sitting position is usually the position of choice. Ensure that the client's feet are firmly on the floor without any crossing of the legs. The back should be supported.
5. Apply the deflated blood pressure (BP) cuff:
    a. Upper arm: Wrap the BP cuff snugly around the bare upper arm. Avoid using an arm that is edematous or that is injured. The bottom of the BP cuff should be 1 to 2 inches above the antecubital fossa. The center of the bladder should be directly above the brachial artery.
    b. Leg: Place the client in a prone position or supine position with the hip and knee slightly flexed. Wrap the BP cuff around the bare thigh, with the bottom of the BP cuff slightly above the knee. The popliteal artery below the cuff is used for BP measurement.
6. Establish a baseline systolic blood pressure (palpating the blood pressure), if needed:
    a. Palpate the brachial or radial artery with the finger pads of your nondominant hand distal to the BP cuff for an arm BP. Use the popliteal artery for a leg BP.

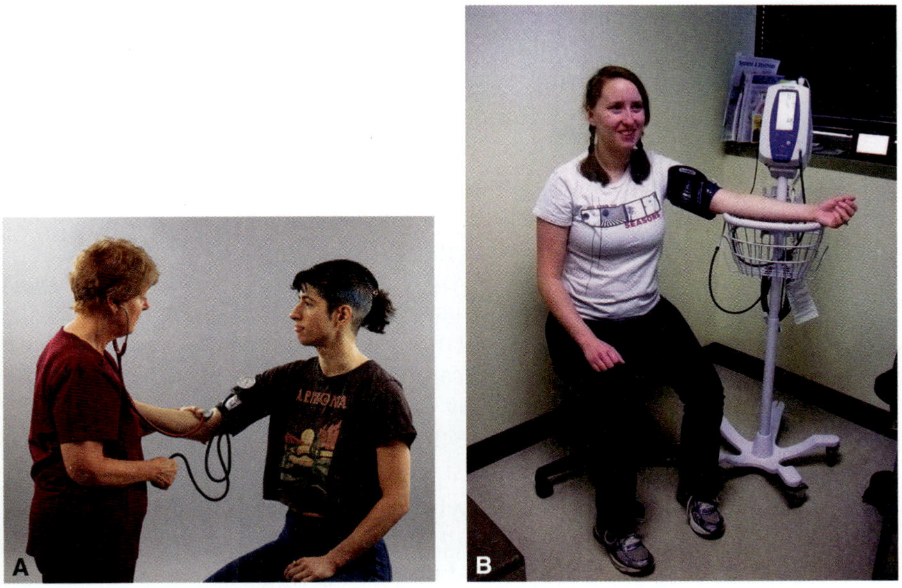

Figure 9-15 Measuring a client's blood pressure. **A.** When taking a blood pressure, the nurse can manually elevate the arm to the level of the client's heart. **B.** The nurse can also rest a client's elevated arm at the level of the heart using equipment. Note that this seated client has her feet resting on the floor.

   b. Inflate the BP cuff, and note when the artery pulsation is no longer palpable.
   c. Release the air from the BP cuff, and wait 1 to 2 minutes.
7. Palpate the pulse distal to the BP cuff.
8. Place the bell of the stethoscope over the blood pressure site (the diaphragm may be used if sounds are hard to hear).
   a. If a Doppler ultrasonic stethoscope is to be used, apply a conducting gel to the site where the pulse was palpated.
   b. Place the Doppler transducer over the site.
9. Inflate the BP cuff to approximately 20 mm Hg above the established baseline blood pressure or 20 mm Hg above where the Korotkoff sounds disappear.
10. Slowly open the valve and release the pressure at a rate of 2 to 3 mm Hg per second.
11. Listen for the Koro tkoff sounds:
    a. Onset of Korotkoff sounds correlates to systolic pressure. Note this reading.
    b. Muffling or disappearance of sounds correlates to diastolic pressures. Note this reading.
12. Deflate the BP cuff completely.
13. Wait 1 to 2 minutes and repeat the blood pressure.
14. Record the average of the blood pressure readings, the extremity used, and the position of the client. Refer to the Nursing Tip, Documenting Blood Pressure.

> **NURSING TIP**
> **Documenting Blood Pressure**
>
> The client's position during the blood pressure measurement should be recorded. Use the following symbols to depict the client's position:
>
> O— supine ♀ sitting ♀ standing
>
> Also, record where the blood pressure was taken. Use the following abbreviations:
>
> RA = right arm LA = left arm
>
> RL = right leg LL = left leg
>
> Examples of blood pressure readings are:
>
> O— 160/122 LL (left leg, supine)
>
> ♀ 98/52 RA (right arm, sitting)
>
> ♀ 118/85 LA (left arm, standing)

Automatic Blood Pressure Measurement

Automatic blood pressure machines are used in many ambulatory settings. They are also used in hospitalized clients and are left in place on the upper arm or leg for frequent blood pressure measurements for clients who require more intensive monitoring. If the client is receiving a drug such as heparin, warfarin, apixaban, rivaroxaban, or another thrombolytic agent, the client is

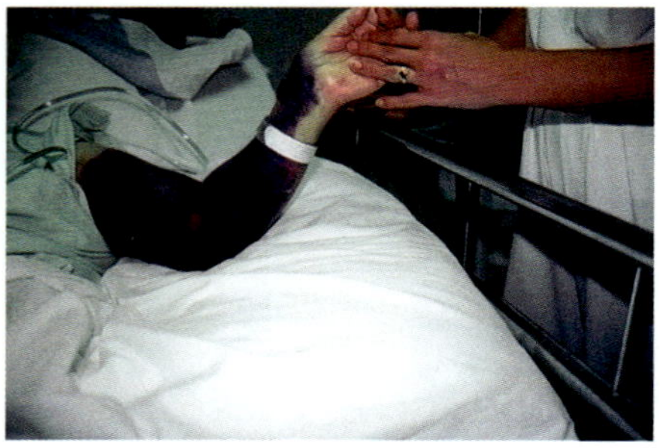

Figure 9-16 Proper placement and monitoring of an automatic blood pressure cuff will reduce the risk of injury or trauma to the client. This client had an automatic blood pressure cuff placed on the left arm while also receiving a heparin infusion in that arm.

> **NURSING TIP**
> **Palpating the Blood Pressure**
> If you are unable to hear a client's blood pressure, and no electronic monitor or amplification device is available, you can use the palpation method. Conduct the blood pressure assessment as described in steps 1 to 6 using the brachial artery. When releasing air from the cuff, note when the brachial artery is palpable. This correlates with systolic pressure. This blood pressure is then documented as a number over palpated (e.g., 115/P)

more susceptible to injury and bleeding (Fig. 9-16). Caution must be observed to prevent any complications from occurring in the arm or leg that is used for noninvasive blood pressure monitoring:

E
1. Follow steps 1 to 5 in Manual Blood Pressure Measurement.
2. Set the frequency for how often the automatic blood pressure cuff will inflate (e.g., every minute, every 5 minutes, every 15 minutes, up to every hour).
3. Activate the automatic blood pressure cuff. Record the reading.
4. Once the client's blood pressure is stable, increase the intervals between measurements. If this is not done, the blood pressure cuff could inflate as often as every minute. Readings can be done as often as needed. A manual button can be activated to obtain a blood pressure at a time not indicated by the set frequency.
5. Whenever permissible, rotate the cuff site and remember to remove the blood pressure cuff at least every shift to assess the client's skin.

N **Normal blood pressure varies with age. As a person ages, blood pressure generally increases. In 2017, the American Academy of Pediatrics (AAP) published new blood pressure guidelines for children and adolescents (Flynn et al, 2017). This built upon the 2004 *Fourth Report on the Diagnosis, Evaluation, and Treatment of High Blood Pressure in Children and Adolescents* from the National, Heart, Lung, and Blood Institute (NHLBI) of the National Institutes of Health (NIH) (NHLBI, 2004). For children under age 13 blood pressure ranges are based on age, height, and sex. Refer to the AAP's Clinical Practice Guideline (Flynn, 2017) for the charts showing blood pressure for sex, age, and height percentile. In children 13 years and older, the blood pressure guidelines more closely parallel those of adults. Table 9-5 shows the AAP classification of blood pressure for children and adolescents.**

Since 1977, NHLBI has established adult blood pressure guidelines. In 2014, The Joint National Committee (JNC) on Prevention, Detection, Evaluation, and Treatment of High Blood Pressure published its eighth report, or JNC 8, for adults. JNC 8 is the last guideline formulated by the NHLBI as they have turned over research and future guidelines to other professional groups. Thus in 2017 and again in 2025 the American College of Cardiology (ACC) and the American Heart Association (AHA) spearheaded new guidelines for the prevention, detection, evaluation, and treatment of high blood pressure in

Table 9-5 AAP Blood Pressure Category for Children and Adolescents

BP Category	Children Aged 1-12 yr (percentile based)	Children ≥13 yr old (mm Hg based)
Normotensive	<90th percentile	<120/<80 mm Hg
Elevated BP	≥90th percentile to <95th percentile or 120/80 mm Hg to <95th percentile (whichever is lower)	120–129/<80 mm Hg
Stage 1 HTN	≥95th percentile to <95th percentile + 12 mm Hg, or 130/80 to 139/89 mm Hg (whichever is lower)	130–139/80–89 mm Hg
Stage 2 HTN	≥95th percentile + 12 mm Hg or ≥140/90 mm Hg (whichever is lower)	≥140/90 mm Hg

BP, Blood pressure; HTN, hypertension; mm Hg, millimeters of mercury.
From Flynn, J. T., Kaelber, D. C., Baker-Smith, C. M., et al. (2017). Clinical practice guideline for screening and management of high blood pressure in children and adolescents. *Pediatrics, 140*(3), e20171904. *https://doi.org/10.1542/peds.2017-1904.*

adults. The 2017 guidelines lowered the criteria for the diagnosis of hypertension or high blood pressure. The ACC/AHA guidelines encourage the use of home blood pressure monitoring as well as ambulatory blood pressure monitoring. Hypertension management of clients with comorbidities such as diabetes, chronic kidney disease, obesity and metabolic syndrome are incorporated into the 2025 blood pressure guidelines. Refer to Table 9-6 for the 2025 ACC/AHA guidelines.

It is not enough to just measure the numeric value of systolic and diastolic blood pressure. The pulse pressure is also a crucial value that provides clues on cardiovascular health and pathology. Recall that the pulse pressure is the difference between the numeric value of the systolic and diastolic readings. The pulse pressure is normally 30 to 40 mm Hg.

An accurate blood pressure reading is vital to understanding the client's health condition. Table 9-7 lists errors in blood pressure measurement that should be avoided.

A Hypertension, or high blood pressure, is confirmed when an adult client has blood pressure readings averaging greater than 120 mm Hg systolic and/or 80 mm Hg diastolic on two or more separate occasions. The 2025 ACC/AHA blood pressure guidelines provide guidance on specific laboratory testing and diagnostic procedures for further evaluation as well as medication management. See Table 9-6 for the classification of hypertension.

P The cause of hypertension in 90% of cases is unknown. This is called essential hypertension. It is thought that the mechanisms that maintain the therapeutic fluid volume in the body (e.g., the heart, kidneys, nervous system, renin-angiotensin-aldosterone system) may be abnormal. The other 10% of the population who have high blood pressure have secondary hypertension.

P Arteriosclerosis reduces arterial compliance. Elastic and muscular tissues of arteries are replaced with fibrous tissue as part of the normal aging process, making the vessels less able to contract and relax in response to systolic and diastolic pressures. When the systolic pressure alone is elevated in an older adult, it is called isolated systolic hypertension.

Table 9-6 2025 ACC/AHA Blood Pressure Categories for Adults*

BP Category	Systolic Blood Pressure	Diastolic Blood Pressure
Normal BP	<120 mm Hg	and <80 mm Hg
Elevated BP	120–129 mm Hg	and <80 mm Hg
Stage 1 HTN	130–139 mm Hg	or 80–89 mm Hg
Stage 2 HTN	≥140 mm Hg	or ≥90 mm Hg
Severe hypertension and hypertensive emergencies**	>180 mm Hg	and/or >120 mm Hg

*Clients who have a BP reading in more than one classification category should be assigned to the higher classification category (e.g., a BP reading of 125/89 mm Hg is Stage 1 HTN).
**Clients with severe hypertension require urgent medication management if there is no acute target organ damage. Clients having a hypertensive emergency with signs of acute target organ damage require immediate hospitalization with intensive treatment.
BP, Blood pressure; HTN, hypertension; mm Hg, millimeters of mercury.
Adapted from Jones, D.W., Ferdinand, K.C., Taler, S.J., Johnson, H.M.et al. (2025). 2025 AHA/ACC/AANP/AAPA/ABC/ACCP/ACPM/AGS/AMA/ASPC/NMA/PCNA/SGIM Guideline for the Prevention, Detection, Evaluation and Management of High Blood Pressure in Adults: A Report of the American College of Cardiology/American Heart Association Joint Committee on Clinical Practice Guidelines. Hypertension, 82(10):e212-e316. doi:10.1161/HYP.0000000000000249

Table 9-7 Errors in Blood Pressure (BP) Measurement

If Reading Shows	Suspect
Inaccurately high blood pressure	• Blood pressure cuff is too short or too narrow (e.g., using a regular-sized blood pressure cuff on an obese arm). • The brachial artery may be positioned below the heart. • The BP cuff may be placed on the arm or leg too loosely or positioned unevenly. • The client may also be stressed, emotional, or have just completed physical activity.
High diastolic blood pressure	• Unrecognized **auscultatory gap** (a silent interval between systolic and diastolic pressures that may occur in hypertensive clients; it can also occur with a rapid deflation of the BP cuff). • Immediate reinflation of the BP cuff for multiple blood pressure readings (resulting venous congestion makes the Korotkoff sounds less audible). • If the client is supporting the arm, the sustained muscular contraction can raise the diastolic blood pressure by 10%.
Inaccurately low blood pressure	• Blood pressure cuff is too long or too wide. • The brachial artery is above the heart.
Low systolic blood pressure	• Unrecognized auscultatory gap (a rapid deflation of the cuff or immediate reinflation of the cuff for multiple readings can result in venous congestion, thus making the Korotkoff sounds less audible, and the pressure appear lower).

P Processes decreasing the size of the arterial lumen cause hypertension. Hyperlipidemia results in deposits of plaque along the inner walls of the vessels, reducing the size of the arterial lumen and increasing blood pressure.

P Processes that increase the viscosity of the blood, such as sickle cell anemia, cause greater friction between molecules of the blood and, thus, higher blood pressure.

P Chronic steroid use, Cushing syndrome, thyroid disease, and parathyroid dysfunction can all cause hypertension.

P High blood pressure may result from diseases affecting other regulatory blood pressure processes. For example, kidney disease, which affects the production of antidiuretic hormone, a hormone that helps control body fluid balance, can cause hypertension. An adrenal gland tumor, or pheochromocytoma, can increase blood pressure because of epinephrine and norepinephrine secretion.

P Overload of fluids from poor renal function or indiscriminate intravenous fluid administration (particularly in children) can result in hypertension.

P Stress can increase blood pressure. Stimulation of the sympathetic nervous system increases cardiac output and vasoconstriction, thus increasing blood pressure.

P A client's stress level can increase when in the presence of a health-care provider. Clients who have elevated blood pressure in an office or hospital environment only are said to have "white coat syndrome." When these clients have their blood pressure measured outside a health-care facility, it is frequently within an acceptable range. The 2025 ACC/AHA guidelines provide direction on how to deal with this condition.

A Blood pressure less than the normal range is called **hypotension**, or low blood pressure, which results in inadequate tissue perfusion and oxygenation. If the standing systolic blood pressure is more than 30 mm Hg below the supine systolic pressure, it may indicate that the person has orthostatic hypotension. Refer to Chapter 17. A slow response by baroreceptors when an individual transitions from a lying to a standing position can result in transitory orthostatic hypotension. When this occurs, the individual may feel dizzy and is at risk for falls.

P Processes drastically reducing circulatory blood volume, such as hypovolemic shock, cause hypotension.

P Medications such as nitroglycerin or antihypertensives lower blood pressure.

P Anaphylactic shock, resulting from massive histamine release, and circulatory collapse cause severe hypotension.

A A difference of greater than 10 to15 mm Hg between the blood pressure in both arms is abnormal.

P This difference in blood pressure between arms can be caused by coarctation of the aorta, aortic aneurysm, atherosclerotic obstruction, and subclavian steal syndrome. These conditions all result in an increased pressure proximal to the narrowing and a decreased pressure distal to the narrowing of the aorta or whatever is causing the obstruction.

A A systolic blood pressure that is greater in the arms than in the legs is abnormal.

P This blood pressure difference between the arms and the legs is caused by constriction or obstruction of the aorta, which can result from an increase in stroke volume ejection velocity, increased cardiac output, peripheral vasodilation, and decreased distensibility of the aorta or major arteries.

A A decreased pulse pressure is abnormal.

P A decreased pulse pressure can result from a decreased stroke volume (cardiac tamponade, shock, and tachycardia) or increased peripheral resistance (aortic stenosis, coarctation of the aorta, mitral stenosis or mitral regurgitation, and cardiac tamponade).

A An increased pulse pressure is abnormal.

P An increased pulse pressure can result from increased stroke volume (aortic regurgitation) or increased peripheral vasodilation (fever, anemia, heat, exercise, hyperthyroidism, and arteriovenous fistula).

Pain

Pain is a complex sensory experience that has received increased clinical attention in the past 50 years. Pain research is conducted as a clinical phenomenon, not just as a symptom of clinical pathology. The International Association for the Study of Pain (IASP) defined pain as "an unpleasant sensory and emotional experience associated with, or resembling that associated with, actual or potential tissue damage" (2017). In 2020, the IASP expanded the definition to include the following key points:

- "Pain is always a personal experience that is influenced to varying degrees by biological, psychological, and social factors.
- Pain and nociception are different phenomena. Pain cannot be inferred solely from activity in sensory neurons.
- Through their life experiences, individuals learn the concept of pain.
- A person's report of an experience as pain should be respected.
- Although pain usually serves an adaptive role, it may have adverse effects on function and social and psychological well-being.
- Verbal description is only one of several behaviors to express pain; inability to communicate does not negate the possibility that a human or a nonhuman animal experiences pain."

Pain is the reason many people seek medical care. Zelaya et al (2020) found that "20.4% of adults had chronic pain and 7.4% of adults had chronic pain that frequently limited life or work activities . . . in the past 3 months." Chronic pain is a leading cause of disability. Pain has been called the "fifth vital sign" because it directly affects the health and well-being of an individual. A pain assessment should be conducted on clients regularly. The Joint Commission (2023) provides pain assessment and management standards for various clinical settings: ambulatory care, behavioral health care, critical access hospitals, hospitals, nursing care centers, office-based surgeries, and home health services. Refer to the Web site for additional information.

Types of Pain

Nociceptive Pain

Nociceptive pain arises from somatic or visceral stimulation. **Nociception**, or pain perception, is a multistep process that involves the nervous system as well as other body systems (Fig. 9-17). A noxious stimulus occurs that stimulates the **nociceptors** (receptive neurons of pain sensation that are located in the skin and various viscera). The noxious stimulus can be many things (e.g., trauma, burn, chemical exposure, internal body inflammation, or internal body growth of tissue). Transduction of the noxious stimulus

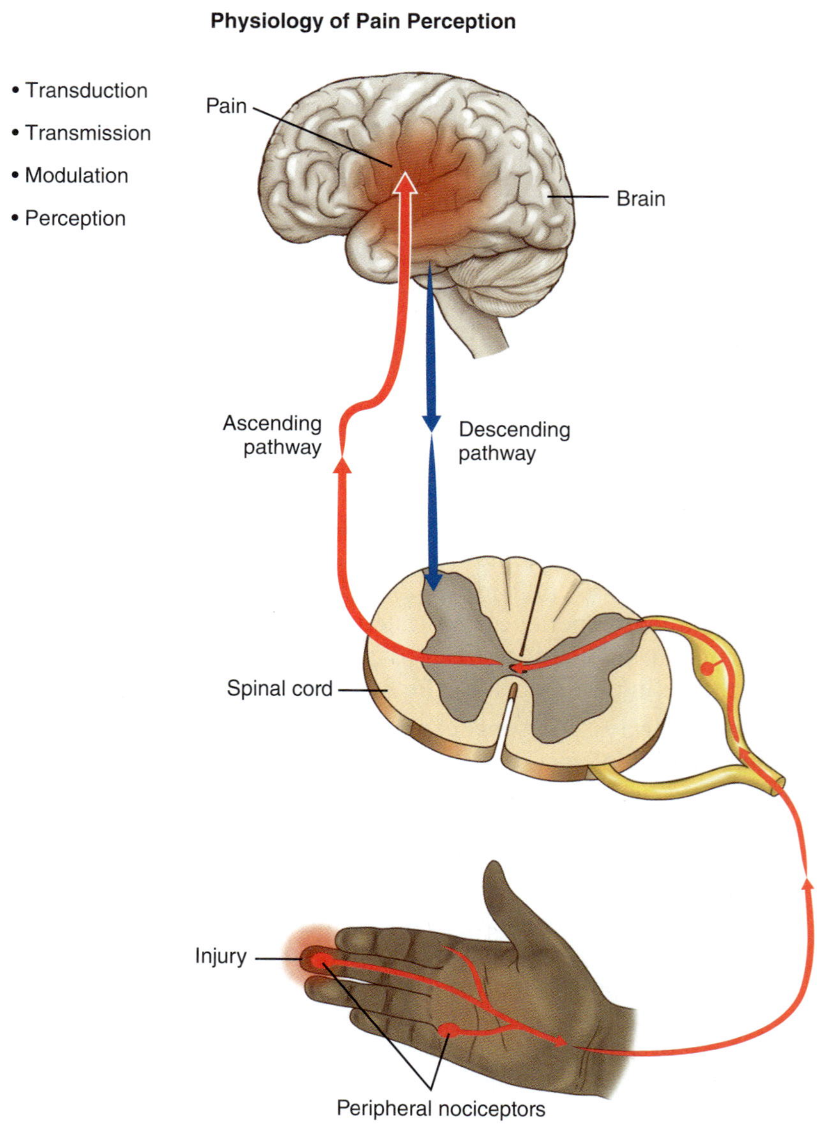

Figure 9-17 Nociception.

travels to the spinal cord via the nociceptors. This transduction causes the conversion of one energy (traveling stimulus) from another (noxious stimulus). Cell damage from the noxious stimulus causes the release of certain chemicals and sensitizing nociceptors. Prostaglandins (PG), bradykinins (BK), serotonin (5 HT), substance P (SP), hydrogen (H^+), potassium (K^+), histamine (H), and leukotrienes are all sensitizing substances. Substance P is unique because it is released only when pain fibers are stimulated.

Activating the sensitizing substances leads to an action potential in which the pain sensation is moved via afferent nerves to the spinal cord. Two types of nerve fibers participate in the action potential: A-delta fibers are myelinated neurons that transmit acute, sharp, shooting, and localized pain; C fibers are nonmyelinated neurons that transmit dull, throbbing, and poorly localized pain. These nerve fibers carry the pain impulse from the spinal cord via the spinothalamic tract to the brainstem and thalamus. The thalamus relays information to the cortex (which can identify past pain memories) and to the limbic system (where the emotional component of pain is formed). It is in these areas of the brain that pain is consciously perceived.

The inhibition of nociceptor impulses occurs in modulation. Neurons from the brainstem release neurotransmitters (e.g., serotonin, norepinephrine [NE], gamma-aminobutyric acid [GABA], 5 HT, and endogenous opioids [e.g., enkephalins, dynorphins, and ß-endorphins]).

Ultimately, the brainstem and thalamus interpret the complex chemical and electrical interactions as the pain message descends to the spinal cord leading to a conscious perception of pain.

Neuropathic Pain

Neuropathic pain can result from lesions in the central nervous system (CNS) or the peripheral nervous system (PNS). It is often characterized as a severe burning or tingling, such as that experienced with herpes zoster (shingles). Neuropathic pain may be difficult to treat clinically.

Nociplastic Pain

Nociplastic pain is a third category of pain that was identified and defined by the IASP in 2017. Nociplastic pain "arises from altered nociception despite no clear evidence of actual or threatened tissue damage causing the activation of peripheral nociceptors or evidence for disease or lesion of the somatosensory system causing the pain." Nociplastic pain may have elements in common with nociceptive pain but not neuropathic pain. The mechanism of nociplastic pain is not fully understood, but it is believed to be related to central sensitization, or the amplification of the neurons that leads to pain hypersensitivity. It is usually a pain that is multifocal and seems more intense than would be expected. Nociplastic pain can be accompanied by symptoms such as fatigue, sleep problems, mood issues, and memory impairment. Fibromyalgia is an example of nociplastic pain. Nociplastic pain can be difficult to treat.

Source of Pain

The source of pain refers to its origin in the body. Cutaneous, somatic, visceral, and referred pain are the types of pain grouped by origin. Cutaneous pain arises from the stimulation of cutaneous nerves. This pain usually has a burning quality. Somatic pain originates from bones, tendons, ligaments, muscles, and nerves and is frequently caused by musculoskeletal injury. Visceral pain arises from the organs. Diseased organs can change size, usually resulting in stretching of the organ, leading to pain. Acute appendicitis is an example of visceral pain. Referred pain is perceived in a location other than where the pathology is occurring. The location of the referred pain is in the dermatome of the spinal cord that is innervating the affected viscera and where the organ was located in its embryonic stage. An example of referred pain is the pain of pancreatitis felt on the left shoulder.

Duration of Pain

Acute, chronic malignant, and chronic nonmalignant pain are examples of pain grouped by their duration. Acute pain has a sudden onset, is of short duration, and is self-limiting. It ranges in intensity from mild to severe. It usually has an identifiable cause, such as surgery or trauma. Chronic malignant pain is pain of more than six months' duration (for example, in a client with cancer). This persistent pain can be due to a tumor, inflammation, blocked ducts, pressure on other body parts, and necrosis. Chronic nonmalignant pain also lasts more than 6 months. It can occur with or without an identifiable cause. The pain can remain even after an initial injury is healed. Chronic back pain and fibromyalgia are examples of chronic nonmalignant pain.

Perception of Pain

Pain is what the client perceives it to be. It is influenced by psychosocial and cultural norms. Pain is a unique, subjective, personal experience that every living person experiences at some time in life. Pain affects a person's physical, emotional, and psychological being. It is vital to remember that not every person experiences the same level of pain in response to similar stimuli. Sometimes the source of the pain cannot be identified, but this does not mean that the client who reports pain is not telling the truth about the pain. The client's pain can be in response to a life crisis, such as the loss of a spouse or child, or another emotional event. Remember that the client's report of pain is the most reliable indicator of pain status.

Variables Affecting Pain

Age

Studies show that pain is perceived by even the youngest members of our society, neonates. As children grow, they learn how to respond to pain by modeling others' behaviors. Pain management is learned via direct and indirect observation. Children learn how to communicate their pain (crying/verbalization), when to seek help, and whom they should seek out for care. As they reach adolescence, children may become more stoic about pain.

Older adults, especially those who have chronic pain, may not complain about their pain until it becomes debilitating, as they think that it is part of the normal aging process. This failure to seek treatment for pain may originate in the client's perception that something is seriously wrong, or in the client's lack of resources to seek treatment. Older adults have a lifetime of experiences with different types of pain, and that greatly influences how they choose to deal with new pain. Conditions such as hearing loss, loss of speech, and aphasia can all hamper communication of needs regarding pain.

Sex

Studies have shown that females have a lower pain tolerance or threshold than males. Females also report pain more frequently (Nasser & Afify, 2019). This may be due to neurohormonal factors in females. Pharmaceutical companies recognize how sexes respond differently to medications and thus include both males and females in clinical trials though females are still underrepresented (Samaei, McGregor, & Jenkins, 2022). The U.S. Food & Drug Administration (2019) also addresses the need for the inclusion of more females in clinical drug trials as well as females of diverse ages, racial and ethnic groups, differing abilities, and those with chronic diseases.

Culture

Cultural norms may determine what the client's pain experience will be. In 1994, the National Institutes of Health mandated that pharmaceutical companies include underrepresented groups in clinical trials to substantiate the efficacy of products for various ethnicities though recruitment of these individuals still proves to be a challenging problem (Clark et al, 2019).

Pain Health History

History of Present Illness

Elicit as much information as possible about the client's pain using the following questions:

- *Location:* Where is the pain located?
- *Radiation:* Does the pain move to another part of the body?
- *Quality:* How does the pain feel?
- *Quantity:* How severe is the pain?
- *Associated manifestations:* What other signs and symptoms are occurring with the pain?
- *Aggravating factors:* What makes the pain worse?
- *Alleviating factors:* What makes the pain better?
- *Setting:* Where were you (physically or emotionally or both) when the pain started?
- *Timing:* When did the pain start? How long does it last? How frequently does it occur?
- *Meaning and impact:* Does this pain have any special significance to you? How has it affected your life?

Past Health History

Past Pain History

- A client's past response to pain, as well as successful pain reduction measures, greatly influence future pain management.
- How have you handled pain in the past?

Medical History

- What medical conditions does the client have?
- Conditions such as diabetic peripheral neuropathy, herpes zoster, rheumatoid arthritis, osteoarthritis, sickle cell disease, multiple sclerosis, and carpal tunnel syndrome can lead to pain.

Surgical History

- What surgeries did the client have?
- Surgery is often performed to alleviate pain. Postoperative pain of varying degrees can result from surgical intervention.

Medications

- What prescription and over-the-counter medications are the client taking?
- Take special note of all medications that can be used to help with pain, especially controlled substances such as narcotics.

Communicable Diseases

- Does the client have any communicable diseases?
- Clients with HIV, herpes zoster, Mpox, and genital herpes may have pain.

Injuries and Accidents

- Has the client had any injuries or accidents that led to the pain?
- Many injuries, such as burns, fractured bones, and trauma from motor vehicle accidents, can lead to pain. Phantom limb pain can occur after limb amputations necessitated by trauma or other conditions.

Differing Abilities

- Does the client have a physical disability that creates pain?
- Assistive devices such as crutches, wheelchairs, and walkers can create pain if not used correctly.

Family Health History

- What is the current health status of family members?
- Has any family member had chronic pain or illnesses?
- Genetics can play a role in pain states. Some chronic pain conditions such as fibromyalgia are familial.

Social History

Alcohol Use

- What quantity of alcohol does the client consume?
- Alcoholism can lead to neuropathy.

Tobacco Use

- Does the client use any tobacco products?
- Some clients use tobacco products as a form of self-medication.

Recreational Drug Use

- Has the client used any illicit drugs?
- Does the client abuse prescribed controlled substances for recreational use?
- Some clients use cannabis and cannabinoids, and other substances to self-medicate for painful conditions.

Sexual Practice

- Has the client had any change in sexual practice with the pain?
- Sexual activity can increase or decrease with pain conditions. Some people with emotional pain use sexual activity as a form of self-medication.

Hobbies and Leisure Activities

- What types of activities does the client do for fun?
- The inability to continue enjoying activities because of pain can lead to depression. Hobbies and leisure activities can also be a form of therapy for some people.

Stress

- How has the client's pain affected their stress level? Physically? Psychologically? Financially?
- Pain places stress on the body that can be detected on examination.

Economic Status

- Does the client have health insurance or resources to properly manage the pain? Has the client been able to maintain a job?
- Lack of resources may cause a client to delay pain treatment.

Roles and Relationships

- Has the pain affected the client's relationships?
- People with chronic pain may have altered relationships, including divorce and isolation. Work relations may be strained.

Health Maintenance Activities

Sleep

- Is the pain affecting the client's sleep?
- Pain can alter sleep habits, which can exacerbate depressive symptoms.

Exercise

- Is the client able to exercise?
- Exercise releases endorphins, which can decrease or alleviate pain.

Stress Management

- What coping strategies have the client used to deal with the pain?
- Positive nonpharmacological pain management strategies are discussed later in the "Pain Management" subsection.

Effects of Pain on the Body

Pain affects everyone in different ways. Acute pain usually manifests differently from chronic pain, although there are some common elements. Physiological responses to pain include:

- *General appearance:* crying, moaning, frowning, anger, irritability, grimacing, rocking motion, pacing, rubbing painful body part, protective splinting, obvious deformities
- *Skin:* diaphoresis
- *Pulmonary:* tachypnea
- *Cardiac:* tachycardia
- *Peripheral vasculature:* hypertension, limb swelling, change in limb color/temperature
- *Gastrointestinal/nutritional:* weight loss/gain
- *Musculoskeletal:* muscle atrophy, muscle hypertrophy, muscle spasms, muscle weakness, pain at trigger points, incoordination, decreased range of motion of joints
- *Mental status:* depression, anxiety, suicidal ideation, altered concentration
- *Neurological:* dilated pupils, paresthesia, dysesthesia, allodynia
- *Immune system:* altered immune response
- *Other:* sleep deprivation, decreased appetite

These responses to pain are by no means all-inclusive. Pain can affect every system in the human body, and unrelieved pain can take its toll on the health of the client over time. Just as pain is a unique experience for the person in pain, so is the client's response to pain.

Assessing Pain

Many pain assessment tools are available for use in clinical settings for clients of various ages. Flow sheets are often used to trend the client's pain and response to pain medication and other interventions.

The easiest pain assessment tools to administer to clients are the rating scales. The Numeric Rating Scale was previously discussed in Chapter 3. It is easily administered because it requires no additional resources. A Visual Analog Scale (VAS) is another easy-to-administer pain assessment tool (Fig. 9-18). The VAS contains a 10-cm line. One end is designated as "no pain," and the other end is labeled "worst pain possible." The client indicates where on this spectrum the pain currently lies. This distance is calculated and used as a reference for current pain status, as well as used to compare future pain.

Categorical scales that can be used with children include the Wong-Baker FACES Pain Rating Scale (Wong-Baker FACES Foundation, n.d.),

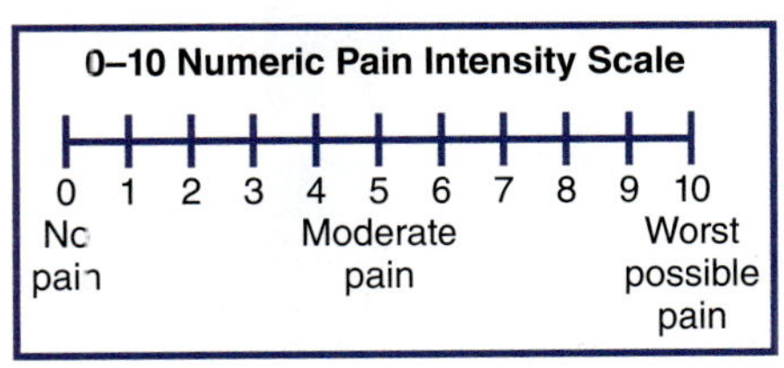

Figure 9-18 Visual Analog Scale for pain assessment.

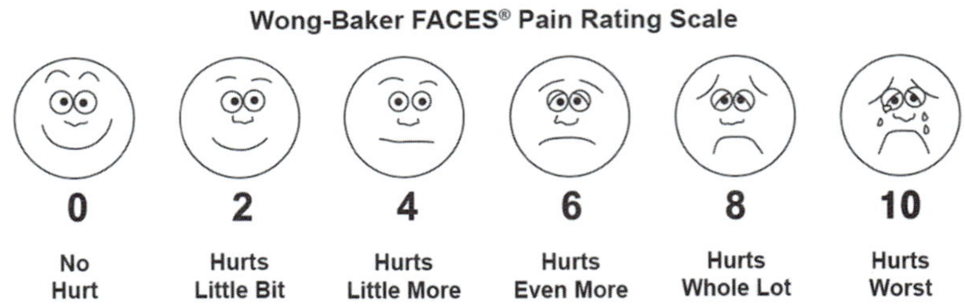

Figure 9-19 Wong-Baker FACES Pain Rating Scale.

and the Oucher Pain Assessment Tool (Beyer, 1983). These scales are easily understood and administered. With each scale, the client has control over each pain assessment encounter. Trending these reports provides information on whether the client's pain is worsening or being alleviated. This information allows the nurse to evaluate the effectiveness of the client's pain regimen.

The Wong-Baker FACES Pain Rating Scale (Fig. 9-19) is recommended for children over the age of 3 years. The nurse needs to explain this scale to the child at each assessment encounter. The Oucher Pain Assessment Tool (Fig. 9-20) is used with children 3–12 years old. The scale should be explained to the child at each assessment. Versions of this tool are available that show White, Hispanic, Black, Asian, and First Nation faces of children.

Additional pain assessment tools include the Brief Pain Inventory (Cleeland & Ryan, 1994), the McCaffrey Initial Pain Assessment Tool (McCaffery & Pasero, 1999), and the McGill Pain Questionnaire (1971). The Brief Pain Inventory, developed by Cleeland and Ryan (1994), is a written tool that is valid and reliable. Published in many languages, its linguistic accuracy has been validated. It is used in both clinical practice and research. McCaffery and Pasero (1999) developed the Initial Pain Assessment Inventory. This visual tool can be completed by the nurse or the client and includes diagrams for noting painful locations. The McGill Pain Questionnaire was developed by Melzack and Torgerson in 1971. Short and long forms of this verbally administered tool are available. It assesses sensory, affective, and evaluative aspects of pain.

Assessing pain in clients who are unable to communicate poses a challenge for nurses. Many pain tools have been developed and tested to assist in these areas. Some examples of these are the CRIES tool, which is used to measure neonatal postoperative pain (Krechel & Bildner, 1995); the FLACC Behavioral Pain Assessment Scale for nonverbal children (Merkel et al, 1997); and the PAINAD Scale for Pain Assessment in Advanced Dementia (Warden, Hurley, & Volicer, 2003). These tools have been found to be valid and reliable pain measurement scales. In addition, many institutions have developed their own pain assessment tools. Many of these include schematics of the human body, which allows the nurse to point out and record areas of pain, incisions, wounds, and so on.

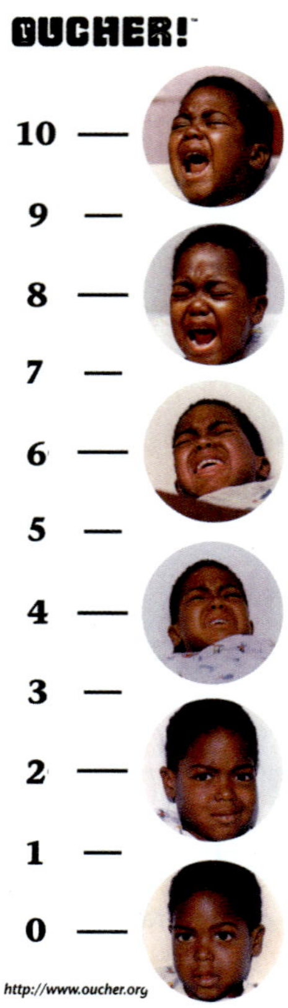

Figure 9-20 Oucher Pain Assessment Tool.

Pain Management

One of the most difficult and challenging clinical practice areas is pain management. Acute pain can often be treated with various interventions and is relatively short-lived. This is not the case with chronic pain from any etiology. Ideally, chronic malignant pain and chronic nonmalignant pain should be managed in an interdisciplinary environment of specialists that incorporates nurses, physicians, physical/occupational/recreational therapists, pharmacists, psychologists/psychiatrists/psychotherapists, social workers, the client's personal support system, and ultimately the client. The goal is to have the client's pain managed with pharmacological and nonpharmacological treatments to allow the client to achieve the highest level of functioning possible.

Medications that are used to control pain include analgesics, antiepileptics, antianxiolytics, gamma aminobutyric acid (GABA) analogues, beta blockers, barbiturates, corticosteroids, ergot alkaloids, muscle relaxants, nonsteroidal anti-inflammatories, opioids, selective 5-HT receptor agonists, serotonin and norepinephrine reuptake inhibitors, sleep aids, topical analgesics/anesthetics, tricyclics, chemotherapy, recreational drugs, alcohol, dietary supplements, herbal products, and probiotics. These medications/substances can be administered by many routes: oral, rectal, intramuscular, intravenous, subcutaneous, sublingual, topical, transdermal, transmucosal, transvaginal, intranasal, inhalation, and intraspinal.

Nonpharmacological treatments for pain include acupuncture/acupressure, aromatherapy, behavior modification, biofeedback, deep breathing exercises, exercise, hot/cold therapy, hypnosis, imagery, light therapy, magnet therapy, massage therapy, music therapy, client education, pet therapy, physical therapy, Pilates, psychotherapy, qi gong, reflexology, Reiki, relaxation techniques, spinal manipulation, surgery, tai chi, TENS units, therapeutic touch, transcendental meditation, and yoga. In addition, many apps are available on mobile phones that can assist clients.

Note that the goal cannot always be to alleviate all of the client's pain. Some pain conditions, such as osteoarthritis, diabetic peripheral neuropathy, migraine headaches, and fibromyalgia, have no cure. In cases such as these, the goal is to decrease the severity of the client's pain symptoms so that the client can lead as normal a life as possible. Whether the client is in a health-care facility or at home, pain assessments must be conducted at regular intervals (the timing depends on the client's condition and other factors), because chronic pain is an ongoing process.

The Opioid Crisis

In the 1990s pharmaceutical companies extolled the virtues and efficacy of effectively controlling pain with controlled substances such as opioids. Similar to the tobacco industry's failure to warn the public of the health risks of tobacco use, manufacturers of opioids assured consumers and health-care providers that their products were safe. Warnings on the risk of addiction were not disclosed (Haffajee & Mello, 2017). This period of time closely aligned with The Joint Commission identifying pain as the "fifth vital sign" in 2001. By 2004 The Joint Commission removed the "fifth vital sign" from its accreditation guidelines though it continues to publish pain assessment and management standards. Due to the proliferation of opioid prescriptions, numerous people were given opioids for legitimate conditions. Unfortunately, the frequent and continued ingestion of opioids turned many of these individuals into opioid abusers. With continued consumption of opioids, the risk increases for misuse, dependency, addiction, overdose, and death.

From 1999 to 2020 approximately 932,000 people died from a drug overdose (CDC, 2023). In 2022 the CDC's National Center for Health Statistics (2022a) estimated that more than 107,000 individuals died from a drug overdose in 2021, and this represented almost a 15% increase from the previous year! The annual increase in the number of opioid overdose deaths poses a major public health concern in the United States.

Opioids were involved in 75% of all drug overdose fatalities. The opioids include prescription medications such as oxycodone and hydrocodone, but also synthetic opioids such as fentanyl. Synthetic opioids have a role in pain management though most of the fentanyl deaths arose from its illegal production and distribution. Synthetic opioids account for almost 82% of all opioid overdose fatalities (CDC, 2022b).

Another source of opioids is from veterinarians (vets). Sadly, some people with pain intentionally injure or cause illness in their pet. When the vet prescribes an opioid or other controlled substance for the pet, the pet's owner instead consumes the medication (American Veterinary Medical Association, n.d.). Just as people can "shop" for opioids from various medical providers, vets must also be aware of pet owners "shopping" vets for opioids.

Clients who have acute or chronic pain expect help from their health-care providers. Thus it is important to remember that used correctly and with caution, opioids do play a role in pain alleviation and management. Clients as well as health-care providers must understand the potential adverse effects of opioids and observe guidelines to help prevent adverse outcomes. Individual states as well as the federal government are recognizing the opioid crisis and are developing strategies to effectively limit the increasing and staggering death tolls.

U.S. Preventive Services Task Force (USPSTF)

Grade A Recommendation:

The USPSTF recommends screening for hypertension in adults 18 years or older with office blood pressure measurement (OBPM). The USPSTF recommends obtaining blood pressure measurements outside of the clinical setting for diagnostic confirmation before starting treatment.

Retrieved October 10, 2025, from *https://www.uspreventiveservicestaskforce.org/uspstf/recommendation-topics/uspstf-a-and-b-recommendations*

Review Questions

Questions 1 to 10 refer to the following situation:

The nurse admits Tyesha, a 44-year-old woman, to the emergency department for an injury to the left knee sustained while playing basketball tonight.

1. The nurse performs a general survey of Tyesha and notes halitosis. Which of the following conditions might Tyesha be experiencing? Select all that apply.
   a. Vaginal infection
   b. Rhinosinusitis
   c. Allergic rhinitis
   d. Kidney disease
   e. Gastroesophageal reflux

2. The nurse counts Tyesha's respiratory rate. Tyesha has a respiratory rate of 32 breaths per minute. The nurse determines that the respiratory rate is:
   a. Within normal limits
   b. Apnea
   c. Bradypnea
   d. Tachypnea

3. The nurse assesses Tyesha's pulse. Which of the following are peripheral pulse sites that can be used? Select all that apply.
   a. Brachial
   b. Carotid
   c. Femoral
   d. Radial
   e. Dorsalis pedis

4. The nurse notes a full, forceful, bounding pulse that is difficult to obliterate with pressure. What might be the etiology of the pulse volume?
   a. Cardiac arrhythmia
   b. Late septic shock
   c. Hyperkinetic state
   d. Aortic stenosis

5. The nurse takes Tyesha's blood pressure in her left arm. The reading is 137/87 mm Hg while sitting. It is unchanged 15 and 30 minutes later. Which of the following accurately describes Tyesha's blood pressure?
   a. Her blood pressure is normal.
   b. Her blood pressure is elevated.
   c. Her blood pressure is Stage 1 hypertension.
   d. Her blood pressure is Stage 2 hypertension.

6. Thirty minutes later the nurse repeats Tyesha's blood pressure with the same cuff. It is now 159/95 mm Hg in her right arm. What conclusion(s) does the nurse make? Select all that apply.
   a. The blood pressure cuff is too wide.
   b. The client is stressed.
   c. The blood pressure cuff is too long.
   d. The brachial artery was above the level of the heart.
   e. A rapid deflation of the cuff occurred.
   f. The client continues to be in pain.

7. The nurse takes Tyesha's temperature. Which method would be the most appropriate and accurate?
   a. Axillary
   b. Forehead infrared
   c. Rectal
   d. Tympanic

8. Which of the following types of pain best describes the pain Tyesha is experiencing in her left knee?
   a. Acute pain
   b. Referred pain
   c. Neuropathic pain
   d. Chronic nonmalignant pain

9. Which of the following pain assessment tools are appropriate to use for assessing Tyesha's pain? Select all that apply.
   a. CRIES
   b. FACES Pain Rating Scale
   c. PAINAD Scale
   d. Numeric Rating Scale
   e. Visual Analog Scale

10. Tyesha tells the nurse that her pain is at a moderate level and is requesting pain relief measures. Which of the following statements accurately depicts appropriate responses?
    a. Acute pain should always be relieved with an opioid.
    b. Physical therapy should be started today to relieve the knee pain.
    c. Women have a lower pain threshold than men so less pain medication should be administered.
    d. A nonsteroidal anti-inflammatory medication, ice pack to the left knee, and left leg elevation should be implemented.

Skin, Hair, and Nails

CHAPTER 10

Learning Outcomes

1. Identify the anatomy and physiology of the skin, hair, and nails.
2. Conduct a complete health history on a client with a skin, hair, and nail condition.
3. Perform a physical examination on a healthy adult and an adult with skin, hair, and nail pathology.
4. Differentiate between normal clinical findings from a client's physical examination and the pathophysiology of abnormal clinical findings.
5. Identify risk factors for basal and squamous cell carcinoma.
6. Identify risk factors for malignant melanoma.
7. Identify the United States Preventive Services Task Force Recommendation for the skin, hair, and nails.
8. Document a complete health history and physical examination of a client with a skin, hair, and nail pathology.

The skin, also known as the **integumentary system**, or cutaneous tissue, is the largest organ system of the body. It shelters most of the other organ systems and, if examined carefully, can provide a noninvasive window to observe the body's level of functioning.

This chapter provides a review of the skin and its appendages: hair and nails. Techniques for examination of the integumentary system are addressed, as is an approach to evaluating skin lesions.

Anatomy and Physiology

The skin, hair, and nails, along with their functions, are discussed.

Skin

The surface area of the skin covers approximately 20 square feet in the average adult, with a thickness varying from 0.2 to 1.5 mm, depending on the region of the body and the client's age. Morphologically speaking, the skin is composed of three main layers: the epidermis, the dermis, and the subcutaneous tissue, or hypodermis (Fig. 10-1).

Epidermis

The **epidermis** is a multilayered outer covering consisting of four layers throughout the body, except for the palms of the hands and soles of the feet, where there are five layers (Fig. 10-2). The deepest layer of the epidermis is the **stratum germinativum**, or basal cell layer. It is composed of columnar-shaped cells that rest on a basement membrane. These

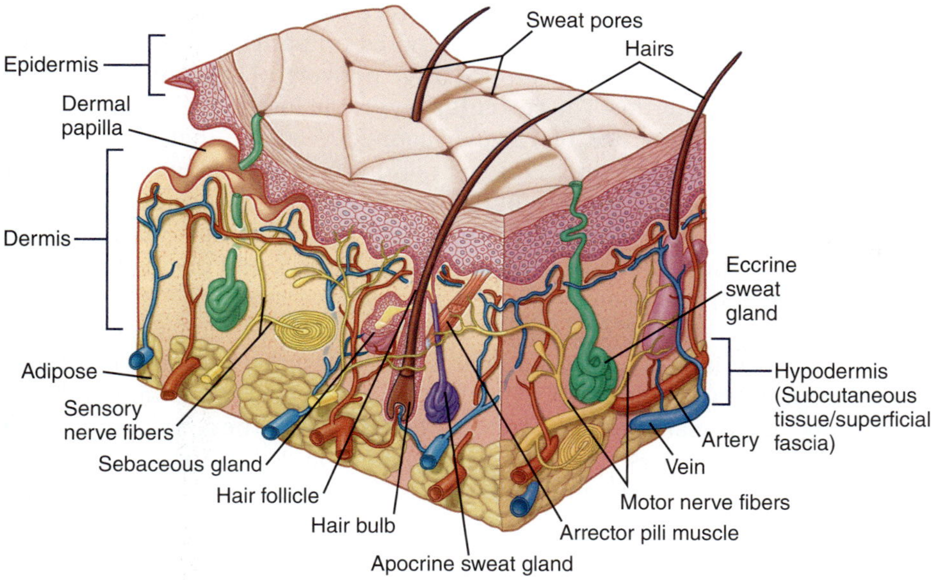

Figure 10-1 Structures of the skin.

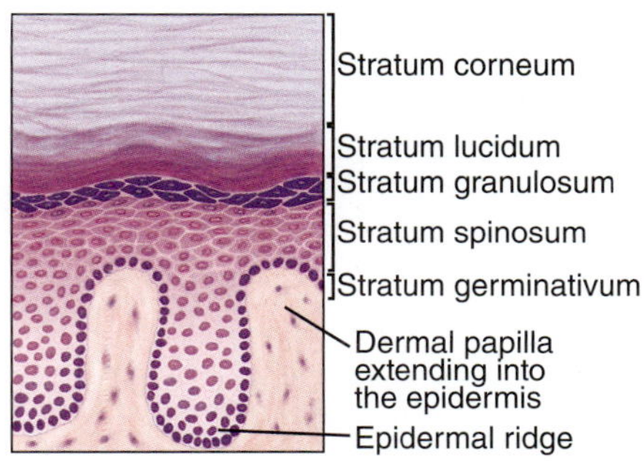

Figure 10-2 Epidermal layers of the skin.

columnar cells undergo continuous mitosis to produce new cells that replace the cells that are lost from the top layer of the epidermis. This layer provides the skin with tone and also creates pigment-producing melanocytes that filter ultraviolet light. The **stratum spinosum** overlays the stratum germinativum. The stratum spinosum consists of layers of polyhedral-shaped cells. Intercellular bridges create an irregular shape. Skin cell death occurs in the **stratum granulosum**, which overlays the stratum spinosum. The stratum granulosum is composed of cells with shriveled nuclei and strands of keratin.

The additional layer, which is found exclusively on the palmar and plantar surfaces, is the stratum lucidum. It contains a thin layer of translucent eleidin that aids in the formation of keratin. Finally, the stratum corneum, also known as the horny layer, completes the epidermis. The stratum corneum is composed of enucleated dead epithelial cells. These cells contain keratin, which provides a waterproof barrier. This layer is in a continual state of desquamation (shedding), as new skin cells are pushed up from the lower layers; a complete turnover of cells occurs every 3 to 4 weeks.

The epidermis, with the exception of the palmar and plantar surfaces, is normally smooth. All epidermal surfaces are devoid of blood vessels. Despite the absence of vessels, pigments in the blood serum can cause changes in the color transmitted to the skin's surface, such as oxyhemoglobin, deoxyhemoglobin, bilirubin, and carotene. Melanin is the pigment responsible for the lightness and darkness of skin tone. The ability of the skin to reflect light, known as the Tyndall effect, can also influence the integumentary color. Skin tones vary and can have yellow, orange, pink, and olive undertones.

In general, epidermal thickness is not dependent on gender or ethnic origin, but instead, on specific skin areas and age. The epidermis is significantly thicker in the plantar aspect of the foot and fingertips. The epidermis is especially thin in areas such as the upper eyelid, pubic area, and penis. Aging skin leads to epidermal thinning (Lintzeri et al, 2022).

Dermis

The **dermis**, or corium, is the second layer of the skin. It is approximately 20 times thicker than the epidermis in certain areas of the body and can be divided into two layers: the papillary layer and the reticular layer. The **papillary layer**, or upper layer, is composed primarily of loose connective tissue, small elastic fibers, and an extensive network of capillaries that serve to nourish the epidermis. The **reticular layer**, the lower layer of the dermis, is formed by a dense bed of vascular connective tissue that also includes nerves and lymphatic tissue. This layer also provides structural support for the skin. In the deeper portions of the reticular layer, collagen fibers in combination with elastic fibers are surrounded by a gelatinous matrix. Intermeshed with the connective tissue are hair follicles, sweat glands, sebaceous glands, and adipose tissue.

The fibrous connective tissue in the dermis gives the skin its strength and elasticity. The fibrous tissues provide structural support for the epidermis and form dermal "ridges" to which the epidermis conforms and anchors, creating epidermal ridges known as fingerprints. These ridges develop during the first trimester of fetal development and although they enlarge with growth, their pattern remains the same throughout life and enhances with age.

Subcutaneous Tissue

Beneath the dermis is the **subcutaneous tissue**, or superficial fascia. It is composed of either loose areolar connective tissue or adipose tissue, depending on its location in the body. The subcutaneous layers attach the skin to the underlying bones. These layers act as a temperature insulator and help regulate body heat; they also encompass fat stores for energy use and contain an extensive venous plexus layer, which acts as a reservoir for the blood that warms the surface of the skin.

Distributed around the dermal blood vessels and the subcutaneous tissue are the skin's mast cells. These cells number from 7000 to 20,000 per cubic centimeter of skin. Mast cells are the body's major source of tissue histamine and trigger the body's reaction to allergens.

Glands of the Skin

The skin has two main groups of glands: the sebaceous glands and the sweat glands.

Sebaceous Glands

The **sebaceous glands** are sebum-producing glands that are found almost everywhere in the dermis except for the palmar and plantar surfaces. They are also part of the apparatus that contains the hair follicle and the **arrector pili muscle**, which causes contraction of the skin and hair, resulting in "goose bumps." The ducts of the sebaceous glands open into the upper part of the hair follicle and are responsible for producing **sebum**, an oily secretion that is thought to retard evaporation and water loss from the epidermal cells. Sebaceous glands are most prevalent in the scalp, forehead, nose, and chin.

Sweat Glands

The two main types of **sweat glands** are **apocrine glands**, associated with hair follicles, and **eccrine glands**, not associated with hair follicles. The secretory apparatus of both types of sweat glands is located in the subcutaneous tissue. Eccrine glands open directly onto the skin's surface and are widely distributed throughout the body. Apocrine glands are found primarily in the axillae, genital and rectal areas, nipples, and navel. These glands become functional during puberty, and secretion occurs during emotional stress or sexual stimulation. After puberty, apocrine glands are responsible for the characteristic body odor that results when sweat mixes with the natural bacterial flora normally present on the skin surface.

Hair

With few exceptions such as the palmar and plantar surfaces, lips, nipples, umbilicus, back of the ear, and the glans penis, hair is distributed over the entire body surface. Its abundance and texture vary. **Vellus hair**, or fine, faint hair, covers most of the body. In general, **terminal hair** is the coarser, darker hair of the scalp, eyebrows, and eyelashes. Terminal hair becomes increasingly evident with the onset of puberty, including the development of coarser, thicker pubic, axillary, chest, and facial hair.

Specialized epidermal cells are located in depressions at the base of each hair follicle and are responsible for the formation of each individual hair shaft. These cells are nourished by blood vessels in the dermis so that they grow and divide, pushing the older cells toward the surface of the skin.

Most hair shafts are composed of three layers: the cuticle, or outer layer; the cortex, or middle layer; and the medulla, or innermost layer. Hair color is determined by the melanocytes produced in the cells at the base of each follicle; an abundance of pigment produces darker hair color, and smaller amounts produce a lighter color.

Nails

Nails are composed of keratinized, or horny, layers of cells that arise from undifferentiated epithelial tissue called the **matrix**. The **nail plate**, tissue that covers the distal portion of the digits and provides protection, is approximately 0.5 to 0.75 mm thick. The nails consist of the **nail root**, which lies posteriorly to the cuticle and is attached to the matrix; the **nailbed**, which is the vascular bed located beneath the nail plate; and the **periungual tissues**, which surround the nail plate and the free edge of the nail (Fig. 10-3). At the proximal end of each nail is a white, crescent-shaped area known as the **lunula**. The **eponychium** is the thickened area at the base of the nails comprised of living cells. The cuticle extends from the eponychium and is comprised of dead cells. The cuticle may be obscured by the lunula in some individuals.

The normally translucent nail plate is given a pinkish cast by the underlying vascular bed in individuals with lighter skin tones and a brownish cast in individuals with darker skin tones. In many disease processes, the color of the nailbed may vary. For instance, a decrease in the oxygen content of the blood will cause the nailbeds to have a blue hue depicting peripheral cyanosis in individuals with lighter skin tones.

The nail plate is formed continuously as the plate is pushed forward by new growth from the germinative layer of the matrix. Normal growth for an adult is 0.1 to 1.0 mm per day, but growth varies with age, season, nutrition, climate, health status, and activity.

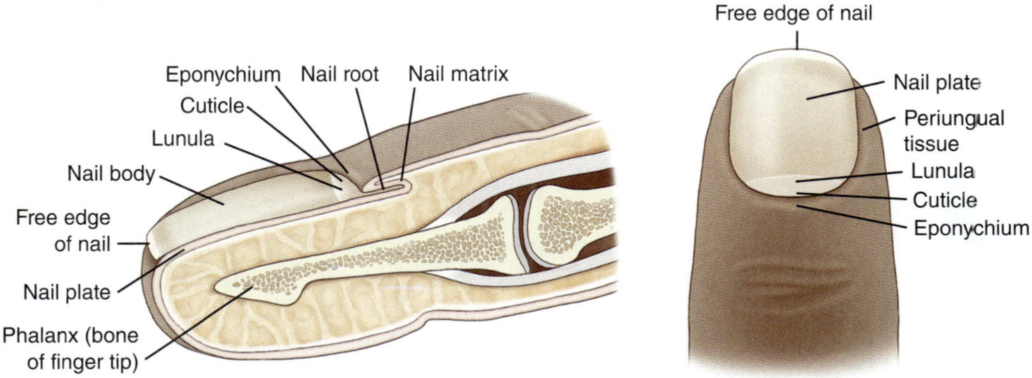

Figure 10-3 Structures of the nail.

Function of Skin

The skin has many functions, but perhaps the most important one is to serve as a protective barrier against invasion from environmental hazards and pathogens. It provides boundaries against materials that might enter the body, such as toxic chemicals, and provides boundaries for fluids and mobile tissues, such as blood, within the body. An intact integument is also responsible for the protection of underlying organs, which would otherwise be vulnerable to injury because of exposure.

Temperature regulation is carried out by the skin through the production of perspiration. During states of increased body temperature, the eccrine glands produce large quantities of sweat. As perspiration reaches the skin's surface, rapid evaporation occurs, and the body temperature decreases. The skin's vascular system also plays a role in heat control. When vasodilation occurs, much body heat can be lost through radiation and conduction. Conversely, vasoconstriction helps to maintain body heat.

The skin contains receptors for pain, touch, pressure, and temperature. These receptors originate in the dermis and terminate as either free nerve endings throughout the skin's surface or as special touch receptors that are encapsulated and found predominantly in the fingertips and lips. Each hair found on the body also contains a basal nerve fiber that acts as a tactile receptor. Sensory signals that help determine precise locations on the skin are transmitted along rapid sensory pathways, and less distinct signals, such as pressure or poorly localized touch, are sent via slower sensory pathways.

The skin acts as an organ of excretion for substances such as water, salts, and nitrogenous wastes. The skin produces cells for wound repair and is the site for the production of vitamin D. The skin is also an indicator of nonverbal language and emotions via blushing and facial expressions. The skin may further be used for identification via fingerprints and birthmarks.

NURSING TIP
SKIN TONE

Dr. Ellis Monk developed the Monk Skin Tone Scale (Fig. 10-4) to advance skin tone evaluation in artificial intelligence (AI). This scale provides a broad representation of the range of skin colors in the form of ten tones. It is available by Google as a free resource: *https://skintone.google/*.

The MST scale demonstrates the variety of human skin tones.

NURSING TIP
Wound Healing and Scar Formation

Wound healing includes **reepithelialization**, which is the migration of epithelial cells inward from the wound edges and from any surrounding hair follicles or eccrine glands. Scab formation may prohibit reepithelialization because of diminished moisture. **Granulation tissue** is a combination of inflammatory cells, new vessels, and white blood cells that form a matrix at the base of the wound. The granulation tissue provides a foundation on which reepithelialization occurs. Scar formation may take several months. New scars are thick, darkened, and vascular in appearance. Over time, the scar tissue flattens and becomes less vascular; however, old scars remain slightly darker or discolored compared with the surrounding tissue.

Figure 10-4 Monk Skin Tone (MST) Scale.

Function of Hair and Nails

Hair provides warmth, protection, and sensation to the underlying systems. Terminal hair of the scalp and face provides warmth, shields against ultraviolet light, and filters dust and particulate matter. Vellus hair enhances tactile sensation and sensory perception. Nails protect the distal surface of the digits and can be used for self-protection. Nails can also contribute to tactile sensation.

HEALTH HISTORY

The skin, hair, and nail health history provides insight into the link between a client's life/lifestyle and skin, hair, and nail information and pathology.

CLIENT PROFILE

Diseases for the skin, hair, and nails are listed.

Age

Skin Fungal infections, diseases of sebaceous glands, such as acne vulgaris (13 to 26); lupus erythematosus, psoriasis, skin tags (acrochordon) (25 to 60 years)

Melanoma (55 to 74)

Basal and squamous cell carcinoma (older adults)

Hair Male pattern alopecia (adolescence to adulthood); thinning, graying, loss of hair in axillary and pubic areas, excessive facial hair (middle to older age)

Sex

Skin Male: Skin pathology is consistently more prevalent among males than females; dermatophyte infections, skin tumors, fungal infections, and increased incidence of tumors related to occupational hazards and hygiene; Kaposi sarcoma associated with immunodeficiency conditions

Hair Female pattern alopecia, increased facial hair with aging; Male alopecia, increased coarse nose and ear hair with aging

Race

Dark Skinned Keloid formation, dermatosis papulosa nigra, hyper- and hypopigmentation, traumatic marginal alopecia, seborrheic dermatitis, pseudofolliculitis barbae, acne keloidalis nuchae, congenital dermal melanocytosis (formerly known as Mongolian spots), albinism, hypopigmented sarcoidosis, granulomatosis skin lesions

Light Skinned Squamous and basal cell carcinoma, actinic keratosis, psoriasis

CHIEF COMPLAINT

Common chief complaints for the skin, hair, and nails are defined, and information on the characteristics of each sign or symptom is provided.

1. **Pruritus** Cutaneous itching that may have a multitude of etiologies

   Location Generalized or localized

   Quality Superficial or deep sensation of itching, intensity of itching, interference with sleep habits

   Associated Manifestations Rashes, lesions, edema, angioedema, anaphylaxis, excoriation or ulcers as the result of scratching, **lichenification** (hyperpigmentation and thickening of the skin), systemic disease

   Aggravating Factors Exposure to chemicals, sunlight, heat, plants, food, animals, stress, climate, parasites, xerosis, drug reaction, systemic disease processes, contact dermatitis, types of clothing (frequently wool)

   Alleviating Factors Dietary changes, medications, antihistamines, biofeedback, cool baths, types of clothing (frequently cotton), increased skin hydration, ultraviolet-band light therapy

   Setting Work, home, school, outside, or recreational environment

   Timing Pre- or postprandial, nocturnal, seasonal, during periods of stress, associated with menstrual cycle

2. **Rash** A cutaneous eruption that may be localized or generalized

   Lesion A circumscribed pathological change in the tissues

   Location Location of where it started and spread, distribution over the body, percent of body involved, following dermatomes

   Quantity "Grouping or arrangement": discrete, grouped, confluent, linear, annular, polycyclic, generalized, zosteriform

Quality "Morphology": macule, patch, papule, plaque, nodule, cyst, wheal, vesicle, pustule, bullae, tumor, lichenification, crust, erosion, fissure, ulcer, or atrophy

Associated Manifestations Edema, angioedema, anaphylaxis, excoriation or ulcers as the result of scratching, lichenification, systemic disease, allergies, fever, induration

Aggravating Factors Exposure to chemicals, sunlight, plants, food, animals, stress, climate, parasites, xerosis, drug reaction, systemic disease processes, contact dermatitis, radiation, types of clothing (frequently wool)

Alleviating Factors Dietary changes, medications, antihistamines, biofeedback, cool baths, types of clothing (frequently cotton), increased skin hydration, ultraviolet-band light therapy, surgery

Setting Work, home, school, or recreational environment, recent insect bite, recent travel, recent COVID-19 infection, exposure to contagious conditions

Timing When it started, pre- or postprandial, nocturnal, seasonal, during periods of stress, associated with menstrual cycle, after using new skincare products/detergents, new foods, new medications

PAST HEALTH HISTORY

The various components of the past health history are linked to skin, hair, and nail pathology and information related to skin, hair, and nails.

Medical History

Skin Specific Acne, contact dermatitis, eczema, atopic dermatitis, melanoma, basal cell carcinoma, squamous cell carcinoma, albinism, vitiligo, psoriasis, fungal infections, birthmarks, body piercing, tattoos, urticaria, excessive bruising, burns, pressure injuries, warts, scabies, rosacea

Non-Skin Specific Renal disease, diabetes mellitus, lupus erythematosus, peripheral vascular disease, idiopathic thrombocytopenia purpura (ITP), Rocky Mountain spotted fever, liver disease, hepatitis, collagen diseases, cardiac dysfunction, sexually transmitted infections, Lyme disease, arthritis, lymphoma, thyroid disease, pregnancy, Addison disease, pernicious anemia, HIV, cytomegalovirus, Epstein-Barr virus, measles, mumps, rubella, coxsackievirus, adenovirus, drug hypersensitivities, varicella, herpes zoster, herpes simplex, Kawasaki disease, toxic shock syndrome, carcinoma, tuberculosis, viral syndromes, asthma, allergic rhinitis, COVID-19, Mpox, poor nutritional status

Hair Specific Allergies, alopecia, lice, bacterial or fungal infections of the scalp, brittle hair, rapid hair loss, trichotillomania, trauma, congenital anomalies

Non-Hair Specific Renal disease, diabetes mellitus, cardiac dysfunction, peripheral vascular disease, thyroid disease, pregnancy, Addison disease, HIV, anemia, malnutrition, stress, chemotherapy, radiation therapy

Nail Specific Allergies, psoriasis, bacterial or fungal infections, trauma, brittle nails, nail-biting, congenital anomalies

Non-Nail Specific Iron deficiency anemia, chronic infection, malnutrition, Raynaud phenomenon, hypoxia, acute infections, syphilis

Surgical History Keloid and scar formation after surgery, plastic surgery, skin grafts, reconstructive surgery, excision biopsy, hair plugs, tattoo removal, laser treatments (used for various conditions)

Allergies Medication, insect stings, foods, soaps, laundry detergent, chemicals, fibers (wool), metals (nickel), animal dander, pollens, grasses, cosmetics, any substance is a possible allergen that can cause a dermatological manifestation

Medications Topical/oral steroids, topical/oral antifungals, topical antibiotics, antivirals, acne medications, retinoids, oral hormone agents, fluorouracil (5-FU), photodynamic therapy, topical agents for pressure ulcers, tumor necrosis factor blockers, interleukin antagonists, over-the-counter skin care products

Communicable Diseases Varicella, roseola, measles, scabies, bacterial or fungal infections, HIV, sexually transmitted infections (STIs): syphilis, gonorrhea, chancroid, genital warts (see Chapters 21, 22, and 23 for additional information), Mpox

Injuries and Accidents Chemical inhalation, trauma, burns, toxin contamination, pressure ulcers

Differing Abilities Poor eyesight can lead to poor hygiene; frequent skin trauma prevents early detection and treatment of skin diseases; bedridden or wheelchair-bound with possibility of pressure trauma and compromised skin integrity

Blood Transfusions Skin eruptions, pruritus

Childhood Illnesses Refer to section on communicable diseases.

FAMILY HEALTH HISTORY

Familial skin, hair, and nail diseases are listed.

Skin Specific Allergies, eczema, melanoma, albinism, vitiligo, psoriasis, nonmelanomatous skin cancer

Hair Specific Allergies, alopecia, brittle hair

Nail Specific Brittle nails

SOCIAL HISTORY

The components of the social history are linked to skin, hair, and nail factors and pathology.

Alcohol Use Hepatotoxicity and subsequent skin manifestations that accompany liver failure, such as jaundice and pruritus; skin bruising and trauma from falls and ataxia while inebriated; telangiectasia of the nose, neck, and upper chest

Tobacco Use Yellow discoloration of fingertips on smoking hand, leathery facial appearance

Recreational Drug Use Skin manifestations from intravenous drug use, such as injection sites or tracks or abscesses; especially prevalent in the forearms, behind the knees, toe webs, finger webs, and under the nails

Sexual Practice Various STIs may manifest in the genital region; these are discussed in Chapters 21, 22, and 23

Travel History

Tropical regions: fungal infections, contact dermatitis, tropical eczema, leishmaniasis

Insect bites: insects indigenous to certain climates, such as the tsetse fly in Africa and the deer tick in wooded areas of the northern and southeastern United States

High-altitude areas: light-sensitive eruptions, dry skin, and eczema

Southeastern United States, Mississippi and Ohio River valleys, and South America: blastomycosis, most likely caused by infected soil

Work Environment

Health-care workers employ frequent hand washing and may have prolonged glove use resulting in skin injury, mechanical/friction dermatitis, and contact dermatitis

Chemical: contact dermatitis and burns

Exposure to toxic substances, dyes, or plants

Sunlight: skin eruptions, increased incidence of basal or squamous cell carcinoma, burns, wrinkles, senile freckles, lightened hair, excessive exposure to ultraviolet radiation

Excessive exposure to water: drying and cracking of skin, pruritus, soft nails, damaged hair shafts

Insect bites: rashes, urticaria, edema, angioedema, pruritus

Operating heavy or sharp equipment: trauma, laceration

Excessive exposure to wind and cold temperatures: aging, drying, and cracking of skin

Pollution: contact dermatitis

Tar and pitch: act as both photosensitizers and carcinogens

Home Environment

Exposure to toxic substances, dyes, or plants

Chemicals used in cleaning can cause contact dermatitis; excessive exposure to water can cause dry, cracked skin, soft nails, and damaged hair shafts; excessive heat in the home can dry skin and cause pruritus; infected kittens and puppies may lead to tinea capitis

Hobbies and Leisure Activities Gardening with exposure to chemicals, sunlight, contact dermatitis (e.g., poison ivy, poison oak), and insect bites; outdoor summer sports or activities increase sun and insect-bite exposure; outdoor winter activities increase frostbite and exposure; excessive exposure to chlorine and saltwater damages hair; excessive use of tanning salons may lead to skin carcinoma

Stress Skin eruptions such as eczema, urticaria, acne, and psoriasis may have a psychological component in some cases; body image disorder as a result of skin disease and hair loss

Economic Status Lower socioeconomic status may result in challenges with proper hygiene related to insufficient resources, which can lead to skin lesions, infestations associated with overcrowding, and infections associated with malnutrition

Ethnic Background

Scandinavian Psoriasis

Hispanics and Non-Hispanic Asians Lupus erythematosus

Tropical Areas Fungal infections related to increased heat and humidity

HEALTH MAINTENANCE ACTIVITIES

This information provides a bridge between health maintenance activities and the skin, hair, and nail function.

Sleep Sleep disturbances caused by symptoms such as itching or burning

Diet Allergies to food can cause skin eruptions such as urticaria; diets high in fat and cholesterol may be connected to the development of xanthelasmatous lesions; vitamin deficiencies result in skin, hair, and nail changes; see Chapter 7 for additional information

Exercise Increased risk for cutaneous trauma associated with contact sports and sun exposure with outdoor sports and activities

Use of Safety Devices Protective garments, hats, and sunblock with appropriate sun protection factor (SPF) to prevent ultraviolet exposure; lotions and creams to prevent drying and cracking of skin; protective gloves when handling harsh, irritating chemicals

Health Checkups Moles and birthmarks assessed for changes in size, shape, or color; skin lesions from sun exposure assessed

NURSING CHECKLIST

Specific Health History Questions Regarding the Skin, Hair, and Nails

Skin Care Habits

- Do you use lotions, perfumes, cologne, cosmetics, soaps, facial skin care products, oils, shaving cream, after-shave lotion, electric or standard razor?
- Do you use any home remedies for skin lesions and rashes?
- How often do you bathe or shower?
- Have you used or do you currently use a tanning bed?
- Have you ever had a reaction to jewelry?
- Do you wear hats, visors, gloves, long sleeves, pants, or sunscreen when in the sun?
- How much time do you spend in the sun?
- How often do you clean your electric razor?
- How often do you replace your standard razor?

Hair Care Habits

- Do you use shampoo, conditioner, hair spray, or other hair products?
- Do you color, dye, bleach, perm, or use relaxants on your hair?
- What products do you use?
- Do you wear a wig or hairpiece?
- Do you have hair extensions?
- Do you have graying hair or hair loss?
- Do you use a hair dryer, heated curlers, hair straightener, or curling iron?
- Do you wear hairstyles that pull on your scalp?

Nail Care Habits

- Do you get manicures or pedicures?
- How do you care for your nails? (trimming, use of polish/gels, acrylics, etc.)?
- Do you bite your nails?
- Do you suffer from nail splitting or discoloration?

NURSING CHECKLIST

General Approach to Skin, Hair, and Nails Examination

1. Observe standard precautions and don personal protective equipment such as gloves, gown, face shield, goggles, N-95 respirator or face mask if your client's status warrants these protective measures.
2. Ensure that the room is well-lit. Daylight is the best source of light, especially when determining skin color.
3. Use a hand-held magnifying glass to aid in inspection when simple visual inspection is not adequate.
4. Explain each step of the examination process to the client.
5. Ensure client privacy by providing drapes.
6. Ensure client comfort by keeping the room at an appropriate temperature.
7. Warm your hands by washing them in warm water before the examination.
8. Gather equipment on a table before initiating the examination.
9. Ask the client to undress completely and put on a client gown, leaving the back untied.
10. Perform the examination in a cephalocaudal fashion.
11. For episodic illness, the skin examination is incorporated into the regional physical examination.

NURSING TIP

Manicures and Pedicures

There is some risk of contracting hepatitis B, hepatitis C, and bacterial and fungal infections in commercial salons from manicures and pedicures if strict sterilization protocols are not followed (Yang et al, 2014). Advise your clients to verify that the facilities in which they obtain these types of cosmetic treatments sterilize the equipment between clients. Also, advise clients to bring their own equipment to be used during the manicures or pedicures.

NURSING TIP

Reducing Exposure to Integumentary Irritants

- In the workplace, always follow Occupational Safety and Health Administration (OSHA) and employer's safety guidelines.
- Follow the directions on the labels of all products; pay special attention to warning labels.
- If using a personal care product for the first time, perform a patch test to evaluate for sensitivity.
- Use gloves when handling toxins or caustic substances.
- Contact a poison control center for treatment guidelines if exposed to toxic or caustic substances.

Assessment in Brief

Skin, Hair, and Nails

Inspection of the Skin

- Color
- Bleeding, ecchymosis, and vascularity
- Lesions

Palpation of the Skin

- Moisture
- Temperature
- Tenderness
- Texture
- Turgor
- Edema

Inspection of the Hair

- Color
- Distribution
- Lesions

Palpation of the Hair

- Texture

Inspection of the Nails

- Color
- Shape and configuration

Palpation of the Nails

- Texture

Equipment

- Appropriate personal protective equipment
- Magnifying glass
- Good source of natural light
- Penlight
- Clean gloves
- Centimeter ruler

Examination of the Skin, Hair, and Nails

Inspection of the Skin

In each area, observe for color, bleeding, ecchymosis, vascularity, lesions, moisture, temperature, tenderness, texture, turgor, and edema.

> **NURSING TIP**
> **Wound Evaluation**
> If a wound is present, remove the dressing and assess the wound for location, color, drainage, odor, size, and depth. Measure the borders of the wound. Some electronic health record systems can incorporate photographs of the wound directly into the client's chart. This can be a helpful tool if different health care personnel examine the wound on different visits to determine whether the wound is healing.

E
1. Facing the client, inspect the color of the skin of the face, eyelids, ears, nose, lips, and mucous membranes.
2. Inspect the anterior and lateral aspects of the neck, then behind the ears.
3. Inspect arms and dorsal and palmar surfaces of the hands. Pay special attention to the webs between the fingers.
4. Have the client move to a supine position with the arms placed over the head.
5. Lower gown to uncover chest and breasts.
6. Inspect intramammary folds and ridges. Pendulous breasts may have to be raised to complete this inspection.
7. Examine axillae, and then cover chest and breasts with gown.
8. Raise gown to uncover abdomen and anterior aspect of the lower extremities; place a sheet over the genital area.
9. Inspect abdomen, anterior aspect of the lower extremities, dorsal and plantar surfaces of the feet, and toe webs.
10. Don gloves and uncover genital area.
11. Inspect inguinal folds and genitalia.
12. Cover genitalia and discard gloves.
13. Have the client turn to a side-lying position on the examination table so the client's back is facing you.
14. Inspect back and posterior neck and scalp. Specifically, look for nevi or other lesions.
15. Inspect posterior aspect of the lower extremities.
16. Don clean gloves and raise the gluteal cleft and inspect the gluteal folds and perianal area; then remove and discard the gloves.
17. Cover the client and assist back to a sitting position.
18. Wash hands.

Color

E Assess for coloration.

N **Normally, the skin is a uniform color depending on the client's exposure to sunlight which can cause increased pigmentation of sun-exposed areas. Freckling of the gums, tongue borders, and lining of the cheeks can be seen in people with darker-pigmented skin. Additionally, the gingiva may appear blue or variegated in color.**

A Lack of oxygenated blood can cause the skin to take on dusky blue undertones (cyanosis) or a gray hue (ashen). Central cyanosis in individuals with lighter skin tones will have a blue hue on the lips, oral mucosa, tongue, conjunctiva, and around the mouth. Individuals with darker skin tones will present with gray-blue hues to the conjunctiva, hard palate, and under the tongue. Cyanotic clients with darker skin tones may also present with hyperpigmentation around the mouth with the skin taking on a gray or pale gray hue. Skin with natural yellow undertones will have a greenish-gray hue with cyanosis. Peripheral cyanosis can be seen in the peripheral skin surfaces and nailbeds of individuals with lighter skin tones and on the palmar and plantar surfaces of individuals with darker skin tones.

P Cyanosis occurs when there is more than 5 g/dL of deoxygenated hemoglobin in the blood. For cyanosis to be an accurate indicator of arterial oxygen (PaO_2), two conditions must be met: The client must have normal hemoglobin and hematocrit as well as normal perfusion. For example, a client with **polycythemia** (elevated number of red

> **NURSING TIP**
> **Tattoos, Body Piercings, and Scarification**
> It is important to inspect the skin and note the presence and location of tattoos and body piercings. Some clients react to the ink used in tattoos and develop various skin disorders (Fig. 10-5A). Body piercing sites should be assessed for signs of allergic reactions or infection (e.g., erythema, purulent discharge, increased skin temperature). Remember to examine all body areas (Fig. 10-5B). The ears, eyebrows, lips, nares, tongue, nipples, umbilicus, and genitalia can be pierced. Scarification is the cutting, burning, or branding to create permanent scars on the skin (Fig. 10-5C). Complications can include infection and keloid formation. Document the location of all permanent body art.

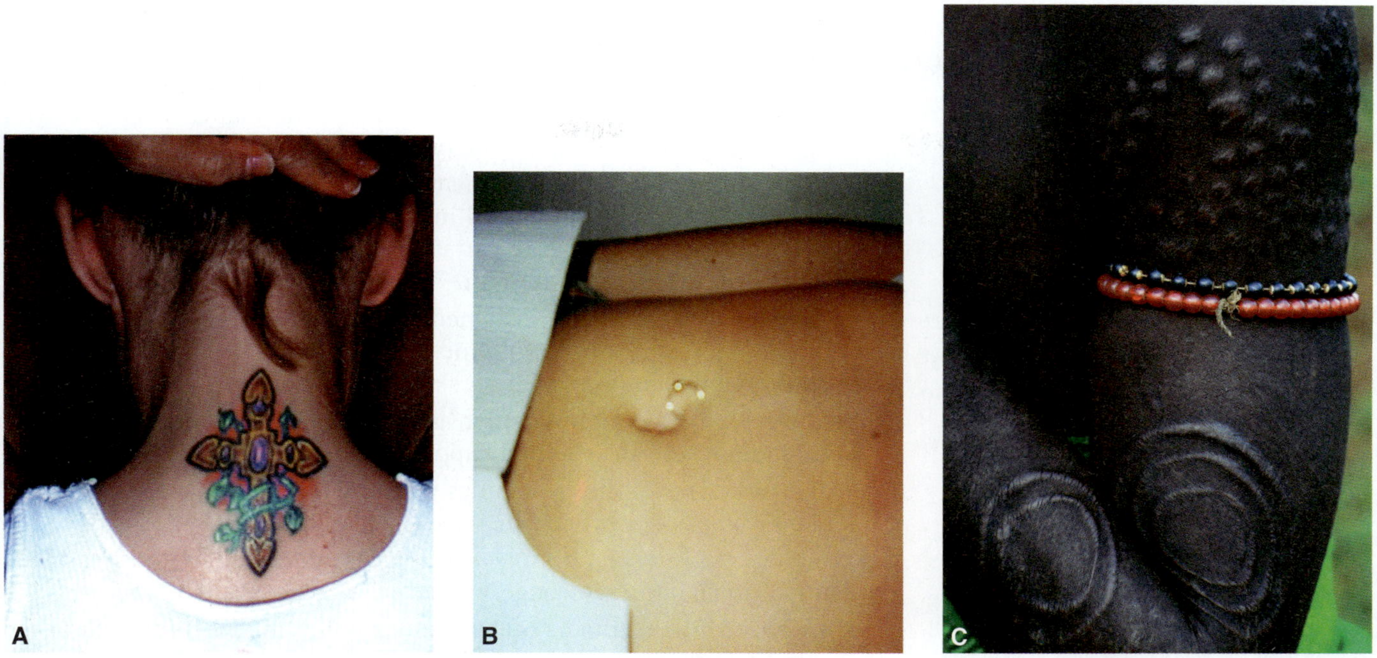

Figure 10-5 Tattoos, body piercings, and scarification. **A.** This client developed cellulitis from the tattoo ink. Note the erythematous areas in the upper half of the tattoo. **B.** Note the presence of all body piercings. Assess the skin at the pierced site. **C.** Scarification is the cutting, burning, or branding to create permanent scars on the skin.

blood cells) can be cyanotic but have adequate oxygenation. The problem lies in the fact that the client has too many red blood cells rather than too little oxygen. Conversely, a client with **anemia** (reduced number of red blood cells) can be hypoxemic but not cyanotic. In this case, the client has too little hemoglobin. Central cyanosis is secondary to marked heart and lung disease; peripheral cyanosis can be secondary to systemic disease, or vasoconstriction stimulated by cold temperatures or anxiety.

A The appearance of **jaundice** (yellow, yellow-green, to orange cast or coloration) of skin, sclera, mucous membranes, fingernails, and palmar or plantar surfaces in the lighter skin tones is abnormal (Fig. 10-6A). Jaundice presenting in darker skin tones may appear as a yellow hue in the sclera, hard palate, and palmar or plantar surfaces (Fig. 10-6B). Of note, yellowing of the sclera can occur naturally with the aging process in individuals with darker skin tones and should not be confused with jaundice.

P Jaundice is caused by an increased serum bilirubin level of greater than 2 mg/dL associated with liver disease or hemolytic disease. Severe burns and sepsis can also produce jaundice.

A A yellow discoloration of the palmar and digital creases is abnormal.

P Xanthoma striata palmaris is caused by hyperlipidemia.

A The orange-yellow coloration of palmar and plantar surfaces and forehead, but no involvement of the mucous membranes, is abnormal.

P **Carotenemia**, elevated levels of serum carotene, results from the excessive ingestion of carotene-rich foods such as carrots.

A A grayish cast to the skin is abnormal.

P A grayish cast is seen in clients with renal disorders and is associated with chronic anemia along with retained urochrome pigments. Slight jaundice may also be found in the renal client.

A Sustained bright red coloration (erythema) in lighter skin tones is abnormal. Darker skin tones may have no underlying change in coloration when erythema is present. Palpation may be used to ascertain signs of warmth, swelling, or induration. The blanch response with light finger pressure will not be present in darker skin tones.

P Hyperemia occurs because of dilated superficial blood vessels, increased blood flow, febrile states, local inflammatory conditions, or excessive alcohol intake. Higher concentration of melanin precludes the visualization of blanching of the skin.

A A bright red to ruddy, sustained appearance that is evident on the integument, mucous membranes, and palmar or plantar surfaces is abnormal in lighter and darker skin tones.

P Polycythemia, as noted earlier, is an increased number of red blood cells and results in this ruddy appearance.

A A dusky rubor of the extremities when in a dependent position, which can be associated with tissue necrosis, is abnormal.

P Venous stasis results from venule engorgement and diminished blood flow, which occurs in congestive heart failure and atherosclerosis.

A Localized skin erythema is abnormal. Erythema appears as pink or red skin in individuals with light skin. In those with darker skin tones, erythema appears as a purplish or a darker skin tone.

P Localized skin erythema can be caused by excessive sun exposure with insufficient or no sunscreen use to exposed areas. This is called sunburn. In addition, localized skin erythema can be caused by sun exposure that is enhanced when the client is taking certain medications. Fluoroquinolones, sulfonamides, tetracyclines, and nonsteroidal anti-inflammatories (NSAIDs) are frequently implicated (Fig. 10-6C). The extent of the erythema ranges from mild to severe. In more severe cases edema and blistering may be present.

A Red to violet or bluish areas on the fingers, toes, legs, or ears that erupt when exposed to cold or damp air is abnormal.

P A vasospasm disorder when exposed to cold or damp air is thought to be the cause of chilblains or pernio. Chilblains can also be associated with systemic diseases such as lupus.

A Pallor is abnormal and causes a pale cast to the skin most evident in the face, mucous membranes, lips, conjunctiva, and nailbeds in lighter skin tones. A gray-brown to ashen-gray cast to the skin, lips, mucous membranes, and conjunctiva is abnormal in darker skin tones. Skin with yellow undertones will have a pale gray or light greenish-gray hue when pallor is present.

P Pallor is due to decreased visibility of the normal oxyhemoglobin. This can occur when the client has decreased blood flow in the superficial vessels, as in shock or syncope, or when there is a decreased amount of serum oxyhemoglobin, as in anemia. Localized pallor may be secondary to arterial insufficiency.

A Hypopigmentation is abnormal and can affect the skin, hair, and eyebrows.

P Hypopigmentation is caused by **albinism**, a congenital inability to form melanin (Fig. 10-6D).

A **Vitiligo** is a condition marked by patchy, symmetrical areas of white on the skin and is abnormal (Fig. 10-6E).

P Vitiligo can be caused by an acquired loss of melanin. Trauma can also lead to hypopigmentation, especially in darker skin tones.

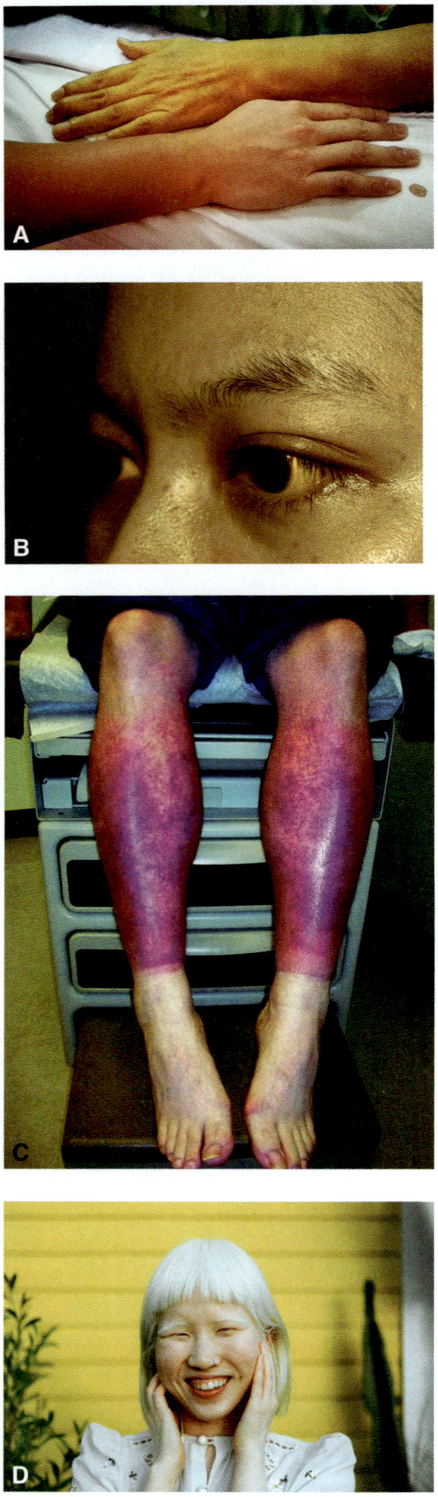

Figure 10-6 Skin color abnormalities. **A.** Note the jaundice in the light-skinned arm on top. **B.** Jaundice may be more prominent in the eyes of clients with darker skin tones. **C.** Note the erythema on the lower legs. **D.** Note the lack of coloration in this woman with albinism.

A Hyperpigmentation in the skin can be generalized or discrete.

P Hyperpigmentation can occur when there is a deposition of melanin, which can be caused by genetic predisposition, pregnancy, Addison disease (deficiency in cortisol leads to enhanced melanin production), café au lait spots (Fig. 10-6F and G), and sunlight.

P Acanthosis nigricans is a condition in which the skin becomes hyperpigmented and thicker, almost leathery in appearance (Fig. 10-6H). This usually occurs in the axillae, groin, neck, and around the umbilicus. Acanthosis nigricans occurs in obesity, diabetes mellitus, and with medications such as steroids.

Bleeding, Ecchymosis, and Vascularity

E Inspect the skin for evidence of bleeding, ecchymosis, or increased vascularity.

N **Normally, there are no areas of increased vascularity, ecchymosis, or bleeding.**

A Bleeding from the mucous membranes, previous venipuncture sites, or lesions should be considered abnormal.

P Spontaneous bleeding can be indicative of clotting disorders, trauma, or the use of anticoagulant medications such as apixaban, rivaroxaban, dabigatran, edoxaban, betrixaban, warfarin, enoxaparin, and heparin.

A **Petechiae** are violaceous (red-purple) discolorations of less than 0.5 cm in diameter (Fig. 10-7A). Petechiae do not blanch. Individuals with darker skin tones should be evaluated for petechiae in the mucous membranes, conjunctiva, and axillae.

P Petechiae can indicate an increased bleeding tendency or embolism; causes include intravascular defects or infections.

A **Purpura** is a condition characterized by the presence of confluent petechiae or confluent ecchymosis over any part of the body (Fig. 10-7B).

P Purpura or peliosis is characterized by hemorrhage into the skin and can be caused by decreased platelet formation. Lesions vary based on the type of purpura; pigmentation changes may become permanent.

A **Ecchymosis** is a violaceous discoloration of varying size, also called a black-and-blue mark (Fig. 10-7C). Dark skin tones can present as areas of hyperpigmentation.

P Ecchymosis is caused by the extravasation of blood into the skin as a result of trauma and can also occur with anticoagulant use or liver dysfunction.

A A localized mass of blood is a hematoma (Fig. 10-7D).

NURSING TIP
Signs of Abuse

Areas of ecchymosis are often signs of trauma that could be the result of physical abuse. Ecchymotic areas at the base of the skull or on the face, buttocks, breasts, or abdomen should warrant a high index of suspicion for abuse, especially if found in children or pregnant clients, as should burns (e.g., cigarettes, iron) and belt buckle or bite marks. In addition, lacerations, scars, hematomas, and puncture wounds should carry a high index of suspicion. Patterned injuries, such as those caused by ropes or chains, should be noted.

Signs of physical abuse can also be present in the hair. Hair that is singed or unusually kinked may have been exposed to fire. Alopecia can be caused by repeated pulling. Any signs of abuse should be investigated further and referred as necessary.

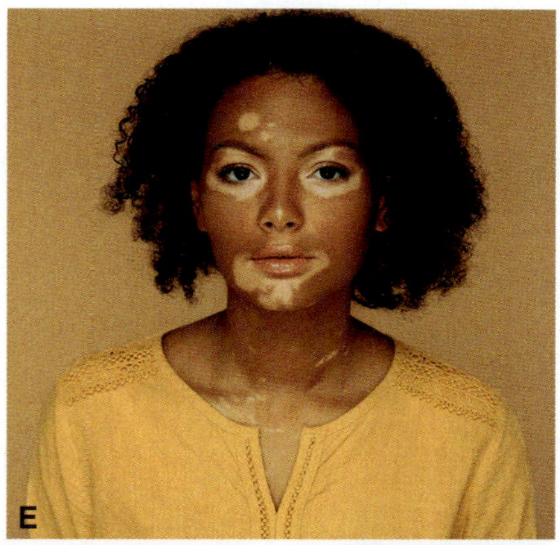

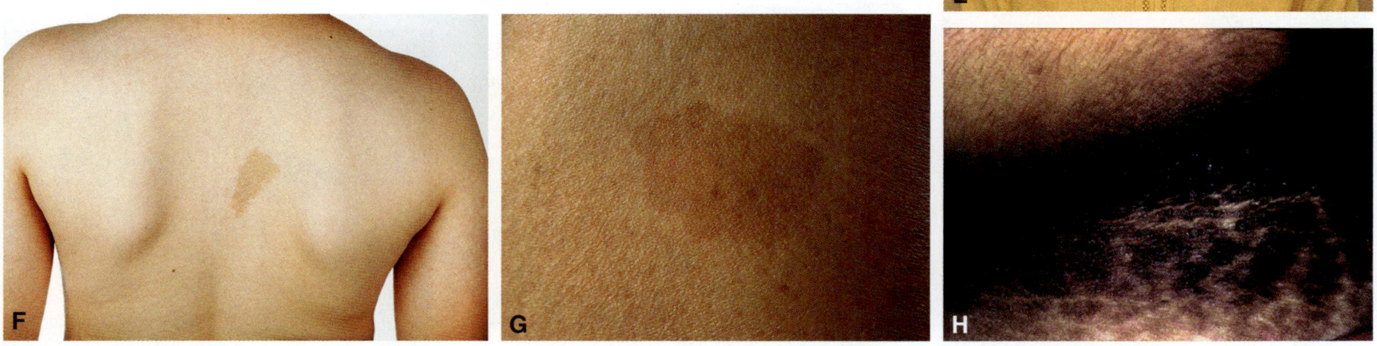

Figure 10-6—cont'd E. Vitiligo. **F.** Café au lait spot in client with lighter skin. **G.** Café au lait spot in client with darker skin. **H.** Acanthosis nigricans.

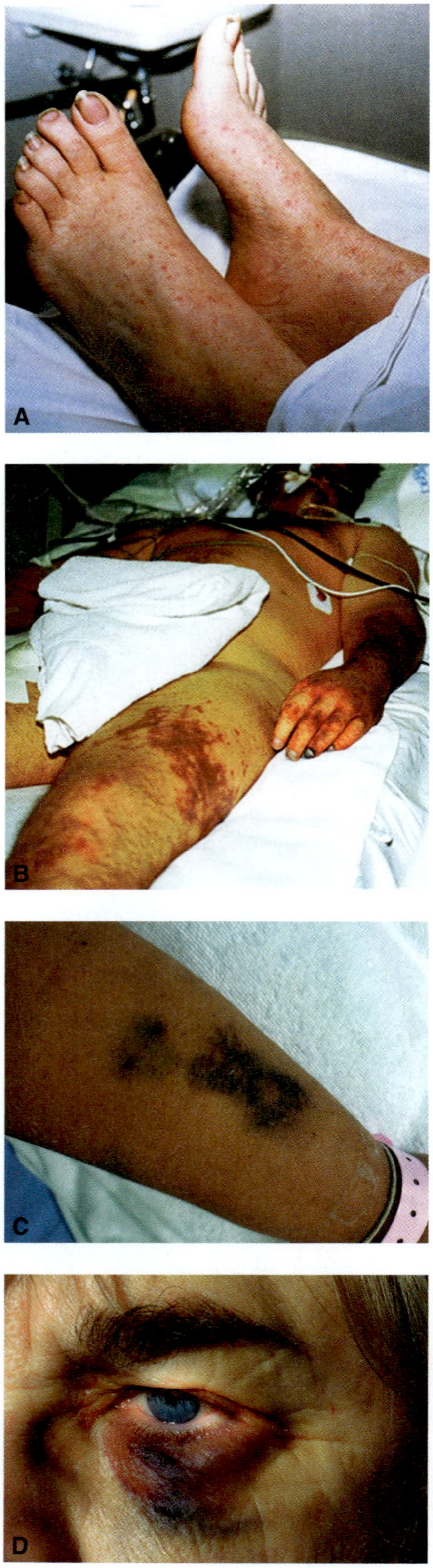

P A hematoma is caused by disease, injury, or trauma to blood vessels where blood extravasates into the surrounding tissue. A hematoma varies in size and occurs both internally and externally.

A An erythematous dilation of small blood vessels is a telangiectasia (Fig. 10-7E).

P A telangiectasia tends to appear on the face and thighs and occurs more frequently in females, such as in rosacea.

A **Spider angiomas** are bright red and star-shaped (Fig. 10-7F). A central pulsation is often noted with pressure, and this pressure results in blanching in the extensions. Most often, these lesions are noted on the face, neck, and chest. They are a type of telangiectasia.

P Causes of spider angiomas include pregnancy, liver disease, and hormone therapy. They are normal in a small percentage of the population and are more prevalent in females.

A **Venous stars** are linear or irregularly shaped, blue vascular patterns that do not blanch with pressure (Fig. 10-7G). These are often noted on the legs near veins or on the anterior chest.

P Venous stars are caused by increased venous pressure in the superficial veins.

A **Cherry angiomas** are bright red, circumscribed areas that may darken with age (Fig. 10-7H). They can be flat or raised and may show partial blanching with pressure. Most often, they are found on the trunk.

P Cherry angiomas are of unknown etiology and are pathologically insignificant except for cosmetic appearance.

A A bright red, raised area that has well-defined borders and does not blanch with pressure describes a strawberry hemangioma (Fig. 10-7I).

P Strawberry hemangiomas, or strawberry marks, are congenital malformations of closely packed, immature capillaries. A strawberry hemangioma is also known as nevus vascularis. They regress as the child grows and are usually gone in a few years.

A A burgundy, red, or violaceous macular/vascular patch that is located along the course of a peripheral nerve is abnormal (Fig. 10-7J).

P This macular/vascular patch is a port-wine stain, or nevus flammeus. The port-wine stain is composed of mature, but thin-walled, capillaries. The lesion is usually present at birth and is frequently located on the face. A port-wine stain can be indicative of underlying disorders, such as Sturge-Weber syndrome.

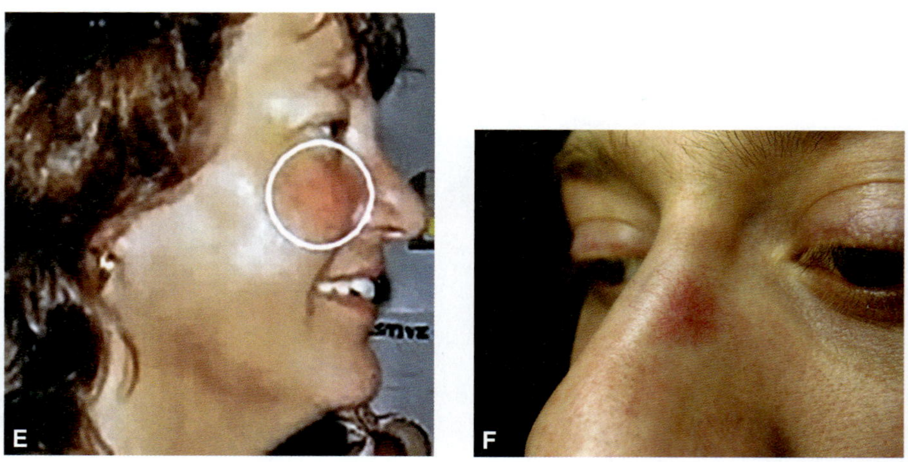

Figure 10-7 Bleeding, ecchymosis, and vascular abnormalities of the skin. **A.** Petechiae. **B.** Purpura. **C.** Ecchymosis. **D.** Hematoma. **E.** Telangiectasia. **F.** Spider angioma.

E Examination N Normal Findings A Abnormal Findings P Pathophysiology

A In lighter skin tones, a purple-to-black discoloration is abnormal (Fig. 10-7K). In darker skin tones, hyperpigmentation is abnormal.

P These findings can indicate different stages of necrosis, or tissue death. Conditions that starve the affected body part of oxygen, whether in acute or chronic situations, can cause necrosis. Diabetes mellitus, disseminated intravascular coagulation, acute hypovolemia, and severe electric charge are some of the conditions that can cause necrosis.

A Dark brown or blackened areas of skin that are edematous and painful are abnormal (Fig. 10-7L). These areas may drain a thin liquid that has a sweet, foul odor. Crepitus may be palpated in the affected areas.

P Gas gangrene, or clostridial myonecrosis, is a gram-positive infection affecting skeletal muscles that have decreased oxygenation. The *Clostridia* organisms are endogenous to the gastrointestinal tract and are also found in the soil. Clients who experience circulatory compromise, such as in diabetes mellitus, arterial insufficiency, trauma, and constricting casts, are at risk for developing gas gangrene. Clients who have contaminated wounds and decreased vascularity in the affected area are also at risk for developing gas gangrene.

NURSING TIP

Enhancement Techniques

Magnification: Use of a magnifying glass may be beneficial in the evaluation of lesions and discolorations for morphology.

Wood's Lamp: Also known as an ultraviolet light, this tool is valuable in the diagnosis of certain skin and hair diseases. Dermatophytosis and erythrasma are easily diagnosed by the fluorescent changes that occur under ultraviolet exposure. Dermatophytosis in the hair shaft will appear green to yellow, and erythrasma will appear coral red.

Diascopy: Consists of pressing a microscope slide over a skin lesion. Diascopy is useful in determining whether a red lesion's coloration is due to erythema, which will blanch, or extravasation of blood, which will not blanch. Diascopy can also be useful in the detection of the glassy, yellow-brown appearance of papules found in tuberculosis of the skin, lymphoma, and sarcoidosis.

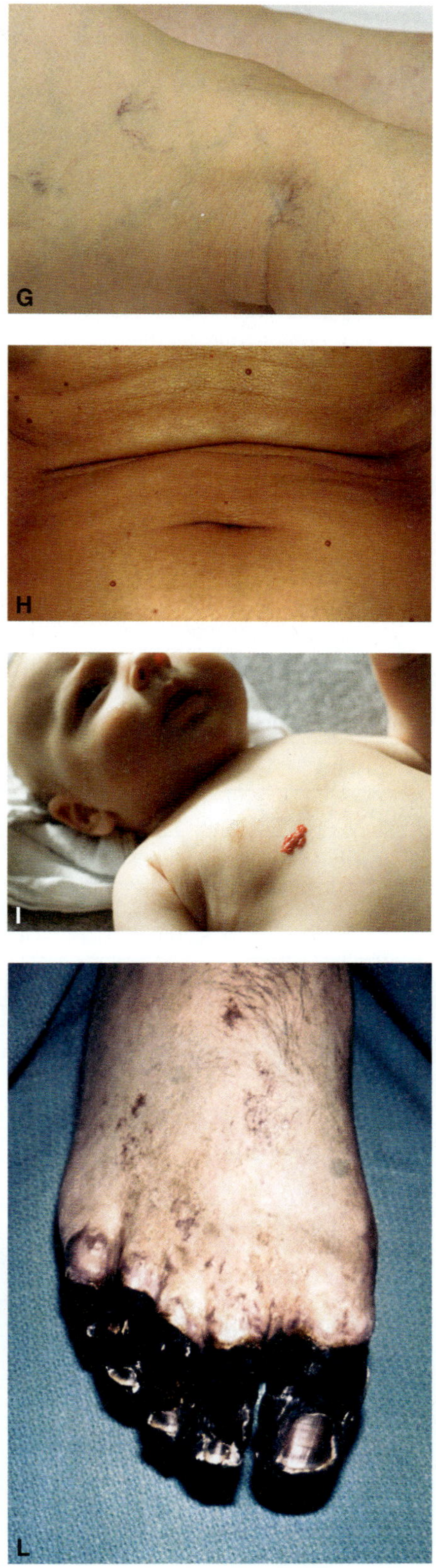

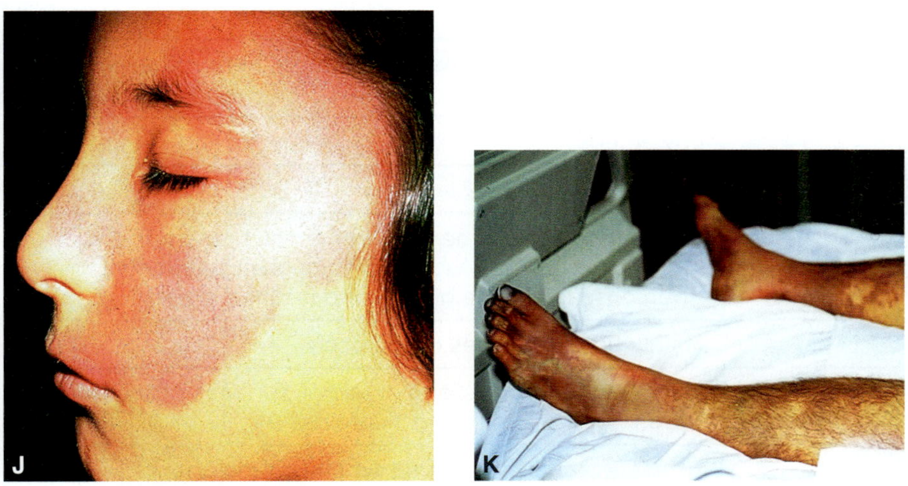

Figure 10-7—cont'd G. Venous star. **H.** Cherry angioma. **I.** Strawberry hemangioma. **J.** Nevus flammeus. **K.** Necrosis. **L.** Gangrene.

Lesions

E

1. Inspect the skin for lesions, noting the anatomic location. Lesions can be localized, regionalized, or generalized (Table 10-1). They can involve exposed areas or skinfolds. A magnifying glass can be used to better visualize a lesion.
2. Note the grouping or arrangement of the lesions: discrete, grouped, confluent, linear, annular, polycyclic, generalized, or zosteriform (Fig. 10-8).
3. Inspect the lesions for elevation (flat or raised).
4. Using a ruler, measure the lesions.
5. Describe the color of the lesions.
6. Note any exudate for color or odor.
7. Note the morphology of the skin lesions. Skin lesions can be primary, originating from previously normal skin, or secondary, originating from primary lesions. For specific descriptions of primary lesion morphology, see Figure 10-9. For specific descriptions of secondary lesion morphology, refer to Figure 10-10.

N

No skin lesions should be present except for freckles, birthmarks, or moles (nevi), which may be flat or elevated.

Table 10-1 Anatomic Locations of Various Skin Lesions

Lesion	Location
Basal cell carcinoma	Medial and lateral canthi and nasolabial fold
Rosacea	Face
Acne vulgaris	Face, back, shoulders, chest
Furuncle	Nose, neck, face, axillae, and buttocks
Lesions resulting from light exposure (squamous cell carcinoma, solar lentigo, solar keratosis)	Forehead, cheeks, tops of the ears, neck, dorsal surface of hands and forearms, and lateral arms
Seborrheic keratosis, spider angioma	Face, trunk, and upper extremities
Impetigo, verruca vulgaris (warts)	Arms, legs, buttocks, face, hands, fingers, and knees
Herpes zoster	Along the cutaneous spinal nerve roots, almost always unilateral
Kaposi sarcoma	Widespread: trunk, head, tip of nose, periorbital, penis, legs, palms, and soles
Erythema nodosum	Lower legs
Stasis dermatitis	Sock area
Cutaneous moniliasis	Moist folds behind the ears, under the breasts, in the axilla, umbilicus, along the inguinal and pudendal regions, and in the gluteal and perineal areas
Adult atopic eczema	Mainly flexor surfaces of the body
Psoriasis	Mainly scalp, elbows, and extensor surfaces of the body (rarely on the face and skinfolds)
Contact dermatitis	Affects surfaces in contact with irritating agents
Pediculosis pubis	Pubic and axillary areas

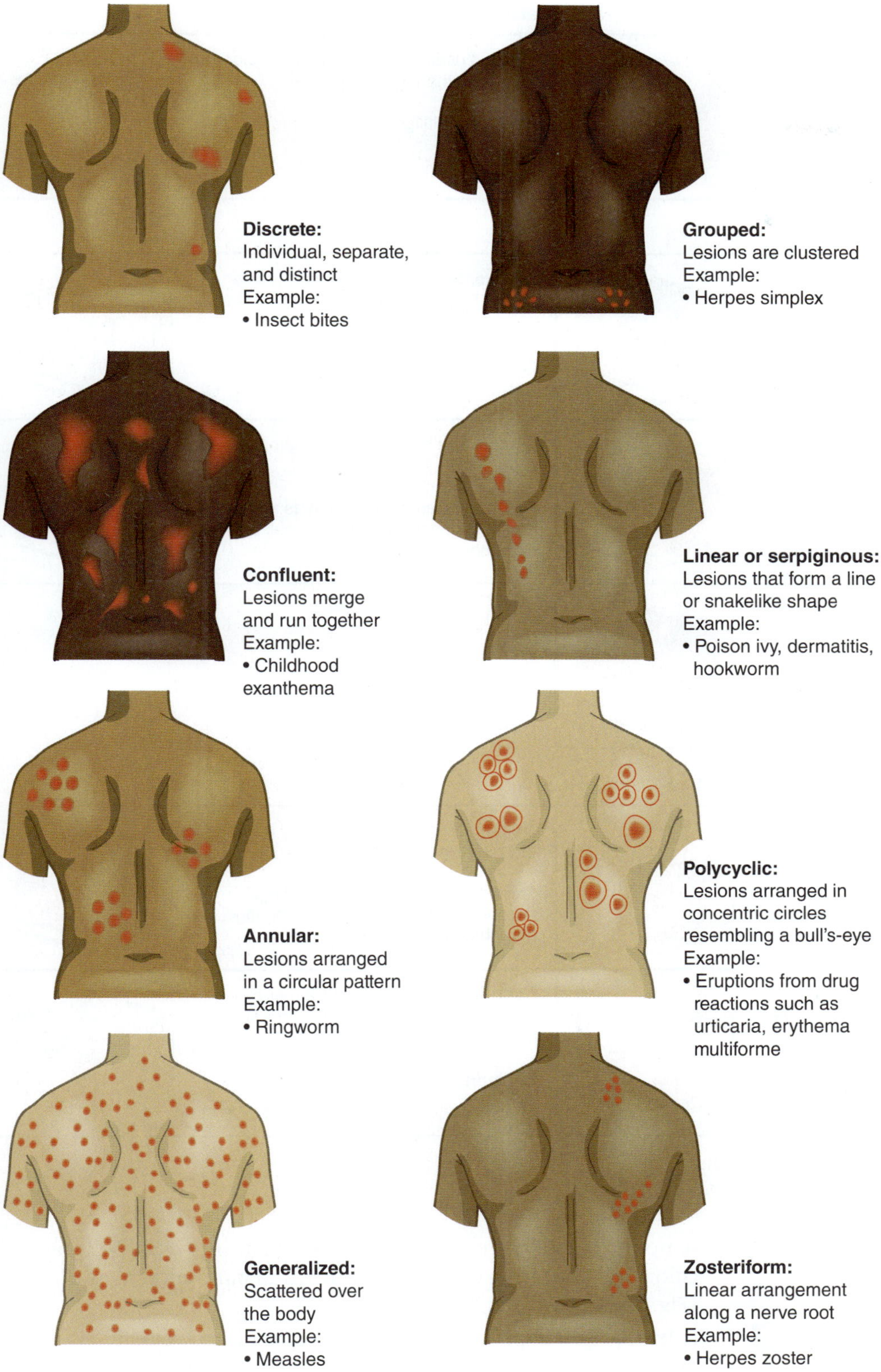

Figure 10-8 Arrangement of lesions.

Nonpalpable

Macule: Localized change in skin color of less than 1 cm in diameter

Example: Freckle

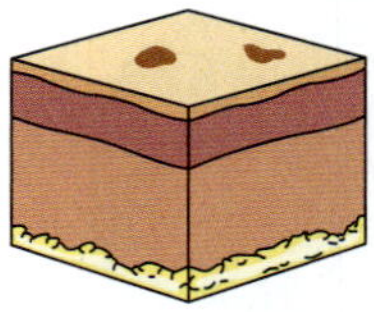

Patch: Localized change in skin color of greater than 1 cm in diameter

Example: Vitiligo, stage 1 of pressure ulcer

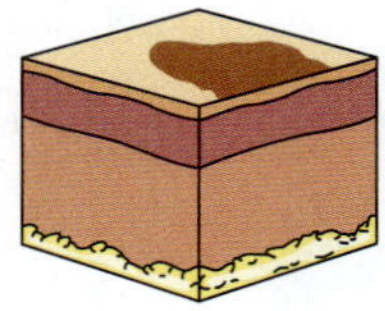

Palpable

Papule: Solid, elevated lesion less than 0.5 cm in diameter

Example: Wart, elevated nevi, seborrheic keratosis

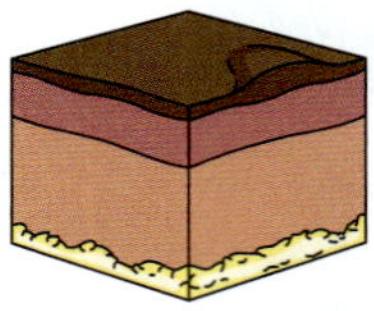

Plaque: Solid, elevated lesion greater than 0.5 cm in diameter

Example: Psoriasis, eczema, pityriasis rosea

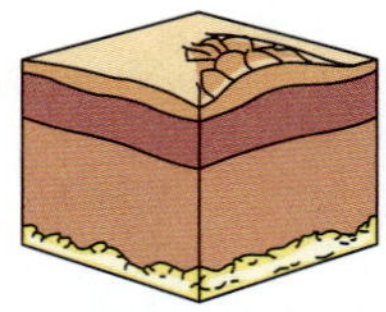

Nodule: Solid and elevated; however, can extend deeper than papules into the dermis or subcutaneous tissues, 0.5–2.0 cm

Example: Lipoma, erythema nodosum, cyst, melanoma, hemangioma

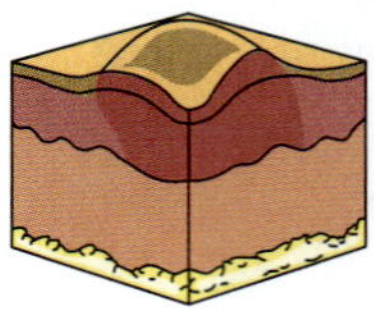

Tumor: The same as a nodule only greater than 2 cm

Example: Carcinoma (such as advanced breast carcinoma); **not** basal cell or squamous cell of the skin

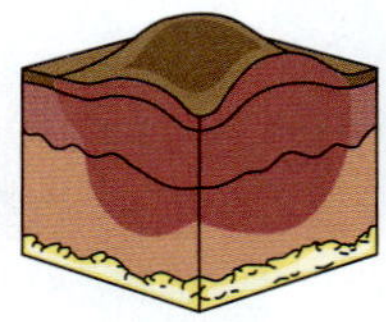

Wheal: Localized edema in the epidermis causing irregular elevation that may be red or pale

Example: Insect bite, hive, angioedema

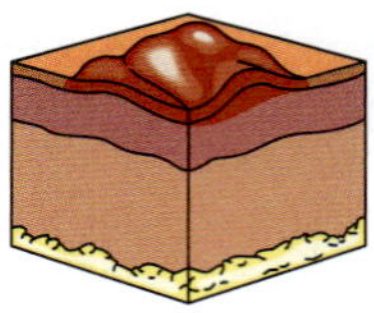

Fluid-Filled Cavities Within the Skin

Vesicle: Accumulation of fluid between the upper layers of the skin; elevated mass containing serous fluid; less than 0.5 cm

Example: Herpes simplex, herpes zoster, chickenpox, scabies

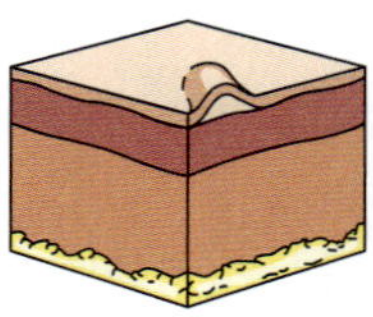

Bullae: Same as a vesicle only greater than 0.5 cm

Example: Contact dermatitis, large second-degree burn, bullous impetigo, pemphigus

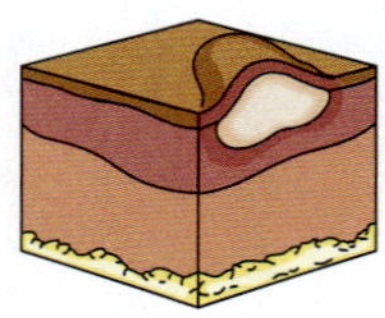

Pustule: Vesicles or bullae that become filled with pus, usually described as less than 0.5 cm in diameter

Example: Acne, impetigo, furuncle, carbuncle, folliculitis

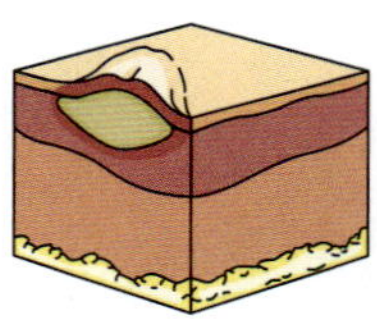

Cyst: Encapsulated fluid-filled or a semi-solid mass in the subcutaneous tissue or dermis

Example: Sebaceous cyst, epidermoid cyst

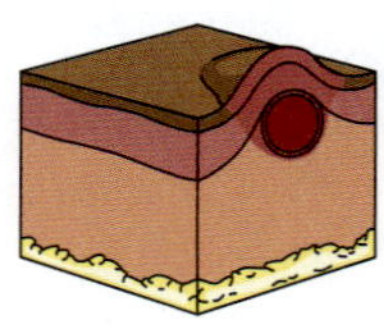

Figure 10-9 Morphology of primary lesions.

A A nonpalpable lesion that is less than 2 cm in size, light brown in color, and appearing on the face, arms, and hands describes a lentigo (Fig. 10-11A).

P A lentigo is a hyperpigmented lesion that occurs in body areas that are exposed to the sun. A lentigo can increase in size as the client ages.

A Intertriginous exudative patches that are beefy red in color, well-demarcated, pruritic, and erythematous are abnormal (Fig. 10-11B).

P Candidiasis, also known as moniliasis, is a yeast infection that may invade numerous areas of the body but normally occurs in the axillae, inframammary areas, groin, and gluteal regions.

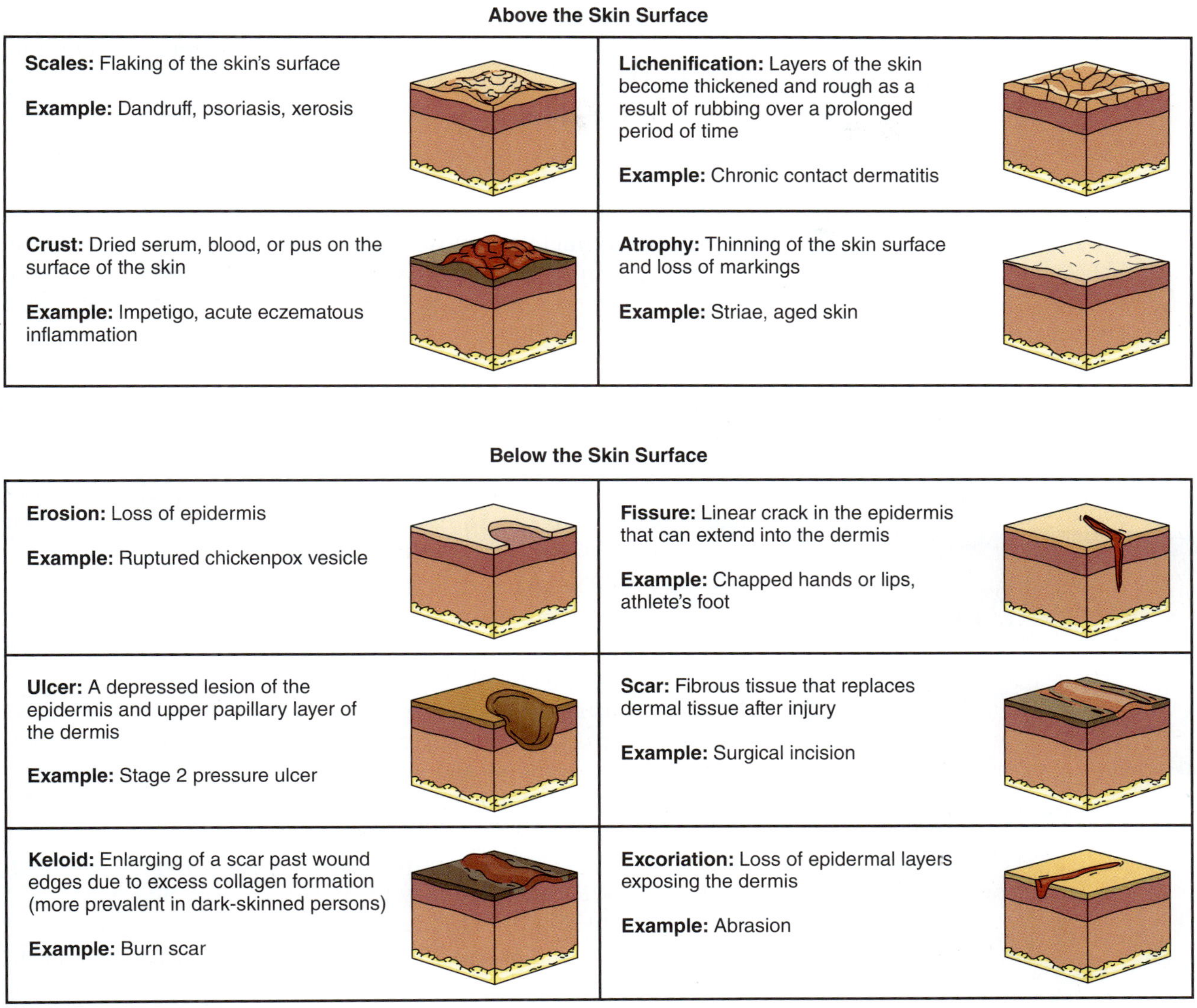

Figure 10-10 Morphology of secondary lesions.

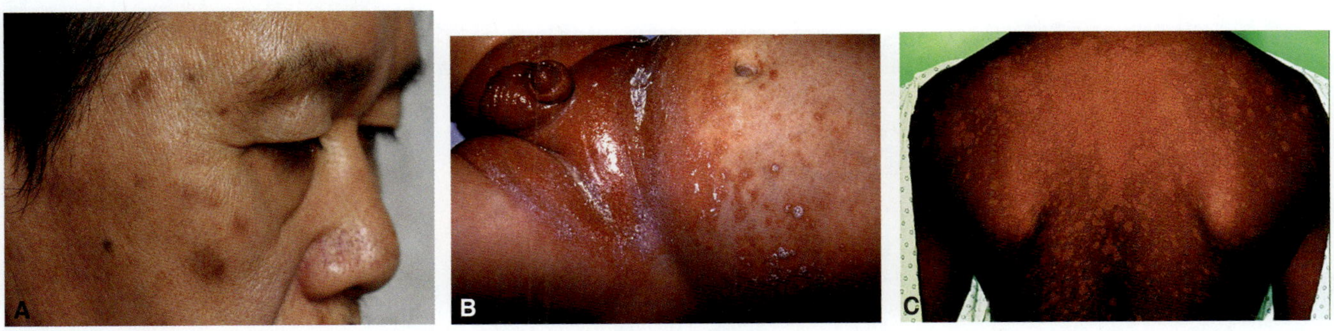

Figure 10-11 Common skin lesions. **A.** Lentigo. **B.** Candidiasis. **C.** Tinea versicolor.

A Scaly macular patches of white, reddish-brown, or tan hyperpigmentation, or hypopigmentation, of the skin are abnormal (Fig. 10-11C).

P Scaly macular patches of white, reddish-brown, or tan hyperpigmentation or hypopigmentation occur in tinea versicolor, which is caused by superficial fungal infections. The lesions usually occur on the trunk and proximal extremities.

A A pink-to-red papulosquamous annular lesion with raised borders that expands peripherally and has a clearing center is abnormal (Fig. 10-11D).

P Tinea corporis is caused by *Trichophyton,* a dermatophyte (fungal) infection.

A Toe web lesions that are macerated and have scaling borders are abnormal (Fig. 10-11E).

P Tinea pedis (athlete's foot) is very common and often erupts in the third and fourth interdigital spaces; with time, the lesions will spread over the plantar surface. Tinea pedis is caused by *Trichophyton mentagrophytes.*

A A slightly erythematous, rose- or fawn-colored, round or oval patch that may have slightly raised borders is abnormal (Fig. 10-11F).

P A herald patch is normally found on the trunk and is indicative of pityriasis rosea. This benign, self-limiting condition is often seen in young adults and may resemble ringworm. The herald patch is normally followed in 5 to 10 days by a generalized eruption of similar lesions. The etiology is thought to be viral.

A Vesicles or bullae that measure 1 to 2 cm and become pustular and rupture easily, discharging straw-colored fluid, are abnormal. The purulent drainage becomes thick as it dries, producing light brown or golden-honey–colored crusts (Fig. 10-11G).

P Impetigo is usually caused by group A streptococcus or *Staphylococcus aureus* and is highly contagious. It is typically found in preschoolers in the late summer and can be associated with poor hygiene, crowding, contact sports, and minor skin trauma that is untreated.

A Red, shiny, indurated (with a peau d'orange appearance), and warm edematous lesions are abnormal. These lesions may be elevated, have defined margins, and may be painful. Vesicles and bullae may also be present (Fig. 10-11H).

P Erysipelas is a type of superficial cellulitis that is usually found in older adults and young children. Erysipelas can originate in cuts or incisions infected by group A streptococcus either from the client's

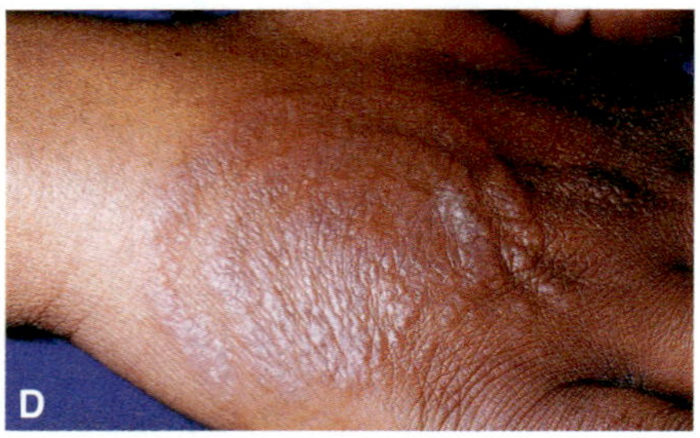

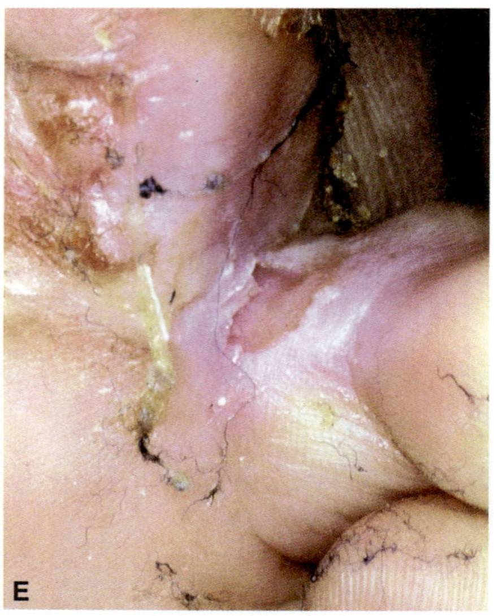

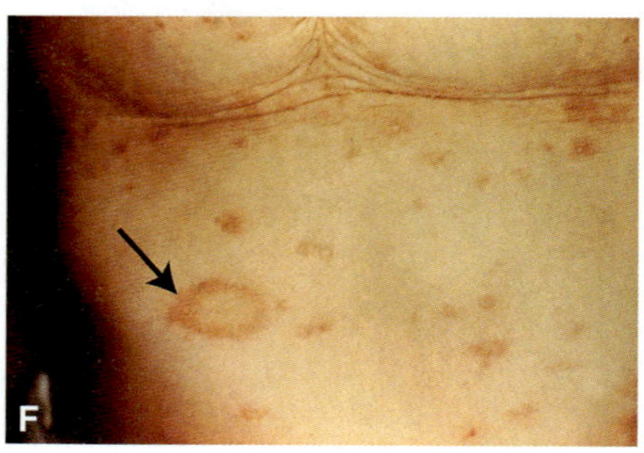

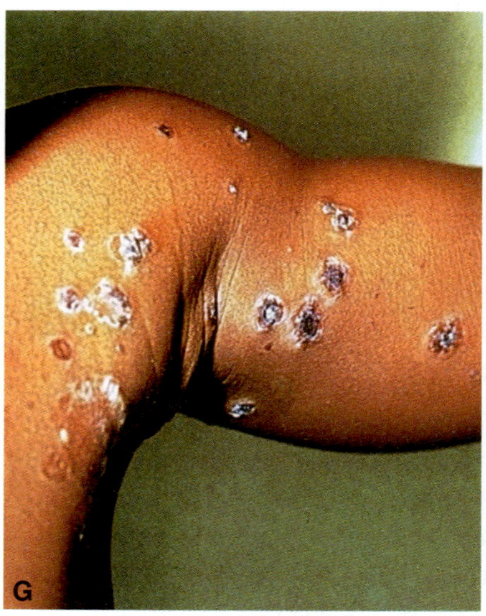

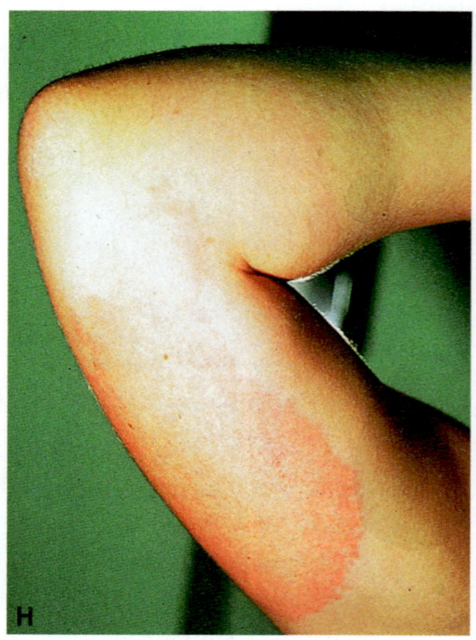

Figure 10-11—cont'd D. Tinea corporis. **E.** Tinea pedis. **F.** Herald patch of pityriasis rosea. **G.** Impetigo. **H.** Erysipelas.

respiratory tract or the respiratory tract of someone who was in close contact with the client.

A A diffuse red area that is warm, edematous, painful, and indurated is abnormal (Fig. 10-11I).

P A diffuse red area that is warm, edematous, painful, and indurated suggests cellulitis, an acute bacterial infection (usually staphylococcal or streptococcal) of the skin and subcutaneous tissues. Cellulitis can result from trauma to the skin, foreign bodies in the skin, and underlying infection.

A A lesion that starts as a tender, deep red papule and develops into a well-defined, erythematous, and painful mass with purulent material (Fig. 10-11J) is abnormal.

P A furuncle, commonly called a boil, can be a firm or fluctuant lesion and is usually caused by a staphylococci infection.

A A flat or raised lesion with a black interior is abnormal.

P A comedo, or blackhead, is usually seen on the face, chest, shoulders, or back (Fig. 10-11K). Comedones are due to increased keratinization in the hair follicle from an unknown etiology. They are associated with acne.

A Comedones accompanied by pustules (with yellow or white centers), red papules (Fig. 10-11L), nodules, and cysts are abnormal.

P Acne vulgaris usually occurs in the middle to late teen years and is caused by an inflammation of the sebaceous follicles. Acne vulgaris is associated with hormonal changes. It can be located on the face, chest, shoulders, and back. Lesions that appear punched out may be present from scarring of previously active acne lesions (Fig. 10-11M).

A Redness, with dilation of the blood vessels on the cheeks and forehead, and acne are abnormal (Fig. 10-11N).

P Acne rosacea is a chronic inflammation seen primarily in middle-aged and older adults. The cause is unknown, although it is aggravated by alcohol, spicy food, hot liquids, sunlight, extremes in temperature, exercise, and stress.

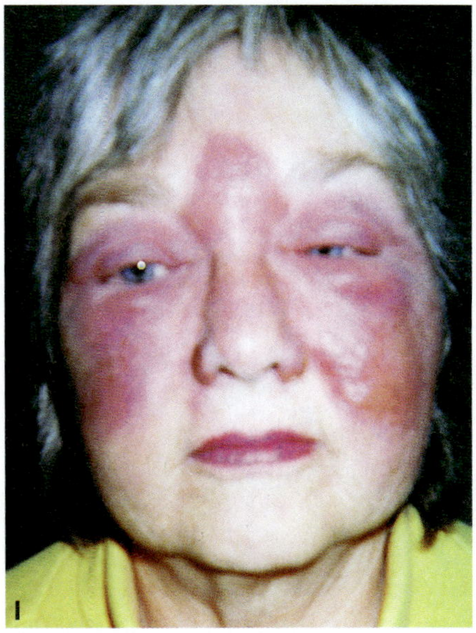

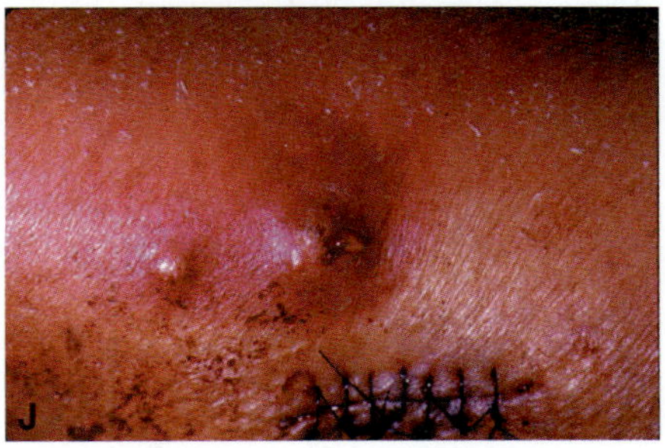

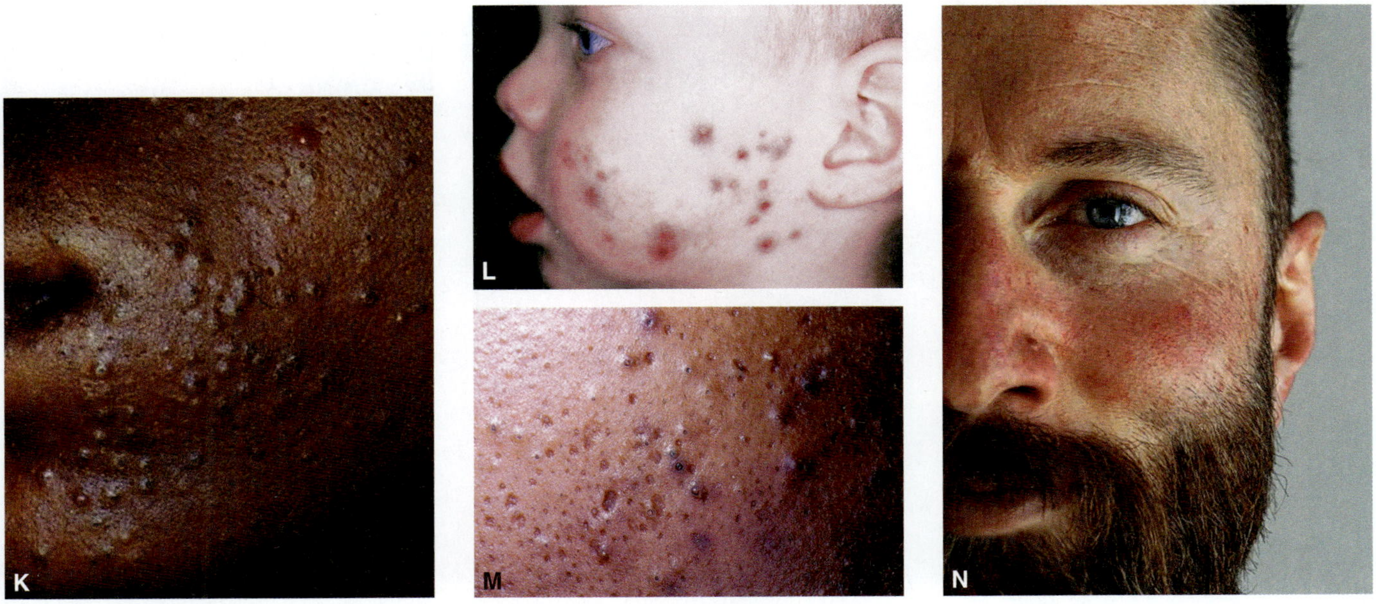

Figure 10-11—cont'd I. Cellulitis. **J.** Furuncle. **K.** Comedomes. **L.** Acne papules and nodules. **M.** Acne scarring. **N.** Acne rosacea.

A Rosacea that is red or purple on the lower nose and is accompanied by thickening of the affected skin and enlargement of the follicular orifices is abnormal (Fig. 10-11O).

P Rosacea that affects the nose is called rosacea rhinophyma. The pathophysiology is the same as for rosacea.

A An erythematous, confluent eruption in a butterfly-like distribution over the face is abnormal (Fig. 10-11P).

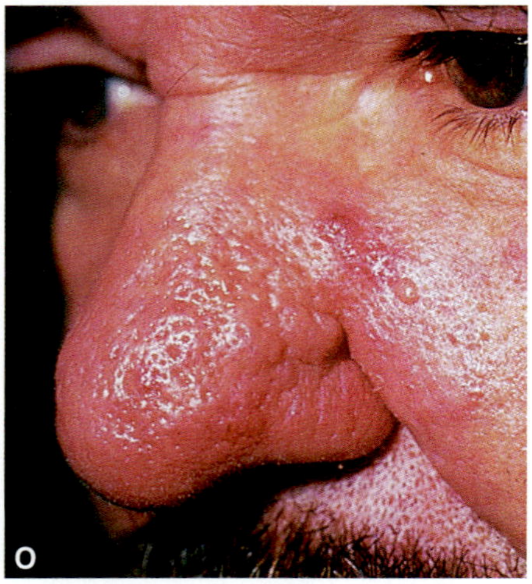

P Systemic lupus erythematosus, an autoimmune connective tissue disorder, is the most likely etiology.

A Reddish-salmon–colored macular lesions as well as elevated purple to brown lesions (in lighter skin tones) and bluish lesions (in darker skin tones) that are spongy, painful, and pruritic are abnormal (Fig. 10-11Q).

P These abnormal findings are typical lesions of Kaposi sarcoma. The reddish-salmon lesions are early findings, and the purplish or bluish lesions are more advanced. Kaposi sarcoma is a neoplastic disorder that is thought to have a genetic, hormonal, and viral etiology. It is frequently found in clients infected with HIV, immunocompromised clients, and older adults.

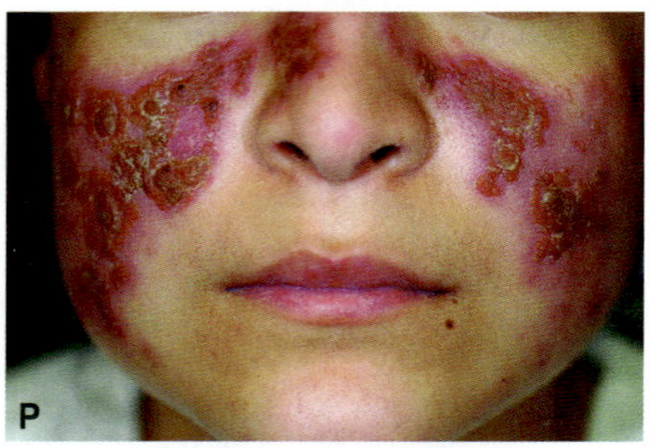

A Pruritic, silvery scales of the epidermis that have clearly demarcated borders and underlying erythema are abnormal. These lesions are circular and are found primarily on the elbows, knees, and behind the ears (Fig. 10-11R).

P The etiology of psoriasis is unknown, but it has a genetic component and may be aggravated by cold weather, trauma, and infection. On rare occasions, psoriasis can progress to pustular psoriasis (Fig. 10-11S). Erythema develops throughout the body, especially in flexural areas. Pustules develop over the erythema and can easily rupture. The client is often febrile. Death can ensue from sepsis.

A A chronic, pruritic rash with red, oozing, crusted lesions on dry skin is abnormal (Fig. 10-11T). In dark-skinned clients the lesions may appear as papules.

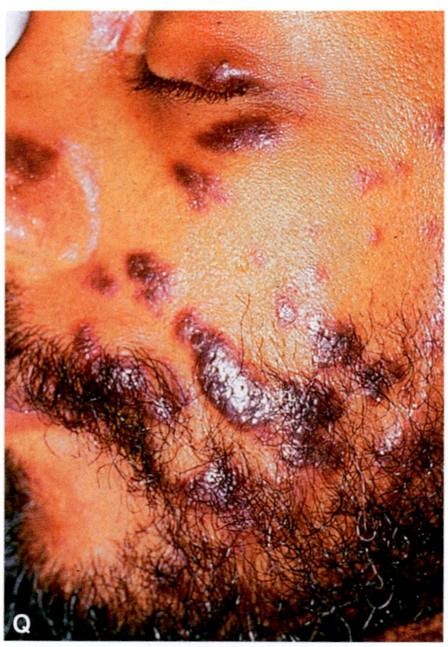

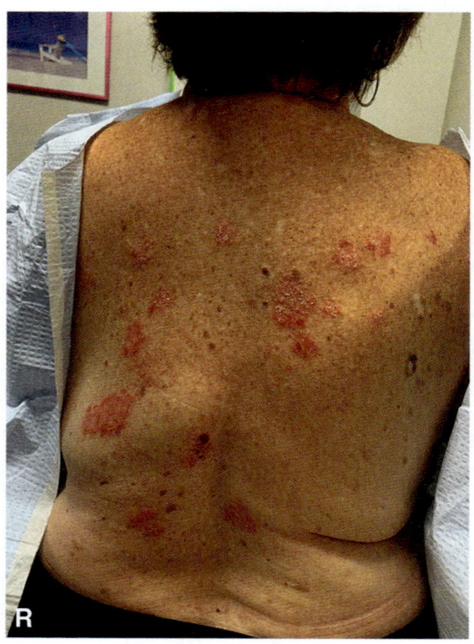

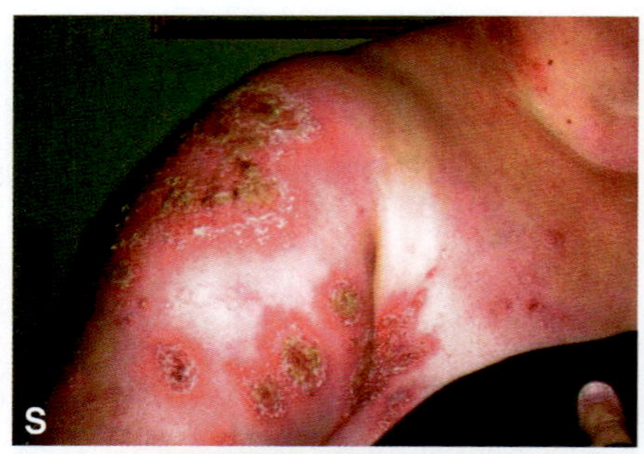

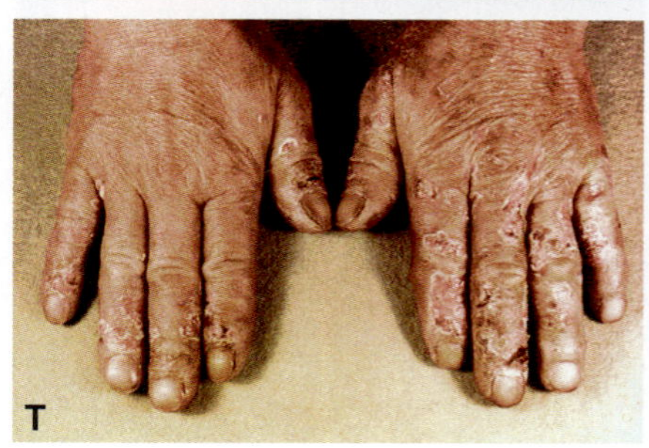

Figure 10-11—cont'd O. Rosacea rhinophyma. **P.** Facial butterfly rash of systemic lupus erythematosus. Note the severe inflammation of lesions with crusting. **Q.** Kaposi sarcoma. **R.** Psoriasis. **S.** Pustular psoriasis. **T.** Eczema.

P Eczema, also known as atopic dermatitis, is a multifaceted disease process that is often associated with asthma and allergic rhinitis. The etiology is unknown, and a family history of related disorders is usually noted.

A It is abnormal to have edema and erythema along with red, pruritic vesicles that may discharge an exudate that leads to crusting (Fig. 10-11U).

P Edema and erythema along with red, pruritic vesicles that may discharge an exudate that leads to crusting describes allergic contact dermatitis. The client must come into direct contact with an irritant/allergen to develop allergic contact dermatitis. In Figure 10-11U, the client reacted to an allergen in a hat. Allergic contact dermatitis can be caused by plants (such as poison oak/ivy), metals such as nickel, detergents, cosmetics, rubber, topical medications, food, shampoo, hair dye, and clothing.

A Red, pruritic papules or vesicles with S-shaped or straight-line burrows are abnormal (Fig. 10-11V). These lesions can be intensely pruritic.

P Scabies is caused by the *Sarcoptes scabiei* mite and may be visible as a small, dark area within the vesicle. It is highly contagious and can sometimes be spread through infected clothing or bedding.

A Red macular and papular lesions that are intensely pruritic are abnormal (Fig. 10-11W).

P Varicella, or chickenpox, usually starts on the trunk and proceeds to the extremities. Papules progress to thin-walled vesicles, pustules, and crusts. The client may exhibit all of the different lesions simultaneously. Varicella is caused by the varicella-zoster virus, which is highly contagious, especially in children.

A Red papules, crusting on the face (Fig. 10-11X), vesicles (Fig. 10-11Y), and open sores in the mouth or on the genitalia are abnormal.

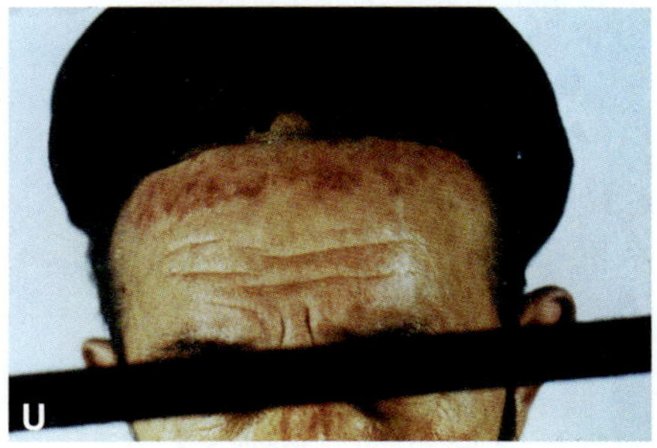

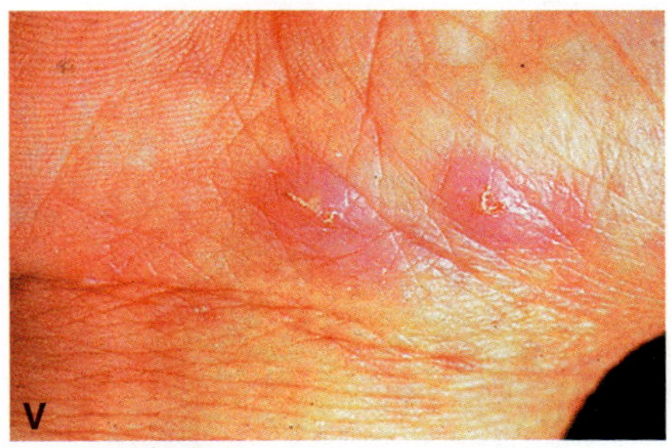

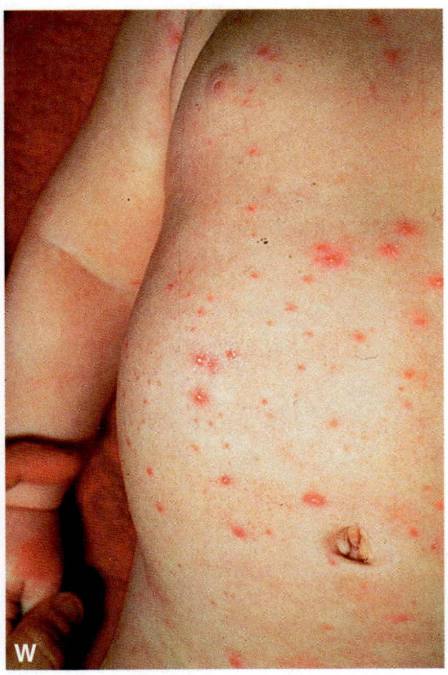

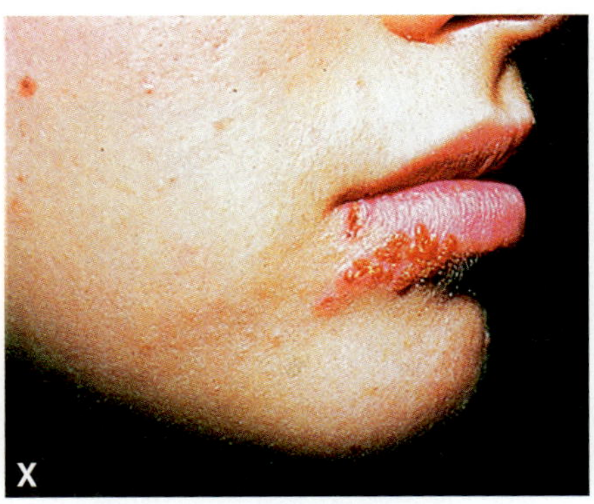

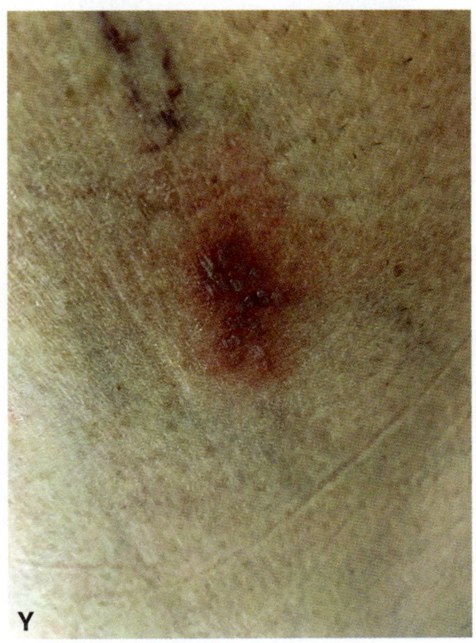

Figure 10-11—cont'd U. Allergic contact dermatitis. **V.** Scabies. **W.** Varicella. **X.** Herpes simplex virus. **Y.** Herpes simplex virus I.

P Herpes simplex virus I is usually responsible for these lesions, which are most common on the face and in the mouth. After the initial exposure, the client can often predict an outbreak because of the presence of numbness, burning, itching, or soreness at the eruption site.

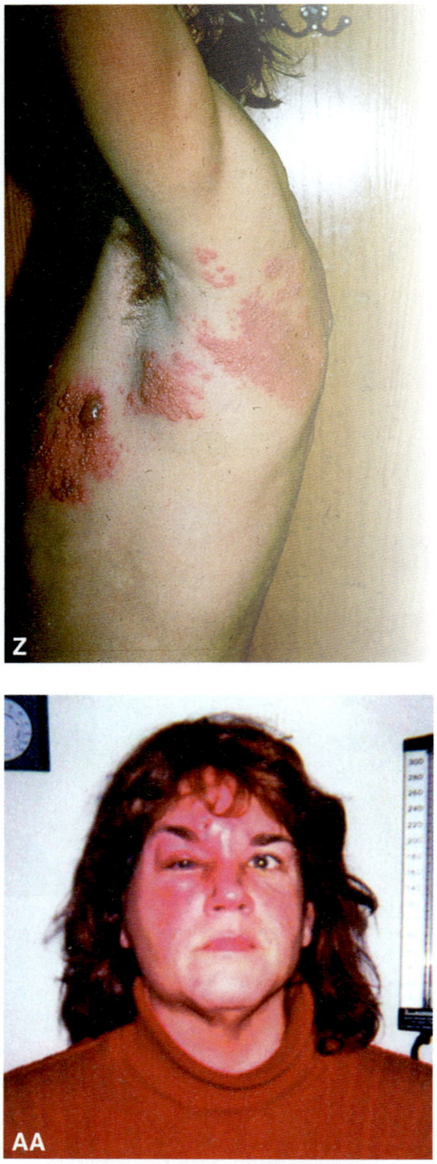

A Red, extremely painful vesicles with paresthesia that are closely grouped in a dermatomal pattern are abnormal (Fig. 10-11Z).

P Herpes zoster, or shingles, is caused by a reactivation of the varicella zoster virus. The virus remains dormant after the initial varicella inoculation. Shingles frequently occurs in older adults. The lesions are similar to those of varicella, but they tend to develop more slowly.

P Herpes zoster which involves the ophthalmic branch of the fifth cranial nerve is called herpes zoster ophthalmicus (Fig. 10-11AA). Anterior uveitis, keratitis, optic neuritis, and retinal necrosis are possible complications of this condition. These clients need to be evaluated by an ophthalmologist within 24 hours.

A Flat, purpuric macules or atypical target lesions that are widespread and/or located on the thorax and progress to blistering are abnormal (Fig. 10-11BB).

P These lesions are characteristic of Stevens-Johnson syndrome. Medications such as phenytoin, sulfonamides, and penicillin are frequently the causative agent. Serious complications can occur with this condition if not diagnosed and treated early.

A An excessive enlarging of a scar past wound edges is abnormal (Fig. 10-11CC).

P Keloids are created by excess collagen formation.

A Discrete pink macules or papular lesions with clear halos are abnormal. These lesions usually start on the trunk and progress to the face, neck, and extremities a few days after the client has had a high fever (Fig. 10-11DD).

P Roseola, or exanthem subitum, is most likely viral in origin.

A A maculopapular rash that is brownish pink and starts around the ears, face, and neck and then progresses over the trunk and limbs is abnormal (Fig. 10-11EE).

P Rubeola (measles) is a highly contagious viral infection that is characterized by high fever, cough, rash, and Koplik spots (whitish-blue spots with a red halo) on the buccal or labial mucosa (Fig. 10-11FF).

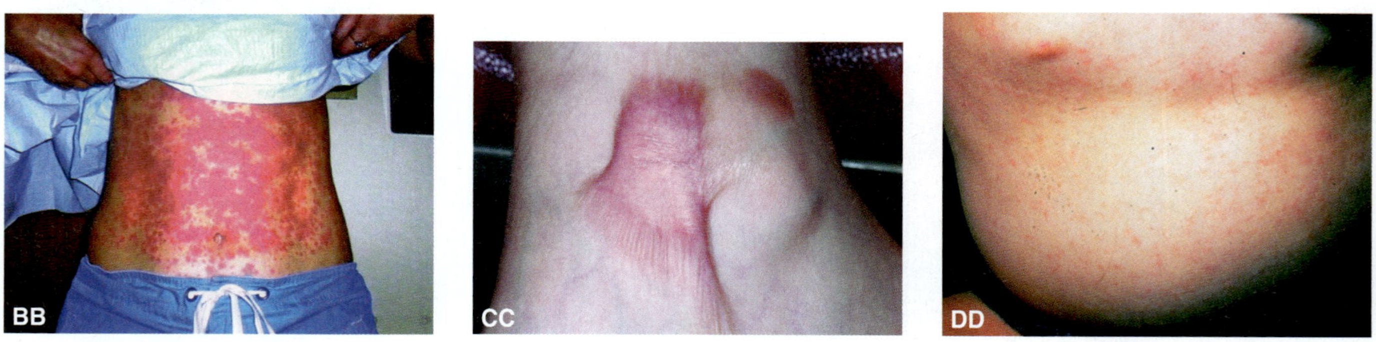

Figure 10-11—cont'd Z. Herpes zoster. **AA.** Herpes zoster ophthalmicus. **BB.** Stevens-Johnson syndrome. **CC.** Keloid. **DD.** Roseola.

The term *morbilliform* refers to a skin outbreak that has a maculopapular rash such as measles.

A Rubella (German measles) displays a fine, pinkish, macular rash that becomes confluent and pinpoint after the second day (Fig. 10-11GG).

P Rubella is caused by an RNA virus and spreads from the face and neck to the trunk.

A A diffuse, pinkish-red flush of the skin that is confluent over the entire body surface is abnormal (Fig. 10-11HH).

P Scarlet fever (scarlatina) is caused by streptococcal bacteria (usually group A) and is associated with a strawberry tongue, circumoral pallor, fever, and chills. Linear petechiae (Pastia sign) may be found in skinfolds such as the antecubital fossa.

A A blotchy, maculopapular rash that may be reticular is abnormal (Fig. 10-11II).

P Erythema infectiosum (fifth disease) usually starts on the cheeks and spreads to the arms and trunk. It gives a "slapped cheek" appearance. Its cause is human parvovirus B19. Erythema infectiosum is usually a benign condition, but it can cause complications in pregnant clients.

A A maculopapular rash with erythemic borders that appears first on the wrists, ankles, palms, soles, and forearms and is associated with a high fever is abnormal (Fig. 10-11JJ).

P Rocky Mountain spotted fever is associated with a history of tick bites. This febrile disease is caused by *Rickettsia rickettsii* and is transmitted by several types of ticks. Severe headaches, myalgia, and vomiting can occur.

A A red papule that progresses to an erythematous circular lesion with central clearing (Fig. 10-11KK) is abnormal.

P Erythema migrans is the characteristic skin lesion of Lyme disease. Lyme disease is caused by the spirochete *Borrelia burgdorferi*. It is transmitted by infected ticks, especially in the northern and mid-Atlantic states. The area of the skin lesion is the site of the tick bite.

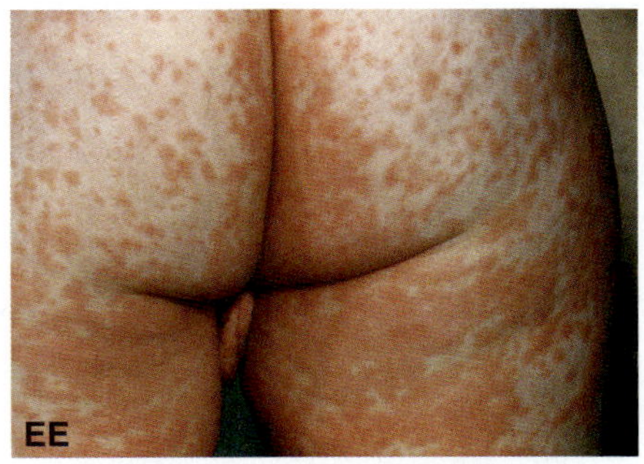

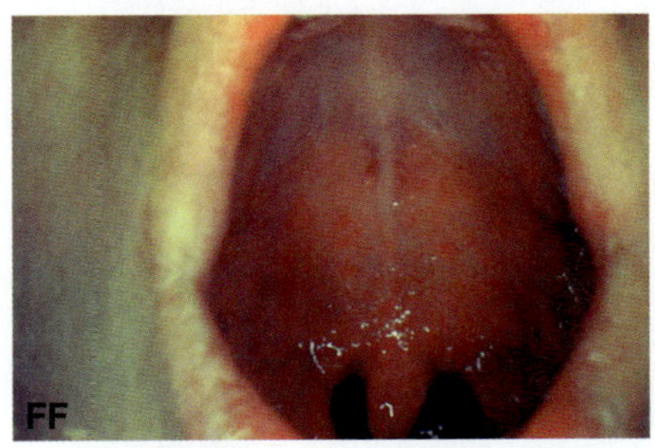

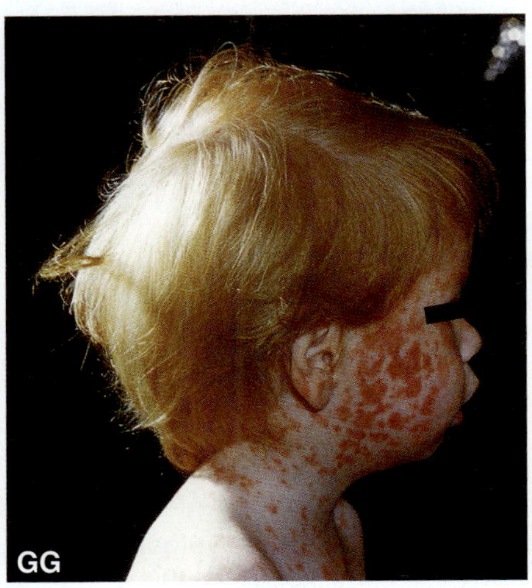

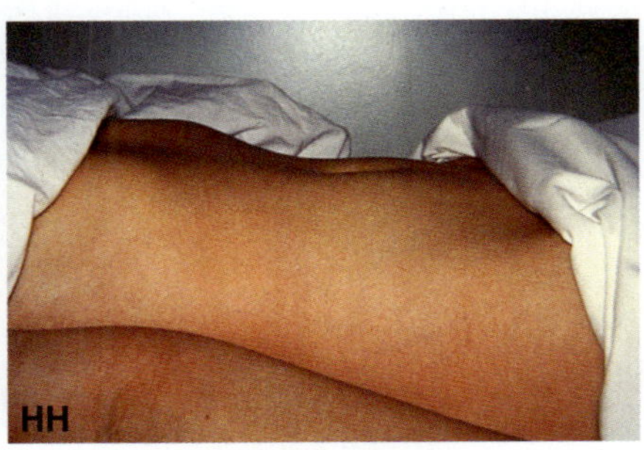

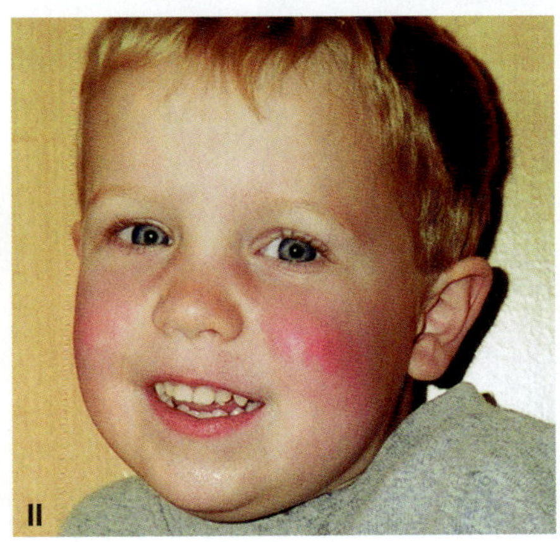

Figure 10-11—cont'd EE. Rubeola. **FF.** Koplik spots. **GG.** Rubella. **HH.** Scarlet fever. **II.** Erythema infectiosum.

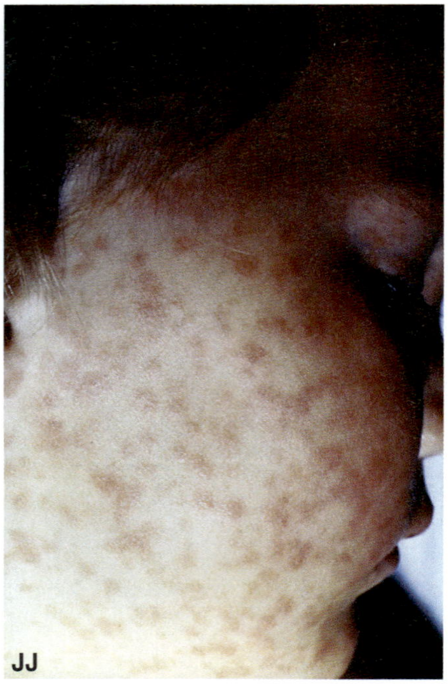

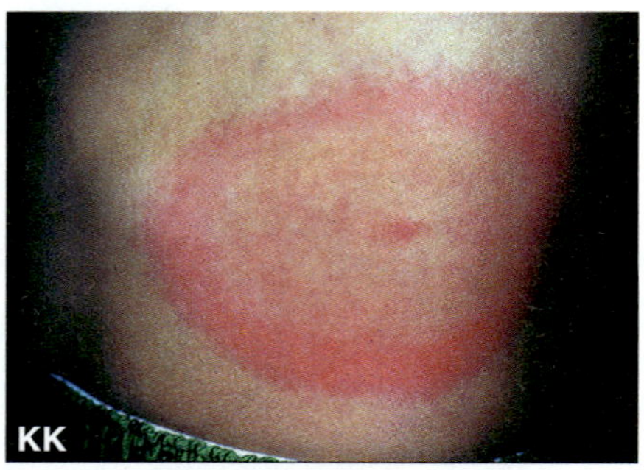

A Flesh-colored, hyperkeratotic papules (Fig. 10-11LL) that may have black dots on them are abnormal.

P Common warts, or verruca vulgaris, are viral in origin. The black dots represent thrombosed blood vessels. Warts that occur on the feet are called plantar warts (Fig. 10-11MM).

A Discrete, flesh-colored, dome-shaped papules that are slightly umbilicated in the center (Fig. 10-11NN) are abnormal.

P Molluscum contagiosum is a self-limiting viral infection. The papules may be found anywhere on the body except the palmar and plantar surfaces. When found on the genitalia of children, sexual abuse must be considered.

A A flesh-colored or brown pedunculated nodule is abnormal (Fig. 10-11OO).

P Skin tags, or acrochordon, are benign nodules. They are frequently removed if they are in an area that receives repeated movement, such as a bra line, or if they are annoying to the client.

A Small, pinkish-brown papules that are slightly raised and retract beneath the skin when compressed are abnormal.

P Dermatofibromas are benign papules that may be scaly. They have no clear etiology.

A Pruritic, red or white wheals (urticarial rash) that vary in size from very small to large and are sometimes accompanied by maculopapular eruptions, vesicles, and bullae are abnormal (Fig. 10-11PP and Figure 10-11QQ).

P Urticaria, or hives, can be acute or chronic in nature. This itchy skin lesion is linked to histamine release within the body. Exposure to food, drugs, infections, chemicals, and physical stimuli (pressure, sun, cold weather or water, exercise) are among the causes of urticaria. In some cases, the cause of urticaria is unknown despite an extensive clinical work-up.

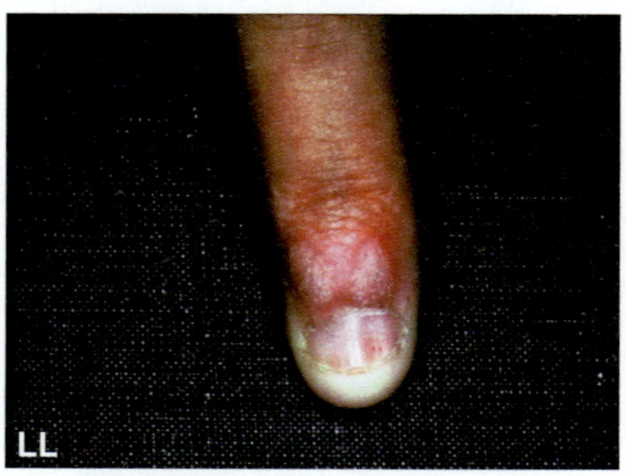

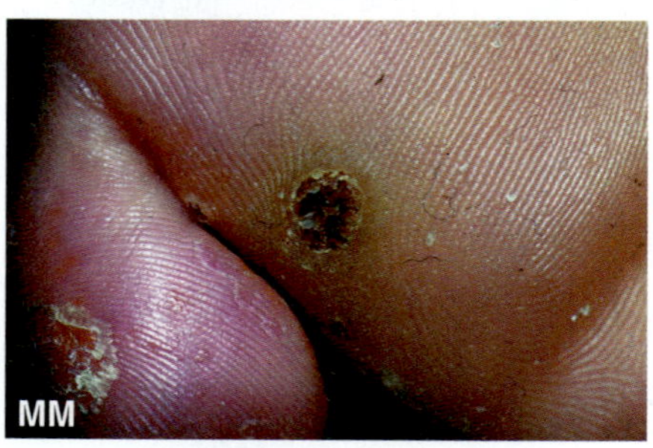

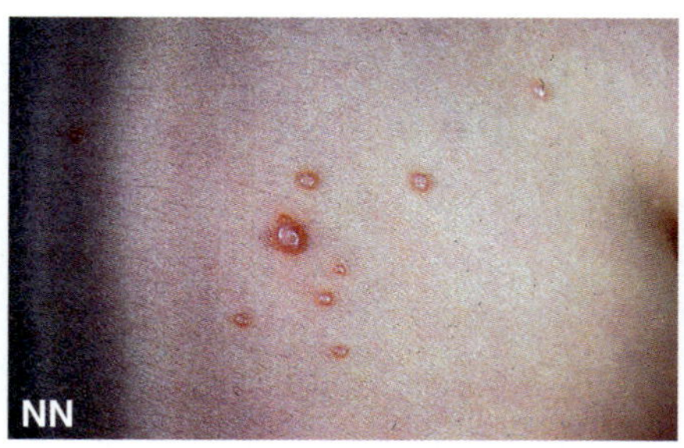

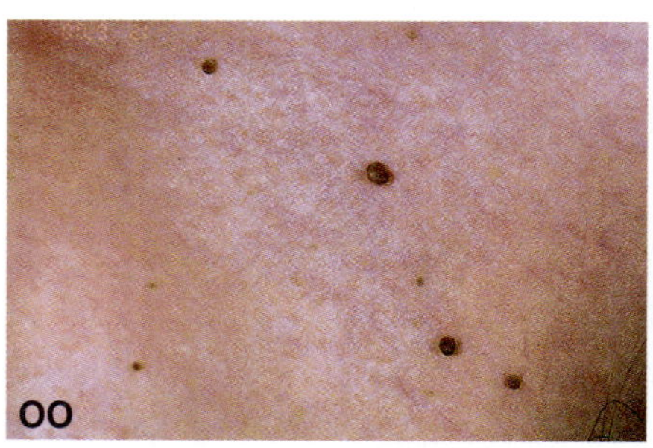

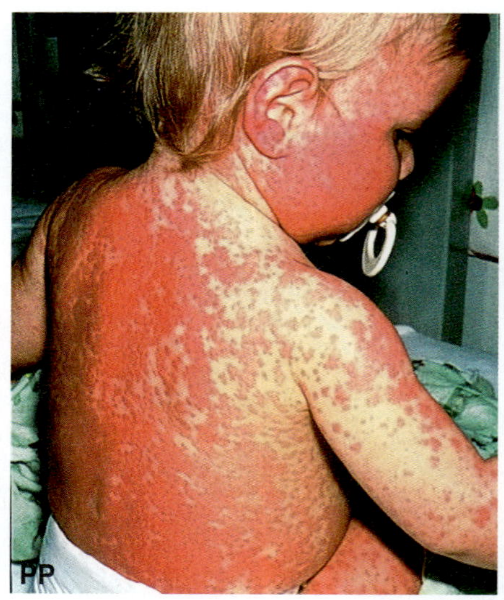

Figure 10-11—cont'd JJ. Rocky Mountain spotted fever. **KK.** Erythema migrans of Lyme disease. **LL.** Verruca vulgaris (wart). **MM.** Plantar wart. **NN.** Molluscum contagiosum. **OO.** Skin tags. **PP.** Urticarial rash: Exanthematous drug eruption.

A A small, hard brownish/tan projection arising from the epidermis is abnormal (Fig. 10-11RR).

P A cutaneous horn is composed of keratin. Actinic keratoses, warts, and squamous cell carcinomas frequently produce cutaneous horns.

A A slightly raised, irregularly shaped erythematous/tannish papule that can be scaly with a yellow crust is abnormal (Fig. 10-11SS).

P An actinic keratosis is usually less than 1 cm in diameter and has a rough texture. It is a premalignant, sun-induced lesion that often appears on the face, ears, and hands. It can occur as a single lesion, or there can be multiple lesions at the same site. Actinic keratoses can evolve into squamous cell carcinomas over time.

A A discrete lesion with a raised, red inflamed base that is mobile is abnormal (Fig. 10-11TT).

P Squamous cell carcinomas (SCC) occur most frequently in the scalp, forehead, superior pinna, and dorsal surface of the hands. SCC can also present as a wart-like, crusting, irregularly shaped lesion (Fig. 10-11UU).

A A pearly white/pinkish irregularly shaped ovoid lesion that may bleed spontaneously is abnormal (Fig. 10-11VV).

P Most basal cell carcinomas (BCC) are located on the head and neck and are due to prolonged sun exposure. BCC can also have a scaly appearance. Some BCC lesions are black, brown, or blue.

NURSING TIP

ABCDE Mnemonic for Evaluating Skin Lesions for Possible Malignancy

A (Asymmetrical): Is the lesion asymmetrical?
B (Borders): Are the borders of the lesion irregular?
C (Color): Is the color of the lesion uneven, irregular, or multicolored?
D (Diameter): Has the diameter of the lesion changed recently? Is it greater than 6 mm? Has it been itchy or bleeding?
E (Evolution): Has the lesion changed?

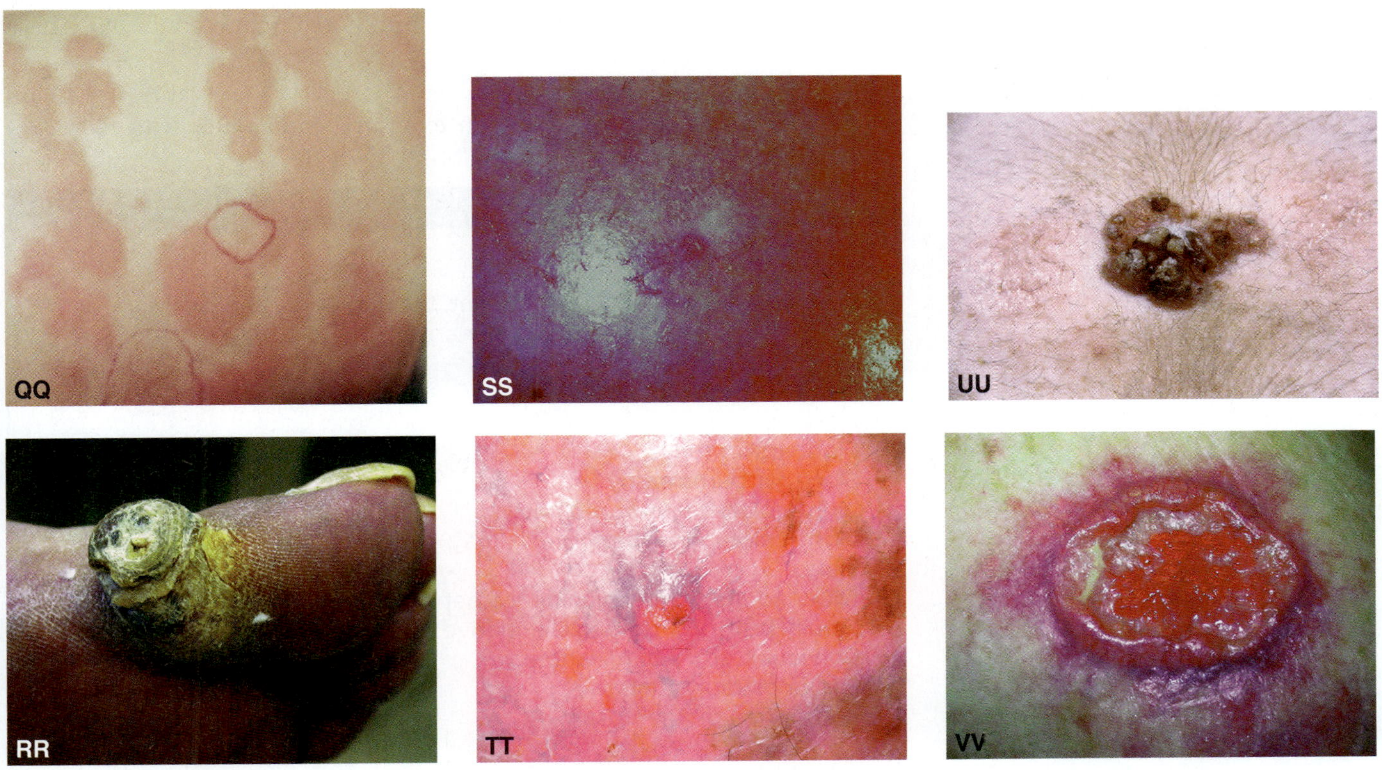

Figure 10-11—cont'd QQ. Urticaria. **RR.** Cutaneous horn. **SS.** Actinic keratosis. **TT.** Early squamous cell carcinoma. **UU.** Squamous cell carcinoma. **VV.** Basal cell carcinoma.

NURSING TIP

Danger Signs in Potentially Cancerous Lesions

1. Rapid change in size
2. Change in coloration
3. Irregular border or butterfly shaped border
4. Multiple colorations in a lesion
5. Change in surface characteristics, such as oozing
6. Change in sensation, such as pain, itching, or tenderness
7. Change in surrounding skin, such as inflammation or induration
8. Bleeding or ulcerative appearance in a mole

Client referral is required for any of these abnormal findings because of the risk of carcinoma.

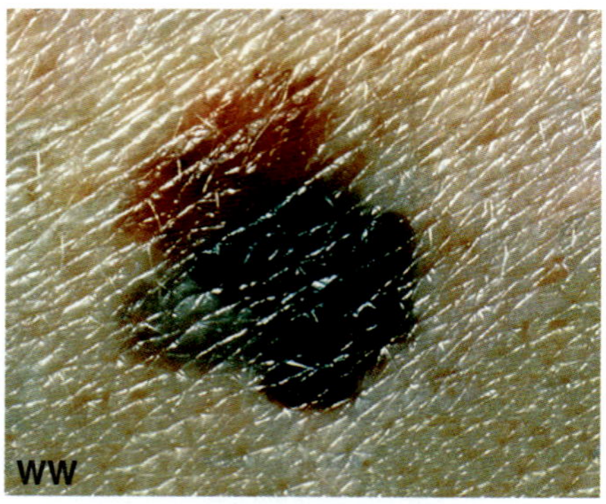

Figure 10-11—cont'd WW. Malignant melanoma.

Risk Factors

Basal and Squamous Cell Carcinoma

- Ultraviolet light (sunlight, tanning beds, and lamps)
- Frequent sunburns as a child or teen
- Lighter skin tones
- Skin that burns easily
- Light-colored hair or red hair
- Light-colored iris (blue/green/gray)
- Adults with lighter skin tones
- Older adults
- Male sex
- Chemical exposure (e.g., arsenic, industrial tar, coal, and paraffin)
- Radiation therapy
- Personal history of skin cancer
- Long-term or severe skin inflammation or injury
- Psoralen and ultraviolet light treatments for psoriasis
- Inherited disorders like xeroderma pigmentosum and basal cell nevus syndrome (Gorlin syndrome)
- Immunosuppression
- Human papillomavirus
- Smoking (risk for squamous cell carcinoma)

Adapted from *https://www.uptodate.com/contents/epidemiology-pathogenesis-clinical-features-and-diagnosis-of-basal-cell-carcinoma* and *https://www.cancer.org/cancer/types/basal-and-squamous-cell-skin-cancer/causes-risks-prevention/risk-factors.html* (Retrieved October 21, 2025).

A Lesions that are brownish-tan, red, white, blue, pink, purple, or gray and that have irregular borders and notching are abnormal. These lesions can be flat or elevated.

P Malignant melanoma (MM) (Fig. 10-11WW) is a cancerous lesion associated with repeated sun exposure. Individuals with light skin

Risk Factors

Melanoma

- Ultraviolet radiation (from sunlight, tanning beds, and lamps)
- Severe sunburns as a teenager or child
- Numerous nevi (>50)
- Dysplastic nevi or atypical nevi
- Nevi increasing in size
- Lighter skin tones
- Skin that burns easily
- Light-colored hair or red hair
- Light-colored iris (blue/green/gray)
- Male
- Older adults (highest incidence between 55 and 74 years old)
- Family history (first-degree relative) of melanoma
- Previous history of melanoma
- Immunosuppression
- Xeroderma pigmentosum

Adapted from *https://www.aad.org/media/stats-skin-cancer; https://seer.cancer.gov/statfacts/html/melan.html;* and *https://www.cancer.org/cancer/melanoma-skin-cancer/causes-risks-prevention/risk-factors.html)* (Retrieved October 21, 2025).

and blue eyes are particularly at risk for MM. These neoplastic lesions can also be related to precancerous lesions such as nevi.

A Perifollicular papules are abnormal.

P Pseudofolliculitis barbae, or ingrown hair, is caused by hair tips that penetrate the skin rather than exiting through the follicular orifice. It usually occurs in the beard area due to the thicker and curlier hair shaft.

A Pustules at the opening of the hair follicle are abnormal.

P Folliculitis is an inflammation of the hair follicle. Figure 10-11XX depicts a staphylococcal folliculitis; however, the causative agent may be fungal and the inflammation is then called tinea barbae (Fig. 10-11YY).

A Multiple pedunculated papules, nodules, or tumors, which are violaceous and soft (Fig. 10-11ZZ), are abnormal.

P A neurofibroma is a hallmark finding of neurofibromatosis, type I (or von Recklinghausen disease). Six or more café au lait spots are concurrently found on the client's skin in neurofibromatosis, type I.

A A raised, circular red or flesh-colored lesion that has a normal or sunken center pattern is abnormal (see Figure 10-11AAA).

P Granuloma annulare is a benign inflammatory condition of unknown etiology but is speculated to be associated with diabetes or thyroid disease. The eruption can occur in a single location or be widespread.

A Any form of self-harm or self-mutilation is abnormal. Any indications of burns, cutting (see Figure 10-11BBB), skin ripping, deep scratches, and other disruptions of the skin is abnormal. The arms, legs, and chest are the areas typically affected.

P Self-harm or self-mutilation is a nonsuicidal injury that a person deliberately inflicts upon themself to deal with extreme stress, emotional pain, anger, frustration, etc. The client who engages in self-harm needs immediate referral to a mental health specialist.

NURSING TIP

Skin Protection Tips

- Use sunscreen daily, even if there is no long exposure to the sun.
- Apply sunscreen of sun protection factor (SPF) 30 or higher to exposed, dry skin 15 to 30 minutes before sun exposure; apply lip balm with an SPF of 30 or greater to the lips.
- Reapply sunscreen every 2 hours after swimming or excessive sweating.
- Wear protective clothing when outside: long-sleeved shirt, long pants, wide-brimmed hat, sunglasses.
- Avoid the sun during peak times, from 10:00 AM to 4:00 PM.
- Avoid tanning beds and lights.
- Use sunscreen and protective measures even if it is cloudy outside; use caution when around water, sand, or snow, as these conditions reflect the sun's rays onto the skin.
- Check with a pediatric provider about sunscreen use on an infant less than 6 months old.
- Perform a skin self-examination regularly (Fig. 10-12).

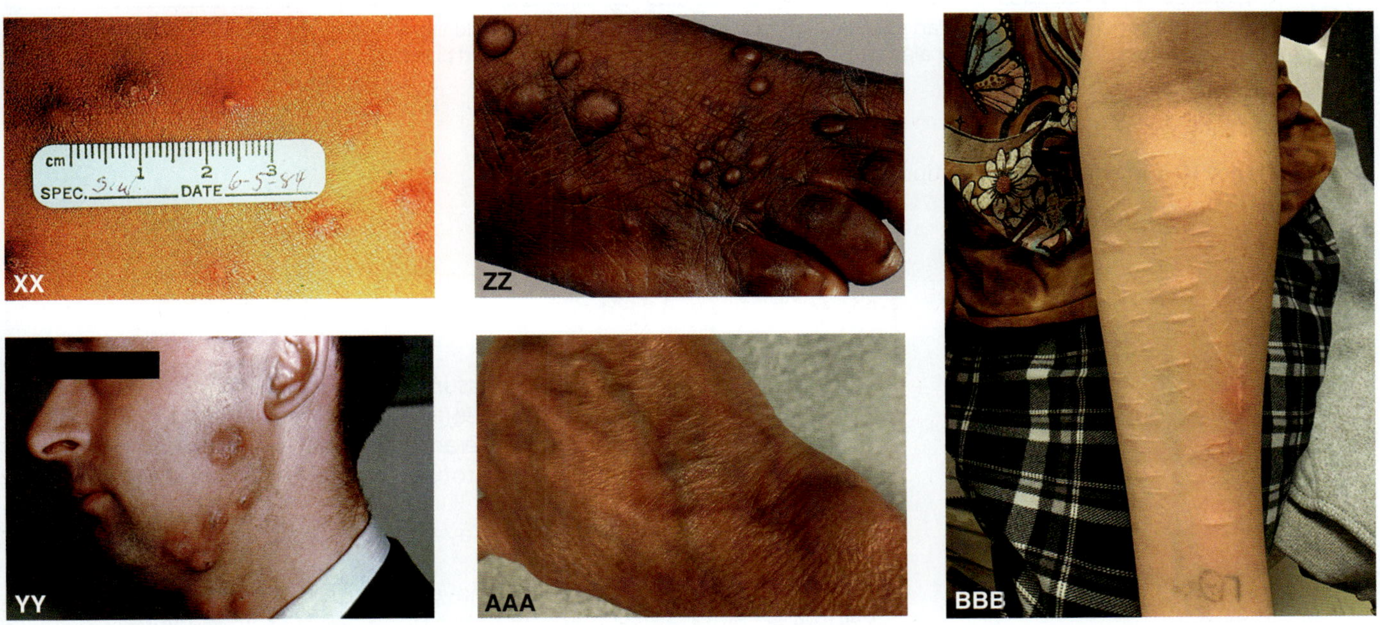

Figure 10-11—cont'd XX. Folliculitis. **YY.** Tinea barbae. **ZZ.** Type I neurofibromatosis (von Recklinghausen disease). **AAA.** Granuloma annulare. **BBB.** Self harm, cutting.

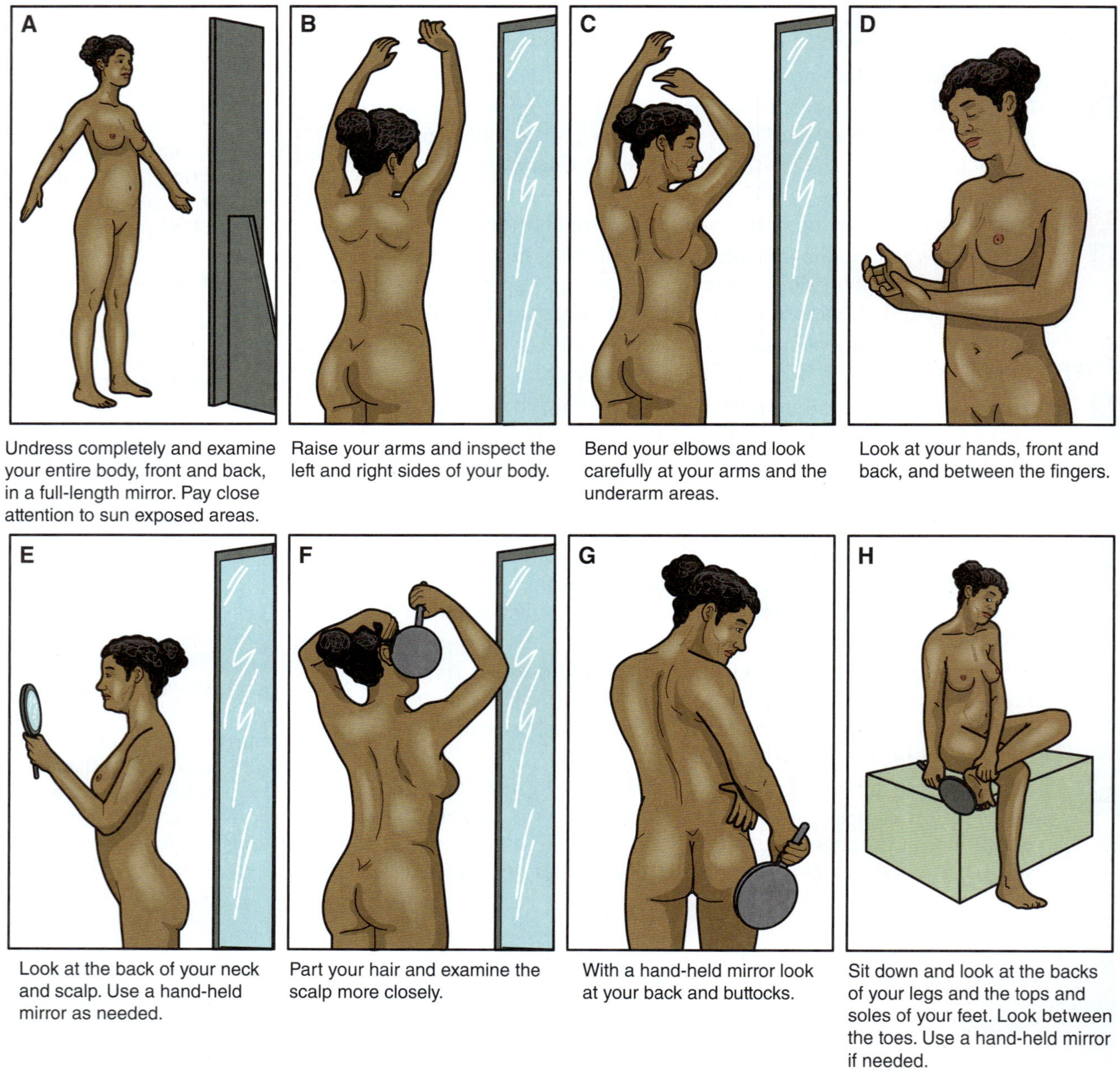

Figure 10-12 Skin self-examination instructions for clients.

NURSING TIP

Stages of Pressure Injuries

Uniform standards for staging pressure injuries are defined by the National Pressure Injury Advisory Panel.

Stage 1 In lighter skin tones, the area is reddened, but skin integrity is intact; in darker skin tones, the pigmentation is enhanced (Fig. 10-13A).

Stage 2 Epidermal and dermal layers have sustained injury, the skin is not intact (Fig. 10-13A).

Stage 3 Subcutaneous tissues have sustained injury (Fig. 10-13B).

Stage 4 Muscle tissue and perhaps bone has sustained injury (Fig. 10-13C).

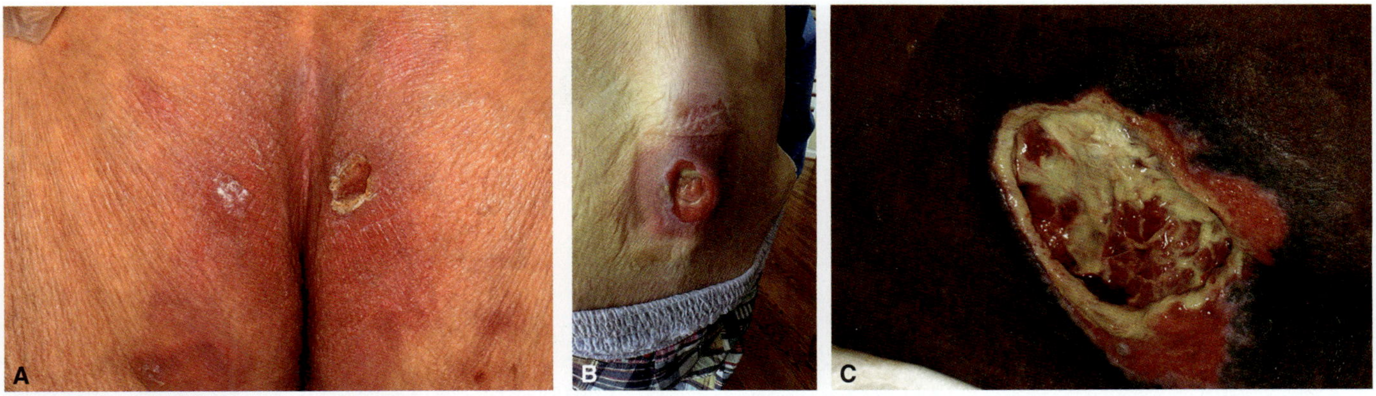

Figure 10-13 Pressure injuries. **A.** Stage 1 (reddened areas) and Stage 2 (broken skin). **B.** Stage 3. **C.** Stage 4.

> **NURSING TIP**
>
> **Identifying Burns**
>
> A client with burns frequently has varying degrees of injury on the body. Parts of the body may have first-degree burns, and other parts may have second-, third-, or fourth-degree burns. The following descriptions and photographs will assist you in identifying burn injuries:
>
> **First-Degree Burn** (superficial thickness) (Fig. 10-14A): The epidermis is injured or destroyed; there may be some damage to the dermis; hair follicles and sweat glands are intact; the skin is red and dry; painful, no blisters.
>
> **Second-Degree Burn** (partial thickness, superficial or deep) (Fig. 10-14B): The epidermis and upper layers of the dermis are destroyed; the deeper dermis is injured; hair follicles, sweat glands, and nerve endings are intact; the skin is red and blistery with exudate; painful, blisters are present.
>
> **Third-Degree Burn** (full thickness) (Fig. 10-14C): The epidermis and dermis are destroyed; subcutaneous tissue may be injured; hair follicles, sweat glands, and nerve endings are destroyed; the skin is white, red, black, tan, or brown with a leathery-looking appearance; painless because nerve endings are destroyed.
>
> **Fourth-Degree Burn** (full thickness) (Fig. 10-14D): The epidermis and dermis are destroyed; subcutaneous tissue, muscle, and bone may be injured; hair follicles, sweat glands, and nerve endings are destroyed; the skin is white, red, black, tan, or brown with exposed and damaged subcutaneous tissue, muscle, or bone; painless.

> **NURSING TIP**
>
> **Braden Scale for Predicting Pressure Injury Risk**
>
> The Braden Scale is a valid and reliable tool to predict who is at risk for developing pressure injuries. This tool can be used to evaluate a client's skin upon admission to a hospital, rehabilitation center, nursing home, or other health care setting. The Braden Scale can also be used to trend skin status over time. The interval of screening depends on the clinical setting and the client's condition. A Braden Scale is also available for home care use. The Braden Scale encompasses six areas that are scored: sensory perception, moisture, activity, mobility, nutrition, and friction and shear. The tool can be viewed at *https://www.in.gov/health/files/Braden_Scale.pdf*

Palpation of the Skin

Use gloves for palpation if there is a probability of contact with body fluids or if the client is in isolation.

Moisture

E Palpate all nonmucous membrane skin surfaces for moisture using the dorsal surfaces of the hands and fingers.

N **Normally, the skin is dry with a minimum of perspiration. Moisture on the skin will vary from one body area to another, with perspiration normally present on the hands, axilla, face, and in between the skinfolds. Moisture also varies with changes in environment,**

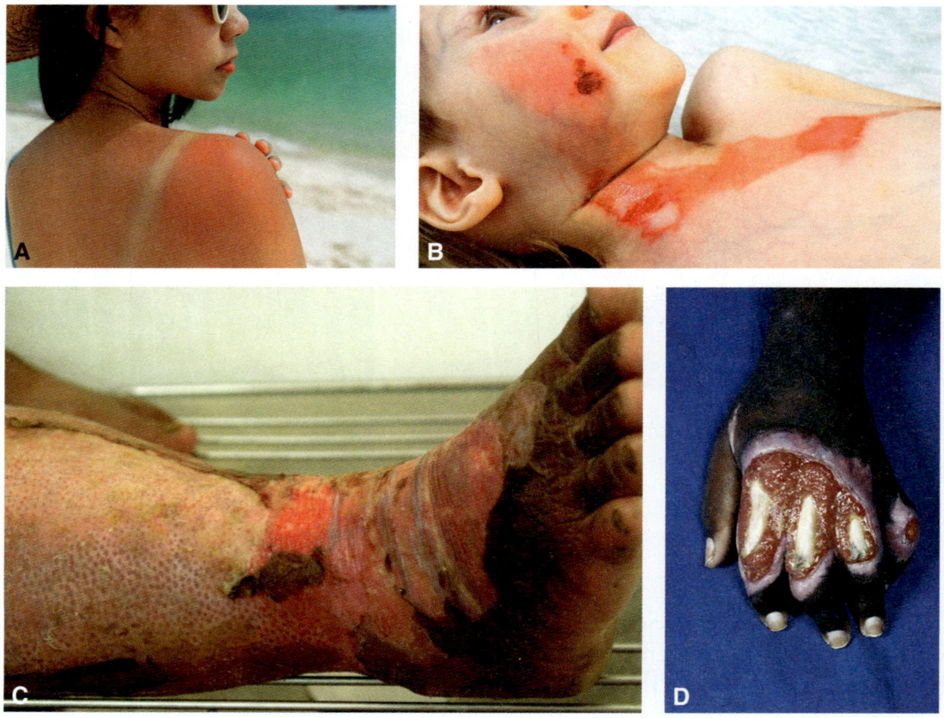

Figure 10-14 Types of burns. **A.** First-degree burn. **B.** Second-degree burn. **C.** Third-degree burn. **D.** Fourth-degree burn.

muscular activity, body temperature, stress, and activity levels. Body temperature is regulated by the skin's production of perspiration, which evaporates to cool the body.

A Excessive dryness of the skin, **xerosis**, as evidenced by flaking of the stratum corneum and associated pruritus, is abnormal.

P Hypothyroidism and exposure to extremely cold and dry climates can lead to xerosis.

A Very dry, large scales that are light-colored or brown are abnormal (Fig. 10-15).

P Ichthyosis vulgaris is a skin abnormality originating from a keratin disorder. It can be associated with atopic dermatitis.

A Diaphoresis is the profuse production of perspiration.

P Causes of diaphoresis include physical activity, hyperthyroidism, increased metabolic rate, sepsis, anxiety, or pain.

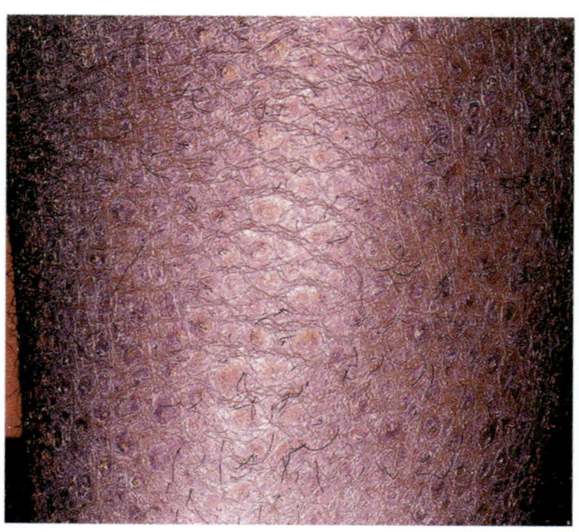

Figure 10-15 Ichthyosis vulgaris.

Temperature

E Palpate all nonmucosal skin surfaces for temperature using the dorsal surfaces of the hands and fingers.

N **Skin surface temperature should be warm and equal bilaterally. Hands and feet may be slightly cooler than the rest of the body.**

A **Hypothermia** is a cooling of the skin and may be generalized or localized.

P Generalized hypothermia is indicative of shock or some other type of central circulatory dysfunction. Localized hypothermia is indicative of arterial insufficiency in the affected area.

A Generalized **hyperthermia** is the excessive warming of the skin and may be generalized or localized.

P Generalized hyperthermia may be indicative of a febrile state, hyperthyroidism, or increased metabolic function caused by exercise. Localized hyperthermia may be caused by infection, trauma, sunburn, or windburn.

Tenderness

E Palpate skin surfaces for tenderness using the dorsal surfaces of the hands and fingers.

N **Skin surfaces should be nontender.**

A Tenderness over the skin structures can be discrete and localized or generalized.

P Discrete tenderness may indicate a localized infection such as cellulitis, and generalized tenderness can indicate systemic illness such as lymphoma or allergic reaction.

Texture

E
1. Evaluate the texture of the skin using the finger pads.
2. Evaluate surfaces such as the abdomen and medial surfaces of the arms first.
3. Compare these areas to areas that are covered with hair.

N **Skin should normally feel smooth, even, and firm except where there is significant hair growth. A certain amount of roughness can be normal.**

A Roughness can occur on exposed areas such as the elbows, the soles of the feet, and the palms of the hands.

P Roughness can be due to wool clothing, cold weather, occupational exposures, or the use of soap. In addition, generalized roughness can be associated with systemic diseases such as scleroderma, hypothyroidism, and amyloidosis. Localized thickening and roughness can be a result of chronic pruritus (lichenification) due to scratching, which causes a thickening of the epidermis.

A Areas of hyperkeratosis and increased roughness that are found in the lower extremities are abnormal.

P Hyperkeratosis and increased roughness may be indicative of peripheral vascular disease, which causes decreased circulation and diminished nourishment of cutaneous layers.

A The skin can feel very soft and silk-like.

P Generalized softness can result from hyperthyroidism secondary to an elevated metabolism.

Turgor

Palpate the skin **turgor**, or elasticity, which reflects the skin's state of hydration.

E
1. Pinch a small section of the client's skin between your thumb and forefinger. Over the sternum or under the clavicle are optimal areas to examine.
2. Release the skin.
3. Observe the speed with which the skin returns to its original contour when released (Fig. 10-16).

N **When the skin is released, it should return to its original contour rapidly.**

A Decreased skin turgor is present when the skin is released and remains pinched and slowly returns to its original contour.

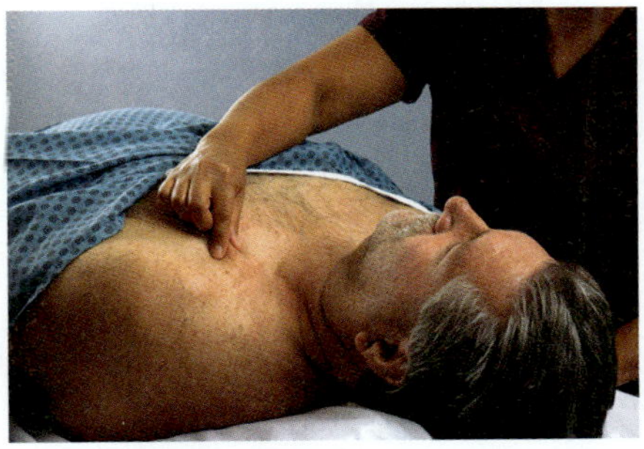

Figure 10-16 Assessment of skin turgor.

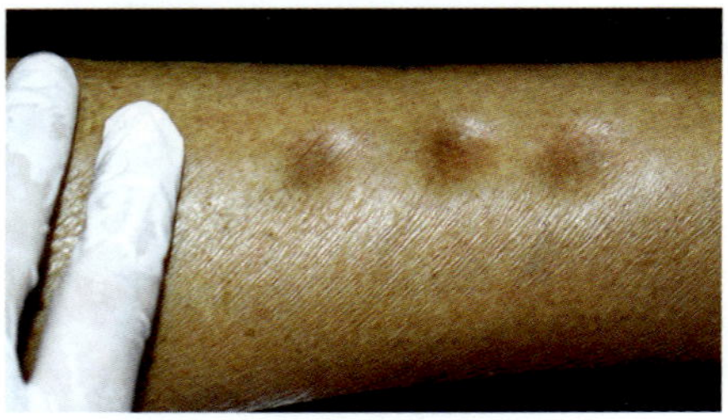

Figure 10-17 Pitting edema.

P **Dehydration**, or lack of fluid in the tissues, is the main cause of decreased skin turgor. The aging process and scleroderma can also decrease the elasticity of the skin.

A Increased turgor or tension causes the skin to return to its original contour too quickly.

P Increased turgor can be indicative of connective tissue disease caused by an increase in granulation tissue.

Edema

Palpate the skin for **edema**, or accumulation of fluid in the intercellular spaces (Fig. 10-17).

E
1. Firmly imprint your thumb against a dependent portion of the body, such as the arms, hands, legs, feet, ankle, or sacrum.
2. Release pressure.
3. Observe for an indentation on the skin.
4. Rate the degree of edema. Pitting edema is rated on a 4-point scale (Fig. 10-18).
5. Check for symmetry and measure circumference of affected extremities.

N **Edema is not normally present.**

A Edema is present if the skin feels puffy and tight. It can be localized in one area (Fig. 10-19) or generalized throughout the body. There are many different types of edema (Table 10-2).

P Localized edema may be due to dependency; however, generalized or bilateral edema is caused by increased hydrostatic pressure, decreased capillary osmotic pressure, increased capillary permeability, or obstruction to lymph flow. This occurs in congestive heart failure or kidney failure.

NURSING TIP
Evaluation of Edema

If the edema is severe enough, it can prohibit the evaluation of pathological conditions that are manifested by coloration changes. Two plus (2+) edema warrants referral if it is new onset. New onset severe edema (3+ or 4+) warrants immediate evaluation.

Inspection of the Hair

Ask the client to remove hair bands and hair pieces or to unbraid hair before the inspection process. If this is not possible, inspect the exposed areas as completely as possible.

Scale	Description
0	No edema
1+	Rebounds immediately
2+	Rebounds in <15 seconds
3+	Rebounds in 30–60 seconds
4+	Rebound takes more than 2 minutes

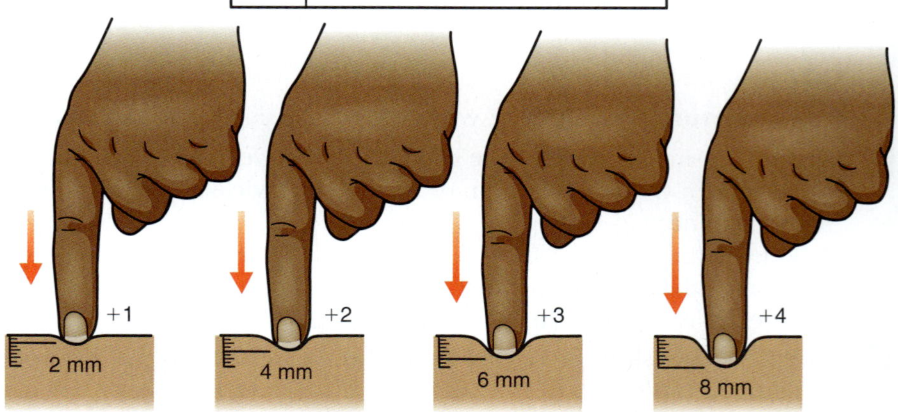

Figure 10-18 Pitting edema grading scale.

Table 10-2 Types of Edema

Type	Description
Pitting	Edema that is present when an indentation remains on the skin after pressure is applied
Nonpitting	Edema that is firm with discoloration or thickening of the skin; results when serum proteins coagulate in tissue spaces
Angioedema	Noninflammatory swelling of any body part in response to a trigger; can affect the face, lips, mucous membranes, extremities, or trunk (Fig. 10-19); may occur in conjunction with hives; onset may be rapid, with resolution requiring hours to days
Dependent	Localized increase of extracellular fluid volume in a dependent limb or area
Inflammatory	Swelling due to an extracellular fluid effusion into the tissue surrounding an area of inflammation
Noninflammatory	Swelling or effusion due to mechanical or other causes not related to congestion or inflammation
Lymphedema	Edema due to the obstruction of a lymphatic vessel

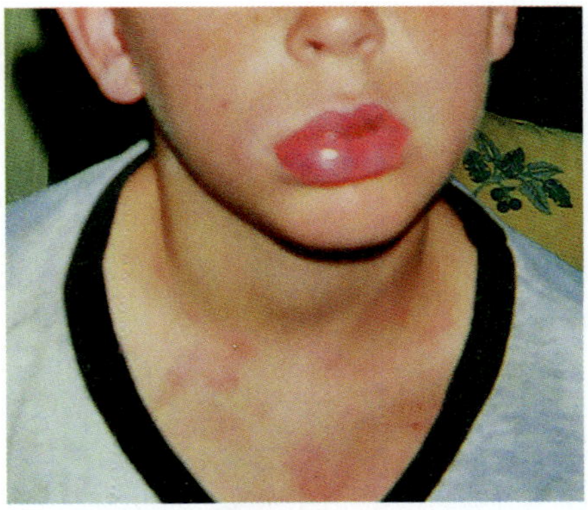

Figure 10-19 Angioedema of the lips. Note the faint urticaria on the anterior chest wall.

Color

E Inspect scalp hair, eyebrows, eyelashes, and body hair for color.

N **Hair color varies from dark black to pale blonde and red based on the amount of melanin present. As melanin production diminishes, hair turns gray. Hair color may also be chemically changed.**

A Patches of gray hair that are isolated or occur in conjunction with a scar are abnormal.

P Patches of gray hair not associated with aging can be indicative of nerve damage.

Distribution

E Evaluate the distribution of hair on the body, eyebrows, face, and scalp.

N **The body is covered in vellus hair. Terminal hair is found in the eyebrows, eyelashes, and scalp, and in the axilla and pubic areas after puberty. Males may experience a certain degree of normal balding and may also develop terminal facial and chest hair.**

A The absence of pubic hair, unless purposefully removed, is abnormal in adults.

P Diminished or absent pubic hair may be indicative of endocrine disorders, such as anterior pituitary adenomas, or chemotherapy.

A Male or female pattern baldness (**alopecia**) may be abnormal in some individuals if associated with pathology. Alopecia areata is a circumscribed bald area (Fig. 10-20A).

P Androgenetic alopecia is a common, progressive hair loss that is caused by a combination of genetic predisposition and androgenetic effects on the hair follicle; however, alopecia may be secondary to chemotherapy and radiation, infection, stress, drug reactions, lupus, and traction. A pathological etiology of alopecia should be ruled out.

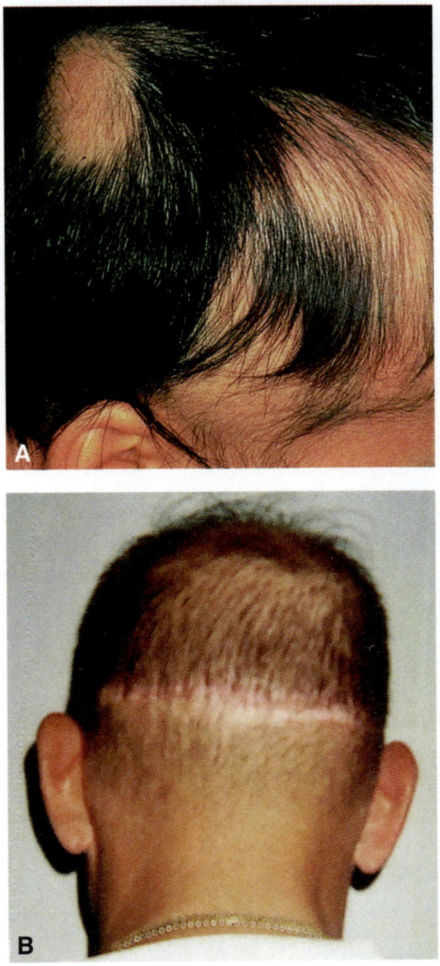

Figure 10-20 Abnormalities of the head and scalp. **A.** Alopecia areata. **B.** Linear alopecia developed in this man from daily wearing of his military uniform cap.

E Examination **N** Normal Findings **A** Abnormal Findings **P** Pathophysiology

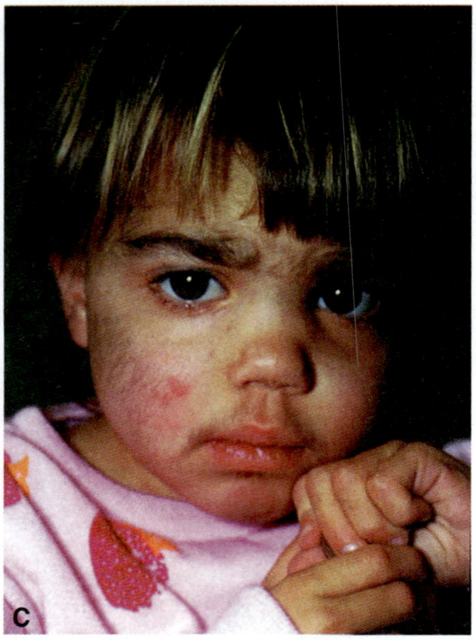

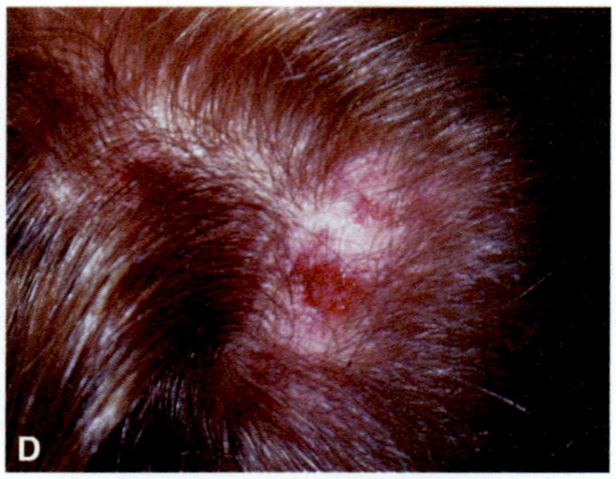

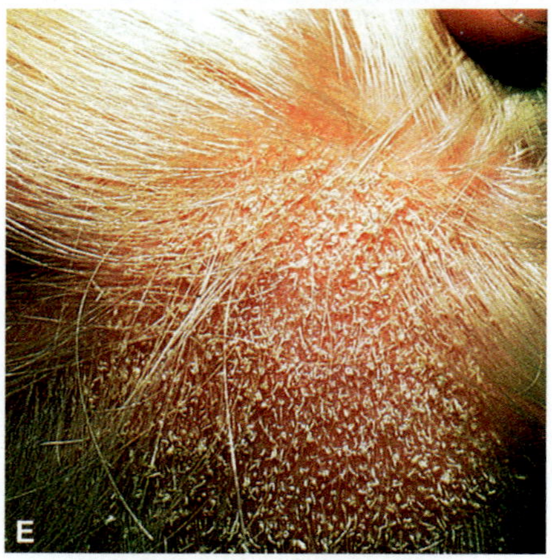

Figure 10-20—cont'd C. Hirsutism caused by the drug cyclosporine. **D.** Trichotillomania. **E.** Tinea capitis.

A Total scalp baldness, or alopecia totalis, is abnormal.

P Autoimmune diseases, emotional crisis, stress, or heredity can cause alopecia totalis.

A Hair loss in linear formations is abnormal (Fig. 10-20B).

P Linear alopecia can be caused by frequent pressure on hair follicles that leads to their inability to produce new hair. In addition, traction alopecia can be caused by the use of curlers and wearing the hair in tightly pulled hair styles whereby traction is continually applied to the hair shaft and scalp.

A Excess facial and body hair is abnormal (Fig. 10-20C).

P **Hirsutism** is manifested by excessive body hair. It is indicative of endocrine disorders such as hypersecretion of adrenocortical androgens, Cushing syndrome, and polycystic ovary syndrome (PCOS). In PCOS, the client may have excess facial and chest hair.

P Hirsutism can also result as a side effect of medications such as cyclosporine, minoxidil, and phenytoin.

A Areas of broken-off hairs in irregular patterns with scaliness, but no infection, are abnormal (Fig. 10-20D).

P Trichotillomania is the manipulation of the hair by twisting and pulling, leading to reduced hair mass. This can be an unconscious action or a sign of a psychiatric condition.

A Broken-off hairs with scaliness and follicular inflammation are abnormal (Fig. 10-20E). The area may be painful and purulent with boggy nodules.

P Tinea capitis (ringworm) is a fungal infection, frequently caused by dermatophytic trichomycosis.

A The scalp is covered with yellow-brown scales and crusts. The scalp may be oily. Edema may be present (Fig. 10-20F).

P Seborrheic dermatitis is caused by increased production of sebum by the scalp.

Lesions

E
1. Don gloves and lift the scalp hair by segments.
2. Evaluate the scalp for lesions or signs of infestation.

N **The scalp should be pale white to pink in lighter skin tones and light brown in darker skin tones. There should be no signs of infestation or lesions. Seborrhea, commonly known as dandruff, may be present.**

A Abnormal manifestations include head lice.

P Head lice (pediculosis capitis) may be distinguished from dandruff in that dandruff can be easily removed from the scalp or hair, whereas nits (Fig. 10-20G), which are the lice larvae, are attached to the hair shaft and are difficult to remove. Both seborrhea and head lice may cause itching.

Palpation of the Hair

Texture

E
1. Palpate the hair between your fingertips.
2. Note the condition of the hair from the scalp to the end of the hair.

N **Hair may feel thin, straight, coarse, thick, or curly. It should be shiny and resilient when traction is applied and should not come out in clumps in your hands.**

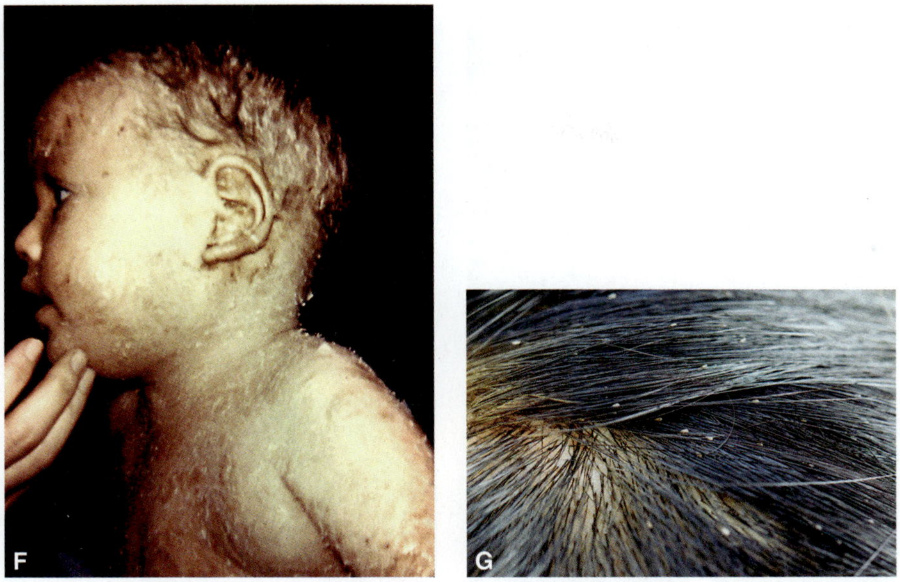

Figure 10-20—cont'd F. Seborrheic dermatitis. **G.** Head lice.

A Brittle hair that easily breaks off when pulled or hair that is listless and dull is abnormal.

P Brittle, dull hair, or hair that is broken off can be indicative of malnutrition, hyperthyroidism, use of chemicals such as permanents, or infections secondary to damage to the hair follicle.

Inspection of the Nails

Color

E
1. Inspect the fingernails and toenails, noting the color of the nails.
2. Check capillary refill by depressing the nail, or the pad of the finger/toe, until blanching occurs.
3. Release the nail and evaluate the time required for the nail to return to its previous color.
4. Perform a capillary refill check on all four extremities.

N **Normally, the nails have a pink cast in clients with lighter skin tones and a brown cast in clients with darker skin tones. Capillary refill is an indicator of peripheral circulation. Normal capillary refill may vary with age, but color should return to normal within 2 to 3 seconds.**

A White striations or dots in the nailbed are abnormal (Fig. 10-21A).

P Leukonychia (Mees bands) may result from trauma, infections, vascular diseases, psoriasis, and arsenic poisoning.

A An entire nail plate that is white is abnormal (Fig. 10-21B).

P Leukonychia totalis may result from hypercalcemia, hypochromic anemia, Hansen disease (leprosy), hepatic cirrhosis, and arsenic poisoning.

A A brown color in the nail plate is melanonychia (Fig. 10-21C).

P Melanonychia can occur in Addison disease and malaria.

P A dark brown/black pigmented area at the proximal end of the nailbed (Hutchinson's sign) is seen in acral lentiginous melanoma (Fig. 10-21D).

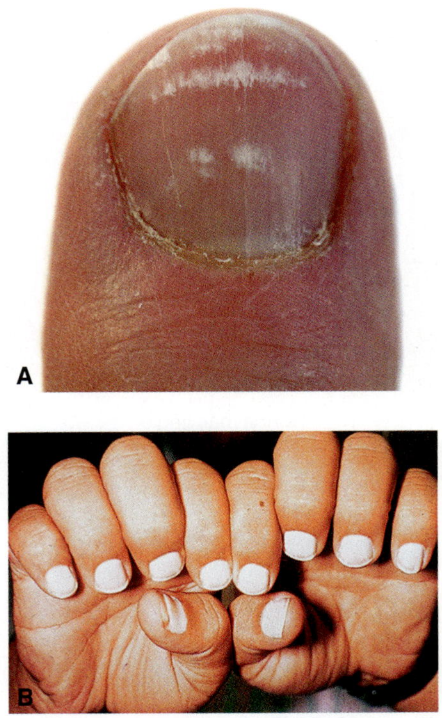

Figure 10-21 Abnormal color changes of the nailbed. **A.** Leukonychia. **B.** Leukonychia totalis.

E Examination **N** Normal Findings **A** Abnormal Findings **P** Pathophysiology

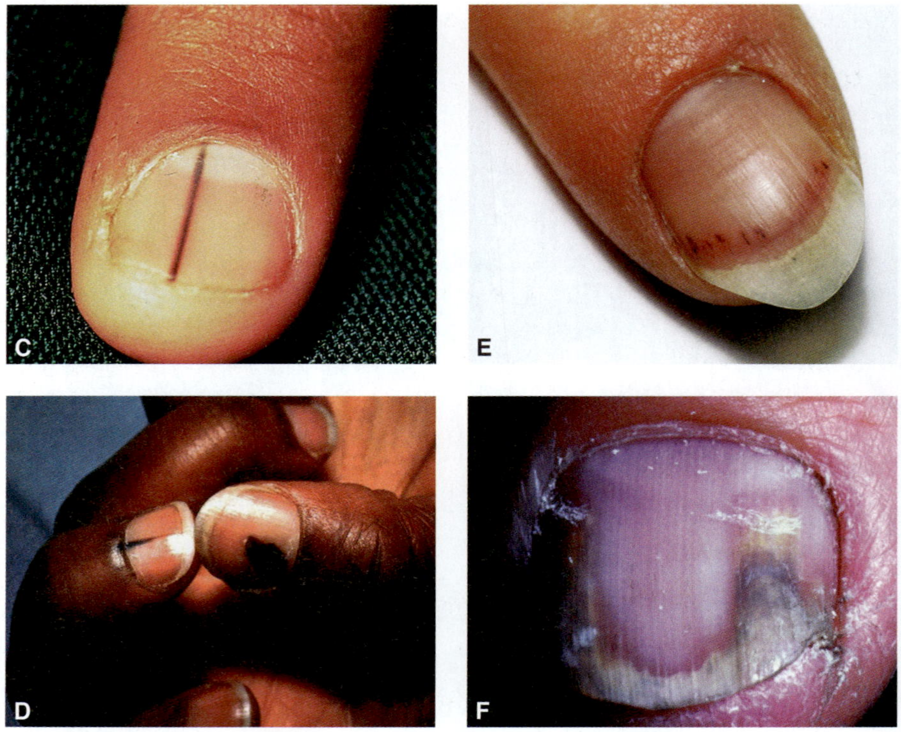

Figure 10-21—cont'd C. Longitudinal melanonychia. **D.** Melanoma. **E.** Splinter hemorrhages. **F.** Onychomycosis.

A Bluish nails are abnormal.

P Bluish nails may result from cyanosis, venous stasis, and sulfuric acid poisoning.

A Red or brown linear streaks in the nailbed are abnormal (Fig. 10-21E).

P Splinter hemorrhages can result from subacute bacterial endocarditis, mitral stenosis, trichinosis, cirrhosis, and nonspecific causes.

A It is abnormal for the proximal end of the nailbed to be white and the distal portion to be pink.

P Lindsey's nails (half-and-half nails) can occur in chronic renal failure and hypoalbuminemia.

A A yellow or white hue in a hyperkeratotic nailbed is abnormal (Fig. 10-21F).

P Onychomycosis is a fungal infection of the nail.

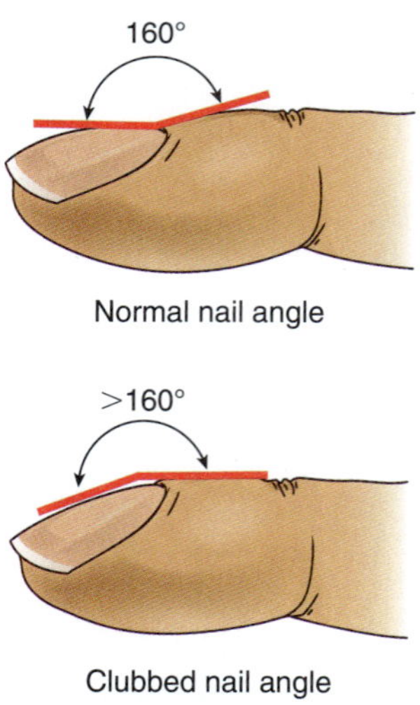

Figure 10-22 Evaluate the angle of the nail base.

Shape and Configuration

E
1. Examine the fingernails and toenails for shape, configuration, and consistency.
2. View the profile of the middle finger and evaluate the angle of the nail base (Fig. 10-22).
3. Have the client bring the distal phalanxes together, as illustrated in Figure 10-23. Note the position of the nailbeds in relation to each other.

N **The nail surface should be smooth and slightly rounded or flat. Curved nails are a normal variant. Nail thickness should**

be uniform throughout, with no splintering or brittle edges. The angle of the nail base should be approximately 160°. Longitudinal ridging is a normal variant. There is a diamond-shaped opening at the base of the nailbeds in nails that are normal when examined, as in Figure 10-23.

A An angle of the nail base greater than 160°, along with sponginess of the nailbed, is abnormal (Fig. 10-24A).

A Nailbeds that do not meet medially and do not have a diamond-shaped opening at their base are abnormal (Fig. 10-24B).

P Clubbing can result from long-standing hypoxia and lung pathology (Fig. 10-24C).

A Thin nail plates with cuplike depressions and concave, or spoon-shaped, nails are abnormal.

P Koilonychia can result from iron-deficiency anemia, chronic infections, malnutrition, or Raynaud phenomenon.

A A transverse (horizontal) furrow in the nail plate is abnormal (Fig. 10-25A).

P Beau lines are caused by an arrest of nail growth at the matrix. It can be associated with an acute phase of infectious disease, malnutrition, anemia, peripheral artery disease, and chemotherapy.

A Separation of the nail from the nailbed is abnormal (Fig. 10-25B).

P Onycholysis can result from hypothyroidism, hyperthyroidism, repeated trauma, Raynaud phenomenon, syphilis, eczema, and acrocyanosis.

A Painful, red swelling of the nail fold is abnormal (Fig. 10-25C).

P Paronychia can be caused by *Candida albicans*, bacteria, and repeated exposure of the nails to moisture.

A Purpura or ecchymosis under the nail plate is abnormal (Fig. 10-25D).

P Subungual hematoma is caused by trauma to the digit and nail, leading to hemorrhage into the matrix and nailbed.

A The distal portion of the nail plate is embedded in periungual tissue. The periungual tissue may become inflamed and have purulent discharge (Fig. 10-25E).

P Onychocryptosis (ingrown nail) is caused by the growth of the distal nail plate into periungual tissue, secondary to increased lateral nail pressure, resulting in trauma to the tissue.

A Nails that become white, thin, and curved under the free edge are abnormal.

P Eggshell nails may be caused by systemic diseases, chemotherapy, iron deficiency, nutritional deficiencies, or sleeping with the hand fisted.

A Nails that atrophy, shrink, and fall off are abnormal.

P Onychatrophia may result from injury to the nail matrix and systemic diseases.

A Nails that hypertrophy (become abnormally thick and overgrown) are abnormal (Fig. 10-25F).

P Onychauxis is caused by systemic infection, electrolyte imbalance, and hereditary predisposition.

A Nails deformed in shape are abnormal (Fig. 10-25G).

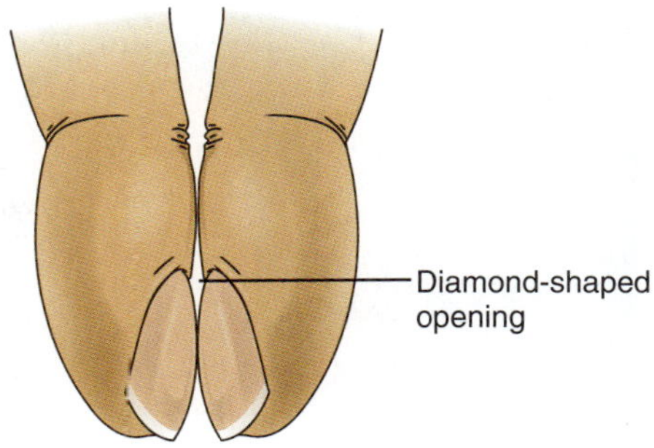

Figure 10-23 Assess the nailbeds' configuration.

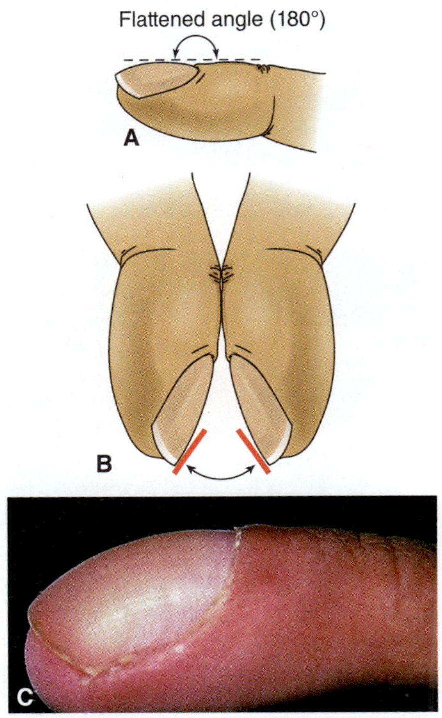

Figure 10-24 Clubbing. **A.** Early clubbing. **B.** Clubbing seen from a lateral view. **C.** Established clubbing.

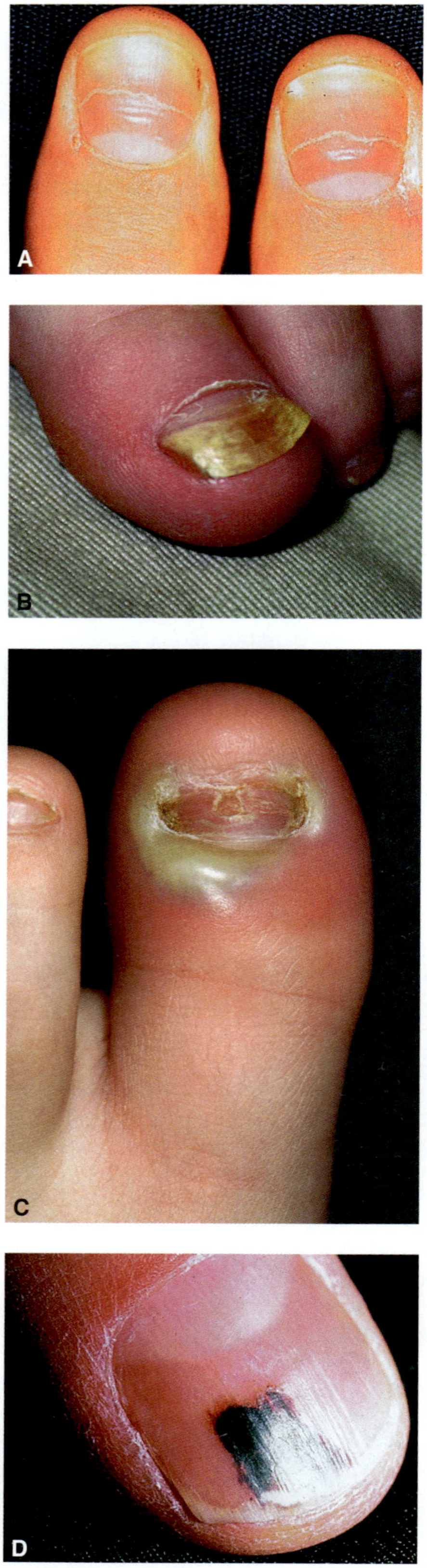

P Onychophagy results from excessive biting of the nails.

A A nail that is split or brittle with lengthwise ridges is abnormal (Fig. 10-25H).

P Onychorrhexis may result from trauma to the nail, toxic exposure to solvents, or harsh nail filing.

A It is abnormal for the cuticle to overgrow the nail and become attached to the nail. The cuticle growth may persist to the free edge.

P Pterygium can occur in Raynaud phenomenon.

A Numerous horizontal depression ridges or a depression down the middle of the nail is abnormal (Fig. 10-25I).

P Habit tic deformity is caused by continuous picking of the cuticle and nail by a finger of the same hand. Trauma ensues to the nail base and nail matrix.

A A soft/thin nail that has horizontal splits or splits at the distal nail edge is abnormal (Fig. 10-25J).

P Onychoschizia refers to a brittle nail. Usually, it is caused by nails that are too "wet" (from frequent exposure to liquids, chemicals, and nail products) or the nails are too "dry" (due to decreased nail moisture). In some instances, onychoschizia can be the result of chronic conditions such as iron deficiency, psoriasis, and Sjögren syndrome.

A A nail that has dimples or depressions can be indicative of systemic disease (Fig. 10-25K).

P Nail pitting can occur in psoriasis, eczema, and autoimmune diseases.

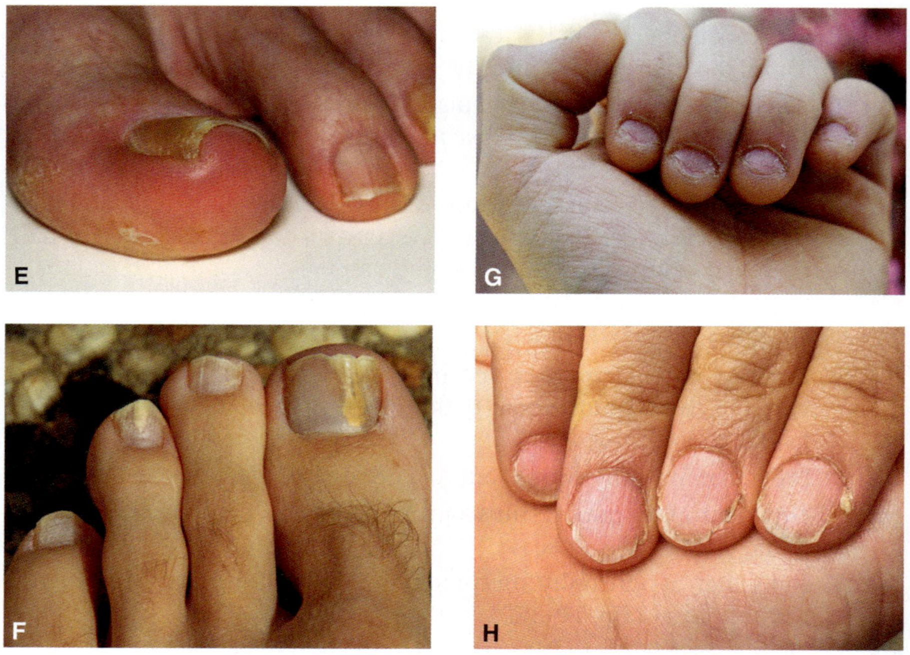

Figure 10-25 Abnormalities of the shape and configuration of the nail. **A.** Beau lines. **B.** Onycholysis. **C.** Paronychia. **D.** Subungual hematoma. **E.** Onychocryptosis. Note the erythema around the ingrown toenail. **F.** Onychauxis. **G.** Onychophagy. **H.** Onychorrhexis.

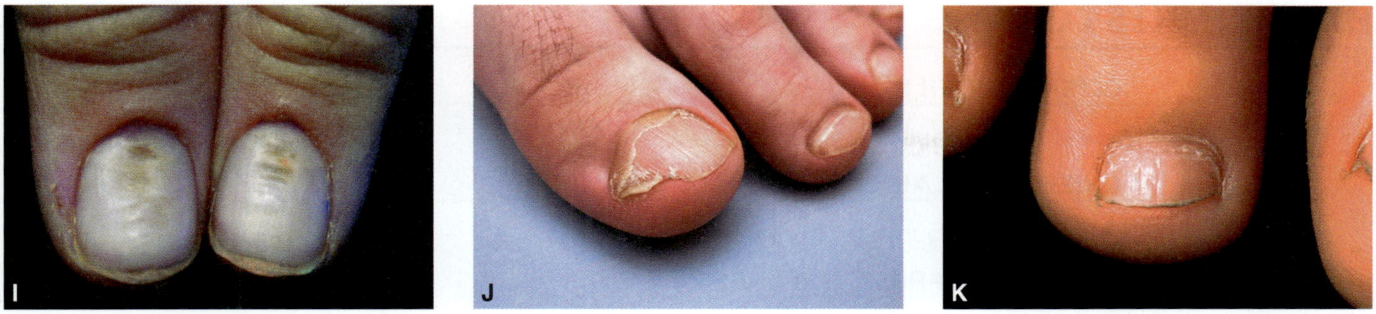

Figure 10-25—cont'd I. Habit tic deformity. **J.** Onychoschizia. **K.** Nail pitting.

Palpation of the Nails

Texture

E
1. Palpate the nail base between your thumb and index finger.
2. Note the consistency.

N **The nail base should be firm on palpation.**

A A spongy nail base is an early indication of clubbing.

P Clubbing is the result of impaired tissue oxygenation over a prolonged period, as in chronic bronchitis, emphysema, and heart disease. See Chapters 15 and 16 for additional information.

U.S. Preventive Services Task Force (USPSTF)

Grade B Recommendation:

The USPSTF recommends counseling young adults, adolescents, children, and parents of young children about minimizing exposure to ultraviolet (UV) radiation for persons aged 6 months to 24 years with fair skin types to reduce their risk of skin cancer.

Retrieved October 20, 2025, from *https:// uspreventiveservicestaskforce.org/uspstf/recommendation-topics/uspstf-a-and-b-recommendations*

CASE STUDY

The Client With a Lip Lesion

This case study illustrates the application and objective documentation of the skin, hair, and nail assessment. Richelle presents with a painful, red rash on her lip. Richelle owns a calligraphy business. With the rising prices of food and gas and the economic recession, customer orders have been decreasing. In addition, Richelle has been stressed about the status of her marriage to husband #3. Richelle is worried about the worsening sores on the lip and goes to a same-day clinic for evaluation.

HEALTH HISTORY

CLIENT PROFILE

48-year-old married female

CHIEF COMPLAINT

"I have a painful bump on my lower lip."

HISTORY OF PRESENT ILLNESS

Client noticed a bump on lower lip 2 days ago that was thought to be a "zit" and tried to "pop it." Felt some tingling in the area before the bump appeared. Now the bump "looks infected" and has been getting bigger. Client was hoping it would go away on its own, but the pain is getting worse. Client reports a dull headache and malaise. Did not take temperature and did not feel feverish. Denies bleeding or drainage. Denies any other lesions. No pain-relieving medications taken. Has taken alprazolam twice a day for 2 days with no effect on the lip, but it made her feel more relaxed. No shortness of breath (SOB), congestion, or cough. Denies nausea, vomiting, diarrhea, constipation (NVDC). Denies any recent trauma to the affected area or previous wound in that area. Has never experienced this before. No new medications/chemical exposure/new clothing. Husband does not have any rash.

PAST HEALTH HISTORY

Medical History

Hypothyroidism diagnosed 10 years ago, controlled on medication

Obstructive sleep apnea (OSA) controlled with continuous positive airway pressure (CPAP) 10 cm at night

Depression and anxiety, diagnosed in early adulthood, sees therapist monthly and psychiatrist every 3 months for medication management; stable with no thoughts of hurting self/others. Has been stable for the past 2 months.

Prediabetes, HbA1c 6.2% 5 months ago

Surgical History

Cesarean section without complications at ages 18 and 25

Open reduction internal fixation (ORIF) of right humerus 7 years ago

Multiple facial reconstructive surgeries to right side of face with the last occurring 5 years ago

Allergies

Denies medication, food, and environmental allergies

Denies allergy to bee stings and latex

Medications

Levothyroxine 125 mcg orally every morning

Duloxetine 60 mg orally daily

Alprazolam 0.5 mg orally every 6 hr as needed

Vitamin D 2,000 IU daily

MVI daily

Communicable Diseases Denies hepatitis/HIV/STIs

Injuries and Accidents Victim of domestic abuse with husband #2—hospitalized 7 years ago with fractured right humerus, crush injury to zygoma, and mandible with right globe rupture

Differing Abilities Right eye blindness and right ear with moderate hearing loss from facial trauma 7 years ago

Blood Transfusions Two units packed red blood cells 7 years ago

Childhood Diseases Chickenpox

Immunizations Up to date with most recent COVID-19 booster and flu vaccine

FAMILY HEALTH HISTORY

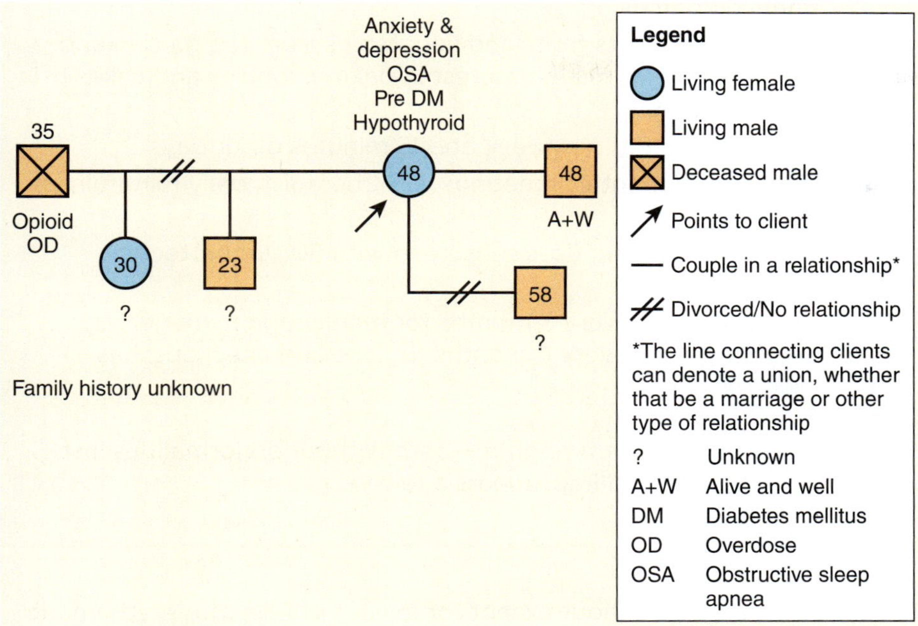

SOCIAL HISTORY

Alcohol Use Drinks 3 to 4 glasses of red wine a week

Tobacco Use Denies ever using

Recreational Drug Use History of cocaine and LSD use in mid-20s

Domestic and Intimate Partner Violence Client reports no abuse in current marriage

Sexual Practice Heterosexual; divorced x2 and remarried last year; sexually active 3 to 4 times a week; engages in vaginal penetration sex and oral sex

Travel History No recent travel with plans of a honeymoon trip to Mexico next month

Work Environment Owns her own online calligraphy business and usually works 20 to 30 hours/week, enjoys her job

Home Environment 1,600-sq-ft townhome that is 50 years old; safe and comfortable

Hobbies and Leisure Activities Geocaching on the weekends and gardening after work on weekdays

Stress Client has evidence that husband has been paying sex workers over the past few months, but she hasn't confronted him yet. "I'm very stressed about whether to confront him or just ignore it. I just can't go through another divorce."

Education Finished high school

Economic Status "I wish we had more money, but there is food on the table and clothes on our backs."

Military Service Denies

Religion Agnostic; does not participate in any faith or spiritual-based communities

Ethnic Background Does not affiliate with any particular ethnic group

Roles and Relationships Lives with her husband, does not feel she has close friends due to her "emotional baggage"; biological family is unknown; does not communicate with family that adopted her related to sustaining sexual abuse from the oldest child while living with them in her early teens (charges were eventually dismissed and she verbalizes still working through the trauma with her therapist). Divorced first husband who then died from an opioid overdose. Divorced second husband after repeated episodes of emotional and physical abuse that resulted in severe injuries. Has no contact with her children.

Characteristic Patterns of Daily Living Client works 3 to 4 days/wk and enjoys being alone in the garden. Has recently started baking. Tries to walk at least 15 min daily.

HEALTH MAINTENANCE ACTIVITIES

Sleep Restful, 6 to 7 hours nightly using CPAP

Diet Does not follow any regimen; eats fruits and vegetables from the garden and enjoys sweet treats, especially with recent interest in baking cookies and cakes using new recipes found on the Internet.

Exercise Walking 30 minutes 2 to 3 times/week and 15 minutes other days

Stress Management Gardening; monthly meetings with therapist; daily mindfulness meditation

Use of Safety Devices Wears seatbelt; uses sunscreen with 50 sun protection factor (SPF)

Health Checkups Sees psychiatrist every 3 months for medication management;

sees primary care provider (PCP) every 6 months for labs and checkups; has appointment for next month

Dentist annually

Up to date with Pap smears and mammogram—both without abnormalities last year. Recalls there were abnormal Pap smears a few years ago.

PHYSICAL EXAMINATION

Inspection of the Skin

Color Light brown pigment throughout except for lower right lip with erythematic lesion

Bleeding, Ecchymosis, and Vascularity None

Lesions Lower right lip lesion 1.5 cm x 1 cm of grouped vesicles on an erythematic base without drainage, no odor

Palpation of the Skin

Moisture Dry

Temperature No areas with increased warmth

Tenderness Lesion painful to light touch; submental lymphadenopathy noted

Texture Nonaffected areas smooth

Turgor Positive skin turgor over anterior chest

Edema Mild inflammatory edema of the affected lip area

Inspection of the Hair

Color Dark brown, graying by ears

Distribution Consistent without alopecia or receding

Lesions No infestations

Palpation of the Hair

Texture Mildly coarse, not brittle

Inspection of the Nails

Color Light brown nailbed; capillary refill less than 2 seconds

Shape and Configuration Smooth and slightly rounded; no splintering or brittle edges; nail base angle approximately 160°

Palpation of the Nails

Texture Firm

CLINICAL JUDGMENT IN ACTION

1. What cues indicate that the client has a skin disorder?
2. What interventions have the highest priority?
3. What assessment findings indicate clinical improvement in this client?

Review Questions

1. Risk factors for developing melanoma include which of the following? Select all that apply.
   a. Previous history of breast cancer
   b. Biological mother treated for melanoma
   c. Fair skin tone
   d. Wearing sunscreen
   e. Using tanning beds

2. Where should the nurse assess for peripheral cyanosis?
   a. Oral mucosa
   b. Conjunctiva
   c. Hard palate
   d. Fingers

3. A condition characterized by the presence of confluent petechiae or ecchymosis is:
   a. Purpura
   b. Venous star
   c. Angioma
   d. Vitiligo

4. A lesion with an accumulation of serous fluid measuring 0.3 cm would best be documented as:
   a. Pustule
   b. Cyst
   c. Bullae
   d. Vesicle

5. A client with chronic dermatitis of both lower legs presents with thickened, rough skin over the affected areas without exudate. How should the nurse document this finding?
   a. Atrophy
   b. Keloid
   c. Lichenification
   d. Crust

6. Education for a parent of a child newly diagnosed with impetigo should include:
   a. Use calamine lotion for the itching.
   b. Refrain from touching the rash and frequently wash hands.
   c. Obtain vaccines to ensure the child is up to date.
   d. Avoid spicy foods, activity, and stress.

7. Danger sign of a potentially cancerous lesion includes:
   a. Consistent color
   b. Border irregularity
   c. Symmetry of the lesion
   d. Nevi without changes for 6 years

8. The client has a burn that affects the epidermis, dermis, and subcutaneous tissue but no involvement of the muscle or bone. How should this burn injury be identified?
   a. First-degree
   b. Second-degree
   c. Third-degree
   d. Fourth-degree

9. The nurse identifies pitting edema that leaves a 6-mm depression that lasts for over a minute. How does the nurse document this edema finding?
   a. 1+
   b. 2+
   c. 3+
   d. 4+

10. Clubbing of the nail can result from:
    a. Chronic hypoxia
    b. Eczema
    c. Paronychia
    d. Diet low in vitamin D

CHAPTER 11

Head, Neck, and Regional Lymph Nodes

Learning Outcomes

1. Identify the anatomy and physiology of the head, neck, and regional lymph nodes.
2. Conduct a complete health history on a client with a head, neck, or regional lymph node condition.
3. Perform a physical examination on a healthy adult and an adult with a head, neck, or regional lymph node pathology.
4. Differentiate between normal clinical findings from a client's physical examination and the pathophysiology of abnormal clinical findings.
5. Identify risk factors for thyroid cancer.
6. Document a complete health history and physical examination of a client with head, neck, and regional lymph node pathology.

Examination of the head, neck, and regional lymph nodes yields a wide range of critical clues about the functions of various body systems. As you examine the head, neck, and regional lymph nodes, you will learn about the skin, endocrine function, musculoskeletal integrity, and neurological and lymphatic functions.

Anatomy and Physiology

The skull, face, neck, thyroid, lymph nodes, and blood supply are discussed in the following sections.

Skull

The skull is a complex bony structure that rests on the superior end of the vertebral column (Fig. 11-1). The skull protects the brain from direct injury and provides a surface for attachment of the muscles that assist with mastication and produce facial expressions.

Cranial bones of the skull are connected by immovable joints called **sutures**. The most prominent sutures are the coronal suture, the sagittal suture, and the lambdoidal suture. The junction of the coronal and sagittal sutures is called the **bregma**.

Face

The face of every individual has its own unique characteristics influenced by factors such as race, state of health, emotions, and environment. Facial structures are symmetrical so that the eyes, eyebrows, nose, mouth, nasolabial folds, and palpebral fissures look the same on both sides.

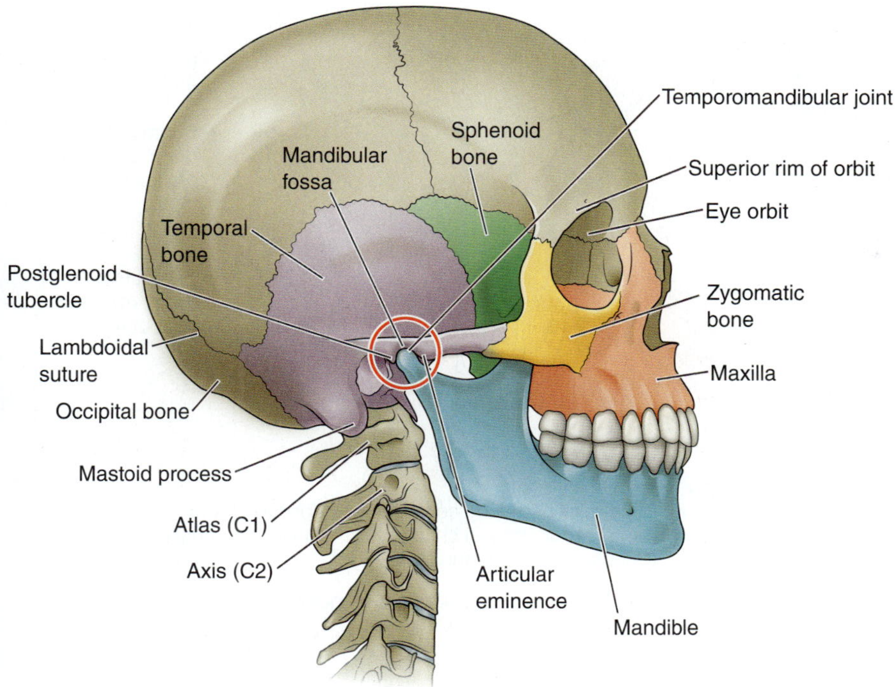

Figure 11-1 Bones of the face and skull (lateral view).

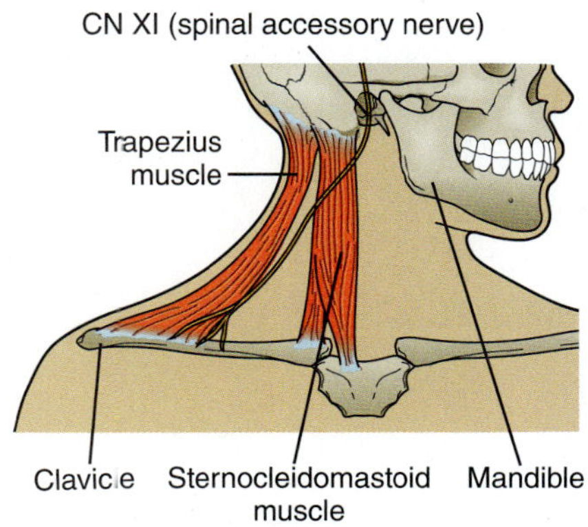

Figure 11-2 Major cervical muscles.

Neck

The neck is made up of seven flexible cervical vertebrae that support the head while allowing maximum mobility. The first cervical vertebra, the **atlas,** articulates with the occipital condyles to support and balance the head. The second vertebra, the **axis,** has an odontoid process that extends into the ring of the atlas, allowing it to pivot as the head is turned from side to side. The seventh cervical vertebra has a long spinous process called the **vertebra prominens,** which serves as a useful landmark during physical examination of the neck and posterior thorax.

The major muscles of the neck are the sternocleidomastoids and the trapezii (Fig. 11-2). The sternocleidomastoid muscles, which extend from the upper portion of the sternum and the clavicle to the mastoid process, allow the head to bend laterally, rotate, flex, and extend. They also divide each side of the neck into two triangles: the anterior cervical and the posterior cervical (Fig. 11-3), which serve as examination landmarks. The **anterior triangle** is formed by the mandible, the trachea, and the sternocleidomastoid muscle and contains the anterior cervical lymph nodes, the trachea, and the thyroid gland. The **posterior triangle,** the area between the sternocleidomastoid and the trapezius muscles with the clavicle at the base, contains the posterior cervical lymph nodes.

The trapezii extend from the occipital bone down the neck to insert at the outer third of the clavicles, at the acromion process of the scapula, and along the spinal column to the level of T_{12}. They allow the shoulders and scapula to move up and down, and rotate the scapula medially.

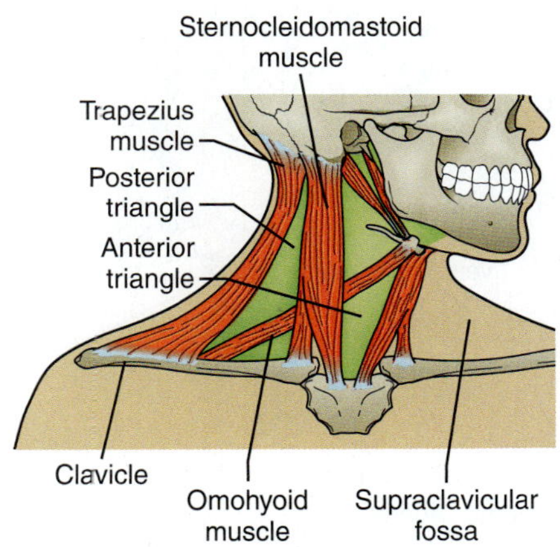

Figure 11-3 Anterior and posterior cervical triangles.

Thyroid

The thyroid gland, the largest endocrine gland in the body, secretes thyroxine (T_4) and triiodothyronine (T_3), which regulate the rate of cellular metabolism. The gland, a flattened, butterfly shaped structure with two lateral lobes connected by the **isthmus,** weighs about 25 to 30 grams and is slightly larger in women (Fig. 11-4). The isthmus rests on top of the trachea, inferior to the cricoid cartilage.

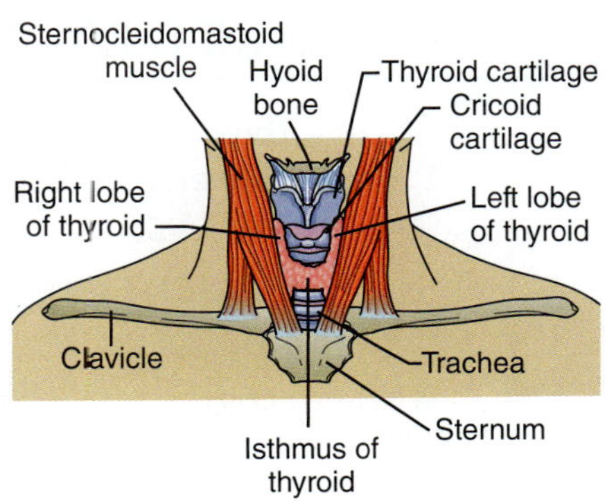

Figure 11-4 Thyroid gland and surrounding structures.

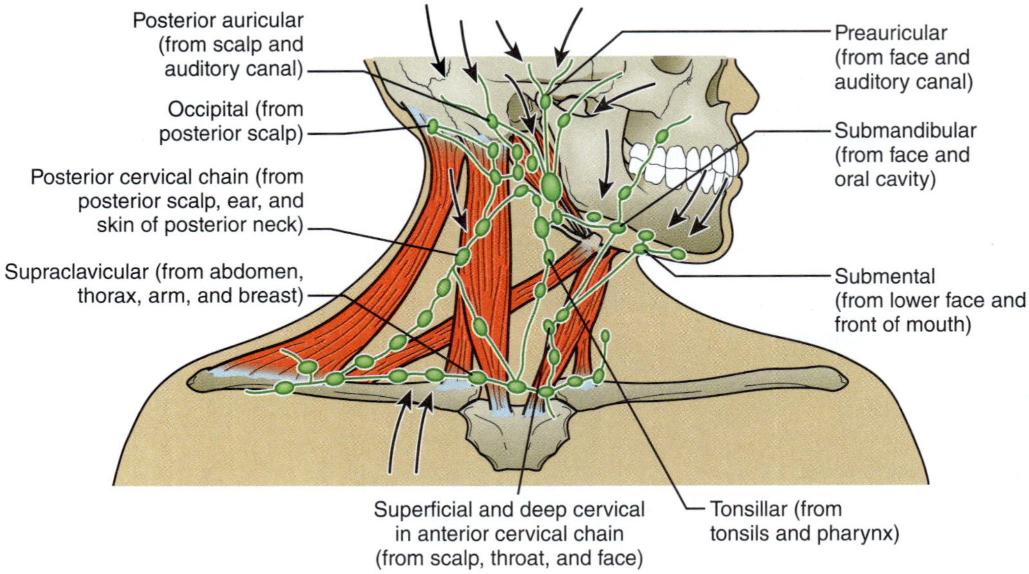

Figure 11-5 Lymph nodes of the head and neck and drainage patterns.

Lymph Nodes

An extensive system of lymphatic vessels drains the head and neck and is an important part of the immune system (Fig. 11-5). Lymphatic tissue in the nodes is responsible for the filtering and sequestration of pathogens and other harmful substances. Lymph nodes are usually less than 1 cm, round or ovoid in shape, and smooth in consistency. When nodes are enlarged or tender, it is important to assess for infection or malignancy. Note the direction in which each node drains (Fig. 11-5). If a tender or enlarged lymph node is found during the clinical examination, assess the entire lymph node area, as well as the area where the involved node drains. For example, if a client's posterior cervical node is enlarged, examine the posterior scalp, the ear (both externally and internally), and the skin of the posterior neck for pathology. Refer to Chapter 17 for additional information on the lymphatic system.

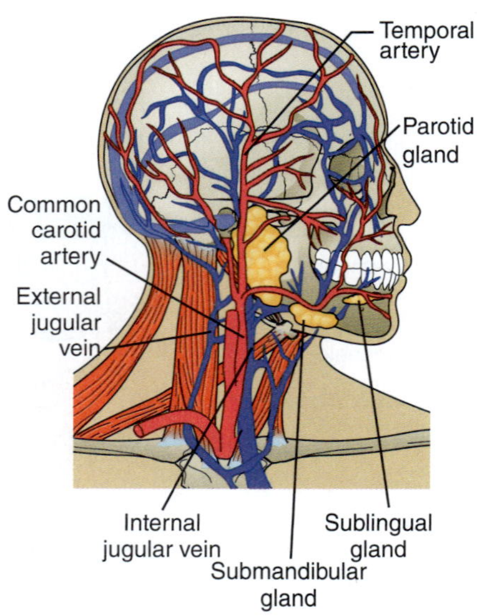

Figure 11-6 Major veins and arteries of the neck.

Blood Supply

The blood supply to the head and neck is quite extensive, with arterial and venous patterns. Major arteries that carry blood to the head and neck include the common carotids (which bifurcate into the internal and external carotid arteries), the brachiocephalic artery (the right common carotid artery branches from this), the subclavian arteries, and the temporal arteries. Deoxygenated blood from the head and neck is returned to the heart via the internal and external jugular veins, the brachiocephalic vein, and the subclavian veins (Fig. 11-6).

HEALTH HISTORY

The head, neck, and regional lymph nodes health history provides insight into the link between a client's life/lifestyle, and head, neck, and regional lymph nodes information and pathology.

CLIENT PROFILE

Diseases that are age- and sex-specific for the head, neck, and regional lymph nodes are listed.

Age

Lymphadenopathies related to Hodgkin disease (11 to 29)
Cervical spine trauma (young adults)

Hyperthyroidism (reproductive years in young women)
Thyroid cancer in women (40 to 50)
Thyroid cancer in men (60 to 70)
Temporal arteritis (older adults)
Decreased mobility of the cervical spine related to an inflammatory or degenerative process (older adults)

Sex

Female Hypo- or hyperthyroidism, thyroid cancer, migraines
Degenerative cervical bone disease
Male Lymphadenopathy related to Hodgkin disease
Trauma-related cervical spine injury

CHIEF COMPLAINT

Common chief complaints for the head, neck, and regional lymph nodes are defined, and information on the characteristics of each sign or symptom is provided.

1. **Stiff Neck** Painful movement of the neck that restricts the range of motion
   - **Quality** Limited range of motion, either passive or active
   - **Associated Manifestations** Headache, neck tenderness, swelling, fever, numbness, and tingling in arms or hands
   - **Aggravating Factors** Position (sitting, standing, lying down), immobilization of position for a prolonged period, mobility, stress, weather
   - **Alleviating Factors** Immobility or rest, certain position, steroids, analgesics, muscle relaxants, heat
   - **Setting** Work, driving, stress
   - **Timing** With all movements, with rotating movements only, with flexion and extension only; with weather changes; after falls, motor vehicle or other accidents; after exposure to meningitis
2. **Neck Mass** Discrete area of swelling found in the neck
   - **Quality** Mobile, nonmobile, smooth, irregular, tender, nontender
   - **Associated Manifestations** Shortness of breath, hoarseness, weight loss, fever and chills, dysphagia, ear pain, prior radiation therapy to head/neck
   - **Aggravating Factors** Eating, talking, movement, tight clothing around the neck, swallowing
   - **Alleviating Factors** Avoidance of tight clothing, analgesic medications, decreased dietary intake
   - **Setting** History of head/neck radiation
   - **Timing** Long-standing, recent
3. **Headache** Pain felt within the head, behind the eyes, or at the nape of the neck (Table 11-1)
   - **Location** Temporal, frontal, occipital, orbital, hemicranial/bilateral, neck, facial pain, behind the eyes, and upper shoulders
   - **Quality** Neck pain: aching, sore, dull, sharp
     Head pain: throbbing, sharp, dull, aching
   - **Associated Manifestations** Neck pain: fever, headache, swelling, tenderness
     Head pain: nausea and vomiting, aura (visual, olfactory, auditory, tactile), diplopia, blurred vision, irritability, sneezing, rhinorrhea, weakness, dizziness, photophobia, phonophobia, use of oral contraceptives, hypertension, nosebleed, cough
   - **Aggravating Factors** Neck pain: stress, trauma, aging, position, mobility, weather changes
     Head pain: stress, fatigue, foods, noxious odors, caffeine intake, coughing, alcohol intake, smoke, hunger, season, menstruation, chemicals, toxins
   - **Alleviating Factors** Medications such as analgesics, anti-inflammatory agents, ergotamine, caffeine or caffeinated medications, antidepressants (e.g., tricyclic antidepressants [TCA]), calcitonin gene-related peptide antagonists (gepants), triptans, opioids, beta blockers, calcium channel blockers, antiseizure medications, Botox injections; position change; rest; sleep; shaking head; food intake

Setting Work, outdoors, relationship to biological events, stressful environment, change in weather, head trauma, sexual activity, after exposure to viral illness, after exposure to meningitis, after head trauma/injury

Timing Acute and sudden onset, at rest, with weather changes

Head pain: constant, intermittent, in the morning, at the end of the day, premenstrual, seasonal

Neck pain: with movement

4. Head Injury

Quality Open, closed

Associated Manifestations Light-headedness, photophobia, phonophobia, poor attention and concentration, sleep disturbances, depression, neck pain, nausea, vomiting, projectile vomiting, dizziness or vertigo, headache, seizure activity, loss of consciousness, amnesia, visual disturbances, gait disturbances, speech disturbances, confusion, drowsiness, abnormal behavior, abnormal movement of extremities, change in respiratory pattern, discharge from nose or ear, head or neck lacerations/abrasions/ecchymoses

Alleviating Factors Ice, analgesics, rest, surgical intervention

Setting Mechanism of injury, use of helmet or protective headgear, use of seat belt, violent activity, fall, sports injury, motor vehicle accident (MVA), alcohol or drug use; concurrent history of seizure disorder, heart disease, or diabetes mellitus

PAST HEALTH HISTORY

The various components of the past health history are linked to head, neck, and regional lymph nodes pathology and head, neck, and regional lymph nodes–related information.

Medical History

Head, Neck, and Regional Lymph Nodes Specific Hypothyroidism, hyperthyroidism, hypoparathyroidism, hyperparathyroidism, history of thyroid nodules, sinus infections, migraines, headaches, head and neck cancer, head injury, skull fracture, Bell palsy, Cushing syndrome, lymphadenopathy, lymphomas

Non-Head, Neck, and Regional Lymph Nodes Specific Pheochromocytoma, recent lumbar puncture

Surgical History Thyroidectomy, parathyroidectomy, facial reconstruction, cosmetic surgery, neurosurgery, and head or neck surgery

Medications Levothyroxine, liothyronine, desiccated thyroid extract, antibiotics, steroids, anticonvulsants, chemotherapy, beta blockers, analgesics, oral contraceptives, radioiodine (^{131}I), propylthiouracil, methimazole

Communicable Diseases Meningitis, encephalitis

Injuries and Accidents Obstruction caused by foreign bodies, trauma to the head or neck, chemical splashes to the face, noxious fumes, sports injuries, motor vehicle accidents

Differing Abilities Tracheostomy, stoma, paralysis

FAMILY HEALTH HISTORY

Familial head, neck, and regional lymph node diseases are listed.

Thyroid disease, migraines, familial medullary thyroid carcinoma, familial nonmedullary thyroid carcinoma, multiple endocrine neoplasia type 2, Cowden syndrome

SOCIAL HISTORY

The components of the social history are linked to head, neck, and regional lymph node factors and pathology.

Alcohol Use Predisposes to accidents and head injury

Work Environment Risk of head injury, exposure to toxins or chemicals, carbon monoxide exposure

Home Environment Risk of falls and head injury due to loose throw rugs or absence of handrails, carbon monoxide exposure

Stress Demands of employment, home, school

HEALTH MAINTENANCE ACTIVITIES

This information provides a bridge between the health maintenance activities and head, neck, and regional lymph node function.

Sleep May be increased due to head injury, may be decreased due to pain

Diet Recent weight gain or loss

Use of Safety Devices Protective headgear for sports and work

Table 11-1 Classification of Headaches

Type of Headache	Clinical Conditions
Vascular Etiologies	Migraine and cluster headache, subarachnoid hemorrhage, subdural hematoma, brain infarction, cerebral aneurysm, temporal arteritis, vasculitis
Muscle Contraction	Tension headache
Intracranial Etiologies	Brain tumor, increased intracranial pressure from hydrocephalus or pseudotumor cerebri, intracranial infection (e.g., meningitis, encephalitis, abscess), ischemic cerebrovascular disease
Systemic Etiologies	Infection, postlumbar puncture, hypertension, exertion from coitus, cough or exercise, postictal, pheochromocytoma, premenstrual syndrome
Food-Related Etiologies	Nitrites (e.g., hot dogs, bacon, processed meats), tyramine (e.g., cheese, chocolate, pickled foods, citrus fruit), monosodium glutamate (e.g., fast food, soups, chips and snacks, processed meats, some ethnic foods), alcohol, ice cream, some artificial sweeteners, food allergy
Facial or Cervical Etiologies	Sinusitis, temporomandibular joint dysfunction, dental lesions, trigeminal neuralgia, cervical spine radiculopathy
Ocular-Related Etiologies	Narrow-angle glaucoma, uveitis, extraocular muscle paralysis, eye strain
Metabolic Etiologies	Hypoxia, hypercapnia, hypoglycemia
Drug Etiologies	Alcohol and alcohol withdrawal, caffeine and caffeine withdrawal, nitrates, oral contraceptives, estrogen, nicotine, side effects of some prescription and over-the-counter medications, acute medication overuse
Environmental Etiologies	Change in barometric pressure from weather or altitude, carbon monoxide poisoning, tobacco smoke, glaring or flickering lights, odors
Miscellaneous Etiologies	Fever, influenza, head trauma, otitis media, parotitis, pregnancy, fatigue and decreased sleep, psychogenic disorders, sexual activity, stress, eye strain

Risk Factors

Migraine Headaches

- Adolescence to age 40
- Female
- Family history of migraines
- Allergies
- Increased stress, anxiety, panic
- Caffeine intake/withdrawal
- Tyramine, MSG, sulfites, or nitrite consumption
- Sleep disorders
- Oral contraceptive and hormone use
- Depression
- Changes in barometric pressure with the weather
- Change in altitude

NURSING CHECKLIST

General Approach to Head, Neck, and Regional Lymph Nodes Examination

1. Observe Standard Precautions and don Personal Protective Equipment (PPE), such as gloves, gown, face shield, goggles, N-95 respirator or face mask, if the client's status warrants these protective measures.
2. Greet the client and explain the examination techniques that you will be using.
3. Ensure that the environment is at a warm, comfortable room temperature to provide the client comfort.
4. Use a quiet room that will be free from interruptions.
5. Ensure that the light in the room is sufficiently bright to allow adequate observation of the client.
6. Place the client in an upright sitting position on the examination table, or gain access to the head of the supine, bedridden client by removing nonessential equipment or bedding (for clients who cannot tolerate the sitting position).
7. If the client is wearing a wig or headpiece, ask the client to remove it.
8. Visualize the underlying anatomic structures during the examination process to permit an accurate description of the location of any pathology.
9. Always compare the right and left sides of the head, neck, and face to one another.
10. Use the same systematic approach every time the examination is performed.

Assessment in Brief

Head, Neck, and Regional Lymph Nodes Examination

Inspection

- Shape of the head
- Scalp
- Face
  - Symmetry
  - Shape and features
- Neck
- Thyroid gland
- Lymph nodes

Palpation

- Head
- Scalp
- Mandible
- Neck
- Thyroid gland
  - Posterior approach
  - Anterior approach
- Lymph nodes

Auscultation

- Mandible
- Thyroid gland

Equipment

- Appropriate PPE
- Stethoscope
- Cup of water
- Tangential light

Examination of the Head and Neck

Inspection of the Shape of the Head

E
1. Have the client sit in a comfortable position.
2. Face the client, with your head at the same level as the client's head.
3. Inspect the head for shape and symmetry.

N **The head should be normocephalic and symmetrical.**

A **Hydrocephalus** is an enlargement of the head without enlargement of the facial structures.

P Hydrocephalus is caused by an abnormal accumulation of cerebrospinal fluid within the skull.

A **Acromegaly** is an abnormal enlargement of the skull with **frontal bossing** (prominent protruding forehead which may occur with protruding eyebrow ridges), mandibular enlargement with **prognathism** (protruding upper jaw, lower jaw, or both), a widened nose, widened space between the lower incisor teeth, and large lips (Fig. 11-7).

P Acromegaly is caused by excessive secretion of growth hormone from the pituitary gland.

A Craniosynostosis is characterized by abnormal shape of the skull or bone growth at right angles to suture lines, exophthalmos, and drooping eyelids.

P Craniosynostosis is caused by the premature closure of one or more sutures of the skull before brain growth is complete.

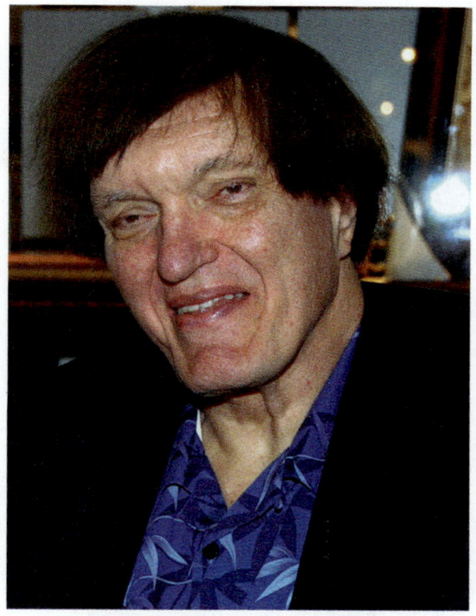

Figure 11-7 Note the enlarged skull and bony facial structures in this man with acromegaly.

Palpation of the Head

E
1. Place the finger pads on the scalp and palpate all of its surfaces, beginning in the frontal area and continuing over the parietal, temporal, and occipital areas.
2. Assess for contour, masses, depressions, tenderness, lesions, symmetry, and trauma
3. Palpate the temporal artery, which is located anterior to the tragus of the ear. Assess for tenderness, hardness, or thickening.

N **The normal skull is smooth, nontender, and without masses or depressions. The temporal artery pulse is usually weaker (1 +/4 + or 1 +/3 +) than the other peripheral pulses of the body. The artery is nontender, smooth, and readily compressible.**

A Masses in the cranial bones that feel hard or soft are abnormal.

P Hard or soft masses may be carcinomatous metastasis from other regions of the body or may result from lymphomas, multiple myeloma, or leukemia.

A Palpation elicits localized edema over the bony frontal portion of the skull.

P Osteomyelitis of the skull may develop following acute or chronic sinusitis if the infection extends out from the sinuses into the surrounding bone.

A Firm palpation reveals a softening of the outer bone layer.

P **Craniotabes** is a softening of the skull caused by hydrocephalus or demineralization of the bone due to rickets, osteogenesis imperfecta, or syphilis.

A A temporal artery that is thickened, hard in consistency, or tender is abnormal.

P A temporal artery that is thickened, hard in consistency, or tender can indicate temporal arteritis. In temporal arteritis, the temporal arteries may also be more torturous.

Inspection and Palpation of the Scalp

E
1. Part the hair repeatedly all over the scalp and inspect the scalp for lesions or masses.
2. Place the finger pads on the scalp and palpate for lesions or masses.

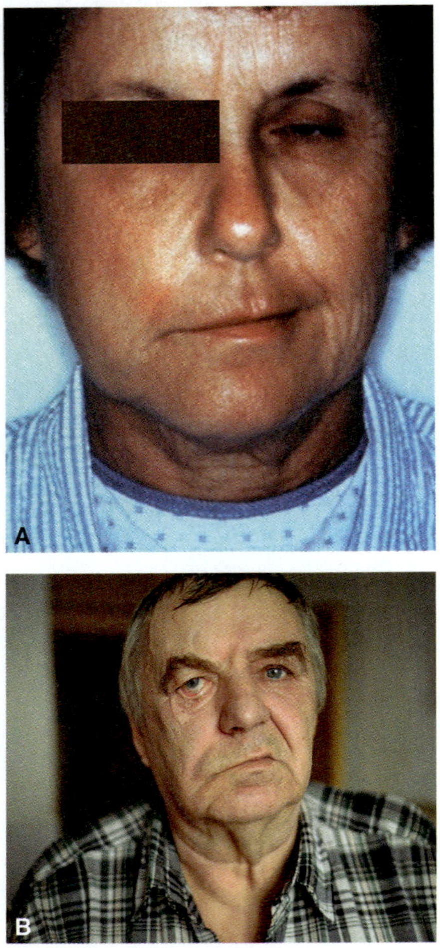

Figure 11-8 Facial asymmetry. **A.** Facial palsy caused by Lyme disease infection. **B.** Bell palsy of the facial nerve (Cranial Nerve VII).

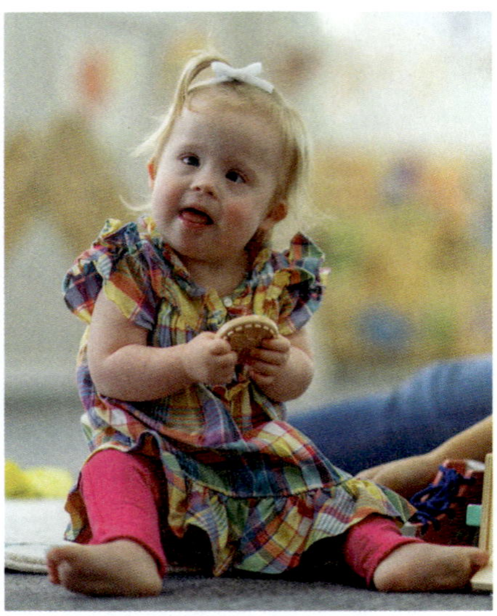

Figure 11-9 Down syndrome.

N **The scalp should be shiny, intact, and without lesions or masses.**

A A laceration or a laceration with bleeding is abnormal.

P Direct trauma can cause lacerations to the scalp.

A A gaping laceration with profuse bleeding is abnormal.

P If the laceration on the scalp is gaping, it indicates a deep wound that may further indicate a compound skull fracture caused by some type of trauma. This requires emergency treatment.

A Palpation reveals a localized, easily movable accumulation of blood in the subcutaneous tissue.

P Hematomas can result from direct trauma to the skull. This can be a life-threatening situation and requires an immediate referral.

A Palpation may reveal either single or multiple masses that are easily movable. They are round, firm, and nontender and arise from either the skin or the subcutaneous tissue.

P These masses are most likely sebaceous cysts that form as a result of the retention of secretions from sebaceous glands.

A Nonmobile, fatty masses with smooth, circular edges may be palpated deeper in the scalp.

P Nonmobile, fatty masses with smooth, circular edges are usually benign fatty tumors known as **lipomas.**

Inspection of the Face

Symmetry

E
1. Have the client sit in a comfortable position facing you.
2. Observe the client's face for expression, shape, and symmetry of the following structures: eyebrows, eyes, nose, mouth, ears.

N **The facial features should be symmetrical. Both palpebral fissures should be equal and the nasolabial fold should present bilaterally. It is important to remember that slight variations in symmetry are common. Eyes with a single epicanthal fold are a normal finding in many clients of Asian descent.**

A Structures are absent or deformed. There is a definite asymmetry of expression, the palpebral fissures, the nasolabial folds, and the corners of the mouth.

P Asymmetry of the palpebral fissures, nasolabial folds, the mouth, and facial expression can be caused by various conditions such as infection (Fig. 11-8A) and damage to the nerves innervating facial muscles (cranial nerve VII), as in stroke or **Bell palsy** (Fig. 11-8B).

Shape and Features

E
1. Face the client.
2. Observe the shape of the client's face.
3. Note any swelling, abnormal features, or unusual movement.

N **The shape of the face can be oval, round, or slightly square. There should be no edema, disproportionate structures, or involuntary movements.**

A Inspection of the face may reveal eyes with a single inner epicanthal fold that gives a "slanted appearance."

P A "slanted" eye appearance likely indicates a chromosomal aberration such as **Down syndrome** (trisomy 21, Figure 11-9), Noonan syndrome, and Turner syndrome, or fetal alcohol syndrome.

A A short, flat nose with a thick, protruding tongue is abnormal.

P A client with Down syndrome may have these findings.

A An abnormally wide distance between the eyes is **hypertelorism**.

P Hypertelorism is caused by a birth defect or chromosomal anomaly such as Noonan syndrome, Apert syndrome, and Crouzon syndrome.

A Facial skin is shiny, contracted, and hard. The face appears to have furrows around the mouth (Fig. 11-10).

P Scleroderma is a collagen disease of unknown cause. Sclerosis of the skin, as well as visceral organs (esophagus, lungs, heart, muscles, and kidneys) occurs.

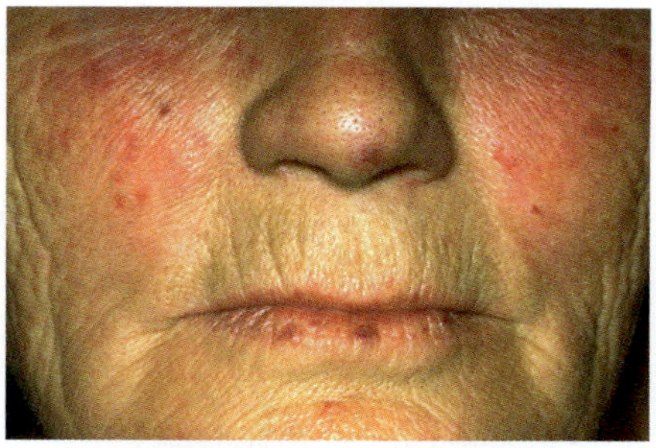

Figure 11-10 Scleroderma.

A The face is thin with sharply defined features and prominent eyes (exophthalmos) in Graves disease (Fig. 11-11).

P Graves disease is an autoimmune thyroid disease.

A The client's face is round and swollen, with characteristic periorbital edema and dry, dull skin.

P This condition is known as myxedema and is associated with hypothyroidism.

A The eyes are sunken and the cheeks are hollow in cachexia.

P Cachexia is a profound wasting of vital tissues that is associated with malignant conditions, malnutrition, and severe chronic illnesses such as HIV.

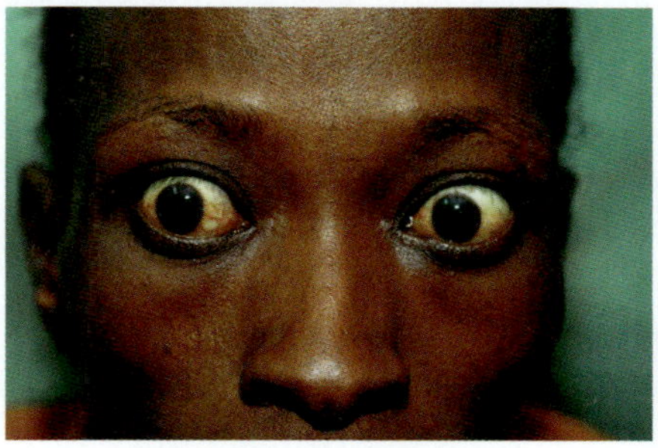

Figure 11-11 Exophthalmos.

A The client's face is immobile and expressionless, with a staring gaze, decreased blinking, and raised eyebrows, in Parkinson disease (Fig. 11-12).

P In Parkinson disease, the basal ganglia degenerate due to a deficiency of the neurotransmitter dopamine.

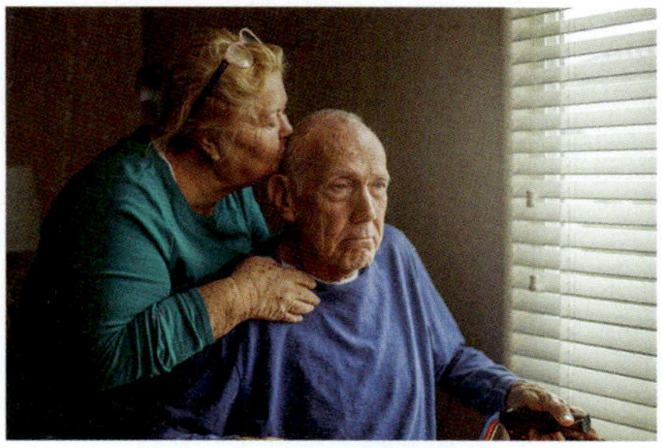

Figure 11-12 Parkinson disease. Note the raised eyebrows and staring gaze.

A The faces of some people of European heritage show a dark or dusky blue discoloration beneath the eyes ("allergic shiners") along with creases below the lower eyelids (Dennie-Morgan lines) and open mouth due to mouth breathing (Fig. 11-13).

P The client with chronic allergies or allergic rhinitis develops this characteristic allergic facies or allergic gape. This can occur in seasonal or perennial allergic rhinitis.

A A transverse crease is noted across the nose.

P This is a characteristic finding in clients with allergies and allergic rhinitis who frequently are observed to do the "nasal salute" or upward wiping of the nose (Fig. 11-14).

A The client has a rounded "moon face" along with red cheeks and excess hair on the jaw and upper lip (Fig. 11-15).

P This is the facies of Cushing syndrome, which is caused by increased production of adrenocorticotropic hormone (ACTH) or prolonged steroid ingestion.

A An enlargement of the cheek is abnormal.

P Salivary gland enlargement can result from an infection, tumor, abscess, or blocked duct. The parotid gland can also be enlarged in mumps (Fig. 11-16).

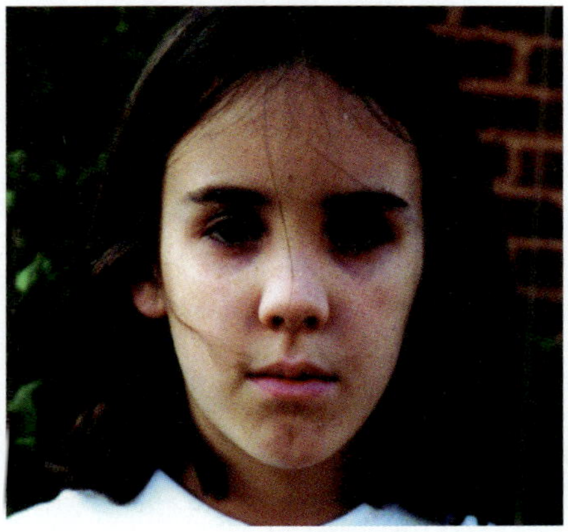

Figure 11-13 Allergic facies.

Palpation and Auscultation of the Mandible

E 1. Use the fingertips of both index and middle fingers to locate the temporomandibular joint anterior to the tragus of the ear on both sides.

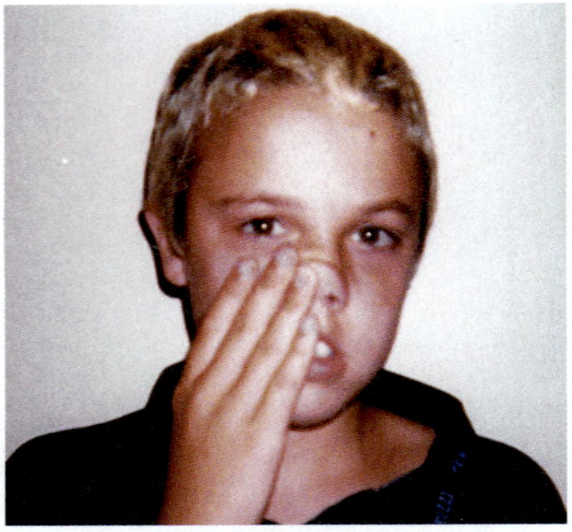

Figure 11-14 This young boy has a characteristic nasal crease from the repeated action of the "nasal salute" caused by allergies.

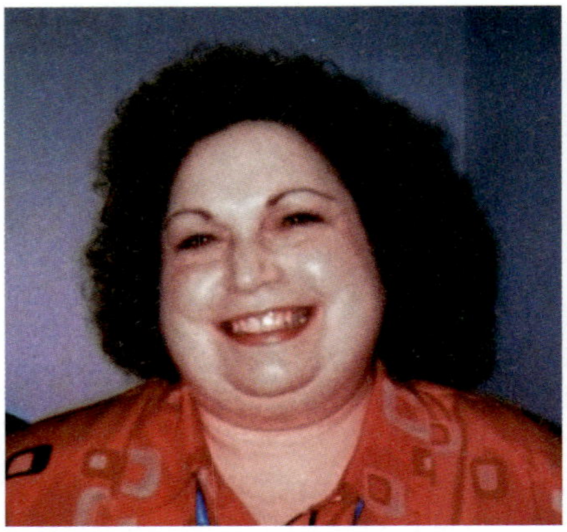

Figure 11-15 Cushing syndrome.

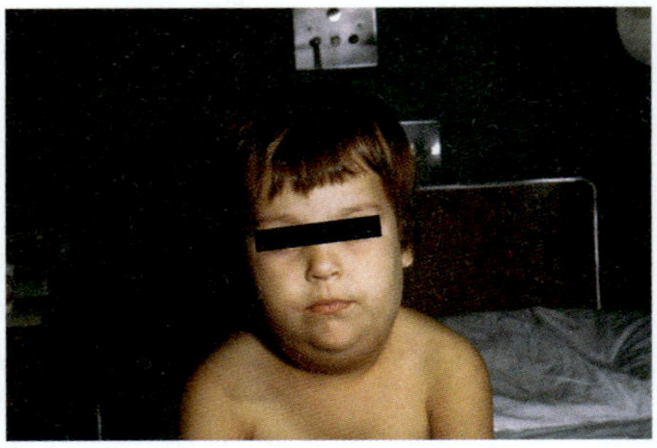

Figure 11-16 A child with mumps.

2. Hold the fingertips firmly in place over the joints and ask the client to open and close the mouth.
3. As the client opens and closes the mouth, observe the relative smoothness of the movement and whether the client notices any discomfort.
4. Remove the hands.
5. Hold the bell of the stethoscope over the joint.
6. Listen for any sound while the client opens and closes the mouth.

N **The client should experience no discomfort with movement. The temporomandibular joint should articulate smoothly and without clicking or crepitus.**

A The client complains of tenderness when the mouth is opened and closed. Palpation or auscultation reveals clicking or crepitus.

P Tenderness in the temporomandibular joint may be from osteoarthritis.

P Crepitus is present from the articulation of irregular bone surfaces found in osteoarthritis.

P Clicking may follow a "snapping" sound if there is displaced cartilage.

A The mouth remains in an open and fixed position.

P Following a wide yawn or trauma to the chin, the temporomandibular joint is dislocated and will not function. This condition requires reduction.

NURSING TIP

Cranial Nerve Examination

The 12 cranial nerves that innervate the head and neck are integrated into the head and neck examination. Additional information is found in Chapters 12 and 20.

Inspection and Palpation of the Neck

Inspection of the Neck

E
1. Have the client sit facing you, with the head held in a central position.
2. Inspect for symmetry of the sternocleidomastoid muscles anteriorly, and the trapezii posteriorly.
3. Have the client touch the chin to the chest, to each side, and to each shoulder.
4. Assess for limitation of motion.
5. Note the presence of a stoma or tracheostomy.
6. Inspect for alignment of the trachea in the neck area. Refer to Chapter 15 for additional information.

N **The muscles of the neck are symmetrical with the head in a central position. The client can move the head through a full range of motion without complaint of discomfort or noticeable limitation. The trachea should be in the midline of the neck. The client may be breathing through a stoma or tracheostomy.**

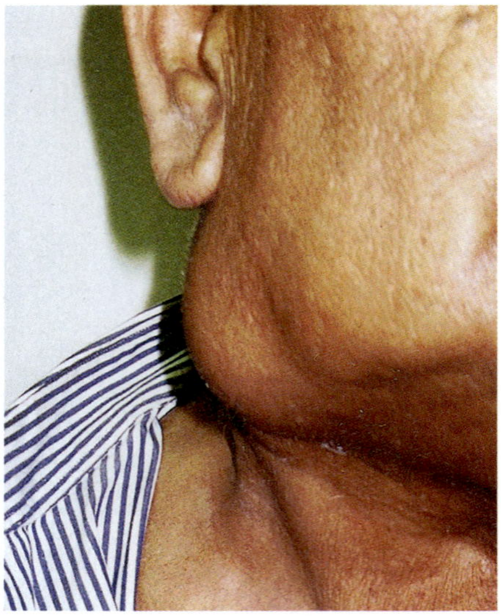

Figure 11-17 This right neck mass was identified as squamous cell carcinoma. *Courtesy of Dr. Daniel D. Rooney.*

A Asymmetry of the neck is abnormal (Fig. 11-17).

E Examination N Normal Findings A Abnormal Findings P Pathophysiology

P Asymmetrical masses can be benign or malignant, but they all must be evaluated further.

A The client complains of pain with flexion or rotation of the head.

P Pain with flexion can be associated with the pain and muscle spasms caused by meningeal irritation of meningitis (see Chapter 20). Generalized discomfort may be related to trauma, spasm, inflammation of muscles, or diseases of the vertebrae.

A There is a slight or prominent lateral deviation of the client's neck. The sternocleidomastoid muscles, and to a lesser extent the trapezius and scalene muscles, may also be prominent on the affected side. The muscles frequently hypertrophy as the result of powerful contractions.

P This condition is called **torticollis** (Fig. 11-18). Causes can be:

1. Congenital: resulting from a hematoma or partial rupture of the sternocleidomastoid at birth, causing a shortening of the muscle.
2. Ocular: a head posture assumed to correct for ocular muscle palsy and resulting diplopia.
3. Acute spasm: commonly associated with the inflammation of viral myositis or trauma such as sleeping with the head in an unusual position.
4. Other: phenothiazine medications and Parkinson disease, as the result of increased cholinergic activity in the brain.

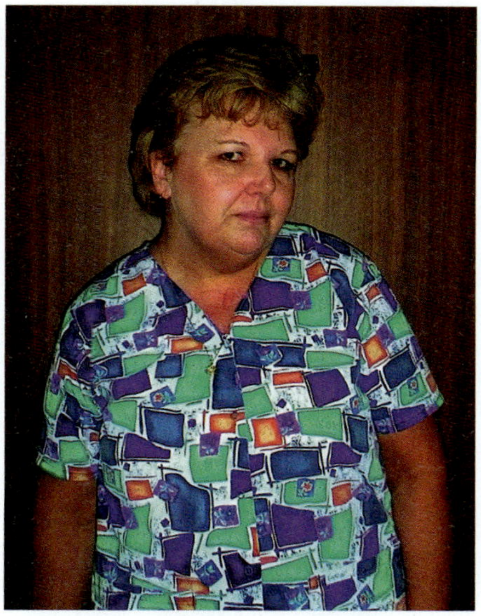

Figure 11-18 Torticollis.

A Range of motion of the neck is reduced.

P Degenerative changes of osteoarthritis may result in a decreased ability for a full range of motion. This condition is usually painless unless nerve root irritation has occurred. Crepitus, or a crunching sound on hyperextension of the neck, may also be observed.

Palpation of the Neck

If a neck injury is suspected, stabilize the neck and do not proceed with the examination. A qualified provider needs to evaluate the extent of the injury.

E

1. Stand in front of the client.
2. With the finger pads, palpate the sternocleidomastoid muscles.
3. Note the presence of masses or tenderness.
4. Stand behind the client.
5. With the finger pads, palpate the trapezius muscles.
6. Note the presence of masses or tenderness.

N **The muscles should be symmetrical, without palpable masses or spasms.**

A A mass is palpated in the musculature.

P A mass may be a tumor, either primary or metastatic.

A A spasm may be felt in the muscles.

P Muscle spasms may be due to varied causes such as infections, trauma, chronic inflammatory processes, or neoplasms.

> **NURSING TIP**
> **Examination of the Neck's Vasculature**
> It is important to examine the carotid arteries and the jugular veins at this point in the examination; refer to Chapter 17 for a description of the technique.

Inspection of the Thyroid Gland

E

1. Secure tangential lighting and shine it at an oblique angle on the client's anterior neck.
2. Face the client.
3. Ask the client to look straight ahead with the head slightly extended.
4. Have the client drink a sip of water and swallow twice.
5. As the client swallows, observe the front of the neck in the area of the thyroid and the isthmus for masses and symmetrical movement.

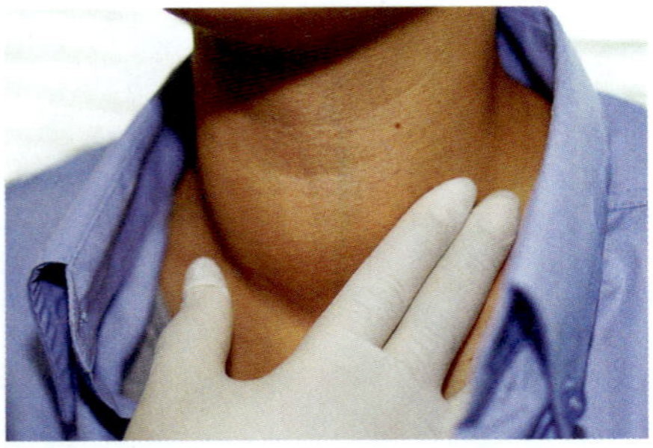

Figure 11-19 Goiter.

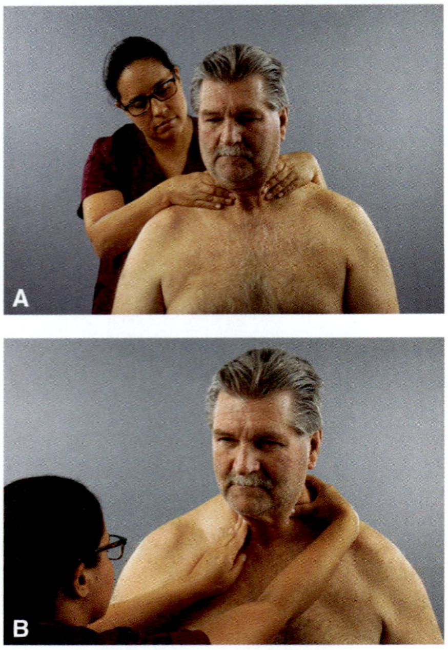

Figure 11-20 Examination of the thyroid gland. **A.** Posterior approach. **B.** Anterior approach.

N **Thyroid tissue moves up with swallowing, but often the movement is so small that it is not visible on inspection. In men, the thyroid cartilage, or Adam's apple, is more prominent than in women.**

A A mass or enlargement of the thyroid that moves upward with swallowing is abnormal.

P Many **goiters** (enlarged thyroid glands) or thyroid nodules are visible and may indicate a variety of thyroid diseases (Fig. 11-19).

Palpation of the Thyroid Gland

Palpation of the thyroid gland may be done using both anterior and posterior approaches (Fig. 11-20).

Posterior Approach

E
1. Have the client sit comfortably. Stand behind the client.
2. Have the client lower the chin slightly to relax the neck muscles.
3. Place the thumbs on the back of the client's neck and bring the other fingers around the neck anteriorly with their tips resting on the lower portion of the neck over the trachea.
4. Move the finger pads over the tracheal rings.
5. Instruct the client to swallow. Palpate the isthmus for nodules or enlargement.
6. Have the client incline the head slightly forward.
7. Press the fingers of the left hand against the left side of the thyroid cartilage to stabilize it while placing the fingers of the right hand gently against the right side.
8. Instruct the client to swallow sips of water.
9. Note consistency, nodularity, and tenderness as the gland moves upward.
10. Repeat on the other side.

N A P Refer to Anterior Approach.

Anterior Approach

E
1. Stand in front of the client.
2. Ask the client to flex the head slightly forward.
3. Place the right thumb on the thyroid cartilage and displace the cartilage to the client's right.
4. Grasp the elevated and displaced right lobe of the thyroid gland with the thumb and index and middle fingers of the left hand.
5. Palpate the surface of the gland for consistency, nodularity, and tenderness.
6. Have the client swallow and then palpate the surface again.
7. Repeat the procedure on the opposite side.

N **No enlargement, masses, or tenderness should be noted on palpation.**

A Palpation reveals the gland to be smooth, soft, and slightly enlarged but less than twice the size of a normal thyroid gland.

P This is referred to as physiological hyperplasia and can be seen premenstrually, during pregnancy, or from puberty to young adulthood in females. Symmetrical enlargement may also be noted in clients who live in areas of iodine deficiency. These are referred to as nontoxic diffuse goiters or endemic goiters.

A Palpation reveals the gland to be two to three times larger than normal size.

P This is diffuse toxic hyperplasia of the thyroid, or Graves disease, an autoimmune disorder that is the most common type of hyperthyroidism. Table 11-2 distinguishes between the signs and symptoms of thyroid disorders. In addition, Table 11-3 identifies the signs and symptoms of parathyroid disease. Because the parathyroid glands can be affected by thyroid manipulation, the examiner must have clinical knowledge of the pathology of the parathyroid glands.

A Asymmetrical enlargement of the thyroid and the presence of two or more nodules are abnormal.

P Thyroid adenomas (benign epithelial tumors) usually occur after the age of 30. A nontoxic, diffuse goiter may become nodular as the client ages. Clients with acromegaly may have a nontoxic multinodular goiter.

A Palpation reveals a solitary nodule in the thyroid tissue.

P A solitary nodule is suggestive of carcinoma (Fig. 11-21).

A Lateral deviation of the trachea is noted on palpation, but you are unable to identify a specific goiter.

P This may be a retrosternal goiter. This type of goiter sometimes occurs in a client with a short neck or may be a goiter with many adenomatous nodules.

A Tenderness of the thyroid is found on palpation.

P Tenderness of an enlarged, firm thyroid suggests thyroiditis.

Table 11-2 Signs and Symptoms of Thyroid Disease

Hypothyroidism and hyperthyroidism are diseases that can occur from birth until later years of life. They can be congenital or acquired. The primary laboratory tests used to screen for these conditions are the thyroid stimulating hormone (TSH), T_3, and T_4.

System	Hypothyroidism	Hyperthyroidism
General	Tired, weak	Fatigue, weak
Skin	Dry, cold, coarse	Sweaty/moist, warm
Hair	Alopecia	Thin hair
Head and Neck	Hoarseness, puffy face	Lid lag, lid retraction, exophthalmos, goiter
Ears and Mouth	Impaired hearing, macroglossia	None
Respiratory	Dyspnea	Tachypnea
Cardiovascular	Bradycardia, cool extremities, peripheral edema	Tachycardia, palpitations
Gastrointestinal	Constipation	Diarrhea
Musculoskeletal	Carpal tunnel syndrome	Muscle weakness
Neurological	Difficulty concentrating, decreased memory, paresthesia, decreased deep tendon reflexes (DTRs)	Hyperactivity, irritability, tremor, insomnia
Reproductive	Amenorrhea	Oligomenorrhea, gynecomastia, decreased libido
Endocrine	Cold intolerance	Heat intolerance
Weight	Weight gain with decreased appetite	Weight loss with increased appetite

Table 11-3 Signs and Symptoms of Parathyroid Disease

Hypoparathyroidism and hyperparathyroidism are diseases that can occur congenitally or can be acquired. Both are primarily conditions of calcium imbalance. In hypoparathyroidism, the client is in a state of hypocalcemia, and in hyperparathyroidism, the client is hypercalcemic. The body has four parathyroid glands, located posterior to the thyroid. Occasionally, they are accidentally removed when a client undergoes thyroid surgery. The parathyroid glands are not accessible for direct physical examination, but parathyroid conditions can be detected by astute history taking, physical examination (for signs and symptoms associated with these conditions), and laboratory data.

Hypoparathyroidism	Hyperparathyroidism
Muscle spasms	Recurrent nephrolithiasis
Facial grimacing	Peptic/duodenal ulcers
Laryngeal spasm	Mental status changes
Seizures	Proximal muscle weakness
Mental status changes	Fatigue
Tetany	Muscle atrophy
Chvostek sign (see Chapter 19)	Osteitis fibrosa cystica
Trousseau sign (see Chapter 19)	
Respiratory arrest	

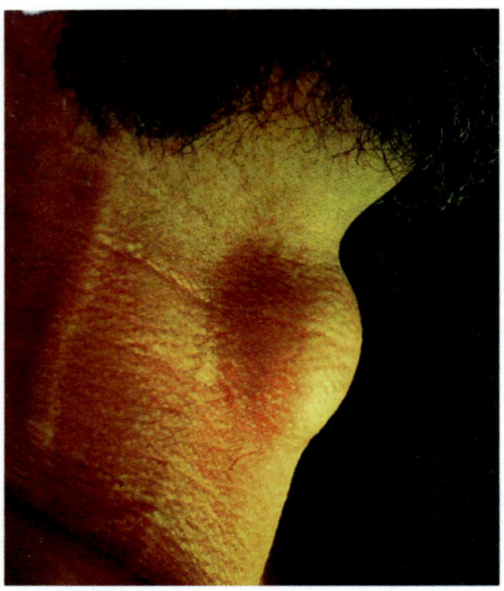

Figure 11-21 Solitary thyroid nodule.

Auscultation of the Thyroid Gland

If the thyroid is enlarged, auscultation should be performed.

E
1. Stand in front of the client.
2. Place the bell of the stethoscope over the right thyroid lobe.
3. Auscultate for bruits.
4. Repeat on the left thyroid lobe.

N **Auscultation should not reveal bruits.**

A Auscultation reveals the presence of a bruit over an enlarged thyroid gland.

P Bruits occur with increased turbulence in blood vessels and are due to the increased vascularization of a thyroid gland that is enlarged due to diffuse toxic goiter.

Risk Factors

Thyroid Cancer

- Diet low in iodine
- History of head or neck radiation, especially in children
- First-degree relative having thyroid cancer
- Elevated BMI (overweight and obese)
- Exposure to nuclear weapons
- Exposure to nuclear power plant accidents (e.g., Chernobyl, Fukushima)
- Genetics (e.g., familial medullary thyroid carcinoma, familial nonmedullary thyroid carcinoma, multiple endocrine neoplasia type 2 (MEN 2), Cowden syndrome, Carney complex, familial adenomatous polyposis)
- Female (approximately 3 times greater than in males)
- Age: 40 to 50 for females, 60 to 70 for males

Adapted from *https://www.cancer.org/cancer/types/thyroid-cancer/causes-risks-prevention/risk-factors.html.* Retrieved September 11, 2025.

E Examination **N** Normal Findings **A** Abnormal Findings **P** Pathophysiology

Inspection of the Lymph Nodes

E
1. Stand in front of the client.
2. Expose the area of the head and neck to be examined.
3. Inspect the nodal areas of the head and neck for any enlargement or inflammation.

N **Lymph nodes should not be visible or inflamed.**

A Enlargement and inflammation are present in specific nodes (Fig. 11-22).

P Lymph nodes can be enlarged and inflamed when there is a localized or generalized infection in the body. This attempt to prevent the spread of infection occurs as a part of the body's immune response to infection.

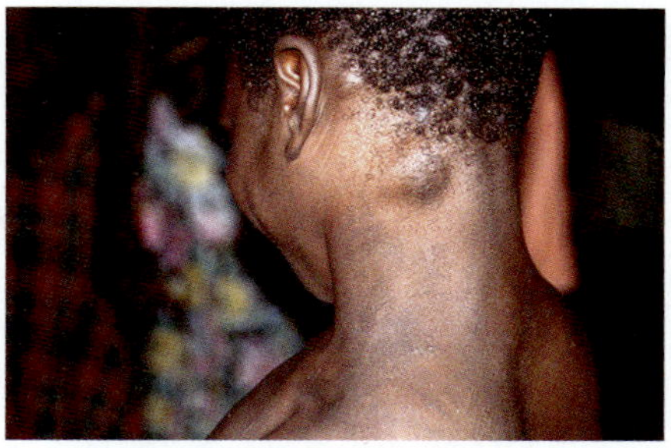

Figure 11-22 This woman is exhibiting lymphadenopathy of an occipital node. *Courtesy of the Centers for Disease Control and Prevention (CDC)/Brian W. J. Mahy, BSc, MA, PhD, ScD, DSc.*

Palpation of the Lymph Nodes

E
1. Have the client sit comfortably.
2. Face the client and examine both sides of the neck simultaneously.
3. Move the pads and tips of the middle three fingers in small circles of palpation using gentle pressure.
4. Follow a systematic, routine sequence beginning with the preauricular, postauricular, occipital, submental, submandibular, and tonsillar nodes. Moving down to the neck, evaluate the anterior cervical chain, the posterior cervical chain, and the supraclavicular nodes (Fig. 11-23).
5. Note size, shape, delimitation (discrete or matted together), mobility, consistency, and tenderness.

N **Lymph nodes should not be palpable in the healthy adult client; however, small, discrete, movable nodes are sometimes present but are of no significance.**

A Palpable lymph nodes are abnormal.

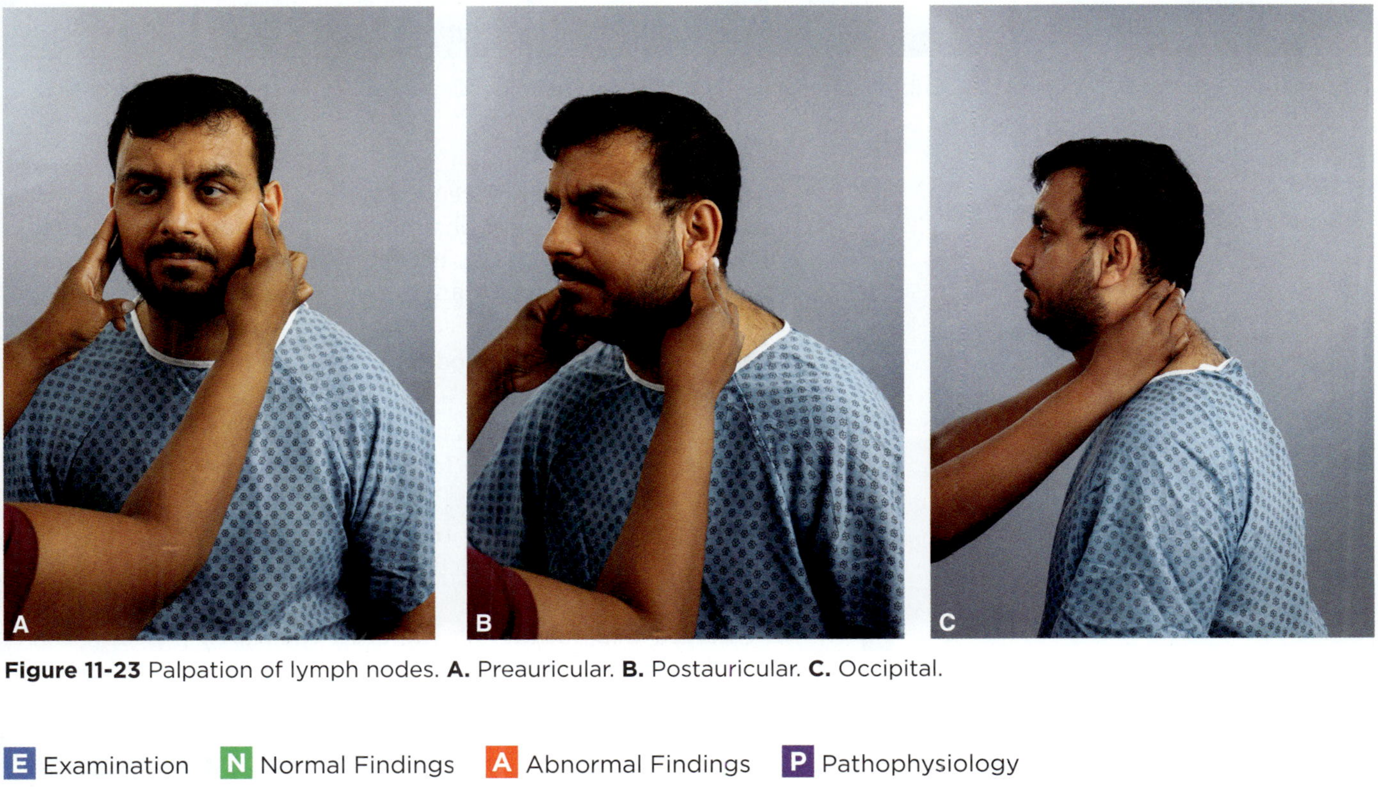

Figure 11-23 Palpation of lymph nodes. **A.** Preauricular. **B.** Postauricular. **C.** Occipital.

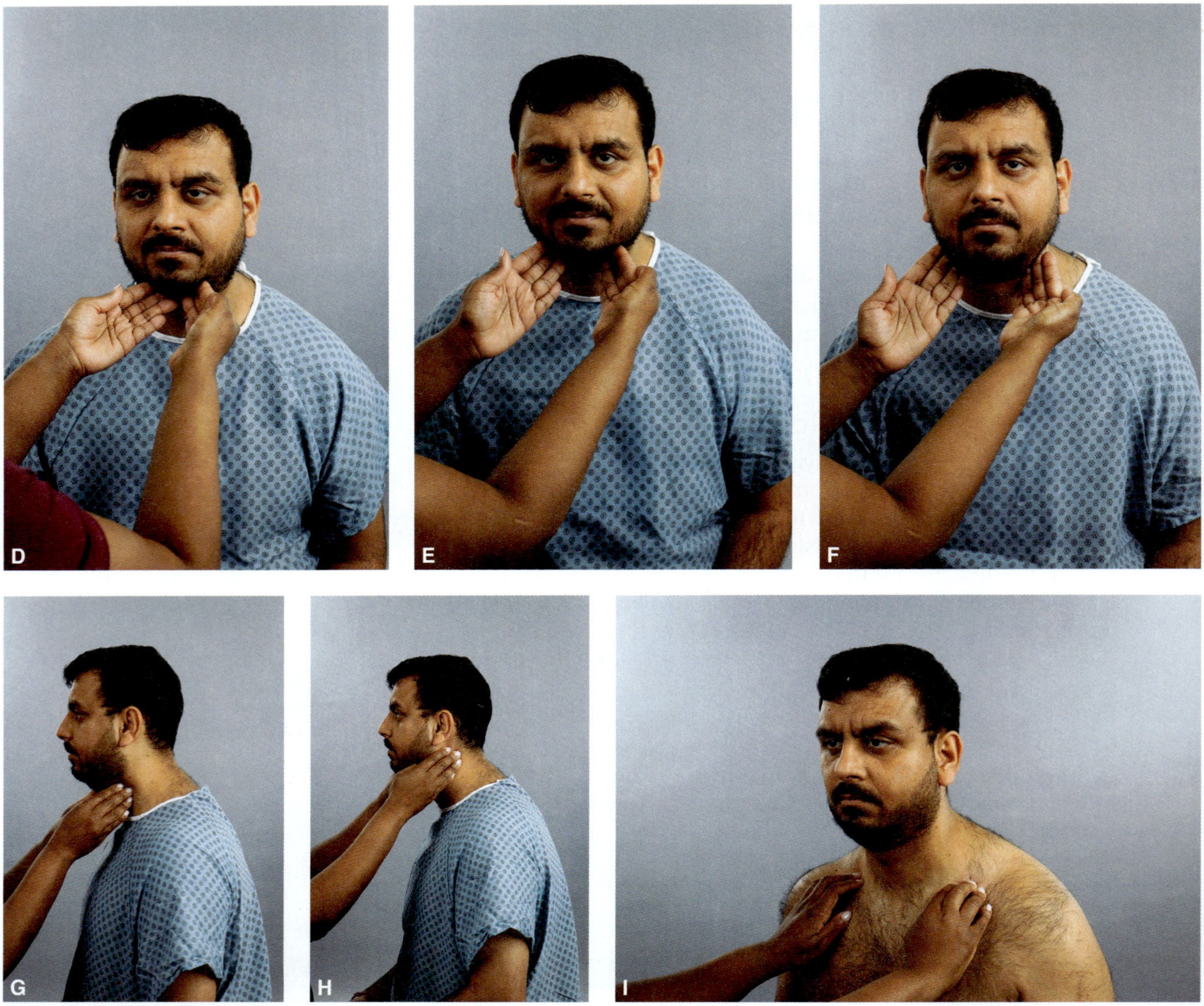

Figure 11-23—cont'd D. Submental. **E.** Submandibular. **F.** Tonsillar. **G.** Anterior cervical chain. **H.** Posterior cervical chain. **I.** Supraclavicular.

P Palpable lymph nodes are frequently seen in acute bacterial infections such as streptococcal pharyngitis. The anterior cervical nodes are usually affected and may be warm, firm, tender, and mobile. A lymph node that is larger than 1 cm in size should be evaluated in greater depth.

P An enlarged postauricular node is sometimes found in clients with ear infections.

P Enlarged, hard, tender nodes are seen in lymphadenitis (inflammation of the lymph nodes). The affected node is the site of the inflammation.

P Enlarged nodes, particularly of the anterior and posterior cervical chains, may be found in infectious mononucleosis. These nodes are usually tender.

P An enlarged node in the left supraclavicular area (Virchow node) may point to malignancy in the abdominal or thoracic regions.

P Nontender, firm, or hard nodes that are nonmobile may indicate a malignancy in the head and neck area, or metastasis from the region that the lymph node drains.

P Clients with malignant lymphomas may also present with nodes that are firm, hard, or rubbery, nontender, and fixed. In Hodgkin disease, the cervical nodes are frequently the first to be palpable.

P Palpable lymph nodes can result from a variety of other pathological processes, including blood dyscrasias, HIV, tuberculosis, surgical procedures that traumatize the nodes, blood transfusions, or chronic illness.

U.S. Preventive Services Task Force (USPSTF)

There are no USPSTF recommendations, Grade A or B Statements, for the head, neck, and regional lymph nodes.

CASE STUDY

The Client With a Thyroid Nodule

This case study illustrates the application and objective documentation of the head, neck, and regional lymph node health history and physical examination. Jia Wong is a 49-year-old woman with a nodule on the left side of her neck for 2 months. The nodule is now tender, and the client is concerned.

HEALTH HISTORY

CLIENT PROFILE

49-year-old married Chinese American woman

CHIEF COMPLAINT

"I have had this big bump on my neck for about 2 months."

HISTORY OF PRESENT ILLNESS

Client reports that over the last 2 months there has been a nodule on the left side of the neck that is tender only when pressing on the area for a few minutes. Denies any fever, cold symptoms, or cough. Denies any recent weight gain or loss, hoarseness, dysphagia, or dyspnea. Has been "feeling cold all the time even in the summer heat" and "having issues with constipation" for the last month and feeling "very tired." Last menstrual period was approximately 2 years ago.

PAST HEALTH HISTORY

Medical History Insomnia × 7 years treated with medication
Osteoarthritis: bilateral hips (started 3 years ago), reports taking celecoxib approximately two times per week for relief.
Vaginal delivery: 25 years ago, no complications

Surgical History Tubal Ligation: 24 years ago, no postoperative complications
Cholecystectomy: 15 years ago, no postoperative complications
Breast augmentation: 11 years ago, no postoperative complications

Allergies Erythromycin: nausea, vomiting, and diarrhea
Denies food allergies or environmental allergies

Medications
Zolpidem 10 mg at bedtime prn (has been using wife's medication)
Celecoxib 100 mg once a day as needed for hip pain
Vitamin D 1,000 IU daily

Communicable Diseases None that client can recall

Injuries and Accidents None

Differing Abilities Denies

Blood Transfusions Denies

Childhood Illnesses Measles, mumps, and chickenpox as a child

Immunizations Tetanus vaccine: 3 years ago; COVID-19 vaccine/2 boosters completed; annual influenza vaccine. Did not receive HPV vaccine.

FAMILY HEALTH HISTORY

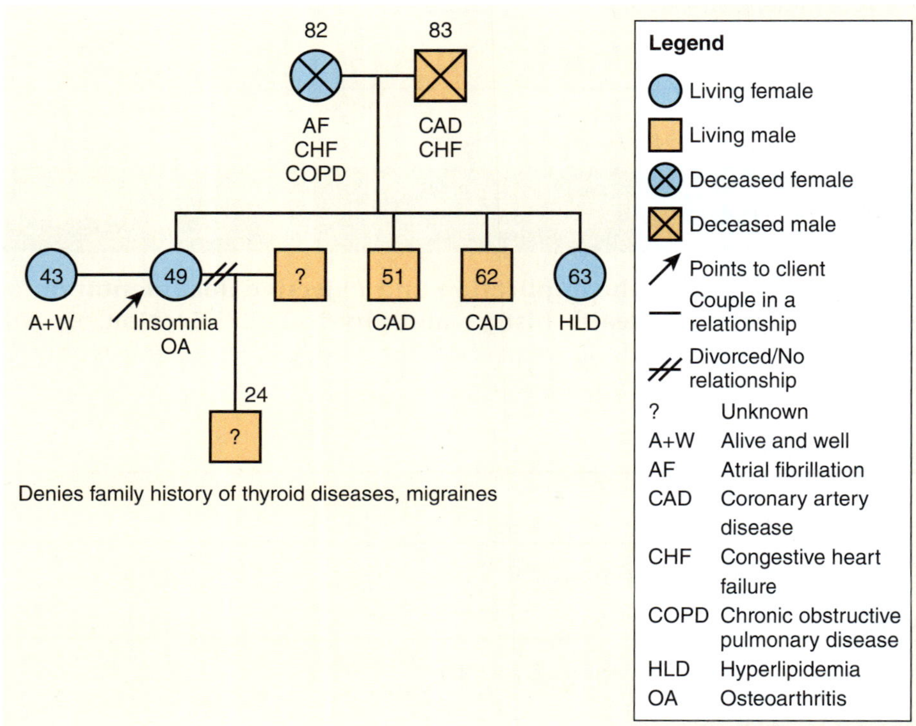

SOCIAL HISTORY

Alcohol Use "Gave up" alcohol 24 years ago, provided no additional information

Tobacco Use Denies any tobacco use

Recreational Drug Use "Never"

Domestic and Intimate Partner Violence Denies

Sexual Practice Lesbian, monogamous for 14 years with wife; 2 prior female partners, 2 prior male partners

Travel History Denies any travel within the past 2 years.

Work Environment Works in the "Mother's Day Out" preschool in town in the infant to 2-year-old department Monday through Friday in the basement of a local church. Facility has smoke detectors. Has a 45-minute commute to work.

Home Environment Lives in a mobile home in a rural area, has well water, feels safe; has 3 dogs

Hobbies and Leisure Activities Walking the dogs; likes to go to garage sales on the weekend with wife and "find treasures"

Stress "I think I need a job change. I am so tired of screaming babies and demanding parents!"

Education High school graduate

Economic Status Declined answering

Military Service Denies

Religion Not affiliated with any organized religion; grew up in a home where parents practiced Buddhism

Ethnic Background Parents emigrated from Hong Kong 50 years ago. Client was born in the U.S.

Roles and Relationships Has been in committed relationship with wife for 14 years. Has no contact with son whom she placed for adoption at birth 24 years ago. This child resulted from a one-night stand relationship with someone she met at a bar and admits to being drunk at the time of intercourse.

Characteristic Patterns of Daily Living Declined answering

HEALTH MAINTENANCE ACTIVITIES

Sleep 6 to 7 hours nightly with zolpidem; denies middle of the night waking or feeling "hung over" in the morning

Diet Eats very few meat products. Currently practicing intermittent 5:2 fasting (eating a normal diet 5 days a week and fasting 2 days a week, only consuming water or calorie-free drinks on fasting days).

Exercise Walks at least 1 mile a day with dogs.

Stress Management Talking with wife, playing with dogs.

Use of Safety Devices Wears seatbelt

Health Checkups No visit to primary care provider (PCP) in past year; last year saw optometrist and dentist

PHYSICAL EXAMINATION

Inspection of the Shape of the Head Normocephalic and symmetrical

Palpation of the Head Skull is smooth, nontender, and without masses or depressions. No hardness or thickening of the temporal arteries

Inspection and Palpation of the Scalp Shiny, intact without lesions/masses

Inspection of the Face

Symmetry Symmetrical

Shape and Features Oval, no edema, no disproportionate structures, or involuntary movements.

Palpation and Auscultation of the Mandible Opens mouth without difficulties. Temporomandibular joint without clicking, crepitus, or tenderness.

Inspection of the Neck Trachea midline, muscles symmetrical, full range of motion without discomfort

Palpation of the Neck Muscles without palpable masses/spasms

Inspection of the Thyroid Gland Moves with swallowing

Palpation of the Thyroid Gland Discrete single nodule 2 cm on the left thyroid lobe, nontender, soft, and mobile. Right thyroid lobe nontender without enlargement/nodules

Auscultation of the Thyroid Gland No bruits

Inspection of the Lymph Nodes No enlargement/inflammation

Palpation of the Lymph Nodes No lymphadenopathy

CLINICAL JUDGMENT IN ACTION

1. What cues indicate that the client is having a disorder of the head and neck?
2. What interventions have the highest priority?
3. What assessment findings indicate clinical improvement or decline in this client?

Review Questions

1. Which of the following risk factors are associated with thyroid cancer? Select all that apply.
   a. Female sex
   b. Diet low in iodine
   c. Females age 20 to 30, Males age 30 to 40
   d. Familial history of medullary thyroid cancer
   e. Head or neck radiation

2. Which of the following physical examination findings might be observed in a client with hyperthyroidism? Select all that apply.
   a. Puffy face
   b. Bradycardia
   c. Moist skin
   d. Tachycardia
   e. Thinning hair

3. The nurse examines a 65-year-old client who is complaining of a sudden onset of drooping of the right side of the face with the right eyelid being affected and the inability to smile properly. What condition or disease do you suspect the client has?
   a. Hypothyroidism
   b. Bell palsy
   c. Hyperparathyroidism
   d. Graves disease

4. During a routine physical examination of the head and neck, which examination finding is cause for concern?
   a. Palpable lymph node, less than 1 cm, mobile with examination
   b. 1-cm lymph node, anterior cervical chain, nontender, soft
   c. No palpable lymph nodes
   d. Palpable hard lymph node, 2 cm, nontender, nonmobile

5. What physical findings would the nurse expect when examining a client with a history of chronic allergies? Select all that apply.
   a. Transverse crease across the nose
   b. Open mouth breathing
   c. Allergic shiners
   d. Creases below the eyelids
   e. Green nasal mucus

6. When performing a physical examination of the muscles in the neck, what examination landmarks are visualized? Select all that apply.
   a. Atlas
   b. Posterior cervical triangle
   c. Vertebra prominens
   d. Anterior cervical triangle
   e. Axis

7. The nurse is conducting a health history on a 23-year-old client with a history of chronic migraine headaches. What health history findings could be related to migraine headaches? Select all that apply.
   a. Family history of migraines
   b. Drinking 6 cups of coffee a day
   c. Taking oral contraceptives
   d. Stressful new job
   e. Family history of thyroid cancer

8. During a physical examination, the nurse palpates an enlarged lymph node behind the client's right earlobe. Which lymph node is enlarged?
   a. Posterior cervical
   b. Superficial cervical
   c. Submandibular
   d. Posterior auricular

9. Facial physical findings that occur with Cushing syndrome are which of the following? Select all that apply.
   a. Round "moon face"
   b. Unusually large lips
   c. Excess of hair on the jaw and upper lip
   d. Large space between the teeth
   e. Wide nose

10. What are the facial physical findings that the nurse would expect to find in a client with Parkinson disease? Select all that apply.
    a. Lack of facial expressions
    b. Raised eyebrows
    c. Staring gaze
    d. Decreased blinking
    e. Unilateral drooping face

CHAPTER

12 Eyes

Learning Outcomes

1. Identify the anatomy and physiology of the eyes.
2. Conduct a complete health history on a client with an eye condition.
3. Perform a physical examination on a healthy adult and an adult with eye pathology.
4. Differentiate between normal clinical findings from a client's physical examination and the pathophysiology of abnormal clinical findings.
5. Identify risk factors for glaucoma.
6. Identify risk factors for cataracts.
7. Identify risk factors for macular degeneration.
8. Document a complete health history and physical examination of a client with eye pathology.

Physical examination of the eyes provides information about the client's nutritional, endocrine, cardiovascular, gastrointestinal, hematologic, and neurological systems. This chapter provides a comprehensive guide to examining the eye and the factors that affect it.

Anatomy and Physiology

External Structures

The external structures of the eyes comprise the eyelids or palpebra, the conjunctiva, the lacrimal glands, and the extraocular muscles. The eyelids consist of smooth muscle covered with a very thin layer of skin; they admit light to the eye while protecting and maintaining lubrication of the eye. The interior surface of the lid muscle is covered with a pink mucous membrane called the **palpebral conjunctiva**. Contiguous with the palpebral conjunctiva is the **bulbar conjunctiva**. The bulbar conjunctiva folds back over the anterior surface of the eyeball and merges with the cornea at the **limbus**, the junction of the sclera and the cornea (Fig. 12-1). The conjunctiva contains blood vessels and pain receptors that respond quickly to outside insult. Eyelashes are evenly spaced along lid margins and curve outward to protect the eye by filtering particles of dirt and dust from the external environment. Eyebrows are symmetrical and evenly distributed above the eyelids.

The opening between the eyelids is called the **palpebral fissure**. Upper and lower eyelids meet at the inner **canthus** on the nasal side and at the outer canthus on the temporal side. Embedded just beneath the lid

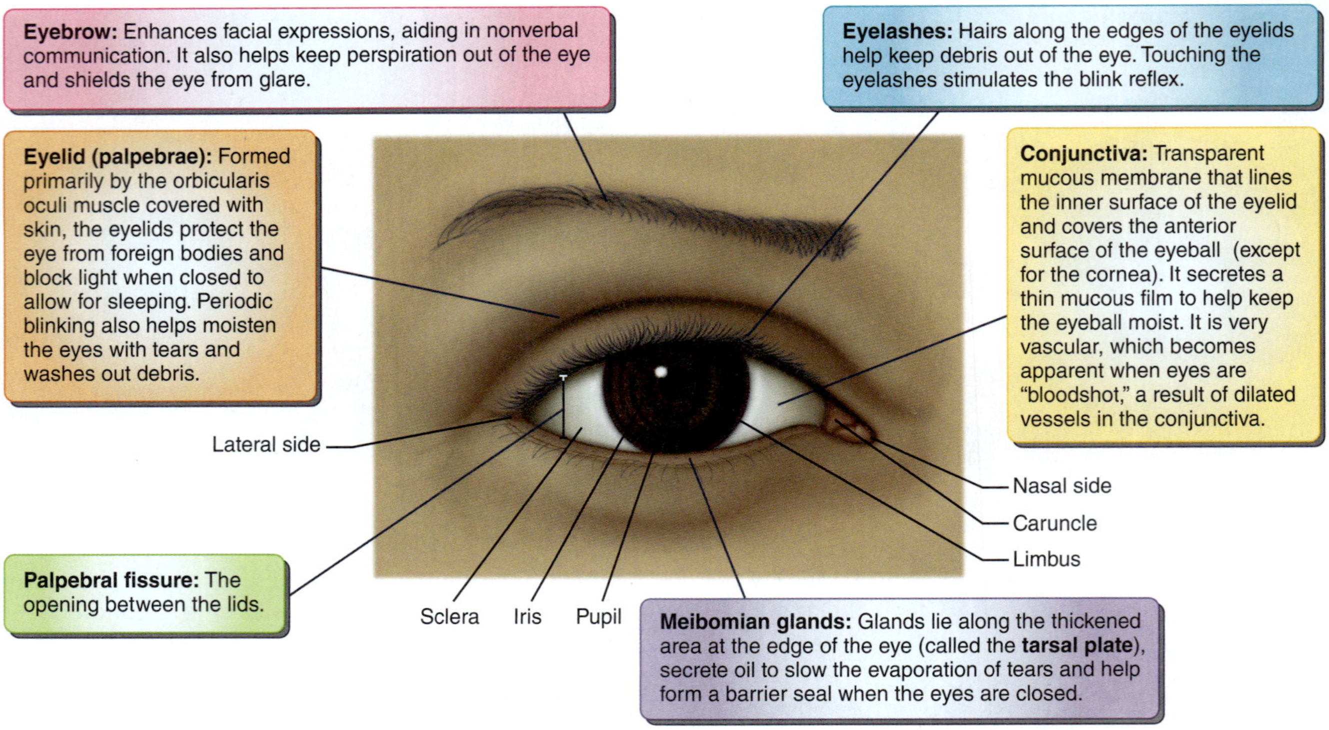

Figure 12-1 External view of the right eye.

margins are the meibomian glands, which secrete a lubricating substance onto the surface of the eye. The **tarsal plates** are connective tissue that gives shape to the upper lids.

Lacrimal Apparatus

The **lacrimal apparatus** is made up of the lacrimal gland and ducts (Fig. 12-2). The lacrimal glands, located above and on the temporal side of each eye, are responsible for the production of tears, which lubricate the eye. Tears drain through the inferior and superior **puncta** at the inner canthus through the nasolacrimal duct and the lacrimal sac to the inferior turbinate in

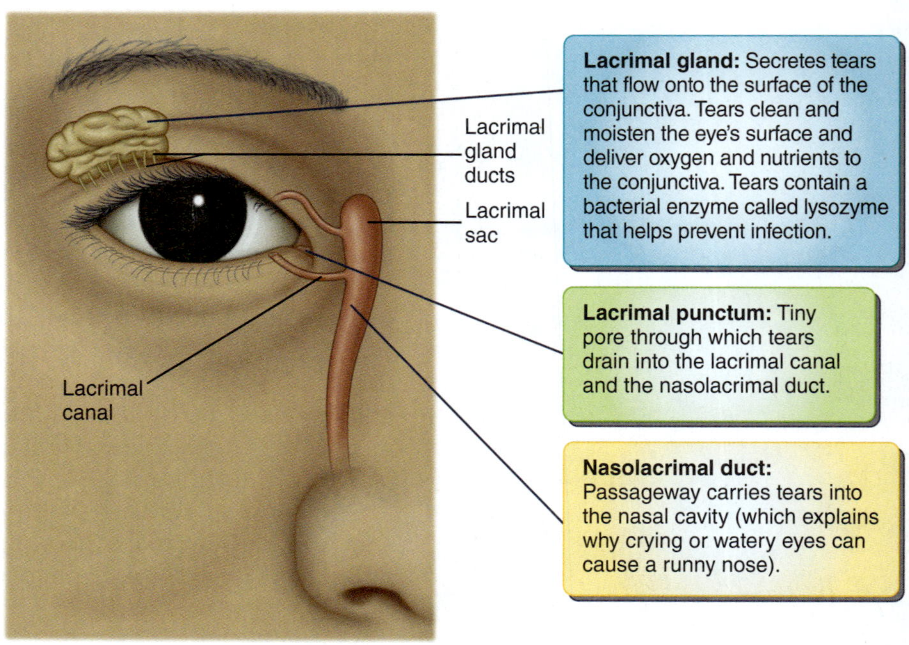

Figure 12-2 Lacrimal apparatus.

the nose. The **caruncle**, which contains sebaceous glands, is the round, red structure in the inner canthus.

Extraocular Muscles

Six extraocular muscles extend from the scleral surface of each eye and attach to the bony orbit. These voluntary muscles work in concert to move the eyes with great precision in several directions to provide a single image to the brain. These muscles are the superior, inferior, medial, and lateral recti, and the superior and inferior obliques.

Internal Structures

The globes of the eyes are spherical structures that are encased in the protective bony orbits of the face along with the lacrimal gland and extrinsic muscles of the eye. Only a small portion of the anterior surface of the eye is exposed. The eye itself is approximately 1 inch in diameter and has three layers: a tough, outer, fibrous tunic (sclera); a middle, vascular tunic; and the innermost layer, which contains the retina (Fig. 12-3).

Outer Layer

The outer tunic consists of the transparent cornea on the outer portion, which is continuous with the **sclera**, an opaque material that appears white and covers the structures inside the eye. The **cornea** is a nonvascular, transparent surface that covers the iris and is continuous with the conjunctival

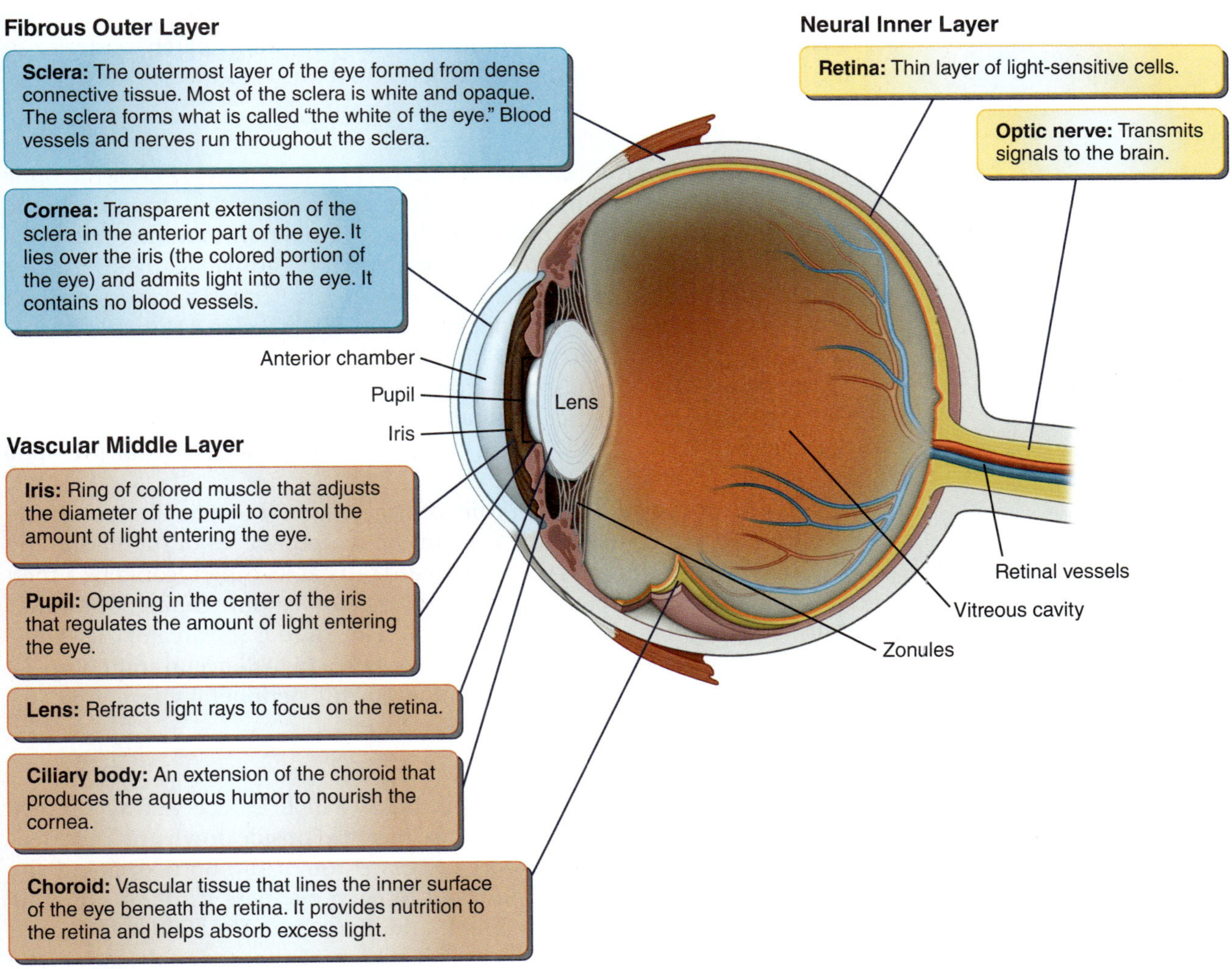

Figure 12-3 Lateral cross-section of the interior eye.

epithelium. The sclera protects the eye and provides a surface for the attachment of the extraocular muscles. The posterior portion of the sclera contains an opening for the entrance of the optic nerve and various blood vessels.

Middle Layer

The pigmented, middle, vascular tunic, or uveal layer, is composed of the choroid, the ciliary body, and the iris. The **choroid** is a vascular tissue that lines the inner surface of the eye just beneath the retina. It provides nutrition to the retinal pigment epithelium and helps absorb excess light.

The **ciliary body** is an anterior extension of the uveal tract; it siphons serum from the systemic blood flow to produce the aqueous humor needed to nourish the corneal endothelium. Zonules are small strands of tissue extending from the ciliary body to the crystalline **lens**. Zonules hold the lens in place and allow it to change shape to refract light from various focusing distances. The **iris**, the most anterior portion of the uveal tract, provides a distinctive color for the eye. It is comprised of smooth muscle that regulates the entrance of light. The **pupil**, an opening in the center of the iris, regulates the amount of light entering the eye. The pupil reacts to light and the closeness of objects by stimulation of the sympathetic nervous system, which dilates it, and the parasympathetic nervous system, which constricts it.

The central cavity of the eye posterior to the lens is filled with a clear, gelatinous material called **vitreous humor**, which helps maintain the shape of the eye and the position of the internal structures.

Visual images pass through the structures and aqueous humor of the **anterior chamber** (the space anterior to the pupil and iris), and the vitreous humor of the **posterior chamber** (the space immediately posterior to the iris), to the fundus of the eye, where the retina is located.

Inner Layer

The innermost layer of the eyeball, the **retina**, is an extension of the optic nerve, which lines the inside of the globe and receives light impulses to be transmitted to the occipital lobe of the brain. Paired retinal arteries and veins branch from the optic disc toward the periphery, growing smaller as they extend outward. Generally, retinal arteries are smaller and a lighter red than veins and often have a silvery-looking "arterial light reflex." Normal arterial-to-venous width is a ratio of 2:3 or 4:5.

The **optic disc** is a round or oval area with distinct margins located on the nasal side of the retina. Retinal fibers join at the optic disc to form the optic nerve. Nerve fibers from the temporal visual fields cross at the optic chiasm.

The **physiological cup** is a pale, central area in the optic disc occupying one-third to one-fourth of the disc. In the temporal area of the retina, the tiny, darker **macula**, with the **fovea centralis** at its center, contains a high concentration of the **cones** necessary for color vision, reading, and other tasks requiring fine visual discrimination. The fovea is the area of the sharpest vision. Other portions of the retina contain a high concentration of **rods**, which provide dark and light discrimination and peripheral vision.

Visual Pathway

Objects in the field of vision reflect light, which is received by sensory neurons in the retina; these images are received upside down and reversed. From there they pass along nerve fibers through the optic disc and the optic nerve. Fibers from the left half of each eye pass through the optic chiasm to the right side of the brain, and fibers from the right side of each eye pass to the left side of the visual cortex of the occipital lobe of the brain (Fig. 12-4).

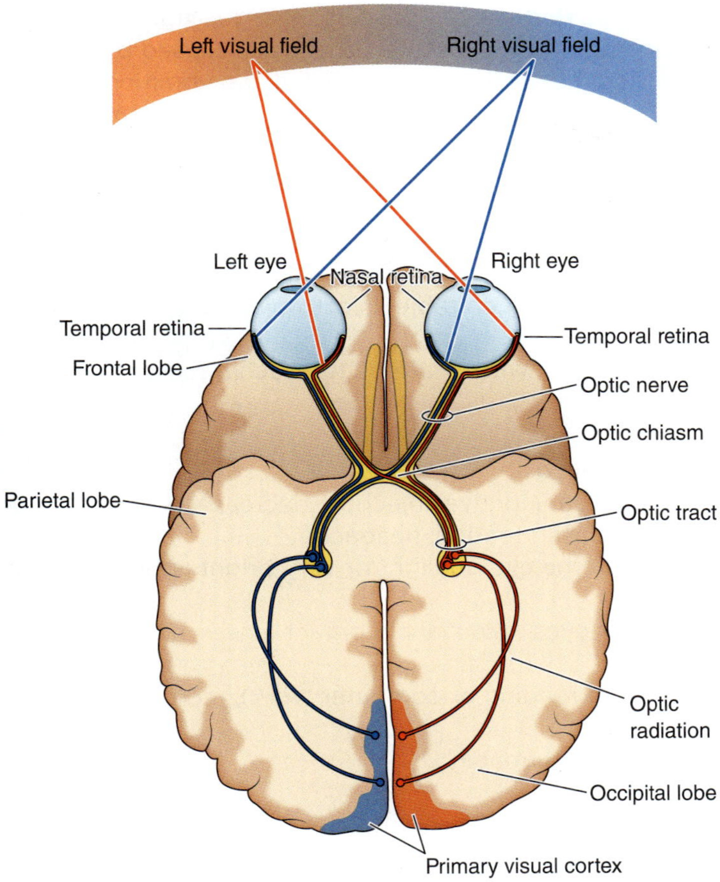

Figure 12-4 Visual pathway.

HEALTH HISTORY

The eye health history provides insight into the link between a client's life/lifestyle and eye information and pathology

CLIENT PROFILE

Diseases that are age-, sex-, and race-specific for the eyes are listed.

Age

Cataract (congenital, older adult)
Presbyopia (>40)
Hypertensive retinopathy (middle age to older adult)
Glaucoma (middle age to older adult)
Macular degeneration (older adult)
Entropion, ectropion (older adult)
Dry eyes (older adult)

Sex Female: age-related macular degeneration, dry eyes, thyroid-related ophthalmopathy

Race Glaucoma (Black [Non-Hispanic] and Asian; Allison et al., 2020), melanoma of the eye in clients with light blue/gray eye color, fair skin (McDonald et al., 2021)

CHIEF COMPLAINT

Common chief complaints for the eyes are defined, and information on the characteristics of each sign or symptom is provided.

1. Changes in Visual Acuity Change in ability to see clearly

Location One eye or both eyes

Quality Dimming of vision, blurred vision, diplopia, visual field loss, legal blindness

Associated Manifestations Headache, rhinorrhea, sneezing, vertigo, "floaters" (spots of different sizes that float across the visual field and are caused by changes in the vitreous humor), flashes of light, aura, nausea and vomiting, generalized muscle weakness, eye pain or pressure, infection (herpes simplex/ herpes zoster or cytomegalovirus)

Aggravating Factors Allergens, stress, lack of sleep, decreased lighting, darkness (night), refractive changes, systemic diseases

Alleviating Factors Improved lighting, medication, corrective glasses, rest or sleep, adequate hydration

Setting Work environment, reading: reading on tablet/electronics versus paper, computer work, night driving

Timing With aging, at night, after trauma, with or after a headache, seasonal, sudden onset, gradual onset

2. **Pain** Discomfort in the eye

Quality Aching, sharp, throbbing, burning

Associated Manifestations Drainage, conjunctival injection, decreased vision, herpes simplex/herpes zoster, increased tearing, headache

Aggravating Factors Foreign body in the eye, sunlight or very bright light, contact lenses, trauma, allergens

Alleviating Factors Closing of eye or eyes, removal of contact lenses, medications, sunglasses, avoiding allergens

Setting Work environment (increased reading or computer work), recreational area, outdoors

Timing Sudden onset, gradual onset, with reading

3. **Drainage** Discharge from the eye

Quality Color, quantity, consistency

Associated Manifestations Crusting on the lids and lashes, pain, itching, redness of the eye or the lids, headache

Aggravating Factors Allergens, eye makeup, chlorine, poor hygiene, upper respiratory infection

Alleviating Factors Medications, hypoallergenic makeup or not wearing eye makeup, avoiding allergens, good hand washing, eye drops

Setting Outdoors, swimming pool

Timing In the morning, continuous, intermittent, seasonal

4. **Itching** Irritation that causes the client to scratch or rub

Quality Mild, severe

Associated Manifestations Rhinitis, sneezing, drainage, burning sensation in the eye, gritty sensation in the eye, conjunctivitis, headache

Aggravating Factors Allergens, contact lenses, eye makeup

Alleviating Factors Medications, cold compresses to the eyes, removal of contacts, avoiding allergens and eye makeup

Setting Indoors, outdoors

Timing Seasonal, intermittent, continuous

5. **Dryness** Reduced amount of lubricating secretions in the eye

Associated Manifestations With systemic disease, redness of the eye, reduced tearing, itching, recent eye surgery

Aggravating Factors Decreased humidity, wind, reading

Alleviating Factors Artificial tears, humidified air, prescription medications

Setting Outdoors, indoors with decreased humidity

Timing With aging, during the winter (decreased humidity), postmenopause, morning, evening

PAST HEALTH HISTORY

The various components of the past health history are linked to eye pathology and eye-related information.

Medical History

Eye Specific Corrective lens: glasses or contact lens for myopia or hyperopia, strabismus, diplopia, astigmatism, glaucoma, cataracts, macular degeneration, diabetic retinopathy, retinal detachment, conjunctivitis, hordeolum, pterygium, blepharitis, chalazion, trachoma, prosthesis, exophthalmos

Non-Eye Specific Diabetes mellitus, renal disease, atherosclerotic disease, hypertension, thyroid disease, inflammatory processes, infections (viral or bacterial), immunosuppressive disease, multiple sclerosis, myasthenia gravis, Sjögren syndrome, scleroderma, lupus, Vitamin A deficiency, collagen vascular diseases

Surgical History Cataract extraction, lens implant, LASIK (laser-assisted in situ keratomileusis [laser vision correction]) or PRK (photorefractive keratectomy), repair of detached retina, neurosurgery, enucleation of eye, optic nerve decompression, prosthesis insertion

Allergies

Pollen: watery or itchy eyes

Animal dander: watery or itchy eyes

Medications Carbonic anhydrase inhibitors, nonselective ß-blockers, mast cell stabilizers, antibiotics, antihistamines, decongestants, corticosteroids, artificial tears, mydriatics, myotics, cholinergics, cyclosporine, hydroxypropyl cellulose, lifitegrast, nasal varenicline

Injuries and Accidents Foreign bodies; trauma to the eyes, corneal abrasions

Differing Abilities Visually impaired, legal blindness

Childhood Illnesses Rubella and visual sequelae (blindness), congenital syphilis, strabismus, amblyopia

FAMILY HEALTH HISTORY

Familial eye diseases are listed.

Myopia, hyperopia, strabismus, color blindness, cataracts, glaucoma, macular degeneration, ocular melanoma, retinitis pigmentosa, retinoblastoma, neonatal blindness secondary to cataracts from mother contracting rubella during pregnancy

SOCIAL HISTORY

The components of the social history are linked to eye factors and pathology.

Alcohol Use Associated with cataract formation and macular degeneration

Tobacco Use Smoking is associated with macular degeneration, cataracts, and glaucoma

Travel History Prolonged facial exposure to sun, facial exposure to contaminated waste, swimming, or facial exposure to stagnant bodies of water

Work Environment Exposure to toxins/chemicals, infections, allergens, eye strain from long hours of reading/computer use

Stress Associated with visual system diseases such as glaucoma and optic neuropathy (Sabel et al., 2018).

HEALTH MAINTENANCE ACTIVITIES

This information provides a bridge between health maintenance activities and eye function.

Diet Vitamin deficiencies may affect vision

Use of Safety Devices Goggles or face shields for sports, job, or home projects; sunglasses in bright ultraviolet light

Health Checkups Eye examination, intraocular pressure measurement

Assessment in Brief

Eye Examination

Visual Acuity
- Distance vision
- Near vision
- Color vision

External Eye and Lacrimal Apparatus
- Eyes, eyelids, eyebrows, and eyelashes
- Lacrimal apparatus
  - Inspection
  - Palpation

Anterior Segment Structures
- Conjunctiva
- Sclera
- Cornea
- Anterior chamber
- Iris
- Pupil
- Lens

Visual Fields
- Confrontation

Extraocular Muscle Function
- Corneal light reflex
- Cover/uncover test
- Cardinal fields of gaze

Posterior Segment Structures
- Retinal structures
- Macula

Advanced Technique
- Amsler grid

Equipment

- Appropriate PPE
- Ophthalmoscope
- Penlight
- Clean gloves
- Snellen chart or Tumbling E chart
- Rosenbaum Near Vision Pocket Screening card
- Vision occluder
- Cotton-tipped swab, 6 inches

Examination of the Eye

Examination of the eyes should be carried out in an orderly fashion, moving from the extraocular structures to the intraocular structures. The eye examination usually includes testing of associated cranial nerves and can be performed in the following order:

1. Determination of visual acuity
2. Determination of visual fields
3. Examination of the external eye and lacrimal apparatus
4. Evaluation of extraocular muscle function
5. Examination of the anterior segment structures
6. Examination of the posterior segment structures

Visual Acuity

The assessment of visual acuity (cranial nerve II) requires testing for central vision and peripheral vision/visual fields. Testing central vision is a noninvasive procedure that is carried out with the use of a Snellen chart and an occluder to cover the client's eye. The **Snellen chart** contains letters of various sizes with standardized visual acuity numbers at the end of each line of letters (Fig. 12-5A). Visual acuity is expressed using two numbers (e.g., 20/70) with 20/20 considered normal vision. The numbers indicate the degree of visual acuity based on what the client can read on that line of letters at a distance of 20 feet. Thus, the numerator will represent the distance of the client to the chart (20 feet) and the denominator reflects the person's vision in comparison to what those with normal vision can see at 20 feet. The higher the denominator, the worse the vision. For instance, a client who has a visual acuity of 20/70 can read at 20 feet what a client with 20/20 vision can read at 70 feet.

Distance Vision

E

1. Ask the client to stand or sit facing the Snellen chart at a distance of 20 feet.
2. Clients should wear corrective lenses during this examination and it should be noted with the findings.
3. Instruct the client to cover one eye with the occluder (Fig. 12-5C) and read the smallest line of print possible. Watch the client for behaviors like squinting, leaning forward, or tilting the head.
4. Note the number at the right hand side end of the line of the Snellen chart where the client was able to identify more than half of the letters. For instance, if the smallest line of printer the client can read is line 7, the client has 20/25 vision in that eye. The visual acuity is written on the left hand side of line 7 of the Snellen Chart.
5. Repeat the test, occluding the other eye. Ask the client to read the line backward (right to left) to prevent memorization (Fig. 12-5D).
6. Repeat the test, using both eyes.
7. If the client is unable to read the letters at the top of the chart, move the client closer to the chart. Note the distance at which the client can read the top line.
8. If the client is unable to read any of the Snellen charts, other gross measures of visual acuity must be used. These include the ability to count the number of fingers the examiner holds up, or if there is a perception of light. In addition, the Tumbling E chart (Fig. 12-5B) can be used to assess visual acuity in clients who do not read English or have low literacy.

N **The client who has a visual acuity of 20/20 is considered to have normal visual acuity.**

A The client is unable to read the chart with an uncorrected visual acuity of 20/30 in one eye, vision in both eyes is different by two lines or more, or acuity is absent.

P The client may have a refractive error related to a difference in the refractive power of the cornea. Figure 12-6A illustrates how light rays focus on the retina in a normal eye. In **myopia** (nearsightedness), the axial length of the globe is longer than normal, resulting in the image not being focused directly on the retina; this condition can be changed with corrective lenses (Fig. 12-6B). If the client is amblyopic, no corrective lenses will improve vision. **Amblyopia** is the permanent loss of visual acuity resulting from strabismus that was not corrected in early childhood, or certain medical conditions (alcoholism, uremia, diabetes mellitus).

P The client may have corneal opacities that are congenital, from lesions that have scarred the cornea (e.g., herpes simplex), from trauma, or from degeneration and dystrophies.

P Visual acuity can be decreased because of opacities of the lens caused by traumatic cataracts or cataracts in the aging client.

NURSING CHECKLIST

General Approach to Eye Examination

1. Observe Standard Precautions and don Personal Protective Equipment (PPE) such as glcves, gown, face shield, goggles, N-95 respirator or face mask if the client's status warrants these protective measures.
2. Greet the client and explain the examination techniques.
3. Ensure the room provides sufficient lighting to allow adequate observation of the client. You may need to alter the lighting for some tests to improve the accuracy of the findings.
4. Place the client in a sitting position.
5. Visualize the underlying structures during the examination to allow an adequate description of the findings.
6. Always compare right and left eyes.
7. Use a systematic approach that is followed consistently each time the examination is performed.

A

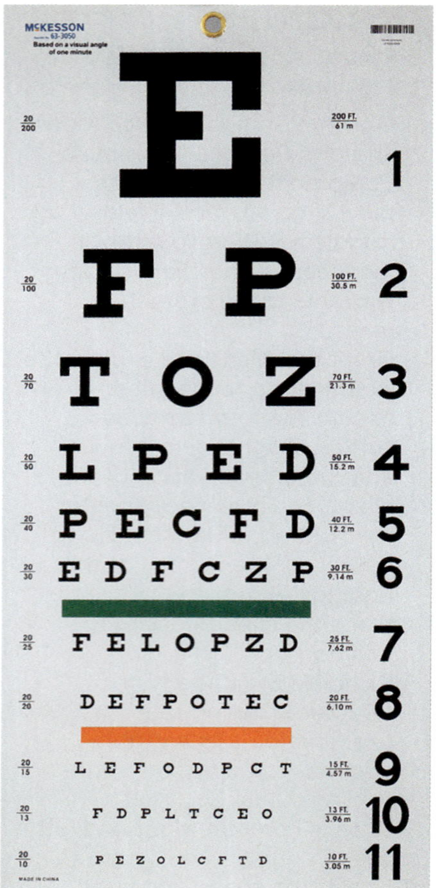

B

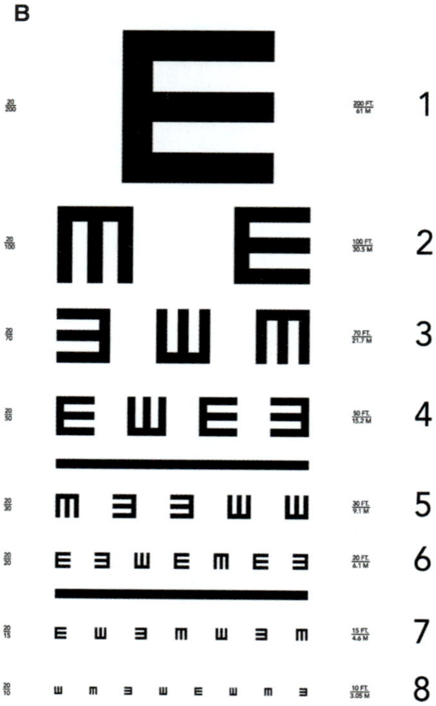

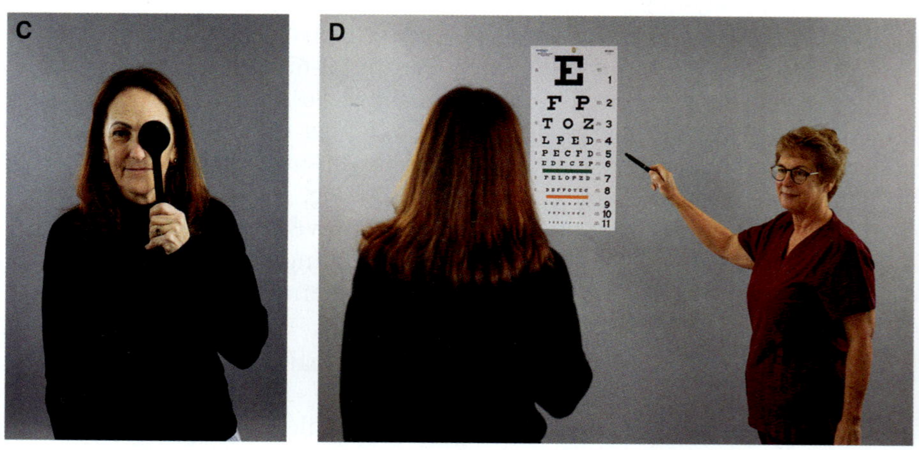

Figure 12-5 Visual acuity testing. **A.** Snellen vision chart. **B.** Tumbling E vision chart. **C.** The client occludes one eye. **D.** Assessing distance vision.

P Systemic autoimmune diseases such as inflammatory bowel disease, rheumatoid arthritis, or other collagen vascular diseases can be associated with inflammation of the iris (iritis), which will affect visual acuity. Iritis can also be idiopathic.

P Inflammation of the retina caused by toxoplasmosis or by the presence of blood in the vitreous humor following hemorrhage can be responsible for decreased visual acuity.

P Systemic diseases, such as hypertension or diabetes mellitus, and trauma may damage the choroid and retina, causing decreased visual acuity.

P Visual acuity can be impaired by pathology affecting the optic nerve, such as multiple sclerosis, tumors or abscesses of the nerve itself, optic atrophy, papilledema resulting from increased intracranial pressure, optic neuritis, or neovascularization of the optic nerve.

Near Vision

E

1. Use a pocket Snellen chart, Rosenbaum card (Fig. 12-7), or any printed material written at an appropriate reading level.
2. If the pocket vision card is available, have the client sit comfortably and hold the card 14 inches from the face without moving it.
3. Ask the client to read the smallest line possible. If other printed material is used, you will be able to gain only a general understanding of the client's near vision.

N **Until the client is in the late 30s to the late 40s, reading is generally possible at a distance of 14 inches.**

A A client in the late 30s to the late 40s who cannot read at 14 inches is considered **presbyopic**. Younger persons may have difficulty seeing up close because they have **hyperopia**, or farsightedness (Fig. 12-6C).

P The normal aging process causes the lens to harden (nuclear sclerosis), decreasing its ability to change shape and therefore focus on near objects.

Color Vision

E Color vision is usually tested in young children. If there is suspicion that the client has a color vision deficit, have the client identify the

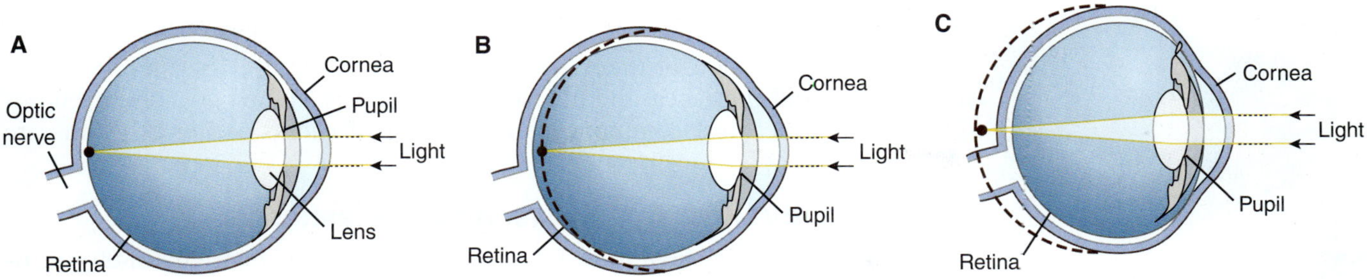

Figure 12-6 Eye refraction. **A.** Normal eye. Light rays focus on the retina. **B.** Myopia (nearsightedness). Light rays focus in front of the retina. **C.** Hyperopia (farsightedness). Light rays focus behind the retina.

primary colors on the Snellen chart or colors in the examining room. For more specific testing, refer to Chapter 25.

N **The client should be able to identify colors correctly.**

A The color vision defect is designated as red/green, blue/yellow, or complete when the client sees only shades of gray.

P Defects in color vision can result from diseases of the optic nerve, macular degeneration, pathology of the fovea centralis, nutritional deficiency, or heredity.

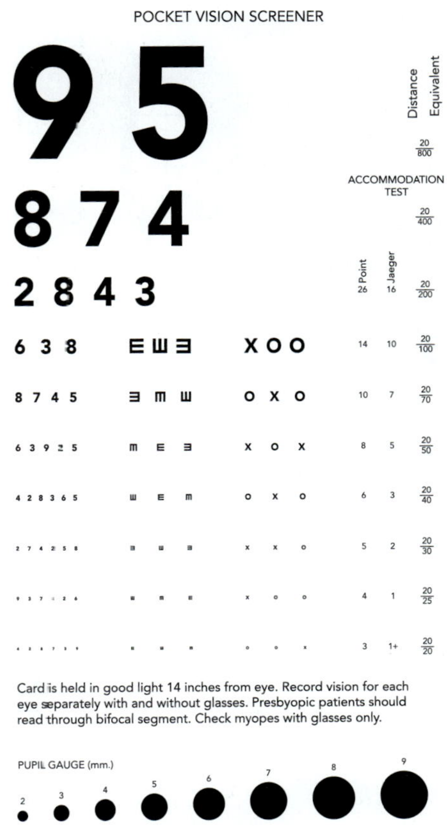

Figure 12-7 Near vision testing with the Rosenbaum Pocket Vision Screener.

Visual Fields

Confrontation is used to test the visual fields to assess peripheral vision. Assuming the examiner has intact peripheral vision, confrontation compares the client's peripheral vision to the examiner to identify areas of deficits. Due to most defects involving the temporal fields, the examiner should start with this field when performing this test.

E
1. Sit or stand approximately two feet away opposite the client, with your eyes at the same level as the client's eyes (Fig. 12-8A).
2. Have the client cover the right eye with an occluder or hand. Cover your left eye with an occluder.
3. Have the client look at the bridge of your nose while you look at the bridge of the client's nose.
4. Extend your right arm just behind the client's head. Wiggle your fingers as you move them into the client's peripheral vision.
5. Ask the client to say "now" when your wiggling fingers are seen moving into the field of vision. Use your own visual fields as the control for comparison to the client's.
6. Starting with the temporal area (lateral fields), slowly move both hands with your wiggling fingers from behind the client centrally until the client reports seeing your fingers. Your fingers should just be moving out of your peripheral vision as the client reports the fingers coming into their periphery.
7. Repeat the process to assess visual fields nasally, superiorly, and inferiorly (Fig. 12-8B).

N **The client can see the stimulus at about 90° temporally, 60° nasally, 50° superiorly, and 70° inferiorly.**

A If the client is unable to identify the movement that you perceive, a defect in the visual field is presumed. The portion of the visual field loss should be noted (Fig. 12-9).

P Defects in the client's visual field can be associated with tumors, strokes, or neurological diseases such as glaucoma or retinal detachment.

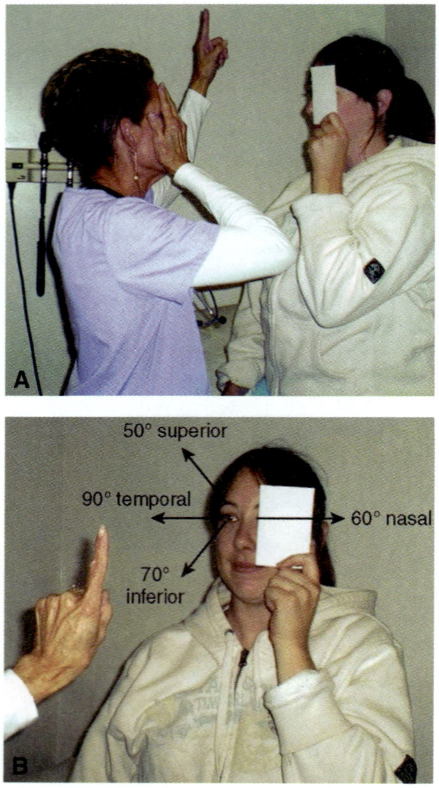

Figure 12-8 Testing visual fields by confrontation. **A.** The nurse and patient should be approximately at an eye-to-eye level. **B.** Range of visual fields.

External Eye and Lacrimal Apparatus

The examination of the external eye includes the eye itself, eyelids, eyebrows and eyelashes, and the lacrimal apparatus. Pathology of the eyelids is among the most common eye complaints of clients seeing a health-care provider.

Eyes, Eyelids, Eyebrows, and Eyelashes

E

1. Ask the client to sit facing you. Note if the eyes are natural or prosthetic.
2. Observe the client's eyelids for drooping, redness, edema, growths, or other abnormalities.
3. Note the distribution and symmetry of the eyelashes and eyebrows. Note any lesions.
4. Instruct the client to focus on an object or a finger held about 10 to 12 inches away and slightly above eye level.
5. Move the object or finger slowly downward and observe for a white space of sclera between the upper lid and the limbus.
6. Observe the blinking of the eyes.
7. Ask the client to elevate the eyelids.

N **Normally the client's natural eyes are present. The eyelids should appear symmetrical without drooping, redness, edema, or growths. When the eyes are focused in a normal frontal gaze, the lids should cover the upper portion of the iris. The client can raise both eyelids symmetrically (CN III). Slight ptosis, or drooping of the lid, can be normal. When the eye is closed, no portion of the cornea should be exposed. Normal lid margins are smooth, with the lashes evenly distributed and sweeping upward from the**

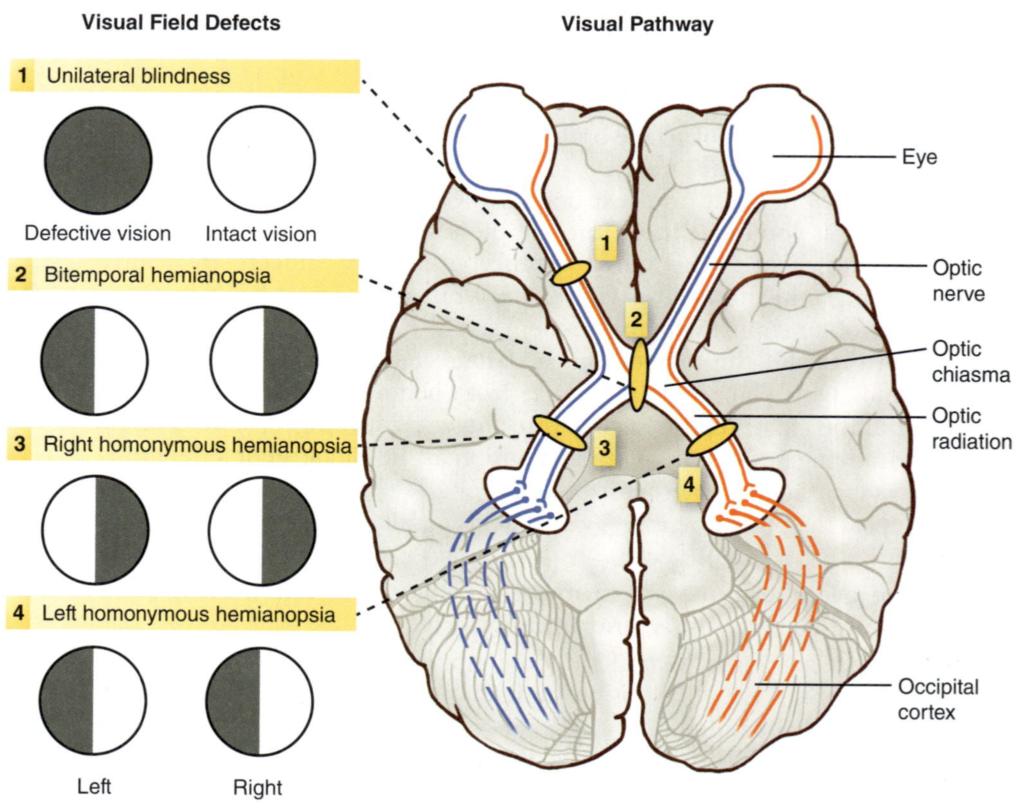

Figure 12-9 Visual field defects.

upper lids and downward from the lower lids. Eyebrows are symmetrical and without lesions or scaling.

A A prosthetic eye is not the natural state of the eyes (Fig. 12-10).

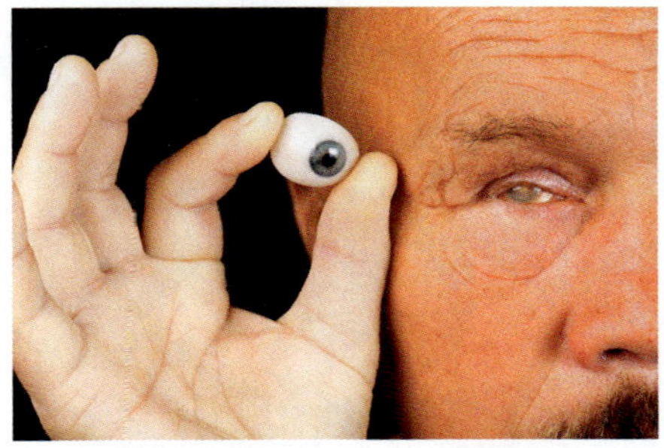

Figure 12-10 Prosthetic eye.

P A prosthetic eye may be worn if the client had an ocular injury, extensive eye disease or surgery for an eye neoplasm (e.g. retinoblastoma). Note any ill-fitting prosthesis or surrounding tissue inflammation.

A The client has either unilateral or bilateral, constant or intermittent ptosis of the lid (Fig. 12-11). If part of the pupil is occluded, there may be wrinkling of the forehead above the affected eye in an attempt to compensate by using the frontalis muscle to lift the lid.

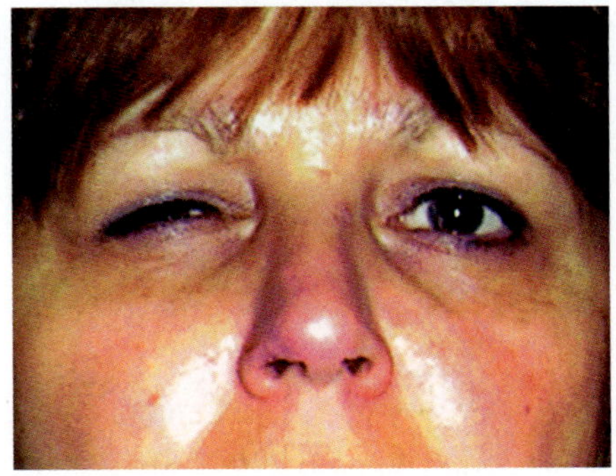

Figure 12-11 Ptosis.

P Ptosis can be either congenital or acquired. In congenital ptosis, the levator muscle fails to develop. This condition may be associated with the pathology of the superior rectus muscle as well. If the ptosis is acquired, it is related to one of three factors:

- *Mechanical:* heavy lids from lesions, adipose tissue, swelling, or edema
- *Myogenic:* muscular diseases such as myasthenia gravis or multiple sclerosis
- *Neurogenic:* paralysis from damage or interruption of the neural pathways

A An area of white sclera appears between the upper lid and the limbus, widening as the object is moved downward.

P An area of white sclera that appears between the upper lid and the limbus, widening as the object is moved downward is called lid lag. Lid lag may indicate the presence of thyrotoxicosis or increased circulating levels of free thyroxine or triiodothyronine.

A The client is unable to bring about complete lid closure. This is generally a unilateral condition.

P The inability to bring about complete lid closure is **lagophthalmos**. It can be associated with Bell palsy, stroke, trauma, or ectropion (everted eyelid).

A During an inspection of the lids, a disparity of the palpebral fissure is noted with apparent lid retraction, indicating a protrusion of the globe. This condition may be unilateral or bilateral.

P A disparity of the palpebral fissure with apparent lid retraction, indicating a protrusion of the globe is **exophthalmos** or proptosis (Fig. 12-12). Unilateral exophthalmos occurs due to orbital tumors, thyroid disease, trauma, or inflammation. Bilateral exophthalmos is related to thyroid disease.

A There is an apparent disparity in the size of the globe, manifested by a narrowing of the palpebral fissure.

P Enophthalmos is a backward displacement of the globe in the orbit, generally caused by orbital blowout fracture due to trauma. When this occurs, the orbital contents herniate through the fracture site.

A The turning inward, or inversion, of the lower lid is referred to as **entropion** and can cause severe discomfort to the client as the eyelashes abrade the cornea (trichiasis) (Fig. 12-13). If left untreated, it can cause inflammation, corneal scarring, and eventual ulceration.

P Entropion is caused by spasms or advancing age (senile entropion). In senile entropion, there is a loss of muscle tone, which causes the lid to fold inward.

NURSING TIP

Blindness Versus Legal Blindness

Be sure to describe visual loss correctly. For example, many more people are legally blind than totally blind (i.e., having no light perception). The definition of legal blindness can vary from state to state, but a commonly used parameter is corrected vision (with corrective glasses/lens) is 20/200 or worse, or peripheral vision is less than 20°.

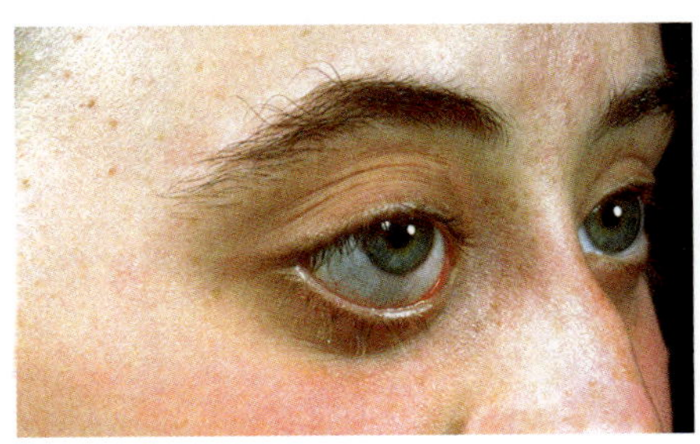

Figure 12-12 Proptosis.

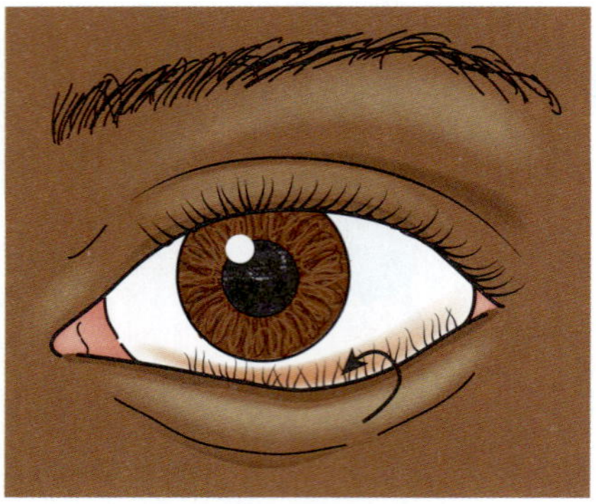

Figure 12-13 Entropion.

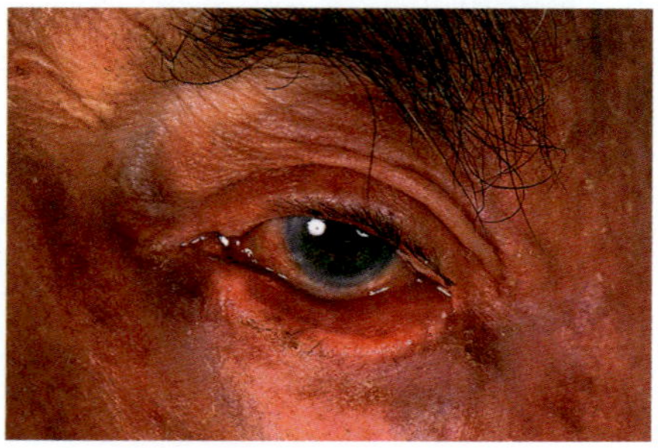

Figure 12-14 Ectropion.

A The turning outward, or eversion, of the lower lid is referred to as **ectropion** and may be unilateral or bilateral (Fig. 12-14). With ectropion, the lower lids appear to be sagging outward.

P The normal aging process can cause the muscles to lose their tone and relax, or they may be affected by Bell palsy.

A The client exhibits excessive blinking that may or may not be accompanied by increased tearing and pain.

P The causes of excessive blinking are both voluntary and involuntary. Voluntary excessive blinking can be caused by irritation to the cornea or the conjunctiva. The blinking frequently disappears when the stimulus is removed. Stress and anxiety can also lead to voluntary blinking. Involuntary excessive blinking is caused by tonic spasms of the orbicularis oculi muscle called blepharospasm. This is often seen in older adults as well as in clients with CN VII lesions, and irritation of the eye. Fatigue and stress can also cause involuntary blinking.

A The lids are black and blue, bluish, yellow, or red, depending on race and skin color.

P Color changes in the lids can result from:

- *Redness:* Generalized redness is nonspecific; however, redness in the nasal half of the lid may indicate frontal sinusitis. Redness adjacent to the lower lid can indicate disease of the lacrimal sac or nasolacrimal duct, such as dacryocystitis; and redness in the temporal portion of the lid can result from dacryoadenitis, an inflammation of the lacrimal gland.
- *Bluish:* Cyanosis can result from orbital vein thrombosis, orbital tumors, or aneurysms in the orbit.
- *Black and blue:* Ecchymosis is caused by bleeding into the surrounding tissues following trauma (black eye).

A Swelling or edema is noted in the eyelid.

P Swelling or edema may be noted in nonocular conditions such as inflammation associated with allergies, conjunctivitis, herpes simplex virus, systemic diseases, medications that contribute to swelling from fluid overload, trichinosis, early myxedema, thyrotoxicosis, or contact dermatitis.

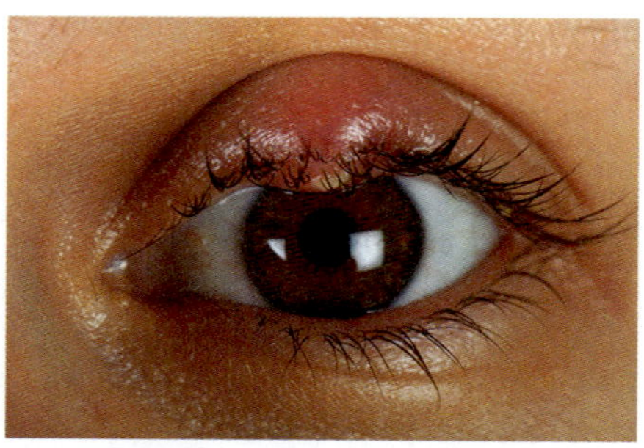

Figure 12-15 Hordeolum.

A There is an acute localized inflammation, tenderness, and redness, with the client complaining of pain in the infected eyelid area. This is called a **hordeolum** (Fig. 12-15).

P Staphylococcus is generally the infecting organism that causes a hordeolum. There are two types of hordeolum:

- *Internal:* Affects the meibomian glands, is usually large, and can point either to the skin or to the conjunctival side of the lid.
- *External:* Often called a stye, an infection of a sebaceous gland that usually points to the skin side of the lid and extends to the lid margin. Infections of the glands of the eyelid can be caused by improper removal of makeup, dry eyes, or seborrhea. There may be some connection between a hordeolum and increased handling of the lids in activities such as inserting and removing contact lenses.

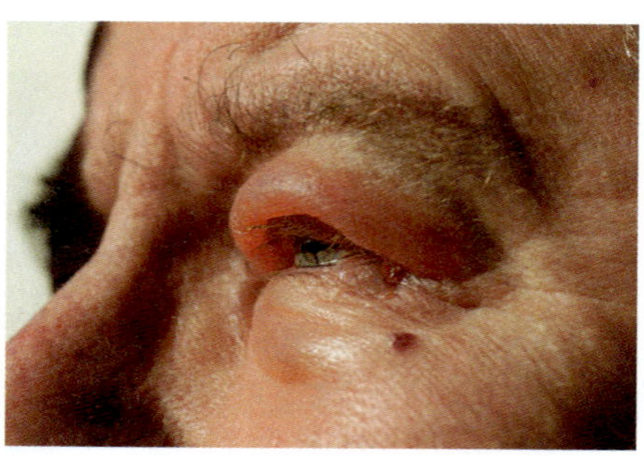

Figure 12-16 Blepharitis.

A The lids are inflamed bilaterally and are red-rimmed, with scales clinging to both the upper and the lower lids. The client complains of itching and burning along the lid margins. There may also be some loss of the eyelashes.

P This is **blepharitis**, which may be either staphylococcal or seborrheic (Fig. 12-16). Often a client has both types simultaneously. If the client has seborrheic infections elsewhere (scalp or eyebrows), it is more likely that the blepharitis is of the seborrheic type.

A There is a chronic inflammation of the meibomian gland in either the upper or the lower lid (Fig. 12-17). It generally forms over several weeks and, in many cases, points toward the conjunctival side of the lid, usually not on the lid margin. There is little or no redness and no tenderness.

P An inflammation of the meibomian gland in either the upper or the lower lid is referred to as a **chalazion**. Its cause is unknown.

A Raised, yellow, nonpainful plaques are present on the upper and lower lids near the inner canthus (Fig. 12-18).

P Raised, yellow, nonpainful plaques on the upper and lower lids near the inner canthus are **xanthelasma**, a form of xanthoma frequently associated with hypercholesterolemia

A The eyebrows have scaling areas.

P Scaling eyebrows can be caused by seborrhea.

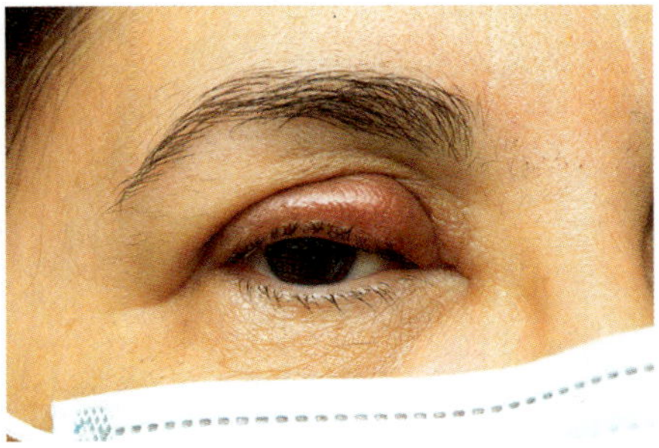

Figure 12-17 Chalazion.

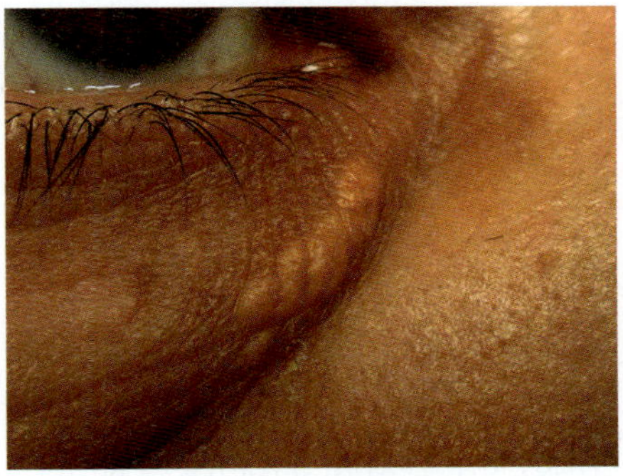

Figure 12-18 Xanthelasma.

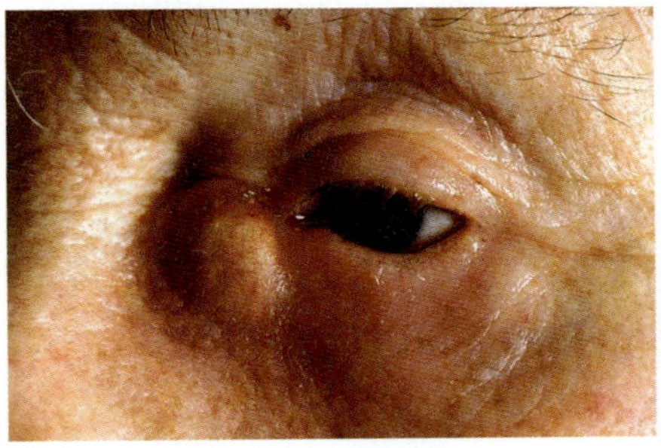

Figure 12-19 Dacrocystitis.

Lacrimal Apparatus

Inspection

E
1. Have the client sit facing you.
2. Identify the area of the lacrimal gland. Note any swelling or enlargement of the gland or elevation of the eyelid. Note any enlargement, swelling, redness, increased tearing, or exudate in the area of the lacrimal sac at the inner canthus.
3. Compare to the other eye to determine whether there is unilateral or bilateral involvement.

N **There should be no enlargement, swelling, or redness; no large amount of exudate; and minimal tearing.**

A There is inflammation and swelling in the upper lateral aspect of one or both eyes, and the client complains of pain in the affected area.

P Acute inflammation of the lacrimal gland is called **dacryoadenitis** and does not occur commonly. Dacryoadenitis may result from trauma or may be found in association with measles, mumps, and mononucleosis.

A There is inflammation and painful swelling beside the nose and near the inner canthus and possibly extending to the eyelid (Fig. 12-19.).

P **Dacryocystitis** is caused by inflammatory or neoplastic obstruction of the lacrimal duct.

Palpation

E
1. To examine the lacrimal sac for obstruction, don gloves.
2. Gently press the index finger near the inner canthus, just inside the rim of the bony orbit of the eye.
3. Note any discharge from the punctum.

N **There should not be excessive tearing or discharge from the punctum.**

A Mucopurulent discharge is noted.

P Obstruction anywhere along the system from the lacrimal sac to the point at which the ducts empty below the inferior nasal turbinate can cause mucopurulent discharge.

A There is an overflowing of tears from the eye.

P An overflowing of tears from the eye is epiphora, which is caused by obstruction of the lacrimal duct.

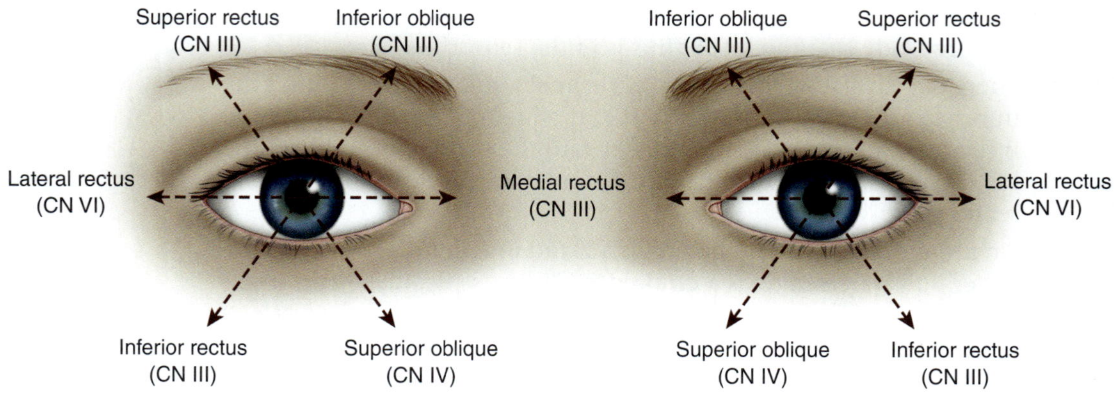

Figure 12-20 Direction of movement of extraocular muscles.

> **NURSING TIP**
> **Extraocular Muscles**
> One method of remembering the names of extraocular muscles and associated cranial nerves (CN) is: LR (lateral rectus) CN VI; SO (superior oblique) CN IV; all others (superior, inferior, and medial rectus and inferior oblique) are CN III.

Extraocular Muscle Function

Six extraocular muscles control the movement of each eye in relation to three axes: vertical, horizontal, and oblique (Fig. 12-20). Examination of extraocular function is carried out by observing corneal light reflex or alignment, using the cover/uncover test, and by testing the six cardinal fields of gaze (cranial nerves III, IV, and VI).

Corneal Light Reflex (Hirschberg Test)

E
1. Instruct the client to look straight ahead.
2. Focus a penlight on the bridge of the nose from a distance of 12 to 15 inches away at the midline.
3. Observe the location of reflected light on the cornea.

N **The reflected light (light reflex) should be seen symmetrically in the center of each cornea.**

A There is a discrepancy in the placement of one of the light reflections.

P Asymmetrical corneal light reflexes indicate an extraocular muscle imbalance that may be related to a variety of causes, depending on the client's age and medical condition: neurological, such as myasthenia gravis, multiple sclerosis, stroke, or neuropathies of diabetes mellitus; uncorrected childhood strabismus; trauma; or hypertension. **Strabismus** is the misalignment or deviation of one eye when looking at an object. Strabismus is due to a weakness in an eye muscle and may also be referred to as a tropia: **esotropia** is an inward turning of the eye; **exotropia** is an outward turning of the eye (Fig. 12-21).

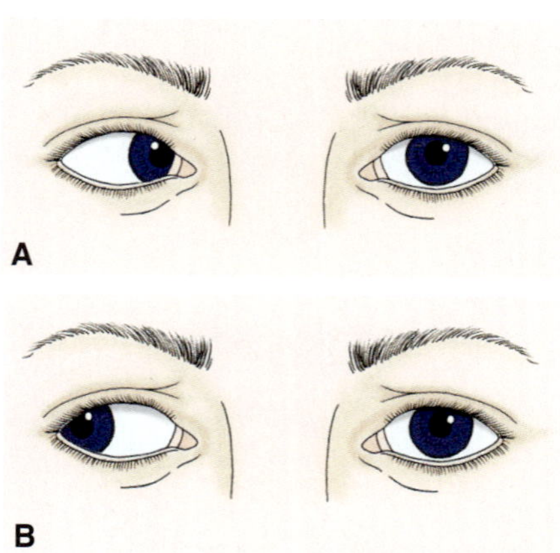

Figure 12-21 Strabismus. **A.** Right esotropia. **B.** Right exotropia.

Cover/Uncover Test

E
1. Ask the client to look straight ahead and to focus on an object in the distance.
2. Place an occluder over the left eye for several seconds and observe for movement in the uncovered right eye.
3. As the occluder is removed, observe the covered eye for movement.
4. Repeat the procedure with the same eye, having the client focus on an object held close to the eye.
5. Repeat on the other side.

N **If the eyes are in alignment, there will be no movement of either eye.**

A If the uncovered eye shifts position as the other eye is covered, or if the covered eye shifts position as it is uncovered, a **phoria**, or latent misalignment of an eye, exists.

E Examination **N** Normal Findings **A** Abnormal Findings **P** Pathophysiology

P Phoria is a mild weakness elicited by the cover/uncover test and has multiple forms: **esophoria**, nasal or inward drift, and **exophoria**, a temporal or outward drift (Fig. 12-22). **Hypophoria**, or a downward turning of the eye, and **hyperphoria**, an upward turning of the eye, can occur.

Cardinal Fields of Gaze (Extraocular Muscle Movements)

E
1. Place the client in a sitting position facing you.
2. Ask the client to follow an object (finger, pencil, or penlight) with the eyes.
3. Move the object through the cardinal fields of gaze (Fig. 12-23) smoothly and steadily, pausing at each extreme position to detect

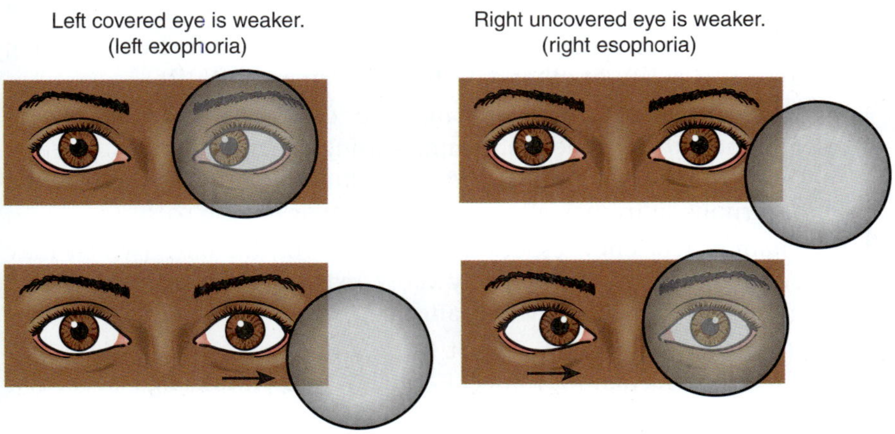

Figure 12-22 Cover/uncover test. Left covered eye is weaker. (Left exophoria) Right uncovered eye is weaker. (Right esophoria)

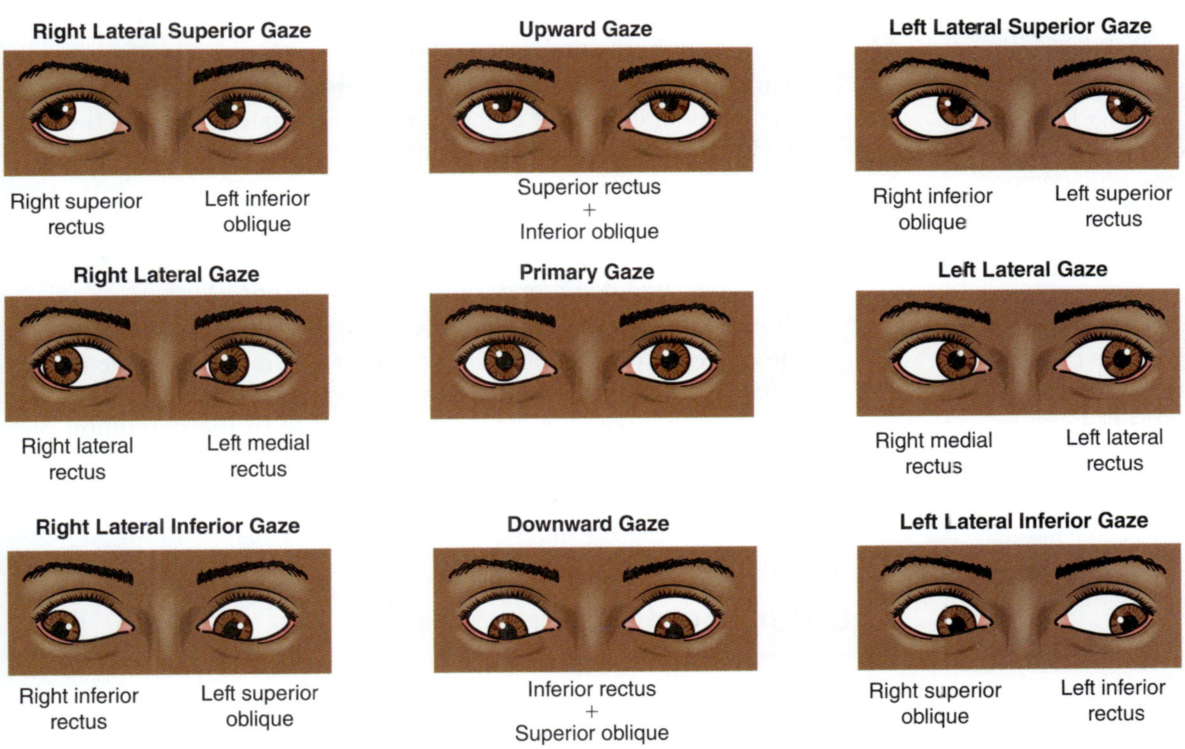

Figure 12-23 Cardinal fields of gaze.

any **nystagmus**, or involuntary movement, and returning to the center after each field is tested.
4. Note the client's ability to move the eyes in each direction.
5. Move the object forward to about five inches in front of the client's nose at the midline.
6. Observe for convergence of gaze.

N **Both eyes should move smoothly and symmetrically in each of the cardinal fields of gaze and converge on the held object as it moves toward the nose. Slight nystagmus can be noted with extreme lateral gaze and can be normal.**

A There is a lack of symmetrical eye movement in a particular direction.

P Inability to move the eye in a given direction indicates a weakness in the muscle responsible for moving the eye in that direction.

A Abnormal eye movements consist of failure of an eye to move lateral (CN VI), the inability of an eye to move downward when deviating inward (CN IV), or other defects in movement (CN III).

P Traumatic ophthalmoplegia may be caused by fracture of the orbit near the foramen magnum, causing damage to the extraocular muscles or CN III, IV, and VI. Basilar skull fractures that involve the cavernous sinus may also cause extraocular muscle palsy.

P Vitamin deficiency, especially of vitamin B_1,thiamine (which may occur in alcohol abuse), may cause extraocular muscle palsy and nystagmus. Usually, CN VI is affected.

P Herpes zoster, syphilis, scarlet fever, whooping cough, or botulism are infections that may affect CN III, IV, and VI, causing extraocular muscle palsy.

A Ophthalmoplegia is paralysis of one or more of the optic muscles.

P Increased intracranial pressure may cause strangulation of CN VI. CN VI palsy occurs late after the onset of increased intracranial pressure.

A Paralysis of horizontal gaze is abnormal.

P Damage to the motor areas of the cerebral cortex causes the loss of the ability of both eyes to look to the contralateral side, so the eyes tend to deviate toward the side of the lesion.

A If one eye deviates down and the other eye deviates up, it is called skew deviation.

P Cerebellar disease or a lesion in the pons on the same side of the eye that is deviated down may cause skew deviation.

A There is a rhythmic, beating, involuntary oscillation of the eyes as the object is held at points away from the midline. Movement is usually lateral, vertical, or rotary. Nystagmus can be jerky, with fast and slow components; or rhythmic, similar to the pendulum of a clock.

P Nystagmus may be caused by a lesion in the brainstem, cerebellum, vestibular system, or along the visual pathways in the cerebral hemispheres.

NURSING TIP
Eye Hygiene

If a client wears contact lenses, inquire what type is worn. Ask the client what the disinfecting criteria are for that type of lens, the frequency of lens replacement, and the daily duration of wear time. Determine whether the client is adhering to these protocols. Failure to comply with contact lens cleaning procedures, wear time, and recommended replacement schedule can lead to corneal abrasions and ocular infections.

Persons who use eye makeup should be sure to replace such items as mascara and eyeliner frequently to avoid the possibility of bacterial colonization. In the event of an episode of conjunctivitis, all items should be discarded to prevent reinfection from makeup, which could be contaminated.

Anterior Segment Structures
Conjunctiva

To examine the bulbar conjunctiva:

E
1. Separate the lid margins with the fingers.
2. Have the client look up, down, and to the right and left.

3. Inspect the surface of the bulbar conjunctiva for color, redness, swelling, exudate, or foreign bodies. Note whether **injection** or redness is around the cornea or toward the periphery.
4. With the thumb, gently pull the lower lid toward the cheek and inspect the surface of the bulbar conjunctiva for color, inflammation, edema, lesions, or foreign bodies.

N **The bulbar conjunctiva is transparent, with small blood vessels visible in it. It should appear white except for a few normal small blood vessels. No swelling, injection, exudate, foreign bodies, or lesions are noted.**

A P Refer to palpebral conjunctiva.

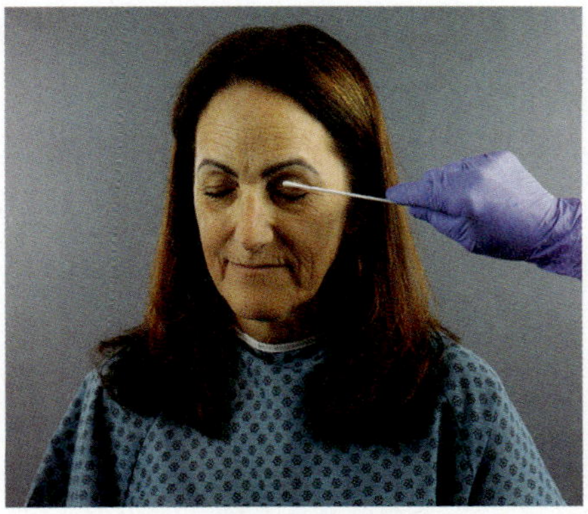

Figure 12-24 Assessing the palpebral conjunctiva.

The palpebral conjunctiva is examined only when there is a concern about its condition. To examine the palpebral conjunctiva of the upper lid:

E
1. Explain the procedure to the client to alleviate the fear of pain or damage to the eye.
2. Don gloves. Have the client look down to relax the levator muscle (Fig. 12-24).
3. Gently pull the eyelashes downward and place a sterile, cotton-tipped applicator about 1 cm above the lid margin.
4. Gently exert downward pressure on the applicator while pulling the eyelashes upward to evert the lid.
5. Inspect the palpebral conjunctiva for injection, swelling or **chemosis**, exudate, and foreign bodies.
6. Return the lid to its normal position by instructing the client to look up and then pulling the eyelid outward and removing the cotton-tipped swab. Ask the client to blink.

N **The palpebral conjunctiva should appear pink and moist. It is without swelling, lesions, injection (reddened or blood shot), exudate, or foreign bodies.**

A Unilateral or bilateral injected conjunctiva with purulent, sticky discharge and lid edema are present (Fig. 12-25A and B).

P Injected conjunctiva with purulent, sticky discharge and lid edema usually indicate the presence of bacterial conjunctivitis.

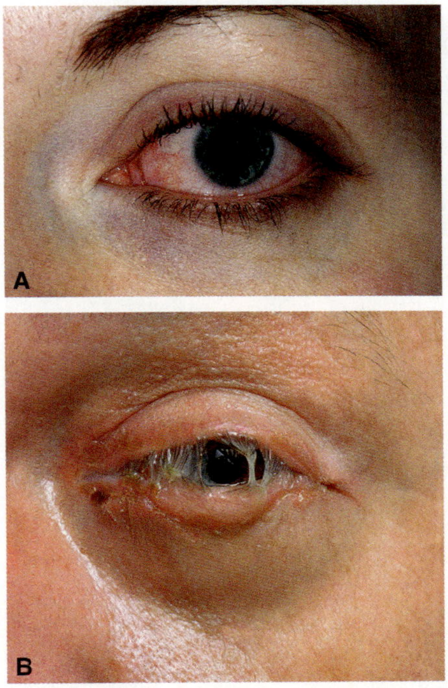

Figure 12-25 Conjunctivitis. **A.** Note the injected eye. **B.** Note the purulent discharge.

A Unilateral injection with moderate pain and without purulent discharge is noted, but the client complains of increased lacrimation.

P These symptoms usually indicate that conjunctivitis is viral. Viral conjunctivitis is most commonly due to adenovirus, which may become epidemic. Herpes simplex virus may also be a viral cause of conjunctivitis. A preauricular node is often felt on palpation.

A Mild inflammation and injection and follicles of palpebral conjunctiva are present with scant discharge. The client reports an itching and burning sensation, as well as increased lacrimation.

P Allergic conjunctivitis and is often associated with seasonal allergies when exposed to allergens such as pollen, ragweed, grasses, and trees.

A A yellow nodule is noted on the nasal side of the bulbar conjunctiva adjacent to the cornea (Fig. 12-26). It may be on the temporal side as well. This lesion is painless unless it becomes inflamed.

P A yellow nodule on the bulbar conjunctiva is called a **pinguecula**. It is a nodular degeneration of the conjunctiva and is thought to be a result of increased exposure to ultraviolet light.

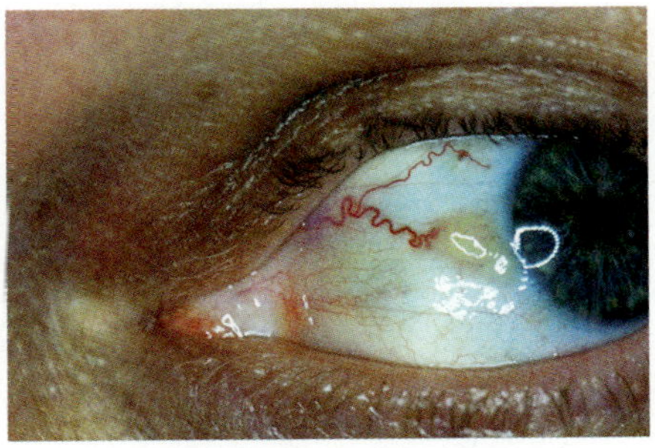

Figure 12-26 Pinguecula

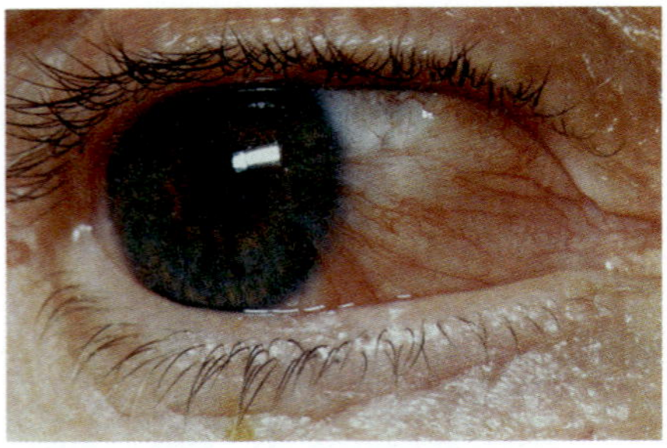

Figure 12-27 Pterygium.

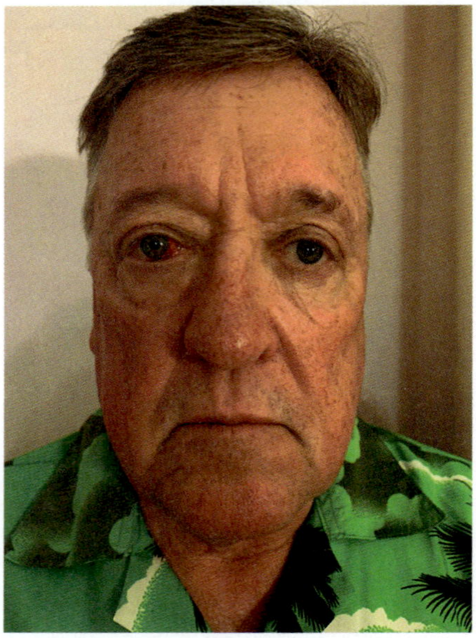

Figure 12-28 Subconjunctival hemorrhage.

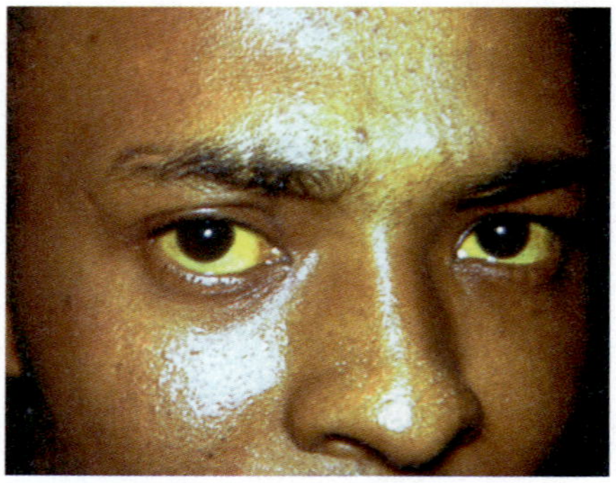

Figure 12-29 Scleral icterus.

A A unilateral or bilateral triangle-shaped encroachment onto the conjunctiva is abnormal (Fig. 12-27). This lesion always occurs nasally and remains painless unless it becomes ulcerated. If the lesion covers the cornea, loss of vision may occur.

P A triangle-shaped encroachment onto the conjunctiva is called a **pterygium** and is also caused by excessive ultraviolet light exposure.

A The client exhibits a sudden onset of a painless, bright-red appearance on the bulbar conjunctiva (Fig. 12-28).

P A painless, bright-red appearance on the bulbar conjunctiva is a subconjunctival hemorrhage. A subconjunctival hemorrhage may result from pressure exerted during coughing, sneezing, or a Valsalva maneuver. Minor trauma can also cause this. A subconjunctival hemorrhage can also be attributed to anticoagulant medications or uncontrolled hypertension.

Sclera

E While examining the conjunctiva, inspect the sclera for color, exudate, lesions, and foreign bodies.

N **Individuals with fair skin should have white sclera with some small, superficial vessels and without exudate, lesions, or foreign bodies. Individuals with darker pigmentation may have tiny brown patches of melanin or a grayish-blue or "muddy" color sclera. Yellowing of the sclera in older adults with darker skin can be a normal finding.**

A The color of the sclera is uniformly yellow (Fig. 12-29).

P A yellow sclera is known as jaundice or scleral icterus and is due to coloring of the sclera with bilirubin, which infiltrates all tissues of the body. This is an early manifestation of systemic conditions such as hepatitis, sickle cell disease, gallstones, and physiological jaundice in the newborn.

A The sclera is blue.

P A blue sclera is a distinctive feature of osteogenesis imperfecta and is due to the thinning of the sclera, which allows the choroid to show through.

Cornea

E
1. Stand in front of the client.
2. Shine a penlight directly on the cornea.
3. Move the light laterally and view the cornea from that angle, noting color, discharge, and lesions.

N **The corneal surface should be moist and shiny, with no discharge, cloudiness, opacities, or irregularities.**

A A grayish or purulent yellow/green, well-circumscribed ulcerated area on the cornea is abnormal (Fig. 12-30).

P Corneal ulceration can result from a bacterial, viral, fungal, or parasitic infection. Corneal ulcers can also result from ocular injuries, ocular burns, corneal abrasions, and injury from contact use or insufficient lens cleaning.

A A treelike configuration on the corneal surface is identified. The client complains of mild discomfort, photophobia, and in some cases blurred vision (depending on the location of the lesions).

P A treelike configuration on the corneal surface is a type of ulceration caused by the herpes simplex virus. The client usually has a history of having had a cold sore (HSV 1 or HSV 2) or herpes zoster (shingles).

A A hazy gray ring about 2 mm in width just inside the limbus is seen (Fig. 12-31).

P A hazy gray ring inside the limbus is called **arcus senilis**. Arcus senilis occurs bilaterally and is a common finding. Arcus senilis is caused by benign degeneration of the peripheral cornea. It can be found at any age but is most common in older adults. If found in a young person, it may be associated with hypercholesterolemia.

A A steamy or cloudy cornea is abnormal. The client may have ocular pain.

P Glaucoma is caused by increased intraocular pressure. Refer to the section on Anterior Chamber examination.

A Any irregularities in the appearance of the cornea are abnormal.

P Keratoconus (Fig. 12-32) is the conical protrusion of the center of the cornea. It is a noninflammatory condition in which the cornea thins, sometimes leading to the need for corneal transplant surgery.

P A corneal scar (Fig. 12-33) can form at the site of past injury or inflammation.

P A corneal laceration (Fig. 12-34) can occur secondary to trauma.

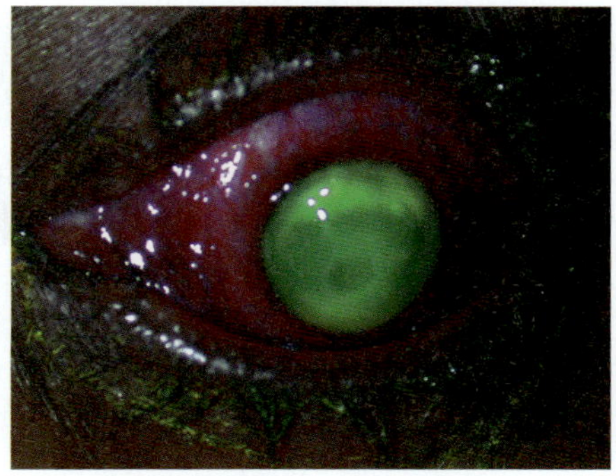

Figure 12-30 Corneal ulceration. Note the injection and hypopyon (purulent material in the anterior chamber), which frequently occur with corneal ulceration.

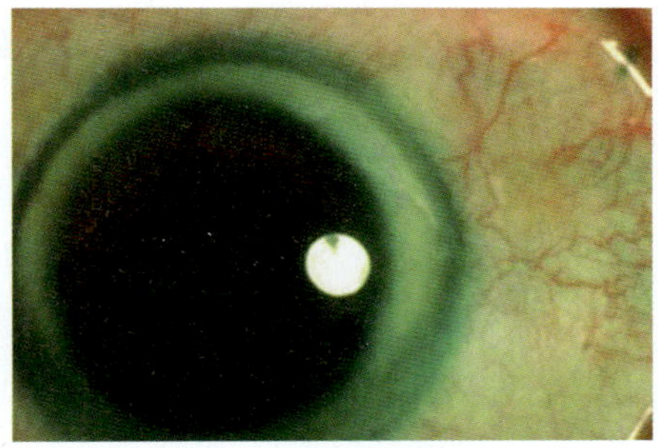

Figure 12-31 Arcus senilis.

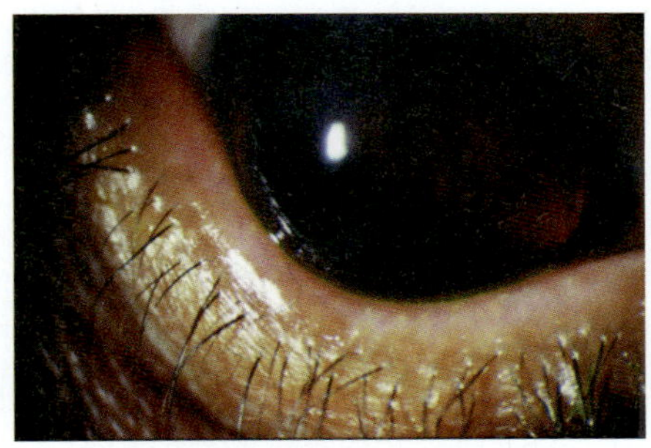

Figure 12-32 Keratoconus.

Anterior Chamber

The anterior chamber is that compartment of the eye found between the cornea and the iris. The space between the flat plane of the iris and the periphery of the cornea must be adequate to allow drainage of aqueous fluid out of the eye. If this angle is too narrow, drainage is inadequate, the pressure of the aqueous fluid in the anterior chamber increases, and **glaucoma** develops. If intraocular fluid pressure remains high, optic nerve damage and visual field loss occur.

To differentiate a normal from a narrowed angle:

E

1. Face the client and shine a light obliquely through the anterior chamber from the lateral side toward the nasal side (Fig. 12-35).
2. Observe the distribution of light in the anterior chamber (Fig. 12-36).
3. Repeat the procedure with the other eye.

N **In a normal eye, the entire iris will be illuminated.**

A The eye has a narrow angle, with the decreased space between the iris and the cornea appearing as a crescent-shaped shadow on the far portion of the iris.

P The narrow angle is an anatomic variant that can predispose an individual to the development of angle-closure glaucoma. As aging progresses, the lens thickens, which may cause even further narrowing of the angle.

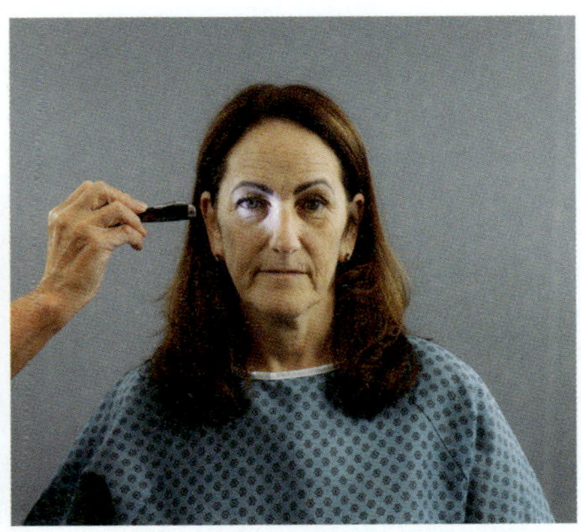

Figure 12-35 Examining the anterior chamber.

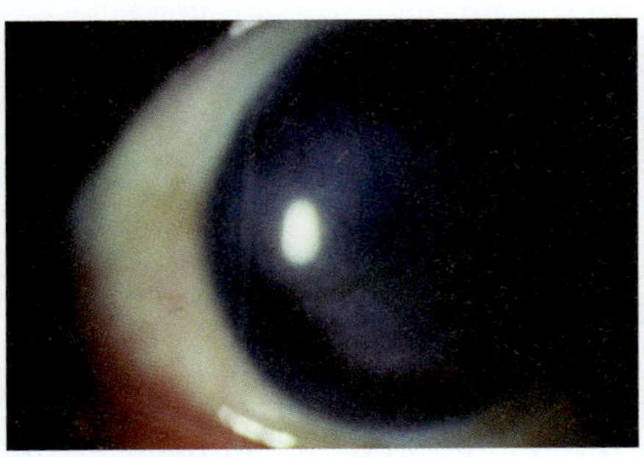

Figure 12-33 Corneal scar.

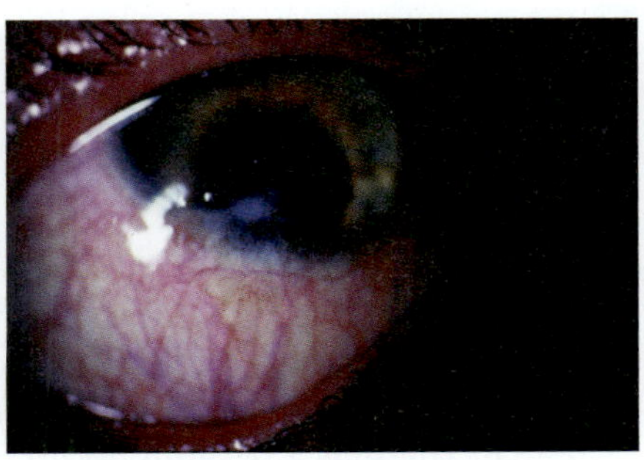

Figure 12-34 Corneal laceration.

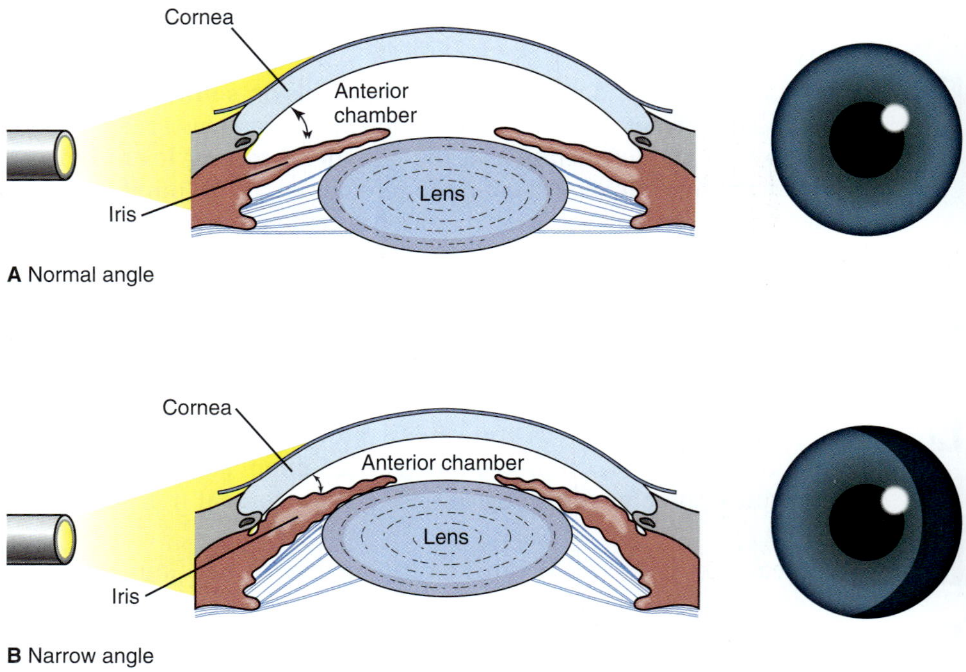

Figure 12-36 Evaluating the angle of the anterior chamber.

Iris

E With the penlight, inspect the iris for color, nodules, and vascularity.

N **Normally, the color is evenly distributed over the iris, although there can be a mosaic variant. It is normally smooth and without apparent vascularity.**

A A heavily pigmented, slightly elevated area is visible in the iris.

P A heavily pigmented, slightly elevated area in the iris can be a benign iris nevus or a malignant melanoma. An iris nevus is much more common than melanoma. Suspected malignant melanoma needs an immediate referral to a qualified specialist.

A The inferior portion of the iris is obscured by blood.

P A **hyphema** is caused by bleeding from vessels in the iris as a result of direct trauma to the globe. It can also occur as a result of eye surgery.

A An absent wedge portion of the iris is abnormal.

P The shape of the iris changes after the surgical removal of a cataract; the pupil may also have an irregular shape.

Pupil

E

1. Stand in front of the client in a darkened room.
2. Note the shape and size of the pupils in millimeters.
3. Move a penlight from the temporal area to the front of one eye without allowing the light to shine on the other eye (Fig. 12-37A and B).
4. Observe the pupillary reaction in that eye. This is the direct light reflex. Note the size of the pupil receiving light stimulus and the speed of pupillary response to light.
5. Move the penlight again to the temporal area and back to the front of the eye, this time observing the opposite eye for pupillary constriction. This is the consensual light reflex.

> **Risk Factors**
>
> **Glaucoma**
>
> - Increasing age
> - Family history
> - Race (especially Black [Non-Hispanic] and Asian)
> - Elevated intraocular pressure
> - Hypertension
> - Diabetes
> - Smoking
> - Sickle cell anemia
> - Extreme myopia
> - Prolonged steroid use
> - Previous eye injury
> - Thin cornea

6. Repeat the procedure on the other eye.
7. Instruct the client to shift the gaze to a distant object for 30 seconds.
8. Instruct the client to then look at your finger or an object held in your hand about 10 cm from the client.
9. Note the reaction and size of the pupils. **Accommodation** occurs when pupils constrict to focus on objects at close range. You may need to increase the light in the room if the pupils are difficult to see.

N **The pupils should be deep black, round, and of equal diameter, ranging from 2 to 6 mm. Pupils should constrict briskly to direct and consensual light and accommodation (CN III). Small differences in pupil size (anisocoria) may be normal in some people.**

A The pupil that constricts to less than 2 mm in diameter is termed **miotic**. The pupil that dilates to more than 6 mm in diameter is termed **mydriatic**.

P Abnormal pupillary size can be caused by medications such as sympathomimetics or parasympathomimetics, iritis, or disorders such as CN III paralysis, which can occur as a result of a carotid artery aneurysm. These abnormalities may also be due to nerve damage or trauma (see Table 12-1 for further pathologies).

A The pupil has an irregular shape.

P An irregularly shaped pupil is usually associated with the surgical removal of cataracts and iridectomy.

A When a light is shone on the pupil, little to no constriction occurs or pupil dilation occurs. The consensual reaction is appropriate. This is called a Marcus Gunn pupil.

P Optic nerve damage in the optic chiasm, such as in trauma, destroys the afferent pathways of the pupillary light reflex (deafferented pupil). Retinal disorders can also cause a Marcus Gunn pupil.

A The hippus phenomenon occurs after the pupil has been stimulated by direct light. Light causes the pupil to constrict, but then the pupil appears to rhythmically vacillate in size from a larger to a smaller diameter.

P Hippus may be caused by a lesion in the midbrain.

A The presence of midposition, round, regular, and fixed (5 to 6 mm) pupils that may show hippus is abnormal.

P These signs usually indicate midbrain damage that interrupts the light reflex but may leave accommodation intact.

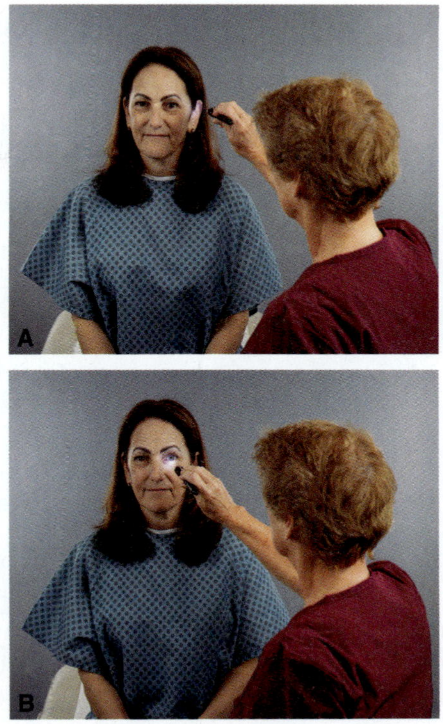

Figure 12-37 Pupil examination. **A.** Starting position with a penlight to the side of the pupil. **B.** Move the penlight directly in front of the pupil.

> **NURSING TIP**
> **Examination of the Lens**
> A detailed examination of the lens requires the use of a slit lamp by an ophthalmologist. Some lens opacities, however, can be seen with the direct ophthalmoscope.

Lens

E
1. Stand in front of the client.
2. Shine a penlight directly on the pupil. The lens is behind the pupil.
3. Note the color.

N **The lens is transparent in color.**

A One or more of the pupils are not deep black.

P In an adult, a pearly gray appearance of one or both pupils may indicate an opacity (cloudiness) in the lens (**cataract**) (Fig. 12-38).

P A senile cataract is the most common type of cataract. Progressively blurred distance vision is the main symptom, although near vision may be improved because of greater convexity of the lens.

P A unilateral cataract may occur soon after an eye injury caused by a foreign body. Along with the lens opacity, there may be intraocular

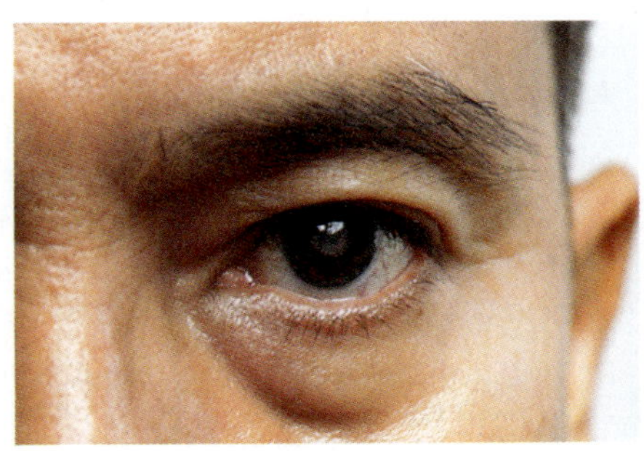

Figure 12-38 Cataract.

Table 12-1 Pupil abnormalities

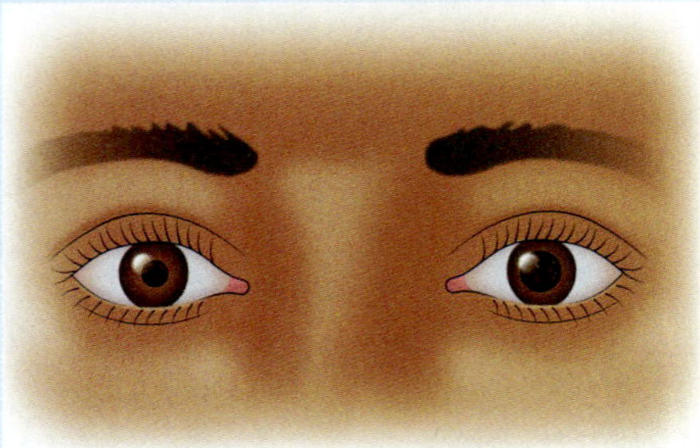

A: The size of pupils is unequal but both pupils react to light and accommodation.

P: Inequality of pupillary size is called **anisocoria** and may be congenital or due to inflammation of ocular tissue or disturbances of neurophthalmic pathways.

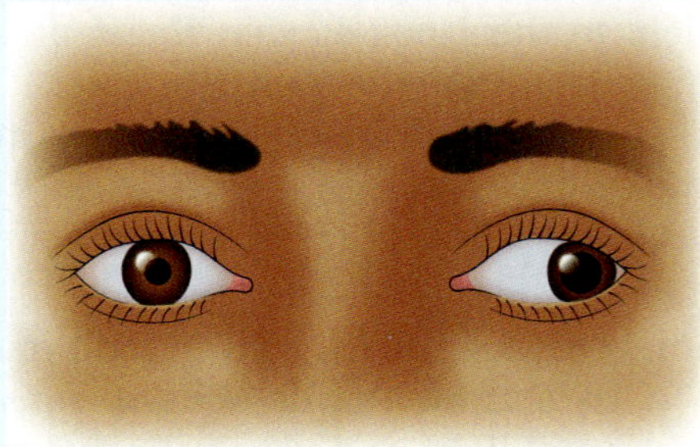

A: A fixed and dilated pupil is observed on one side. The abnormal pupil does not react to direct or consensual light stimulation and does not accommodate. Ptosis and lateral downward deviation may also be noted.

P: This abnormality is caused by oculomotor nerve damage due to head trauma and increased intracranial pressure. Atropine-like agents applied topically may cause an even more widely fixed and dilated pupil.

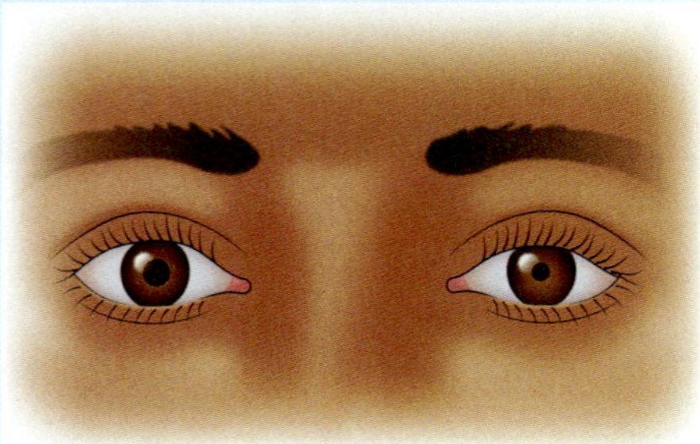

A: A unilateral, small, regularly shaped pupil is observed. Both pupils react directly and consensually and accommodate. Ptosis and diminished or absent sweating on the affected side may also be noted.

P: This finding is Horner's syndrome, which is caused by a lesion of the sympathetic nerve pathway.

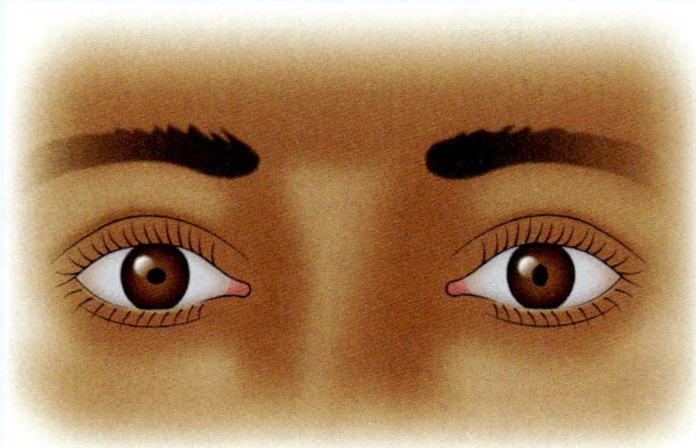

A: Pupils are bilaterally small and irregularly shaped. They react to accommodation but sluggishly or not at all to light.

P: These abnormalities are Argyll Robertson pupils and are usually caused by central lesions of late-stage neurosyphilis. Other causes include encephalitis, multiple sclerosis, diabetes, brain tumors, and alcoholism.

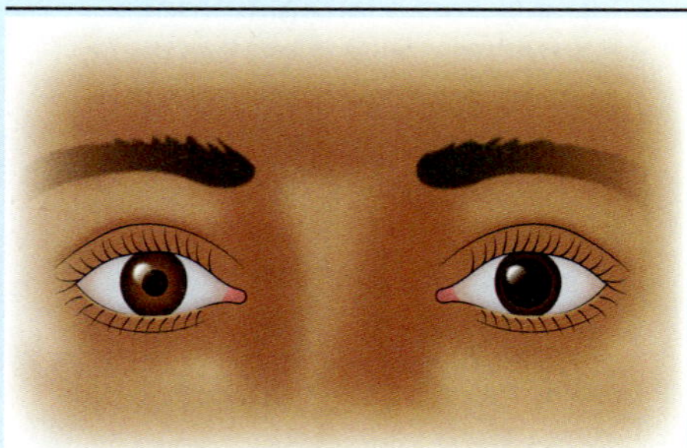

A: A unilateral, large, regularly shaped pupil is noted. The affected pupil's reaction to light and accommodation is sluggish or absent. The client may report blurred vision because of the slow accommodation. You may observe diminished patellar and Achilles deep tendon reflexes.

P: This abnormality, a tonic or Adie's pupil, is thought to result from a bacterial or viral infection or autoimmune condition.

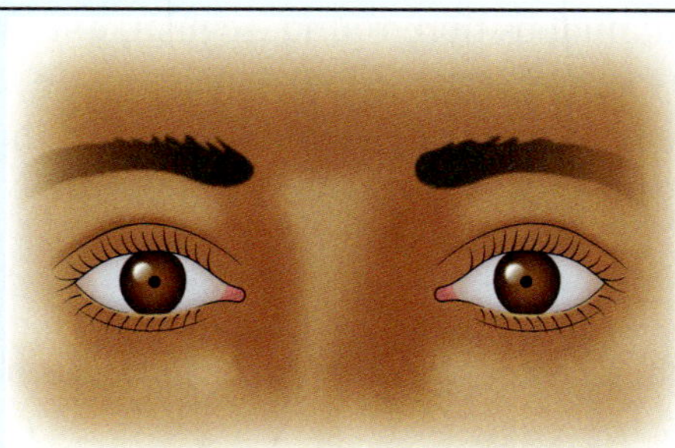

A: Both pupils are small, fixed, regularly shaped, and do not react to light or accommodation.

P: This abnormality may be caused by opiate ingestion, topical application of miotic drops, or lesions in the brain.

A: Pupils are small, equal, and reactive.

P: Diencephalic injury or metabolic coma may cause these findings.

Table 12-1 Pupil abnormalities—cont'd

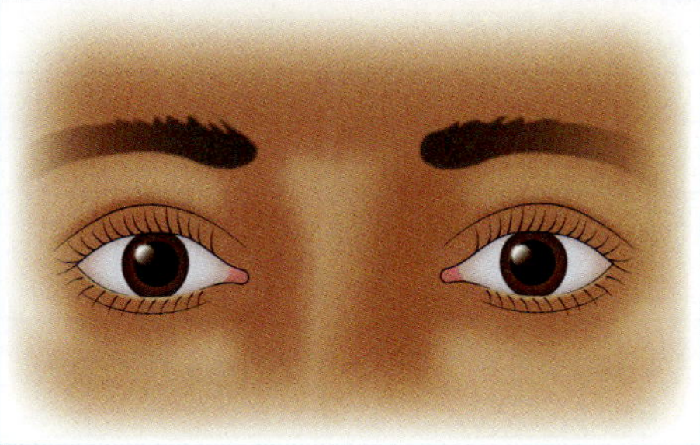

A: Both pupils are dilated and fixed and do not react to light or accommodation.

P: Severe head trauma, brainstem infarction, and cardiopulmonary arrest (after 4 to 6 minutes) can lead to these findings.

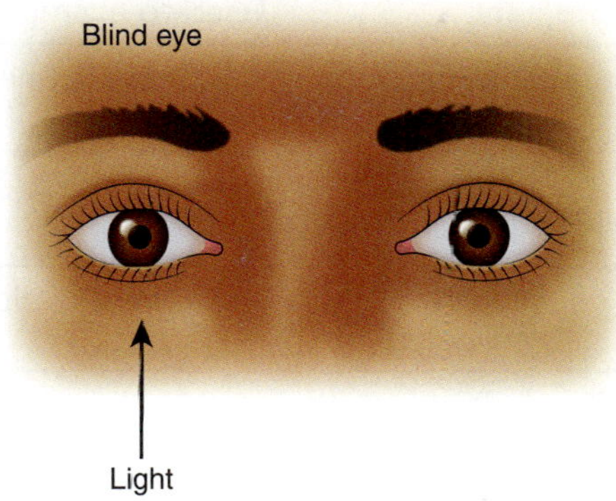

A: Light shone into a blind eye (amaurotic pupil) will cause no reaction (direct or consensual) in either pupil. If light is shone in the other eye, and CN III is intact, both pupils should constrict.

P: Due to a lesion in the retina or the optic nerve, the light stimulus shown in the amaurotic pupil is unable to pass along the sensory pathway; therefore, the oculomotor response in both eyes is absent.

hemorrhage or aqueous or vitreous humor leaking from the globe. The client reports an immediate blurring of vision.

P Bilateral cataracts found in infants or young children are congenital cataracts. These cataracts are probably genetically determined, although maternal rubella in the first trimester can also be responsible.

Posterior Segment Structures

The funduscopic examination (CN II) requires the use of a direct ophthalmoscope to assess the structures in the posterior segment of the eye (Fig. 12-39). The ophthalmoscope consists of two parts: the head and the handle. To activate the light source in the head, depress the rheostat button and move it as far as possible. Move the aperture selector to produce the largest beam of light that can be visualized by focusing the beam of light on the palm of the hand. The larger beam is preferred when examining an average-sized pupil, and the smaller beam makes the examination of a smaller pupil easier. Table 12-2 lists the various apertures of the ophthalmoscope and their uses. The lens selector allows you to choose lenses of varying power for different parts of the examination. These lenses are marked with red and black numbers, signifying different focal lengths. These numbers are called **diopters**, a unit of refractive measurement. The 0 lens sits between the red- and black-numbered lenses and has no correction. In some ophthalmoscopes, there is no color designation (red or black), and the lens power is signified by + or – signs in front of the numbers. A + sign, or diopter, is equivalent to black and focuses closer to the ophthalmoscope. This is used to correct for farsightedness, or hyperopia. A – sign, or diopter, is equivalent to red and focuses farther from the instrument. This is used to correct nearsightedness or myopia. These lenses compensate for the refractive error of both the client and the nurse.

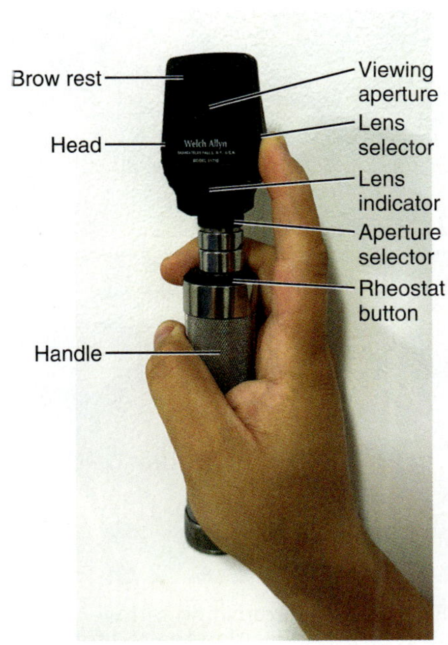

Figure 12-39 Ophthalmoscope.

Table 12-2 Apertures of the Ophthalmoscope

○	Small round light	Used to examine eyes with small, undilated pupils
◯	Large round light	Used for routine eye examinations and examination of dilated eyes
▦	Grid	Used to assess size and location of funduscopic lesions
▯	Slit light	Assesses anterior eye and determines elevation of funduscopic lesions
●	Green light (red-free filter)	Used to assess retinal hemorrhages (which appear black) and small vessel changes

Risk Factors

Cataracts

- Increasing age
- Family history
- Hypertension
- Diabetes
- Smoking
- Alcohol use
- Ultraviolet light exposure
- Malnutrition
- Obesity
- History of eye injury
- Previous eye surgery
- Prolonged steroid use

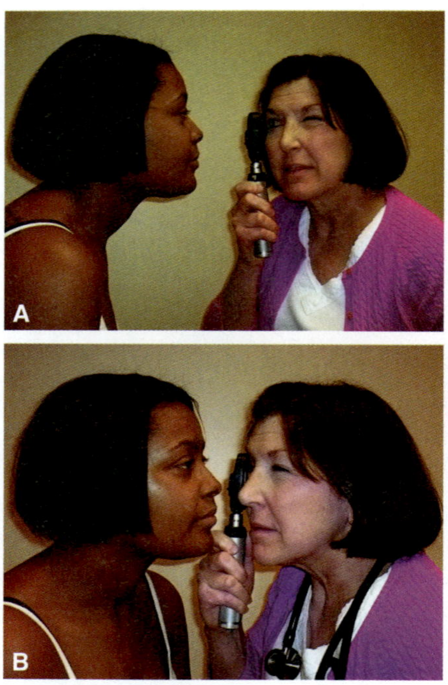

Figure 12-40 Examining retinal structures. **A.** Eliciting the red reflex. **B.** Funduscopic examination.

NURSING TIP

Comprehensive Eye Examination

Clients should be referred to a qualified eye specialist for a comprehensive eye examination according to their age if there are no other risk factors for eye disease. Clients under 40 should seek care every 5 to 10 years, ages 40 to 54 every 2 to 4 years, ages 55 to 64 every 1 to 3 years, and age 65 and older every 1 to 2 years. Clients with type 1 diabetes should start examinations 5 years after onset, then yearly. Clients with type 2 diabetes should seek care at the time of diagnosis, then yearly.

Retinal Structures

In a darkened room, ask the client to remove eyeglasses; contact lenses may be left in place.

E

1. Instruct the client to look at a distant object across the room. This will help to dilate the eyes.
2. Set the ophthalmoscope on the 0 lens and hold it in front of your right eye with your index finger on the lens selector.
3. From a distance of 8 to 12 inches from the client and about 15° to the lateral side, shine the light into the client's right pupil, eliciting a light reflection from the retina; this is called the **red reflex** (Fig. 12-40A).
4. While maintaining the red reflex in view, move closer to the client and move the lens selector from 0 to the 1, or black, numbers to focus on the anterior ocular structures.
5. For optimum visualization, keep the ophthalmoscope within an inch of the client's eye (Fig. 12-40B).
6. At this point, move the lens selector from the 1, or black, numbers, through 0, and into the –, or red, numbers to focus on structures progressively more posteriorly.
7. Focus on the optic disc at the nasal side of the retina by following any retinal vessels centrally.
8. You may need to reverse direction along the vessel if the disc does not appear.
9. Observe the retina for color and lesions; the retinal vessels for configuration and characteristics of their crossing; and the optic disc for color, shape, size, margins, and comparison of cup-to-disc ratio.

10. Describe the size, position, and location of any abnormality. Use the diameter of the disc (DD) as a guide to describe the distance of the abnormality from the optic disc. View the optic disc as a clock face for a reference point to describe the location of the abnormality. Describe the size of the abnormality in relation to the size of the optic disc.
11. Repeat on the left side, using the ophthalmoscope in your left hand to examine the client's left optic fundus.

N **Refer to Table 12-3. The red reflex is present. The optic disc is pinkish-orange in color, with a yellow-white excavated center known as the physiological cup (Fig. 12-41). The ratio of the cup diameter to that of the entire disc is 1:4 to 1:3. The border of the disc may range from a sharp, round demarcation from the surrounding retina to a more blended border, but should be on the same plane as the retina. In general, four main vascular branches emanate from the disc, each branch consisting of an arteriole and a venule. The venules are approximately four times the size of the accompanying arterioles and are darker in color. Light often produces a glistening "light reflex" from the arteriolar vessel. Normal arterial-to-venous width is a ratio of 2:3 or 4:5.**

A The red reflex is absent.

P The presence of cataracts can prevent the red reflex from being observed due to the opacity of the lens.

A The red reflex is absent and the pupil appears white.

P Leukocoria, or white reflex, is found in retinoblastoma (Fig. 12-42), congenital cataracts, and retinal detachment. This is often referred to as the cat's eye reflex.

A The optic disc is pale.

P Pallor is due to optic atrophy caused by increased intracranial pressure or from congenital syphilis, an intracranial space-occupying lesion (e.g., meningioma), or end-stage glaucoma.

Table 12-3 Retinal Color Variations

Findings	Characteristics
Fair-skinned client	• Retina appears a lighter red-orange color • Tessellated appearance of the fundi (pigment does not obscure the choroid vessels)
Dark-skinned client	• Fundi appear darker in color; grayish-purple to brownish (from increased pigment in the choroid and retina) • No tessellated appearance • Choroidal vessels usually obscured
Older adult client	• Vessels are straighter and narrower • Choroidal vessels are easily visualized • Retinal pigment epithelium atrophies and causes the retinal color to become paler

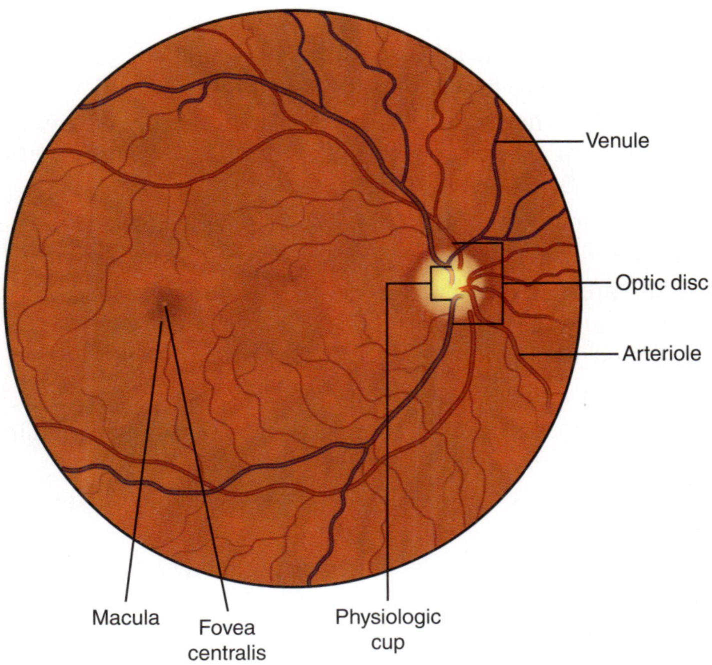

Figure 12-41 Optic disc of the right eye.

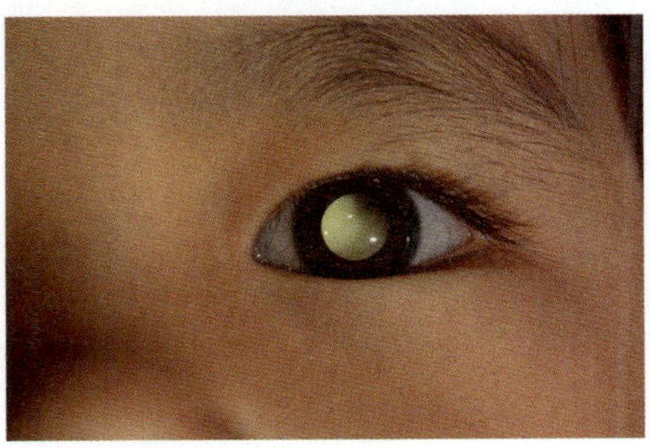

Figure 12-42 Leukocoria.

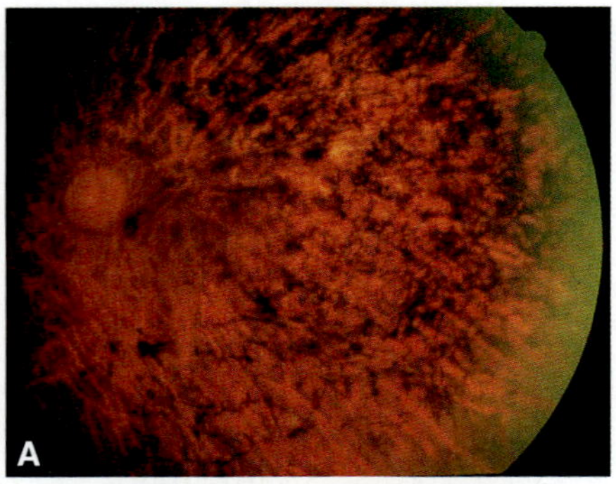

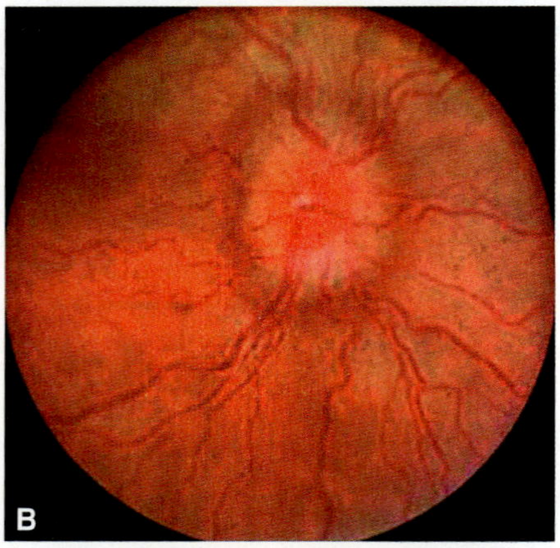

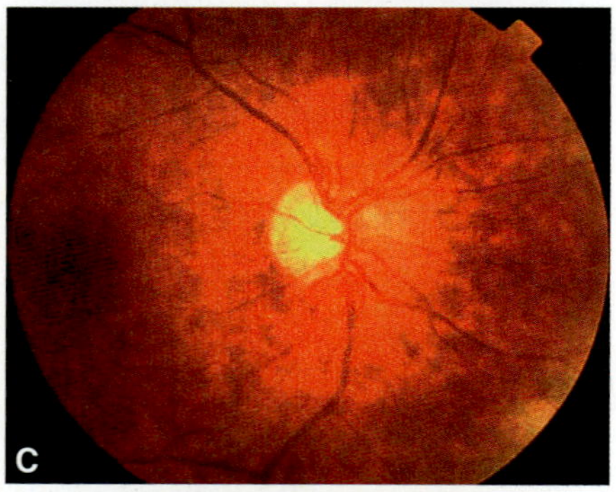

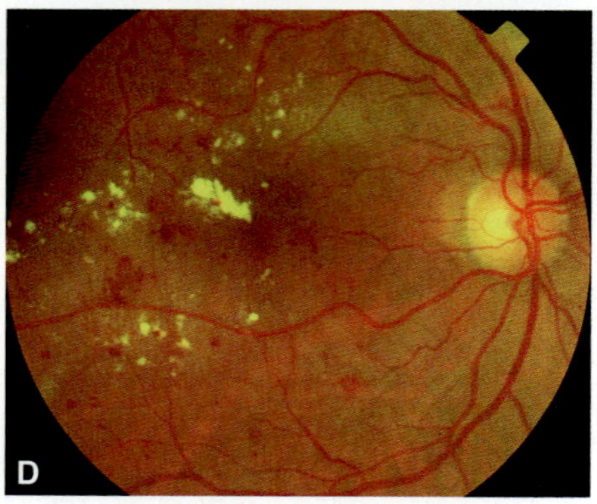

Figure 12-43 Retinal abnormalities. **A.** Retinitis pigmentosa. **B.** Papilledema. **C.** Glaucomatous cupping. **D.** Microaneurysms with exudate and dot hemorrhages.

A Optic disc atrophy is abnormal.

P Optic disc atrophy occurs in retinitis pigmentosa (Fig. 12-43A). Arteriole narrowing and "bone spicule" are also noted on the fundus. There is a loss of central and/or peripheral vision, night blindness, and glare sensitivity in this familial condition.

A The physiological cup exceeds the 1:3 ratio. The disc appears elevated above the plane of the surrounding retina.

P Disc edema and loss of vision are caused by papillitis resulting from optic neuritis. The disc is hyperemic, the margins are blurred, and the disc surface is elevated.

P Disc edema and an elevated disc without loss of vision are found in papilledema (Fig. 12-43B), which is caused by increased intracranial pressure obstructing return blood flow from the eye. This is also called a choked disc.

P Glaucomatous cupping (Fig. 12-43C) occurs due to increased intraocular pressure. The physiological cup is enlarged and may extend to the edge of the optic disc. Blood vessels are displaced nasally.

A The normal red stripe of retinal arteries appears instead as a copper-colored stripe.

P This copper-wire appearance of retinal arteries is characteristic of hypertensive changes.

A At the crossing of retinal arteries over veins, the vein is not seen on either side of the overlying artery.

P Arteriovenous (A-V) nicking, is a sign of retinal arteriolar sclerosis that occurs as the arterial walls become thickened and obscure portions of the veins that lie underneath. This can also occur in hypertension.

A Superficial retinal hemorrhages are flame-shaped hemorrhages found in the fundi, or they may appear as red hemorrhages with white centers called Roth spots. These hemorrhages form a pattern related to the nerve fibers that radiate from the optic disc.

P Superficial retinal hemorrhages may be due to severe hypertension, occlusion of the central retinal vein, and papilledema. Roth spots are sometimes associated with infective endocarditis.

A Deep retinal hemorrhages, or dot hemorrhages, appear as small red dots or irregular spots in the deep layer of the retina (Fig. 12-43D).

P Deep retinal hemorrhages can be associated with diabetes mellitus.

A Diffuse preretinal hemorrhages occur in the small space between the vitreous and the retina.

P Preretinal hemorrhages may occur in conjunction with a sudden increase in intracranial pressure.

A Microaneurysms are tiny, round, red dots that can be seen in peripheral and macular areas of the retina (Fig. 12-43E).

P Microaneurysms are small retinal vessels that dilate in diabetic retinopathy.

A Neovascularization is the formation of new vessels that are very narrow and disorderly in appearance. The new vessels may extend into the vitreous. These vessels may bleed, resulting in a loss of vision.

P Neovascularization occurs in proliferative diabetic retinopathy.

A Fluffy white or gray, slightly irregular areas that appear on the retina and are ovoid in shape are abnormal (Fig. 12-43F).

P Cotton wool spots represent microscopic infarcts of the nerve fiber layer and are due to diabetic or hypertensive retinopathy.

A Drusen are small white dots in the fundus that are arranged in an irregular pattern (Fig. 12-44). They may also occur on the optic disc and may become shiny with calcification.

P Drusen are findings of the normal aging process. They may cause loss of vision if they occur in the macular region.

A Hard exudates are yellow with distinct borders and are small unless they coalesce (Fig. 12-45). They are arranged in round, linear, or star-shaped patterns.

P Hard exudates are associated with diabetes mellitus or hypertension.

A A cleft defect of the choroid and retina is abnormal. The size ranges from medium to large.

P **Coloboma** is a congenital, pathological, or surgically induced abnormality.

A The red-orange retinal reflex is absent in the area of a retinal detachment. The area appears pearly gray and is elevated and wrinkled.

P A detached retina may be associated with severe myopia, cataract surgery, or diabetic retinopathy, or it may be caused by trauma.

A Fibrous white bands that obscure the retinal vessels are abnormal. Neovascularization may also be present.

P Fibrous white bands that obscure the retinal vessels occur in proliferative diabetic retinopathy.

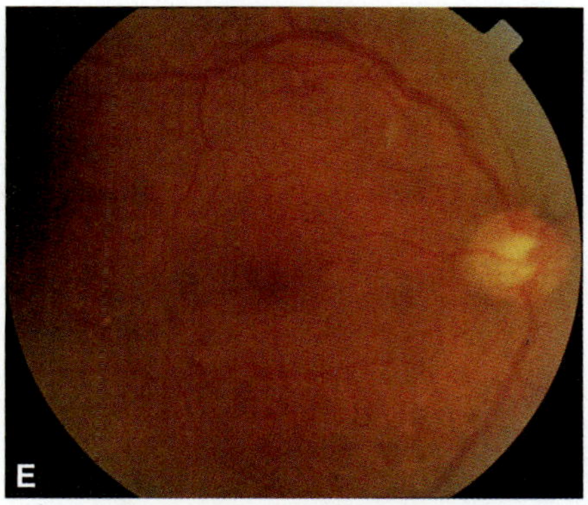

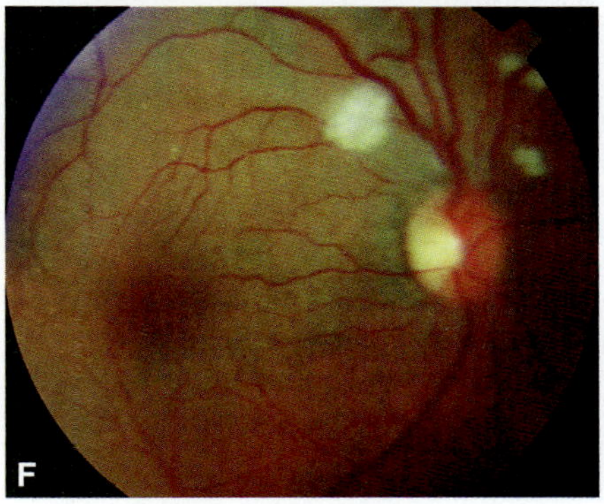

Figure 12-43—cont'd E. Microaneurysms in diabetic retinopathy. **F.** Cotton wool spots.

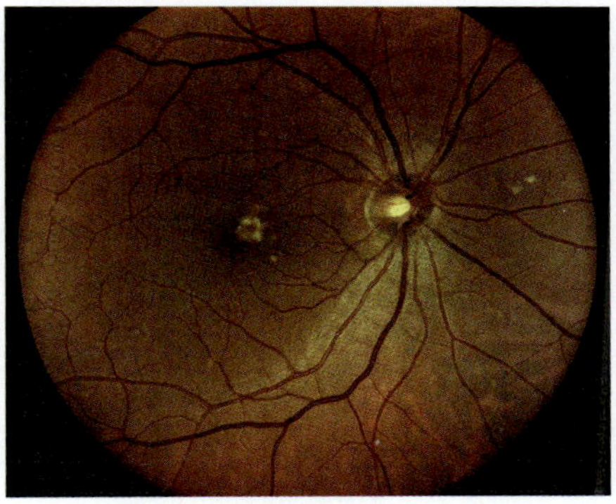

Figure 12-44 Drusen.

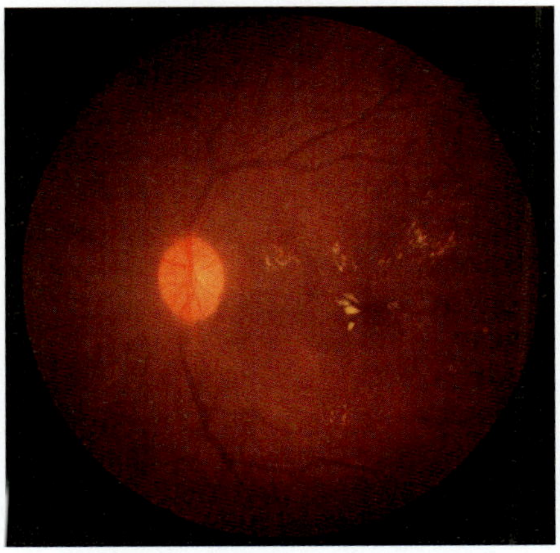

Figure 12-45 Hard exudates.

Risk Factors

Macular Degeneration

- Increasing age
- Sex: Female
- Smoking
- Family history
- High dietary intake of vegetable fat
- Genetic variants
- Light-colored iris
- History of macular degeneration in the other eye
- Low dietary intake of antioxidants and zinc
- Obesity
- Fair skin
- Ultraviolet light exposure
- Alcohol use
- Cardiovascular disease

Macula

When the retinal structures and the optic disc have been examined:

E 1. Move the ophthalmoscope approximately two disc diameters temporally to view the macula, or ask the client to look at the

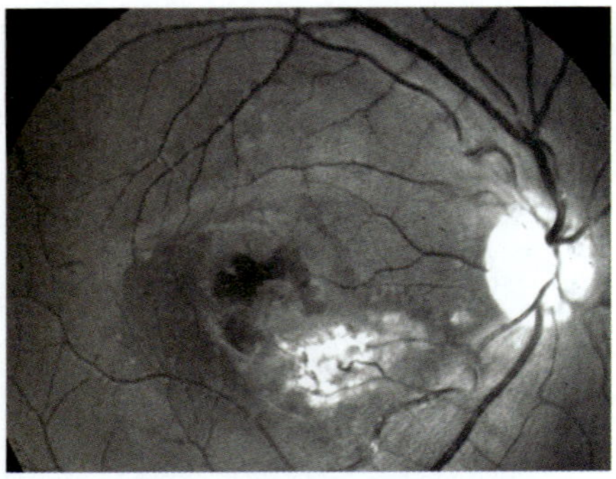

Figure 12-46 Macular edema with bleeding.

light. The red-free filter lens of the ophthalmoscope may also help examine the macula. Because the macula is not clearly demarcated, and because it is very light-sensitive, you may have difficulty examining it.

2. Note the macula's color, shape, and the presence of any lesions.
3. Note the foveal light reflex. This is a small white light in the center of the macula (fovea centralis) that is reflected from the ophthalmoscope's light. The client tends to turn away when the light strikes the fovea centralis, making it difficult to examine details of the macular area.
4. Repeat with the other eye.

N **The macula is a darker, avascular area with a pinpoint reflective center known as the fovea centralis. The fovea centralis is present.**

A The retina is pale with the macular region appearing as a cherry red spot.

P A central retinal artery occlusion is an indication of Tay-Sachs disease.

A An enlarged macula is abnormal (Fig. 12-46).

P Macular edema is caused by the leakage of fluid from retinal blood vessels. This can occur in diabetes mellitus, hypertension, age-related macular degeneration, and retinal blood vessel obstruction.

A Sharply defined, small red spots are found in and around the macula.

P These microaneurysms are pathognomonic of diabetes mellitus.

A Macular borders are blurred, with a few spots of pigment near the macula; a hole may appear to be present in the center of the region, or a hemorrhage may have occurred.

P This finding is characteristic of age-related macular degeneration. Hemorrhages, patches of retinal atrophy, and pigmented areas may also be associated with this condition.

ADVANCED TECHNIQUE

Assessing for Macular Degeneration

The Amsler Grid (Fig. 12-47) is used to assess the central 10 degrees of the visual field for each eye and for macular degeneration.

E
1. If the client uses reading glasses, they should be worn. Hold the Amsler Grid at the usual distance used for reading, about 14 inches from the face.
2. Have the client cover one eye and focus on the dark dot in the middle of the grid.
3. Ask the client if any of the lines appear wavy, blurred, or distorted.
4. Ask the client if there are any missing or dark areas on the grid.
5. Repeat the procedure with the other eye.

N **Grid lines are all seen as straight and without distortion. All areas of the grid should be seen.**

A The straight lines in the grid pattern appear wavy (metamorphopsia) or are absent (scotomata) to the client.

P Abnormal findings can be seen in macular degeneration.

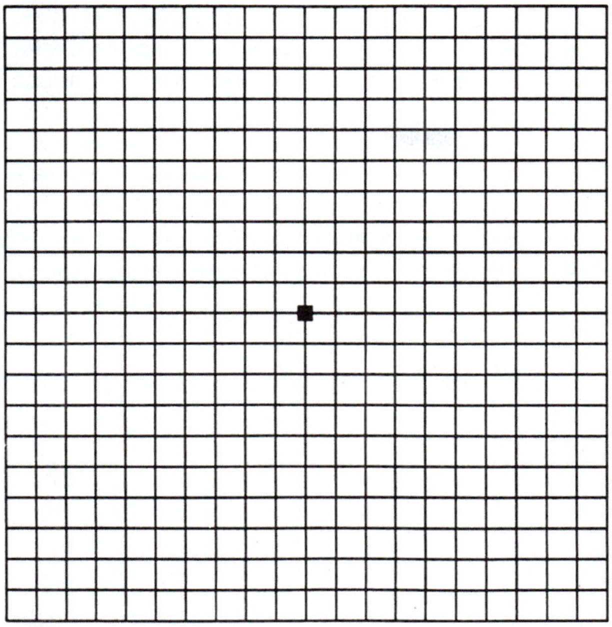

Figure 12-47 Amsler grid.

U.S. Preventive Services Task Force (USPSTF)

There are no USPSTF Grade A or B Recommendations for the eyes.

CASE STUDY

The Client With a Stye, Conjunctivitis, and Diabetic Retinopathy

This case study illustrates the application and objective documentation of the eye examination.

Carter is a 48-year-old who identifies as nonbinary. Carter has a history of diabetes, hypertension, and hyperlipidemia. Carter ran out of all prescription medications a few months ago and just never got around to making an appointment for refills. Client is not monitoring blood pressure or blood sugar at home. Has had no blood work in over 1 year.

Carter has not had a comprehensive eye examination in 4 years. Carter presents today with eye problems.

HEALTH HISTORY

CLIENT PROFILE

48-year-old nonbinary

CHIEF COMPLAINT

"My left eye is swollen and has been getting worse over the past 2 days and I have a bump on the other eye."

HISTORY OF PRESENT ILLNESS

Client with left eye swelling and pain for 2 days. Noticed a small red bump on the right lower eyelid 2 days ago and it is getting bigger. Has increased redness, swelling, and discomfort when blinking. Client has been unable to wear contacts due to the pain and has been wearing glasses. No changes to vision other than not being able to open the left eye due to the swelling. Moderate yellow crusting "glued-closed" noted in the morning. Tried warm compresses at night without relief. Client has 17-year history of type 2 diabetes and is not monitoring glucose levels at home. Denies previous eye problems and eye surgery/procedures. Last optometrist visit was over 4 years ago; gets contacts and glasses online. Denies: history of head or eye trauma, visual changes, diplopia, changes in peripheral vision, or flashes of light. Admits occasional "floaters." Denies: fever, headaches, rhinorrhea, vertigo, nausea, vomiting, or neurological changes.

PAST HEALTH HISTORY

Medical History

Type 2 diabetes diagnosed at age 31. Hypertension diagnosed at age 35. Hyperlipidemia diagnosed at age 35. Dysmenorrhea with menorrhagia at age 39.

Surgical History

Tonsillectomy, age 5.

Total hysterectomy with bilateral salpingo-oophorectomy, age 41.

Allergies

Cephalexin: body-wide rash and itching

Medications

Metformin 500 mg twice daily

Dapagliflozin 5 mg daily

Enalapril 20 mg daily

Hydrochlorothiazide 25 mg daily

Rosuvastatin 10 mg daily

Communicable Diseases Pertussis 5 years ago treated with azithromycin; gonorrhea in college treated at student health center.

Injuries and Accidents Burned 1-inch area on left forearm while cooking last month, healed without complications.

Differing Ability None identified

Blood Transfusions Two RBC transfusions at age 41 with GYN surgery.

Childhood Illnesses Chickenpox age 4

Immunizations Tdap 5 years ago, flu vaccine annually, two doses Moderna COVID-19 vaccine, no boosters; has not received hepatitis B vaccine series or HPV vaccines.

FAMILY HEALTH HISTORY

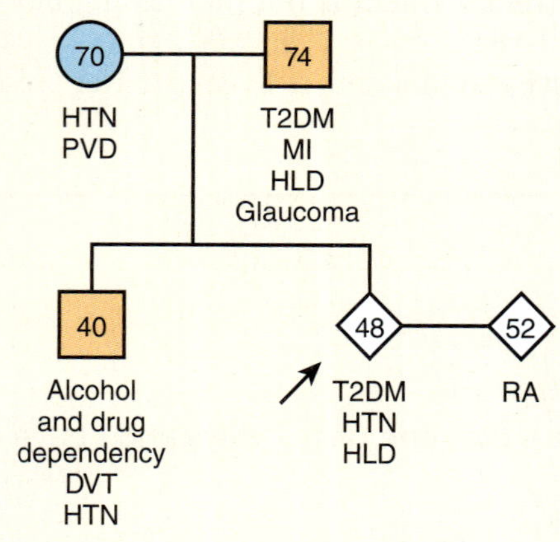

Denies family history of color blindness, cataracts, macular degeneration, ocular melanoma, retinitis pigmentosa, retinoblastoma

Legend

Living female

Living male

Nonbinary

Points to client

Couple in a relationship*

*The line connecting clients can denote a union, whether that be a marriage or other type of relationship

DVT	Deep vein thrombosis
HLD	Hyperlipidemia
HTN	Hypertension
MI	Myocardial infarction
PVD	Peripheral vascular disease
RA	Rheumatoid arthritis
T2DM	Type 2 diabetes mellitus

SOCIAL HISTORY

Alcohol Use 3 to 4 glasses of wine per week on the weekend

Tobacco Use ½ PPD while in college and graduate school, quit 10 years ago

Recreational Drug Use Smoked marijuana in college.

Domestic and Intimate Partner Violence Denies

Sexual Practice Monogamous with partner

Travel History Travels to see extended family in Ashdod, Israel yearly; has not been yet this year.

Work Environment Works as a public relations director for a large nonprofit organization; mostly works from home with occasional domestic business travel.

Home Environment Lives in a single-family home with partner with 3 bedrooms, 3 baths, built 5 years ago. Gas heat, air-conditioned

Hobbies and Leisure Activities Enjoys strategy board games and crafting/painting. Has a pet cockatoo.

Stress Worries about aging parents' health—mother has hypertension and doesn't believe in taking medication and father recently had a myocardial infarction and gained weight, which has made it more difficult to manage his blood sugar. Parents live over 6 hours away and they do not have family or friends nearby to support them. Reports having one brother who is in and out of rehab facilities for alcohol and drug dependency. Brother called to ask for money 6 months ago and client and parents haven't heard from him since.

Education Master's degree in marketing

Economic Status Reports steady income and does not worry about finances

Military Service Denies

Religion Active leader in Reform Judaism

Ethnic Background Mother and her family are from Israel. Mother emigrated to the U.S. at age 15. Father was born in New York City and grew up in an Italian neighborhood.

Roles and Relationships Reports being in a healthy, mutually monogamous relationship of 5 years.

Characteristic Patterns of Daily Living Works 60 to 70 hours a week sitting at a computer; Attends religious functions twice weekly and has regular leadership meetings every Monday and Thursday nights.

HEALTH MAINTENANCE ACTIVITIES

Sleep About 5 to 6 hours nightly and sleeps well until the alarm goes off; sleeps about 10 hours on weekends.

Diet Admits to only liking pasta, chicken nuggets, and pizza. Doesn't like many fruits or vegetables and doesn't like to cook. Partner doesn't like to cook either, so they get take-out food often.

Exercise Walking around the house to do chores.

Stress Management Prays, attends religious services twice weekly; Unwinds in crafting room or watching crime documentaries on TV with a glass of wine; has a small group of confidants they talk to once a week.

Use of Safety Devices Wears seat belt; wears sunblock when going outside.

Health Checkups Has not been to provider in past year due to time constraints; would like to make health a priority this year. Last comprehensive eye examination was 4 years ago.

PHYSICAL EXAMINATION

Visual Acuity

Distance vision:
Without correction (glasses):
- Bilaterally: 20/100
- Right eye: 20/100
- Left eye: 20/100

With correction (glasses):
- Bilaterally: 20/30
- Right eye: 20/25
- Left eye: 20/40

Near vision: reads newspaper with several errors without glasses
Color vision: intact

Visual Fields Intact bilaterally

External Eye and Lacrimal Apparatus

Eyes, eyelids, eyebrows, and eyelashes: no prostheses; left upper lid mildly edematous and erythematous without lesions, scaling, or ptosis, right lower lid with 3-mm pink lesion without odor or discharge; eyebrows without lesions; eyelashes evenly distributed with scant yellow discharge on left

Lacrimal apparatus: no enlargement, swelling, redness, or exudates; no excessive tearing

Extraocular Muscle Function

Corneal light reflex: symmetric without strabismus
Cover/uncover test: no movement of either eye
Cardinal fields of gaze: extraocular movements smooth without nystagmus

Anterior Segment Structures

Conjunctiva: transparent, without swelling, injection, exudates, or lesions
Sclera: white without exudates or lesions on right, left with mild injection
Cornea: without opacities
Anterior chamber: iris illuminates
Iris: brown, uniform color without vascularity
Pupils: black, equal, round with diameter 3 mm, react briskly to direct and consensual light and accommodation
Lens: transparent

Posterior Segment Structures

Retinal structures: Numerous preretinal dot and flame hemorrhages, deep retinal hemorrhages, and cotton wool spots; venous dilation noted with neovascularization
Macula: enlarged with sharply defined, small red spots around macula; positive foveal light reflex

CLINICAL JUDGMENT IN ACTION

1. What cues indicate that the client is having an eye disorder?
2. What interventions have the highest priority?
3. What assessment findings indicate clinical improvement or decline in this client?

Review Questions

1. 55-year-old Nahuel complains of recent changes to vision while reading. Nahuel used to have no problem seeing up close but recently there is a need to hold the book farther away to be able to see the words clearly. This ocular condition is best described as which of the following?
   a. Myopia
   b. Presbyopia
   c. Strabismus
   d. Hyperopia
2. The nurse tests the extraocular muscle movements by assessing the cardinal fields of gaze. What cranial nerves (CN) are being tested? Select all that apply.
   a. CN II
   b. CN III
   c. CN IV
   d. CN V
   e. CN VI
   f. CNVII
3. For which ocular condition is the nurse assessing when conducting the corneal light reflex?
   a. Strabismus
   b. Presbyopia
   c. Hyperopia
   d. Myopia
4. The nurse determines that the client has 20/40 vision bilaterally after performing a visual acuity screening using the Snellen chart. The client asks what the result means. The nurse's best response is:
   a. You don't need glasses, so we will check again next year for any changes.
   b. You can read at 40 feet what a person with perfect vision can read at 20 feet.
   c. You can read at 20 feet what a person with 20/20 vision can read at 40 feet.
   d. Your eyes are hyperopic.
5. The client reports being born with an underdeveloped levator muscle. What finding does the nurse expect to find upon assessment of the eyes?
   a. Ptosis of the left eye
   b. Amblyopia of the right eye
   c. Ectropion of the right eye
   d. Nystagmus of the left eye
6. To determine whether the conjunctiva is inflamed, the nurse will:
   a. Have the client cover one eye while reading the Snellen chart with the other eye.
   b. Shine the penlight into the center of the cornea.
   c. Inspect the eyebrows and eyelashes for hair distribution.
   d. Gently pull down on the lower lids.
7. The nurse notes that the client has anisocoria. The nurse recognizes that anisocoria can be caused by which of the following? Select all that apply.
   a. Cranial Nerve III deficit
   b. Cataracts
   c. Parasympathetic medications
   d. Trauma
   e. Corneal abrasions
   f. Iritis
8. The nurse inspects for a red reflex with the ophthalmoscope. The red reflex occurs due to which of the following?
   a. Light reflecting from the retina
   b. The pupil widening
   c. Inflammation of the iris
   d. Optic disc swelling
9. Risk factors for macular degeneration include which of the following? Select all that apply.
   a. Low-fat diet
   b. Older age
   c. Alcohol abuse
   d. Family history
   e. Ultraviolet light exposure
   f. High intake of zinc
10. The nurse is providing client education on glaucoma for a 31-year-old client. Which of the following statements would the nurse include?
    a. Managing high blood pressure can reduce the chance of developing glaucoma.
    b. A 31-year-old with diabetes and a history of prolonged steroid use has a decreased risk of developing glaucoma.
    c. Family history of glaucoma does not increase the risk for a 31-year-old client until middle age.
    d. There isn't much one can do to prevent glaucoma.

Ears, Nose, Mouth, and Throat

CHAPTER

13

Learning Outcomes

1. Identify the anatomy and physiology of the ears, nose, mouth, and throat.
2. Conduct a complete health history on a client with an ear, nose, mouth, or throat condition.
3. Perform a physical examination on a healthy adult and an adult with ear, nose, mouth, or throat pathology.
4. Differentiate between normal clinical findings from a client's physical examination and the pathophysiology of abnormal clinical findings.
5. Identify risk factors for otitis media.
6. Identify risk factors for hearing loss.
7. Identify risk factors for mouth and throat cancer.
8. Document a complete health history and physical examination of a client with an ears, nose, mouth, or throat pathology.

Physical examination of the ears, nose, sinuses, mouth, and throat provides a wealth of information about the integrity of many body systems and serves as the foundation for assessment of the neurological, respiratory, endocrine, gastrointestinal, musculoskeletal, and cardiovascular systems.

Anatomy and Physiology

Ear

The ear has three sections: the external, the middle, and the inner ear.

External Ear

The external ear, which is also called the **auricle** or **pinna**, extends through the auditory canal to the tympanic membrane. The auricle receives sound waves and funnels them through the auditory canal to produce vibrations on the tympanic membrane. The auricle is composed of cartilage (Fig. 13-1).

The external auditory canal is an S-shaped tube approximately 2.5 cm in length, with the outer third made up of cartilage and the remainder of bone covered by a thin layer of skin (Fig. 13-2). The canal is lined with tiny hairs and modified sweat glands that secrete a thick, waxlike substance called **cerumen**, which can vary in consistency from dry and flaky to wet and waxy. Cerumen ranges from a pale, honey color in light-skinned individuals to dark brown or black in dark-skinned people.

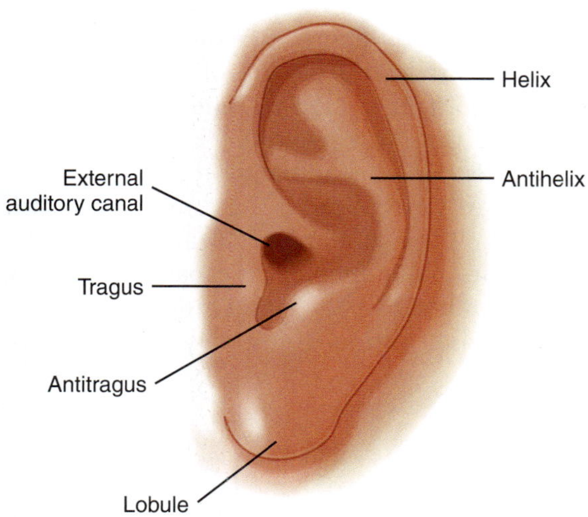

Figure 13-1 External ear.

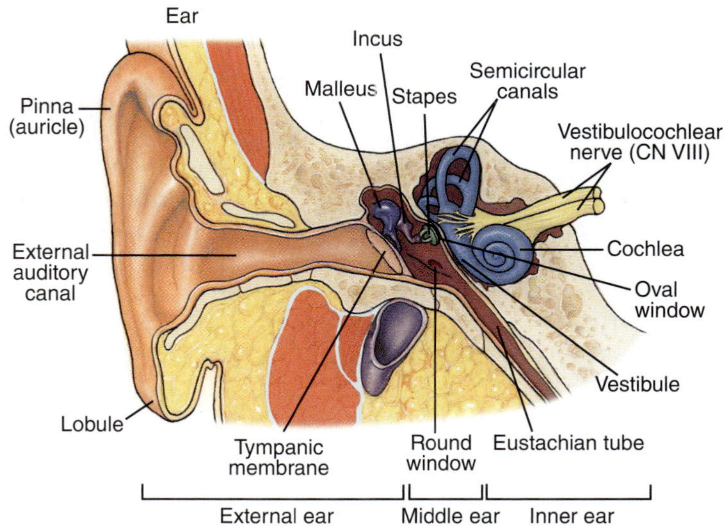

Figure 13-2 Cross section of the ear. CN = cranial nerve.

Middle Ear

The middle ear is composed of the tympanic membrane, the ossicles, and the tympanic cavity. The cavity is an air-filled compartment that separates the external ear from the internal ear. The tympanic membrane, which is circular or oval and is about an inch in diameter, sits in an oblique position in the external canal so that it leans slightly forward. The rim of the tympanic membrane is called the annulus, the superior portion is the pars flaccida, and the tighter, largest area of the drum is the pars tensa (Fig. 13-3).

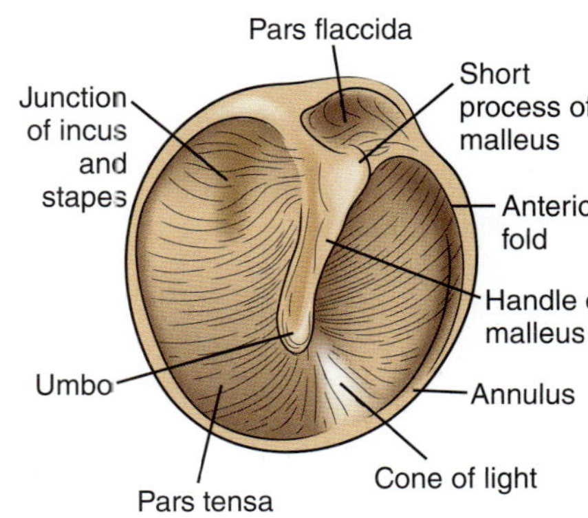

Figure 13-3 Landmarks of the right tympanic membrane.

The **ossicles** are three tiny bones—the malleus (hammer), the incus (anvil), and the stapes (stirrup)—that play a crucial role in the transmission of sound. The long handle, or manubrium, of the malleus extends downward from the short process and meets the tympanic membrane at the umbo. The stapes is held against the wall of the tympanic membrane at the oval window by tiny ligaments. The head of the malleus articulates with the incus, which in turn articulates with the stapes; they work as a unit when the tympanic membrane begins to vibrate. Vibrations set up in the tympanic membrane by sound waves reaching it through the external auditory canal are transmitted to the inner ear by the rapid movement of the ossicles.

The tensor tympani and the stapedius are two tiny muscles involved in the movement of the ossicles. The tensor tympani maintains the tension of the tympanic membrane and pulls the malleus inward when it contracts. The stapedius works in opposition by pulling the stapes outward. This coordinated movement is an important mechanism in reducing the intensity of loud sounds that might otherwise result in serious damage to hearing receptors in the inner ear.

The middle ear is connected to the nasopharynx by the auditory or **eustachian tube**, which serves as a channel through which air pressure within the cavity can be equalized with the air pressure outside to maintain normal hearing. Equalization of pressure is aided by yawning or swallowing, which causes the opening of valvelike flaps that cover the openings of the eustachian tubes.

Inner Ear

The inner ear is a complex, closed, fluid-filled system of interconnecting tubes called the **labyrinth**, which is essential for hearing and equilibrium. The labyrinth has bony and membranous portions. The bony labyrinth is composed of the cochlea, the semicircular canals, and the vestibule. The

vestibule is located between the cochlea and the **semicircular canals** and is important in both hearing and balance. The three semicircular canals located at right angles to each other provide balance and equilibrium for the body. The **cochlea** is a snail-shaped structure made up of three compartments. The first two compartments contain perilymph, and the third contains endolymph. As sound waves travel through the ear, they cause the perilymph and the endolymph to vibrate, stimulating the thousands of hearing-receptor cells of the organ of Corti. Nearby nerve fibers transmit impulses along the cochlear branch of the vestibulocochlear nerve to the brain, allowing the individual to hear. The human ear is capable of hearing within a frequency range of 20 to 20,000 Hz and a decibel range of 0 to 140. Figure 13-4 illustrates the decibel levels of various commonly heard sounds.

Nose

The nose consists of the external or outer nose and the nasal fossae, or internal nose (Fig. 13-5). The outer nose is made up of bone and cartilage and is divided internally into two nasal fossae by the nasal septum, and externally by the columella. Anterior openings into the nasal fossae are nostrils, or nares. Each fossa has a lateral extended "wing" portion, called the ala nasi, on the outside and a vestibule just inside the nostril. Superior, middle, and inferior meatuses or grooves are located on the lateral walls of the nostrils just below the corresponding **conchae**, or **turbinates**. The nasal turbinates are covered by mucous membranes and greatly increase the surface area of the mucous membranes in the nose because of their shape. Kiesselbach's plexus is a vascular area on the nasal septum and a common site of nosebleeds.

Air enters the anterior nares, passes through the vestibule, and enters the fossa. The vestibule contains nasal hairs and sebaceous glands. The fossae have both olfactory and respiratory functions. To protect the lungs from noxious agents, these structures of the nose clean, filter, humidify, and control the temperature of inspired air. The mucous covering in the nose and sinuses traps fine dust particles, and lysosomes kill most of the bacteria. The

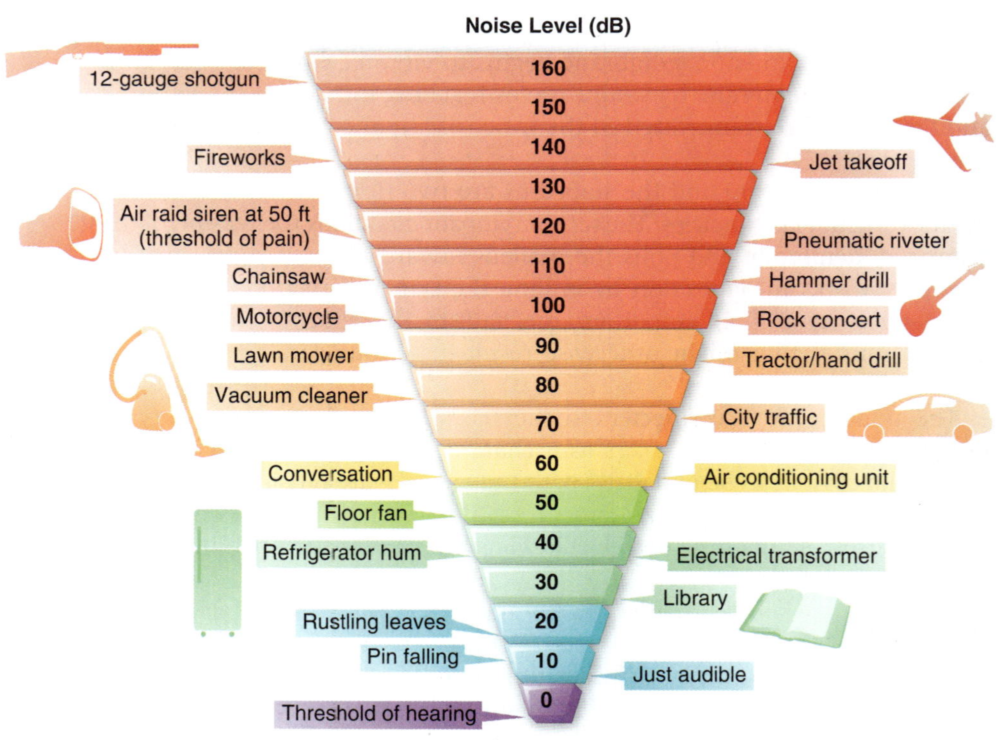

Figure 13-4 Decibel scale of frequently heard sounds.

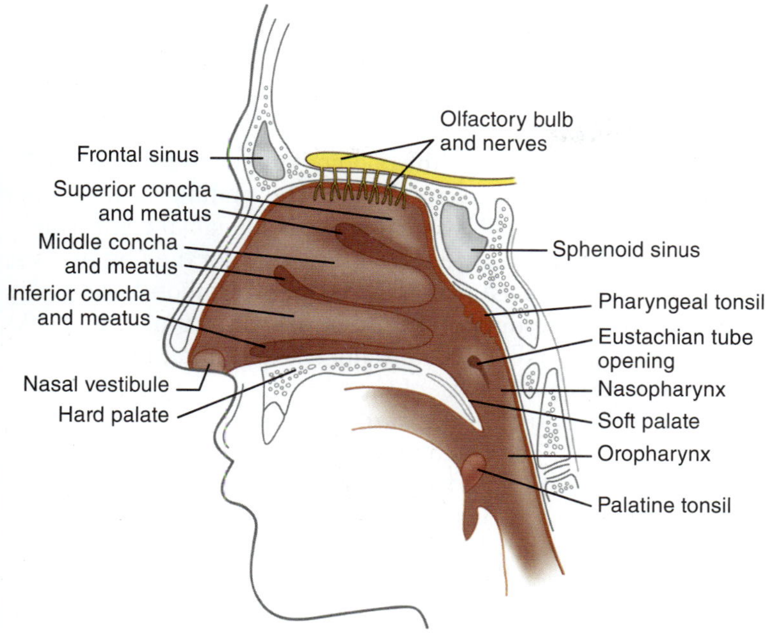

Figure 13-5 Lateral cross section of the nose.

tiny hairs of the nose (cilia) transport the mucus and the particles to the pharynx to be swallowed.

The nasal mucosa can add large amounts of water to inspired air through evaporation from its surface. The rich vascular supply to the turbinates radiates heat to the incoming air as it passes through the nasal cavity.

Olfactory receptor cells are located in the upper parts of the nasal cavity, the superior nasal conchae, and on parts of the nasal septum. These cells are covered by hairlike cilia that project into the cavity. The chemical component of odors binds with the receptors, causing nerve impulses to be transmitted to the olfactory cortex, located in the base of the frontal lobe.

Sinuses

Air-filled cavities lined with mucous membranes are present in some of the cranial bones and are referred to as **paranasal sinuses** (Fig. 13-6). These air-filled sinuses lighten the weight of the skull and add resonance to the quality of the voice. The frontal, maxillary, ethmoid, and sphenoid paranasal

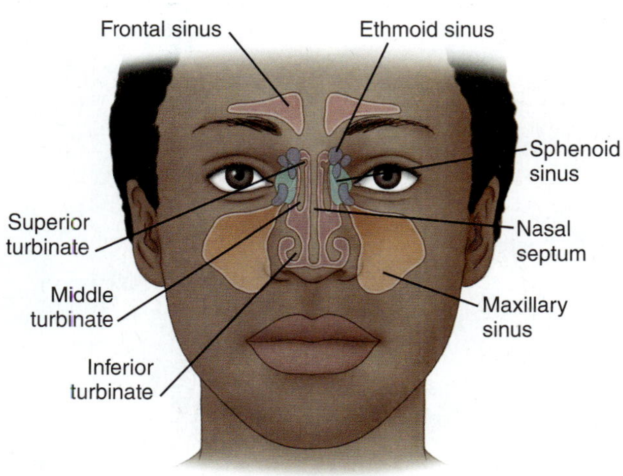

Figure 13-6 Location of the sinuses (the sphenoid sinuses are directly behind the ethmoid sinuses).

sinuses open into the nose. Only the frontal and maxillary sinuses can be assessed in the physical examination.

Mouth and Throat

The lips are sensory structures found at the opening of the mouth (Fig. 13-7). The labial tubercle is the small projected area in the midline of the upper lip. The area where the upper and lower lips meet is the labial commissure. The vermilion zone is the reddish or reddish-brown area of the lips, and the area where the lips meet the facial skin is called the vermilion border. The median groove superior to the upper lip is called the philtrum. The cheeks form the lateral walls of the mouth and are lined with buccal mucosa. The posterior pharyngeal wall is at the back of the mouth.

The roof of the mouth consists of the hard palate anteriorly and the soft palate posteriorly (Fig. 13-8). The **linear raphe** is a linear ridge in the middle of the hard palate that is formed by two palatine bones and part of the superior maxillary bone. The mucous membrane on either side of the linear raphe is thick, pale, and corrugated, while the posterior mucous membrane is thin, a deeper pink, and smooth.

Situated on the floor of the mouth, the tongue is a muscular organ connected to the hyoid bone posteriorly and to the floor of the mouth anteriorly by the **frenulum**. The tongue assists with mastication, swallowing, speech, and mechanical cleansing of the teeth.

The mucous membrane covering the upper surface of the tongue has numerous projections called **papillae**, which assist in handling food and contain taste buds. Five qualities of taste are found in taste buds distributed over the surface of the tongue: Bitter is located at the base, sour along the sides, and salty and sweet near the tip. Umami is now recognized as the fifth quality of taste. Taste buds for umami are located throughout the tongue.

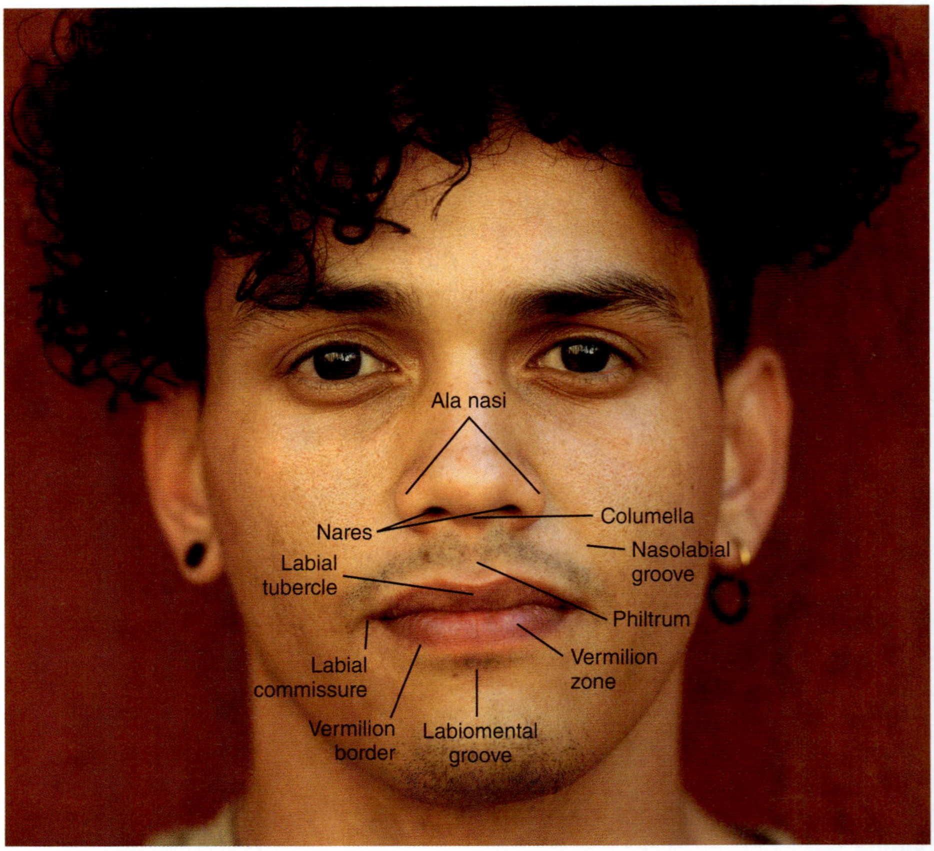

Figure 13-7 Landmarks of the area around the mouth.

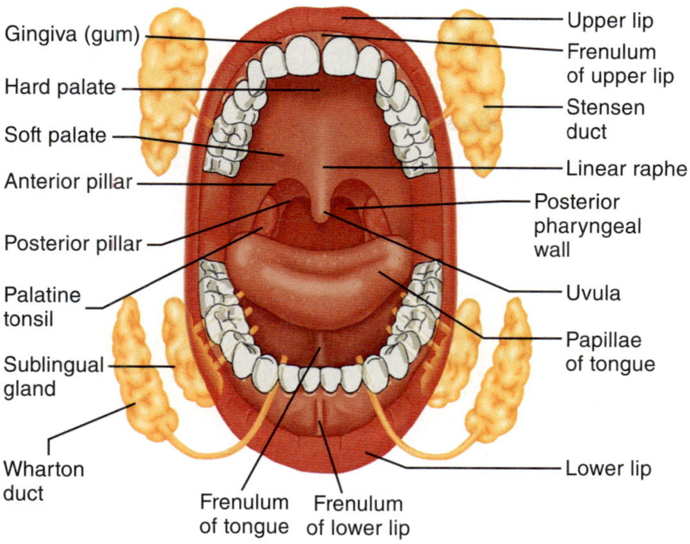

Figure 13-8 Structures of the mouth.

Umami is a Japanese word that describes a meaty, delicious, pleasant, and savory taste. The umami taste is derived from ribonucleotides and glutamate in food. The **sulcus terminalis** is the midline depression that separates the anterior two-thirds of the tongue from the posterior one-third.

Two of the three pairs of salivary glands open into the mouth on the ventral surface of the tongue. Submaxillary glands secrete fluid through **Wharton's ducts**, located on both sides of the frenulum. Sublingual glands open into the floor of the mouth posteriorly to Wharton's ducts. The larger parotid glands are located in the cheeks and secrete their amylase-rich fluid through **Stensen's ducts**, located just opposite the upper second molars.

These salivary glands produce 1,000 to 1,500 mL of saliva per day to assist with the digestion of food and the maintenance of oral hygiene. Saliva prevents dental caries and bacterial damage to healthy oral tissue by washing away bacteria and destroying them with antibodies and proteolytic enzymes.

Gums, or gingivae, appear pink or coral in light-skinned individuals and brown with a darker melanotic line along the edges in dark-skinned individuals. Gums hold the teeth in place.

Adults have 32 permanent teeth: four incisors, two canines, four premolars, and six molars in each half of the mouth (Fig. 13-9). The three parts of the tooth are the top, or the crown; the root, which is embedded in the gum; and the neck, which connects the root and the crown. The teeth are well designed for chewing. Incisors provide strong cutting action, and molars provide strong grinding action.

The soft palate is suspended from the posterior border of the hard palate and extends downward as folds called palatine arches or pillars, forming an incomplete septum between the mouth and the nasopharynx. The **uvula** is a fingerlike projection of tissue that hangs down from the center of the soft palate. Two palatine tonsils containing primarily lymphoid tissue are connected to the palatine arches; they vary greatly in size from one individual to another. Lymphoid tissue in the tonsils plays a role in the control of infection.

NURSING TIP

Tooth Numbering System

When examining the client's teeth, it is best to document tooth anomalies using the tooth numbering system. Figure 13-10 illustrates this system in the adult mouth. For example, the left mandibular central incisor is tooth number 24.

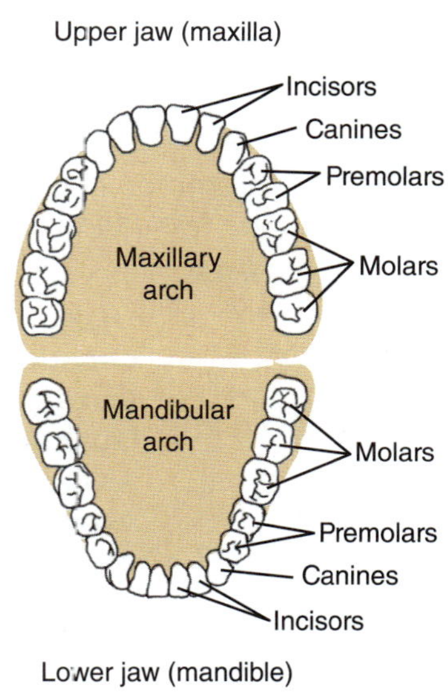

Figure 13-9 Permanent teeth.

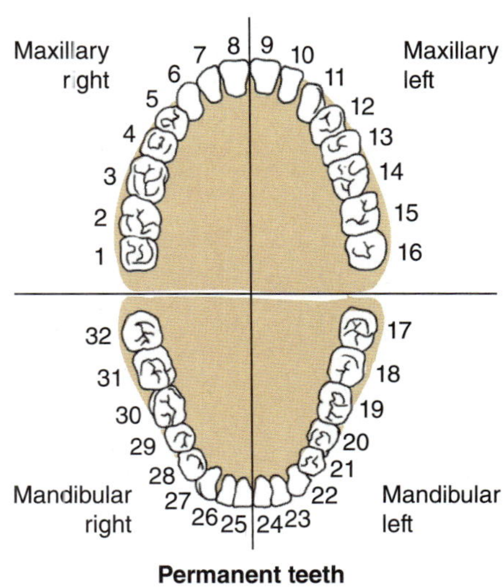

Figure 13-10 Tooth numbering system.

HEALTH HISTORY

CLIENT PROFILE

The ears, nose, mouth, and throat health history provides insight into the link between a client's life/lifestyle and ears, nose, mouth, and throat information and pathology.

Diseases that are age- and sex-specific for the ears, nose, mouth, and throat are listed.

Age

Ears Hearing loss related to presbycusis, sensorineural degeneration, or otosclerosis (older adult)

Excessive or impacted cerumen (older adult)

Nose Decrease in ability to smell (older adult)

Mouth and Throat Mouth and throat cancer >55

Orthodonture (middle age)

Tooth loss and gum disease (older adult)

Thrush related to immunosuppression (older adult)

Decrease in ability to taste (older adult)

Sex

Ears Female: Calcifications of the ossicles

Nose Male: Rhinophyma, deviated septum related to trauma, polyps

Mouth and Throat Male: Mouth/throat cancer, cancer of the larynx, leukoplakia of the tongue, gums, and buccal mucosa

CHIEF COMPLAINT

Common chief complaints for the ears, nose, mouth, and throat are defined, and information on the characteristics of each sign or symptom is provided.

EAR

1. Change in or Loss of Hearing Reduction in the perception of sound

Location Unilateral, bilateral

Quality Loud sounds heard, soft sounds heard

Quantity Partial or complete

Associated Manifestations Tinnitus, vertigo, drainage, swelling, fever, ear pain

Aggravating Factors Loud noises, excessive or impacted cerumen, swimming

Alleviating Factors Hearing aid, removal of excessive cerumen, turning up volume when possible, cupping the ear, facing the speaker

Setting Work (occupations with loud background noise or machinery); long-term exposure to loud sounds/music

Timing Constant, intermittent, after drug therapy, onset sudden, gradual, or slow

2. Otalgia Discomfort in the ear

Location Unilateral or bilateral, in jaw region, in pinna region

Quality Aching, dull, sharp

Associated Manifestations Drainage, tinnitus, dysphagia, sore throat, vertigo, diminished hearing, fever, reddened/edematous external auditory canal

Aggravating Factors Tooth infection, upper respiratory infection (URI), perforated tympanic membrane (TM), insect bite in the ear, upright or supine position, foreign body in an ear, change in barometric air pressure, change in altitude

Alleviating Factors Analgesics, upright or supine position, avoiding swimming, avoiding barometric air pressure changes, removal of objects, change in air pressure, change in altitude

Setting Outdoors, high altitudes, airplane travel, noisy environments, scuba diving/skydiving

Timing Continuous, intermittent, after swimming, following trauma to the head or ear, following loud noises, after pressure changes, flying

3. Tinnitus "Ringing" in the ears

Location Unilateral or bilateral

Quality Pulsatile, buzzing, high-pitched ringing

Associated Manifestations Vertigo, drainage, pain, nausea, fullness or pressure in the ears, hearing loss, URI, allergies, otitis media, serous otitis, inner ear lesions, eustachian tube dysfunction (ETD)

Aggravating Factors Medications, serous otitis, perforation of the TM, position, pressure on the neck, excessive cerumen

Alleviating Factors Discontinuing medications, position change, avoiding allergens

Setting Work (high noise levels), outdoors, medications (e.g., nonsteroidal anti-inflammatory drugs [NSAIDs], loop diuretics, antidepressants, antibiotics, chemotherapy, antimalarial)

Timing Long-standing, recent, constant, intermittent, following drug therapy, after exposure to loud noises

4. Otorrhea Drainage of liquid from the ear

Location Unilateral or bilateral

Quality Painful or nontender, watery, bloody or purulent, foul odor

Associated Manifestations Hearing loss, otalgia, headache, fever, vertigo, URI

Aggravating Factors Upright or supine position

Alleviating Factors Upright or supine position

Timing Following trauma, after high altitude exposure, especially with coexisting allergies, coryza, or URI, continuous, intermittent

NOSE

1. Pain Discomfort in the nose

Quality Aching, throbbing, sharp

Associated Manifestations Fever, chills, visual changes, swelling, sneezing, nasal discharge (note color)

Aggravating Factors Exposure to allergens, decreased humidity indoors, cocaine use, improper nasal steroid administration

Alleviating Factors Use of medications (decongestant or antihistamine), removal of allergens, humidification of the environment, discontinuation of cocaine, correct nasal steroid administration

Setting Outdoors, dry heat, low humidity

Timing Seasonal, in the morning

2. Drainage Excessive discharge of nasal secretions

Quality Unilateral or bilateral, amount, viscosity, color, odor, blood-tinged

Associated Manifestations Fever, sneezing, pain, mouth breathing, swelling, skin irritation around nose, itchy eyes

Aggravating Factors Allergens, infections

Alleviating Factors Medication, hydration, avoiding allergens

Setting Outdoors, indoors

Timing In the morning, seasonal, after trauma, with sinusitis

3. Blockage or Congestion Reduced ability to move air through the nose secondary to obstruction

Quality Complete, partial

Associated Manifestations Mouth breathing, snoring, pain, disfigurement, sneezing, itchy eyes, sinus infection

Aggravating Factors Infection, allergens, medications, foreign bodies in nose, deviated septum

Alleviating Factors Mouth breathing, medications, avoidance of allergens, removal of foreign bodies

Setting Outdoors, indoors

Timing Following drug therapy, trauma, after nasal surgery

MOUTH AND THROAT

1. Halitosis Unpleasant odor of the breath

Quality Ammonia, acetone, newly mown grass or old wine odor, foul

Associated Manifestations Gum disease, dental caries, systemic disease, sinusitis, pharyngitis, GERD, smoking

Aggravating Factors Poor oral hygiene, poor nutrition, uncontrolled diabetes mellitus, alcohol consumption, decreased hydration, decreased renal function
Alleviating Factors Good oral hygiene, control of systemic diseases, breath mints, proper nutrition, adequate dental care, treatment of infection
Timing Associated with systemic disease or acute infectious process

2. **Lesions** Disruptions in the mucosa of the mouth or tongue
Quality Tender, nontender
Associated Manifestations Malnutrition, odor, pain, swelling, fever, stress
Aggravating Factors Eating, drinking, spicy foods, tobacco use, hot or cold stimuli, alcohol, dehydration
Alleviating Factors Medications, avoiding eating, hydration, proper nutrition, avoiding smoking and alcohol
Timing Associated with systemic disease, intermittent, continuous

3. **Swelling** Edema of the oropharynx
Quality Mild, moderate, severe
Associated Manifestations Dysphagia, urticaria, wheezing, pruritus, rhinorrhea, difficulty breathing, lesions, chills, sweats, fever, sneezing, itchy eyes, erythematous oropharynx
Aggravating Factors Exposure to allergens, heat
Alleviating Factors Medications, avoiding allergens, ice, saltwater gargles
Timing Following drug therapy, after eating, after an insect bite, after trauma, during or after an infectious process

PAST HEALTH HISTORY

The various components of the past health history are linked to ears, nose, mouth, and throat pathology and ears-, nose-, mouth-, and throat-related information.

Medical History

Ear Specific Acute otitis media, acute otitis externa, serous otitis media, past rupture of TM, furunculosis, exostoses, myringosclerosis, hemotympanum, cholesteatoma, hearing difficulties
Nose Specific Epistaxis, polyps, septal deviation, septal perforation, rhinosinusitis, allergic rhinitis, vasomotor rhinitis, anosmia
Mouth and Throat Specific Tonsillitis, dental caries, herpes simplex virus, oral *Candida* infections, strep throat, tonsillar abscess, bruxism, gum recession, bleeding gums, gingivitis, leukoplakia, sialadenitis
Non-Ear, Nose, Mouth, and Throat Specific Diabetes mellitus, renal disease, atherosclerotic disease, hypertension, inflammatory processes, infections (viral or bacterial), immunosuppressive disease, dental pathology, blood dyscrasias, STIs, anaphylaxis, nutritional deficiencies

Surgical History Neurosurgery (e.g., transsphenoidal) , tonsillectomy, adenoidectomy, tumor removal, cosmetic surgery of head or neck, repair of septal deviation, oral surgery, tympanostomy tube placement, cochlear implant

Allergies Pollen: sneezing, nasal congestion, watery or itchy eyes, cough
Insect stings: swelling of the throat and/or around the eyes
Animal dander: sneezing, nasal congestion, watery or itchy eyes, cough

Medications Antibiotics, oral and nasal antihistamines, nasal anticholinergics, decongestants, oral and nasal steroids, immunotherapy (allergy shots), leukotriene modifiers, immunosuppressive drugs, chemotherapy

Injuries and Accidents Foreign bodies; trauma to the ears, nose, mouth, throat; noxious fumes; sports injuries to the face; motor vehicle accidents

Differing Needs Decreased hearing, deafness, speech disorders

Childhood Illnesses Frequent tonsillitis, frequent ear infections

FAMILY HEALTH HISTORY

Familial ears, nose, mouth, and throat diseases are listed.
Hearing loss, otitis media, otosclerosis, allergic rhinitis

SOCIAL HISTORY

The components of the social history are linked to ears, nose, mouth, and throat factors and pathology.

Alcohol Use Predisposes the patient to cancer of the oral cavity as well as decreased nutrition leading to angular cheilosis

Tobacco Use Smoking (tobacco or marijuana), snuff, or chewing tobacco predispose the client to mouth, lip, and throat cancer

Recreational Drug Use Snorting cocaine may cause perforation of the nasal septum; methamphetamine abuse may lead to dental disease (e.g., meth mouth)

Sexual Practice Herpes simplex viruses (HSV) I and II, human papillomavirus (HPV), and gonorrhea can be contracted from oral sex

Work Environment Exposure to toxins, chemicals, infections, excess noise, allergens

Home Environment Exposure to loud noise may cause hearing loss; exposure to allergens may cause allergic rhinitis

Hobbies and Leisure Activities Hunting, skeet shooting, and other activities (e.g., attending rock concerts, listening to loud music with ear/headphones), that are associated with loud noise conducted without proper ear protection may cause hearing loss; scuba diving/skydiving may cause ear barotrauma

Stress Relationship to frequent URIs, decreased hearing
Bruxism (grinding of teeth)

Ethnic Background Nasopharyngeal cancer: Southeast Asians, Northern Africans (Lang et al, 2019)

HEALTH MAINTENANCE ACTIVITIES

This information provides a bridge between the health maintenance activities and ears, nose, mouth, and throat functions.

Sleep Deprivation may be associated with frequent URIs, sleep apnea

Diet Deficiencies may affect integrity of nasal and oral mucosa

Use of Safety Devices Use of mouth guard for sports participants or bruxism; face shields for sports, job, or home projects; ear protection when around loud noise to prevent damage to hearing

Health Checkups Hearing evaluation, dental examination

NURSING CHECKLIST

General Approach to Ears, Nose, Mouth, and Throat Examination

1. Observe Standard Precautions and don personal protective equipment (PPE) such as gloves, gown, face shield, goggles, N-95 respirator or face mask if the client's status warrants these protective measures.
2. Greet the client and explain the examination techniques that you will be using.
3. Use a quiet room that will be free from interruptions.
4. Ensure that the light in the room provides sufficient brightness to allow adequate observation of the client.
5. Place the client in an upright sitting position on the examination table; for clients who cannot tolerate the sitting position, gain access to the client's head so that it can be rotated from side to side.
6. Visualize the underlying structures during the examination to allow an adequate description of the findings.
7. Always compare the right and left ears, as well as the right and left sides of the nose, sinuses, mouth, and throat.
8. Use a systematic approach that is followed consistently each time the examination is performed.

Assessment in Brief

Ears, Nose, Mouth, and Throat Examination

Ears

- Auditory screening
  - Voice-whisper test
  - Tuning fork tests
    - Weber test
    - Rinne test
- External ear
  - Inspection
  - Palpation
- Otoscopic examination

Mouth and Throat

- Mouth
  - Breath
  - Lips
    - Inspection
    - Palpation
  - Tongue
  - Buccal mucosa
  - Gums
  - Teeth
  - Palate
- Throat

Nose

- External inspection
- Patency
- Internal inspection

Sinuses

- Inspection
- Palpation and percussion

Advanced Technique

- Transillumination of the sinuses

Assistive Devices

- Hearing aids
- Oral appliances
- Nasal rinse devices

Equipment

- Appropriate PPE
- Otoscope with earpieces of different sizes and pneumatic attachment
- Nasal speculum
- Penlight
- Tuning fork, 512 Hz
- Tongue blade
- Watch
- Gauze square
- Clean gloves
- Transilluminator
- Cotton-tipped applicator

Examination of the Ear

Physical examination of the ear consists of three parts:

1. Auditory screening (CN VIII)
2. Inspection and palpation of the external ear
3. Otoscopic examination

Auditory Screening

Voice-Whisper Test

E

1. Instruct the client to occlude one ear with a finger.
2. Stand 2 feet behind the client's other ear and whisper a two-syllable word (e.g., *baseball*) or phrase that is evenly accented.

3. Ask the client to repeat the word or phrase.
4. Repeat the test with the other ear.

N **The client should be able to repeat words whispered from a distance of 2 feet.**

A The client is unable to repeat the words correctly or states the inability to hear anything.

P These findings indicate a hearing loss in the high-frequency range that may be caused by excessive exposure to loud noises (Fig. 13-11).

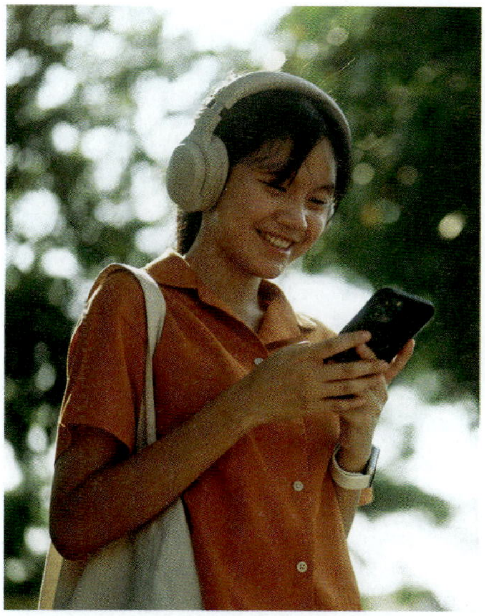

Figure 13-11 Consistently listening to loud music can lead to hearing loss.

Tuning Fork Tests

Weber and **Rinne tests** help to determine whether the type of hearing loss the client is experiencing is conductive or sensorineural. To understand how these tests are evaluated, it is important to know the difference between air and bone conduction. Air conduction refers to the transmission of sound through the ear canal, tympanic membrane, and ossicular chain to the cochlea and auditory nerve. Bone conduction refers to the transmission of sound through the bones of the skull to the cochlea and auditory nerve.

Weber Test

E
1. Hold the handle of a 512 Hz (vibrates 512 cycles per second to create a specific frequency) tuning fork and strike the tines on the ulnar border of the palm to activate it.
2. Place the stem of the fork firmly against the middle of the client's forehead, on the top of the head at the midline, or on the front teeth (Fig. 13-12).
3. Ask the client if the sound is heard centrally or toward one side.

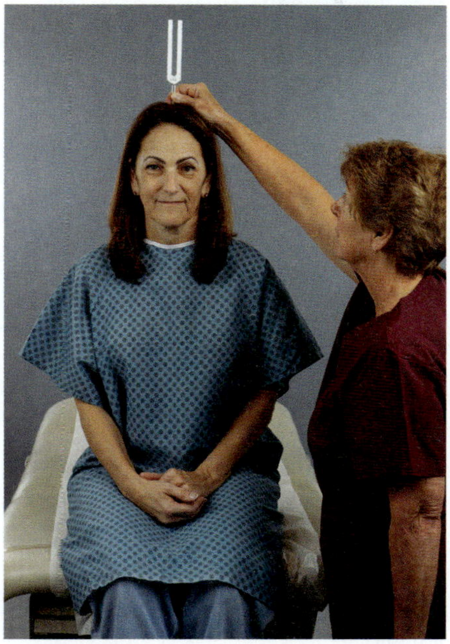

Figure 13-12 Weber test.

N **The client should perceive the sound equally in both ears or "in the middle." No lateralization of sound is known as a "negative" Weber test.**

A The sound lateralizes to the affected ear.

P Sound lateralizing to the affected ear occurs with unilateral conductive hearing loss because the sound is being conducted directly through the bone to the ear. Conductive hearing loss occurs when there are external or middle ear disorders such as impacted cerumen, perforation of the tympanic membrane, serum or pus in the middle ear, or a fusion of the ossicles.

A The sound lateralizes to the unaffected ear.

P Sound lateralizing to the unaffected ear occurs with sensorineural loss related to nerve damage in the impaired ear. Sensorineural hearing loss occurs when there is a disorder in the inner ear, the auditory nerve, or the brain; disorders include congenital defects, effects of ototoxic drugs, and repeated or prolonged exposure to loud noise.

NURSING TIP

The Client With Decreased Hearing

Observe the client for signs of hearing difficulty and deafness during the health history and physical examination. Turning the head to facilitate hearing, lip reading, speaking in a loud voice, or asking you to write words are signs of hearing difficulty. If the client is wearing a hearing aid, ask if it is turned on, when the batteries were last changed, and if the device causes any irritation of the ear canal.

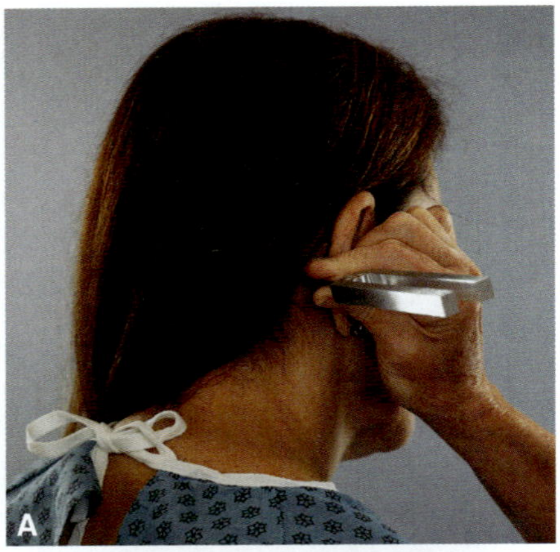

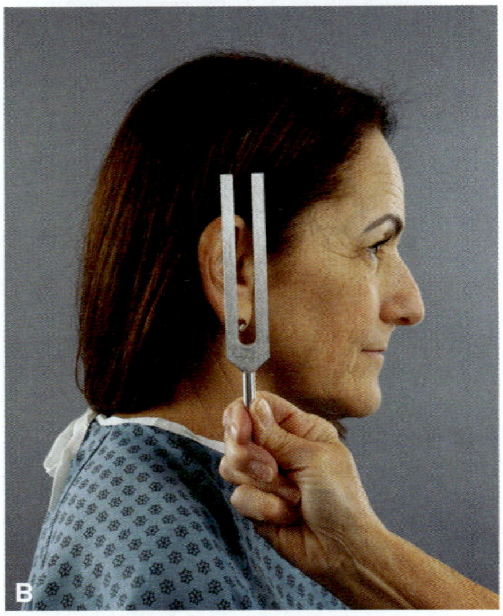

Figure 13-13 Rinne test. **A.** Assessing bone conduction. **B.** Assessing air conduction.

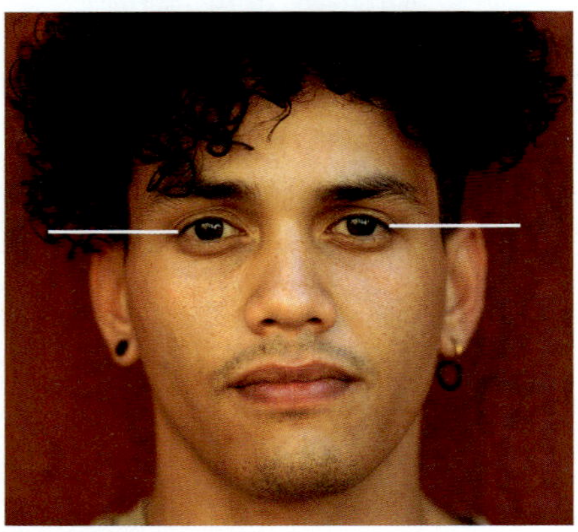

Figure 13-14 Normal ear alignment.

Rinne Test

E

1. Stand behind or to the side of the client and strike the tuning fork.
2. Place the stem of the tuning fork against the client's right mastoid process to test bone conduction (Fig. 13-13A).
3. Instruct the client to indicate if the sound is heard.
4. Ask the client to tell you when the sound stops.
5. When the client says that the sound has stopped, move the tuning fork, with the tines facing forward, in front of the right auditory meatus, and ask the client if the sound is still heard. Note the length of time the client hears the sound (testing air conduction) (Fig. 13-13B).
6. Repeat the test on the left ear.

N **Air conduction is heard twice as long as bone conduction when the client hears the sound through the external auditory canal (air) after it is no longer heard at the mastoid process (bone). This is denoted as AC > BC, or a positive Rinne test.**

A The client reports hearing the sound longer through bone conduction; that is, bone conduction is equal to or greater than air conduction. This is a negative Rinne test.

P A negative Rinne test occurs when there is conductive hearing loss resulting from disease, obstruction, or damage to the outer or middle ear.

A Bone conduction is prolonged in the context of a normal tympanic membrane, patent eustachian tube, and middle ear disease.

P These findings are typical of otosclerosis.

External Ear

Inspection

E

1. Inspect the ears and note their position, color, size, and shape.
2. Note any deformities, nodules, inflammation, or lesions.
3. Note color, consistency, and amount of cerumen.

N **The ear should match the flesh color of the rest of the client's skin and should be positioned centrally and in proportion to the head. The top of the ear should cross an imaginary line drawn from the outer canthus of the eye to the occiput (Fig. 13-14). Cerumen should be moist and not obscure the tympanic membrane. There should be no foreign bodies, redness, drainage, deformities, nodules, or lesions.**

A The ears are pale, red, or cyanotic.

P Vasomotor disorders, fevers, hypoxemia, and cold weather can account for various color changes of the external ear.

A The ears are abnormally large or small.

P Abnormally large or small ears can be congenital or the result of trauma. Figure 13-15 depicts microtia (an unusually small external ear). Frequently, this is accompanied by an absent external ear canal and middle ear, but an intact inner ear.

A An ear that is swollen and deformed resembling a "cauliflower" is abnormal (Fig. 13-16).

P Perichondrial hematoma (cauliflower ear) is a condition common among wrestlers and boxers that is caused by blunt trauma to the external ear resulting in blood clot formation and fluid collection under the perichondrium, which leads to fibrosis and deformity of the external ear.

A An external ear that is erythematous, edematous, warm to the touch, and painful is abnormal.

P Perichondritis is an inflammation of the fibrous connective tissue that overlies the cartilage of the ear (Fig. 13-17).

A A skin lesion or tumor on the external ear is abnormal.

P Basal cell and squamous cell carcinoma are the most common external ear tumors. Prolonged sunlight exposure is a predisposing factor for these tumors.

A Purulent drainage is abnormal.

P Purulent drainage usually indicates otitis media with tympanic membrane perforation.

A Bloody drainage is present.

P Bloody drainage may result from head trauma or surgery.

A Clear ear drainage is present. The clear drainage must be differentiated from water or other substances.

P Clear ear drainage may result from head trauma or surgery and may indicate a leakage of cerebrospinal fluid (CSF). CSF tests positive for glucose on test strips. A client with a CSF leak needs an immediate referral to a neurosurgeon or otolaryngologist.

A A hematoma behind an ear over the mastoid bone is abnormal.

P This is called Battle's sign and indicates head trauma to the temporal bone of the skull

A A hard, painless, irregular-shaped nodule on the pinna is abnormal (Fig. 13-18).

P Tophi are uric acid crystals and may indicate the presence of gout. These are usually located near the helix. Many other nodules are benign fibromas.

A Sebaceous cysts are abnormal.

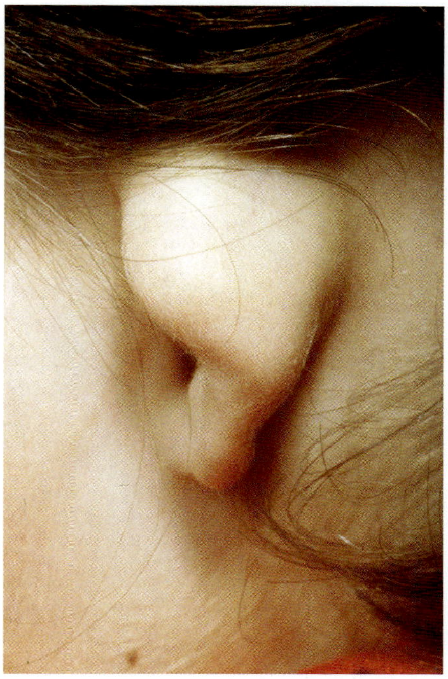

Figure 13-15 Microtia.

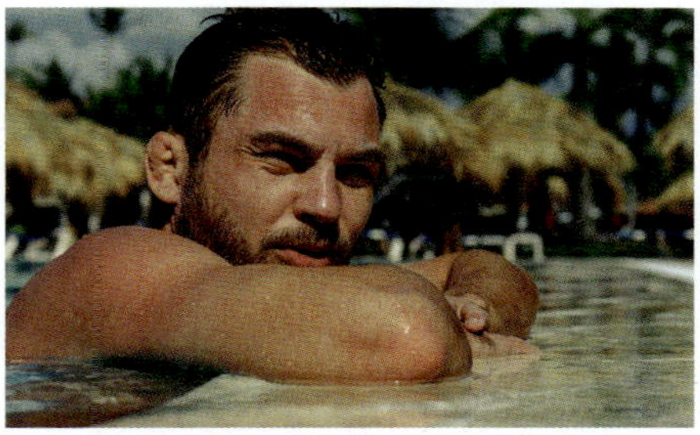

Figure 13-16 This man acquired a perichondrial hematoma (cauliflower ear) on the right ear after years of wrestling.

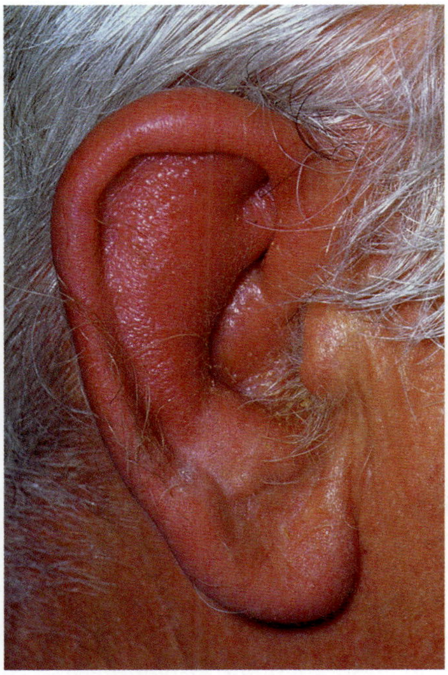

Figure 13-17 Perichondritis.

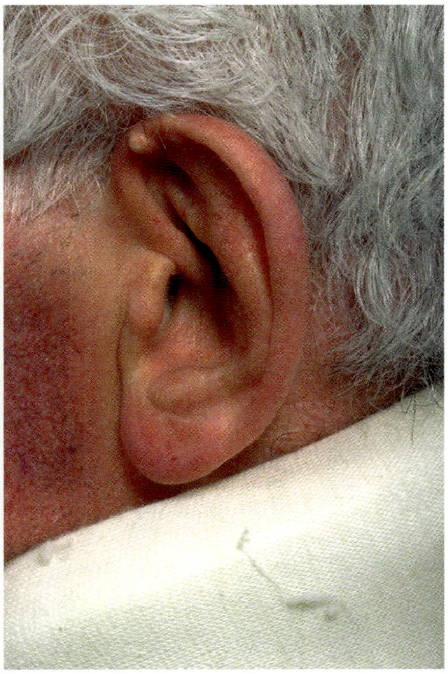

Figure 13-18 Auricular tophi.

P Sebaceous cysts or retention cysts form as a result of blockage of the ducts to the sebaceous gland.

A Lymph nodes anterior to the tragus or overlying the mastoid are abnormal.

P Lymph nodes may be enlarged due to a malignancy or an infection such as acute otitis media and otitis externa.

Palpation

E
1. Palpate the auricle between the thumb and the index finger, noting any tenderness or lesions. If the client has ear pain, examine the unaffected ear first, then cautiously examine the affected ear.
2. Using the tips of the index and middle fingers, palpate the mastoid tip, noting any tenderness.
3. Using the tips of the index and middle fingers, press inward on the tragus, noting any tenderness.
4. Hold the auricle between the thumb and the index finger and gently pull up and down, noting any tenderness.

N **The client should not complain of pain or tenderness during palpation.**

A Auricular pain or tenderness is noted.

P Auricular pain is a common finding in otitis externa, an external ear infection.

A Tenderness over the mastoid part of the temporal bone or mastoid process is abnormal. Erythema may be present.

P Mastoid tenderness and erythema are associated with middle ear inflammation and mastoiditis.

A The tragus is edematous or sensitive.

P This finding may indicate inflammation of the external or middle ear.

Otoscopic Examination

E
1. Ask the client to tip the head away from the ear being examined.
2. Select the largest speculum that will comfortably fit the client.
3. Hold the otoscope securely in the dominant hand, with the handle held like a pencil between the thumb and the forefinger.
4. Rest the back of the dominant hand on the right side of the client's head (Fig. 13-19).
5. Use the free hand to pull the right ear in a manner that will straighten the canal. In adults and children over 3 years old, pull the ear up and back. Refer to Chapter 25 for the examination of children.
6. If hair obstructs visualization, moisten the speculum with water or a water-soluble lubricant.
7. If wax obstructs visualization, it should be removed by a skilled practitioner, either by curettement (if the cerumen is soft or the tympanic membrane is ruptured) or by irrigation (if the cerumen is dry and hard and the tympanic membrane is intact).
8. Slowly insert the speculum into the canal, looking at the canal as the speculum passes.
9. Examine the canal for inflammation, exudates, lesions, and foreign bodies.
10. Continue to insert the speculum into the canal, following the path of the canal until the tympanic membrane is visualized.
11. If the tympanic membrane is not visible, gently pull the pinna slightly further; this straightens the canal to allow adequate visualization.

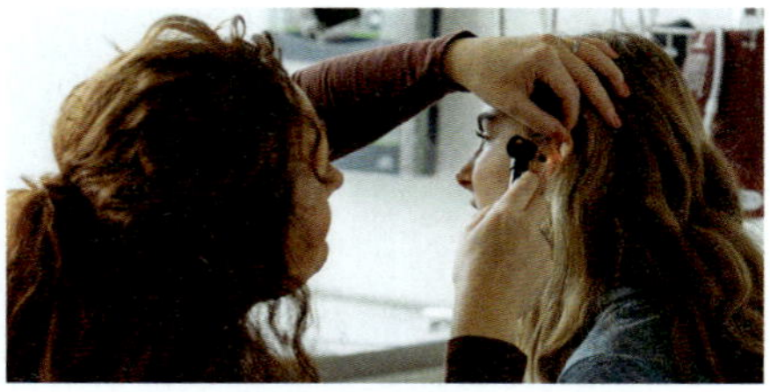

Figure 13-19 Position for otoscopic examination of the left ear.

12. Identify the color, light reflex, umbo, the short process, and the long handle of the malleus. Note the presence of perforations, lesions, bulging or retraction of the tympanic membrane, dilation of blood vessels, bubbles, or fluid.
13. Ask the client to close the mouth, pinch the nose closed, and blow gently while you observe for movement of the tympanic membrane. A pneumatic attachment may be used to create this movement if one is available.
14. Gently withdraw the speculum and repeat the process with the left ear.

N **The ear canal should have no redness, swelling, tenderness, lesions, drainage, foreign bodies, or scaly surface areas. Cerumen varies in amount, consistency, and color. The tympanic membrane should be pearly gray with clearly defined landmarks and a distinct cone-shaped light reflex extending from the umbo toward the anteroinferior aspect of the membrane. This light reflex is seen at 5 o'clock in the right ear and at 7 o'clock in the left ear. Blood vessels should be visible only on the periphery, and the membrane should not bulge, be retracted, or have any evidence of fluid behind it (Fig. 13-20). The tympanic membrane should move when the client blows against resistance.**

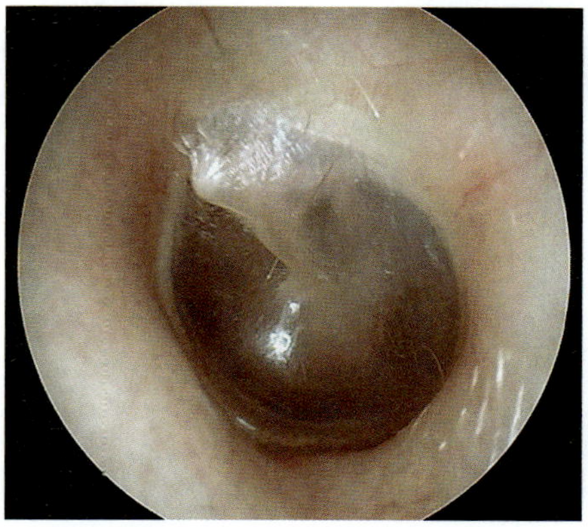

Figure 13-20 Normal tympanic membrane.

NURSING TIP

Clearing the EAC of Cerumen

Various methods can be used to remove cerumen from the external auditory canal (EAC) to allow visualization of the tympanic membrane: manual removal and irrigation. Manual removal involves the use of a curette. This method is quick and does not expose the EAC to moisture; therefore, it may reduce the risk of infection. However, it requires a cooperative client and skilled practitioner to reduce the risk of trauma to the EAC.

Irrigation with water and saline or diluted hydrogen peroxide at body temperature can be performed with a 20 to 30 mL syringe with a plastic catheter or a bulb syringe. The liquid should be instilled gently, and the canal should be checked intermittently for clearance of cerumen. Oral jet irrigators are fast and portable; however, they have been associated with trauma. Liquid irrigation should be avoided in clients with tympanic membrane perforation, acute otitis media, otitis externa, myringotomy tubes, ear surgery, or vertigo.

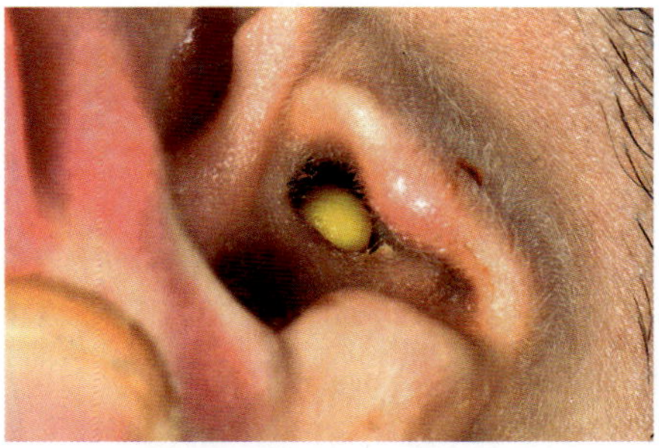

Figure 13-21 EAC foreign body (toy gun pellet).

A A foreign body in the external auditory canal is abnormal (Fig. 13-21).

P Both adults and children can have foreign bodies in the EAC. Some objects are more difficult to remove than others; for instance, vegetables in the EAC can swell with time and make removal challenging.

P Tympanostomy tubes, or pressure equalization (PE) tubes (Fig. 13-22), are surgically placed for prolonged or frequent occurrences of otitis media with effusion (OME). The tubes allow drainage of the effusion, normal vibration of the ossicles, and equalization of pressures across the tympanic membrane. When a myringotomy has been performed with tympanostomy tube placement, the presence of the tubes (or lack of) should be documented.

A A painful, boil-like pustule in the EAC is abnormal.

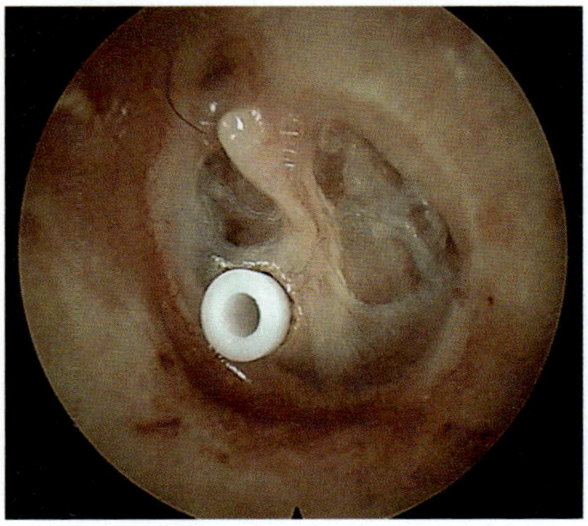

Figure 13-22 PE tube.

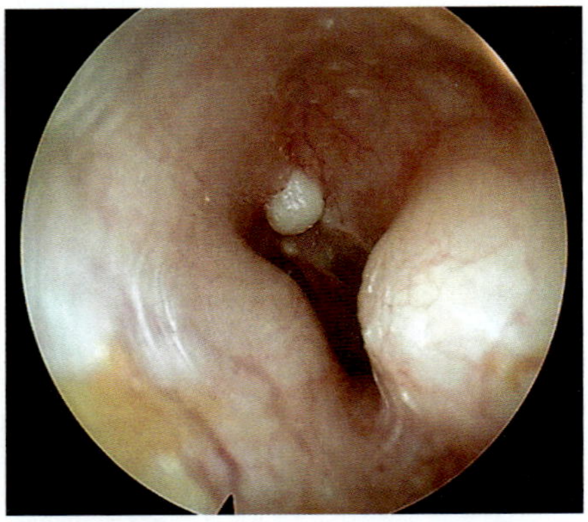

Figure 13-23 Exostoses.

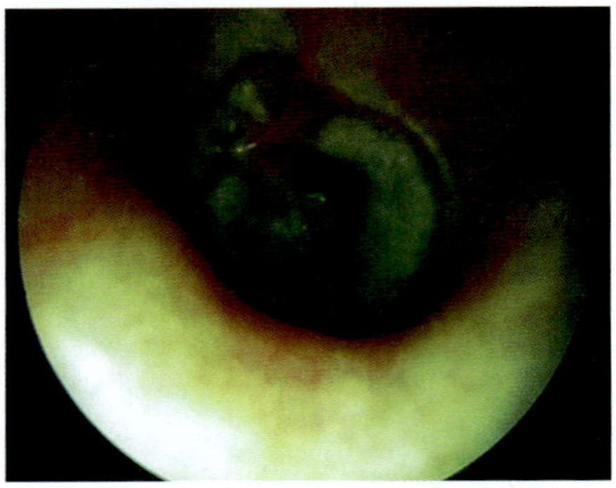

Figure 13-24 Myringosclerosis and otitis media with effusion.

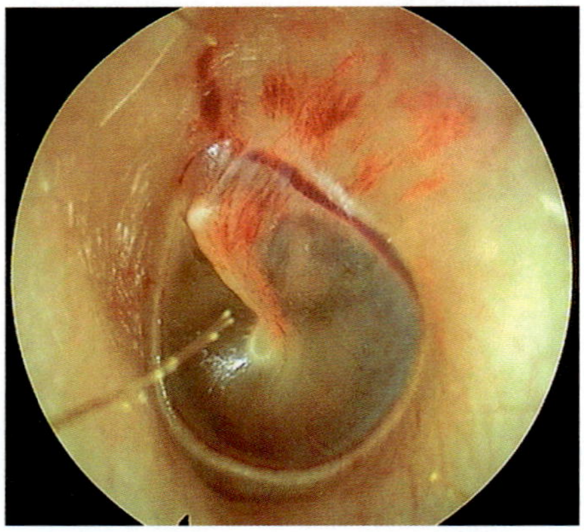

Figure 13-25 Barotrauma caused by scuba diving.

P Furunculosis is an infection of a hair follicle in the ear. EAC edema and otorrhea may also be present.

A Black or brown spores, yellow or orange spores, or white fluffy hyphae in the EAC are abnormal.

P Prolonged use of aural antibiotics can cause otomycosis, or a fungal infection, in the ear. Different strains of fungi cause variations in appearance.

A Bony, hard lesions in the EAC (Fig. 13-23) are abnormal.

P Bony overgrowths in the EAC are exostoses. Clients who frequently participate in cold-water activities (e.g., swimming, scuba diving, surfing) are at risk for developing them. If an exostosis becomes large enough, it can block the EAC and trap debris between it and the tympanic membrane. This can lead to infection.

A Severe pain accompanied by erythema deep into the EAC and on the tympanic membrane, along with serous-filled blebs, is abnormal.

P Deep EAC and TM erythema with serous-filled blebs describe viral bullous myringitis. This can easily be mistaken for acute otitis media.

A The appearance of chalky-white patches on the tympanic membrane (Fig. 13-24) is abnormal.

P Chalky-white patches on the tympanic membrane are calcifications found in myringosclerosis, which can occur after tympanic membrane surgery, infection, or inflammation. Myringosclerosis can be associated with gradual hearing loss. The involvement of the entire tympanic membrane is called tympanosclerosis.

A Air bubbles on the tympanic membrane (Fig. 13-25) are abnormal.

P Conditions such as coryza, influenza, allergies, and changes in extratympanic pressure (such as in scuba diving/skydiving and airplane travel) can lead to eustachian tube failure and air bubbles on the tympanic membrane.

A The presence of blood in the middle ear is abnormal (Fig. 13-26).

P Hemotympanum occurs as a result of trauma to the head. The tympanic membrane can have a bluish hue or can be red in appearance.

A A severely retracted tympanic membrane has exaggerated landmarks (Fig. 13-27). Mobility of the tympanic membrane is decreased.

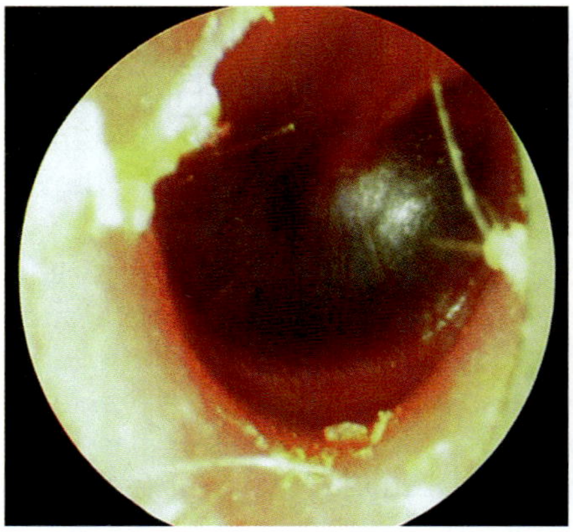

Figure 13-26 Hemotympanum.

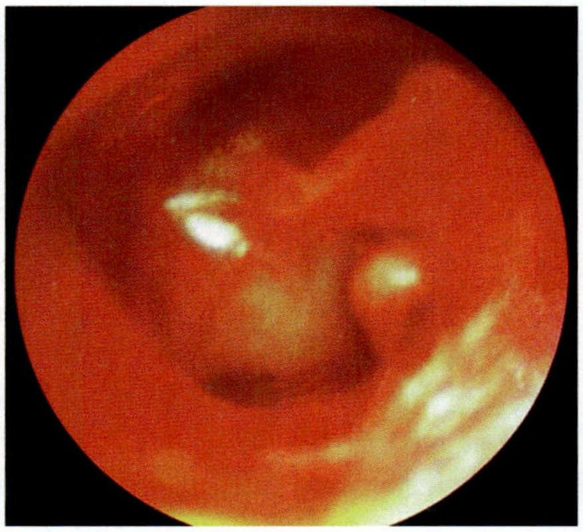

Figure 13-27 Severe tympanic membrane retraction.

P Retraction of the tympanic membrane can occur when the intratympanic membrane pressures are reduced, as in eustachian tube blockage caused by otitis media with effusion or allergies. Repeated negative pressure in the middle ear sucks in the tympanic membrane and leads to retractions. Over time, keratinized epithelial debris deposits itself in these retraction pockets and leads to ossicle fixation. This leads to cholesteatoma (Fig. 13-28). A foul-smelling ear discharge, as well as deafness, may accompany cholesteatoma.

A There is redness, swelling, narrowing, and pain in the external ear (Fig. 13-29). Drainage may be present.

P Acute otitis externa is caused by infectious organisms or allergic reactions. Predisposing factors include excessive moisture in the ear related to swimming, humid environments, trauma from cleansing the ears with a sharp instrument, or allergies to substances such as hairspray.

A Hard, dry, and very dark yellow-brown cerumen is abnormal.

P Old cerumen is harder and drier and may become impacted if not removed. This can lead to ear pain and decreased hearing.

A The tympanic membrane is red, with decreased mobility and possible bulging (Fig. 13-30).

P A tympanic membrane that is red, with decreased mobility and possible bulging is seen in **acute otitis media** (AOM), or an inflammation/infection of the middle ear. Pain and fever may accompany the ear infection. Otalgia, fever, decreased hearing, irritability, disturbed sleep, and otorrhea may accompany the middle ear infection. *Streptococcus pneumoniae, Haemophilus influenzae,* and *Moraxella catarrhalis* are the major pathogens that cause AOM.

A Along with a bulging eardrum and decreased mobility, the landmarks are diffuse, displaced, or absent.

P The late stage of acute otitis media causes landmarks to become progressively obscured.

A Amber-yellow fluid on the tympanic membrane is abnormal. It may be accompanied by a fluid line or bubbles behind the membrane. Bulging may be present and mobility of the eardrum may be decreased (Figs. 13-31 and 13-32). The client may complain of ear popping, pain, and decreased hearing.

P Otitis media with effusion (OME), or serous otitis media, can be caused by allergies, infections, and a blocked eustachian tube. Table 13-1 compares AOM, OME, and otitis externa.

A The tympanic membrane appears to have a darkened area or a hole.

P A perforated eardrum is caused by an untreated ear infection secondary to increasing pressure. Trauma to the ear canal can also cause a perforation (Fig. 13-33).

A The tympanic membrane is pearly gray and has dark patches.

P These patches are usually old perforations in the tympanic membrane.

A The tympanic membrane is pearly gray and has dense white plaques.

P These plaques represent calcific deposits of scarring of the tympanic membrane from frequent past episodes of otitis media and past tympanic membrane perforation.

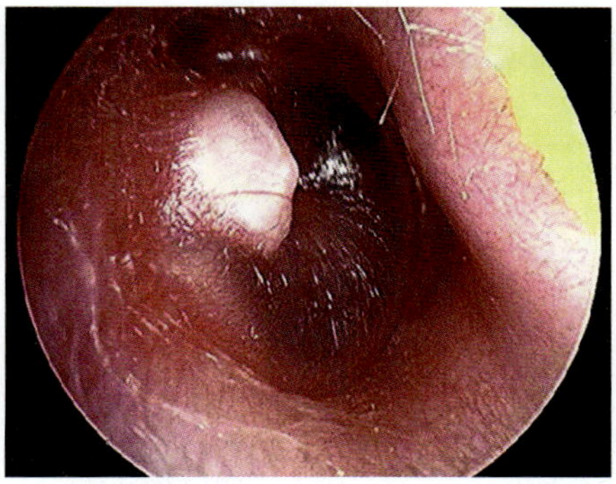

Figure 13-28 Cholesteatoma.

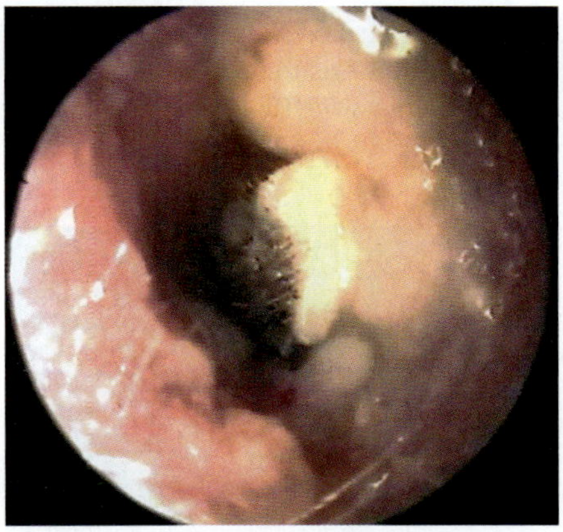

Figure 13-29 Acute otitis externa.

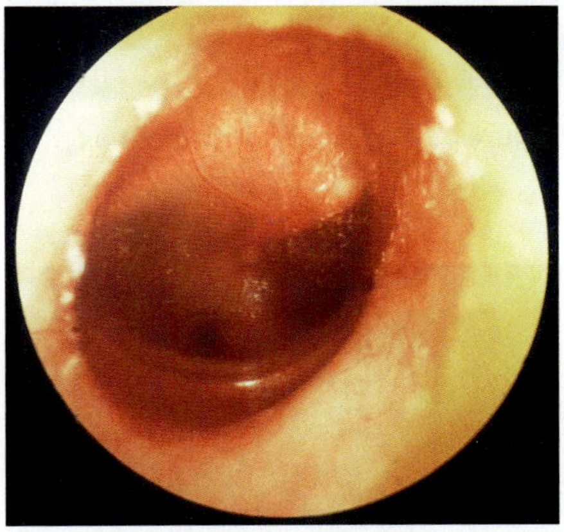

Figure 13-30 Acute otitis media. Note the bulging TM.

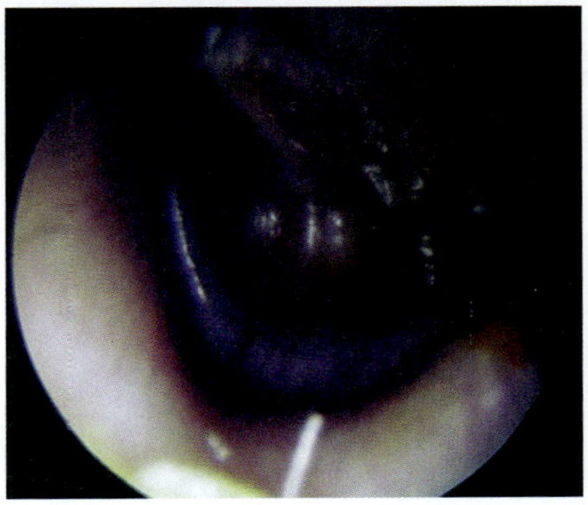

Figure 13-31 Otitis media with effusion.

Table 13-1 Comparison of AOM, OME, and Otitis Externa

	AOM	OME	Otitis Externa
TM color	Diffuse red, dilated peripheral vessels	Yellowish	WNL
TM appearance	Bulging	Bubbles, fluid line	WNL
TM landmarks	Decreased	Retracted with prominent malleus	WNL
Movement of tragus	Painless	Painless	Painful
Hearing	WNL/decreased	WNL/decreased	WNL
EAC	WNL	WNL	Erythematous, edematous

AOM = acute otitis media; EAC =external auditory canal; OME = otitis media with effusion; TM = tympanic membrane; WNL = within normal limits.

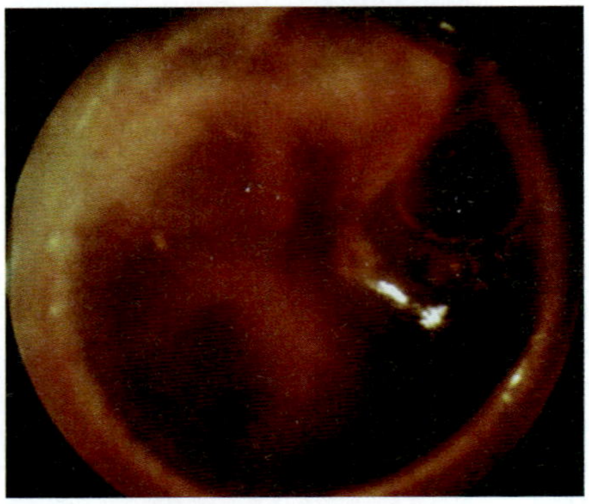

Figure 13-32 Serous otitis media.

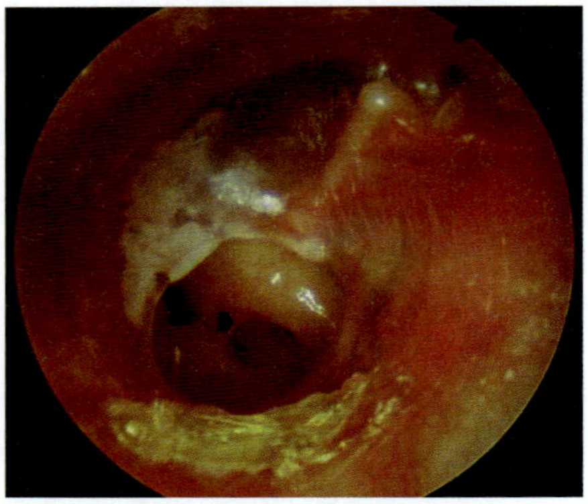

Figure 13-33 Tympanic membrane perforation.

Risk Factors

Otitis Media

- Less than 2 years of age
- Frequent URIs and colds
- Seasonal: fall, winter
- Female
- Whites, Native Americans, Alaskan natives
- Family history (parents, siblings)
- Smoky environment
- Group day care
- Bottle-fed
- Craniofacial disorders (e.g., cleft palate)
- Chronic illnesses (e.g., sinusitis, asthma, allergies, cystic fibrosis, immunodeficiencies, immunocompromised status)

Risk Factors

Hearing Loss

- Loud noise exposure
- Smoking
- Ototoxic drugs (e.g., aspirin, gentamicin, vancomycin, tobramycin, furosemide, torsemide, quinine)
- Congenital or hereditary
- Aging
- Tumors
- Trauma
- Chronic ear infections
- Ruptured tympanic membrane
- Cerumen or otic foreign body
- Systemic disease
- Tympanic membrane perforation
- Ménière disease
- Barotrauma from extreme atmospheric pressure changes

Examination of the Nose

External Inspection

E Inspect the nose, noting any trauma, bleeding, lesions, masses, swelling, or asymmetry.

N **The shape of the external nose can vary greatly among individuals. Normally, it is located symmetrically in the midline of the face and is without swelling, bleeding, lesions, or masses.**

A The nose is misshapen, broken, or swollen (Fig. 13-34).

P The shape of the nose is determined by genetics; however, changes can occur because of trauma or cosmetic surgery.

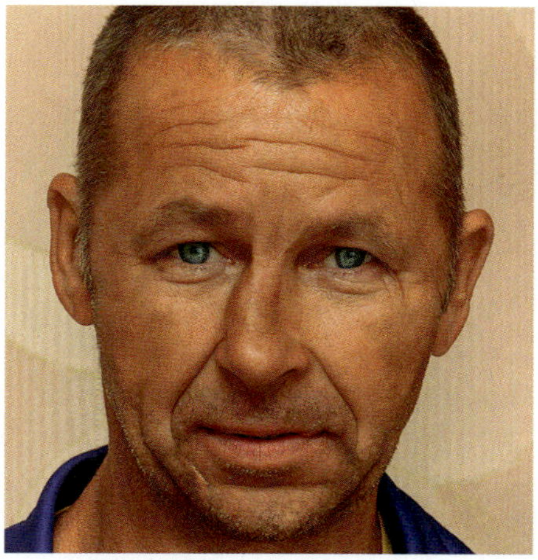

Figure 13-34 Misshapen nose.

Patency

E
1. Have the client occlude one nostril with a finger.
2. Ask the client to breathe in and out through the nose as you observe and listen for air movement in and out of the nostril.
3. Repeat on the other side.

N **Each nostril is patent.**

A You observe or the client states that air cannot be moved through the nostril(s).

P Occlusion of the nostrils can occur with a deviated septum, foreign body, upper respiratory infection, allergies, or nasal polyps.

A Nasal drainage is observed from only one side of the nose.

P Unilateral nasal drainage may be a sign of nasal obstruction.

> **NURSING TIP**
>
> **Assessing Patency of the Nose**
>
> The sense of smell (CN I) is evaluated during the testing of cranial nerves. Refer to Chapter 20.

Internal Inspection

E
1. Position the client with the head in an extended position.
2. Place the nondominant hand firmly on top of the client's head.
3. Using the thumb of the same hand, lift the tip of the client's nose.
4. Gently insert a nasal speculum or an otoscope with a short, wide nasal speculum (Fig. 13-35A and B). If using a nasal speculum, use a penlight to view the nostrils.

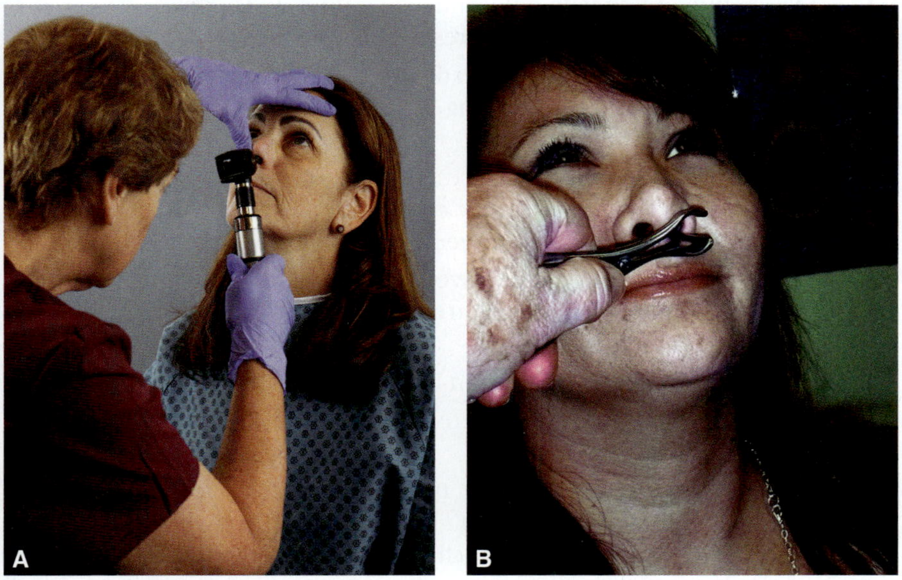

Figure 13-35 Internal inspection of the nose. **A.** Using an otoscope for nasal inspection. **B.** Using a nasal speculum for nasal inspection.

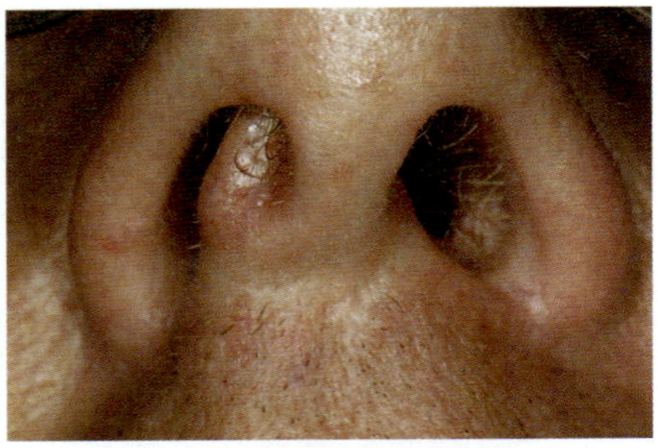

Figure 13-36 Deviated nasal septum.

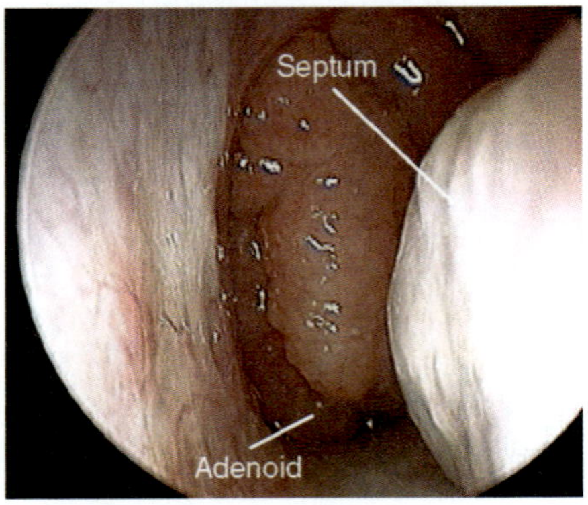

Figure 13-37 Nasal cavity blocked by adenoid.

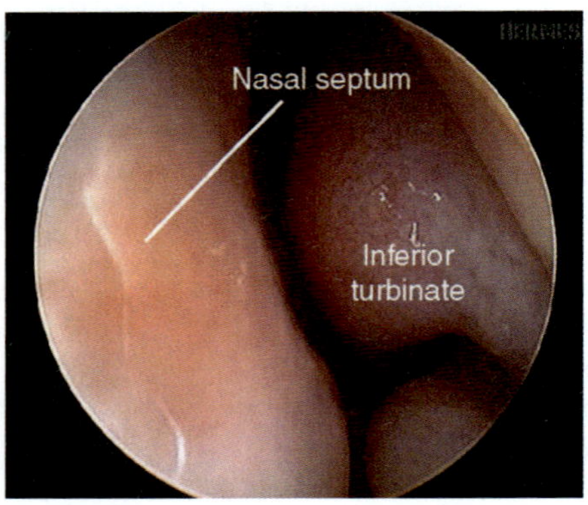

Figure 13-38 Edematous inferior turbinate causing almost total occlusion of the nasal cavity. Note the slight difference in color between the septum and the turbinate. These findings can occur in clients with allergic rhinitis.

5. Examine each nostril separately.
6. Inspect the mucous membranes for color and discharge.
7. Inspect the middle and inferior turbinates and the middle meatus for color, swelling, drainage, lesions, and polyps.
8. Observe the nasal septum for deviation, perforation, lesions, and bleeding.

N **The nasal mucosa should be pink or dull red without swelling or polyps. The septum is at the midline and without perforation, lesions, or bleeding. A small amount of clear, watery discharge is normal.**

A A nasal septum that is "pushed" to one side can be an abnormal finding (Fig. 13-36).

P A deviated septum can occur naturally, or it can be caused by trauma to the face and nasal area.

A A nasal septum with a hole or fissure is abnormal.

P A perforated nasal septum may be caused by nasal insufflation (snorting) of cocaine, which can lead to necrosis of the septal cartilage. Long-term intranasal corticosteroid use can also result in a perforated nasal septum if the administration technique is incorrect.

A An occluded nasal cavity is abnormal.

P There are many causes of an occluded nasal cavity. Foreign bodies may be present, especially in children. Trauma may induce nasal edema. A sinus infection may produce copious discharge. An adenoid may be so large that it occludes the nasal cavity (Fig. 13-37). Allergies can lead to edematous turbinates that occlude a nasal passage (Fig. 13-38).

A The nasal mucosa is red and swollen with copious clear, watery discharge. This is called rhinitis, an inflammation of the nasal mucosa.

P Nasal mucosa that is red and swollen with copious clear, watery discharge indicates coryza (the common cold) when there is an acute onset of symptoms. Discharge may become purulent if a secondary bacterial infection develops.

A Nasal mucosa is pale and edematous with clear, watery discharge.

P Nasal mucosa that is pale and edematous with clear, watery discharge usually indicate the presence of allergies or hay fever.

A Following trauma to the head, there is a clear, watery nasal discharge with normal-appearing mucosa. This discharge tests positive for glucose.

P These findings indicate the presence of cerebrospinal fluid. This may occur following a head injury or complications of nose or sinus surgery or dental work. An immediate referral is warranted.

A Nasal mucosa is red and swollen with purulent nasal discharge (Fig. 13-39). These findings are usually worse on one side but may be found bilaterally.

P These are common findings in bacterial sinusitis.

A Smooth, round masses that are pale and shiny are noted protruding from the middle meatus.

P Pale, smooth, round, shiny masses protruding from the middle meatus are nasal polyps (Fig. 13-40), which may obstruct air passages. They are often seen in clients who have chronic allergic rhinitis, asthma, and cystic fibrosis. They are usually found bilaterally. A unilateral polyp is suspect for a malignancy until proven otherwise.

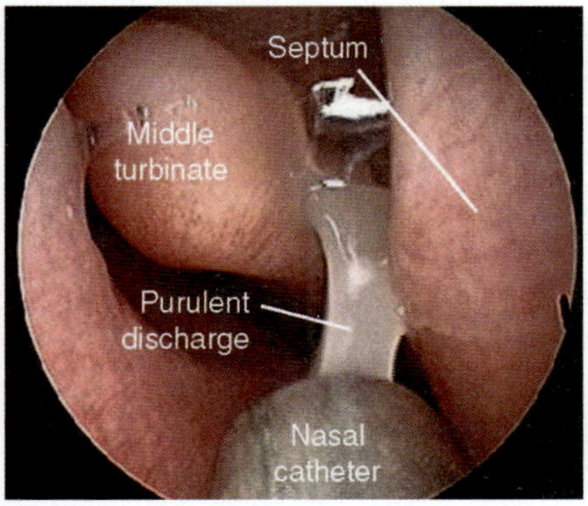

Figure 13-39 Purulent discharge in the nasal cavity at the middle turbinate.

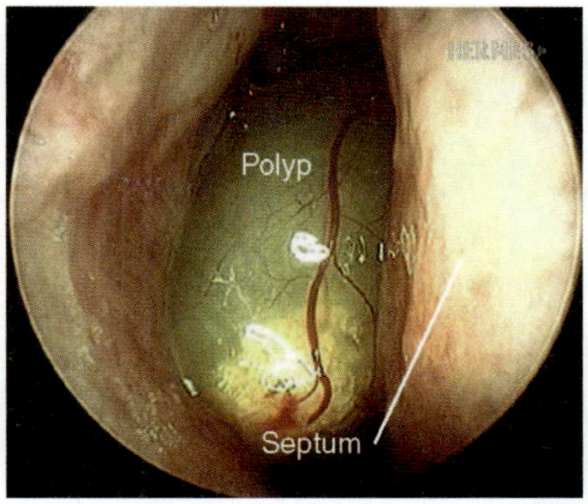

Figure 13-40 Nasal polyp.

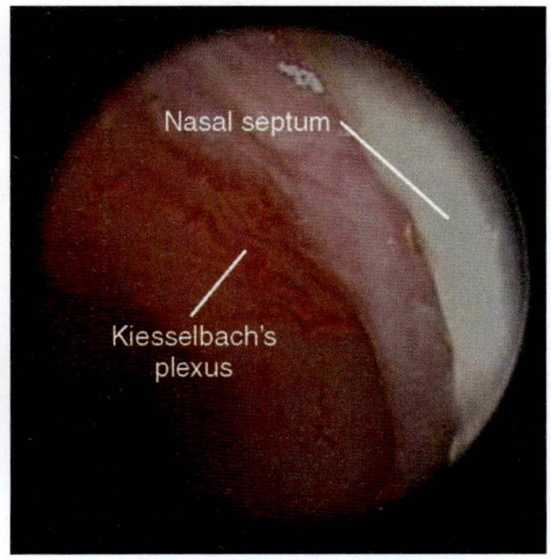

Figure 13-41 Kiesselbach's plexus.

A Bleeding is noted from an area of the lower portion of the nasal septum.

P Kiesselbach's plexus, a vascular area on the septum, is the site of most nosebleeds (Fig. 13-41). Repeated nosebleeds warrant attention for blood dyscrasias, environmental causes, medication use (e.g., anticoagulants), and malignancies, among other etiologies.

A There is unilateral purulent discharge; however, the client does not experience other symptoms of an upper respiratory infection. Nasal mucosa on the unaffected side appears normal.

P Unilateral purulent discharge without other findings of an upper respiratory infection indicates the development of a local infection. A common cause of localized infection is the presence of a foreign body.

A Nasal mucosa are inflamed and friable with possible septal perforation. No infection is present.

P These findings may indicate nasal inhalation of cocaine or amphetamines or the overuse of decongestant or corticosteroid nasal sprays.

Examination of the Sinuses

Inspection

E Observe the client's face for any swelling around the nose and eyes.

N **There is no evidence of swelling around the nose and eyes.**

A Swelling is noted above or below the eyes.

P Acute sinusitis may result in swelling of the face around the eyes due to inflammation and accumulation of purulent material in the paranasal sinuses.

Palpation and Percussion

To palpate and percuss the frontal sinuses:

E
1. Stand facing the client.
2. Gently press the thumbs under the bony ridge of the upper orbits (under the eyebrows) (Fig. 13-42A). Avoid applying pressure on the globes themselves.
3. Observe for the presence of pain.
4. Percuss the areas using the middle or index finger of the dominant hand (direct percussion).
5. Note the sound.

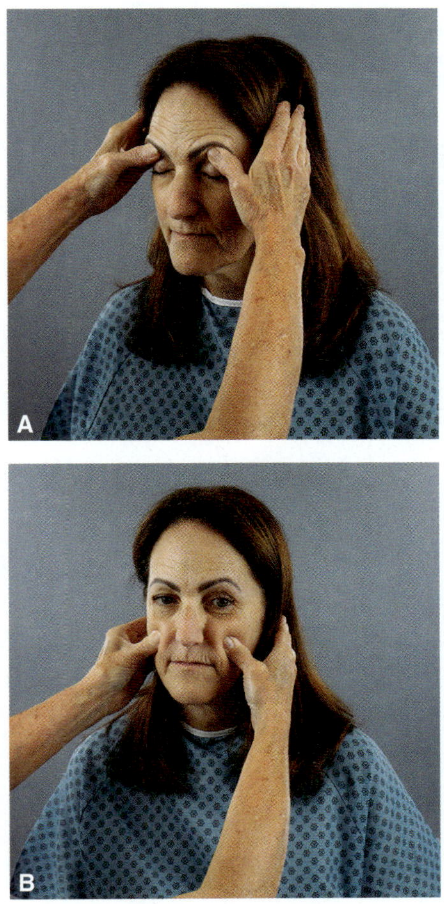

Figure 13-42 Palpation of sinuses. **A.** Palpation of frontal sinuses. **B.** Palpation of maxillary sinuses.

N A P Refer to maxillary sinuses.

To palpate and percuss the maxillary sinuses:

E
1. Stand in front of the client.
2. Apply gentle pressure in the area under the infraorbital ridge using the thumb or middle finger (Fig. 13-42B).
3. Observe for the presence of pain.
4. Percuss the area using the dominant middle or index finger.
5. Note the sound.

N **The client should experience no discomfort during palpation or percussion. The sinuses should be filled with air and therefore resonant to percussion.**

A The client complains of pain or tenderness at the site of palpation or percussion.

P Sinusitis can be due to viral, bacterial, fungal, or allergic processes that cause inflammation of the mucous membranes and obstruction of the drainage pathways.

A Percussion of the sinuses elicits a dull sound.

P Dullness can be caused by fluid or cells present in the sinus cavity from an infectious or allergic process, or congenital absence of a sinus.

ADVANCED TECHNIQUE

Transillumination of the Sinuses

If palpation and percussion of the sinuses suggest sinusitis, transillumination of the frontal and maxillary sinuses should be performed.

To evaluate the frontal sinuses:

E
1. Place the client in a sitting position facing you in a dark room.
2. Place a strong light source, such as a transilluminator, penlight, or tip of an otoscope with the speculum, under the bony ridge of the upper orbits (Fig. 13-43A).
3. Observe the red glow over the sinuses and compare the symmetry of the two sides.

To evaluate the maxillary sinuses:

E
1. Place the client in a sitting position facing you in a dark room.
2. Place the light source firmly under each eye and just above the infraorbital ridge (Fig. 13-43B).
3. Ask the client to open the mouth; observe the red glow on the hard palate (Fig. 13-43C).
4. Compare the two sides.

N **The glow on each side is equal, indicating air-filled frontal and maxillary sinuses.**

A Absence of glow is abnormal.

P Absence of glow suggests sinus congestion or the congenital absence of a sinus.

A An extremely bright glow is abnormal.

P This finding may be present in an older adult client with decreased subcutaneous fat.

Examination of the Mouth and Throat

Physical examination of the mouth includes the breath, lips, tongue, buccal mucosa, gums and teeth, hard and soft palates, and throat (oropharynx). Examination of the temporomandibular joint is discussed in Chapter 19. If the client is wearing dentures or removable orthodontia, ask that they

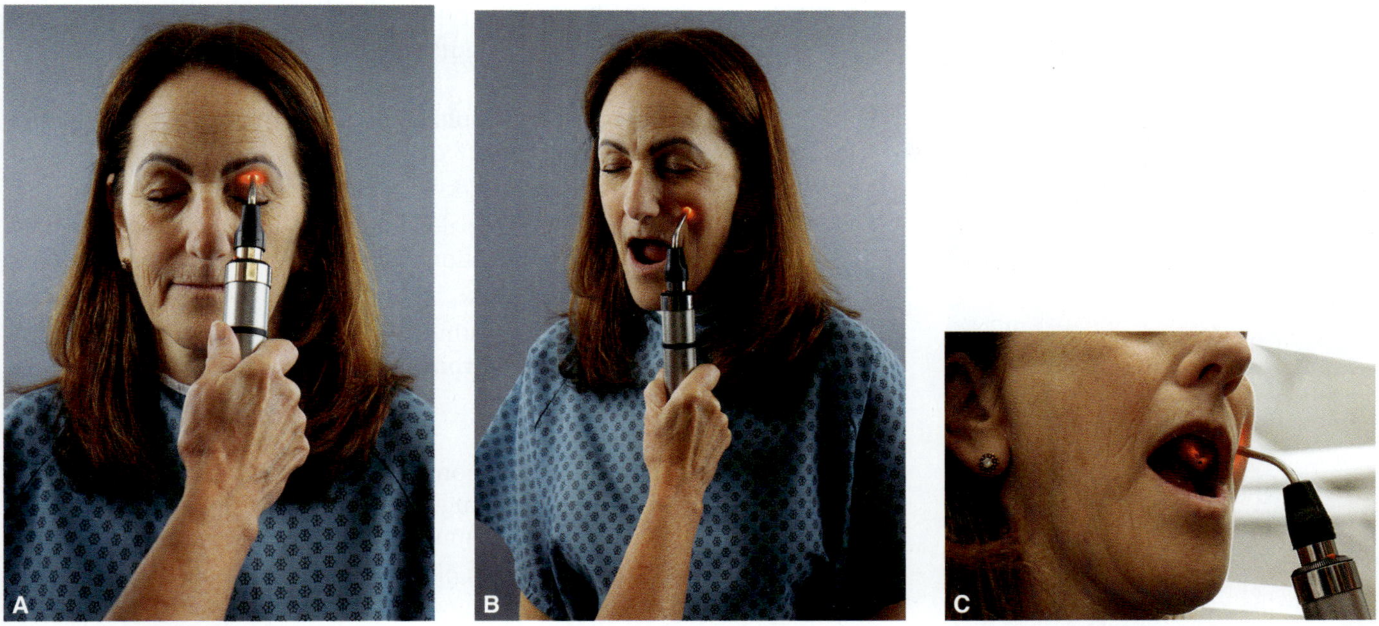

Figure 13-43 Transillumination of sinuses. **A.** Frontal sinus. **B.** Maxillary sinus. **C.** Transillum nation is visualized in the mouth.

be removed before the examination begins. Use gloves and a good light source (such as a penlight) for optimum visualization of the oral cavity and pharynx.

Examination of the Mouth

Breath

E
1. Stand facing the client and about 12 inches away.
2. Smell the breath.

N **The breath should smell fresh.**

A The breath smells foul.

P The foul smell of halitosis can be a symptom of gastroesophageal reflux disease, tooth decay, poor oral hygiene, or diseases of the gums, tonsils, or sinuses.

A The breath smells of acetone.

P Acetone or "fruity" breath is common in clients who are malnourished or who have diabetic ketoacidosis. The client may also be on a low-carbohydrate diet.

A The breath smells musty.

P Fetor hepaticus is the musty smell of the breath of a client with liver failure and is caused by the breakdown of nitrogen compounds.

A The breath smells of ammonia.

P The smell of ammonia can be detected in a client with end-stage renal failure (uremia) because of the inability to eliminate urea.

Lips

Inspection

E
1. Observe the lips for color, moisture, swelling, lesions, or other signs of inflammation.
2. Instruct the client to open their mouth.

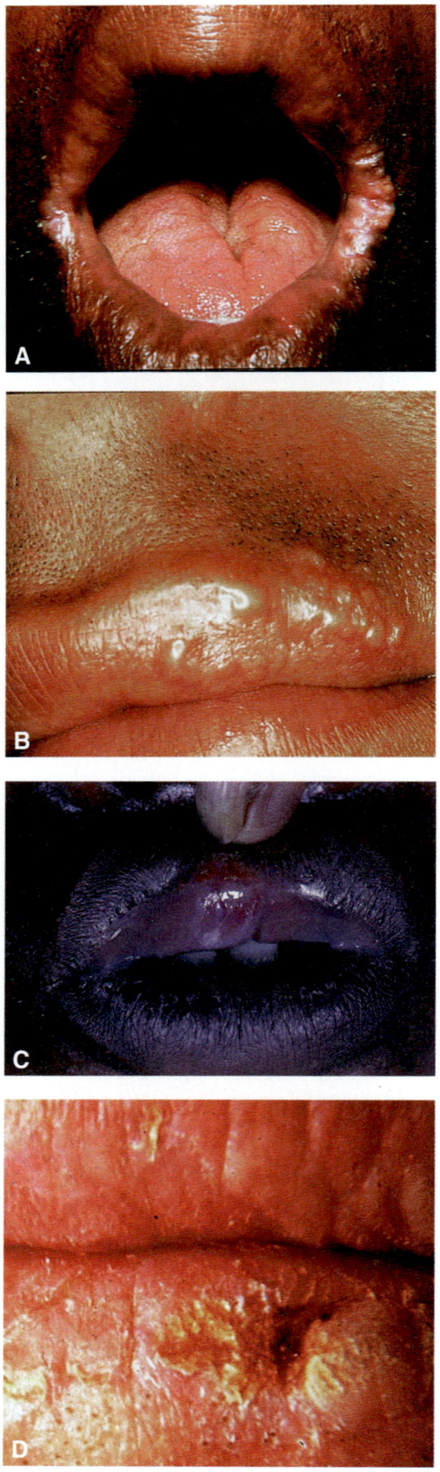

Figure 13-44 Lip abnormalities. **A.** Angular cheilosis. **B.** Fever blister (herpes simplex virus). **C.** Chancre from primary syphilis. **D.** Squamous cell carcinoma.

3. Use a tongue blade to inspect the membranes that connect the upper and lower lips to the gums for color, inflammation, lesions, and hydration.

N **The lips and membranes should be pink and moist with no evidence of lesions or inflammation.**

A The lips are pale or cyanotic.

P Many conditions can lead to pale or cyanotic lips such as vitamin deficiency, anemia, and oxygenation deficits. Refer to Chapters 7 and 17.

A The lips are dry and cracked.

P Chapping or superficial cracking of the lips may be due to exposure to wind, sun, or a dry environment, dehydration of the client, or persistent licking of the lips.

A Swelling of the lips is noted.

P Allergic reactions to medications, foods, or other allergens can result in swelling of the lips. Swelling of the lips due to an allergic reaction is called angioedema and is a medical emergency.

A The skin at the outer corners of the mouth is atrophic, irritated, and cracked (Fig. 13-44A).

P Angular cheilosis may be due to increased accumulation of saliva in the corners of the mouth or constant drooling from the mouth. This may be caused by nutritional deficiencies (such as riboflavin deficiency), poorly fitting dentures, and deficiencies in the immune system. *Candida* infections may also be present.

A Vesicles on erythematous bases with serous fluid are found on the lips, gums, or hard palate, either singly or in clusters. They can later rupture, crust over, and become painful (Fig. 13-44B).

P These findings are characteristic of herpes simplex lesions, which are commonly called cold sores or fever blisters. This common viral infection may be precipitated by febrile illness, sunlight, stress, or allergies.

A A round, painless lesion with central ulceration (Fig. 13-44C) is noted. This lesion may become crusted.

P A round, painless lesion with central ulceration on the lip describes a chancre, the primary lesion of syphilis.

A A plaque, wart, nodule, or ulcer is noted, usually on the lower lip.

P A plaque, wart, nodule, or ulcer on the lip may be squamous cell carcinoma, the most common form of oral cancer, which is more frequent in males (Fig. 13-44D).

P Basal cell carcinoma lesions can have pearly borders, crusting, and central ulcerations (Fig. 13-44E).

A Persistent, painless, white, painted-looking patches are noted on the lips (Fig. 13-44F).

P White, painted-looking patches on the lips are called leukoplakia and are considered premalignant lesions. They are associated with heavy smoking and the use of chewing tobacco. They often occur at sites of chronic irritation from dentures, tobacco, or excessive alcohol intake.

A A soft, pearly, round mass on the lip is abnormal (see Figure 13-45).

P A mucocele is caused by trauma to the mouth/lip such as being hit by a ball. It can also be caused by chronic lip biting. In a mucocele the damaged salivary ducts become obstructed. The drainage from the salivary duct then begins to form a cyst-like mass into the obstructed area in the lip.

Palpation

E
1. Don clean gloves.
2. Gently pull down the client's lower lip with the thumb and index finger of one hand and pull up the client's upper lip with the thumb and index finger of the other hand.
3. Note the tone of the lips as they are manipulated.
4. If lesions are present, palpate them for consistency and tenderness.

N **Lips should not be flaccid and lesions should not be present.**

A P See inspection of the lips for pathologies.

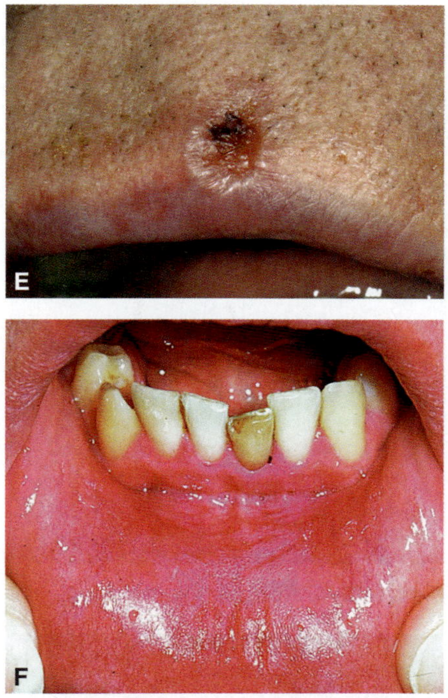

Figure 13-44—cont'd E. Basal cell carcinoma. **F.** Leukoplakia.

Tongue

E
1. Ask the client to stick out the tongue (CN XII assesses tongue movement).
2. Observe the dorsal surface for color, hydration, texture, symmetry, fasciculations, atrophy, position in the mouth, and the presence of lesions. Note the presence of any piercings (see Figure 13-46).
3. Ask the client to move the tongue from side to side and up and down.
4. With the client's tongue back in the mouth, ask the client to press it against the cheek. Provide resistance with your finger pads held on the outside of the cheek. Note the strength of the tongue and compare it bilaterally.
5. Ask the client to touch the tip of the tongue to the roof of the mouth. You may also grasp the tip of the tongue with a gauze square held between the thumb and the index finger of the gloved hand (Fig. 13-47).
6. Inspect the ventral surface of the tongue, the frenulum, and Wharton's ducts for color, hydration, lesions, inflammation, and vasculature.
7. With the gauze square, pull the tongue to the left and inspect and palpate the tongue using the finger pads.
8. Repeat with the tongue held to the right side.

N **The tongue is in the midline of the mouth. The dorsum of the tongue should be pink, moist, rough (from the taste buds), and without lesions. The tongue is symmetrical and moves freely. The strength of the tongue is symmetrical and strong. The ventral surface of the tongue has prominent blood vessels and should be moist and without lesions. Wharton's ducts are patent and without inflammation or lesions. The lateral aspects of the tongue should be pink, smooth, and lesion free.**

A The tongue is enlarged.

P An enlarged tongue may be associated with myxedema, acromegaly, Down syndrome, or amyloidosis. Transient enlargement may be associated with glossitis, stomatitis, cellulitis of the neck, angioneurotic edema, hematoma, or abscess.

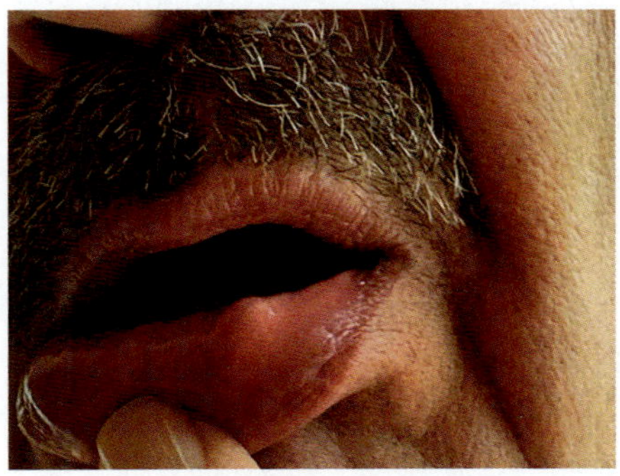

Figure 13-45 Mucocele.

A The tongue is red and smooth with absent papillae.

P A tongue that is red and smooth with absent papillae indicates glossitis, a tongue inflammation. Glossitis can be caused by a vitamin B_{12}, iron, or niacin deficiency. It may also be a side effect of chemotherapy.

A There is a thick, white, curd-like coating on the tongue that leaves a raw, red surface when it is scraped off (Fig. 13-48A).

P Candidiasis, or thrush, may also be red in the absence of the coating. Thrush can result from changes in the normal oral flora due to chemotherapy, radiation therapy, disorders of the immune system such as HIV, antibiotic therapy, or excessive use of alcohol, tobacco, or cocaine.

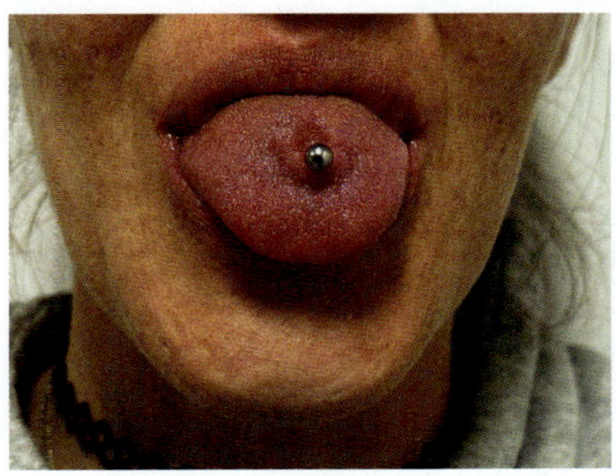

Figure 13-46 Tongue piercing.

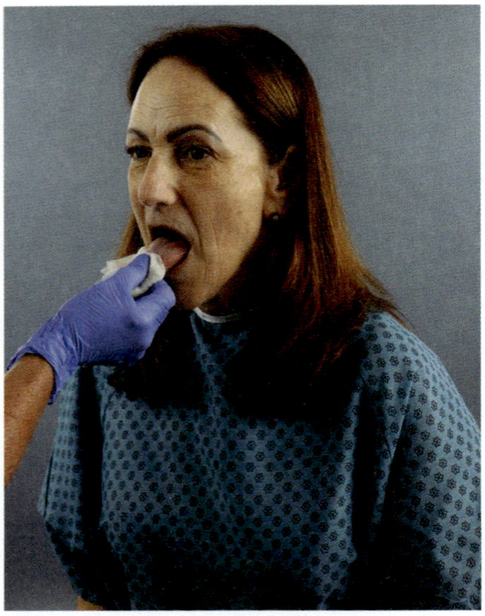

Figure 13-47 Tongue examination.

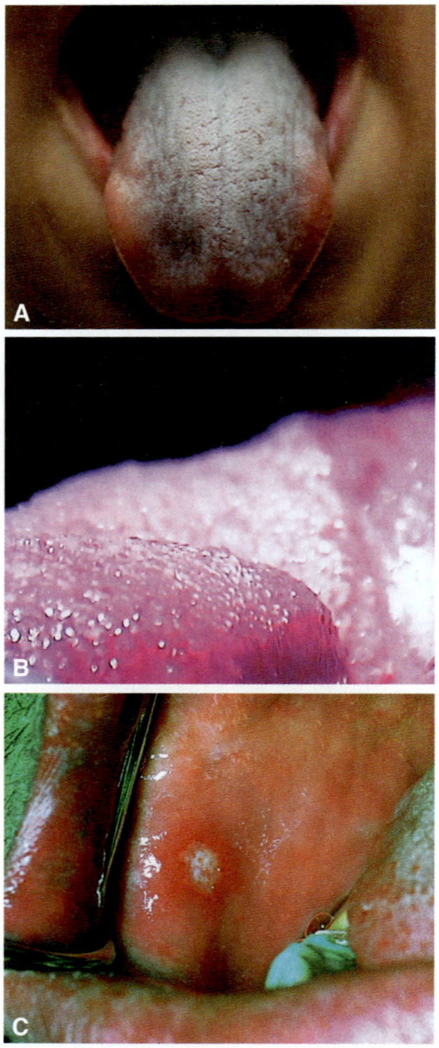

Figure 13-48 Tongue conditions. **A.** Candidiasis (thrush). **B.** Leukoplakia. **C.** Aphthous ulcer (canker sore).

A Thin, pearly white lesions that coalesce and become thick and palpable are noted on the sides of the tongue. These white lesions are firmly attached to the underlying tissue and will not scrape off.

P Leukoplakia (Fig. 13-48B) is considered a premalignant lesion. Some leukoplakia progresses from dysplasia to a malignancy.

A A painful, small, round white ulcerated lesion with erythematous borders is abnormal (Fig. 13-48C).

P An aphthous ulcer (canker sore) can be associated with stress, extreme fatigue, food allergies, and oral trauma.

A A short lingual frenulum is observed (Fig. 13-48D).

P Ankyloglossia is a congenital abnormality.

A The tongue has a hairy appearance and is yellow, black, or brown (Fig. 13-48E).

P Oral hairy leukoplakia, or hairy tongue, is a benign condition that can result from antibiotic therapy. The hairy appearance is caused by elongated papillae.

A Lesions are noted on the ventral surface of the tongue.

P The ventral surface of the tongue is an area where malignancies are likely to develop, especially in clients who drink alcohol and smoke or use smokeless tobacco.

A Indurations, or ulcerations (Fig. 13-48F), are present on the lateral surfaces of the tongue.

P Most lingual cancers are located in this area and are associated with the use of alcohol and tobacco.

A Patches of red denuded areas on the lingual surface of the tongue, frequently at the papillae, surrounded by ridges of pale yellow epithelium, are abnormal (Fig. 13-48G).

P Geographic tongue is a harmless condition and has no known cause. Its name is derived from the patterns of regular and irregular surfaces on the tongue that resemble a map.

A Numerous furrows or grooves are observed, often radiating horizontally from the midline of the dorsal surface of the tongue (Fig. 13-48H).

P Fissured or scrotal tongue is a harmless and often inherited condition. It is different from syphilitic glossitis, which is characterized by longitudinal furrows.

A Engorged blood vessels of the tongue are abnormal (Fig. 13-48I).

P A hemangioma of the tongue is a benign overgrowth of vascular tissue.

A Deviation of the tongue toward one side, atrophy, and asymmetrical shape of the tongue are abnormal.

P Unilateral paralysis of the tongue muscles will cause the tongue to deviate toward the affected side because the muscles on the paralyzed side are unable to oppose the strong muscles of the unaffected side. The client is unable to push the tongue toward the nonparalyzed side. Lesions of the hypoglossal nucleus or nerve fiber cause these unilateral symptoms.

A Atrophy of the tongue and the inability to protrude the tongue are abnormal.

P Bilateral paralysis of the tongue muscles will prevent the client from protruding the tongue. Syringobulbia or trauma to CN XII may cause hypoglossal nerve paralysis.

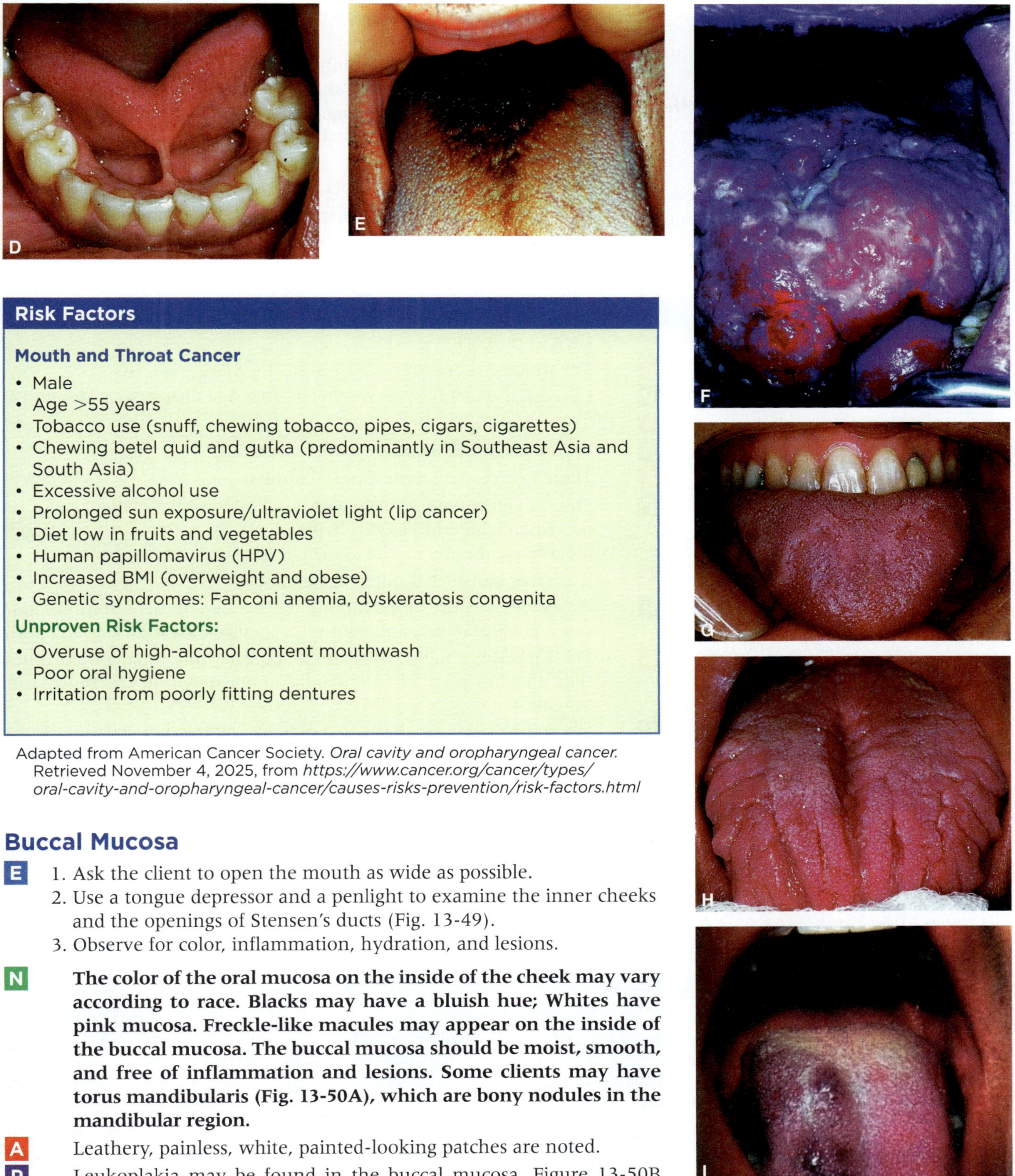

Figure 13-48—cont'd **D.** Ankyloglossia. **E.** Oral hairy leukoplakia. **F.** Carcinoma of the tongue. **G.** Geographic tongue. **H.** Fissured tongue (scrotal tongue). **I.** Hemangioma.

Risk Factors

Mouth and Throat Cancer

- Male
- Age >55 years
- Tobacco use (snuff, chewing tobacco, pipes, cigars, cigarettes)
- Chewing betel quid and gutka (predominantly in Southeast Asia and South Asia)
- Excessive alcohol use
- Prolonged sun exposure/ultraviolet light (lip cancer)
- Diet low in fruits and vegetables
- Human papillomavirus (HPV)
- Increased BMI (overweight and obese)
- Genetic syndromes: Fanconi anemia, dyskeratosis congenita

Unproven Risk Factors:

- Overuse of high-alcohol content mouthwash
- Poor oral hygiene
- Irritation from poorly fitting dentures

Adapted from American Cancer Society. *Oral cavity and oropharyngeal cancer.* Retrieved November 4, 2025, from *https://www.cancer.org/cancer/types/oral-cavity-and-oropharyngeal-cancer/causes-risks-prevention/risk-factors.html*

Buccal Mucosa

E
1. Ask the client to open the mouth as wide as possible.
2. Use a tongue depressor and a penlight to examine the inner cheeks and the openings of Stensen's ducts (Fig. 13-49).
3. Observe for color, inflammation, hydration, and lesions.

N **The color of the oral mucosa on the inside of the cheek may vary according to race. Blacks may have a bluish hue; Whites have pink mucosa. Freckle-like macules may appear on the inside of the buccal mucosa. The buccal mucosa should be moist, smooth, and free of inflammation and lesions. Some clients may have torus mandibularis (Fig. 13-50A), which are bony nodules in the mandibular region.**

A Leathery, painless, white, painted-looking patches are noted.

P Leukoplakia may be found in the buccal mucosa. Figure 13-50B shows leukoplakia caused by snuff.

A Yellow patches on the buccal mucosa are present.

P Yellow patches on the buccal mucosa are Fordyce spots, which are small sebaceous glands (Fig. 13-50C).

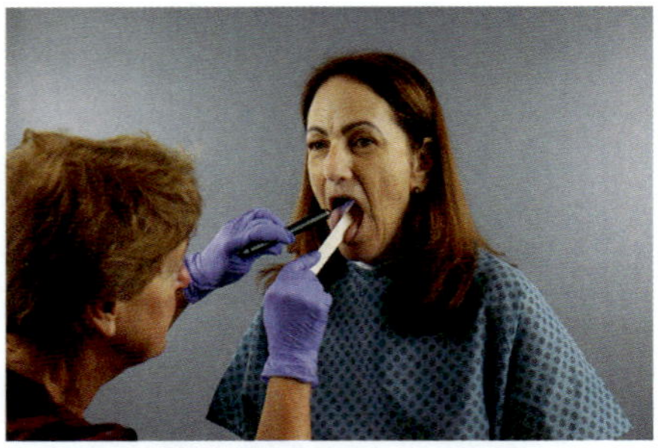

Figure 13-49 Examination of the buccal mucosa.

A The orifice of Stensen's duct is erythematous and edematous. It may be tender to palpation.

P This is seen in parotitis, an inflammation of the parotid gland. The area between the ear lobule and the angle of the mandible may not be visible due to the swelling of the parotid gland (Fig. 13-50D). Acute unilateral swelling may be seen in mumps.

A Small, round, white ulcers, surrounded by a halo of reddened mucosa, are found on the buccal mucosa.

P Small, round, white ulcers, surrounded by a halo of reddened mucosa, on the buccal mucosa are aphthous ulcers. Refer to Figure 13-48C.

A The mucosa is pale.

P Pale buccal mucosa can be caused by anemia or vasoconstriction that may occur when the sympathetic nervous system is stimulated, such as in shock.

A The mucosa is cyanotic.

P Cyanosis can indicate systemic hypoxemia. See Chapters 10, 16, and 17.

A The mucosa is erythematous.

P Erythema can be associated with stomatitis.

A There is excessive dryness of the mucosa.

P This is xerostomia, which occurs when salivary gland activity is decreased when the client is hypovolemic, or with mouth breathing, Sjögren syndrome, or salivary gland obstruction.

A Excessive moisture is noted in the mouth.

P Excessive moisture in the mouth may be seen in oral infections, gastroesophageal reflux, and with some medications (e.g., clonazepam).

A Flat-topped papules with thin, bluish-white spider-web lines (Fig. 13-50E) resembling leukoplakia are noted on the mucosa or tongue.

P Wickham's striae are the lesions of lichen planus, which is an inflammatory and pruritic disease of the skin and mucous membranes. It is usually a benign disease, and the cause is unknown.

Gums

E

1. Instruct the client to open their mouth.
2. Observe dentures or orthodontics for fit.
3. Remove any dentures or removable orthodontia.
4. Shine the penlight in the mouth.

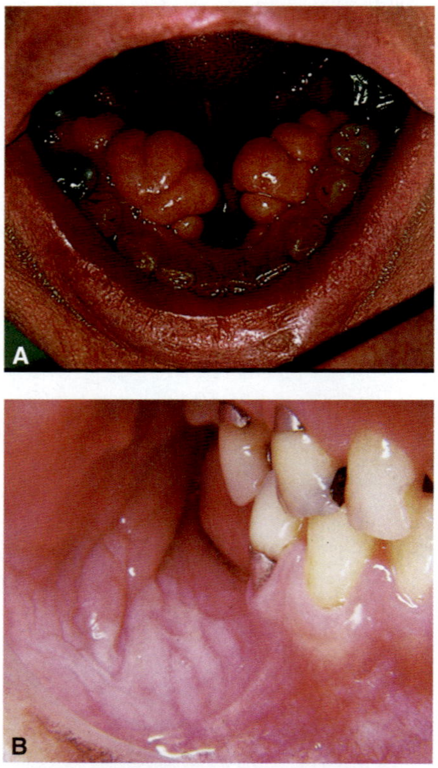

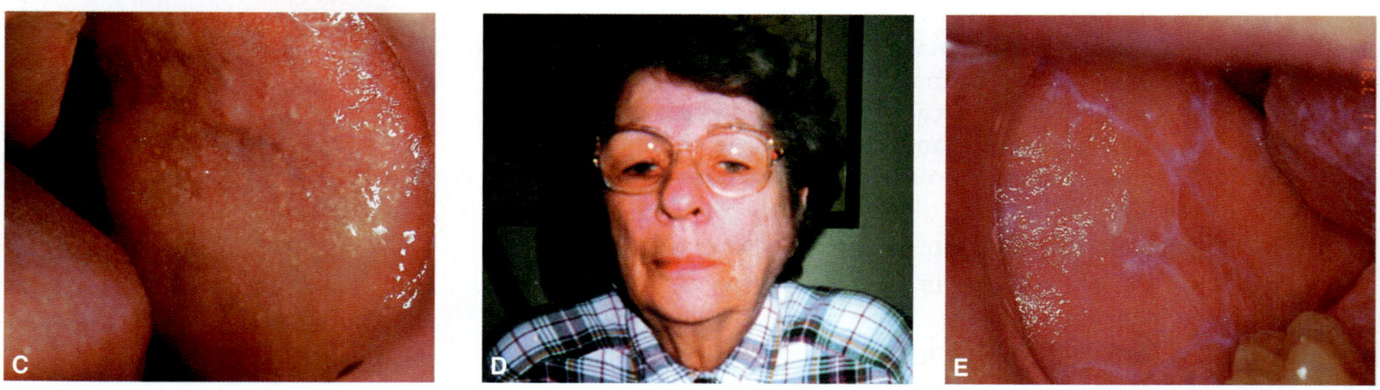

Figure 13-50 Buccal mucosa conditions. **A.** Torus mandibularis. **B.** Leukoplakia caused by snuff. **C.** Fordyce spots. **D.** Left parotitis. **E.** Lichen planus.

5. Use the tongue depressor to move the tongue to visualize the gums.
6. Observe for redness, swelling, bleeding, retraction from the teeth, or discoloration.

N **In light-skinned individuals, the gums have a pale red, stippled surface. Patchy brown pigmentation may be present in dark-skinned clients. The gum margins should be well defined with no pockets existing between the gums and the teeth and no swelling or bleeding.**

A The gingiva are red, tender, and swollen and bleed easily (Fig. 13-51).

P Red, tender, and swollen gingiva that bleed easily may be present in gingivitis, a gum inflammation. Gingivitis may be caused by poor dental hygiene, improperly fitted dentures, and scurvy. Gingivitis can also occur with stomatitis that occurs in mouth infections and upper respiratory tract infections.

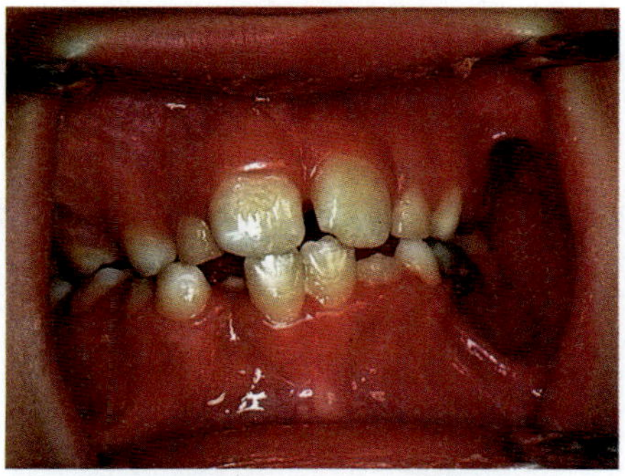

Figure 13-51 Gingivitis with herpes simplex.

A Gingival borders are red, and there is an infection of the pockets formed between receding gums and teeth. Purulent drainage may be present.

P Periodontitis is an inflammation of the periodontium due to chronic gingivitis. This condition is caused by infrequent brushing of the teeth and poor oral hygiene.

A Blue lines are noted approximately 1 mm from the gingival margin.

P Blue lines close to the gingival margin are lead bismuth lines caused by chronic exposure to lead or bismuth.

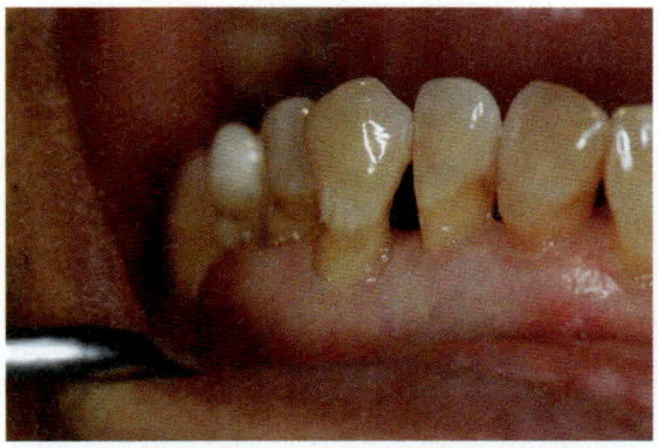

Figure 13-52 Gingival recession.

A The gums are brownish.

P Brownish gums can occur in Addison disease, an adrenal insufficiency.

A A grayish membrane is noted over an inflamed and ulcerated area of the mucosa.

P This condition is Vincent stomatitis, or trench mouth, a bacterial infection of the gums that may extend into pharyngeal structures and bones.

A A nontender, immobile tumor lighter in color than the gums is present.

P This lesion is epulis, a fibrous tumor of the gums.

A The gums are retracted from the teeth (Fig. 13-52), sometimes exposing the roots of the teeth.

P This recession of the gums often occurs in older adults due to poor oral hygiene and in those who aggressively brush their teeth. Gum recession is also seen in clients who grind their teeth. Wearing a nighttime mouthguard can slow gum recession in clients who grind their teeth.

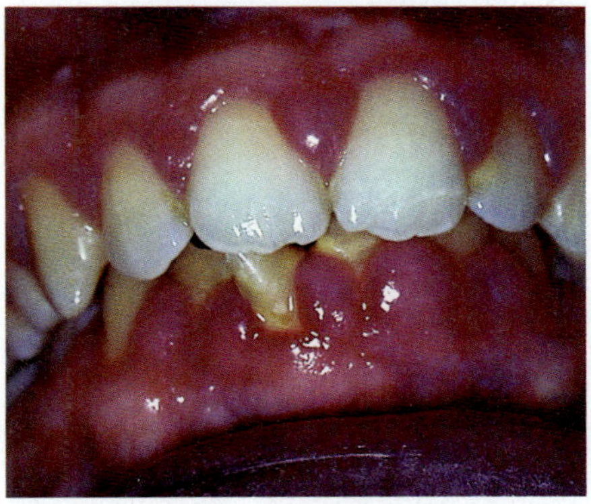

Figure 13-53 Gingival hyperplasia.

A Hypertrophy of gum tissue is abnormal (Fig. 13-53).

P This is called gingival hyperplasia and is usually painless; it occurs in pregnancy, in wearers of orthodontic braces, because of dental plaque, or with the use of some medications such as phenytoin.

A Small ulcers or folds of excess tissue are noted on the gums under an ill-fitting denture. Inflamed and swollen nodules may be seen in the area of the palate.

P Continued irritation of the gums by ill-fitting dentures results in hyperplasia.

Teeth

E
1. Instruct the client to open their mouth.
2. Count the upper and lower teeth.

3. Observe the teeth for discoloration, loose or missing teeth, caries, malocclusion, and malformation.

N **The adult normally has 32 teeth, which should be white with smooth edges, in proper alignment, and without caries.**

A Teeth are absent.

P Absent teeth may be due to a failure of development. Trauma can lead to absent teeth as well as nutritional deficits and poor oral hygiene. The client's nutritional status may be seriously impaired when the number of teeth is reduced.

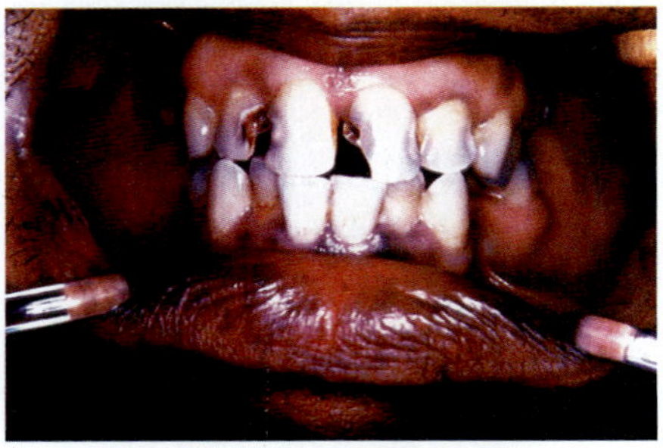

Figure 13-54 Dental caries.

A There are white or black patches on the surface of a tooth. These patches may become eroded as damage progresses (Fig. 13-54).

P These are dental caries, or cavities, resulting from poor oral hygiene.

A The teeth are worn at an angle.

P Biting surfaces of the teeth may become worn down by repetitive biting on hard substances or objects or grinding of teeth, called bruxism, especially at night.

A A tooth is dark in color, and the client reports insensitivity to cold.

P This is usually a dead tooth, which results in a darkening of the enamel.

A Teeth that are blackened, broken off at the gum line, and highly sensitive to temperature change are abnormal.

P Methamphetamine addiction results in decreased salivary production and poor dental hygiene. This condition is referred to as "meth mouth" (Fig. 13-55).

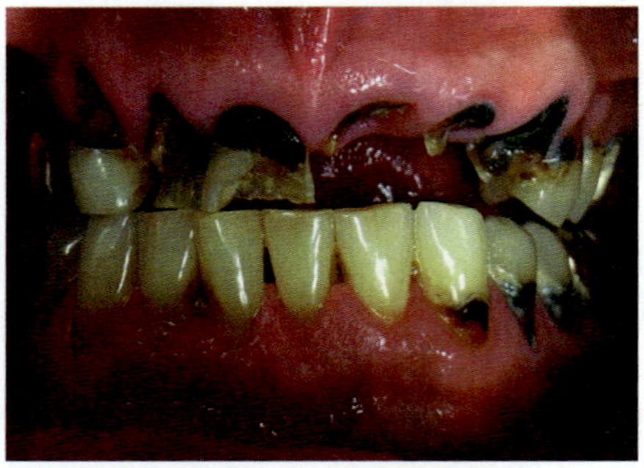

Figure 13-55 Meth mouth.

A Teeth that have serrated edges (Fig. 13-56) are abnormal.

P These are called Hutchinson's incisors. The infants of pregnant women with syphilis can have abnormal fetal dentition because of the effects of the disease on tooth development.

Palate

E
1. Ask the client to tilt the head back and open the mouth as wide as possible.
2. Shine the penlight in the client's mouth.
3. Observe both the hard and the soft palates.
4. Note the palate's shape and color and the presence of any lesions or malformations.

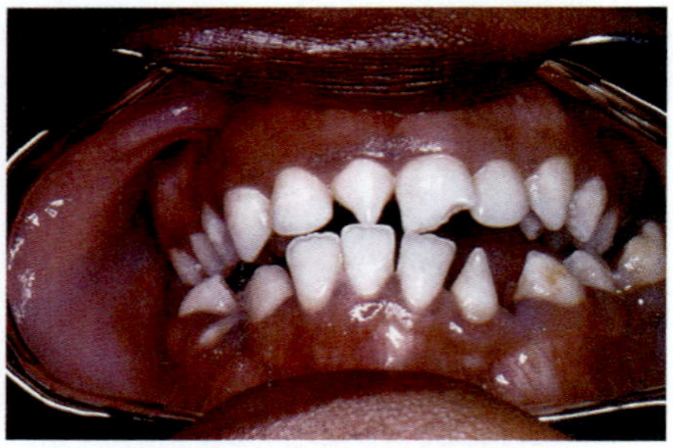

Figure 13-56 Hutchinson's incisors.

N **The hard and soft palates are concave and pink. The hard palate has many ridges; the soft palate is smooth. No lesions or malformations are noted.**

A The palates are red, swollen, tender, or with lesions.

P A palate that is red, swollen, tender, or with lesions may be infected.

A There is a bony ridge in the midline of the hard palate (Fig. 13-57).

P A bony ridge in the midline of the hard palate is a benign condition called torus palatinus, which develops in adulthood.

A A fibrous, encapsulated tissue growth on the palate is abnormal (Fig. 13-58).

P A fibroma may be idiopathic or neoplastic in origin. Chronic trauma can also lead to fibroma formation.

A A lesion that has become eroded is noted on the palate.

P An eroded lesion may be a cancerous lesion in the epithelium of the hard palate.

A The palate is highly arched.

P A highly arched palate is associated with Turner syndrome and Marfan syndrome.

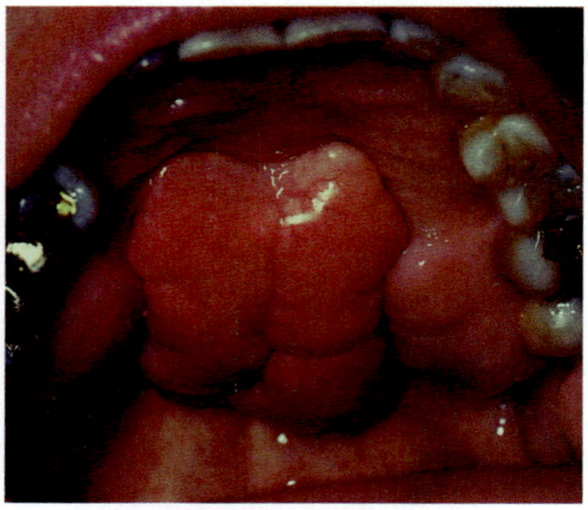

Figure 13-57 Torus palatinus.

A There is a hole in the hard palate (Fig. 13-59).

P Palatine perforation is related to syphilis or radiation therapy.

Inspection of the Throat

E

1. Ask the client to tilt the head back and to open the mouth widely. The client can either stick out the tongue or leave it resting on the floor of the mouth. Asking the client to yawn may allow better visualization of the posterior oral pharynx.
2. With the right hand, place the tongue blade on the middle third of the tongue.
3. With the left hand, shine a light at the back of the client's throat.
4. Ask the client to say "ah."
5. Observe the position, size, color, and general appearance of the tonsils and uvula.
6. Touch the posterior third of the tongue with the tongue blade.
7. Note the movement of the palate and the presence of the gag reflex.
8. Examine the color of the oropharynx. Note the presence of swelling, exudate, or lesions.

N **When the client says "ah," the soft palate and the uvula should rise symmetrically (CN IX and X). The uvula is midline. The throat is normally pink and vascular and without swelling, exudate, or lesions. Normal tonsillar size is evaluated as 1 + to 2 +. This indicates that both tonsils are behind the pillars. Refer to Figure 13-60 for a tonsillar grading scale. A variant of a normal tonsil is the cryptic tonsil—a tonsil that contains small folds and pockets. Cryptic tonsils can harbor food debris, bacteria, and sloughed cells that place the client at risk for tonsillitis. The client's gag reflex should be present but is congenitally absent in some clients (CN IX and X).**

A The posterior pharynx is red with white patches. The tonsils are large and red with white patches, and the uvula is red and swollen.

P Viral pharyngitis and tonsillitis are common illnesses with these findings. It is not uncommon to have these clinical findings in a client with infectious mononucleosis.

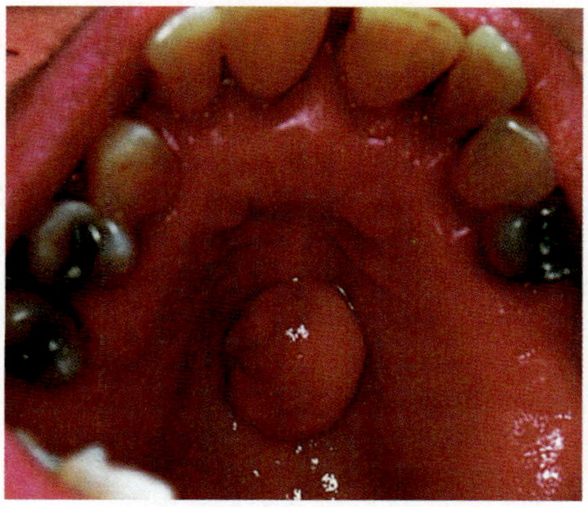

Figure 13-58 Fibroma.

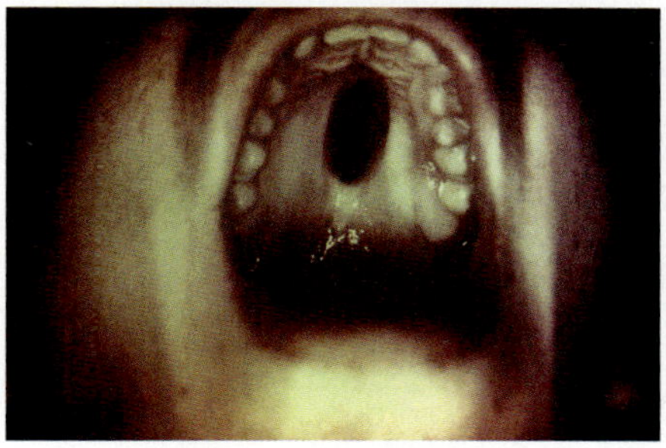

Figure 13-59 Palatine perforation caused by a congenital syphilis infection.

> **NURSING TIP**
> **Eliciting the Gag Reflex**
> Before eliciting the gag reflex, be sure to warn the client about what to expect during your examination. It may not be necessary to elicit the gag reflex if the palate and uvula rise symmetrically with phonation.

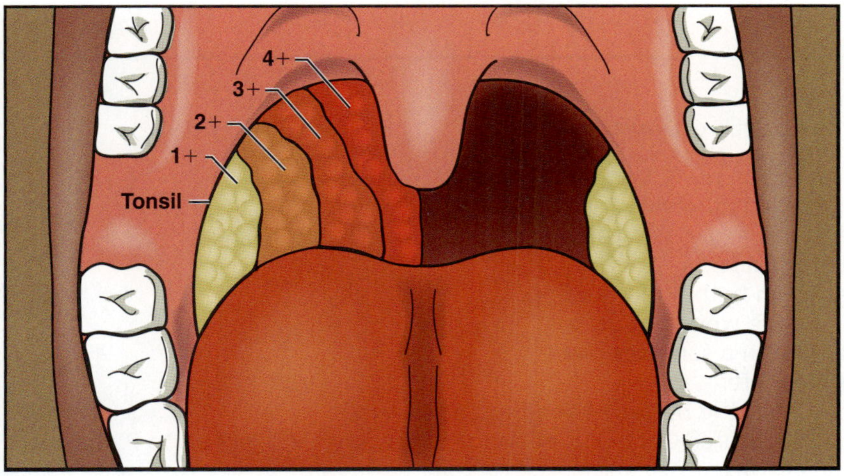

Figure 13-60 Grading of tonsils: 1 + tonsils are visible, 2 + tonsils are between the pillars and uvula, 3 + tonsils extend beyond the pillars but do not touch the uvula, and 4 + tonsils extend to the midline of the oropharynx.

E Examination **N** Normal Findings **A** Abnormal Findings **P** Pathophysiology

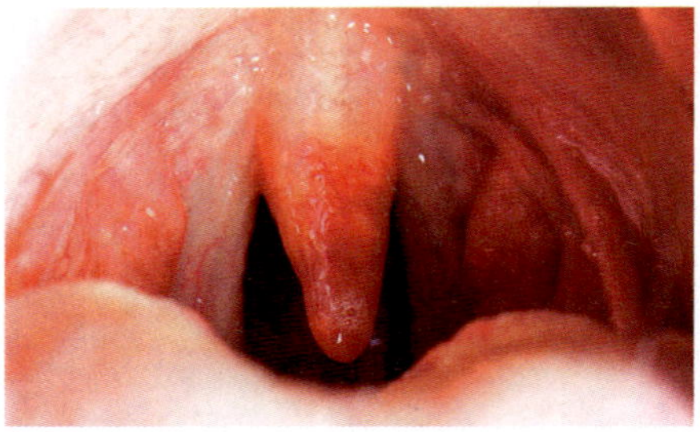

Figure 13-61 Streptococcal pharyngitis.

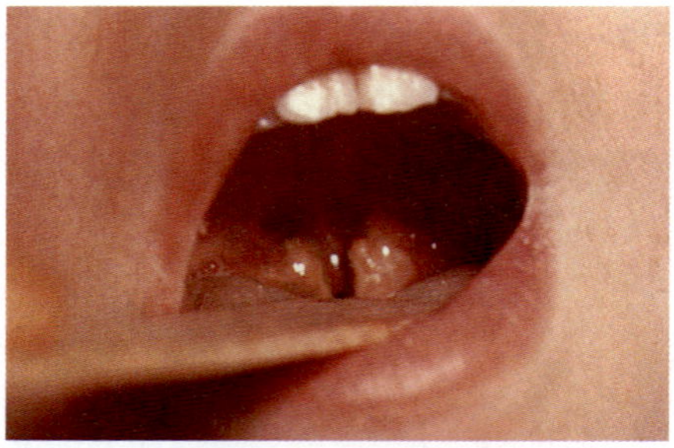

Figure 13-62 A grayish membrane can form over the mucous membranes in the mouth and oropharynx in diphtheria.

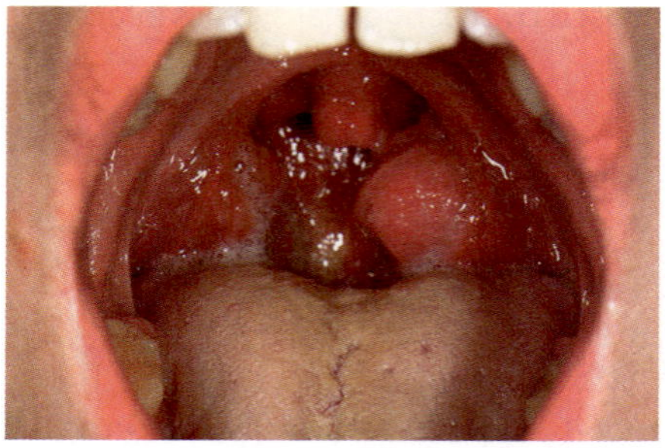

Figure 13-63 Left tonsil is 4 + and right tonsil is 3 +.

A Tonsils, pillars, and uvula are very red and swollen, with patches of white or yellow exudate on the tonsils (Fig. 13-61). The posterior pharynx is bright red. The client reports soreness of the throat with swallowing.

P Streptococcal pharyngitis and tonsillitis are usually associated with significant lymphadenopathy. However, the diagnosis requires a throat culture or rapid strep test.

A There is a grayish membrane covering the tonsils, uvula, and soft palate (Fig. 13-62).

P A grayish membrane covering the oropharynx, tonsils, uvula, and soft palate are typical of diphtheria, acute tonsillitis, or infectious mononucleosis.

A The debris in cryptic tonsils can harden and turn yellow or white and create a tonsil stone.

P The tonsil stone is called a tonsillolith. It is a painless and harmless clinical finding that can cause pharyngitis and halitosis. Usually there is no treatment for the tonsillolith unless it becomes infected.

A The client speaks with a hoarse voice and the oropharynx is red.

P Causes of hoarseness are varied and may include overuse of the voice, inflammation due to viral or bacterial infection, lesions of the larynx, foreign bodies, and pressure on the larynx from masses or an enlarged thyroid gland.

A The client has difficulty opening the mouth (trismus) and is noted to have unilateral tonsillar swelling. Unusual phonation is also observed.

P Peritonsillar abscess is most commonly seen in older children and young adults with a history of frequent tonsillitis.

A Chronic 3 + or 4 + tonsils (Fig. 13-63) are abnormal.

P Large tonsils frequently lead to loud snoring and obstructive sleep apnea.

A The client has a small oropharynx and a history of snoring.

P Obstructive sleep apnea occurs when muscles in the nasopharynx and pharynx relax during sleep, resulting in pauses in breathing. Typically, clients are overweight, middle-aged males who complain of excessive daytime sleepiness.

NURSING CHECKLIST

Assessing Clients With Hearing and Oral Assistive Devices

Hearing Aids

- Hands need to be clean and dry when handling hearing aids.
- Clean hearing aids per manufacturer's directions; avoid using alcohol, solvents, or cleaning agents.
- Avoid getting hairspray and makeup on hearing aids.
- Avoid getting the hearing aids wet; remove when bathing/swimming.
- Always place the hearing aids in a protective case when not using.
- Follow a daily routine and keep the hearing aids in a safe, dry place.
- Turn off when not in use to preserve the battery life.
- Be aware of the beeping sounds that indicate that the batteries need to be changed.
- Change the batteries as indicated by the manufacturer. Generally, hearing aid batteries will last up to 22 days.
- Have a health-care professional remove any ear wax.

Oral Appliances

- Clean oral appliance per manufacturer's directions.
- Let the oral appliance dry completely before storing; clean the storage container regularly.
- Clean the oral appliance if it falls on the ground.
- Take the oral appliance to dental visits for the dentist to evaluate its condition.

Nasal Rinse Devices

Nasal saline rinses are used to irrigate the nasal passages. This helps to decrease nasal congestion that is related to allergies, environmental irritants, and the common cold. Neti pots, NeilMed rinses, bulb syringes, squeeze bottles, and battery-operated pulsed water devices are considered safe and effective nasal rinse devices if used and cleaned properly.

Client Instructions for Usage:

- Advise the client that only distilled water, sterile water, or water that has been boiled for at least 3 to 5 minutes and cooled, or water that was properly boiled within the past 24 hours should be used.
- Do not use tap water as it can contain harmful organisms.
- Follow the instructions provided for proper usage of the device.
- Wash and dry the device after each use and store it in a dry place.
- Clean the device according to the manufacturer's directions.
- Advise the client to consult a health-care provider for the frequency and duration in which the nasal rinsing can be performed.
- Advise the client to discontinue the nasal rinsing if they experience pain, bleeding, or persistent nasal congestion.

Adapted from U.S. Food & Drug Administration. Is rinsing your sinuses with neti-pots safe? Retrieved on November 4, 2025, from *https://www.fda.gov/consumers/consumer-updates/rinsing-your-sinuses-neti-pots-safe*

U.S. Preventive Services Task Force (USPSTF)

There are no USPSTF recommendations, Grade A or B Statements, for the ears, nose, mouth, or throat.

CASE STUDY

The Client With Streptococcal Pharyngitis

This case study illustrates the application and the objective documentation of the ears, nose, mouth, and throat examination. Mandi is complaining of a sore throat for a few days. Mandi is concerned that she picked up a "bug" at a party last weekend. Mandi and her husband have an autistic son, Jake, who attends school full time. Jake requires a lot of Mandi's attention when the school bus drops him off in the afternoon.

HEALTH HISTORY

CLIENT PROFILE

34-year-old White female

CHIEF COMPLAINT

"I have had a sore throat and fever for 2 days. I need to be well to look after my autistic son."

HISTORY OF PRESENT ILLNESS

The client was in her usual state of good health until 3 days ago when she developed sore throat, nasal congestion, rhinorrhea with clear to yellow drainage. Client started with a low-grade temperature of 100°F, yesterday the temperature rose to 102.5°F. Client reports that the sore throat has increased in intensity over the past 2 days, from 4/10 to 8/10 intensity now. Also reporting headache and fatigue for the past 3 days. Mandi denies cough, wheezing, dyspnea, abdominal pain. She has been taking acetaminophen 1,000 mg every 12 hours for the past 2 days, and it has eased the sore throat pain and headache and decreased the temperature to 101.5°F.

PAST HEALTH HISTORY

Medical History Treated for streptococcal pharyngitis with azithromycin pack 4 times within the last 2 years; never had mononucleosis
Vitamin D deficiency

Surgical History Laparoscopy cholecystectomy age 30
C-Section age 28 with bilateral tubal ligation

Allergies Penicillin (reports a rash, nausea, and vomiting)

Medications Acetaminophen 1,000 mg every 12 hours for the last 2 days
Vitamin D 1,000 IU daily

Communicable Diseases Denies

Injuries and Accidents None

Differing Needs None

Blood Transfusions None

Childhood Illnesses Chickenpox age 4

Immunizations Up to date; annual flu vaccine, COVID-19 Vaccine × 4, Tdap 6 years ago

FAMILY HEALTH HISTORY

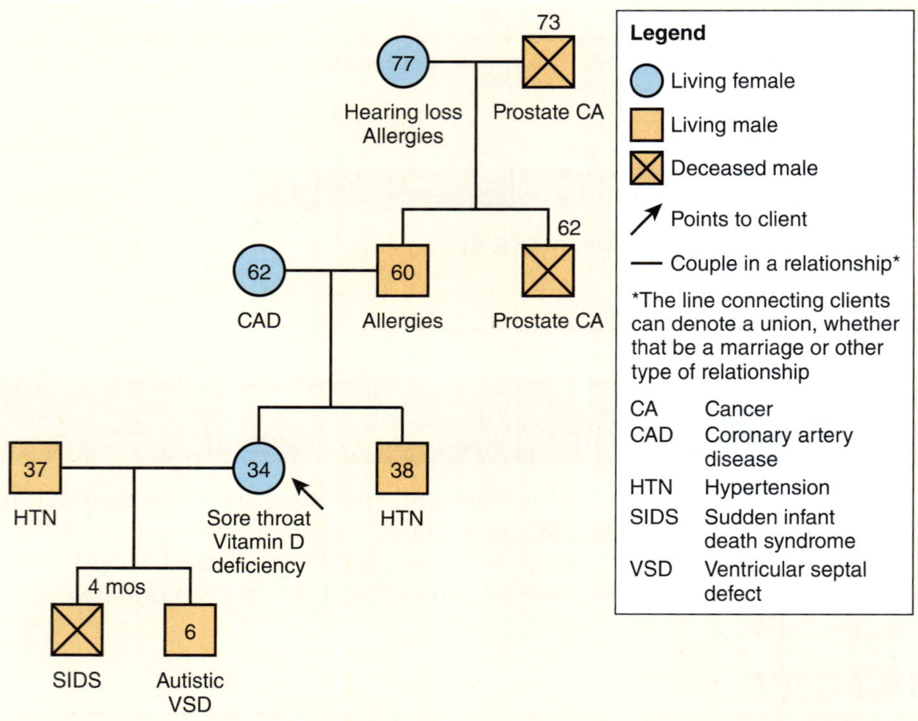

Denies family history of otitis media, otosclerosis.

SOCIAL HISTORY

Alcohol Use Denies

Tobacco Use Denies use of cigarettes, chewing tobacco, pipes, cigars, snuff

Recreational Drug Use Denies

Domestic and Intimate Partner Violence Denies

Sexual Practice Heterosexual relationship—one partner (husband), married 10 years

Travel History Never been out of the country

Work Environment Works from home as a medical coder, full time

Home Environment Lives with husband and 6-year-old son in a two-story home. Home equipped with smoke detectors and carbon monoxide detectors. Denies firearms in home

Hobbies and Leisure Activities Gardening, playing with son; participates in a monthly book club

Stress Assisting with the care of grandparents who live 45 minutes away and taking care of autistic son after school and on weekends; client and husband share care of son. Jake has bouts of poor health and client does everything she can to keep him well.

Education Associate Degree in Marketing and certificate in Medical Coding

Economic Status Middle class; husband works outside the home as a soft drink vendor salesperson

Military Service None

Religion Baptist, nonpracticing

Ethnic Background Uncertain of ethnic background

Roles and Relationships Reports an excellent relationship with husband, son, parents, and grandparents

Characteristic Patterns of Daily Living Wakes at 5:00 AM Monday–Friday for work. Her husband helps son get on the school bus so client can start working early and be done by the time son gets off the school bus at 4:20 PM

HEALTH MAINTENANCE ACTIVITIES

Sleep 7 to 8 hours of sleep during the week; 9 hours on the weekends

Diet No special diet

Exercise Walks at least 1 mile, 2 times a week with husband and son

Stress Management Talks with friends and family

Use of Safety Devices Uses seat belts in car

Health Checkups Has annual well-women examinations by GYN; dental checkup every 6 months

Only urgent care visits when sick, does not have a regular health-care provider

PHYSICAL EXAMINATION

Ears

Auditory Screening

Voice-whisper test: intact

Tuning fork tests

Weber: no lateralization of sound

Rinne: AC > BC

External Ear No redness, drainage, deformities, nodules, or lesions. Nontender, EAC clear without inflammation, no mastoid tenderness

Otoscopic Examination Bilateral TMs intact with mild erythema, mobile with visible light reflex, without bulging or perforation

Nose

External Inspection Midline without swelling, bleeding, lesions, or masses

Patency Both nares patent

Internal Inspection Mucosa is erythemic, with clear nasal discharge bilaterally

Sinuses

Inspection No swelling around nose and eyes

Palpation and Percussion Minimal tenderness to palpation of the maxillary sinuses. Resonant to percussion

Mouth

Breath No odor noted

Lips Pink, moist without lesions, nontender

Tongue Midline, pink, well papillated without fasciculations; no lesions, swelling, or bleeding; symmetrical movement

Buccal Mucosa Pink, moist without lesions

Gums Pink and moist without swelling or bleeding

Teeth 32 present with proper alignment, no caries
Palate Intact, rises with phonation

Throat Posterior pharynx erythematous without exudate; grade + 3/4 + erythematous, cryptic tonsils with white exudative patches bilaterally; uvula midline, gag reflex present

Diagnostic procedures

Rapid Strep Test: positive group A beta-hemolytic streptococcus
Monospot: negative

CLINICAL JUDGMENT IN ACTION

1. What cues indicate that the client is having a disorder of the ears, nose, mouth, and throat?
2. What interventions have the highest priority?
3. What assessment findings indicate clinical improvement or decline in this client?

Review Questions

1. Which of the following factors contribute to halitosis? Select all that apply.
   a. Gum disease
   b. Uncontrolled diabetes mellitus
   c. Decreased hydration
   d. Sinusitis
   e. Oral candidiasis
2. Which of the following physical examination findings would a client with acute otitis media (AOM) exhibit? Select all that apply.
   a. Tympanic membrane—TM bulging
   b. Pain with movement of the tragus
   c. Tympanic membrane—TM landmarks diffuse and/or displaced
   d. Tympanic membrane—TM is yellowish in color
   e. Pain with movement of the ear antihelix
3. When performing an auditory screening, which examination finding is cause for concern?
   a. Negative Weber test
   b. Whisper words repeated at 2 feet
   c. Negative Rinne test
   d. Air conduction is heard twice as long as bone conduction
4. The nurse examines a 70-year-old client and notes that the tongue is red and smooth without papillae. What are the causes that could be associated with this finding? Select all that apply.
   a. Iron deficiency
   b. Vitamin B_{12} deficiency
   c. A side effect of chemotherapy
   d. Niacin deficiency
   e. Oral candidiasis
5. Trauma to which cranial nerve (CN) can cause hypoglossal nerve paralysis?
   a. CN I and II
   b. CN V
   c. CN X
   d. CN XII
6. What are the physical findings that the nurse would expect to find in a client with pharyngitis? Select all that apply.
   a. The posterior pharynx is erythematous.
   b. The uvula is erythematous and edematous.
   c. Tonsils are +3 with white patches of exudate.
   d. The gingiva is erythematous, tender, and swollen.
   e. A bony ridge is present in the hard palate.
7. During a physical examination, the nurse finds a lesion on the upper lip that is crusting with pearly borders and central ulceration. This finding is consistent with which condition?
   a. Basal cell carcinoma
   b. Squamous cell carcinoma
   c. Herpes simplex
   d. Chancre
8. Which of the following are risk factors for oral cancer? Select all that apply.
   a. Age >45 years old
   b. Male sex
   c. Chewing gum
   d. History of leukoplakia
   e. Oral human papillomavirus

9. Which of the following statements regarding the ear is correct? Select all that apply.
   a. The external ear, known as the pinna, extends through the auditory canal to the tympanic membrane.
   b. The ear comprises three sections: external, middle, and inner ear.
   c. The external auditory canal is an S-shaped tube approximately 2.5 cm in length.
   d. The ossicles have no necessary function.
   e. A decibel reading of 130 dB is heard with conversation.

10. During the examination of the nose, you note that the nasal mucosa is red and swollen. Purulent nasal discharge is seen in the right naris. These findings are commonly associated with which of the following?
    a. Hay fever
    b. Rhinitis
    c. Bacterial sinusitis
    d. Nasal inhalation of cocaine or amphetamines

CHAPTER

14

Breasts and Regional Lymph Nodes

Learning Outcomes

1. Describe the anatomy and physiology of the breasts and regional lymph nodes.
2. Conduct a complete health history on a client with breast and regional lymph node pathology.
3. Identify risk factors for breast cancer.
4. Perform a physical examination of a client's breasts and regional lymph nodes.
5. Differentiate normal breast and regional lymph node physical examination clinical findings from abnormal clinical findings.
6. Describe male breast cancer screening and how to conduct a clinical breast examination on a male client.
7. Identify the United States Preventive Services Task Force recommendations for breast cancer screening.
8. Document a complete history and physical examination of a client with breast and regional lymph node pathology.

The breasts hold significant symbolism in our society. In females, they are an external symbol of sexuality, femininity, and nurturance. In males, they symbolize strength, fitness, and masculinity. Breast disease and its devastating effects have come to the forefront of public attention in recent years. Breast cancer incidence rates have increased significantly over the past 50 years, with Blacks dying exponentially faster than Whites from the disease; however, survival rates remain constant despite increased research dollars and public attention to preventative screening. The current 5-year survival rate is 91% compared with 75% in 1975 due to improvements in breast cancer treatment (National Cancer Institute, n.d.).

Long-term survival rates have a direct correlation with early detection of breast cancer. Nurses can have a major impact on a client's health by encouraging breast self-awareness and by supporting a client in achieving healthier lifestyles, which are believed to minimize breast cancer risk.

This chapter focuses primarily on the female breast because it is a more complicated structure than the male gland and because of the higher incidence of breast disease. Of the number of breast cancer cases, 99% occur in women and 1% in men (American Cancer Society, 2019, 2024). Examination of the male breast and breast cancer screening will also be discussed.

Anatomy and Physiology

Breasts

The female breasts are a pair of mammary glands located on the anterior chest wall, extending vertically from the second to the sixth rib and laterally from the sternal border to the axilla. Anatomically, the breast may be divided into four quadrants: the upper inner quadrant, the lower inner quadrant, the upper outer quadrant, and the lower outer quadrant (Fig. 14-1). The upper outer quadrant, which extends into the axilla, is known as the tail of Spence. The breasts are supported by a bed of muscles: the pectoralis major and minor, latissimus dorsi, serratus anterior, rectus abdominis, and external oblique muscles, which extend vertically from the deep fascia (Fig. 14-2). Cooper's ligaments, which extend vertically from the deep fascia through the breast to the inner layer of the skin, provide support for the breast tissue (Fig. 14-3).

In the center of each breast is the nipple, a round, hairless, pigmented protrusion of erectile tissue approximately 0.5 to 1.5 cm in diameter. The nipple becomes more erect during sexual excitement, pregnancy, lactation, cold temperatures, and certain phases of the menstrual cycle. There are 12- to 20-minute openings on the surface of the nipple. These are openings of the lactiferous ducts through which milk and colostrum are excreted.

The milk line, or ectodermal galactic band, shown in Figure 14-4A, develops from the axilla to the groin during the fifth week of fetal development. Most of the band atrophies except in the thoracic area, where it forms a mammary ridge. Incomplete atrophy of the galactic band results in the development of extra nipples or breast tissue known as supernumerary nipples, shown in Figure 14-4B. The additional nipples or mammary tissue develop along the milk lines and are a normal variant in a small percentage of adult women. This may also occur in men.

Surrounding the nipple is the areola, a pigmented area approximately 2.5 to 10 cm in diameter. The size and pigmentation vary from patient to patient. Several sebaceous glands (Montgomery's tubercles) are present on the surface of the areola. These glands lubricate the nipple, helping to keep it supple during lactation. Hair follicles punctuate the border of the areola.

The breast is composed of glandular, connective (Cooper's ligaments), and adipose tissue. The glandular tissue is arranged radially in the form of 12 to

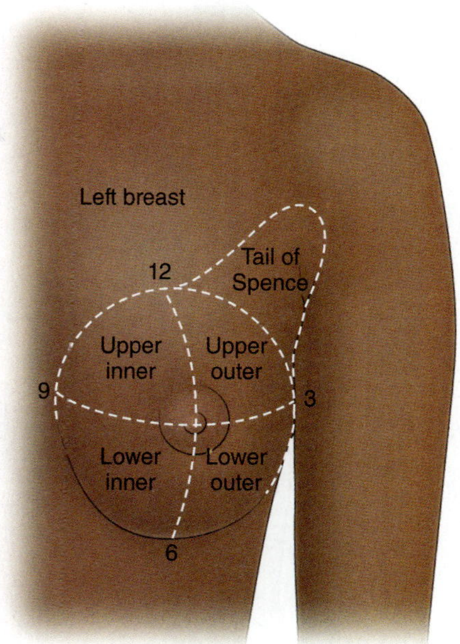

Figure 14-1 Quadrants of the left breast. Note the numbers on the breast. They represent the hours of a clock face that can be used to specify the location of a finding on the circular breast. The right breast clock notation is a mirror image of the left breast.

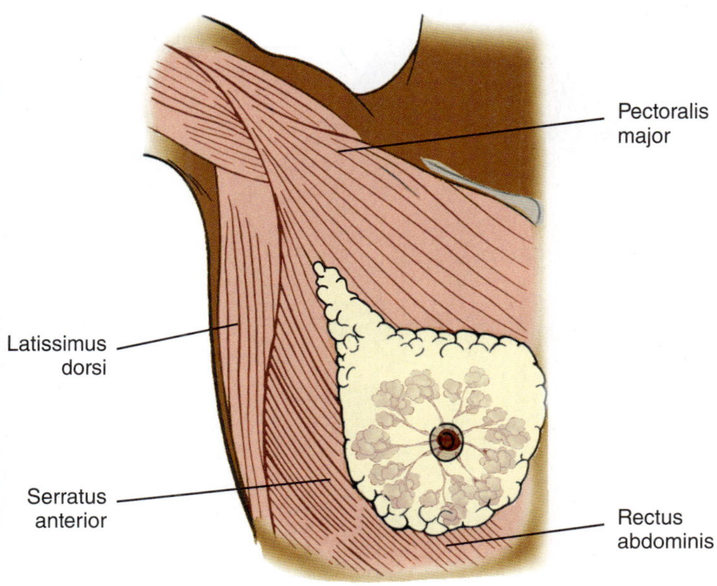

Figure 14-2 Muscles supporting the breast.

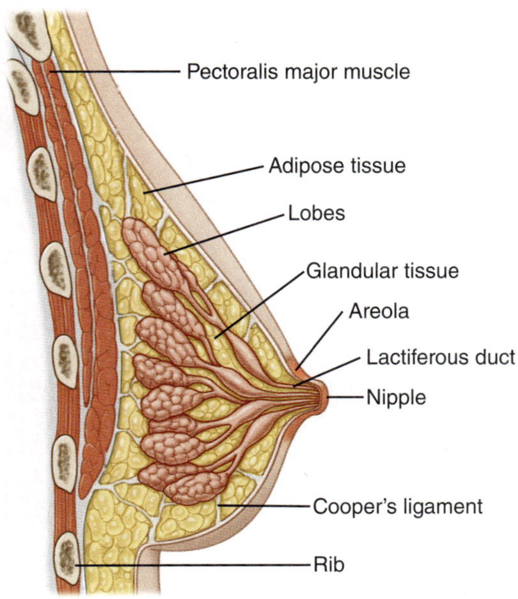

Figure 14-3 Cross section of the breast.

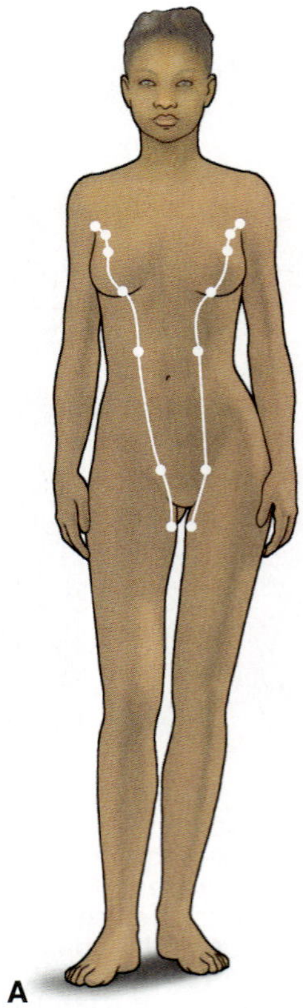

A

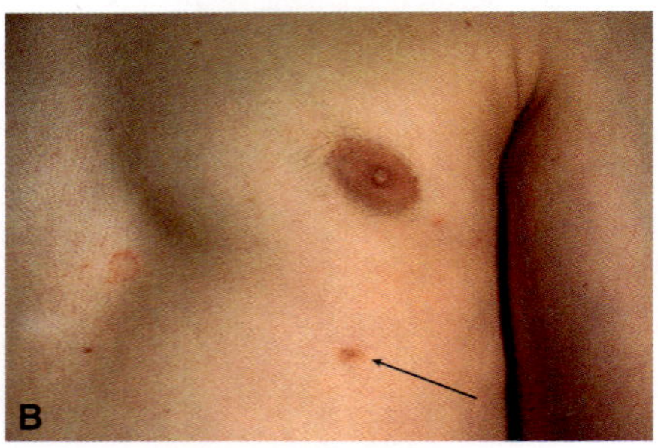

B

Figure 14-4 Ectodermal galactic bands. **A.** These bands develop in utero and later atrophy. **B.** Supernumerary nipple.

20 lobes. This disbursement is similar to a bicycle wheel; each lobe represents a spoke of the wheel and extends from a central point (the nipple) to the outermost border (Fig. 14-5). Each lobe is composed of 20 to 40 lobules that contain milk-producing glands called alveoli or acini. The lobules are arranged in grapelike bunches and are clustered around several ducts. These ducts gradually form one main lactiferous (excretory) duct per lobe. Each lactiferous duct widens to form a sinus that acts as a reservoir for milk during lactation. The duct opens onto the surface of the nipple. The lobes are lodged in tissue composed of subcutaneous and retromammary adipose tissue, and it is this tissue that composes the bulk of the breast.

The function of the female breast is to produce milk for the nourishment and protection of neonates and infants. In many cultures, breasts provide sensual pleasure during sexual foreplay and breastfeeding. The breasts also provide some protection to the anterior thoracic chest wall.

Regional Lymph Nodes

The lymphatic drainage (the yellow alkaline drainage composed primarily of lymphocytes) of the breast uses a complex network of lymph vessels and nodes. It is estimated that a majority of the lymph from the breast flows to the axillary nodes. The axillary nodes are composed of four groups: brachial nodes (lateral), central axillary nodes (midaxillary), pectoral nodes (anterior), and subscapular nodes (posterior). The central axillary nodes receive lymph from the three other nodal groups. The lymph is then channeled from the central axillary nodes to the infraclavicular and supraclavicular nodes. The remainder of the lymph flows into the internal mammary chain or directly to the infraclavicular chain via the Rotter's nodes, deep into the chest or abdominal cavity, or to the other breast. The pattern of lymph drainage is illustrated in Figure 14-6.

The axillary nodes are easily accessible by palpation because of their superficial location. The internal mammary nodes are very deep in the chest wall and are inaccessible by palpation.

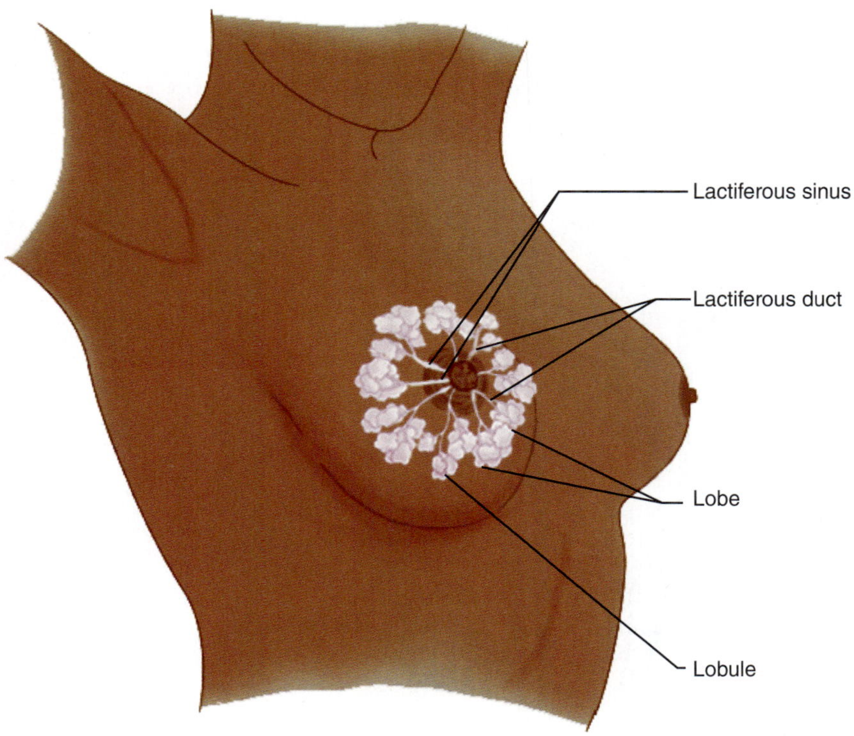

Figure 14-5 Glandular tissue of the right breast.

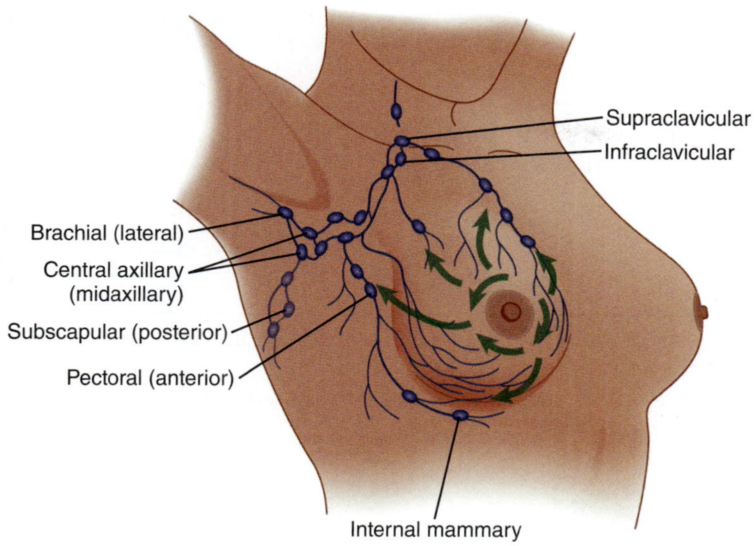

Figure 14-6 Regional lymph nodes and drainage patterns of the right breast.

Breast Development Throughout the Life Span

Female breast development usually begins at 8 to 10 years of age and is stimulated by estrogen release during puberty (thelarche). Enhanced fat deposition increases the size of the breasts, while the ductal system, lobes, and lobules increase in number and size. Asymmetry in breast development is not abnormal. Tanner staging, or sexual maturity ratings, describe the pattern of adolescent breast development for females (Table 14-1).

The female breasts go through multiple developmental changes throughout the life span. During pregnancy, the lactiferous ducts begin to proliferate. The alveoli increase in size and number, thus increasing the breast size 2 to 3 times the prepregnancy size. The areolae become more erect and darker in pigment. Montgomery tubercles develop as the sebaceous glands hypertrophy. There is also an increase in vascularization. In preparation for lactation, colostrum is produced. During lactation, colostrum is secreted in the first few days after delivery. Milk replaces colostrum and is produced 2 to 4 days after delivery. Breasts become fuller due to the filling of the alveoli and lactiferous ducts. Engorgement will occur if milk is not released. Involution occurs over a period of 3 months after lactation has been discontinued. Breast size decreases, although it rarely returns to prepregnancy size.

Later in life, during menopause, glandular tissue atrophies and is replaced by fatty tissue. The breasts become more pendulous as a result of the tissue changes and the relaxation of the suspensory ligaments. The nipples become smaller and flatter, losing their erectile ability, and the skin may appear dry and have a thin texture.

NURSING TIP

Breast Health in a Transgender Man

In a client assigned female at birth who elects to undergo hormonal and/or surgical means to affirm their gender identity who has not completed a bilateral mastectomy or who has completed breast reduction surgery, breast cancer screening guidelines for female breasts should be followed. For transgender men who have completed a mastectomy, annual chest wall examinations, ultrasounds, and MRIs have been suggested for breast cancer screening, but further research is needed to establish evidence-based guidelines for this population.

Table 14-1 Sexual Maturity Rating (SMR) for Female Breast Development

	Developmental Stage
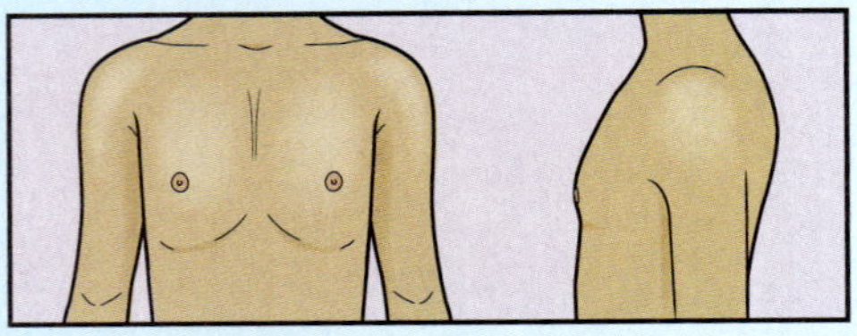	Preadolescent stage (before age 8). Nipple is small, slightly raised.
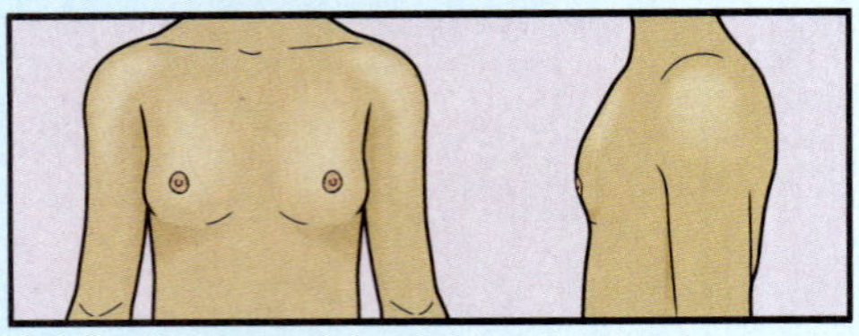	Early adolescent stage. Breast bud development (after age 8). Nipple and breast form a small mound. Areola enlarges. Height spurt begins.
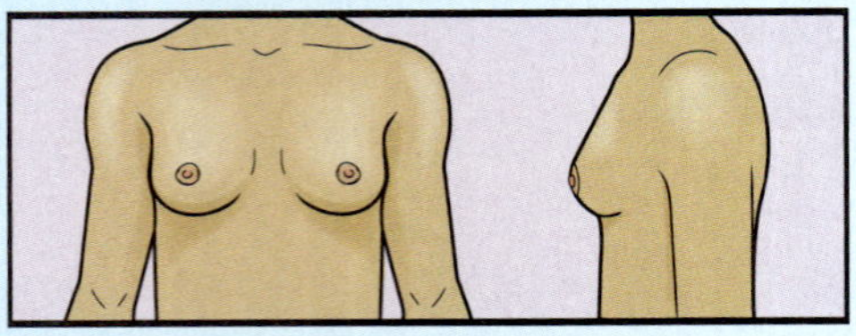	Adolescent stage (10 to 14 years). Nipple is flush with breast shape. Breast and areola enlarge. Menses begin. Height spurt peaks.
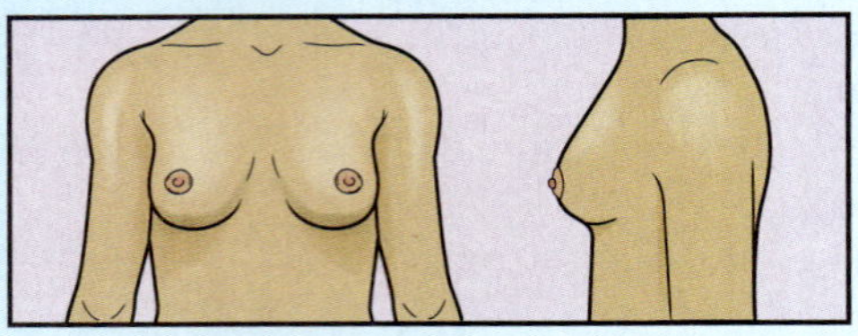	Late adolescent stage (14 to 17 years). Nipple and areola form a secondary mound over the breast. Height spurt ends.
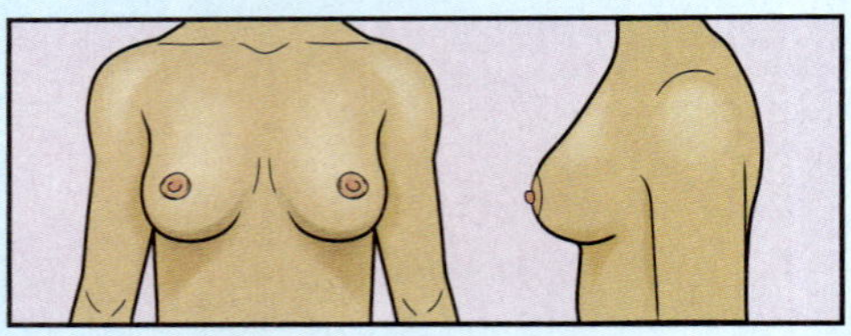	Adult stage. Nipple protrudes. Areola is flush with the breast shape.

HEALTH HISTORY

The breasts' and regional lymph nodes' health history provides insight into the link between a client's life/lifestyle and breast and lymph node information and pathology.

CLIENT PROFILE

Diseases that are age-, sex-, and race-specific for the breasts and regional lymph nodes are listed.

Age Early menarche increases the risk of breast cancer (puberty)
Gynecomastia (adolescent males and older adult males)
Fibroadenoma (15 to 20)
Benign breast disease (30 to 55)
Mastitis and plugged milk ducts (childbearing years)
Increasing risk of breast cancer (first pregnancy after 30, or nulliparous)
Paget disease (postmenopausal)
Incidence of breast cancer increases (50 or older)

Sex

Female An estimated 310,720 new cases of breast cancer were expected to occur among women in the United States during 2024 (American Cancer Society, 2024).

99% of all breast disease occurs in women; refer to Table 14-2 for breast cancer risk factors.

One in every eight women in the United States will develop breast cancer; breast cancer is second only to skin cancer in new cases in women, and it is the second leading cause of cancer death.

Male 2,790 new cases of breast cancer are expected in males in 2024 (American Cancer Society, 2023, 2024).

Gynecomastia (adolescent and older adult males)

Race Breast cancer death rate is higher for Black females than for White females in the United States.

CHIEF COMPLAINT

Common chief complaints for the breasts and regional lymph nodes are defined, and information on the characteristics of each sign or symptom is provided.

1. Breast Mass Presence of a lump in the breast

Location Anywhere in the breast or axilla; usually in the upper outer quadrant, unilateral or bilateral

Quality Size, size in relationship to menstrual cycle, shape, consistency, mobility, delineation of borders

Quantity Number of masses

Associated Manifestations Tenderness, presence of dimpling, nipple retraction, nipple discharge, tender palpable lymph nodes

Aggravating Factors Methylxanthines, recent injury to breast

Alleviating Factors Aspiration, biopsy, surgery, radiation, chemotherapy

Timing Incidence rises with age, in relation to menses and ovulation

2. Breast Tenderness Sensation of discomfort in the breast

Location Pinpoint, discrete, generalized, unilateral, or bilateral

Quality Sharp, dull, pulling

Associated Manifestations Mass, dimpling, nipple retraction, breast swelling, premenstrual syndrome symptoms (refer to Chapter 21), induration, discharge, palpable nodes, fever, breastfeeding

Aggravating Factors Recent injury to breast, palpation, vigorous exercise, oral contraceptives, chlorpromazine, or methyldopa

Alleviating Factors Warm compresses, analgesics, massage, support bras, aspiration, biopsy, surgery, breastfeeding, cessation of aggravating medications

Timing In relation to menses or ovulation, pregnancy, lactation, activity

3. Breast Discharge Abnormal substance expressed from the breast

Location From the nipple or sebaceous gland, unilateral or bilateral

Quality Color, odor, consistency

Associated Manifestations Redness, swelling, induration, mass, dimpling, nipple retraction, breast swelling, palpable nodes, lactation, headaches, history of pituitary disorders, fever, excessive breast stimulation

Aggravating Factors Trauma to breast, breastfeeding, pituitary tumor, hyperthyroidism, medications, papillomas, carcinomas of the ducts

Alleviating Factors Breastfeeding, biopsy, surgery, cessation of medications

Timing In relation to pregnancy, menses, lactation, ovulation, medications

PAST HEALTH HISTORY

The various components of the past health history are linked to breasts and regional lymph nodes pathology and related information.

Medical History

Breast Specific Benign breast disease, cysts, fibroadenomas, intraductal papillomas, mammary duct ectasia, mastitis, areas of greater density, breast cancer, breast mass, breast abscess, Paget disease, inflammatory breast disease

Non-Breast Specific Thyroid disorders, pituitary tumor, chest radiation, cancer of ovary or endometrium, obesity, and lifetime weight gain associated with increased risk of postmenopausal breast cancer

Surgical History Breast biopsy, lumpectomy, quadrantectomy, partial mastectomy, radical mastectomy, breast reduction or augmentation

Allergies Localized rashes of breast, contact dermatitis

Medications Chlorpromazine, methyldopa, diuretics, oral contraceptives, risperidone, tricyclic antidepressants, selective serotonin reuptake inhibitors, metoclopramide, verapamil, codeine, and morphine may precipitate nipple discharge; use of hormone replacement therapy has been linked with increased incidences of some breast cancers

Injuries and Accidents May cause hematoma or edema; lumps may result from previous trauma to soft tissue

Childhood Illnesses Varicella scarring of cutaneous tissue

FAMILY HEALTH HISTORY

Familial breast and regional lymph node diseases are listed.

5% to 10% of breast cancers are thought to have a familial link via a primary relative (mother, father, brother, sister, or child) (American Cancer Society, 2021).

BRCA 1 or BRCA 2 gene mutation, Cowden or Hamartoma syndrome (*PTEN* gene mutation), Li-Fraumeni (*TP53* and *CHEK 2* gene mutations), Peutz-Jeghers syndrome (*STK 11* gene mutation), ataxia telangiectasia (ATM)

Benign breast disease

SOCIAL HISTORY

The components of the social history are linked to breasts and regional lymph node factors and pathology.

Alcohol Use More than two drinks per day is associated with some risk; recurrent/current use increases risk rather than past use; research shows a dose-response relationship.

Tobacco Use Cigarette smoking of long duration is a risk factor for breast cancer.

Recreational Drug Use Heroin may cause galactorrhea.

Work Environment Radiation exposure

Home Environment Increased incidence of breast cancer noted in urban dwellers

Economic Status Increased incidence of breast cancer in females of upper and lower socioeconomic status

Ethnic Background Incidence of breast cancer among American and European females is higher than that in Japanese and Middle Eastern females; it is estimated that 1 in 100 females of Ashkenazi Jewish origin is at greater risk of breast cancer due to a mutation of the *BRCA 1* gene.

HEALTH MAINTENANCE ACTIVITIES

This information provides a bridge between the health maintenance activities and breasts and regional lymph nodes' function.

Diet No longer accepted that there is a correlation between a high-fat diet and incidence of breast cancer; increased incidence of benign breast disease with caffeine use

Exercise Strong correlation between obesity and incidence of breast cancer; multiple studies show a breast cancer reduction with increased activity

Use of Safety Devices Use of restraining devices in motor vehicles to prevent chest trauma

Health Checkups Refer to Table 14-3 for breast cancer screening guidelines. Some women experience axillary lymphadenopathy after receiving the COVID-19 vaccine. It is recommended that women do not delay breast cancer screening after receiving the COVID-19 vaccine. However, some radiological facilities ask women clients to wait 4 to 6 weeks postvaccine injection before having breast cancer screening to avoid callbacks with abnormal results as well as the fear of breast cancer being present (Mema, et al, 2023, Robinson et al, 2021).

Table 14-2 Breast Cancer Risk Factors in Women

Nonmodifiable Risk Factors	Modifiable Factors	Red Flags for High-Risk Factors
Female gender	Increased alcohol consumption	Early age of onset of breast cancer (<50 in client or family member)
Age greater than 50	Obesity	Multiple family members with breast cancer
Personal history of breast cancer	Physical inactivity	Autosomal dominant pattern
Family history of breast cancer, ovarian cancer, prostate cancer, pancreatic cancer	Smoking	Individual with more than one primary breast cancer
Prior thoracic radiation (e.g., Hodgkin disease)	Postmenopausal hormonal therapy (use of estrogen and progesterone)	Radiation therapy to chest between ages 10–30 years
Number and result of prior breast biopsies (e.g., atypical hyperplasia, lobular carcinoma in situ)	Childbearing history	Male breast cancer at any age
Hereditary breast cancer syndromes: • *BRCA1* and *BRCA2* are the majority of breast cancer syndromes • Cowden or Hamartoma syndrome (*PTEN* gene mutation) • Li-Fraumeni (*TP53* and *CHEK2* gene mutations) • Peutz-Jeghers syndrome (*STK11* gene mutation) • Ataxia telangiectasia (*ATM*)	Recent oral contraceptive use Not breastfeeding	Family member with known hereditary mutation (e.g., *BRCA1, BRCA2, TP53, PTEN*) Family history of a first-degree relative (parent, brother, sister, or child) with breast cancer and ovarian cancer on same side of family
Reproductive history (earlier age at menarche<12, nulliparity, first child after age 30, late onset of menopause (after age 55)		
African American/Ashkenazi Jewish heritage		
Dense breast tissue		
High postmenopausal bone density		
Personal history of endometrial, ovarian, or colon cancer		
Taking diethylstilbestrol (DES) or exposure in utero		

Table 14-3 Breast Cancer Screening Guidelines

Population	Recommendation	Grade
Women age 40 to 74 years	The USPSTF recommends biennial screening mammography for women ages 40 to 74 years.	B
Women 75 years or older	The USPSTF concludes that the current evidence is insufficient to assess the balance of benefits and harms of screening mammography in women 75 years or older.	I
Women with dense breasts	The USPSTF concludes that the current evidence is insufficient to assess the balance of benefits and harms of supplemental screening for breast cancer using breast ultrasonography or magnetic resonance imaging in women identified to have dense breasts on an otherwise negative screening mammogram.	I

USPSTF = U.S. Preventive Services Task Force.
Retrieved November 5, 2025, from *https://www.uspreventiveservicestaskforce.org/uspstf/recommendation/breast-cancer-screening*

NURSING CHECKLIST

General Approach to Breast Examination

Before the Examination

1. Observe standard precautions and don Personal Protective Equipment (PPE) such as gloves, gown, face shield, goggles, or N-95 respirator or face mask if the client's status warrants these protective measures.
2. When possible, instruct the client not to use creams, lotions, or powders, nor to shave underarms 24 to 48 hours before the scheduled examination. The application of toiletry products may mask or alter the nature of the surface integument of the breasts, and shaving the underarms may cause folliculitis, which may result in pain upon palpation.
3. Encourage the client to express any anxieties and concerns about the physical examination. Acknowledge anxieties and validate concerns. Many females avoid having their breasts examined because they fear abnormal findings. Assure the client that this is a positive step in owning personal health care by having the breasts examined.
4. Inform the client that the examination should not be painful but may be uncomfortable at times. This is especially true if the client is currently experiencing menses, ovulation, or pregnancy.
5. Adopt a nonjudgmental and supportive attitude.
6. Be aware of the impact of culture on breast examination and breast self-examination. In Asian cultures, breast self-examination may be considered a form of masturbation. In some Middle Eastern cultures, baring the breasts to a man is taboo, even if the man is a health-care provider.
7. Instruct the client to remove any jewelry that might interfere with the examination.
8. Ensure that the room is warm enough to prevent chilling and provide additional draping material as necessary.
9. Warm your hands with warm water or by rubbing them together before the examination.
10. Ensure that privacy will be maintained during the examination. Provide screens, closed doors, and a door sign stating that an examination is in progress.

During the Examination

1. Inform the client of what you are going to do before you do it.
2. Use this time to educate the client about the body.
3. Offer the client the opportunity to ask questions about the body and sexuality.
4. Keep areas not being examined appropriately draped.
5. Always compare right and left breasts.
6. Wear gloves if the client has had any discharge from the breast.

After the Examination

1. Assess whether the client needs assistance in dressing.
2. After the client is dressed, discuss the experience, invite questions and comments, listen carefully, and provide information regarding the examination.

Assessment in Brief

Breasts and Regional Lymph Nodes Examination

Inspection

- Color
- Vascularity
- Thickening/edema
- Size and symmetry
- Contour
- Lesions/masses
- Discharge

Palpation

- Supraclavicular and infraclavicular lymph nodes
- Breasts: Client in sitting position
- Axillary lymph node region
- Breasts: Client in supine position

Equipment

- Appropriate PPE
- Towel
- Drape
- Centimeter ruler
- Teaching aid for breast self-examination

Examination of the Female Breasts and Regional Lymph Nodes

Physical examination produces feelings of fear, anxiety, embarrassment, and loss of control in many women. These feelings may be reduced by the sensitivity of the nurse before, during, and after examination of the breasts. Examination of the female breasts and regional nodes includes inspection and palpation.

Inspection

E
1. Position the client uncovered to the waist, seated at the edge of the examination table, and facing you.
2. Instruct the client to let their arms relax by their sides as shown in Figure 14-7.
3. Inspect the breasts, axillae, areolar areas, and nipples for color, vascularity, thickening, edema, size, symmetry, contour, lesions, masses, and exudates.
4. Repeat this inspection sequence with the client's arms raised above the head (Fig. 14-8). This will accentuate any retraction (tissue drawn back) if present.
5. Repeat the inspection sequence with the client pressing hands into hips, which will contract the pectoral muscles (Fig. 14-9). Once again, if retraction is present, it will be more pronounced with this maneuver.
6. Have the client lean forward to allow the breasts to hang freely away from the chest wall, as shown in Figure 14-10, and repeat the inspection sequence. Provide support to the client as necessary.

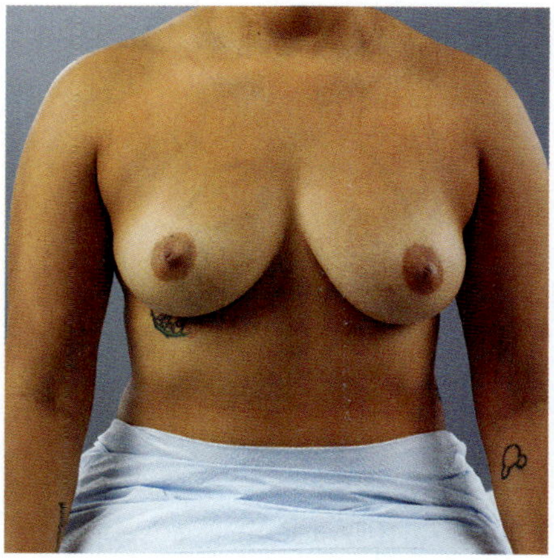

Figure 14-7 Position of client for breast inspection: Arms at side.

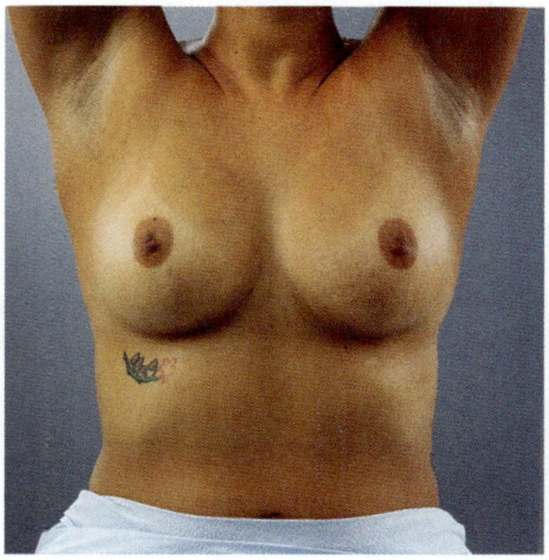

Figure 14-8 Position of client for breast inspection: Arms overhead.

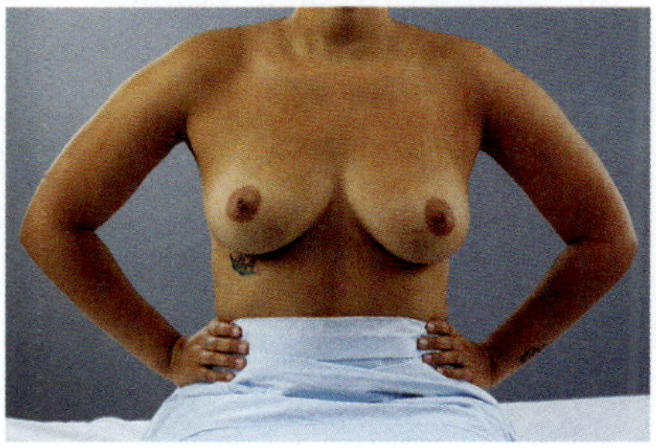

Figure 14-9 Position of client for breast inspection: Hands pressed against hips.

Color

E Inspect the breasts, areolar areas, nipples, and axillae for coloration.

N **The breasts and axillae are flesh-colored, and the areolar areas and nipples are usually darker in pigmentation. The color of the nipples and areola ranges from a light beige to pale pink to dark brown. This pigmentation is normally enhanced during pregnancy. Moles and nevi are normal variants, and terminal hair may be present on the areolar areas.**

A Reddened areas of the breasts, nipples, or axillae require further assessment.

P Redness may be an indication of inflammation, an infection such as mastitis, or carcinoma (Fig. 14-11). Table 14-4 outlines the five major types of breast cancer.

A Striae are streaks over the breasts or axillae and are abnormal. In light-skinned individuals, new striae are red and become silver to white in coloration with age. In dark-skinned individuals, new striae are a ruddy, dark brown color, and older striae become lighter than the skin color.

P Striae are caused by rapid stretching of the skin, which damages the elastic fibers found in the dermis. Though normal in pregnancy, striae are often observed with obesity.

Vascularity

E Observe the entire surface of each breast for superficial vascular patterns.

E Examination N Normal Findings A Abnormal Findings P Pathophysiology

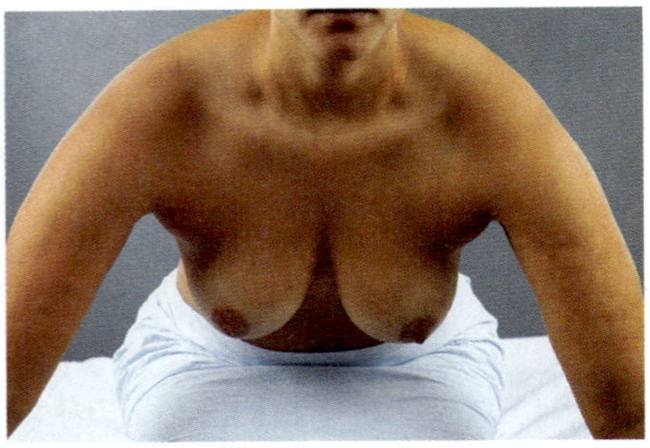

Figure 14-10 Position of client for breast inspection: Leaning forward.

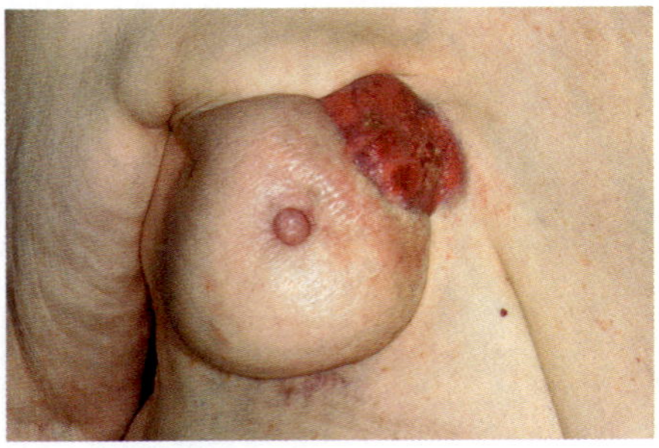

Figure 14-11 Erythema in advanced stage breast cancer.

N **Normal superficial vascular patterns are diffuse and symmetrical.**

A Abnormal patterns of vascularity are focal or unilateral.

P Focal or unilateral superficial vascular patterns occur as the result of an increased blood supply and may indicate tumor formation, which requires increased vascularization and an increased blood supply.

Thickening/Edema

E Observe the breasts, axillae, and nipples for thickening and edema.

N **Normally, thickening or edema is not found in the breasts, axillae, or nipples.**

A Thickening or edema of the breast tissue or nipple may present itself as enlarged skin pores that give the appearance of an orange rind (**peau d'orange**). It may be more prevalent in the dependent or inferior portions of the breast.

P A peau d'orange appearance may be indicative of obstructed lymphatic drainage due to a tumor or inflammatory breast cancer.

Size and Symmetry

E Observe the breasts, axillae, areolar areas, and nipples for size and symmetry.

N **It is not unusual for there to be some difference in the size of the breasts and areolar areas, with the breast on the side of the dominant arm being larger (Fig. 14-12). Bilateral hypertrophy of the breasts may be normal for some clients (Fig. 14-13). Nipple inversion, which is present from puberty, is a normal variant and is of no clinical consequence except for difficulty in breastfeeding. Nipples can point upward and laterally, or they may point outward and downward (Fig. 14-14A). Nipples should be symmetrical on the same horizontal plane. Supernumerary nipples are a variant of normal and have no pathological significance in either males or females.**

Table 14-4 Breast Cancer Types

Type of Breast Cancer	Description
Ductal Carcinoma In Situ (DCIS)	Cancer cells confined to the milk ducts. DCIS may present as microcalcifications on mammography. There is no invasion to outlying tissue or lymph nodes.
Infiltrating (Invasive) Ductal Carcinoma (IDC)	Cancer cells that have invaded tissues beyond the milk ducts. IDC usually presents as a discrete, solid breast mass on mammography.
Infiltrating (Invasive) Lobular Carcinoma (ILC)	Cancer cells that started in the lobules and milk ducts, and have invaded outlying tissue. This cancer may present as a thickened area rather than a mass.
Inflammatory Breast Cancer (IBC)	Cancer cells that have rapid tumor growth with an erythemic, thickened skin or diffuse edema (peau d'orange). It is diagnosed via core biopsy or punch biopsy.
Paget Disease	Presents as an eczematous rash on the nipple. Pruritus, erythema, and nipple discharge may be present. Paget disease can coexist with DCIS or IDC.

A Asymmetry in the directions in which the nipples are pointed is an abnormal finding (Fig. 14-14B).

P Asymmetrical nipple direction is suggestive of an underlying invasive process that is contorting nipple tissue. Often the direction of nipple deviation is toward the underlying process.

A Significant differences in the size or symmetry of the breasts, axillae, areolar areas, or nipples are abnormal.

P Significant enlargement of one breast, axilla, or areola may be indicative of tumor formation.

A Recent inversion, flattening, or depression of a nipple is abnormal.

P A sudden onset of nipple inversion, flattening, or depression is indicative of nipple retraction, which is suggestive of underlying cancer.

A Nipples that have been inverted since puberty and become broader or thicker are abnormal.

P Additional broadening or thickening of a previously inverted nipple may be indicative of tumor formation.

A Lack of breast tissue unilaterally is abnormal.

P Unilateral reduction of breast tissue or structures may result from trauma, mastectomy, or breast reduction.

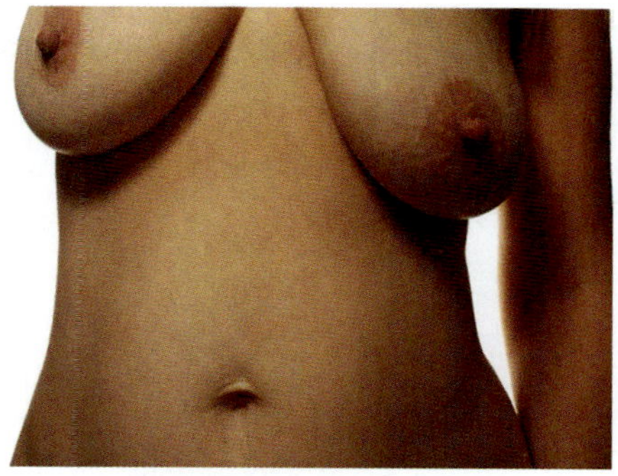

Figure 14-12 Breast asymmetry.

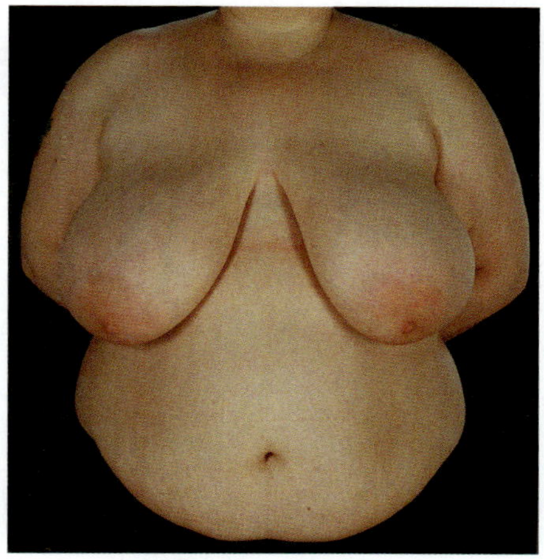

Figure 14-13 Breast Hypertrophy.

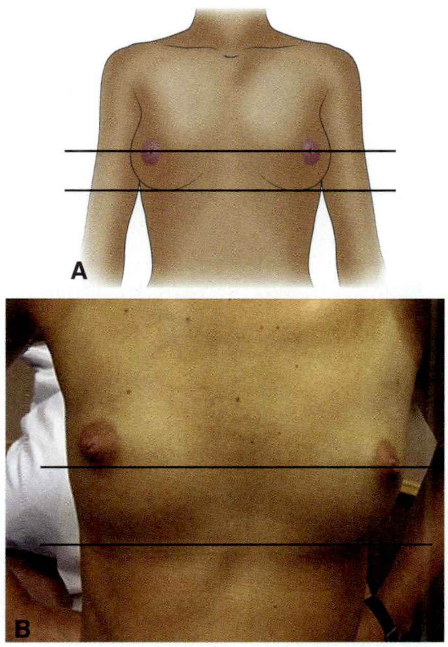

Figure 14-14 Nipple symmetry.
A. Symmetrical without deviation.
B. Asymmetrical with deviation.

Contour

E
1. Examine the contour of the breasts.
2. Compare the breasts to each other.

N **The breast is normally convex, without flattening, retractions, or dimpling.**

A Dimpling, retractions, flattening, or other changes in breast contour are abnormal.

P Changes in contour are highly suggestive of cancer. The invasive process that causes the contour changes is the result of fibrotic shortening and disablement of the Cooper's ligament. Fat necrosis and mammary duct ectasia may also cause retraction, dimpling, and puckering.

Lesions/Masses

E Inspect the breasts, axillae, areolar areas, and nipples for lesions and masses.

N **The breasts, axillae, areolar areas, and nipples are free of masses, tumors, and primary or secondary lesions.**

A Breast masses, tumors, nodules, or cysts of any kind are abnormal.

P Table 14-5 lists common pathologies of breast masses.

A A scaly, eczema-like erosion of the nipple, or persistent dermatitis of the areola and nipple, is abnormal.

P Persistent eczematous dermatitis of the areola and nipple region is suggestive of Paget disease, a malignant neoplasm, which is usually unilateral in its involvement.

Discharge

E Observe for spontaneous discharge from the nipples or other areas of the breast.

N **In the female breast of a client that is nonpregnant and is not lactating, there should be no discharge. During pregnancy and up through the first week after birth, there may be a yellow discharge known as colostrum coming from the nipple of the female breast. During lactation, there is a white discharge of breast milk.**

A The presence of nipple discharge in the female breast of a nonpregnant, nonlactating client is abnormal.

P Nipple discharge may be caused by the use of medications such as tranquilizers and oral contraceptives, manual stimulation, pituitary tumor, or infection. It may also be indicative of malignant or benign breast disease.

Table 14-5 Characteristics of Common Breast Masses

	Gross Cyst	Fibroadenoma	Carcinoma
	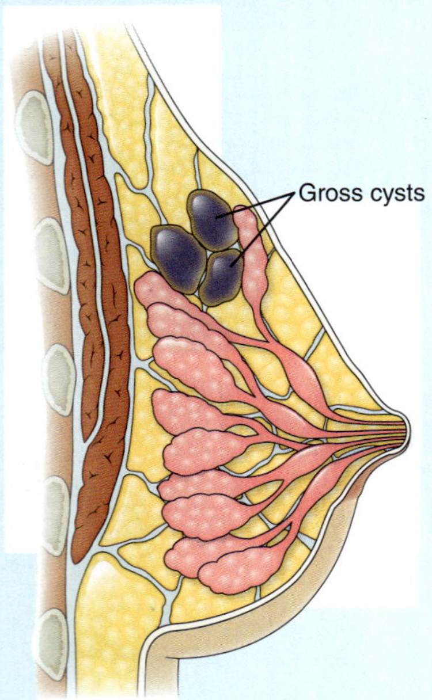	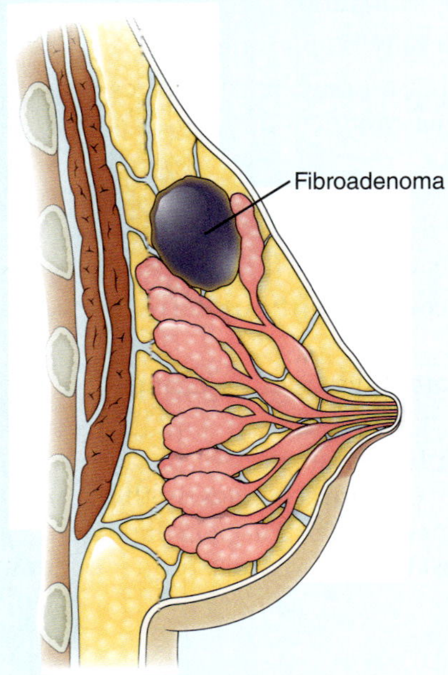	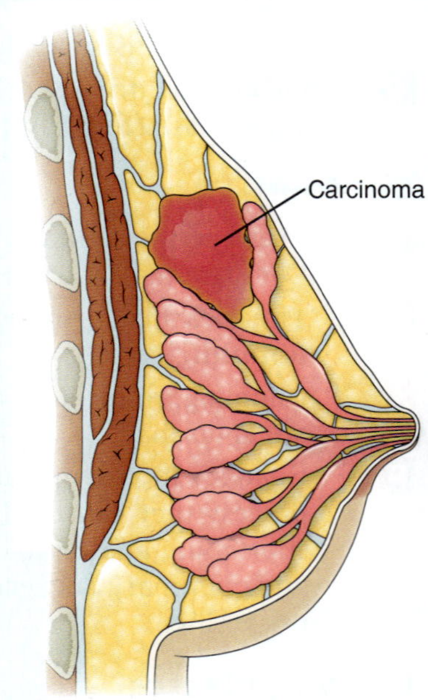
Age	30 to 50; diminishes after menopause	Puberty to menopause; peaks between ages 20 to 30	Most common after 50 years
Shape	Round	Round, lobular, or ovoid	Irregular, stellate, or crab-like
Consistency	Soft to firm	Usually firm	Firm to hard
Discreteness	Well defined	Well defined	Not clearly defined
Number	Single or grouped	Most often single	Usually single
Mobility	Mobile	Very mobile	May be mobile or fixed to skin, underlying tissue, or chest wall
Tenderness	Tender	Nontender	Usually nontender
Erythema	No erythema	No erythema	May be present
Retraction/ dimpling	Not present	Not present	Often present

Risk Factors

Benign Breast Disease

- Caffeine use
- Imbalance between estrogen and progesterone
- Estrogen excess
- Hyperprolactinemia
- Age 20 to 50 years
- Family history of benign breast disease

NURSING TIP

Clinical Breast Examinations in Women

The clinical breast examination (CBE) is a physical examination of the breasts performed by a health-care professional. In the past, routine CBE and mammography were thought to reduce the risk of dying from breast cancer. More recently, there has been insufficient evidence on the benefits of routine CBE in early breast detection due to improvements in mammography and female breast awareness in response to changing breast developments. Some evidence shows CBE along with mammography increases the rate of false positives. However, CBE is still recommended for clients who present with complaints of nipple discharge or a suspected breast mass.

Palpation

If the client has a known/suspected mass or irregularity in one breast, begin palpation on the unaffected breast. The unaffected breast should indicate the client's normal physiological state. Palpation is performed sequentially:

1. Supraclavicular and infraclavicular lymph node areas
2. Breasts, with the client in sitting position
   a. Arms at side
   b. Arms raised over head
3. Axillary lymph node regions
4. Breasts, with the client in supine position

Supraclavicular and Infraclavicular Lymph Nodes

E
1. Have client seated and uncovered to the waist.
2. Encourage the client to relax the muscles of the head and neck, because this pulls the clavicles down and allows a thorough exploration of the supraclavicular area.
3. Flex the client's head to relax the sternocleidomastoid muscle.
4. Standing in front of the client, in a bilateral and simultaneous motion, place the finger pads over the client's clavicles, lateral to the tendinous portion of the sternocleidomastoid muscles.
5. Using a rotary motion of the palmar surfaces of the fingers, probe deeply into the scalene triangles to palpate the supraclavicular lymph nodes (Fig. 14-15).
6. Palpate the infraclavicular nodes using the same rotary motion of the palmar surfaces of the fingers (Fig. 14-16).

N **Palpable lymph nodes less than 1 cm in diameter are usually considered normal and clinically insignificant, provided that there are no additional enlarged lymph nodes found in other regions such as the axilla. Palpation should not elicit pain.**

A Fixed, firm, immobile, irregular lymph nodes more than 1 cm in diameter are considered abnormal.

P Fixed, firm, immobile, irregular lymph nodes more than 1 cm in diameter are considered suspicious for metastasis from a variety of sources or primary lymphoma.

A Enlarged, painful, or tender nodes that are matted together are abnormal.

P Tender, enlarged nodes may indicate systemic infection or carcinoma.

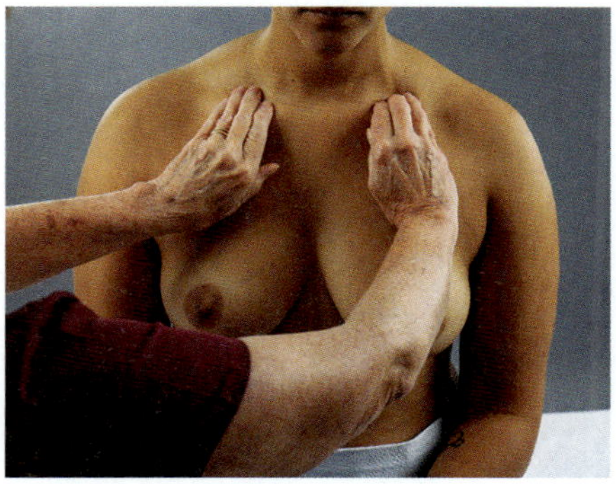

Figure 14-15 Palpation of supraclavicular lymph nodes.

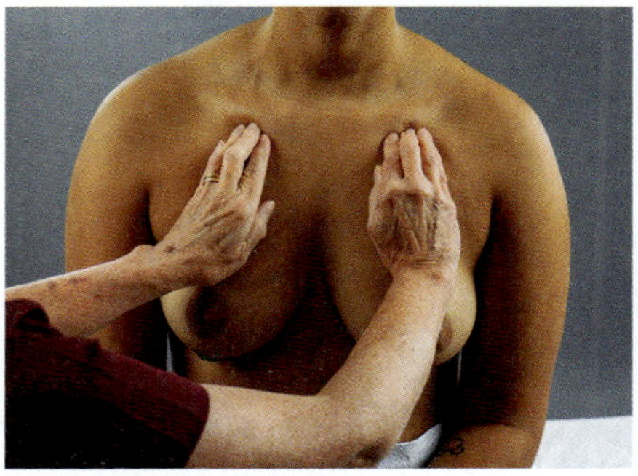

Figure 14-16 Palpation of infraclavicular lymph nodes.

Breasts: Client in Sitting Position

E
1. Place the client in a sitting position with arms at sides.
2. Stand to the client's right side, facing the client.

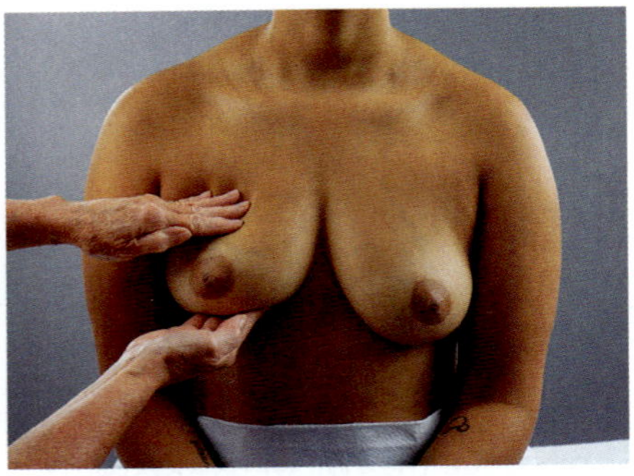

Figure 14-17 Bimanual palpation of the breasts while client is sitting.

3. Using the palmar surfaces of the fingers of the dominant hand, begin the palpation at the outer quadrant of the client's right breast.
4. Use the other hand to support the inferior aspect of the breast.
5. In small-breasted clients, the dominant hand can palpate the tissue against the chest wall, but if the breasts are pendulous, use a bimanual technique of palpation as shown in Figure 14-17.
6. Palpate in a downward fashion, sweeping from the outer quadrants to the sternal border of each breast.
7. Repeat this sequence on the other breast.
8. Repeat the entire examination with the client's arms raised over their head to enhance any potential retraction.

N **The consistency of the breasts is widely variable, depending on age, time in menstrual cycle, and proportion of adipose tissue. The breasts may have a nodular or granular consistency that may be enhanced before the onset of menses. The inferior aspect of the breast will be somewhat firmer due to a transverse inframammary ridge. Palpation should not elicit significant tenderness, although the breasts and especially the nipples may become full and slightly tender premenstrually. Breasts that feel fluid-filled or firm throughout with accompanying inferior suture-line scars are indicative of breast augmentation.**

A The presence of any lump, mass, thickening, or unilateral granulation that is noticeably different from the rest of the breast tissue should be considered suspicious and abnormal.

P For a description of breast masses and their pathologies, refer to Table 14-5.

A Significant breast tenderness is abnormal and may indicate mammary duct ectasia.

P Mammary duct ectasia is a benign condition in which lactiferous ducts become thickened and inflamed.

A Erythema and swelling of the breast with possible pitting edema are abnormal and usually indicate mastitis.

P Mastitis is usually seen postpartum and is an inflammation of the breast usually caused by *Staphylococcus aureus*.

Axillary Lymph Node Region

E
1. Stand on the client's right side, facing the client.
2. Tell the client to take a deep breath and relax the shoulders and arms (this relaxes the areas to be palpated).
3. Using your left hand, adduct the client's right arm so that it is close to the chest wall. This maneuver relaxes the muscles.
4. Support the client's right arm with your left hand.
5. Using the palmar surfaces of the finger pads of your right hand, place your fingers into the apex of the axilla. Your fingers will be positioned behind the pectoral muscles.
6. Gently roll the tissue against the chest wall and axillary muscles as you work downward.
7. Locate and palpate the four axillary lymph node groups:
   a. Brachial (lateral) at the inner aspect of the upper part of the humerus, close to the axillary vein.
   b. Central axillary (midaxillary) at the thoracic wall of the axilla.
   c. Pectoral (anterior) behind the lateral edge of the pectoralis major muscle.
   d. Subscapular (posterior) at the anterior edge of the latissimus dorsi muscle.

8. Repeat this method of palpation with the client's arm abducted (i.e., instruct the client to remain in the same position while you lift their upper arm and elbow away from the body). Support the client's abducted arm on your left shoulder, as shown in Figure 14-18.
9. Palpate the client's left axilla using the same technique.

N **Palpable lymph nodes less than 1 cm in diameter are usually considered normal and clinically insignificant provided that no additional enlarged lymph nodes are found in other regions. Palpation should not elicit pain.**

A Fixed, firm, immobile, irregular lymph nodes more than 1 cm in diameter are clinically significant.

P Fixed, firm, immobile, irregular lymph nodes more than 1 cm in diameter are considered suggestive of metastasis from a variety of sources or primary lymphoma.

A Enlarged, painful, or tender nodes that are matted together are abnormal.

P Tender, enlarged nodes may be indicative of a systemic infection or carcinoma.

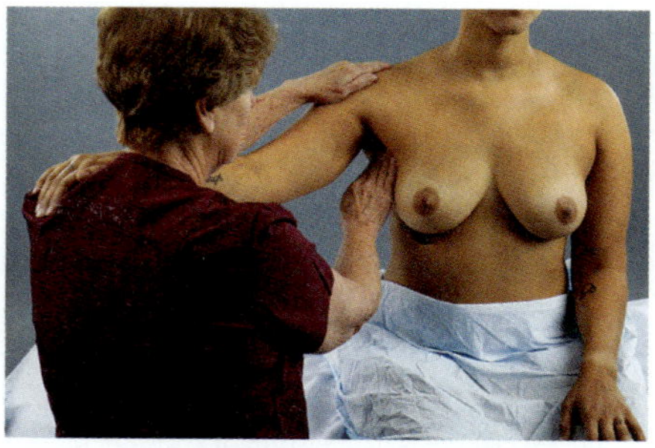

Figure 14-18 Palpation of axillary lymph nodes.

Breasts: Client in Supine Position

E

1. Keep the client uncovered to the waist.
2. Instruct the client to assume a supine position. This position spreads the breast tissue thinly and evenly over the chest wall. Palpation is more accurate when there is the least amount of breast tissue between the skin and the chest wall.
3. If the breasts are large, place a small towel or folded sheet under the client's right shoulder. This helps to flatten the breast more.
4. Stand on the right side of the client. Palpation can be performed with the client's arms at their sides or with their right arm above their head.
5. Using the palmar surfaces of the fingers, palpate the right breast by compressing the mammary tissues gently against the chest wall. Do not press too hard. You may mistake a rib for a hard breast mass. Palpation may be performed in wedge sections, concentric circles, or parallel horizontal, or vertical lines (Fig. 14-19A–D). Using two out of the four palpation methods is acceptable to ensure thoroughness of palpation.
6. Palpation must include the tail of Spence, periphery (Fig. 14-20A). Don gloves and palpate the areola (Fig. 14-20B).

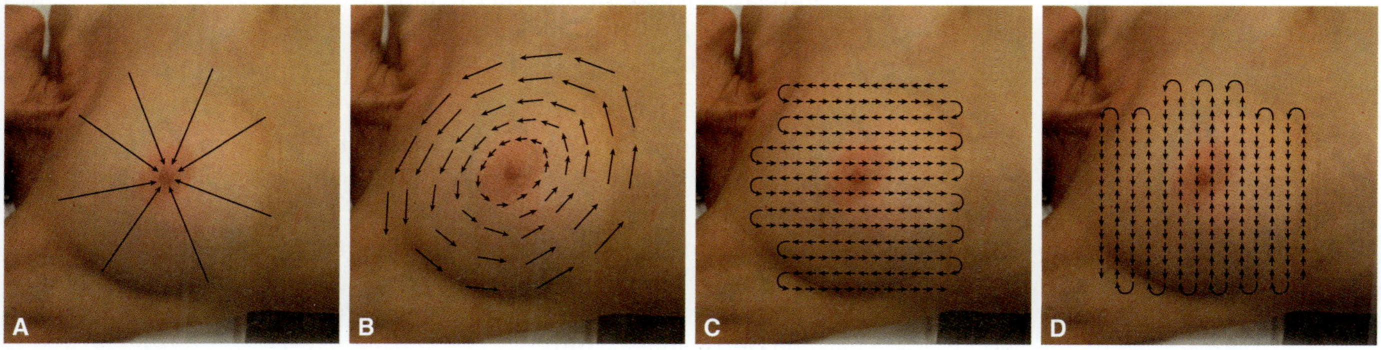

Figure 14-19 Breast palpation methods. **A.** Wedge. **B.** Concentric circles. **C.** Parallel lines, horizontal. **D.** Parallel lines, vertical.

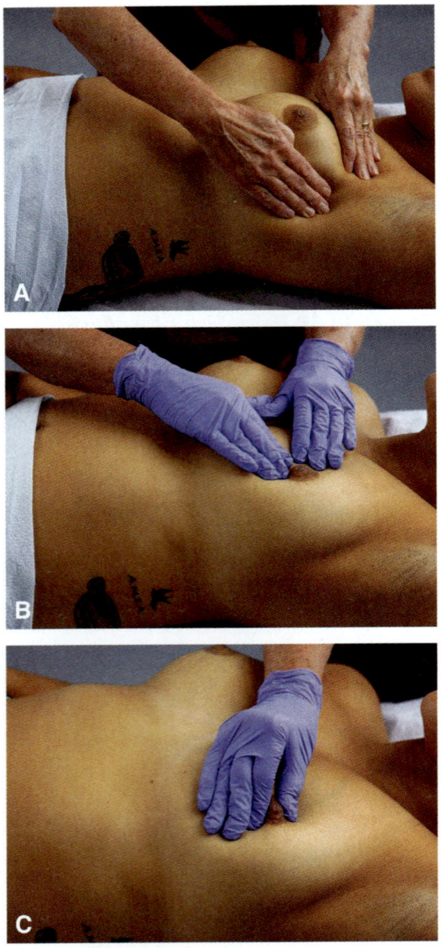

Figure 14-20 Palpation of the breasts while client is supine. **A.** Palpation of the glandular tissue. **B.** Palpation of the areola. **C.** Compression of the nipple.

7. Compress the nipple to express any discharge, as shown in Figure 14-20C. If discharge is noted, palpate the breast along the wedge radii to determine from which lobe the discharge is originating. Once you have identified which lobe the discharge originated from, obtain a specimen, using a glass slide and cytological fixative, sterile culture swab, or other preparation as dictated by your institution's policy. Note the color, odor, and consistency of the discharge. The discharge can also be evaluated for occult blood.
8. Repeat the procedure on the opposite breast.

N **See the previous section on normal breast tissue findings upon palpation. The nipple should be elastic and return readily to its previous shape. No discharge should be expressed in the nonpregnant, nonlactating client.**

Refer to Table 14-5 for a description of breast masses. The Nursing Tip, Documenting Breast Mass Characteristics, lists breast mass characteristics that need to be evaluated and documented for abnormal clinical findings.

NURSING TIP

Breast Examination in the Pregnant and Breastfeeding Client

Physical examination of the breast is a very important part of breast assessment both for breast cancer screening and when approaching breast lesions. Examination during pregnancy and breastfeeding follows the same method as in nonpregnant clients. Physical changes that occur in the breast during pregnancy and breastfeeding are due to hormonal effects and may cause alterations that conceal some pathological disorders; however, breast changes may appear as pathological while being purely physiological. Additional testing and imaging may be necessary.

A Loss of nipple elasticity or nipple thickening is abnormal.

P Loss of elasticity in the nipple may indicate tumor formation.

A Milky-white discharge in a nonpregnant, nonlactating client may be nonpuerperal galactorrhea.

P Nonpuerperal galactorrhea is either hormonally induced from lesions of the anterior pituitary gland or drug-induced.

A Nonmilky discharge from the nipple, which may be green, brown, straw-colored, or gray, is abnormal.

P Nonmilky discharge may be indicative of benign or malignant breast disease such as intraductal carcinoma.

A Bleeding from the nipple is abnormal.

P Bleeding from the nipple is often seen in the benign condition of intraductal papilloma.

A An excision of the breast (**mastectomy**) is an abnormal finding (Fig. 14-21A and B). Refer to Table 14-6 for the types of mastectomy surgeries.

P A woman with a breast malignancy may have a mastectomy. In addition, some women with a history of breast cancer in the other breast or a strong family history of breast cancer may have a prophylactic mastectomy.

Table 14-6 Types of Mastectomy Surgeries

Mastectomy Surgery	Description
Simple	Only the breast is removed
Modified radical (Figs. 14-21A and 14-21B)	The breast and lymph nodes from the axilla are removed
Radical	The breast, lymph nodes from the axilla, and pectoral muscles are removed
Subcutaneous	The skin and nipple are left intact, but the underlying breast tissue and lymph nodes are removed. This procedure is rarely performed.

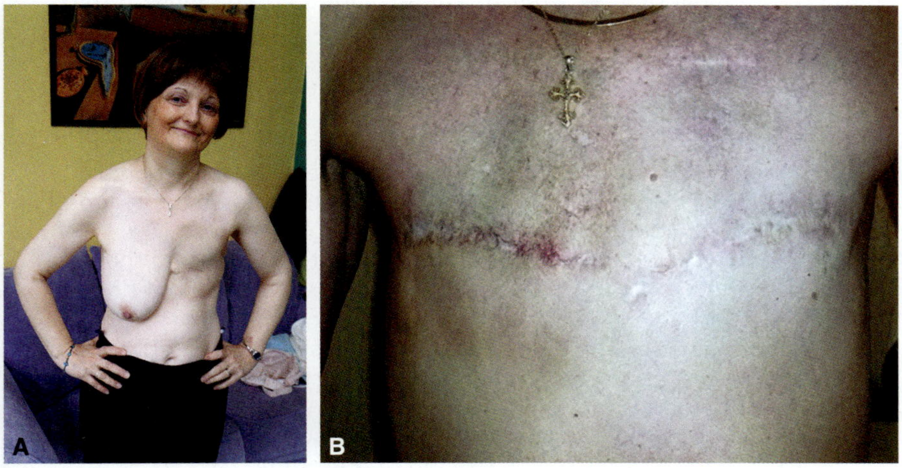

Figure 14-21 Mastectomy clients. **A.** Left-sided modified radical. **B.** Bilateral modified radical.

Examination of the Client Who Has Undergone a Mastectomy and Breast-Augmentation

Examination of the client who has undergone a mastectomy will be guided by the type of mastectomy and the presence or absence of breast augmentation. Follow the standard examination procedures and modify your technique to suit the amount of breast tissue. Always begin the examination on the unaffected breast. Inspect the scar(s) for swelling, lumps, thickening, redness, rash, and irritation. Palpating the surgical scar should include using two finger pads to perform small, circular motions assessing for swelling, lumps, thickening, and tenderness. Clients who have undergone a mastectomy should continue to perform monthly breast self-examinations to determine whether masses have returned to the excised area. Annual clinical evaluations and mammography are also recommended.

A client undergoing a mastectomy may elect to have reconstruction of the affected breast. Reconstruction techniques include synthetic implants, tissue expansion techniques (a temporary inflatable device is placed in a

NURSING TIP

Documenting Breast Mass Characteristics

Any mass found on the clinical breast examination requires documentation including the following characteristics:

- **Location:** Identify the right or left breast and quadrant involved. To document the mass, visualize the breast with the face of a clock superimposed upon it. The nipple represents the center of the clock. Note where the mass lies in relation to the nipple (e.g., left breast mass, 3 cm from the nipple in the 2 o'clock position, upper outer quadrant). The mass may be singular or there may be multiple masses. Each mass requires examination and documentation.
- **Size:** Measure the size in centimeters in all three planes (height, width, and depth).
- **Shape:** A mass may be round, ovoid, matted, or irregular.
- **Consistency:** The consistency of the mass may be firm, hard, soft, fluid, or cystic.
- **Borders:** The borders of the mass may be discrete or irregular.
- **Mobility:** The mass may be fixed or freely movable in relation to the chest wall.
- **Tenderness:** Note if pain occurs with palpation.
- **Erythema:** Note any erythema over the involved area.
- **Dimpling or Retraction:** Note any dimpling or retraction when the client raises their arms overhead and presses their hands into their hips.
- **Lymphadenopathy:** Note any enlarged regional lymph nodes.

subpectoralis-subserratus position between the anterior chest wall and skin and inflated with saline over a period of weeks), and latissimus dorsi myocutaneous flap breast reconstruction. A myocutaneous flap reconstruction involves transferring skin from the back or the abdomen to the anterior chest wall.

NURSING TIP

Breast Self-Awareness

Breast self-examination (BSE) used to be a routine monthly examination encouraged for women. Recent evidence has not shown BSE to be more effective than CBE in reducing the number of deaths or improving survival rates from breast cancer. Health organizations are no longer recommending the client perform monthly BSE as a part of breast cancer screening. However, it is encouraged for the client to be breast aware (to be familiar with one's breast for early detection of changes) of what the breasts look and feel like in the normal state so the client can promptly report any changes if they occur.

For clients who choose to be breast self-aware, the following can be taught:

- Stand in front of a mirror with arms at the side (Fig. 14-22A), then with arms raised over the head (Fig. 14-22B), and with the hands pressed into the hips (Fig. 14-22C). Observe the breasts for symmetry, retractions, dimpling, and nipple deviations.
- Palpate the breasts while in the standing position by raising the left arm over the head and palpating the left breast with the right hand (Fig. 14-22D), moving in concentric circles from the periphery inward, including the tail of Spence and areola. Reverse the procedure to palpate the right breast. The client should become familiar with the feel of the breasts.
- Repeat the palpation process with the client supine and a small towel placed under the breast being examined (Figure 14-22E).

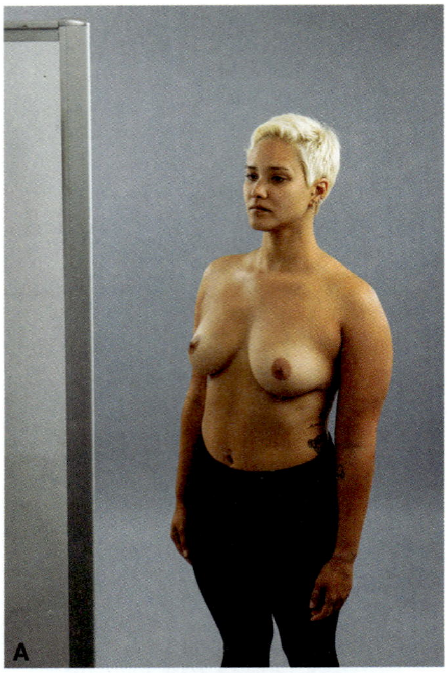

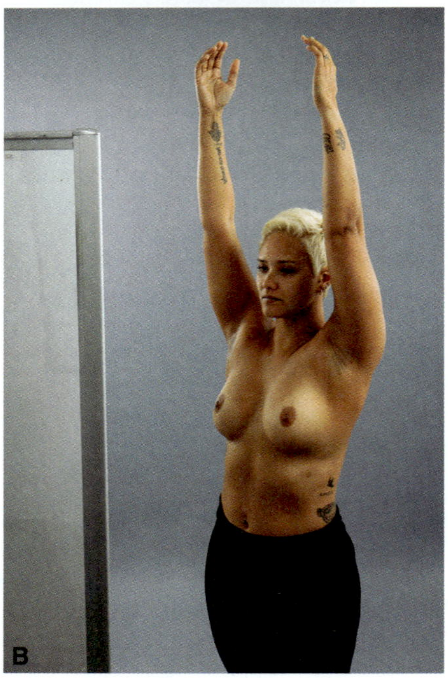

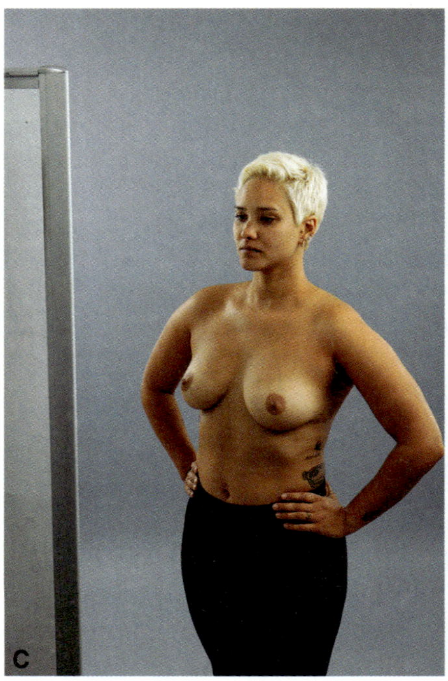

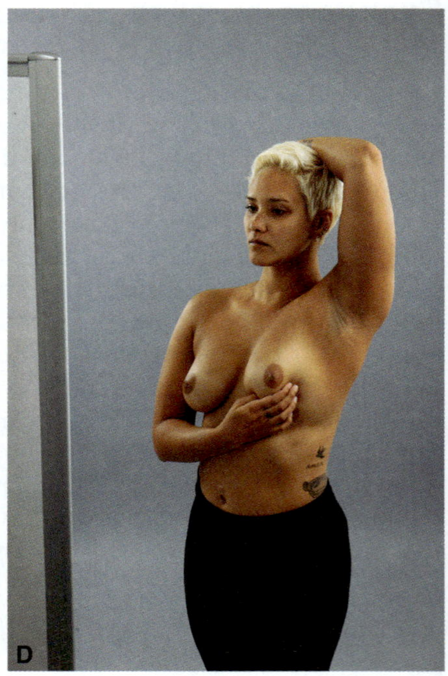

Figure 14-22 Breast self-awareness technique. **A.** Inspection before a mirror: Arms at side. **B.** Inspection before a mirror: Arms overhead. **C.** Inspection before a mirror.: Hands pressed into hips. **D.** Palpation: Arm overhead while standing.

Breast augmentation, or augmentation mammoplasty, using synthetic implants is the second most popular surgical procedure among women in the United States. There are three types of synthetic implants: the gel-filled implant, the saline inflatable implant, and the polyurethane-covered implant filled with silicone. When examining a client, ask if the breasts have been augmented, what type of implant was used, and when they were inserted.

Incision sites from breast augmentation can be found in the axillae, circumareolar areas, and inframammary creases. Potential complications from augmentation include hematoma, infection, scarring, loss of nipple or skin sensation, pain from engorgement, asymmetry, malpositioning, and breakage of the implant. Breakage can lead to a granulomatous reaction in the breasts in which small, nodular, inflammatory lesions develop, and a capsular membrane forms over the breasts. The augmented breast will feel firmer upon palpation, and the nipples may remain more erect when the client is supine.

Before augmentation, a baseline mammogram should be performed to provide a reference for future mammography. The guidelines for breast self-examination, clinical examination, and mammography are the same for the client who has undergone augmentation as they are for the client who has not undergone breast surgery.

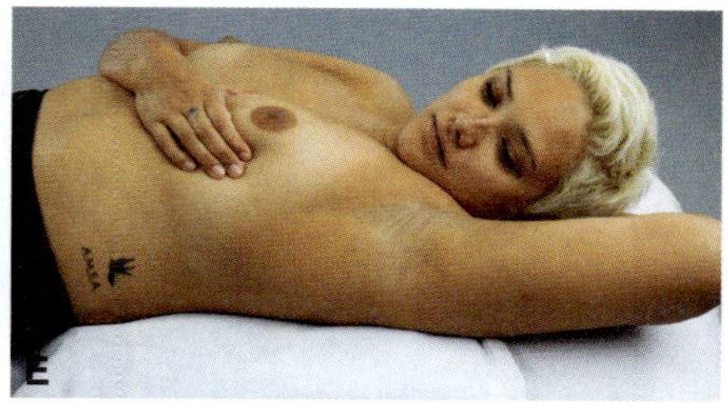

Figure 14-22—cont'd E. Palpation: Arm overhead while supine.

The Male Breasts

Anatomy

The male breast is composed of a well-developed areola and a small nipple that has immature tissue underneath. **Gynecomastia**, the enlargement of male breast tissue (Fig. 14-23), may occur normally in adolescent and elderly men.

Gynecomastia must be differentiated from breast enlargement caused by fat deposits (lipomastia) seen in overweight men. Up to 70% of early to midpuberty boys experience gynecomastia due to normal pubertal hormonal changes. It is reported to be due to an imbalance in estrogen and androgen production, hormonal action, or both (Braunstein & Anawalt, 2021).

Up to 65% of middle-aged and older males experience gynecomastia. Common causes of gynecomastia in adult males include unresolved pubertal gynecomastia, medications such as spironolactone, ketoconazole, and cimetidine, or idiopathic reasons (Braunstein & Anawalt, 2021). The appearance of enlarged breasts may cause anxiety, psychosocial discomfort, and fear of breast cancer.

Breast Cancer Screening in Men

With 1% of all breast cancers found in males, breast cancer screening is only recommended for males at increased risk of breast cancer due to a *BRCA1* or *BRCA2* inherited gene mutation (American Cancer Society, 2024).

The National Comprehensive Cancer Network (NCCN) recommends males who have a *BRCA1* or *BRCA2* inherited gene mutation get breast cancer screening starting at age 35. The NCCN recommends these males should:

- Have a clinical breast examination every year
- Learn how to do breast self-examination

The NCCN recommends that males with a *BRCA1 or BRCA2* inherited gene mutation have an annual mammogram, beginning 10 years before the earliest known breast cancer in a male family member or at age 50 (whichever age comes first) (Daly et al, 2021).

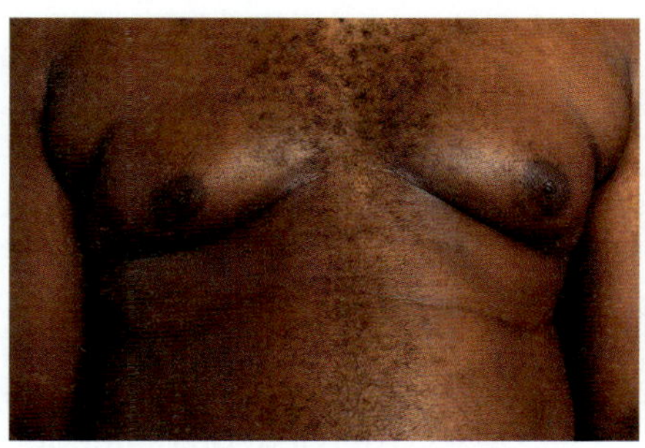

Figure 14-23 Gynecomastia.

Examination of the Male Breasts

Examination of the male breasts is completed in essentially the same manner as that of the female breasts. Modify your technique for a smaller breast with less tissue bulk. Having the client lean forward is usually not necessary unless gynecomastia is present. If gynecomastia is present, a thorough clinical breast examination should be performed to determine whether the enlarged breast tissue is fatty or glandular. Glandular tissue has ducts that are designed to secrete substances, such as milk or hormones. Breast imaging may be needed if there is difficulty determining whether a client has gynecomastia. Early diagnostic evaluation is critical.

U.S. Preventive Services Task Force (USPSTF)

Grade B Recommendations:

- The USPSTF recommends that primary care clinicians assess women with a personal or family history of breast, ovarian, tubal, or peritoneal cancer or who have an ancestry associated with breast cancer susceptibility 1 and 2 *(BRCA1/2)* gene mutations with an appropriate brief familial risk assessment tool. Women with a positive result on the risk assessment tool should receive genetic counseling and, if indicated after counseling, genetic testing.
- The USPSTF recommends biennial screening mammography for women aged 40 to 74 years.
- The USPSTF recommends that clinicians offer to prescribe risk-reducing medications, such as tamoxifen, raloxifene, or aromatase inhibitors, to women who are at increased risk for breast cancer and low risk for adverse medication effects.

Retrieved November 5, 2025, from *https://www.uspreventiveservicestaskforce.org/uspstf/recommendation-topics/uspstf-a-and-b-recommendations*

CASE STUDY
The Client With a Breast Mass

This case study illustrates the application and objective documentation of the breasts and regional lymph nodes examination. Tiffany Brown is a 20-year-old college student who is home for the summer break leading into senior year. She is preparing to complete her last year of college as an electrical engineering major and is planning for a summer internship. She presents to the provider's office for her well-woman visit and contraceptive pill prescription refill.

HEALTH HISTORY

CLIENT PROFILE

20-year-old single, Black, female

REASON FOR SEEKING HEALTH CARE

"I am doing fine. I need a new prescription for my birth control pill."

PRESENT HEALTH

Ms. Brown has been taking a combined oral contraceptive pill for 2 years. She denies any side effects or problems with her birth control pill. In a monogamous relationship with a partner of 2 years who is also a college student at her school. Uses condoms along with birth control pills. She is fearful of becoming pregnant while in college and having to tell her parents. Lifetime sexual partners is one. Denies any chest pain, shortness of breath, abdominal pain, headaches, visual changes, breast tenderness, and breakthrough uterine bleeding. Client started menses at age 11.

PAST HEALTH HISTORY

Medical History Denies any medical conditions; menses regular, has never been pregnant

Surgical History Denies

Allergies No known allergies to medication, foods, insect bites/stings

Medications Desogestrel/ethinyl estradiol 0.15 mg/0.03 mg every morning

Communicable Diseases Denies ever having any STI or other communicable diseases

Injuries and Accidents May 2021 motor vehicle accident—Client was driver, was stopped at a red light when she was hit by another car at approximately 35 mph, airbag did not deploy. Denies injuries. No emergency care sought

Differing Abilities Denies

Blood Transfusions Denies

Childhood Illnesses Chickenpox as a child, unsure of age

Immunizations Had all required vaccines before starting college including HPV, meningitis, and hepatitis A; COVID-19 vaccine x 2 in 2021-none since

FAMILY HEALTH HISTORY

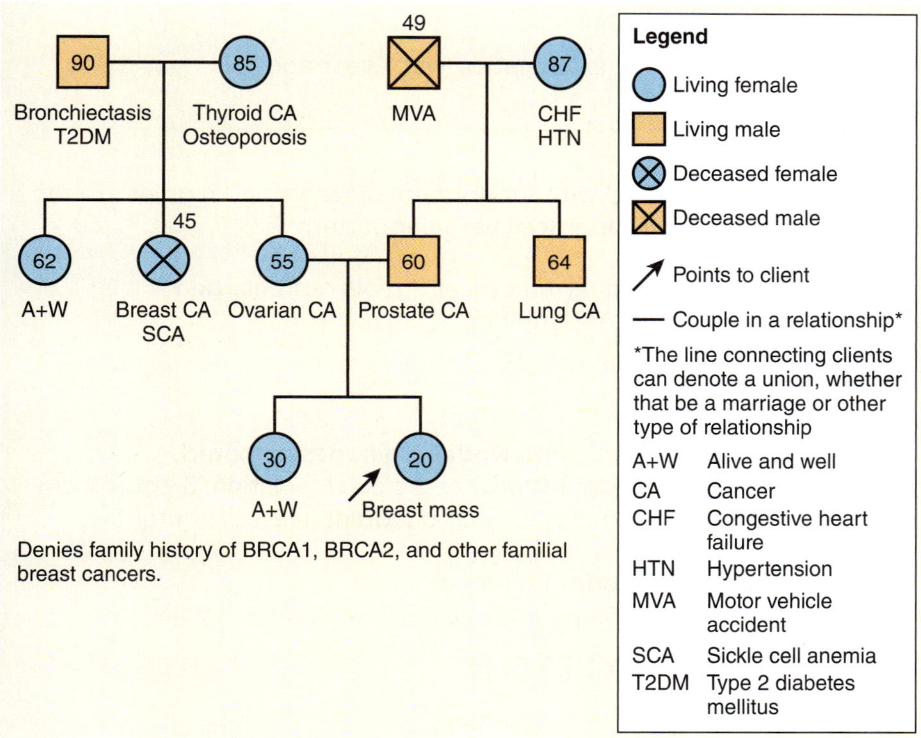

SOCIAL HISTORY

Alcohol Use Social drinker on weekends, one glass of beer

Tobacco Use Denies

Recreational Drug Use Denies

Domestic and Intimate Partner Violence Denies

Sexual Practice Heterosexual, same partner x 2 years, uses condoms with each act

Travel History Completed study abroad in China last year, no acute illnesses

Work Environment College student. Lives on campus in dormitory with female roommate

Home Environment Lives with mother and father when not in college. Has one older sister who lives 10 miles away

Hobbies and Leisure Activities Running and yoga, hanging out with friends

Stress Concerned with completing her last year of school and doing well in her summer internship.

Education Undergraduate electrical engineering student - rising senior

Economic Status Middle socioeconomic status. Comfortable as student, dependent on family for living expenses while a student

Military Service Denies

Religion Baptist

Ethnic Background Black

Roles and Relationships In monogamous relationship with boyfriend for 2 years. She is the first of her generation in her family to go to college. She works/studies hard to make her family proud. Gets along with family

Characteristic Patterns of Daily Living Takes college classes 5 days a week, works out after classes. Eats healthy diet at school cafeteria

HEALTH MAINTENANCE ACTIVITIES

Sleep Regular sleep cycle 5 to 8 hours each night during academic year

Diet Low fat/low carb 2,500-kcal diet

Exercise Daily cardio—running 3 miles, yoga on weekends

Stress Management Works out after classes, talks with her partner and roommate

Use of Safety Devices Wears seat belts.

Health Checkups Last gynecological examination was 1 year ago

PHYSICAL EXAMINATION

Inspection

Color Bilateral breasts flesh colored without erythema. Areola and nipples are tan

Vascularity No focal or unilateral superficial vascular pattern

Thickening/Edema None

Size and Symmetry Bilateral breasts symmetrical. Areola not enlarged

Contour No flattening, retractions, or dimpling

Lesions/Masses None visible

Discharge No discharge

Palpation

Supraclavicular and Infraclavicular Lymph Nodes No nodes palpated

Breasts: Client in Sitting Position Right breast at 2 o'clock position: 3 cm × 2 cm × 1 cm firm, mobile breast mass in upper-inner quadrant. Mass is nontender, round, and smooth

Axillary Lymph Node Region No nodes palpated

Breasts: Client in Supine Position Same as in sitting position

CLINICAL JUDGMENT IN ACTION

1. What cues indicate that the client is having a breast disorder?
2. What interventions have the highest priority?
3. What assessment findings indicate clinical improvement or decline in this client?

Review Questions

1. A client visits the clinic for a well-woman examination. The client complains of having right breast pain when the health history is conducted. What would be the nurse's most appropriate response?
   a. Tell the client it is probably nothing to worry about.
   b. Reassure the client that she has the same pain during her menstrual cycle and it is probably normal.
   c. Refer the client for a mammogram.
   d. Ask the client for more information about the pain in the right breast.

2. The nurse is reviewing the history of a female client during a routine gynecological visit. The nurse recognizes what risk factor(s) in the client's history increases the risk for breast cancer? Select all that apply.
   a. History of ovarian cancer in her mother
   b. History of prostatic hypertrophy in her father
   c. Menarche at age 16
   d. Obesity
   e. White race
   f. Cigarette smoker
   g. First child at age 26

3. A mother brings her 7-year-old daughter to the clinic with concerns about suspected abnormal breast development and breast tenderness in the child. Upon examination, the daughter is found to have left breast bud development with slight areola enlargement. The right breast nipple is small and slightly raised. The nurse's best response to the mother and child would be:
   a. The daughter should be examined further since this is abnormal breast development.
   b. Reassure the mother that breast development may be asymmetrical during the early stages of breast development and tenderness is not uncommon.
   c. Ask if there is a family history of breast cancer since this may be an early sign.
   d. Tenderness is uncommon and may be a sign of something more serious.

4. Which of the following clients should the nurse identify as having an increased risk of breast cancer? Select all that apply.
   a. A 40-year-old woman with three children
   b. A 25-year-old woman with a father diagnosed with breast cancer
   c. A 55-year-old woman who never had children
   d. A 33-year-old postpartum mother breastfeeding her second child
   e. A 45-year-old woman with a sister diagnosed with breast cancer
   f. A 35-year-old woman with breast augmentation

5. A 35-year-old breastfeeding mother calls the nurse with complaints of a fever of 101°F, pain, redness, and engorgement in the left breast. The nurse suspects which of the following diagnoses?
   a. Benign breast disease
   b. Ductal carcinoma in situ
   c. Mastitis
   d. Fibroadenoma

6. A 35-year-old client with dense breasts is concerned with developing breast cancer. She does not have a family history of breast cancer. The nurse tells the client the most effective method to identify early breast lumps to evaluate for breast cancer for someone with her history is:
   a. Yearly clinical breast examination starting at age 25
   b. Monthly self-breast examination
   c. Mammograms every 3 years starting at age 35
   d. Becoming breast aware of one's breasts

7. The nurse is completing the health history of a client with a complaint of a breast lump. What information should the nurse ask the client? Select all that apply.
   a. In which breast is the lump located?
   b. What time of day did you notice the lump?
   c. Does the lump move?
   d. What size is the lump?
   e. Is the lump painful?

8. A 52-year-old transmasculine client presents for an annual wellness examination. What breast cancer screening should be recommended to this client?
   a. Schedule a breast ultrasound
   b. Schedule a screening mammogram
   c. Schedule a breast MRI
   d. Perform self-breast examination every month

9. A female client has the left breast and left axillary lymph nodes removed due to a diagnosis of breast cancer. This description describes which type of mastectomy?
   a. Simple
   b. Modified radical
   c. Radical
   d. Subcutaneous

10. A 55-year-old female client informs the nurse that she does not get her mammograms since she has breast implants and does not want them to become damaged during the procedure. The nurse's best response is:
    a. Document the client's refusal to have the mammogram.
    b. Explain to the client, females with breast implants should continue to get mammograms as recommended unless they had a bilateral mastectomy.
    c. Thank the client for her honesty and letting the nurse know.
    d. Agree with the client telling her she would not want anything to happen to the implants during the procedure as well.

CHAPTER

15 Thorax and Lungs

Learning Outcomes

1. Identify the anatomic landmarks of the thorax and lungs.
2. Explain the physiology of ventilation.
3. Conduct a complete health history on a client with a lung condition.
4. Perform inspection, palpation, percussion, and auscultation on a healthy adult and on an adult with lung pathology.
5. Differentiate between normal clinical findings from a client's physical examination and the pathophysiology of abnormal clinical findings.
6. Identify risk factors for lung cancer.
7. Identify the United States Preventive Services Task Force recommendations for the thorax and lungs.
8. Document a complete health history and physical examination on a client with a thorax and lung pathology.

The respiratory system extends from the nose to the alveoli (Fig. 15-1). The normal air pathway is nose, pharynx, larynx, trachea, mainstem bronchus, right and left main bronchi, lobar/secondary bronchi, tertiary/segmental bronchi, terminal bronchioles, respiratory bronchioles, alveolar ducts, alveolar sacs, and alveoli.

The respiratory system is divided into the upper and lower tracts. The upper respiratory tract comprises the nose, pharynx, larynx, and upper trachea. The nose and pharynx are discussed in Chapter 13. The lower respiratory tract is composed of the lower trachea to the lungs. This chapter deals only with the components of the respiratory system that are located in the thorax.

Anatomy

Thorax

The **thorax** is a cone-shaped structure (narrower at the top and wider at the bottom) that consists of bones, cartilage, and muscles. Of these, the bones are the supportive structure of the thorax. On the anterior thorax, these bones are the 12 pairs of ribs and the sternum. Posteriorly, there are the 12 thoracic vertebrae and the spinal column.

Sternum

The sternum, or breastbone, is a flat, narrow bone approximately 15 cm long (Fig. 15-2). It is located at the median line of the anterior chest wall and is divided into three sections: the **manubrium** (the upper bone of

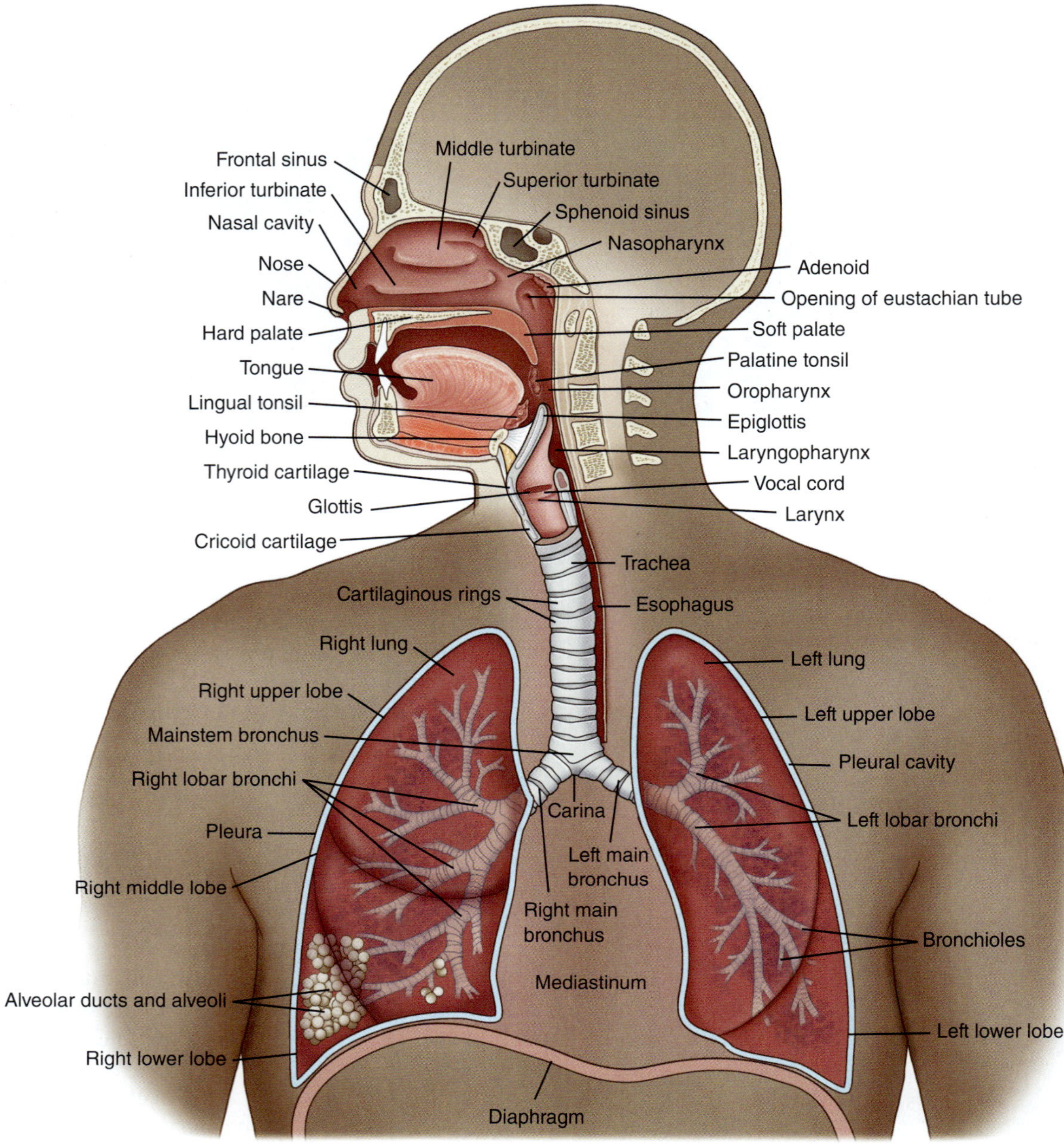

Figure 15-1 The respiratory tract.

the sternum that articulates with the clavicles and the first pair of ribs), the body, and the **xiphoid process** (a cartilaginous process at the base of the sternum that does not articulate with the ribs).

Ribs

The first seven pairs of ribs are articulated to the sternum via the costal cartilages and are called the **vertebrosternal** or **true ribs.** The **false ribs** or rib pairs 8–10, articulate with the costal cartilages just above them. The remaining two pairs of ribs (11 and 12) are termed **floating ribs** and do not articulate at their anterior ends. The 10th rib is the lowest rib that can be palpated anteriorly. The 11th rib is palpated on the lateral thorax, and the 12th rib is palpated on the posterior thorax. All ribs articulate posteriorly to the vertebral column. When a rib is palpated, the costal cartilage cannot be distinguished from the rib itself (Fig. 15-2).

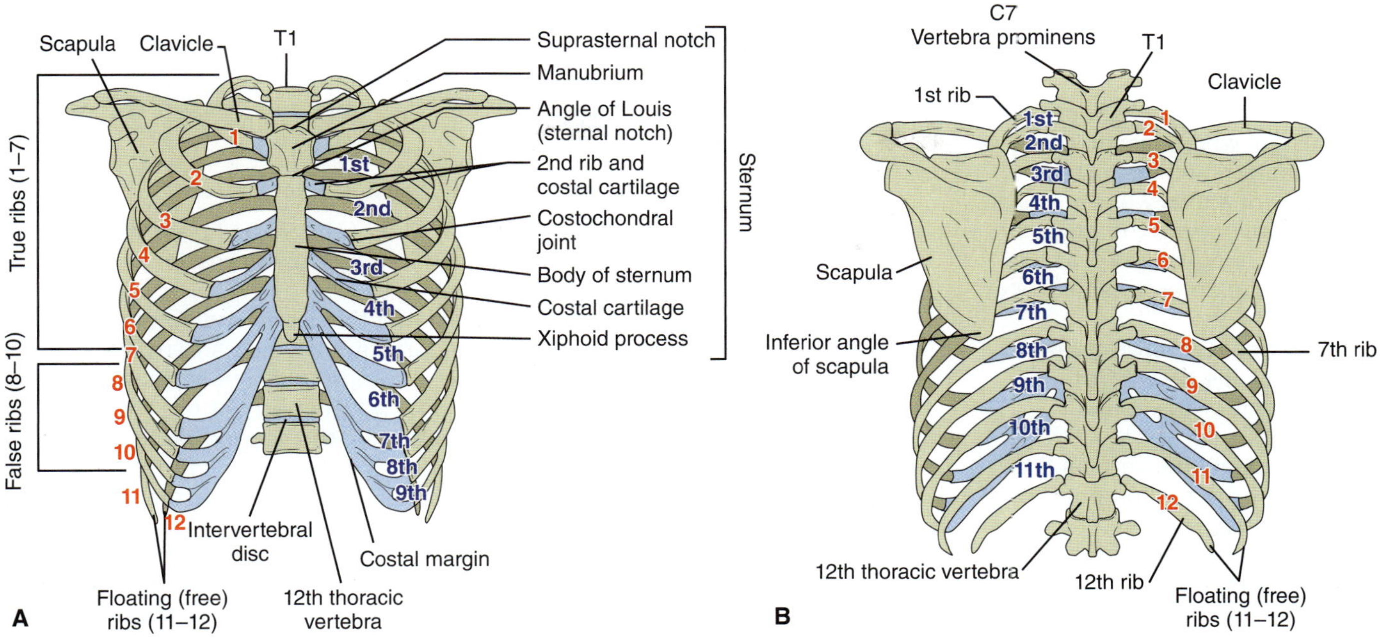

Figure 15-2 Thorax: Rib number is shown on the client's right; intercostal space number is shown on the client's left. **A.** Anterior view. **B.** Posterior view.

Intercostal Spaces

Each area between the ribs is called an **intercostal space** (ICS). There are 11 ICSs.

Lungs

The lungs are cone-shaped organs that fill the lateral chambers of the thoracic cavity. The lower outer surface of each lung is concave where it meets the convex diaphragm. Likewise, the medial aspect is concave to allow room for the heart, with the left lung having a more pronounced concavity (cardiac notch). The lungs lie against the ribs anteriorly and posteriorly.

The right lung is broader than the left lung because of the position of the heart. Inferiorly, the right lung is about 2.5 cm shorter than the left lung because of the upward displacement of the diaphragm by the liver. The right lung consists of three lobes (upper, middle, and lower), whereas the left lung has two lobes (upper and lower). In the lung, the **apex** denotes the top of the lung and the **base** refers to the bottom of the lung. Anteriorly, the apices of the lung extend 2.5 to 4 cm superior to the inner third of the clavicles; posteriorly, the apices lie near the T1 process. On deep inspiration posteriorly, the lower lung border extends to the level of T12, and to T10 on deep expiration (Fig. 15-3).

The lobes of the right and left lungs are divided by grooves called **fissures.** It is important to know the locations of the fissures to describe clinical findings. Figures 15-3 and 15-4 illustrate the right oblique (or diagonal) fissure, the right horizontal fissure, and the left oblique (or diagonal) fissure.

When assessing the thorax, it is helpful to envision it as a rectangular box, with the four sides being the anterior, posterior, right lateral, and left lateral thoraxes. For example, the anterior inferior border of the lungs is at the sixth rib at the **midclavicular line** (MCL: vertical line drawn from the midpoint of the clavicle) and at the eighth rib at the **midaxillary line** (MAL: vertical line drawn from the apex of the axillae and lying midway between the anterior and the posterior axillary lines). Figure 15-5 illustrates the imaginary thoracic lines on the anterior, posterior, and left lateral sides. These landmarks are helpful in discussing clinical findings.

> **NURSING TIP**
> **Counting Anterior Intercostal Spaces**
> Use the angle of Louis as a landmark for identifying the rib number. Count the ribs in the midclavicular line. Each intercostal space (ICS) is named for the number of the rib directly above it. For example, the space between the third and fourth ribs would be called the third ICS.

NURSING TIP
Thoracic Anatomic Topography

Additional landmarks that are useful when describing examination findings are:

- **Anterior axillary line**: vertical line drawn from the origin of the anterior axillary fold and along the anterolateral aspect of the thorax.
- **Midspinal (vertebral) line**: vertical line drawn from the midpoint of the spinous process.
- **Midsternal line**: vertical line drawn from the midpoint of the sternum.
- **Posterior axillary line**: vertical line drawn from the posterior axillary fold.
- **Scapular line**: vertical line drawn from the inferior angle of the scapula.

NURSING TIP
Identifying Thoracic Landmarks

Anterior

- Sternum
- Clavicles
- Nipples
- **Suprasternal notch**: With the finger pad of the index finger, feel in the midsternal line above the manubrium; the depression is the suprasternal notch.
- **Angle of Louis** (or **manubriosternal junction** or **sternal angle**): With the finger pads, feel for the suprasternal notch and move your finger pads down the sternum until they reach a horizontal ridge (the junction of the manubrium and the body of the sternum); this is the angle of Louis (or sternal angle); the second rib articulates with this landmark and serves as a convenient reference point for counting the ribs and ICSs (the first rib is difficult to palpate).
- **Costal angle**: Place your right finger pads on the bottom of the client's anterior left rib cage (10th rib); place your left finger pads on the bottom of the anterior right rib cage (10th rib); move both hands horizontally toward the sternum until they meet in the midsternal line; the angle formed by the intersection of the ribs creates the costal angle.

Posterior

- **Vertebra prominens**: Flex the neck forward; palpate the posterior spinous processes; if two processes are palpable, the superior process is C7 (vertebra prominens) and the inferior is T1; this landmark is useful in counting ribs to the level of T4; beyond T4 the spinous processes project obliquely and no longer correspond to the rib of the same number as the vertebral process.
- **Inferior angle of scapula**: Locate the inferior border of the scapula; this level corresponds to the seventh rib or seventh ICS.
- Spine
- **Twelfth rib**: Palpate the lower thorax in the scapular line. Move your hand laterally to palpate the free tip of the 12th rib.

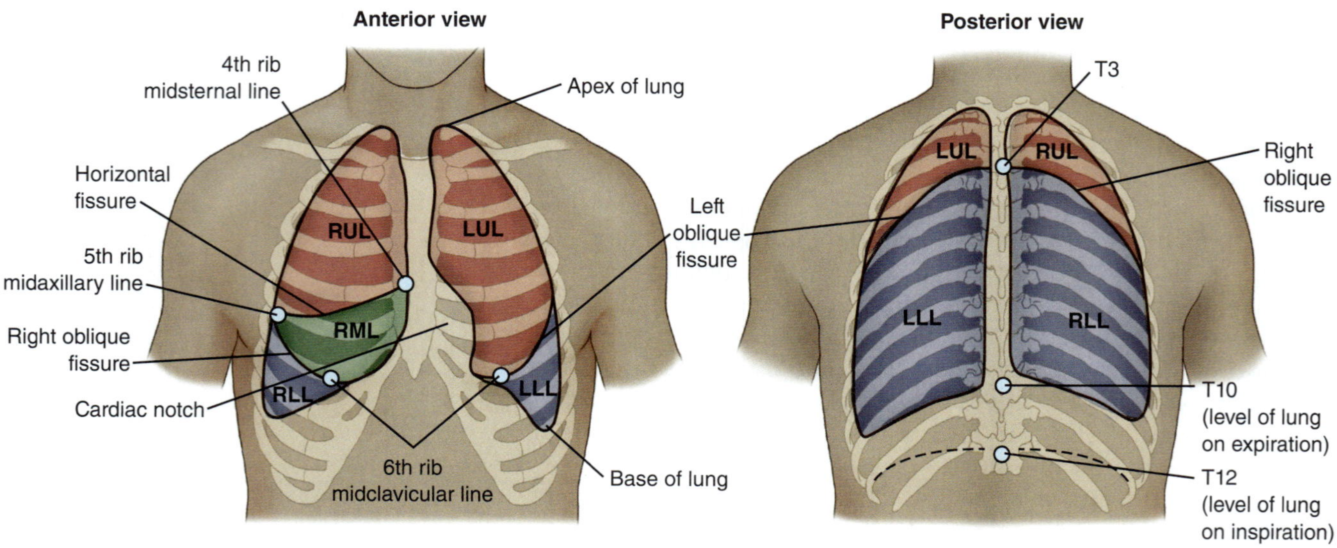

Figure 15-3 Lungs: Anterior view (left) and posterior view (right). RUL = right upper lobe, RML = right middle lobe, RLL = right lower lobe, LUL = left upper lobe, LLL = left lower lobe.

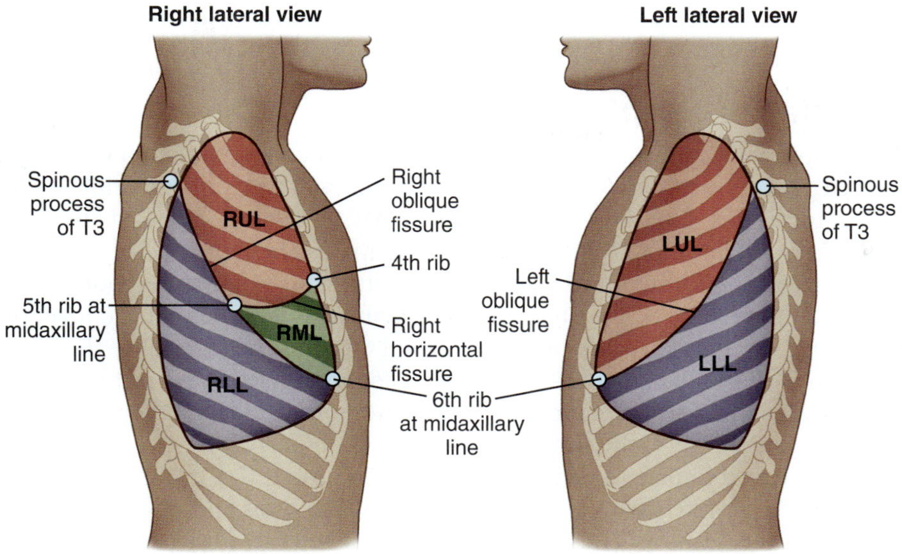

Figure 15-4 Lung fissures: Right and left lateral views. RUL = right upper lobe, RML = right middle lobe, RLL = right lower lobe, LUL = left upper lobe, LLL = left lower lobe.

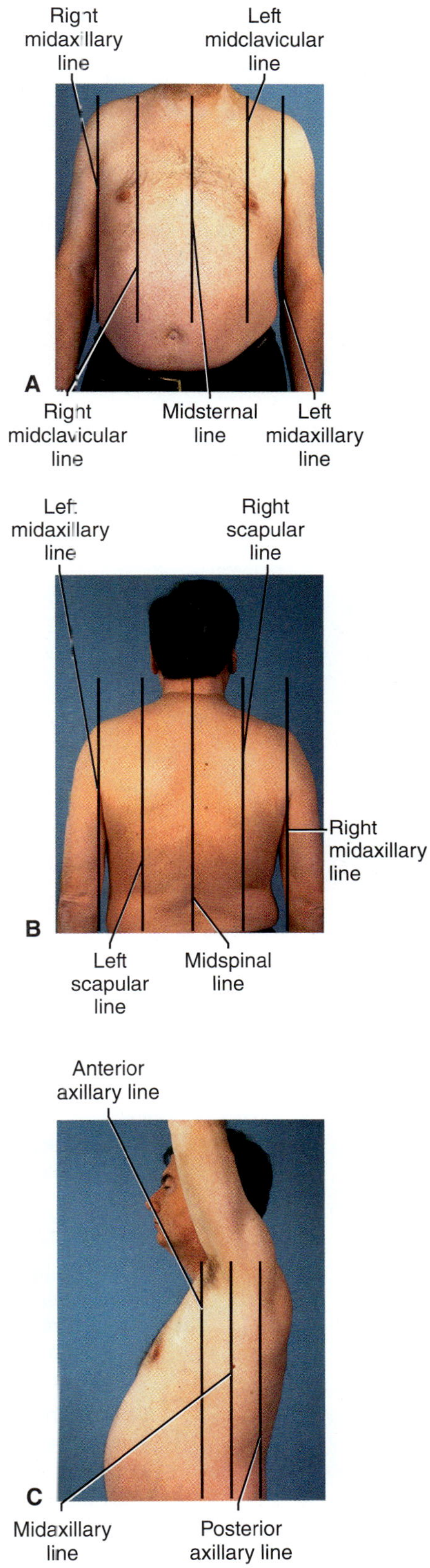

Figure 15-5 Imaginary thoracic lines. **A.** Anterior view. **B.** Posterior view. **C.** Left lateral view. Note that the right lateral view is similar.

Pleura

Each lung is encased in a serous sac, or **pleura**. The **parietal pleura** lines the chest wall and the superior surface of the diaphragm. The **visceral pleura** lines the external surface of the lungs. Usually, a small amount of fluid is found in the space between these two pleurae; this fluid prevents the pleurae from rubbing against each other and acts as a cushioning agent for the lungs.

Mediastinum

The **mediastinum**, or **interpleural space**, is the area between the right and left lungs. It extends from the sternum to the spinal column and contains the heart, great vessels, trachea, esophagus, and lymph vessels. The only respiratory structures in the mediastinum are the trachea and the pulmonary vasculature. The trachea is a fibromuscular hollow tube located in the anterior thorax in the median plane. It is 11 to 13 cm in length and 2 to 3 cm in width. The trachea lies anterior to the esophagus.

Bronchi

The cartilaginous projection at the last tracheal ring is the **carina**. It is at the carina that the trachea bifurcates into the left and right mainstem bronchi. Anatomically this is at the level of the fourth or fifth vertebral process posteriorly and the sternal angle anteriorly. The right mainstem bronchus is wider, shorter, and more vertical than the left. This anatomic difference is critical because it makes the right mainstem bronchus more susceptible to aspiration and endotracheal intubation. The mainstem bronchi further divide into lobar or secondary bronchi. Each lobar bronchus supplies a lobe of the lung. The bronchi transport gases and trap foreign particles in their mucus. Cilia aid in sweeping the foreign particles upward in the respiratory tract for possible elimination. Culmination of the tracheobronchial tree is in the alveoli.

Alveoli

The **alveoli** are the smallest functional units of the respiratory system. It is here that gas exchange occurs. It is estimated that approximately 300 million alveoli are present in each lung. This aerating surface is about equal to 100 times the body surface area of an adult. Each alveolus has its own blood supply and lymphatic drainage. Branches of the pulmonary artery carry blood to the capillaries surrounding the alveoli to be oxygenated. Branches of the pulmonary vein transport oxygenated blood from the alveoli to the heart.

Muscles of Respiration

The diaphragm, which is innervated by the phrenic nerve, is a dome-shaped muscle that forms the inferior border of the thorax. Anteriorly, its right edge is located at the fifth rib—fifth ICS at the MCL. The left dome of the diaphragm is at the sixth rib—sixth ICS at the MCL. The presence of the liver below the right dome of the diaphragm accounts for the elevated border on that side. On expiration posteriorly, the diaphragm is located at the level of the 10th vertebral process, and at T12 on inspiration. Laterally, the diaphragm is found at the eighth rib at the midaxillary line. The diaphragm is the principal muscle of respiration. Contraction of the diaphragm leads to an increase in volume in the thoracic cavity.

The external intercostal muscles are located in the ICS. During inspiration, the external intercostal muscles elevate the ribs, thus increasing the size of the thoracic cavity. The internal intercostal muscles draw adjacent ribs together, thereby decreasing the size of the thoracic cavity during expiration.

Accessory respiratory muscles are used to accommodate increased oxygen demand. Exercise and some diseases lead to the use of accessory muscles. The inspiratory accessory muscles are the trapezius, sternocleidomastoid, scalene, pectoralis, serratus anterior, and serratus posterior. The expiratory muscles of respiration are the rectus abdominis, external and internal obliques, and the transversus abdominis (Fig. 15-6).

Physiology

Ventilation

The primary function of the respiratory system is to deliver oxygen to the lungs and to remove carbon dioxide from the lungs. The breathing process

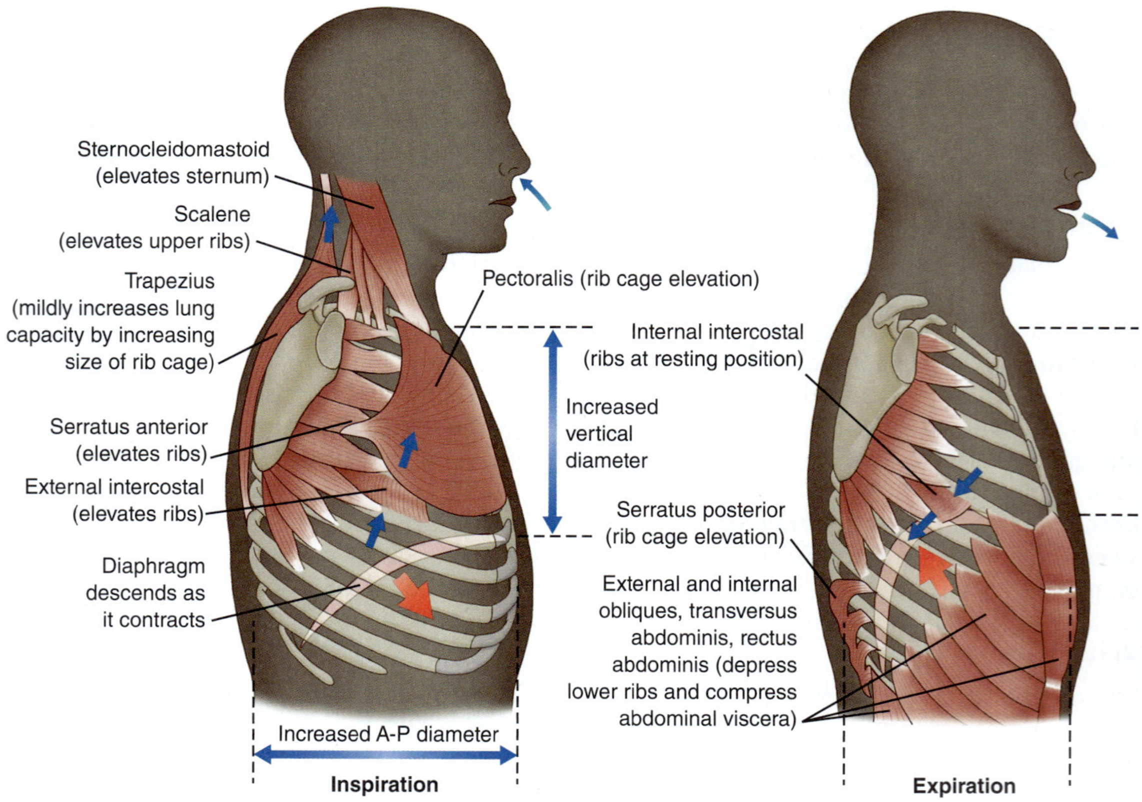

Figure 15-6 Muscles of respiration.

includes inspiratory and expiratory phases. During inspiration (inhalation), the pressure inside the lungs becomes subatmospheric when the diaphragm and external intercostal muscles contract. The diaphragm lowers and the ribs elevate, thus increasing the intrapulmonic volume. As a result of the negative intra-alveolar pressure, atmospheric air is pulled into the respiratory tract until intra-alveolar pressure equals atmospheric pressure. The lungs increase in size with the air.

Expiration (exhalation) is a passive process and occurs more rapidly than inspiration. During expiration, the diaphragm and external intercostal muscles relax, decreasing the volume of the thoracic cavity. The diaphragm rises. The intrapulmonic volume decreases, and the intrapulmonic pressure increases above the atmospheric pressure. The lungs possess elastic recoil capabilities that allow air to be expelled until intrapulmonic pressure equals atmospheric pressure.

External Respiration

External respiration is the process by which gases are exchanged between the lungs and the pulmonary vasculature. Oxygen diffuses from the alveoli into the blood, and carbon dioxide diffuses from the blood to the alveoli. Diffusion is a passive process in which gases move across a membrane from an area of higher concentration to an area of lower concentration. In the lungs, the membrane is the alveolar-capillary network.

Internal Respiration

Internal respiration is the process by which gases are exchanged between the pulmonary vasculature and the body's tissues. Oxygen from the lungs diffuses from the blood into body tissue. Carbon dioxide diffuses from the tissue into the blood. This blood is then carried back to the right side of the heart for reoxygenation.

Control of Breathing

Control of breathing is influenced by neural and chemical factors. The pons and medulla are the central nervous system structures primarily responsible for involuntary respiration. The stimulus for breathing is an increased carbon dioxide level, a decreased oxygen level, or an increased blood pH level.

HEALTH HISTORY

The thorax and lungs health history provides insight into the link between a client's life/lifestyle and thorax and lungs information and pathology.

CLIENT PROFILE

Diseases that are age-, sex-, and race-specific for the thorax and lungs are listed.

Age Respiratory syncytial virus (RSV) (premature infants–12 mo)
- Bronchiectasis (birth–20)
- Cystic fibrosis (birth–30)
- Scheuermann kyphosis (10–15, around puberty)
- Pneumothorax (20–40)
- Sarcoidosis (30–40)
- Chronic obstructive pulmonary disease (COPD) (>40)
- Pneumonia (>60)
- RSV (>60)
- Idiopathic pulmonary fibrosis (60–70)
- Lung cancer (>65)

Sex

Female Sarcoidosis, kyphosis

Male Obstructive sleep apnea (OSA), mesothelioma, idiopathic pulmonary fibrosis, pneumothorax

Race

Black Lung cancer, sarcoidosis

White Cystic fibrosis

CHIEF COMPLAINT

Common chief complaints for the thorax and lungs are defined, and information on the characteristics of each sign or symptom is provided.

1. **Dyspnea** Subjective feeling of shortness of breath (SOB)

   Quantity The number of steps that can be climbed before SOB occurs; distance that can be walked; number of pillows needed to sleep comfortably

   Associated Manifestations Palpitations, leg pain, faintness, anxiety, panic attack, fatigue, cough, sputum, wheezing, diaphoresis, cyanosis, pain, fever

   Aggravating Factors Smoking, exercise, poorly ventilated rooms, cold weather, wind, outdoor/indoor allergens, specific foods, animals, prolonged wearing of N-95 respirator or face mask

   Alleviating Factors Pillow orthopnea, side-lying position, tripod position, fresh air, medications (e.g., bronchodilators), supplemental oxygen, resting

   Timing Nighttime (paroxysmal nocturnal dyspnea)

2. **Cough** Stimulation of afferent vagal endings, which helps clean the airway of extraneous material by producing a sudden, forceful, and noisy expulsion of air from the lungs

   Quality Dry, wet, hacking, barking, congested, harsh, brassy, high-pitched, whooping, bubbling, productive/nonproductive

   Associated Manifestations SOB, wheezing, sputum, pleuritic pain, chest pain, fever, hemoptysis, coryza, anxiety, diaphoresis, gastroesophageal reflux disease (GERD) symptoms, postnasal drip, hoarseness

   Aggravating Factors Position of client, exposure to noxious stimuli, exercise, outdoor/indoor allergens, specific foods, animals

   Alleviating Factors Medications (e.g., nebulizer, inhaler, cough suppressant medications, steroids), humidity, cool air, cool liquids

   Setting Temperature and humidity of environment, exertion

   Timing Winter weather, early morning, bedtime, middle of the night, after eating, before fainting, continuous

3. **Sputum** Substance produced by the respiratory tract that can be expectorated or swallowed; it is composed of mucus, blood, purulent material, microorganisms, cellular debris, and, occasionally, foreign objects

   Quality Color: white or clear, purulent, blood-tinged, yellow or green, mucoid, rust, black, pink

   Consistency: thick, thin, moderate; frothy (separates into layers)

   Odor: malodorous

   Quantity Normal daily sputum production is 60 to 90 mL (normally little is expectorated; it is eliminated into the gastrointestinal tract); small, moderate, copious

   Associated Manifestations Cough, fever, dyspnea

   Aggravating Factors Exposure to indoor/outdoor allergens, smoking

   Alleviating Factors Medications (e.g., guaifenesin), liquids

   Setting Sleep, exposure to allergen

   Timing Early morning

4. **Chest Pain** Pain can have a pulmonary, cardiac, gastrointestinal, or musculoskeletal etiology. Chapter 16 differentiates types of chest pain.

PAST HEALTH HISTORY

The various components of past health history are linked to thorax and lung pathology and thorax- and lung-related information.

Medical History

Respiratory Specific Asthma, bronchitis, COPD, croup, frequent coryza, cystic fibrosis, pulmonary fibrosis, epiglottitis, OSA, RSV, pleurisy, pneumonia, pneumothorax, pulmonary edema, pulmonary embolus, lung cancer, tuberculosis, pertussis, pleural effusion, bronchiectasis, pulmonary hypertension, hypersensitivity pneumonitis, interstitial lung disease, tracheal intubation

Nonrespiratory Specific Lupus, drug-induced respiratory pathology, rheumatoid arthritis, congenital musculoskeletal chest defects, severe scoliosis, immunosuppression, multiple sclerosis, amyotrophic lateral sclerosis, and other neuromuscular disorders

Surgical History Lobectomy, pneumonectomy, tracheostomy, wedge resection, bronchoscopy, bronchial thermoplasty, lung biopsy, chest tube insertion

Allergies Asthma is the predominant manifestation of allergies in the client with respiratory conditions. Hypersensitivity to medications, food, pets, cigarette smoke, perfume, indoor allergens (such as dust/dust mites) or outdoor allergens (such as pollen and ragweed) are possible triggers. In addition, any common signs of allergies, such as cough, sneeze, nasal discharge, and sinusitis, should be closely evaluated.

Medications Beta agonist, inhaled corticosteroid, inhaled anticholinergic, mast cell stabilizer, leukotriene modifiers, IgE blocker, biologics, antibiotics, cough expectorant, cough suppressant, oxygen, oral corticosteroids, immunotherapy (allergy shots)

Communicable Diseases Coryza: sneezing, coughing

RSV: cough, wheezing, bronchiolitis, pneumonia
Tuberculosis (TB): pulmonary fibrosis and calcification
Influenza: pneumonia
HIV: *Pneumocystis carinii* pneumonia
COVID-19: pneumonia, bronchitis, acute respiratory distress syndrome (ARDS)
Hantavirus: bilateral pulmonary infiltrates, respiratory failure

Injuries and Accidents Chest trauma (e.g., rib fractures, pneumothorax, penetrating wounds), near-drowning

Differing Abilities Oxygen dependent, phrenic pacer dependent, ventilator dependent

Childhood Illnesses Pertussis and measles: bronchiectasis

FAMILY HEALTH HISTORY

Familial thorax and lung diseases are listed.

Allergies, alpha-1 antitrypsin deficiency, asthma, bronchiectasis, cancer, cystic fibrosis, emphysema, sarcoidosis, TB, pulmonary emboli, OSA

SOCIAL HISTORY

The components of social history are linked to thorax and lung factors and pathology.

Alcohol Use Decreases efficiency of lung defense mechanisms, predisposes to aspiration pneumonia; clients with carbon dioxide retention are more sensitive to alcohol's depressant effect

Tobacco Use Cigarette smoking is the primary risk factor for chronic bronchitis, emphysema, and lung cancer, as well as other disorders. Vaping, electronic cigarettes, and marijuana are equally harmful to the lungs.

Recreational Drug Use Heroin: pulmonary edema

Barbiturates or narcotic overdose: respiratory depression
Cocaine: tachypnea

Travel History Prolonged exposure to confined space with recirculated air (e.g., airplane)

TB (Asia, Eastern Europe, sub-Saharan Africa): poor sanitation and rural conditions
San Joaquin Valley fever or coccidioidomycosis (Southwest United States and Mexico): agent is in dirt and dusty winds

Work Environment Repeated exposure to materials in the workplace can create respiratory complications that range from minor problems to life-threatening events. Numerous categories of respiratory diseases have been identified, from repeated exposure to toxic substances. These diseases are listed along with the industries and agents related to them.

Silicosis: glassmaking, tunneling, stonecutting, mineral mining, insulation work, quarrying, cement work, ceramics, foundry work, semiconductor manufacturing

Asbestosis: mining, shipbuilding, construction

Coal worker's pneumoconiosis: coal mining

Pneumoconioses: tin and aluminum production, welding, insecticide manufacturing, rubber industry, fertilizer industry, ceramics, cosmetic industry

Occupational asthma: electroplating, grain working, woodworking, photography, printing, baking, painting

Chronic bronchitis: coal mining, welding, firefighting

Byssinosis: cotton mill dust, flax

Extrinsic allergic alveolitis (hypersensitivity pneumonia): animal hair, contamination of air-conditioning or heating systems, moldy hay, moldy grains, moldy dust, sugarcane

Toxic gases and fumes: welding, cigarette smoke, auto exhaust, chemical industries, firefighting, hair spray

Pulmonary neoplasms: radon gas, mustard gas, printing ink, asbestos, chromium (from chrome plating, stainless steel welding)

Pneumonitis: furniture polish, gasoline, or kerosene ingestion; mineral oil, olive oil, and milk aspiration

Home Environment Air pollution, cigarette smoke, wood-burning stoves, gas stoves and heaters, kerosene heaters, radon gas, pet hair and dander

Hobbies and Leisure Activities Birds (bird breeder's lung), mushroom growers (mushroom grower's lung), scuba diving (lung rupture, oxygen toxicity, decompression sickness), high-altitude activities (e.g., skiing, mountain climbing: pulmonary edema and pulmonary embolus)

Stress Asthma can be exacerbated by stress.

Economic Status Poor sanitation and densely populated areas are ideal conditions for the spread of TB.

HEALTH MAINTENANCE ACTIVITIES

This information provides a bridge between the health maintenance activities and thorax and lung function.

Sleep OSA: absence of inspiratory muscle activation; upper-airway occlusion

COPD or neuromuscular disease: nocturnal oxygen desaturation caused by hypoventilation without apnea

Diet Obesity: chronic hypoventilation, OSA

Exercise Regular exercise improves pulmonary function

Use of Safety Devices Mask worn when exposed to toxic substances, other occupational precautions as mandated by Occupational Safety and Health Administration (OSHA); knowledge of Heimlich maneuver

Health Checkups Respiratory rate, lung auscultation, chest X-ray, sputum analysis, pulmonary function test, nitric oxide testing, methacholine challenge, TB testing, influenza, RSV, and pneumococcal vaccines, allergy testing, immunotherapy

NURSING CHECKLIST

General Approach to Thorax and Lung Examination

1. Greet the client and explain the examination techniques you will be using.
2. Ensure the examination room is at a warm, comfortable temperature to prevent client chilling and shivering.
3. Use a quiet room that will be free from interruptions.
4. Ensure the light in the room provides sufficient brightness to adequately observe the client.

5. Instruct the client to remove all street clothes from the waist up and to don an examination gown.
6. Place the client in an upright sitting position on the examination table.
7. Observe Standard Precautions and don personal protective equipment (PPE), such as gloves, gown, face shield, goggles, N-95 respirator or face mask if the client's status warrants these protective measures.
8. Expose the entire area being assessed. Provide a drape to clients to cover their breasts (if desired).
9. When palpating, percussing, or auscultating the anterior thorax of a client with large breasts or a client with obesity, ask the client to displace the breast tissue. Assessing directly over breast tissue is not an accurate indicator of underlying structures.
10. Visualize the underlying respiratory structures during the examination process to assist in accurate description of the location of any pathology.
11. Always compare the right and the left sides of the anterior thorax and the posterior thorax to one another, as well as the right lateral thorax to the left lateral thorax.
12. Use a systematic approach each time the examination is performed. Proceed from the lung apices to the bases, right to left to lateral.
13. If the client is an older adult, frail, weak, or unable to sit for a short period of time and must be assessed while in a supine position, a second person may be needed to help you roll the client from side to side to perform the examination.

NURSING TIP

Influenza Vaccine

The Centers for Disease Control and Prevention (CDC) recommends that all persons from age 6 months receive the annual influenza vaccine. Various types of "flu" vaccines are available: Influenza inactivated (IIV3, ccIV3, aIIV3, HD-IIV3), Influenza recombinant (RIV3), Influenza live, attenuated (LAIV3). Refer to the CDC Web site for guidance on which vaccine is appropriate for a client's age and health status (CDC, 2025).

Retrieved November 5, 2025, from *https://www.cdc.gov/vaccines/hcp/imz-schedules/adult-age.html.*

Assessment in Brief

Thorax and Lung Examination

Inspection

- Shape of thorax
- Symmetry of chest wall
- Presence of superficial veins
- Costal angle
- Angle of the ribs
- Intercostal spaces
- Muscles of respiration
- Respirations
  - Rate
  - Pattern
  - Depth
  - Symmetry
  - Audibility
  - Client position
  - Mode of breathing
- Sputum

Palpation

- General palpation
  - Pulsations
  - Masses
  - Thoracic tenderness
  - Crepitus
- Thoracic expansion
- Tactile fremitus
- Tracheal position

Percussion

- General percussion
- Diaphragmatic excursion

Auscultation

- Breath sounds
- Adventitious sounds
- Voice sounds

Advanced Technique

- Forced expiratory time

Assistive Devices

- Oxygen
- Bilevel positive airway pressure (BiPAP)
- Endotracheal tube
- Tracheostomy tube
- Mechanical ventilation
- Pulse oximeter

Equipment

- Appropriate PPE
- Stethoscope
- Centimeter ruler or tape measure
- Washable marker
- Watch with second hand

Examination of the Thorax and Lungs

Inspection

Shape of the Thorax

E
1. Stand in front of the client.
2. Visually estimate the transverse diameter of the thorax.
3. Move to either side of the client.
4. Visually estimate the width of the anteroposterior (AP) diameter of the thorax.
5. Compare the estimates of these two visualizations.

N **In the normal adult, the ratio of the AP diameter to the transverse diameter is approximately 1:2 to 5:7. In other words, the normal adult is wider from side to side than from front to back. The normal thorax is slightly elliptical in shape. A barrel chest is normal in infants and sometimes in older adults. Refer to Chapter 25 for a discussion of the pediatric client.**

A In **barrel chest,** the ratio of the AP diameter to the transverse diameter is approximately 1:1. The client's chest is circular or barrel shaped in appearance.

P The client with COPD has a barrel chest due to air trapping in the alveoli and subsequent lung hyperinflation. Lung volume thus increases, and the diaphragm flattens over time. The ribs are forced upward and outward. Collectively, these changes result in the barrel-chest appearance (Fig. 15-7).

A **Pectus carinatum**, or pigeon chest, is a marked protrusion of the sternum. This increases the AP diameter of the thorax (Fig. 15-8A).

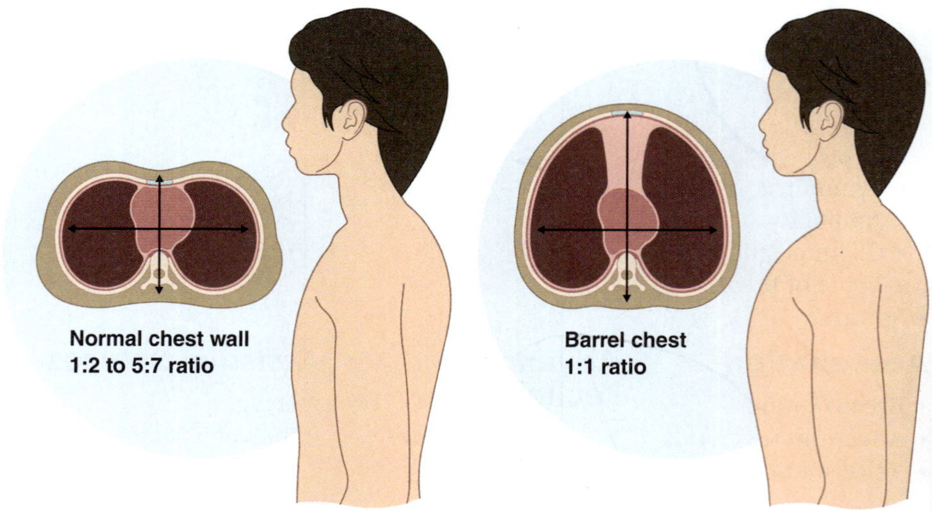

Figure 15-7 Chest configurations: Normal adult, barrel chest.

P Pectus carinatum can result from a congenital anomaly. A client with severe pectus carinatum may exhibit respiratory difficulty.

P Rickets results from a vitamin D deficiency. In this condition, the bones become demineralized and weak. The loss of bone strength allows the intercostal muscles to pull the ribs and sternum forward, resulting in pectus carinatum.

A **Pectus excavatum**, or funnel chest (Fig. 15-8B), is a depression in the body of the sternum. This indentation can compress the heart and cause myocardial disturbances. The AP diameter of the chest decreases.

P Pectus excavatum results from a congenital anomaly. Respiratory insufficiency can ensue from the compression of the lungs in marked pectus excavatum.

A **Kyphosis**, or humpback, is an excessive convexity of the thoracic vertebrae. See Chapter 19 for additional information.

P The majority of kyphosis cases are idiopathic from conditions such as degenerative disc disease, osteoporosis, vertebral fracture, birth defects, and syndromes such as Marfan. Respiratory compromise is manifested only in severe cases.

A **Scoliosis** is a lateral curvature of the thoracic or lumbar vertebrae. See Chapter 19 for further discussion.

P The majority of the cases of scoliosis are idiopathic, although scoliosis can also result from neuromuscular diseases, connective tissue diseases, and osteoporosis. Marked scoliosis can interfere with normal respiratory function. The total lung capacity and vital capacity decline in proportion to the severity of the scoliosis.

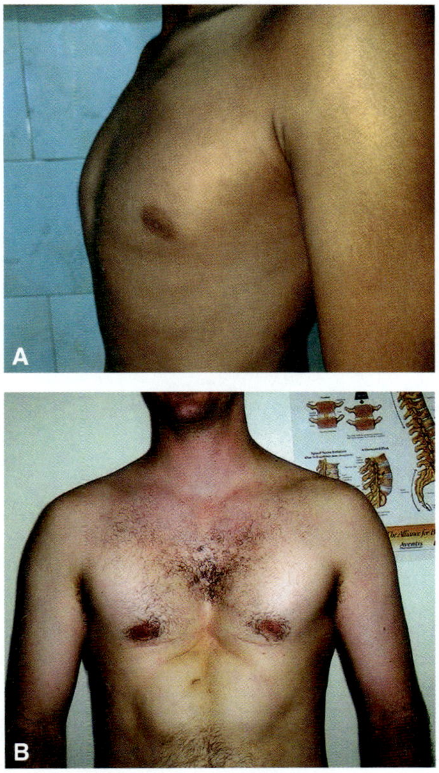

Figure 15-8 Chest configuration variations. **A.** Pectus carinatum. **B.** Pectus excavatum.

Symmetry of Chest Wall

E
1. Stand in front of the client.
2. Inspect the right and the left anterior thoraxes.
3. Note the shoulder height. Observe any differences between the two sides of the chest wall, such as the presence of masses.
4. Move behind the client.
5. Inspect the right and the left posterior thoraxes, comparing right and left sides.
6. Note the position of the scapula.

N **The shoulders should be at the same height. Likewise, the scapula should be the same height bilaterally. There should be no masses.**

A Having one shoulder or scapula higher than the other is abnormal.

P The presence of scoliosis can lead to a shoulder or a scapula that is higher than its corresponding part (Fig. 15-9). Marked scoliosis impairs lung function.

A The presence of a visible mass is abnormal.

P A visible chest mass is always abnormal. Likely etiologies are mediastinal tumors or cysts. If large enough, they can compress lung tissue and impair normal lung function.

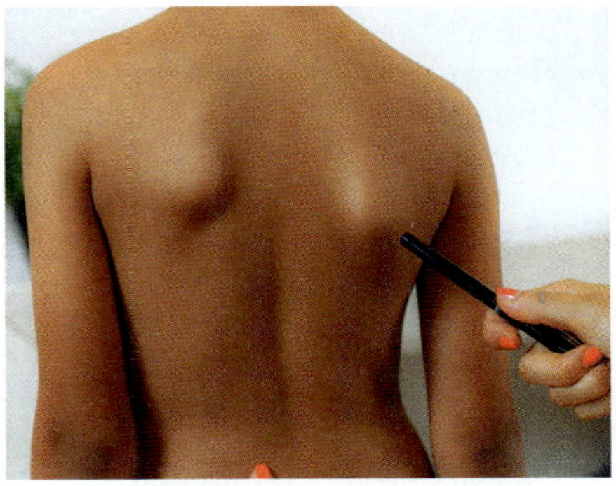

Figure 15-9 Scoliosis. Note the uneven height of the shoulders and scapula.

Presence of Superficial Veins

E
1. Stand in front of the client.
2. Inspect the anterior thorax for the presence of dilated superficial veins.

N **In the normal adult, dilated superficial veins are not seen.**

A The presence of dilated superficial veins on the anterior chest wall is an abnormal finding.

P Dilated veins on the anterior thorax may be indicative of superior vena cava obstruction. Due to the obstruction, the superficial veins and collateral vessels become engorged with blood and dilate. Venous return to the heart is diminished, compromising oxygenation. A client may present with dyspnea.

> **NURSING TIP**
>
> **Assessing Oxygenation in the Thorax Examination**
>
> When the chest is exposed, remember to examine the color and temperature of the thoracic skin as well as the color of the client's lips and nailbeds. Note any nasal flaring. The presence of nailbed clubbing provides information on long-term oxygen status. Capillary refill, skin color, and temperature indicate present oxygenation status. The presence of nasal flaring indicates respiratory distress. Examination techniques are described in Chapters 10, 17, and 25.

> **NURSING TIP**
>
> **Maintaining Respiratory Health**
>
> - Never smoke. Encourage smokers living with you to quit.
> - If you live with a smoker, insist that smoking be conducted outside.
> - Never smoke around infants and children.
> - Never smoke in bed.
> - If dust and mold are allergy triggers or aggravating factors for other respiratory ailments, clean house frequently, avoid wall-to-wall carpeting, use easily washed curtains, and avoid having a cluttered room.
> - Change filters on furnace, heaters, air conditioners, exhaust systems, and range hoods as frequently as the manufacturer specifies.
> - Have chimneys cleaned at the beginning of each season and more frequently if used heavily.
> - Have home inspected for radon and take remedial steps as needed.
> - Check carbon monoxide and smoke detectors monthly.
> - If oxygen is used in the home, use and store away from heat; avoid contact with open flames and cigarettes.

Costal Angle

E
1. Stand in front of the client.
2. In a client whose thoracic skeleton is easily viewed, visually locate the **costal margins** (medial borders created by the articulation of the false ribs).
3. Estimate the angle formed by the costal margins during exhalation and at rest. This is the costal angle (Fig. 15-10).
4. If you are unable to visualize the costal margin, such as in a client with obesity, place your fingertips on the lower anterior borders of the thoracic skeleton.
5. Gently move your fingertips medially to the xiphoid process.
6. As your hands approach the midline, feel the ribs as they meet at the apex of the costal margins. Visualize the line created by your fingers as they move up the floating ribs toward the sternum. This is the costal angle (Fig. 15-10A). Approximate this angle.

N **The costal angle is less than 90° during exhalation and at rest. The costal angle widens slightly during inhalation due to expansion of the thorax.**

A A costal angle greater than 90° is abnormal (Fig. 15-10A).

P Processes in which hyperinflation of the lungs (emphysema) or dilation of the bronchi (bronchiectasis) occurs also result in a costal margin angle greater than 90°. The diaphragm flattens out and the ribs are forced upward and outward, leading to the change in the costal margin angle.

Angle of the Ribs

E
1. Stand in front of the client.
2. In a client whose thoracic skeleton is easily viewed, visually locate the midsternal area.
3. Estimate the angle at which the ribs articulate with the sternum.
4. If you are unable to visually locate the angle of the ribs, such as in a client with obesity, place your fingertips on the midsternal area.

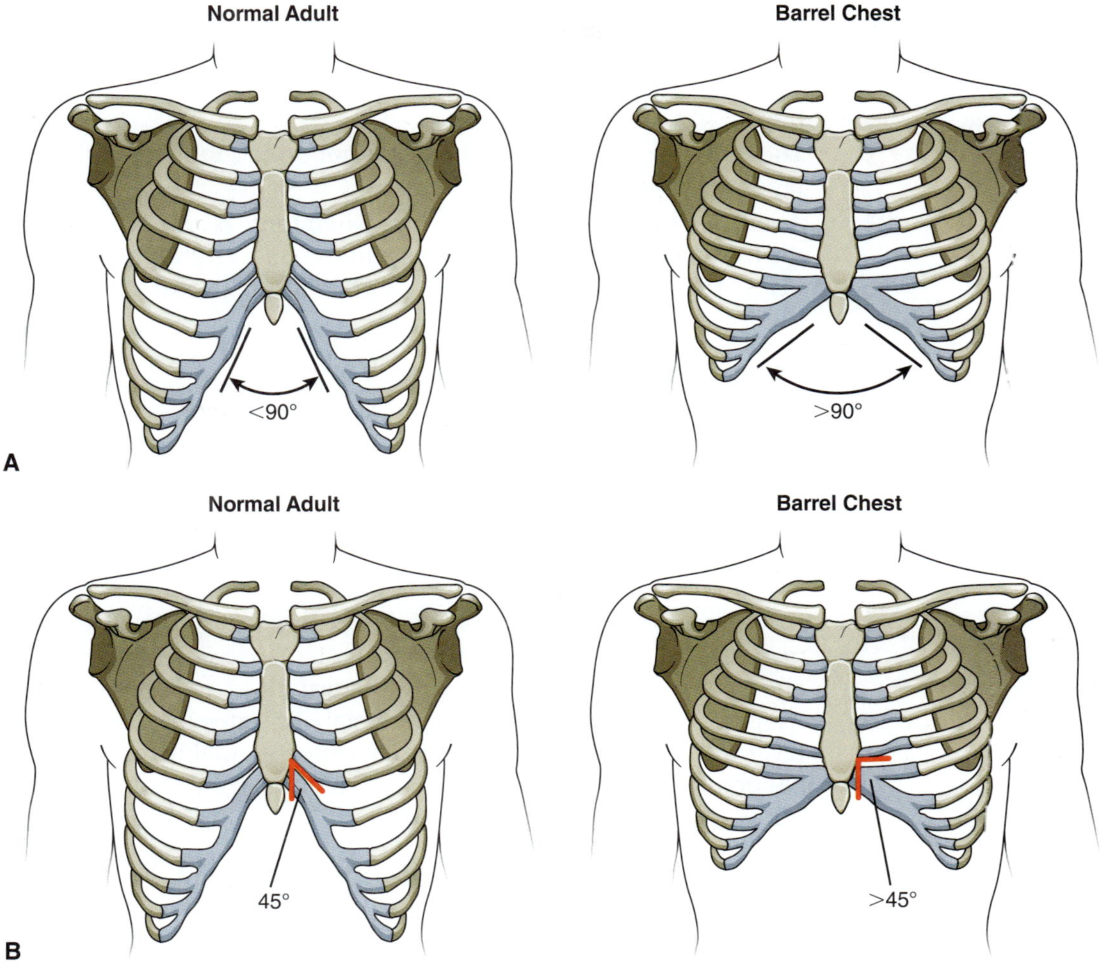

Figure 15-10 Rib cage angles. **A.** Costal angle. **B.** Angle of ribs.

5. Move your fingertips along a rib laterally to the anterior axillary line. Visualize the line created by your hand as it traces the rib. Approximate this angle.

N **The ribs articulate at a 45° angle with the sternum.**

A An angle greater than 45° is considered abnormal (Fig. 15-10B). Clients with respiratory pathology may have ribs that are nearly horizontal and perpendicular to the sternum.

P Conditions characterized by an increased AP diameter, such as emphysema, bronchiectasis, and cystic fibrosis, result in an angle greater than 45° because the lungs are forced out due to hyperinflation or dilation of the bronchi.

Intercostal Spaces

E
1. Stand in front of the client.
2. Inspect the ICS throughout the respiratory cycle.
3. Note any bulging of the ICS and any retractions.

N **There should be an absence of retractions and of bulging of the ICS.**

A The presence of retractions is abnormal. Retractions occur during inspiration.

P Conditions that obstruct the free inflow of air may lead to retractions. These include emphysema, asthma, tracheal or laryngeal obstruction, and the presence of a foreign body or tumor that compresses the respiratory tract.

A The presence of bulging of the ICS is abnormal. Bulging of the ICS tends to occur during expiration.

P Abnormal bulging of the ICS occurs when there is an obstruction to the free exhalation of air, such as in emphysema, asthma, an enlarged heart, aortic aneurysm, massive pleural effusion, tension pneumothorax, and tumors.

Muscles of Respiration

E
1. Stand in front of the client.
2. Observe the client's breathing for a few respiratory cycles, paying close attention to the anterior thorax and the neck.
3. Note all of the muscles that the client is using.

N **No accessory muscles are used in normal breathing.**

A Use of accessory muscles is a pathological finding.

P Any condition that creates a state of hypoxemia or hypermetabolism may lead to the use of accessory muscles. Accessory muscles are attempting to create an extra respiratory effort to inhale needed oxygen. Clients experiencing hypermetabolic states such as exercise, fever, or infection, or hypoxic events such as COPD, pneumonia, pneumothorax, pulmonary edema, or pulmonary embolus, usually present with accessory muscle use.

> **NURSING TIP**
> **Respiratory Rate Emergencies**
> Extreme tachypnea (more than 30 breaths per minute in an adult), bradypnea, and apnea are emergency conditions. Immediate intervention is necessary to prevent complications.

Respirations

The inspection of the respiration process includes seven components: rate, pattern, depth, symmetry, audibility, client position, and mode.

Rate

E
1. Stand in front of the client or to the right side (Fig. 15-11).
2. Observe the client's breathing without stating what you are doing, because the client may change the respiratory rate (increase or decrease it) if aware that you are watching the chest rising and falling. This assessment can be conducted simultaneously with the pulse rate assessment.
3. Count the number of respiratory cycles that the client has for one full minute. A respiratory cycle consists of one inhaled and one exhaled breath.

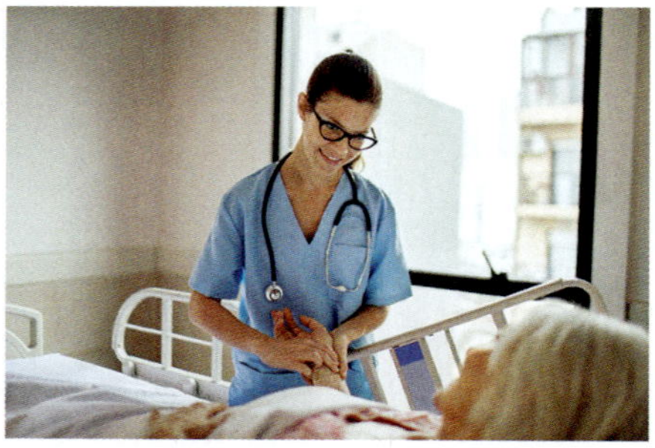

Figure 15-11 Nurse standing to the client's right side to observe respirations.

N **In the resting adult, the normal respiratory rate is 12 to 20 breaths per minute. This type of breathing is termed eupnea, or normal breathing.**

A A respiratory rate greater than 20 breaths per minute is termed **tachypnea**. Extreme tachypnea (more than 30 breaths per minute in an adult) is an emergency condition.

P Tachypnea is frequently present in hypermetabolic and hypoxic states. By increasing the respiratory rate, the body is trying to supply additional oxygen to meet the body's demands. Tachypnea occurs in many disease states, such as pneumonia, bronchitis, asthma, and pneumothorax.

P Tachypnea can be a sign of anxiety and stress. In anxious or stressful situations, the body releases catecholamines that elevate the respiratory rate to supply sufficient oxygen.

A In **hyperventilation** the respirations are rapid and deep.

P **Hyperventilation** can occur in cardiac and lung conditions, stress, anxiety, panic attacks, traumatic brain injury, pain, infection, and at high altitudes.

A A respiratory rate lower than 12 breaths per minute is termed **bradypnea**. Nonsleep related bradypnea is frequently a medical emergency.

P Injury to the brain may cause bradypnea because of excessive intracranial pressure applied to the respiratory center in the medulla oblongata.

P In drug overdoses (barbiturates, alcohol, and opiates), bradypnea is a sign of the drug's depressant effect on the respiratory center.

P Bradypnea occurs in sleep because of the lowered metabolic state of the body. The respiratory rate also slows in nonrapid eye movement (REM) sleep due to changes in the response of the respiratory center to chemical signals.

A **Apnea** is the lack of spontaneous respirations for 10 or more seconds. Nonsleep related apnea is a medical emergency.

P Traumatic brain injury may lead to apnea because of herniation of the brainstem.

P Sleep apnea can be central or obstructive in nature. In central sleep apnea, the respiratory drive is altered, leading to periods of respiratory cessation. In obstructive sleep apnea, enlarged upper-airway anatomy leads to a physical blockage in the oropharynx.

Pattern

E
1. Stand in front of the client.
2. While counting the respiratory rate, note the rhythm or pattern of the breathing for regularity or irregularity (Fig. 15-12).

N **Normal respirations are regular and even in rhythm.**

A **Cheyne-Stokes respirations** occur in crescendo and decrescendo patterns interspersed between periods of apnea that can last 15 to 30 seconds. This can be a normal finding in older adult clients and in young children. Cheyne-Stokes respiration is an example of a regularly irregular respiratory pattern, that is, the respirations predictably or regularly become irregular.

P Central cerebral or high brainstem lesions that occur in brain injury produce Cheyne-Stokes respirations.

P Cheyne-Stokes respirations can also appear in sleep due to alterations in the respiratory center's ability to accurately perceive chemical and mechanical stimuli.

A **Biot respirations**, or **ataxic respirations**, is an example of an irregularly irregular respiratory pattern. In an irregularly irregular rhythm, there is no identifiable pattern to the respiratory cycle. There is an absence of a crescendo and decrescendo pattern. Deep and shallow breaths occur at random intervals interspersed with short and long pauses. Periods of apnea can be long and frequent.

P Biot respirations indicate damage to the medulla or pons caused by a stroke or trauma.

A **Apneustic respirations** are characterized by a prolonged gasping during inspiration followed by a very short, inefficient expiration. These pauses can last 30 to 60 seconds.

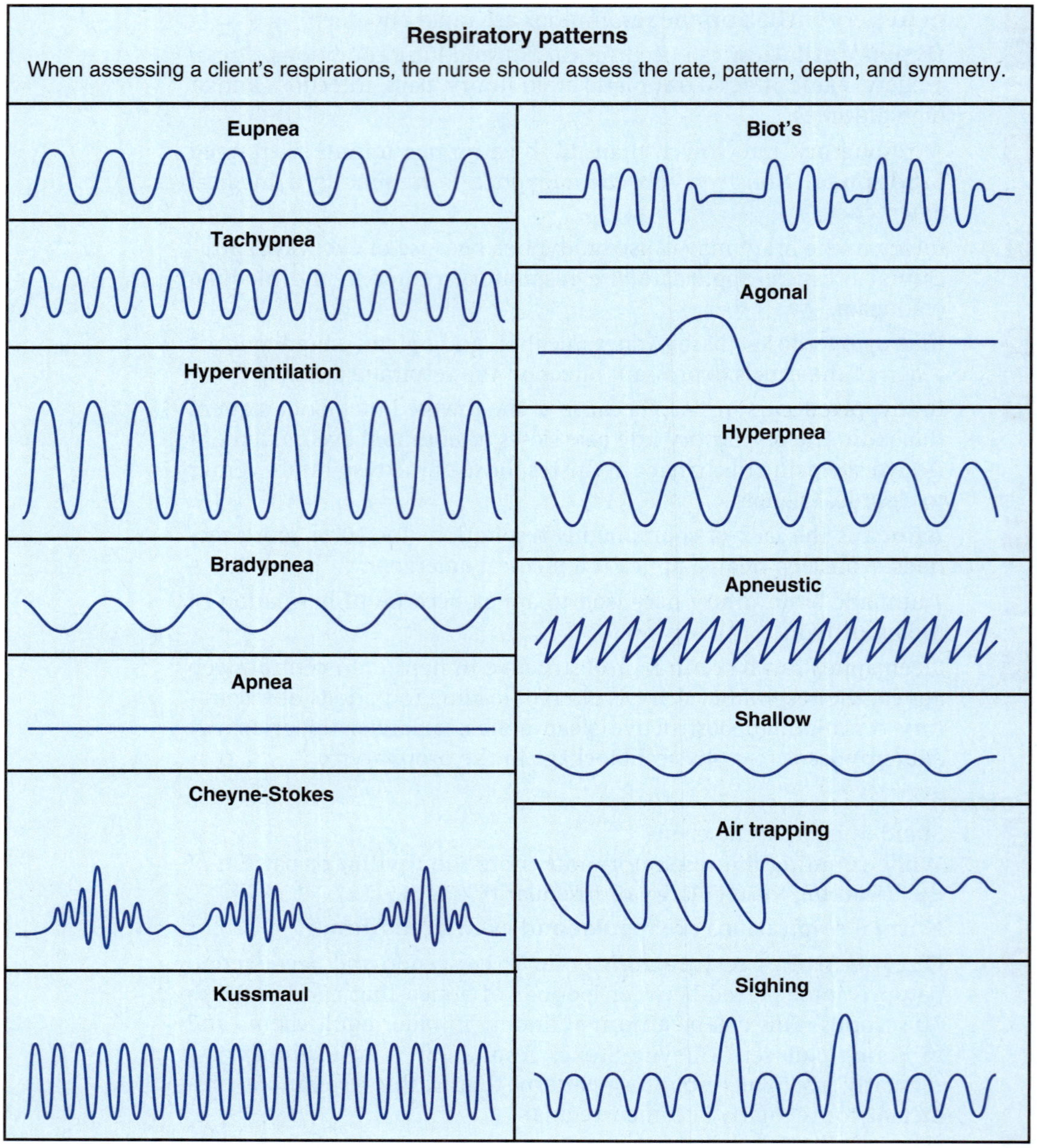

Figure 15-12 Respiratory patterns.

P Injury to the upper portion of the pons such as in a stroke or trauma can lead to apneustic breathing.

A **Agonal respirations** are irregularly irregular respirations. They are of varying depths and patterns.

P Impending death, where there is little or no oxygen supplying the brain, or compression of the respiratory center may lead to agonal breaths.

Depth

E
1. Stand in front of the client.
2. Observe the relative depth with which the client draws a breath during inspiration.

N **The normal depth of inspiration is nonexaggerated and effortless.**

A In hypoventilation, or shallow respirations, the chest wall is moved minimally during inspiration and expiration. A small tidal volume is being inspired.

P A client with obesity may have a small tidal volume due to the sheer weight of the chest wall and the effort required to move it with each breath.

P The client in pain or with a recent abdominal or thoracic incision may have shallow respirations due to the discomfort of moving the rib cage, the integument, and the respiratory muscles with each breath.

P Shallow respirations are also seen in conditions where lung pathology exists and breathing is painful: pulmonary embolus, pneumonia, pneumothorax.

A **Hyperpnea** is a breath that is greater in volume than the resting tidal volume. The respiratory rate is normal and the pattern is even in hyperpnea.

P In the warm-up and cool-down periods of exercise, hyperpnea is present. The deep breath is drawn to meet the increased metabolic needs of the body.

P Clients in highly emotional states exhibit hyperpnea as the body attempts to meet the increased oxygen demand.

P Clients who are thrust into high-altitude regions may become hyperpneic due to the decreased partial pressure of oxygen. Deep breaths and tachypnea represent an attempt to supply the oxygen needs of the body.

A **Air trapping** is an abnormal respiratory pattern with rapid, shallow respirations and forced expirations.

P Clients with COPD have difficulty exhaling. When these clients exercise or experience increased heart rate, they have insufficient time to fully exhale. As a result, air is trapped in the lungs, and, over time, the chest overexpands. Likewise, a client experiencing an acute asthma attack has difficulty exhaling due to increased mucus and bronchial constriction. Air trapping ensues.

A **Kussmaul respirations** are characterized by extreme, increased depth and rate of respirations without pauses. These respirations are regular, and the inspiratory and expiratory processes are both active.

P Diabetic ketoacidosis and metabolic acidosis may result in Kussmaul respirations. The body is lowering its $PaCO_2$ level, thereby raising the pH and attempting to correct the acidosis.

A **Sighing** is characterized by normal respirations interrupted by a deep inspiration and followed by a deep expiration. This occurs naturally to help expand alveoli and maintain respiratory health. It may be accompanied by an audible sigh. Sighing is pathological if it occurs frequently.

P Excessive sighing can occur in central nervous system lesions.

P Sighing is often associated with emotional responses as in anxiety states and stressful situations.

Symmetry

E
1. Stand in front of the client.
2. Observe the symmetry with which the chest rises and falls during the respiratory cycle.

N **The healthy adult's thorax rises and falls in unison in the respiratory cycle. There is no paradoxical movement.**

A Unilateral expansion of either side of the thorax is abnormal.

P Conditions in which the lung is absent or collapsed (pneumonectomy, pneumothorax) are characterized by unilateral thoracic expansion, secondary to the lack of active alveolar expansion on inspiration.

P Absence of expansion is evident on the affected lung side in a client with pulmonary fibrosis, due to the thickening of the lung and decreased elasticity.

P Acute pleurisy and massive atelectasis are pathologies in which pain and collapsed alveoli, respectively, interfere with the respiratory process and prevent adequate bilateral and equal chest symmetry.

A Paradoxical, or seemingly contradictory, chest wall movement is always abnormal. In paradoxical chest wall movement, the unaffected part of the thorax will rise during inspiration while the affected area will fall. Conversely, during expiration the unaffected part of the thorax will fall while the affected area will rise.

P Broken ribs from trauma to the chest wall or flail chest interfere with the normal rib cage dynamics during the respiratory process and may lead to paradoxical chest wall movement.

A Hoover sign is the paradoxical inward movement of the lower ICS during inspiration. This occurs when the diaphragm is flat instead of its normal dome shape. Muscle fibers are horizontal, and diaphragmatic contraction pulls the rib cage inward rather than down.

P Broken ribs from trauma to the chest wall or flail chest interfere with the normal rib cage dynamics during the respiratory process and may lead to the presence of Hoover sign.

Audibility

E
1. Stand in front of the client.
2. Listen for the audibility of the respirations.

N **Respirations are normally heard by the unaided ear a few centimeters from the client's nose or mouth.**

A It is abnormal to hear breathing when standing a few feet from the client. Upper airway sounds may also be heard. These should not be confused with pulmonary sounds.

P Any condition in which air hunger exists has the potential to create audible and noisy breathing. The body is attempting to meet its oxygen demands. Examples of these states are exercise, COPD, pneumonia, and pneumothorax.

P Loud and persistent coughing can indicate asthma, COPD, and many other pulmonary conditions. Be alert to a "whooping" sound because of the increasing incidence of pertussis. To hear an example of a "whooping" cough, perform an Internet search for "whooping cough video." Look for examples from trusted sources, such as the Mayo Clinic.

> **NURSING TIP**
>
> **Pertussis Trends**
>
> During the COVID-19 pandemic, the CDC reported fewer cases of pertussis, perhaps because of isolation and mask wearing. In 2024 the CDC reported that pertussis cases were increasing and approximating prepandemic levels. Some areas experienced regional outbreaks of pertussis (Virginia Department of Health, 2024). People of all ages can become infected with pertussis. Severe illness can occur at any age, although infants are the most vulnerable population. The best protection is for children to receive the DTaP vaccine and adults the Tdap vaccine. In addition, pregnant clients should receive Tdap in their third trimester. Additional information can be found at *https://www.cdc.gov/pertussis/php/public-health-strategy/*.

Client Position

E
1. Ask the client to sit upright for the respiratory examination.
2. View the client either before or after the examination and note the assumed position for breathing. Ask if the assumed position is required for respiratory comfort.
3. Note if the client can breathe normally when in a supine position.
4. Note if pillows are used to prop the client upright to facilitate breathing.

N **The healthy adult breathes comfortably in a supine, prone, or upright position.**

A **Orthopnea** is difficulty breathing in positions other than upright.

P COPD, congestive heart failure, and pulmonary edema exemplify conditions in which orthopnea may be present. The upright position maximizes the use of the respiratory muscles in clients who might otherwise be unable to breathe in a supine position, secondary to fluid in the lungs. Clients with COPD may assume the tripod position to breathe easier (Fig. 15-13). The tripod position allows for easier use of accessory muscles.

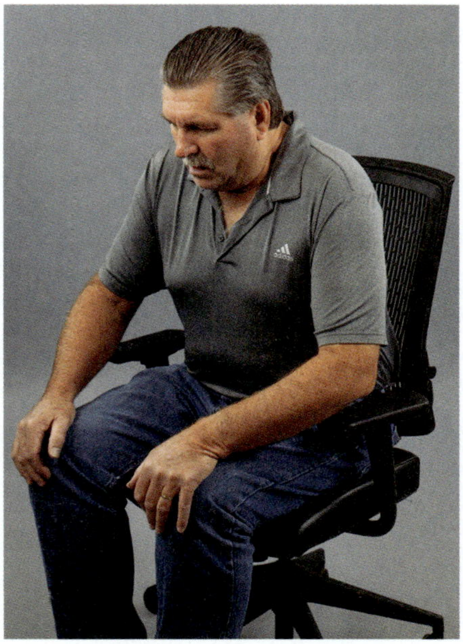

Figure 15-13 Tripod position.

Mode of Breathing

E
1. Stand in front of the client.
2. Note whether the client is using the nose, the mouth, or both to breathe.
3. Note for which part of the respiratory cycle each is used.

N **Normal findings vary among individuals but, generally, most people inhale and exhale through the nose.**

A Continuous mouth breathing is usually abnormal.

P Any type of nasal or sinus blockage obstructs the normal breathing passageway and leads to mouth breathing.

A Pursed-lip breathing is performed by clients who need to prolong the expiration phase of the respiratory cycle. This type of breathing gives the appearances that the client is trying to blow out a candle or is preparing for a kiss.

P Pursed-lip breathing is performed by clients with COPD. It is the client's innate mechanism to apply positive-pressure breathing to prevent total alveolar collapse with every breath. Less energy is expended with each breath because the alveoli do not completely collapse after expiration.

A Clients may breathe through a stoma or tracheostomy (Fig. 15-14).

P Clients with laryngeal cancer who have had a surgical removal of the larynx breathe initially through a tracheostomy and then through a stoma. This is their normal mode of breathing.

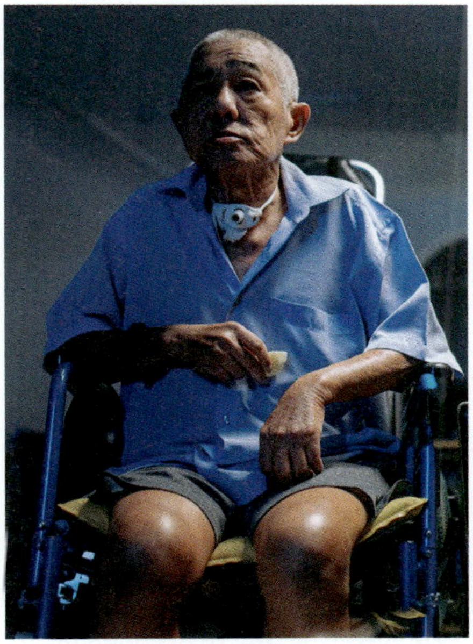

Figure 15-14 Tracheostomy.

Sputum

To ease sputum collection, it is best to increase the client's fluid intake and humidify the environment. For clients with copious secretion, such as in cystic fibrosis, it may be helpful to first use postural drainage and chest physiotherapy. Postoperative clients and those who have pain may benefit from splinting the painful area with a pillow during the expectoration.

E
1. Ask the client to expectorate a sputum sample.
2. If the client is unable to expectorate, ask the client for a recent sputum sample from a handkerchief or tissue.
3. Note the color, odor, amount, and consistency of the sputum.

N **A small amount of sputum is normal in every individual. The color is light yellow or clear. Normal sputum is odorless. Depending on the client's hydration status, the sputum can be thick or thin.**

A Abnormal colors of sputum are mucoid, yellow or green, rust or blood-tinged, black, and pink (and frothy).

P Table 15-1 lists the pathologies associated with different colors of sputum.

A Foul-smelling sputum is always abnormal.

P Anaerobic infections produce foul-smelling sputum.

A A large amount of sputum can be pathological.

Risk Factors

Lung Cancer

Known Risk Factors for Lung Cancer:

- Smoking tobacco
- Secondhand tobacco smoke exposure
- Air pollution exposure
- Radiation therapy to chest
- Personal history of lung cancer
- Family history of lung cancer
- Occupational or environmental exposure to known carcinogens (e.g., asbestos, radon, arsenic, diesel exhaust, uranium, beryllium, cadmium, silica, coal products, vinyl chloride, nickel compounds, chromium compounds, mustard gas, chloromethyl ether)

Uncertain/Unproven Risk Factors for Lung Cancer:

- Marijuana smoking
- E-cigarette smoking

Adapted from *https://www.cancer.org/cancer/types/lung-cancer/causes-risks-prevention/risk-factors.html* (retrieved November 5, 2025).

P Chronic bronchitis produces a large amount of sputum as a result of the irritation to the respiratory tract.

P Clients with pneumonia may expectorate large quantities of sputum. The sputum is produced in reaction to the infectious process.

P A large quantity of pink and frothy sputum is found in pulmonary edema, from the fluid that has leaked from pulmonary capillary membranes into large airways.

A Very thick sputum can be abnormal.

P Water is a normal component of the sputum. Therefore, when a client is dehydrated, the sputum will be thicker because the mucus, blood, purulent material, and cellular debris form the bulk of the sputum.

A Sputum that has a thin consistency can be abnormal.

P In overhydration, the extra fluid tends to dilute the remaining components of the sputum. In pulmonary edema, the sputum is thin, pink, and frothy.

Table 15-1 Pathologies Associated With Different Colors of Sputum

Sputum Color	Pathology
Mucoid	Tracheobronchitis, asthma, coryza, viral infection
Yellow or green	Bacterial infection
Rust or blood-tinged	Pneumococcal pneumonia, pulmonary infarction, tuberculosis, lung cancer
Black	Black lung disease
Pink	Pulmonary edema

NURSING CHECKLIST

Assessing Clients With Respiratory Assistive Devices

Oxygen

- Mode of delivery (e.g., nasal cannula [Figure 15-15A], face mask)
- Percentage of oxygen being delivered (e.g., 25%, 40%)
- Flow rate of the oxygen (e.g., 2 liters per minute, 4 liters per minute)
- Temperature of the humidification
- Temperature of the oxygen

Bilevel Positive Airway Pressure (BiPAP)

- Inspiratory positive airway pressure setting
- Expiratory positive airway pressure setting
- Rate
- FiO_2 setting
- Alarm settings

Endotracheal Tube

- Size of endotracheal tube
- Nasal or oral insertion
- Tube secured to the client
- Length of the endotracheal tube as it exits the nose or the mouth (e.g., 24 cm at the lips or 27 cm at the tip of the left naris)
- Cuff inflated or deflated

Tracheostomy Tube

- Size of tracheostomy tube
- Cuff present; if yes, cuff inflated or deflated
- Tracheostomy ties secure the tube

Mechanical Ventilation

- FiO_2 setting
- Mode used (e.g., assist, synchronized intermittent mandatory ventilation)
- Amount of positive end-expiratory pressure (PEEP) or continuous positive airway pressure (CPAP)
- Rate and tidal volume
- Peak inspiratory pressure
- Temperature of the humidification
- Alarm settings

Pulse Oximeter

- Determine the monitor settings (if using an institutional device).
- The monitor alarms are on. The appropriate limits are set (if using an institutional device).
- If using the probe on a nail, the client's nail polish should be removed. Apply the pulse oximeter to the client's finger. (Fig. 15-15B).
- If using the probe on the ear, the skin should be intact and earrings are not interfering.
- Read the pulse oximeter 15 to 30 seconds after it has been applied to the body.

NURSING TIP

Accuracy of Pulse Oximetry in Dark-Skinned People

While pulse oximetry is easily conducted in the health-care setting, many studies report its inaccuracy in clients with dark skin. Melanin is increased in people with dark skin tones, and this may alter the pulse oximeter's ability to accurately measure the oxygen saturation. Especially in low perfusion states such as shock where hypoxemia exists, the validity of the oxygen saturation may not truly reflect the client's actual clinical status (Khanna et al, 2024).

Risk Factors

Tuberculosis

Tuberculosis (TB) is an infectious and dangerous communicable disease that primarily affects the lungs. TB is spread via droplet nuclei into the respiratory tract. In 2023 Williams et al reported that the incidence of TB has increased annually in the United States from 2020 to 2023 in both U.S.-born and non-U.S.-born persons. In 2025 the Center for Infectious Disease Research and Policy reported a large, yearlong outbreak of tuberculosis in the United States in Kansas City. Clinicians need to be cognizant of risk factors for pulmonary tuberculosis so high-risk clients can be screened and a treatment regimen started:

- Age: Infants, young children, and older adults
- Living with or in close contact with others who have active TB
- Malnourishment
- Immunosuppressed status (HIV, cancer, chemotherapy, chronic steroid use, immunosuppressive drugs, low body weight, silicosis, organ transplants)
- Working or living in a shelter for people who are unhoused or living in a refugee camp
- Working or living in a correctional facility
- Working or residing in a long-term care facility
- Chronic diseases leading to decreased resistance (kidney disease, COPD, alcoholism, substance abuse, diabetes mellitus)
- Clients who have immigrated from areas where TB is common

Adapted from *https://www.cdc.gov/tb/about/?CDC_AAref_Val=https://www.cdc.gov/tb/topic/basics/default.htm#cdc_disease_basics_risk-risk-factors* (retrieved November 5, 2025). Center for Infectious Disease Research and Policy (2025): *https://www.cidrap.umn.edu/tuberculosis/kansas-tuberculosis-outbreak-now-largest-us* (retrieved January 29, 2025).

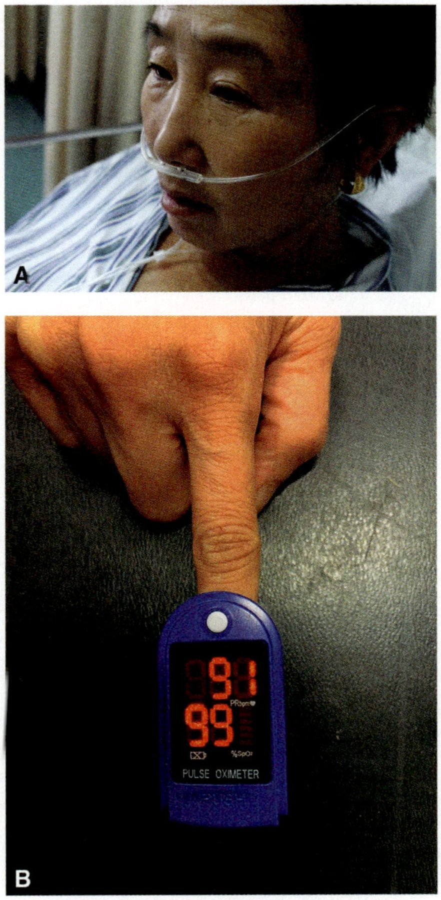

Figure 15-15 Respiratory assistive devices. **A.** Oxygen is being delivered to this client using a nasal cannula. **B.** Pulse oximeter.

Palpation

General Palpation

General palpation assesses the thorax for pulsations, masses, thoracic tenderness, and crepitus.

To perform anterior palpation:

E
1. Stand in front of the client.
2. Place the finger pads of the dominant hand on the apex of the right lung (above the clavicle).
3. Using light palpation, examine the integument of the thorax in that area.

> **NURSING TIP**
> **Assessing the Thoracic Skin**
> When palpating the thorax, remember to assess the skin's temperature, turgor, moisture, texture, and edema. Refer to Chapter 10 for additional information.

4. Move the finger pads down to the clavicle and palpate.
5. Proceed with the palpation, moving down to each rib and ICS of the right anterior thorax. Palpate any area(s) of tenderness last.
6. Repeat the procedure on the left anterior thorax.

To perform posterior palpation:

E
1. Stand behind the client.
2. Place the finger pads of the dominant hand on the apex of the right lung (approximately at the level of T1).
3. Using light palpation, examine the integument of the thorax in that area.
4. Move the finger pads down to the first thoracic vertebra and palpate.
5. Proceed with the palpation, moving down to each thoracic vertebra and ICS of the right posterior thorax.
6. Repeat the procedure on the left posterior thorax.

To perform lateral palpation:

E
1. Stand to the client's right side.
2. Have the client lift the arms overhead.
3. Place the finger pads of the dominant hand beneath the right axillary fold.
4. Using light palpation, examine the integument of the thorax in that area.
5. Move the finger pads down to the first rib beneath the axillary fold.
6. Proceed with the palpation, moving down to each rib and ICS of the right lateral thorax.
7. Move to the client's left side.
8. Repeat steps 2–6 for the left lateral thorax.

Pulsations

N **No pulsations should be present.**

A The presence of pulsations on the thorax is abnormal.

P A thoracic aortic aneurysm that is large may be seen pulsating on the anterior chest wall.

Masses

N **No masses should be present.**

A The presence of a thoracic mass is abnormal.

P The presence of a thoracic tumor or cyst should be closely evaluated and malignancy ruled out.

Thoracic Tenderness

N **No thoracic tenderness should be present.**

A Fractured ribs may cause thoracic tenderness.

P Blunt chest trauma can affect any component of the respiratory tract, as well as the heart and great vessels. The region involved, the type of injury, and the impact of the injury dictate the amount of internal damage.

Crepitus

N **Crepitus should be absent.**

A The presence of **crepitus**, also referred to as subcutaneous emphysema, is always an abnormal finding. Fine beads of air escape the lung and are trapped in the subcutaneous tissue. As this area is palpated, a crackling sound may be heard. This air is slowly absorbed by the body.

Crepitus is usually felt earliest in the clavicular region, but it can easily be found in the neck, face, and torso. It can also be described as feeling similar to bubble packing material that can be palpated and popped.

P Any condition that interrupts the integrity of the pleura and the lungs has the potential to lead to crepitus. Pathologies where crepitus is frequently found are pneumothorax, chest trauma, thoracic surgery, mediastinal emphysema, alveolar rupture, and tearing of pleural adhesions.

Thoracic Expansion

Thoracic expansion assesses the extent of chest expansion and the symmetry of chest wall expansion. Anterior and posterior thoracic expansions can be assessed (Fig. 15-16).

To perform anterior thoracic expansion:

E

1. Stand directly in front of the client. Place the thumbs of both hands on the costal margins and pointing toward the xiphoid process. Gather a small fold of skin between the thumbs to assist with seeing the results of this technique.
2. Lay your outstretched palms on the anterolateral thorax.
3. Instruct the client to take a deep breath.
4. Observe the movement of the thumbs, both in direction and in distance.
5. Ask the client to exhale.
6. Observe the movement of the thumbs as they return to the midline.

To perform posterior thoracic expansion:

E

1. Stand directly behind the client. Place the thumb of each hand at the level of the 10th spinal vertebra, equidistant from the spinal column and approximately 1 to 3 inches apart. Gather a small amount of skin between the thumbs as directed for anterior expansion.
2. Place your outstretched palms on the posterolateral thorax.
3. Instruct the client to take a deep breath.
4. Observe the movement of the thumbs, both in direction and in distance.
5. Ask the client to exhale.
6. Observe the movement of the thumbs as they return to the midline.

N **The thumbs separate an equal amount from the spinal column or xiphoid process (distance) and remain in the same plane of the 10th spinous vertebra or costal margin (direction). The normal distance for the thumbs to separate during thoracic expansion is 3 to 5 cm.**

A Unilateral decreased thoracic expansion is abnormal.

P Unilateral decreased thoracic expansion on the affected or pathological side occurs in pneumothorax, pneumonia, atelectasis, lower lobe lobectomy, pleural effusion, and bronchiectasis. In these conditions, the alveoli are either not present or not fully expanding on the affected side due to pathology inside or outside the lung.

A Bilateral decreased thoracic expansion is an abnormal finding.

P Bilateral disease external or internal to the lungs is present if bilateral decreased thoracic expansion is present. Hypoventilation, emphysema, pulmonary fibrosis, and pleurisy exemplify diseases in which the alveoli do not fully expand. Musculoskeletal pain from strain/sprain, fractures, or postoperative pain can decrease chest expansion.

A Displacement of thumbs from the 10th spinal vertebra region (thumbs will not meet in the midline when the client exhales) is abnormal.

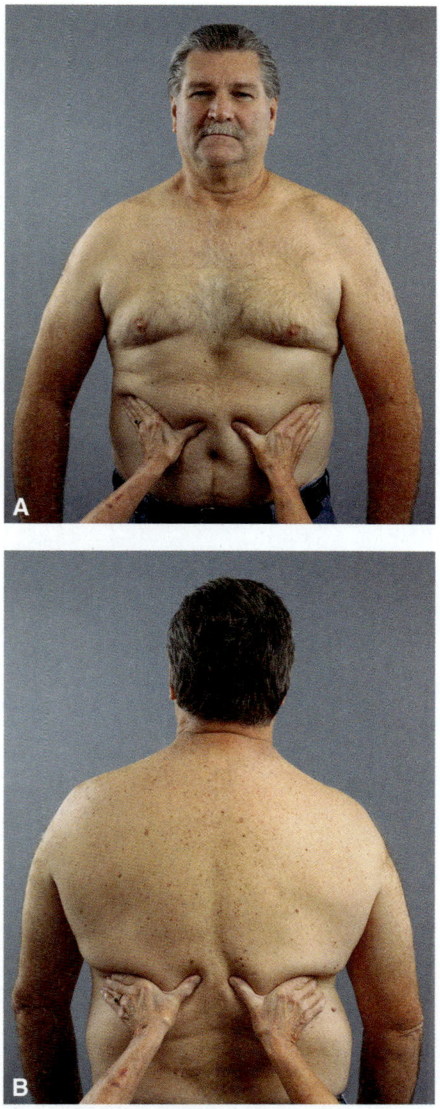

Figure 15-16 Thoracic expansion. **A.** Anterior. **B.** Posterior.

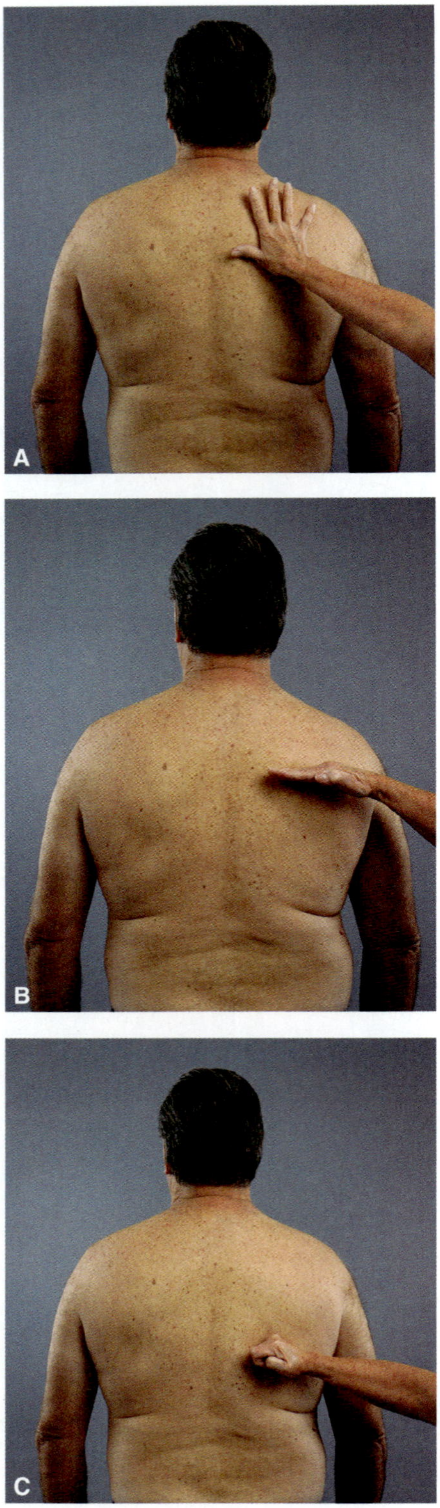

Figure 15-17 Tactile fremitus. **A.** Using palmar base of fingers. **B.** Using ulnar aspect of hand. **C.** Using ulnar aspect of closed fist.

P In scoliosis, the spine is laterally deviated to a particular side. Thus, when the client takes a deep breath, there can be a slight or markedly unequal expansion of the lungs due to the compression of the lungs by the spine.

Tactile Fremitus

Tactile or **vocal fremitus** is the palpable vibration of the chest wall produced by the spoken word. This technique is useful in assessing the underlying lung tissue and pleura. The anterior, posterior, and lateral chest walls are assessed. Three different aspects of the hand can be used to perform this skill: the palmar bases of the fingers, the ulnar aspect of the hand, and the ulnar aspect of a closed fist (Fig. 15-17). The nurse may wish to experiment with each technique and decide which is the most comfortable. It is recommended that the ulnar aspect of the hand be used initially because this exposes the least amount of surface area; therefore, more discrete areas can be assessed.

To perform tactile fremitus:

E

1. Firmly place the ulnar aspect of an open hand (or palmar base of the fingers or ulnar aspect of a closed fist) on the client's right anterior apex (remember that this is above the clavicle).
2. Instruct the client to say the words "99" or "1, 2, 3" with the same intensity every time you place your hand on the thorax.
3. Feel any vibration on the ulnar aspect of the hand as the client phonates. If no fremitus is palpated, you may need to have the client speak more loudly.
4. Move your hand to the same location on the left anterior thorax.
5. Repeat steps 2 and 3.
6. Compare the vibrations palpated on the right and left apices.
7. Move the hand down 2 to 3 inches and repeat the process on the right and then on the left. Ensure that your hand is in the ICS in order to avoid the bony structures. Minimal or no fremitus will be felt over the ribs, because they lie on top of the lungs. Avoid performing tactile fremitus over large breasts or breast implants.
8. Continue this process down the anterior thorax to the base of the lungs.
9. Repeat this procedure for the lateral chest wall and compare symmetry. Either do the entire right then the entire left thorax, or alternate right and left at each ICS.
10. Repeat this procedure for the posterior chest wall. Figure 15-18 illustrates the progression of the examination.

N **Normal fremitus is felt as a buzzing on the ulnar aspect of the hand. The fremitus will be more pronounced near the major bronchi (second ICS anteriorly, and T1 and T2 posteriorly) and the trachea, and it will be less palpable in the periphery of the lung. The diaphragm is approximately at the level of T10–T12 posteriorly, and it is slightly higher on the right because of the presence of the liver.**

A Increased tactile fremitus is abnormal.

P Diseases that involve consolidation, such as pneumonia, atelectasis, and bronchitis, also involve increased tactile fremitus in the affected area. A compressed lung will also exhibit increased tactile fremitus because solids conduct sound better than does air.

A Decreased or absent tactile fremitus is a pathological finding.

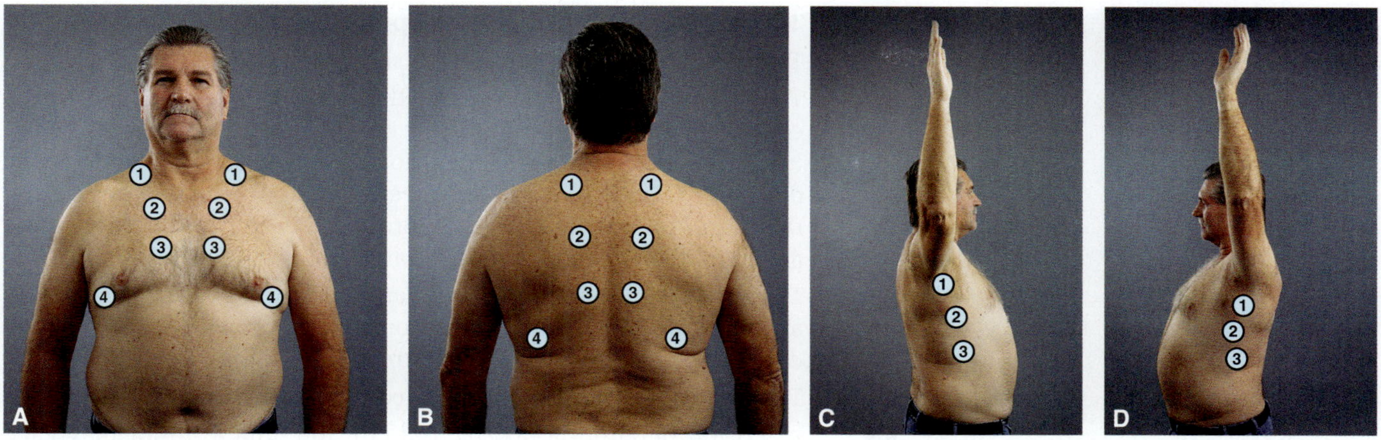

Figure 15-18 Pattern for tactile fremitus. **A.** Anterior thorax. **B.** Posterior thorax. **C.** Right lateral thorax. **D.** Left lateral thorax.

P Because porous materials conduct vibrations less effectively than do fluids and solids, decreased tactile fremitus will be present in pneumothorax, emphysema, and asthma.

P In a pleural effusion, the exudate is external to the alveoli and therefore blocks the transmission of sound waves. This results in decreased tactile fremitus.

P A client with obesity or a large chest wall may have decreased tactile fremitus, because the sound waves are dampened as they pass through a greater distance.

A A high diaphragm level is abnormal.

P The diaphragm level is abnormally high in a client with a lower-lobe lobectomy. Tactile fremitus will be present above the surgical site.

A Three additional findings can be revealed during tactile fremitus: pleural friction fremitus, tussive fremitus, and rhonchal fremitus.

P **Pleural friction fremitus** is a palpable grating sensation that feels more pronounced on inspiration when there is an inflammatory process between the visceral and the parietal pleura.

P **Tussive fremitus** is the palpable vibration produced by coughing.

P **Rhonchal fremitus** is a coarse, palpable vibration produced by the passage of air through thick exudate in large bronchi or the trachea. This can clear with coughing.

Tracheal Position

To assess the position of the trachea:

E
1. Place the finger pad of the index finger on the client's trachea in the suprasternal notch (Fig. 15-19).
2. Move the finger pad laterally to the right and gently move the trachea in the space created by the border of the inner aspect of the sternocleidomastoid muscle and the clavicle.
3. Move the finger pad laterally to the left and repeat the procedure.

Another method by which the trachea can be palpated is:

E
1. Gently place the finger pad of the index finger in the midline of the suprasternal notch.
2. Palpate for the position of the trachea.

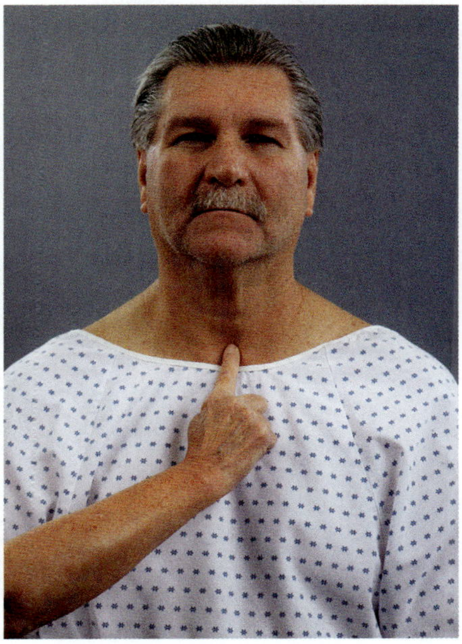

Figure 15-19 Assessing tracheal position.

N **The trachea is midline in the suprasternal notch.**

A Tracheal deviation to the affected side is abnormal.

P The normal midline position of the trachea is maintained by the counterbalancing forces of the air in the alveoli in the right and left lungs. In atelectasis and pneumonia, alveoli are closed to some degree or filled with exudate. Fewer aerating alveoli are present and therefore the trachea is slightly pushed by the healthy lung to the affected side, which contains less air.

P The mechanical pulling force of ventilator tubing that is attached to an endotracheal tube or tracheostomy for a prolonged period of time can cause tracheal deviation toward the side of the pulling.

A Tracheal deviation to the unaffected side is abnormal.

P A tension pneumothorax, pleural effusion, and a tumor may each generate sufficient pressure to force the trachea toward the unaffected side.

P An enlarged thyroid may also deviate the trachea via its space-occupying capacity.

Percussion

Indirect or mediate percussion is used to further assess the underlying structures of the thorax. Remember that percussion reverberates a sound generated from structures approximately 5 cm below the chest wall. Deep pathological conditions will not be revealed during the percussion process.

There is no harm in repeating the percussion strike in a given area if you are uncertain about the sound that was produced or if you would like to compare it to the sound from another area. Always remember to visualize the underlying structures being assessed.

General Percussion

Figure 15-20 demonstrates the percussion pattern for the anterior, posterior, right lateral, and left lateral thoraxes.

To perform anterior thoracic percussion:

E 1. Place the client in an upright sitting position with the shoulders back.

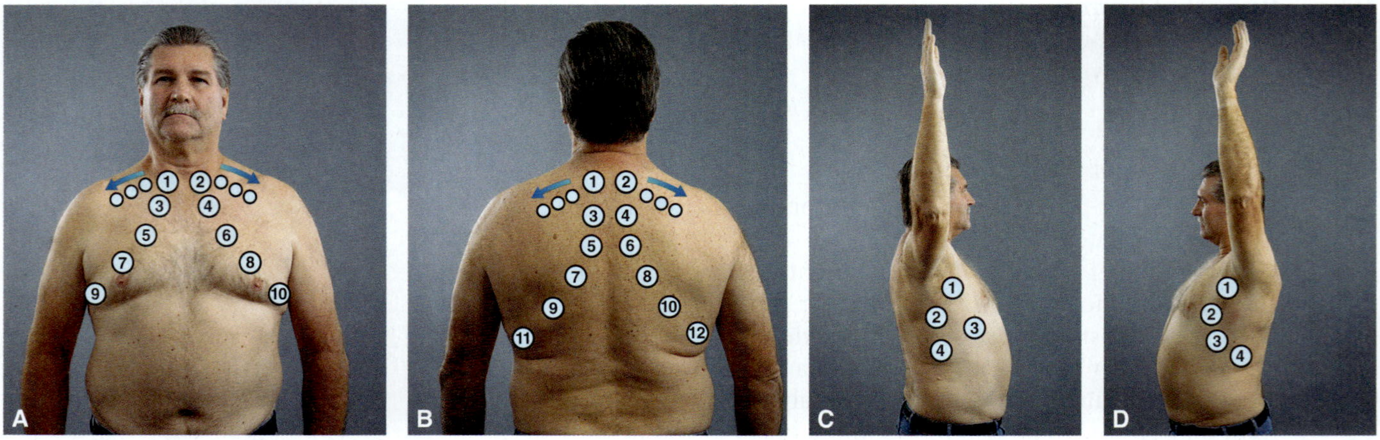

Figure 15-20 Percussion patterns. **A.** Anterior thorax. **B.** Posterior thorax. **C.** Right lateral thorax. **D.** Left lateral thorax.

2. The client may use a drape to cover the anterior thorax during posterior percussion. The entire chest must be exposed for anterior and lateral percussions.
3. Percuss two or three strikes along the right lung apex.
4. Repeat this process at the left lung apex.
5. Note the sound produced from each percussion strike and compare the sounds from each. If different sounds are produced, or if the sound is not resonant, then pathology is suggested.
6. Move down approximately 5 cm, or every other ICS, and percuss in that area. Avoid percussing over large breasts or breast implants.
7. Percuss in the same position on the contralateral side.
8. Continue to move down until the entire lung has been percussed.

To perform posterior thoracic percussion:

E 1. Place the client in an upright sitting position with a slight forward tilt. Have the client bend the head down and fold the arms in front at the waist. These actions move the scapula laterally and maximize the lung area that can be percussed (Fig. 15-21). The anterior thorax can be covered.
2. Percuss the left lung apex located along the top of the shoulder. Perform approximately three percussion strikes along this area.
3. Repeat the process on the left lung apex.
4. Note the sound produced from each percussion strike and compare the sounds from each. If different sounds are produced, or if the sound is not resonant, then pathology is suggested.
5. Move down approximately 5 cm, or every other ICS, and percuss in that area.
6. Percuss in the same position on the contralateral side.
7. Continue to move down the thorax until the entire posterior lung field has been percussed.

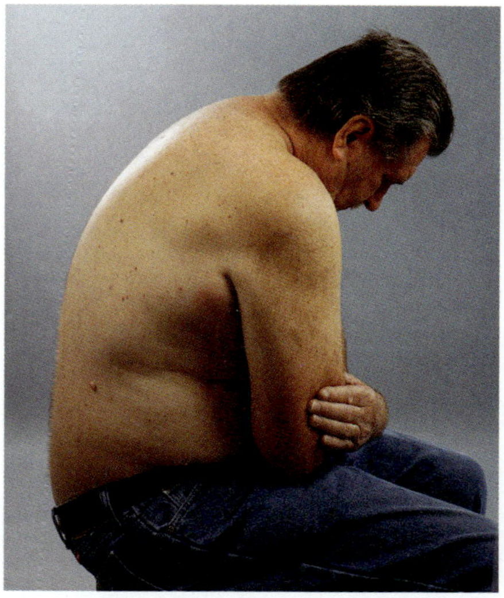

Figure 15-21 Client position for posterior percussion.

To perform lateral thoracic percussion:

E 1. Place the client in an upright sitting position, with hands and arms raised directly overhead. This position allows the greatest exposure of the thorax.
2. Either percuss the entire right lateral thorax and then the entire left lateral thorax, or alternate right and left sides. Start to percuss in the ICS directly below the axilla.
3. Note the sound produced from that strike.
4. Percuss approximately 5 cm below the original location, or about every other ICS.
5. Percuss down to the base of the lung.

N **Normal lung tissue produces a resonant sound. The diaphragm and the cardiac silhouette emit dull sounds. Rib sounds are flat. Hyperresonance is normal in thin adults and in clients with decreased musculature.**

A The presence of hyperresonance in the majority of adults is abnormal.

P Hyperresonance is percussed in air-filled spaces. It can be elicited in pneumothorax, emphysema, asthma, and an emphysematous bulla.

A The healthy human lung never produces a dull sound.

P Dullness is found in solid or fluid-filled structures. Pneumonia, atelectasis, pulmonary edema, pleural effusion, pulmonary fibrosis, hemothorax, empyema, and tumors are dull to percussion.

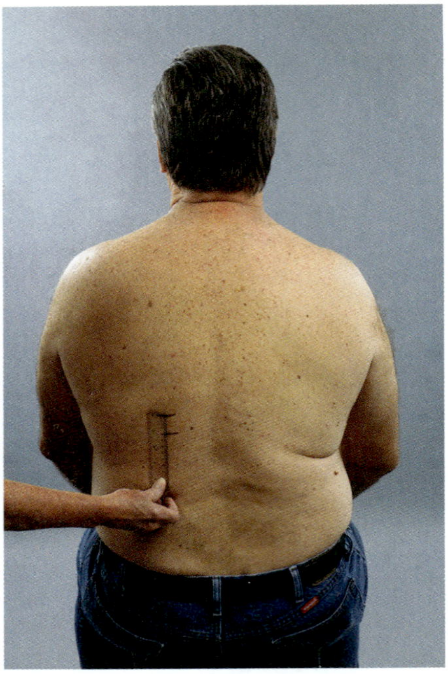

Figure 15-22 Diaphragmatic excursion.

Diaphragmatic Excursion

Diaphragmatic excursion provides information on the client's depth of ventilation. This is accomplished by measuring the distance the diaphragm moves during inspiration and expiration.

To perform diaphragmatic excursion:

E

1. Position the client for posterior thoracic percussion.
2. With the client breathing normally, percuss the right lung from the apex (resonance in healthy adults) to below the diaphragm (dull). Note the level at which the percussion changes quality to orient your examination to the client's percussion sounds. If full posterior thoracic percussion has already been performed, this step can be eliminated.
3. Instruct the client to inhale as deeply as possible and hold that breath.
4. With the client holding the breath, percuss the right lung in the scapular line from below the scapula to the location where resonance changes to dullness.
5. Mark this location and tell the client to exhale and breathe normally.
6. When the client has recovered, instruct the client to inhale as deeply as possible, exhale fully, and hold this exhaled breath.
7. Repercuss the right lung below the scapula in the scapular line in a caudal direction. Mark the spot where resonance changes to dullness.
8. Measure the distance between the two marks.
9. Repeat steps 1–8 for the left posterior thorax. Figure 15-22 illustrates diaphragmatic excursion.

N **The measured distance for diaphragmatic excursion is normally 3 to 5 cm. The level of the diaphragm on inspiration is T12, and T10 on expiration. The right side of the diaphragm is usually slightly higher than the left.**

A A diaphragmatic excursion that is less than 3 cm is abnormal.

P Conditions involving hypoventilation, where the client is unable to inhale deeply or hold that breath, can lead to a reduction in the diaphragmatic excursion. Pain, obesity, lung congestion, emphysema, asthma, and pleurisy are examples.

A A high diaphragm level suggests lung pathology.

P Surgical intervention can elevate the diaphragm. If a lower-lobe lobectomy is performed, the diaphragm will move upward to partially fill the empty space. Likewise, after a pneumonectomy the paralyzed diaphragm will move upward, leading to a high diaphragm level.

P Space-occupying states such as ascites and pregnancy will lead to an elevated diaphragm due to the upward displacement of the lungs and diaphragm.

P If atelectasis or a pleural effusion is present in a lower lobe, then the diaphragm will seem abnormally high because these conditions are dull to percussion, as is the diaphragm. The border between the diaphragm and the dull lung will thus be indistinguishable.

Auscultation

The aim of respiratory auscultation is to identify the presence of normal breath sounds, abnormal lung sounds, adventitious (or added) lung sounds,

NURSING TIP
Smoking Cannabis

People smoke cannabis or marijuana for many reasons. Frequently it is for the euphoria or its "high" effect but marijuana is also smoked for medicinal purposes. Cannabis use can have negative side effects such as paranoia, sedation, and dizziness. Like tobacco, marijuana contains many inert ingredients and remains an irritant to the throat and lungs. According to the American Cancer Society (2024) marijuana smoking is an uncertain/unproven risk factor for lung cancer. The National Institute on Drug Abuse (2020) poses that marijuana smoking may lead to large airway inflammation, lung hyperinflation, and increased airway resistance. Smoking cannabis may possibly increase a person's risk for developing respiratory tract infections. As marijuana laws relax throughout the country and more people smoke it, future research will provide more definitive clinical data.

American Cancer Society (2024). Lung cancer risk factors. *https://www.cancer.org/cancer/types/lung-cancer/causes-risks-prevention/risk-factors.html* (retrieved November 5, 2025).

National Institute on Drug Abuse (September, 2024). Cannabis (Marijuana). *https://nida.nih.gov/research-topics/cannabis-marijuana#long-term-health-cannabis* (retrieved November 5, 2025).

NURSING TIP
Electronic Cigarette Use

Electronic cigarettes, or e-cigarettes, are another delivery system of toxic substances to the lungs. The use of e-cigarettes is often referred to as "vaping." Most e-cigarettes contain nicotine, flavoring, heavy metals, and other chemicals. E-cigarette delivery systems can take the form of a cigarette, pipe, cigar, pen, and even a flash drive. The e-cigarette unit heats the chemical substances, and the user inhales the aerosolized product. These devices can sometimes be used to smoke marijuana and other harmful substances. JUUL is a commonly used type of e-cigarette. Some JUUL products are reported to contain as much nicotine in one JUUL as in an entire box of cigarettes! Whatever form of vaping is selected, the exhaled air from its use poses harm to anyone in close proximity to the e-cigarette user.

E-cigarette use can replace tobacco-filled cigarettes in nonpregnant adults. The CDC states this switch has the potential to benefit smoking adults if used as a total nicotine replacement to decrease the harmful effects of tobacco-filled cigarettes by inhaling less nicotine and fewer toxic substances. E-cigarettes should never be used by children, young adults, and pregnant women.

E-Cigarette Use Among Youth. *https://cdc/gov/tobacco/e-cigarettes/youth.html* (retrieved November 5, 2025). E-Cigarettes (Vapes). *https://www.cdc.gov/tobacco/e-cigarettes/* (retrieved November 5, 2025).

and adventitious pleural sounds. The anterior, posterior, and lateral aspects of the chest are auscultated. A stethoscope is required for this assessment. If an acoustic stethoscope is used, the diaphragm, which transmits high-pitched sounds, is the headpiece of choice.

General Auscultation

Watch the client closely for signs of hyperventilation during auscultation, such as dizziness. If the client complains of dizziness, normal breathing should be resumed. Continue the examination when the client's dizziness is gone and the client's breathing has returned to baseline. If the client has secretions in the oropharynx (upper airway), the respirations may be loud and gurgling. It may sound as if the client is having difficulty breathing. Ask the client to clear the throat, then reassess the breath sounds.

To perform anterior thoracic auscultation:

E

1. Place the client in an upright sitting position with the shoulders back.
2. Instruct the client to breathe only through the mouth. Mouth breathing, compared with nasal breathing, decreases air turbulence, which can interfere with the interpretation of breath sounds. Have the client inhale and exhale deeply and slowly every time the stethoscope is felt or when instructed to do so.
3. Place the stethoscope on the apex of the right lung and listen for one complete respiratory cycle (one inhalation and one exhalation).
4. Note the sound that is auscultated.
5. Repeat on the left apex.
6. Note the breath sound auscultated in each area and compare one side to the other.
7. Continue to move the stethoscope down approximately 5 cm, or every other ICS, comparing contralateral sides. Remember to visualize the anatomic topography of the chest during auscultation.

> **NURSING TIP**
> **Factors Affecting Auscultation**
> - Chest hair: Coarse or dense chest hair can be dampened to prevent the distortion of auscultatory findings (coarse or dense chest hair can make a crackling sound).
> - Rustling of paper gowns or drapes: Instruct the client to remain still while you are auscultating the lungs.
> - Mechanical ventilator tubing: Water accumulation in mechanical ventilator tubing can produce a gurgling sound. Clear all tubing of moisture before auscultation.
> - Shivering or chattering teeth: Ascertain why the client is shivering or chattering the teeth (e.g., hypothermia) and intervene to correct the etiology.

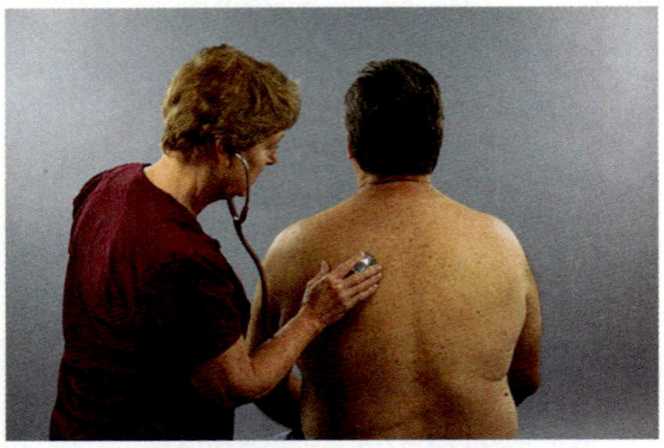

Figure 15-23 Posterior thorax lung auscultation.

To perform posterior thoracic auscultation:

E
1. Place the client as shown in Figure 15-21, in an upright sitting position with a slight forward tilt, head bent down, and arms folded in front at the waist. These actions move the scapula laterally and maximize the lung area that can be auscultated.
2. Place the stethoscope firmly on the client's right lung apex. Ask the client to inhale and exhale deeply and slowly every time the stethoscope is felt on the back.
3. Repeat this process on the left lung apex.
4. Move the stethoscope down approximately 5 cm, or every other ICS, and auscultate in that area (Fig. 15-23).
5. Auscultate in the same position on the contralateral side.
6. Continue to move inferiorly with the auscultation until the entire posterior lung has been assessed. Refer to Figure 15-20 from the percussion section for the recommended stethoscope location for each auscultation.

To perform lateral thoracic auscultation:

E
1. Place the client in an upright sitting position with the hands and arms directly overhead.
2. Auscultate the entire right thorax first, then the entire left thorax, or auscultate the right and left lateral thoraxes by comparing side to side. The stethoscope should initially be placed in the ICS directly below the axilla.
3. Instruct the client to breathe only through the mouth. Have the client inhale and exhale deeply and slowly every time the stethoscope is felt on the lateral thorax.
4. Note the sound that is auscultated and continue to move the stethoscope inferiorly approximately every 5 cm, or every other ICS, until the entire thorax has been auscultated.

Breath Sounds

N **Air rushing through the respiratory tract during inspiration and expiration generates different breath sounds in the normal client. There are three distinct types of normal breath sounds (Fig. 15-24):**

1. Bronchial (or tubular)
2. Bronchovesicular
3. Vesicular

Each breath sound is unique in its pitch, intensity, quality, and relative duration in the inspiratory and expiratory phases of respiration, and its location. Table 15-2 depicts this information. It is abnormal to auscultate these breath sounds in locations other than where they are usually found. For example, a client with emphysema may have bronchial breath sounds in the peripheral lung parenchyma, where vesicular sounds are expected to be found. Also keep in mind that heart sounds may obscure some of the breath sounds during the anterior chest auscultation.

Breath sounds that are not normal can be classified as either abnormal or adventitious breath sounds. Abnormal breath sounds are characterized by decreased or absent breath sounds. **Adventitious breath sounds** are sounds superimposed on the normal bronchial, bronchovesicular, and vesicular breath sounds.

There are six adventitious breath sounds:

1. Fine crackle
2. Coarse crackle

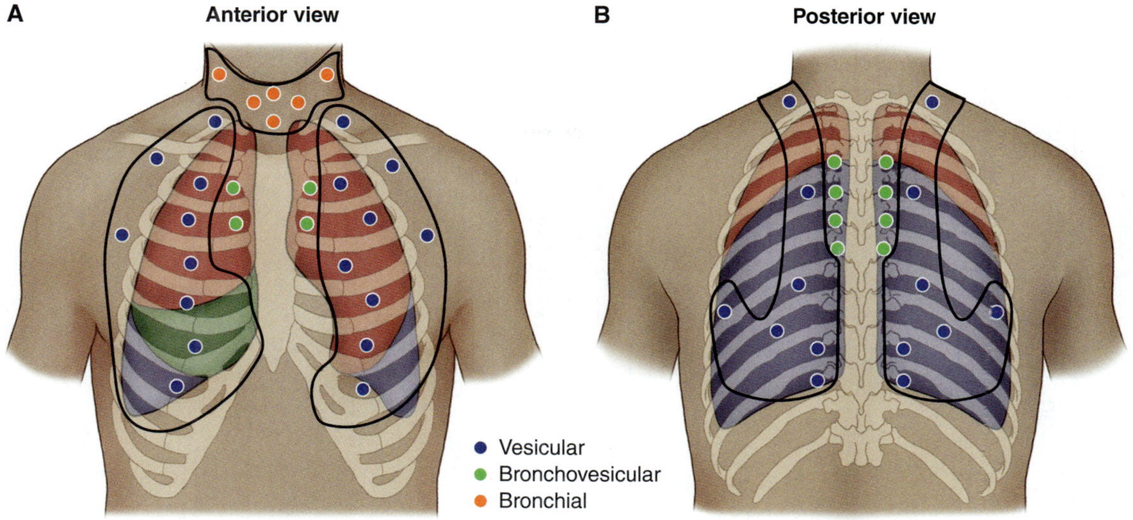

Figure 15-24 Location of breath sounds. **A.** Anterior thorax. **B.** Posterior thorax.

Table 15-2 Characteristics of Normal Breath Sounds

Breath Sound	Pitch	Intensity	Quality	Relative Duration of Inspiratory and Expiratory Phases	Location
Bronchial	High	Loud	Blowing or hollow	I < E	Trachea
Bronchovesicular	Moderate	Moderate	Combination of bronchial and vesicular	I = E	Between scapulae, first and second ICS lateral to the sternum
Vesicular	Low	Soft	Gentle rustling or breezy	I > E	Peripheral lung

3. Sonorous wheeze
4. Sibilant wheeze
5. Pleural friction rub
6. Stridor

Table 15-3 depicts general characteristics of adventitious breath sounds.

A Decreased breath sounds are abnormal.

P Decreased breath sounds may be noted when auscultating a large chest because of the distance between the lungs, where the sounds are generated, and the chest wall.

P A client with emphysema may have decreased breath sounds due to the inability to inhale and exhale deeply.

P Conditions such as bronchial obstruction and atelectasis may lead to decreased breath sounds because a foreign object or sputum occludes some portion of the respiratory tract, thus blocking the passage of air.

A Absent breath sounds are always a pathological finding.

Table 15-3 Characteristics of Adventitious Breath Sounds

Breath Sound	Respiratory Phase	Timing	Description	Clear with Cough	Etiology	Conditions
Fine crackle 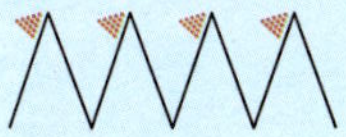	Predominantly inspiration	Discontinuous	Dry, high-pitched crackling, popping, short duration; roll hair near ears between your fingers to simulate this sound	No	Air passing through moisture in small airways that suddenly reinflate	COPD, congestive heart failure (CHF), pneumonia, COVID-19, pulmonary fibrosis, atelectasis
Coarse crackle 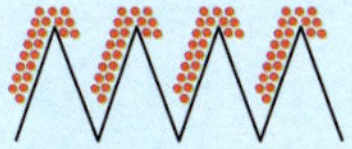	Predominantly inspiration	Discontinuous	Moist, low-pitched crackling, gurgling; long duration	Possibly	Air passing through moisture in large airways that suddenly reinflate	Pneumonia, COVID-19, pulmonary edema, bronchitis, atelectasis
Sonorous wheeze (rhonchi) 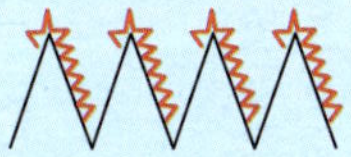	Predominantly expiration	Continuous	Low pitched; snoring	Possibly	Narrowing of large airways or obstruction of bronchus	Asthma, bronchitis, airway edema, tumor, bronchiolar spasm, foreign body obstruction
Sibilant wheeze 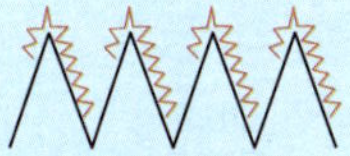	Predominantly expiration	Continuous	High pitched; musical	Possibly	Narrowing of large airways or obstruction of bronchus	Asthma, chronic bronchitis, emphysema, tumor, foreign body obstruction
Pleural friction rub 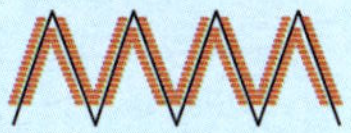	Inspiration and expiration	Continuous	Creaking, grating	No	Inflamed parietal and visceral pleura; can occasionally be felt on thoracic wall like two pieces of dry leather rubbing against each other	Pleurisy, tuberculosis, pulmonary infarction, pneumonia, lung abscess
Stridor 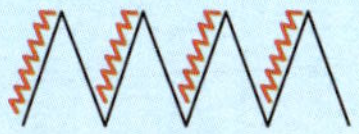	Predominantly inspiration	Continuous	Crowing	No	Partial obstruction of the larynx, trachea	Croup, foreign body obstruction, large airway tumor

NURSING TIP

Preventing Aspiration

Aspiration, or the inhalation of fluids (e.g., mucus, vomitus) or foreign bodies (e.g., food, beverages, other items) into the respiratory tract, places the client at risk for airway obstruction and pneumonia. To prevent respiratory complications, employ these practices:

- Place the client in an upright position for eating and medication administration
- Advise the client to avoid talking and laughing while eating/drinking
- Cut food into a size that the client with dysphagia can easily swallow. Direct the client to chew thoroughly before swallowing. Alternate the intake of solid food and liquids.
- Place a client who is unconscious or intoxicated in an upright or side-lying position
- Minimize the administration of sedatives and hypnotics
- Place a client who is vomiting into an upright position; if unconscious or weak, place the client into a side-lying position
- Place a client receiving intermittent tube feedings in an upright position and maintain that position for 30 minutes after the completion of the tube feeding
- Place a client receiving continuous tube feedings in an upright position
- Hold a client's tube feeding for the specified period of time if the gastric residual is greater than the prescribed amount (this varies per the volume and frequency of the tube feedings which is based on the client's calculated nutritional needs)
- Suction the client's mouth and oropharynx before deflation of a tracheostomy cuff

P A pleural effusion, tumor, pulmonary fibrosis, empyema, hemothorax, and hydrothorax lead to absent breath sounds. These states occupy or displace normal aerating lung space internally or externally to the lungs.

P A client with a large pneumothorax can present with absent breath sounds due to collapse of the lung.

P Breath sounds will be absent when the lung has been removed (pneumonectomy).

P Blocked passageways in the respiratory tract explain the etiology for absent breath sounds in pulmonary edema, massive atelectasis, and complete airway obstruction.

Voice Sounds

The assessment of **voice sounds** will reveal whether the lungs are filled with air, with fluid, or are solid. This auscultation need be performed only if an abnormality is detected during the general auscultation, percussion, or palpation. There are three techniques by which voice sounds can be assessed:

1. Bronchophony
2. Egophony
3. Whispered pectoriloquy

Only one of these techniques needs to be performed, as they all are variations on the same physical principle and assessment technique, and they all provide the same information. The voice sound findings will parallel those

NURSING TIP

Lung Auscultation Practice

In addition to practicing auscultation in the clinical setting, it is possible to refine these skills using resources on the Internet. Web sites—such as the R.A.L.E. Repository at *www.rale.ca*—allow you to hear a variety of normal and pathological breath sounds.

> **NURSING TIP**
> **The 6-Minute Walk Test**
> In 2002 the American Thoracic Society established guidelines for the 6-Minute Walk Test. It is conducted to evaluate cardiopulmonary status in clients with COPD, pulmonary hypertension, interstitial lung disease, heart failure, coronary arterial disease, and peripheral arterial disease. It is easily administered and requires no sophisticated equipment or technical expertise. Results provide information on functional exercise capacity and response to current treatment regimen.
> Agarwala, P., & Salzman, S. H. (2019). Six-minute walk test. Clinical role, technique, coding, and reimbursement. Chest, 157(3), 603–611. Retrieved November 5, 2025 from *https://www.ncbi.nlm.nih.gov/pmc/articles/PMC7609960*

obtained during tactile fremitus. Thus, voice sounds will be heard loudest over the trachea and softest in the lung's periphery.

To perform **bronchophony**:

E
1. Position the client for posterior, lateral, or anterior chest auscultation. The area to be auscultated will be that in which an abnormality was found during percussion or palpation or in which adventitious breath sounds were heard.
2. Place the stethoscope in the appropriate location on the client's chest.
3. Instruct the client to say the words "99" or "1, 2, 3" every time the stethoscope is placed on the chest or when told to do so.
4. Auscultate the transmission of the client's spoken word.

To perform **egophony**:

E
1. Repeat steps 1 and 2 from the bronchophony procedure.
2. Instruct the client to say the sound "ee" every time the stethoscope is placed on the chest or when told to do so.
3. Auscultate the transmission of the client's spoken word.

To perform **whispered pectoriloquy**:

E
1. Repeat steps 1 and 2 from the bronchophony procedure.
2. Instruct the client to whisper the words "99" or "1, 2, 3" every time the stethoscope is placed on the chest or when told to do so.
3. Auscultate the transmission of the client's spoken word.

N **The normal finding when performing tests for bronchophony, egophony, and whispered pectoriloquy is an unclear transmission or muffled sounds.**

A Positive (or present) voice sounds are:

Bronchophony: clear transmission of "99" or "1, 2, 3" with increased intensity.

Egophony: transformation of "ee" to "ay" with increased intensity; the voice has a nasal or bleating quality.

Whispered pectoriloquy: clear transmission of "99" or "1, 2, 3" with increased intensity.

P Any type of consolidation process, such as pneumonia, will produce positive voice sounds. Remember the principle that sound is transmitted reasonably well by a fluid medium.

P Pneumonia is frequently the presenting condition for COVID-19. COVID-19 can be a serious risk in a healthy adult and poses an even greater risk for the person who has a preexisting pulmonary condition or is immunocompromised.

A Voice sounds are absent or even more decreased than in the normal lung in conditions where the lung is more air filled than usual.

P Air conducts sound poorly. Therefore, air-filled lungs (emphysema, asthma, pneumothorax) will produce absent voice sounds.

Table 15-4 compares physical examination findings for 12 respiratory conditions. Figure 15-25 illustrates each of these 12 respiratory conditions.

Table 15-4 Comparison of Physical Examination Findings in Selected Respiratory Conditions

Inspection

Condition	Shape of Thorax	Skin Color: Lips and Nails	Clubbing, Angle of Ribs
A. Normal lung	1:2 to 5:7	Pink in individuals with light skin; darker than other areas in individuals with dark skin	No clubbing, rib angle 45°
B. Asthma	If chronic, may have barrel chest	Pale or cyanotic in acute attack	No clubbing, rib angle 45°
C. Atelectasis (patent bronchus)	1:2 to 5:7	Pale or cyanotic	No clubbing, rib angle 45°
D. Atelectasis (obstructed bronchus)	1:2 to 5:7	Pale or cyanotic	No clubbing, rib angle 45°
E. Bronchiectasis	1:1 (barrel chest)	Pale or cyanotic if severe	Clubbing possible, rib angle >45°
F. Bronchitis	1:2 to 5:7	Possibly pale	No clubbing, rib angle 45°
G. Congestive heart failure	1:2 to 5:7	Pale or cyanotic	Clubbing possible, rib angle 45°
H. Emphysema	1:1 (barrel chest)	Pale	Clubbing, rib angle >45°
I. Pleural effusion	1:2 to 5:7	Pale or cyanotic	No clubbing, rib angle 45°
J. Pneumonia with lobar consolidation	1:2 to 5:7	Pale or cyanotic	No clubbing, rib angle 45°
K. Pneumothorax	1:2 to 5:7	Pale or cyanotic	No clubbing, rib angle 45°
L. Pulmonary edema	1:2 to 5:7	Pale or cyanotic	No clubbing, rib angle 45°

Inspection

Condition	Capillary Refill	Retractions or Bulging of ICS	Respiratory Rate
A. Normal lung	Brisk	Absent	12 to 20/min eupnea
B. Asthma	Sluggish in acute attack	Retractions	>20/min tachypnea
C. Atelectasis (patent bronchus)	Sluggish to moderate	Absent	>20/min tachypnea
D. Atelectasis (obstructed bronchus)	Sluggish	Absent	>20/min tachypnea
E. Bronchiectasis	Sluggish if severe	Retractions if severe	>20/min tachypnea
F. Bronchitis	Sluggish to moderate	Absent	>20/min tachypnea
G. Congestive heart failure	Sluggish	Retractions	>20/min tachypnea
H. Emphysema	Sluggish	Both present	>20/min tachypnea
I. Pleural effusion	Sluggish	Bulging	>20/min tachypnea
J. Pneumonia with lobar consolidation	Sluggish	Absent	>20/min tachypnea
K. Pneumothorax	Sluggish	Bulging	>20/min tachypnea
L. Pulmonary edema	Sluggish	Absent	>20/min tachypnea

Continued

Table 15-4 Comparison of Physical Examination Findings in Selected Respiratory Conditions—cont'd

Palpation

Condition	Thoracic Expansion	Tactile Fremitus	Tracheal Position
A. Normal lung	3–5 cm	Moderate (normal)	Midline
B. Asthma	Decreased in attack	Decreased	Midline
C. Atelectasis (patent bronchus)	Decreased	Increased	Shifts to affected side
D. Atelectasis (obstructed bronchus)	Decreased	Increased	Shifts to affected side
E. Bronchiectasis	Decreased on affected side	Increased	Midline or deviated toward affected side
F. Bronchitis	Possibly decreased	Moderate or increased	Midline
G. Congestive heart failure	May be decreased	Moderate	Midline
H. Emphysema	Decreased	Decreased	Midline
I. Pleural effusion	Decreased	Decreased	Shifts to unaffected side
J. Pneumonia with lobar consolidation	Decreased	Increased	Shifts to affected side
K. Pneumothorax	Decreased	Absent or decreased	Shifts to unaffected side
L. Pulmonary edema	Decreased	Increased	Midline

Percussion

Condition	General Percussion	Diaphragmatic Excursion
A. Normal lung	Resonant	3 to 5 CM
B. Asthma	Hyperresonant	Decreased
C. Atelectasis (patent bronchus)	Dull	Decreased
D. Atelectasis (obstructed bronchus)	Dull	Decreased
E. Bronchiectasis	Resonant to dull	Decreased
F. Bronchitis	Resonant	Decreased if severe
G. Congestive heart failure	Resonant	Decreased
H. Emphysema	Hyperresonant	Decreased
I. Pleural effusion	Dull	Decreased
J. Pneumonia with lobar consolidation	Dull	Decreased
K. Pneumothorax	Hyperresonant	Decreased
L. Pulmonary edema	Dull	Decreased

Table 15-4 Comparison of Physical Examination Findings in Selected Respiratory Conditions—cont'd

Auscultation

Condition	Breath Sounds	Adventitious Sounds	Voice Sounds
A. Normal lung	Vesicular in periphery	Absent	Muffled
B. Asthma	Decreased or absent in severe obstruction	Wheezes	Decreased
C. Atelectasis (patent bronchus)	Bronchial	Crackles or wheezes	Increased or muffled
D. Atelectasis (obstructed bronchus)	Absent or decreased	Absent	Absent or muffled
E. Bronchiectasis	Vesicular or bronchial if severe	Crackles or wheezes	Muffled or decreased
F. Bronchitis	Vesicular or bronchial	Crackles or wheezes	Increased or muffled
G. Congestive heart failure	Vesicular	Crackles	Muffled
H. Emphysema	Bronchial and decreased	Wheezes	Decreased
I. Pleural effusion	Absent or decreased	Possible friction rub	Decreased or absent
J. Pneumonia with lobar consolidation	Bronchial	Crackles or occasional friction rub	Increased
K. Pneumothorax	Absent or decreased	Absent	Decreased or absent
L. Pulmonary edema	Absent or decreased	Crackles	Increased

ADVANCED TECHNIQUE

Forced Expiratory Time

Forced expiratory time is a gross measurement of the forced expiratory volume (FEV).

To perform this assessment:

E
1. Place your stethoscope over the client's trachea.
2. Instruct the client to inhale as deeply as possible and then exhale forcefully through the mouth (as if blowing out a candle).
3. Time the exhalation phase.

N **Normal exhalation occurs in less than 4 seconds.**

A The forced expiratory time is abnormal if it is greater than 4 seconds.

P Clients with COPD have a prolonged forced expiratory time and FEV because of air trapping in the lungs. A complete exhalation is difficult to achieve.

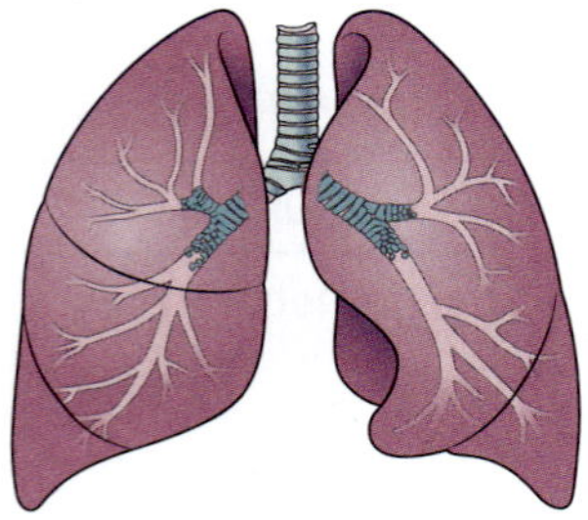

A. Normal lung

Shape of thorax: 1:2 to 5:7
Tracheal position: Midline
Percussion: Resonant
Adventitious sounds: Absent

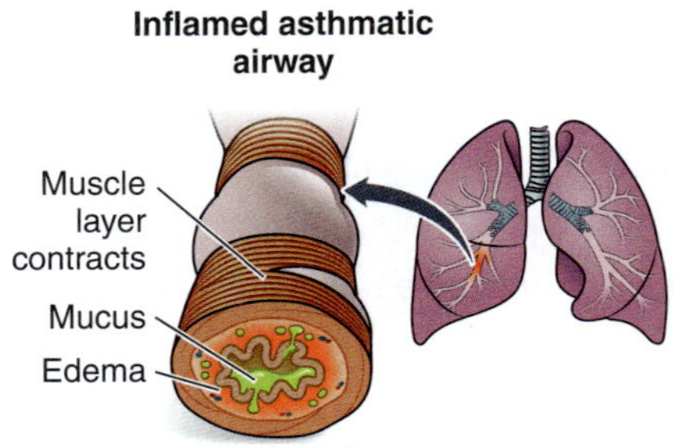

B. Asthma

Shape of thorax: 1:2 to 5:7 unless chronic may have barrel chest
Tracheal position: Midline
Percussion: Hyperresonant
Adventitious sounds: Wheezes

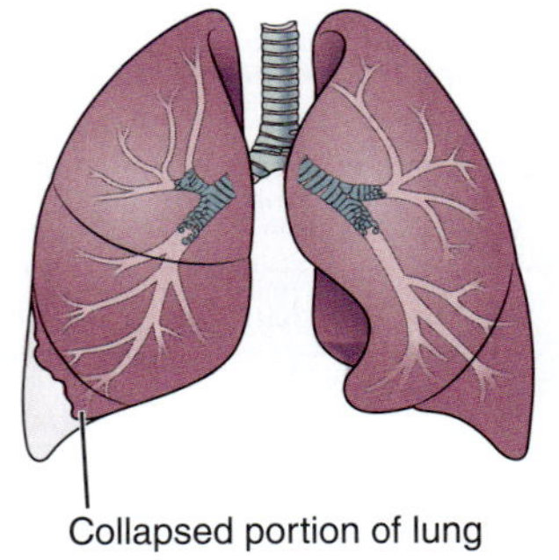

C. Atelectasis (patent bronchus)

Shape of thorax: 1:2 to 5:7
Tracheal position: Shifts to affected side
Percussion: Dull
Adventitious sounds: Crackles or wheezes

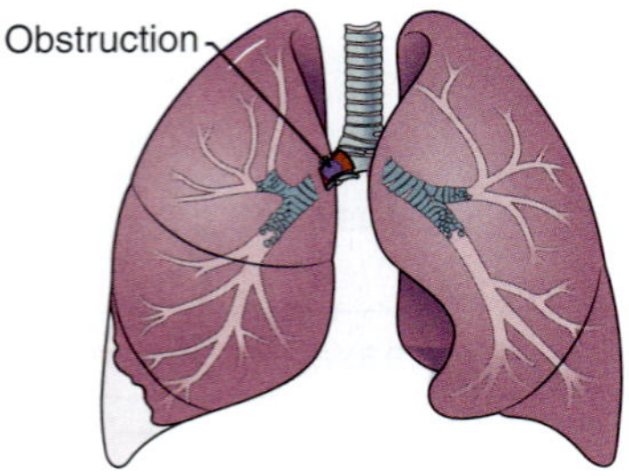

D. Atelectasis (obstructed bronchus)

Shape of thorax: 1:2 to 5:7
Tracheal position: Shifts to affected side
Percussion: Dull
Adventitious sounds: Absent

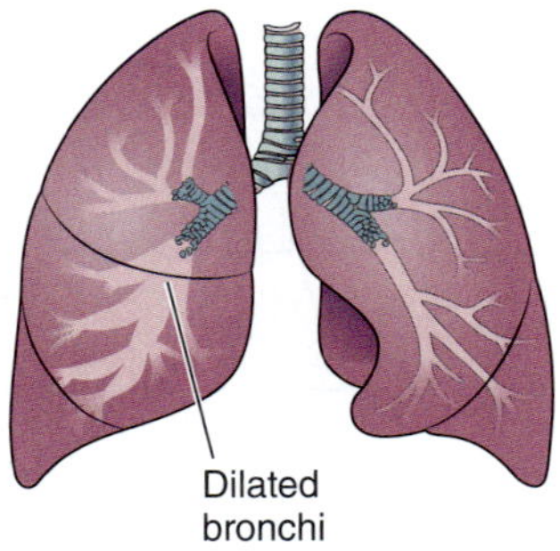

E. Bronchiectasis

Shape of thorax: 1:1
Tracheal position: Midline or deviated toward affected side
Percussion: Resonant to dull
Adventitious sounds: Crackles or wheezes

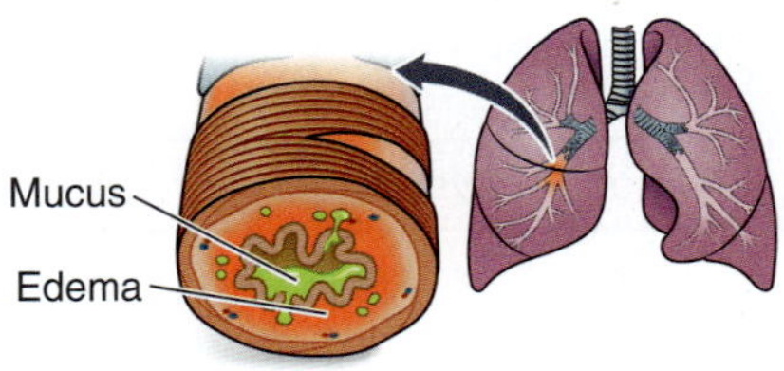

F. Bronchitis

Shape of thorax: 1:2 to 5:7
Tracheal position: Midline
Percussion: Resonant
Adventitious sounds: Crackles or wheezes

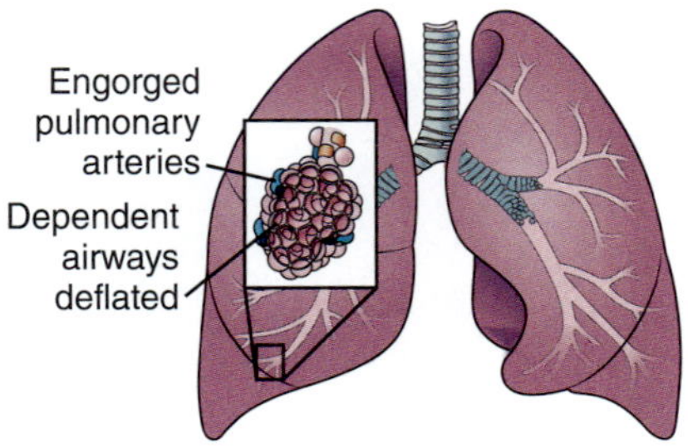

G. Congestive heart failure

Shape of thorax: 1:2 to 5:7
Tracheal position: Midline
Percussion: Resonant
Adventitious sounds: Crackles

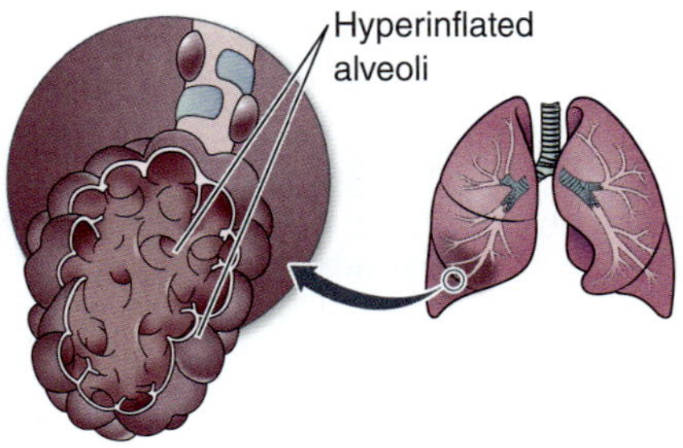

H. Emphysema

Shape of thorax: 1:1
Tracheal position: Midline
Percussion: Hyperresonant
Adventitious sounds: Wheezes

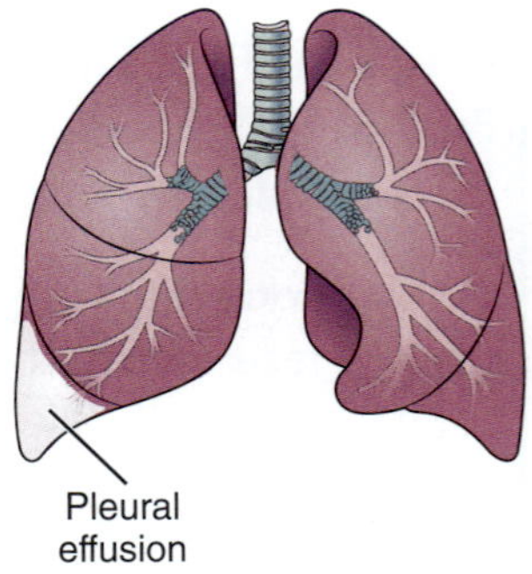

I. Pleural effusion

Shape of thorax: 1:2 to 5:7
Tracheal position: Shifts to unaffected side
Percussion: Dull
Adventitious sounds: Possible friction rub

Figure 15-25A-L Comparison of selected respiratory conditions.

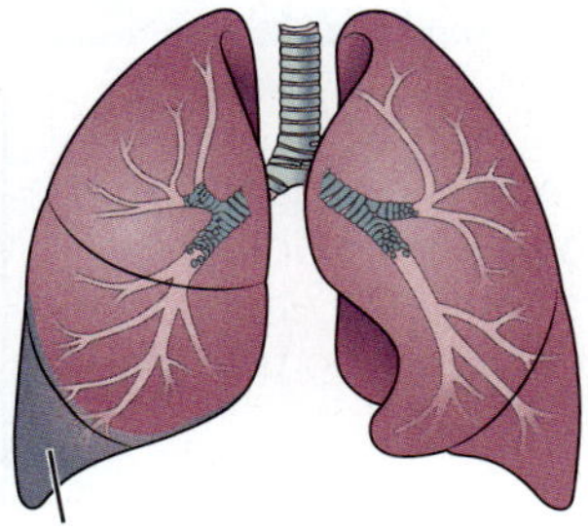

J. Pneumonia with lobar consolidation
Shape of thorax: 1:2 to 5:7
Tracheal position: Shifts to affected side
Percussion: Dull
Adventitious sounds: Crackles or occasional friction rub

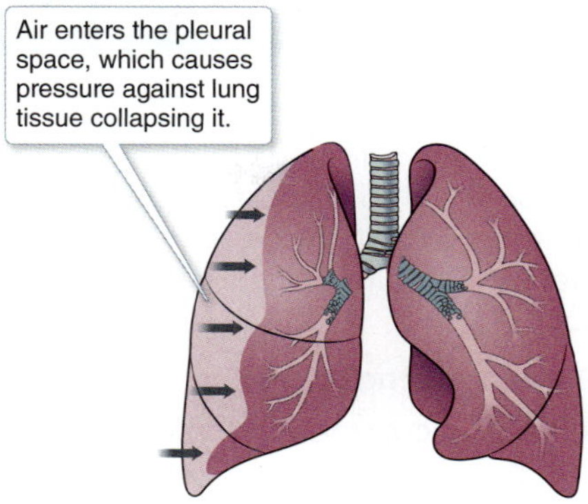

K. Pneumothorax
Shape of thorax: 1:2 to 5:7
Tracheal position: Shifts to unaffected side
Percussion: Hyperresonant
Adventitious sounds: Absent

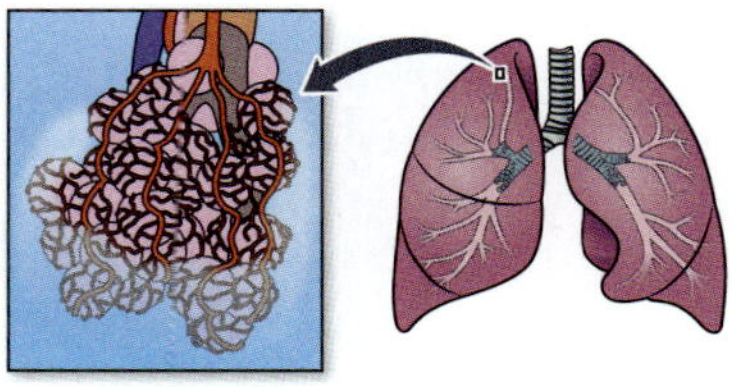

L. Pulmonary Edema
Shape of thorax: 1:2 to 5:7
Tracheal position: Midline
Percussion: Dull
Adventitious sounds: Crackles

Figure 15-25A-L—cont'd

Risk Factors

Pneumonia

- Smoking/secondhand smoke exposure
- Age <2 years old and >65 years old
- Underlying lung disease (e.g., COPD, asthma, interstitial lung disease, cystic fibrosis)
- Chronic diseases (e.g., kidney disease, heart failure, liver disease, diabetes mellitus, sickle cell disease)
- Malnutrition
- Alcohol and drug use
- Bedridden status
- Client in intensive care unit
- Mechanical ventilation
- Oxygen therapy
- Postoperative status
- Immunosuppressed status (chemotherapy, HIV, chronic steroid use, organ transplant recipients)
- Decreased cough reflex
- Sedated or decreased consciousness
- Swallowing disorders (cerebral vascular accident (CVA), Parkinson disease, traumatic brain injury, multiple sclerosis, amyotrophic lateral sclerosis, dementia, Alzheimer disease)
- Close living quarters (college dormitory, military barracks, long-term care facilities, shelters)

U.S. Preventive Services Task Force (USPSTF)

Grade A Recommendation:

- The USPSTF recommends that clinicians ask all adults about tobacco use, advise them to stop using tobacco, and provide behavioral interventions and US Food and Drug Administration (FDA)-approved pharmacotherapy for cessation to nonpregnant adults who use tobacco.

Grade B Recommendations:

- The USPSTF recommends screening for latent tuberculosis infection (LTBI) in populations at increased risk.
- The USPSTF recommends annual screening for lung cancer with low-dose computed tomography (LDCT) in adults aged 50 to 80 years who have a 20-pack-year smoking history and currently smoke or have quit within the past 15 years. Screening should be discontinued once a person has not smoked for 15 years or develops a health problem that substantially limits life expectancy or the ability or willingness to have curative lung surgery.

Retrieved November 5, 2025 from *https:// www.uspreventiveservicestaskforce.org/uspstf/recommendation-topics/uspstf-a-and-b-recommendations*

CASE STUDY
The Client With COVID-19 and Pneumonia

This case study illustrates the application and objective documentation of the thorax and lungs examination. Aarush Gupta is a 72-year-old man who emigrated to the United States from Pakistan 50 years ago to attend graduate school. He has resided in the United States since that time to work, marry, raise children, and retire. Aarush was diagnosed with COPD 10 years ago and takes medication daily for it. One week ago he was a science fair judge at his grandson's school where he interacted with numerous students and faculty. Aarush presents with a high fever, shortness of breath, and fatigue. His son, Guneet, has brought him to your office today to be evaluated.

HEALTH HISTORY

CLIENT PROFILE

72-year-old widowed man

CHIEF COMPLAINT

"I feel so sick."

HISTORY OF PRESENT ILLNESS

Aarush's symptoms started 2 days ago: fever of 100°F, mild sore throat, chills, and myalgia. He took acetaminophen 1,000 mg twice that day which brought his temperature down to 98.5°F. The following day client woke at 4 a.m. with a severe headache and worsening fever and chills. His temperature was 101.5°F. He started having a harsh, nonproductive cough. He uses tiotropium bromide 18 mcg, 2 inhalations daily; he also used his rescue inhaler, albuterol HFA, 2 inhalations every 6 hours, which helped his cough "a little." His temperature never went below 100°F that day despite acetaminophen 1,000 mg taken 4 times. He tried to nap some during the day but never really fell asleep. He went to bed at 10 p.m. last night after taking diphenhydramine 50 mg but woke with a 102.5°F fever and has used the albuterol inhaler every 2 to 3 hours since then to help his worsening cough. He was unable to sleep in a supine position due to cough, wheezing, and shortness of breath. Client reports having palpitations, diaphoresis, chest pain, and a feeling of suffocation. Aarush denies hemoptysis, leg edema, abdominal pain, rash, and change in urination. Client lives alone in his apartment in a retirement community and was exposed to many people 1 week ago when he volunteered at his grandson's school science fair. Aarush called his son this morning to ask him to take him to his primary care provider's office, as he was too ill to drive.

PAST HEALTH HISTORY

Medical History COPD diagnosed age 62
Hypertension diagnosed age 47

Surgical History Appendectomy age 15 without complications
Wisdom teeth extraction age 16 without complications

Allergies Penicillin caused a rash

Medications Albuterol HFA 1 to 2 inhalations every 4 to 6 hours, prn; typically uses 1 to 2 times a week
Tiotropium bromide 18 mcg/cap, two inhalations daily
Olmesartan 40 mg daily
MVI daily

Communicable Diseases Influenza last winter, recovered without problems

Injuries and Accidents Left humerus fracture age 62 when he tripped over his dog and fell onto his arm; casted, no sequelae

Differing Abilities Denies

Blood Transfusions Denies

Childhood Illnesses Chickenpox age 7

Immunizations Up to date per Aarush but did not get the RSV vaccine, 'I didn't know about it"; had BCG vaccine as a child

FAMILY HEALTH HISTORY

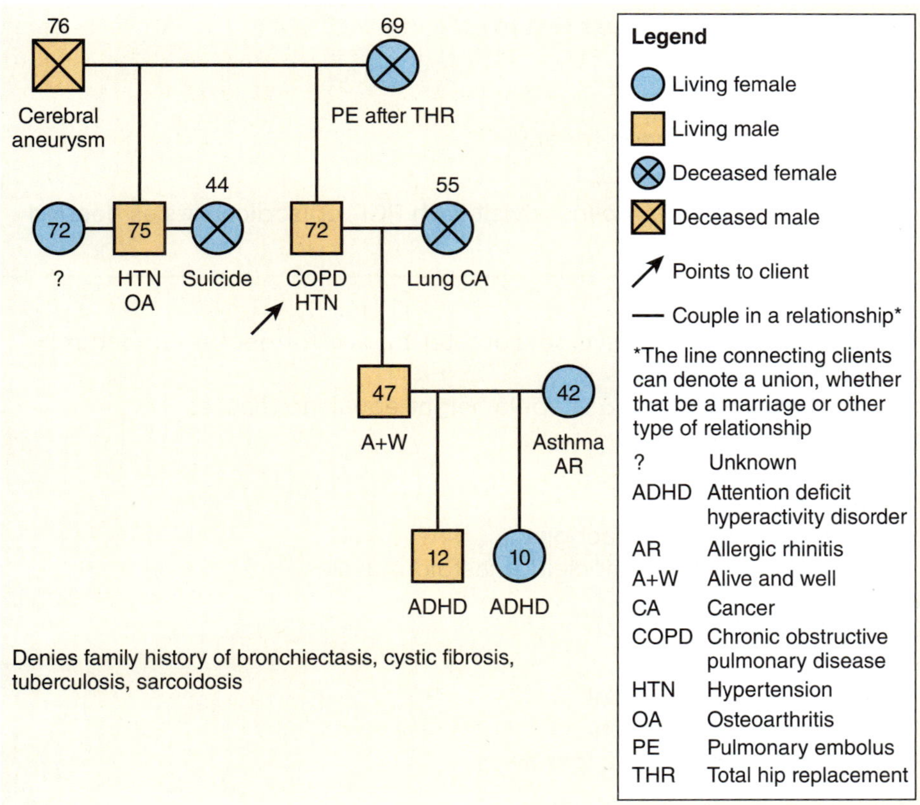

SOCIAL HISTORY

Alcohol Use Denies

Tobacco Use Smoked 1 PPD for 45 years, quit 11 years ago

Recreational Drug Use Denies use, including marijuana/THC products

Domestic and Intimate Partner Violence Denies

Sexual Practice Not sexually active for many years, his wife died 15 years ago

Travel History No recent travel; typically he visits relatives in Pakistan every 5 to 10 years, last visit was in early 2019

Work Environment Retired

Home Environment Lives in an older adult community, has his own 1,000 square-foot apartment, has weekly cleaning service

Hobbies and Leisure Activities Golfs 1 to 2 days a week with the same group of men

Stress "Not since I retired!"

Education PhD clinical virologist

Economic Status "No worries ... thankfully."

Military Service Denies

Religion Nonpracticing Hindu

Ethnic Background Aarush came to the U.S. for graduate school and identifies as a Pakistani-born American citizen

Roles and Relationships Has son, Guneet, who lives 30 minutes away; client spends most Sundays at son's house for lunch and playing with the grandchildren. Has positive relationships with son, son's wife, and 2 grandchildren

Characteristic Patterns of Daily Living Typically wakes at 7 a.m., prepares breakfast and then goes for 45-minute walk; prepares lunch at noon, plays golf some afternoons, runs errands or reads a book; meets his friends for dinner at 6 p.m. at the community dining room; occasionally participates in group activities at his community in the evening; retires about 10 p.m.

HEALTH MAINTENANCE ACTIVITIES

Sleep Typically 9 hrs per night and feels rested

Diet Low salt

Exercise Walking/golf

Stress Management Denies the need for any

Use of Safety Devices Wears seat belt

Health Checkups Medicare annual wellness visit with PCP, episodic visits as needed

PHYSICAL EXAMINATION

Inspection

Shape of Thorax AP diameter/transverse diameter 1:1; neg for pectus carinatum/pectus excavatum/kyphoscoliosis

Symmetry of Chest Wall Shoulder & scapula height equal, no masses

Presence of Superficial Veins None

Costal Angle Greater than 90°

Angle of the Ribs Greater than 45°

Intercostal Spaces No bulging/retractions

Muscles of Respiration Use of sternocleidomastoid muscles

Respirations

Rate: 32

Pattern: regular/even

Depth: shallow, little chest movement

Symmetry: no paradoxical movement

Audibility: respirations heard from 2 feet away

Client position: sitting upright

Mode of breathing: open-mouthed breathing with intermittent gasping

Sputum None

Palpation

General Palpation

Pulsations: none

Masses: none

Thoracic tenderness: none
Crepitus: none

Thoracic Expansion Anterior and posterior expansion 1 to 2 cm
Tactile Fremitus Positive bilateral bases
Tracheal Position Midline

Percussion

General Percussion Bibasilar dullness, hyperresonance other lobes
Diaphragmatic Excursion Deferred due to client's condition

Auscultation

Breath Sounds Bronchial, bronchovesicular, and vesicular breath sounds present in expected locations
Adventitious Sounds Bibasilar inspiratory coarse crackles
Voice Sounds Positive bronchophony bilateral bases

Assistive Devices Pulse oximeter: 90% on room air (normal = 97–99%)

Rapid Strep Test Negative for Group A beta-hemolytic streptococcus; throat culture sent

Rapid Influenza Test Negative for strains A & B

Rapid COVID-19 Antigen Test Positive for COVID-19

Chest X-ray PA and Lateral views obtained. Bibasilar opacity. Other lobes are clear. No pneumothorax or pleural effusion. Mild cardiomegaly.

CLINICAL JUDGMENT IN ACTION

1. What cues in the health history indicate that the client is having respiratory distress?
2. What interventions have the highest priority?
3. What assessment findings indicate clinical improvement or decline in this client?

Review Questions

1. The nurse auscultates the lungs of a healthy adult. The nurse identifies the breath sound as having a high pitch and being loud in intensity with a blowing quality. The expiratory phase of respiration is longer than the inspiratory phase. Where is it most likely that the nurse auscultates these breath sounds?
   a. Between the scapula
   b. Lateral to the sternum at the first and second intercostal spaces
   c. Over the trachea
   d. Peripheral lung

2. The client flexes the neck forward for posterior percussion. The nurse identifies the vertebra prominens. What is the significance of identifying this landmark?
   a. The vertebra prominens is used to identify the inferior angle of the scapula.
   b. The vertebra prominens is used to identify the manubriosternal junction.
   c. The vertebra prominens is used to identify the costal angle.
   d. The vertebra prominens is used to identify the posterior ribs to the level of T_4.

3. Inspecting the shape of the thoracic cavity, the nurse notes that the chest configuration is circular with the anteroposterior diameter to the transverse diameter in an approximate 1:1 ratio. What pulmonary conditions can lead to this finding? Select all that apply.
   a. Vitamin D deficiency
   b. Osteoporosis
   c. COPD
   d. This is the normal finding in a healthy adult
   e. This is a normal finding in a healthy infant

4. Which of the following physical assessment findings illustrates what a client with emphysema might exhibit?
   a. Pectus carinatum, costal angle <90°, angle of ribs >45°
   b. Barrel chest, costal angle >90°, angle of ribs >45°
   c. Pectus excavatum, costal angle >90°, angle of ribs <45°
   d. Elliptical chest, costal angle <90°, angle of ribs >45°

5. Bradypnea may occur in which of the following conditions? Select all that apply.
   a. Drug overdose
   b. Non-REM sleep
   c. Anxiety
   d. Pneumothorax
   e. Injury to the medulla oblongata

6. The nurse suctions the client's endotracheal tube and notes large quantities of pink, frothy sputum. What is the most likely etiology of this clinical finding?
   a. Asthma
   b. Bronchitis
   c. Pneumonia
   d. Pulmonary edema

7. The nurse auscultates an adventitious breath sound that is heard continuously in inspiration and expiration. It has a grating quality, and it does not clear with coughing. The nurse suspects that the client has which of the following clinical conditions?
   a. Asthma
   b. Atelectasis
   c. Croup
   d. Pleurisy

8. Which of the following clients are at risk for contracting TB? Select all that apply.
   a. A 6-month-old baby recently adopted from China
   b. A 3-year-old with a fractured humerus
   c. A 17-year-old high school student with anorexia nervosa who has a BMI of 15
   d. A 42-year-old correctional officer who has ulcerative colitis
   e. A 55-year-old salesclerk who recently had a lung transplant
   f. A 72-year-old retired plumber who had a stroke and is intubated in the intensive care unit

9. A nonsmoking, previously healthy client with pneumonia with lobar consolidation may exhibit which of the following physical examination findings? Select all that apply.
   a. Barrel chest
   b. Pale skin
   c. Clubbing
   d. Tachypnea
   e. Decreased tactile fremitus
   f. Dull percussion

10. A diaphragmatic excursion of 4 cm is seen in which of the following clients?
    a. An adult with normal ventilation depth
    b. An adult with a BMI of 52
    c. An adult who had a pneumonectomy 12 hours ago
    d. An adult experiencing respiratory distress

CHAPTER

16 Heart

Learning Outcomes

1. Identify the anatomy and physiology of the heart.
2. Conduct a complete health history on a client with a cardiac condition.
3. Perform a physical examination on a healthy adult and an adult with cardiac pathology.
4. Differentiate between normal clinical findings from a client's physical examination and the pathophysiology of abnormal clinical findings.
5. Identify risk factors for cardiac disease.
6. Assess if a client's Cardiac Assistive Devices are adversely affecting a client's cardiac health.
7. Identify the United States Preventive Services Task Force recommendations for the heart.
8. Document a complete history and physical examination of a client with cardiac pathology.

The heart's primary function is to pump blood to all parts of the body. The circulating blood not only brings oxygen and nutrients to the body's tissues but also helps to take away the body's waste products. The body's activities determine the amount of blood that is pumped. The heart will beat faster or slower and the blood vessels will expand or relax to properly distribute the blood that the body demands.

Anatomy and Physiology

Heart

In a resting, healthy adult, the heart contracts 60 to 100 times while pumping 4 to 5 liters of blood per minute. An individual's heart is about the size of a clenched fist. The human heart is remarkably efficient considering its size in relation to the rest of the body.

The heart is located in the thoracic cavity between the lungs and above the diaphragm in an area known as the mediastinum (Fig. 16-1). The **base** of the heart is the uppermost portion, which includes the left and right atria, the aorta, pulmonary arteries, and the superior and inferior venae cavae. These structures lie behind the upper portion of the sternum. The **apex**, or lower portion of the heart, extends into the left thoracic cavity, causing the heart to appear as if it is lying on its right ventricle.

Pericardium

The heart and roots of the great vessels lie within a sac called the pericardium, which is composed of fibrous and serous layers. The fibrous layer is the outermost layer and is connected to the diaphragm and

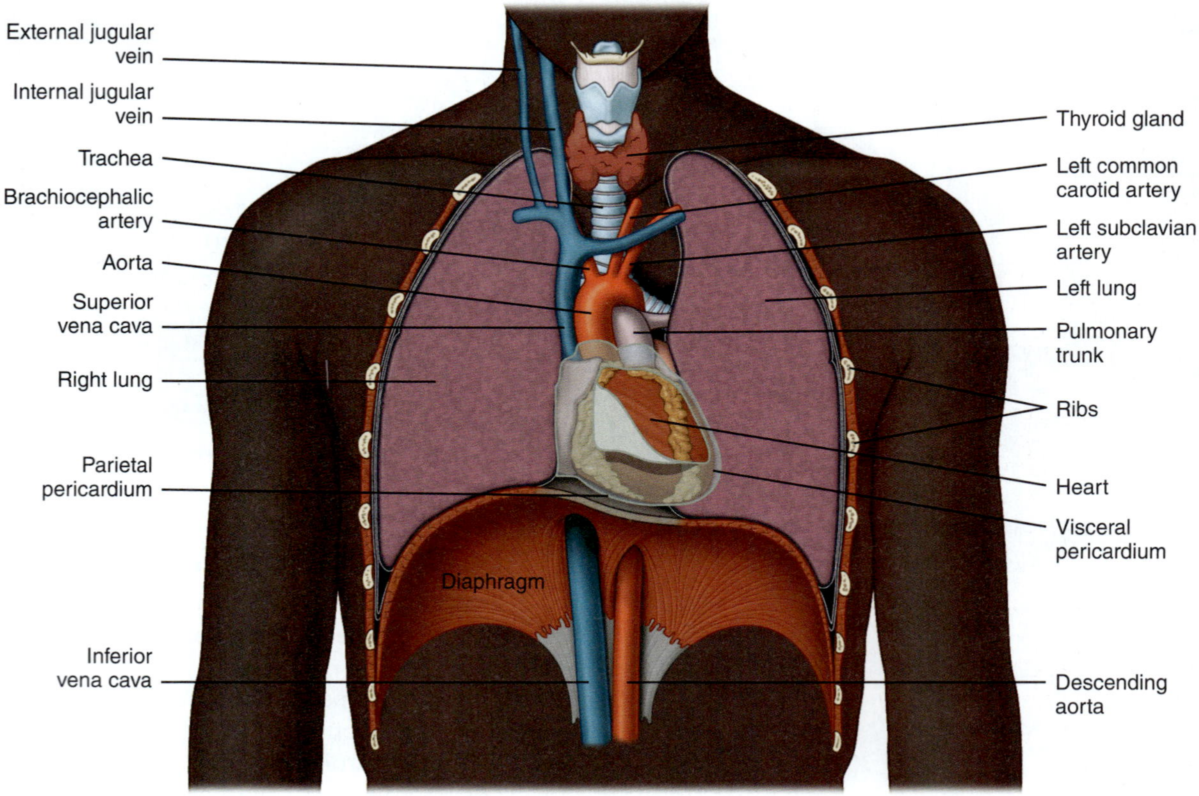

Figure 16-1 Position of the heart in the thoracic cavity.

sternum by ligaments and tendons. Its major role is to limit the stretching of the myocardial muscle, especially in the setting of strenuous activity or hypervolemia.

There are two serous layers of the pericardium: the **parietal** layer, which lies close to the fibrous tissues, and the **visceral** layer, which lies against the actual heart muscle. This visceral layer is often referred to as the epicardium. Between the two serous layers is a small space that contains approximately 20 to 50 mL of pericardial fluid. This pericardial fluid facilitates the movement of the heart muscle and protects it via a lubricant effect.

Chambers of the Heart

The heart is divided into four chambers, which are separated laterally by walls known as vertical **septa**. These vertical septa divide the heart into the right and the left atria (interatrial septum) and the right and the left ventricles (interventricular septum). The right atrium is the collection point for the blood returning from systemic circulation for reoxygenation in the lungs. The left atrium receives its freshly oxygenated blood via the four pulmonary veins, which are the only veins in the body that carry oxygenated blood.

The walls of the left ventricle are three times thicker than those of the right ventricle because of its greater workload as it pumps blood through the high-pressure systemic arterial system. Left ventricular pressures are five times greater than those in the right ventricle. Figure 16-2 shows the configuration of the heart's chambers, the pressures, and the normal oxygen content of the blood contained therein.

Heart Valves

As blood empties into the two atria, the **atrioventricular (A-V) valves** prevent it from prematurely entering the ventricles. The A-V valve between the right atrium and the right ventricle is known as the tricuspid valve,

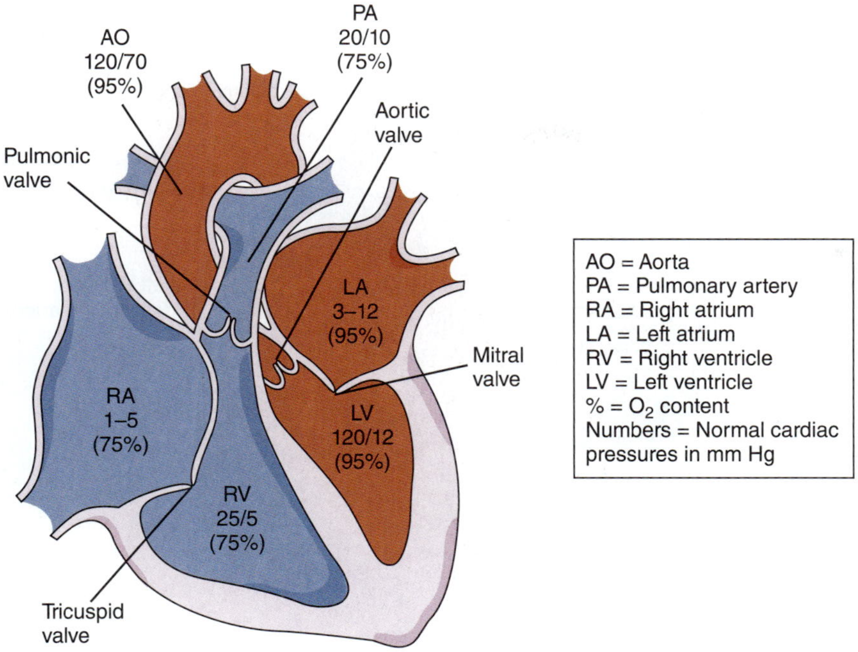

Figure 16-2 The configuration, normal pressures, and oxygen content of the heart chambers.

named for its three flaps or cusps. The A-V valve between the left atrium and the left ventricle is the bicuspid valve, named for its two flaps or cusps; it is commonly known as the mitral valve. When the tricuspid and mitral valves are closed, blood cannot flow from the atria into the ventricles. In a normal heart, they open only as atrial pressures increase with progressive filling.

The semilunar valves are also known as outflow valves because blood exits the heart through them. Blood flows from the right ventricle to the pulmonary vasculature for oxygenation by way of the pulmonic valve. Blood is pumped from the left ventricle into the systemic and coronary circulation through the aortic valve.

Coronary Circulation

The exterior surface of the heart muscle contains a very important and intricate blood supply. Two major coronary arteries arise from the small openings in the aorta known as the sinuses of Valsalva, located just behind the aortic valve. Figure 16-3 shows the position of the coronary arteries as they exit from the aorta to cover the myocardium with an arterial network. The left and right coronary arteries run superficially across the heart muscle, but the smaller branches of these two main arteries actually penetrate deeply into the myocardium, carrying with them a rich, nutritive blood supply. Blood flow to the coronary arteries is greatest during diastole because the force of the ventricular contraction during systole actually impedes flow through the sinuses of Valsalva.

The myocardium is extremely dependent on a constant supply of oxygen that is delivered through the coronary arterial system. The heart's oxygen requirements increase when it is stimulated by conditions such as exercise. If the coronary blood supply is not sufficient to meet the needs of the heart, the result may be **ischemia** (local and temporary lack of blood supply to the heart), injury (beyond ischemia but still reversible), or an **infarction** (necrosis) of the heart muscle itself. Myocardial ischemia is often manifested as chest, neck, or arm pain known as **angina**.

The left main coronary artery branches into the left circumflex coronary artery and the left anterior descending (LAD) coronary artery and supplies

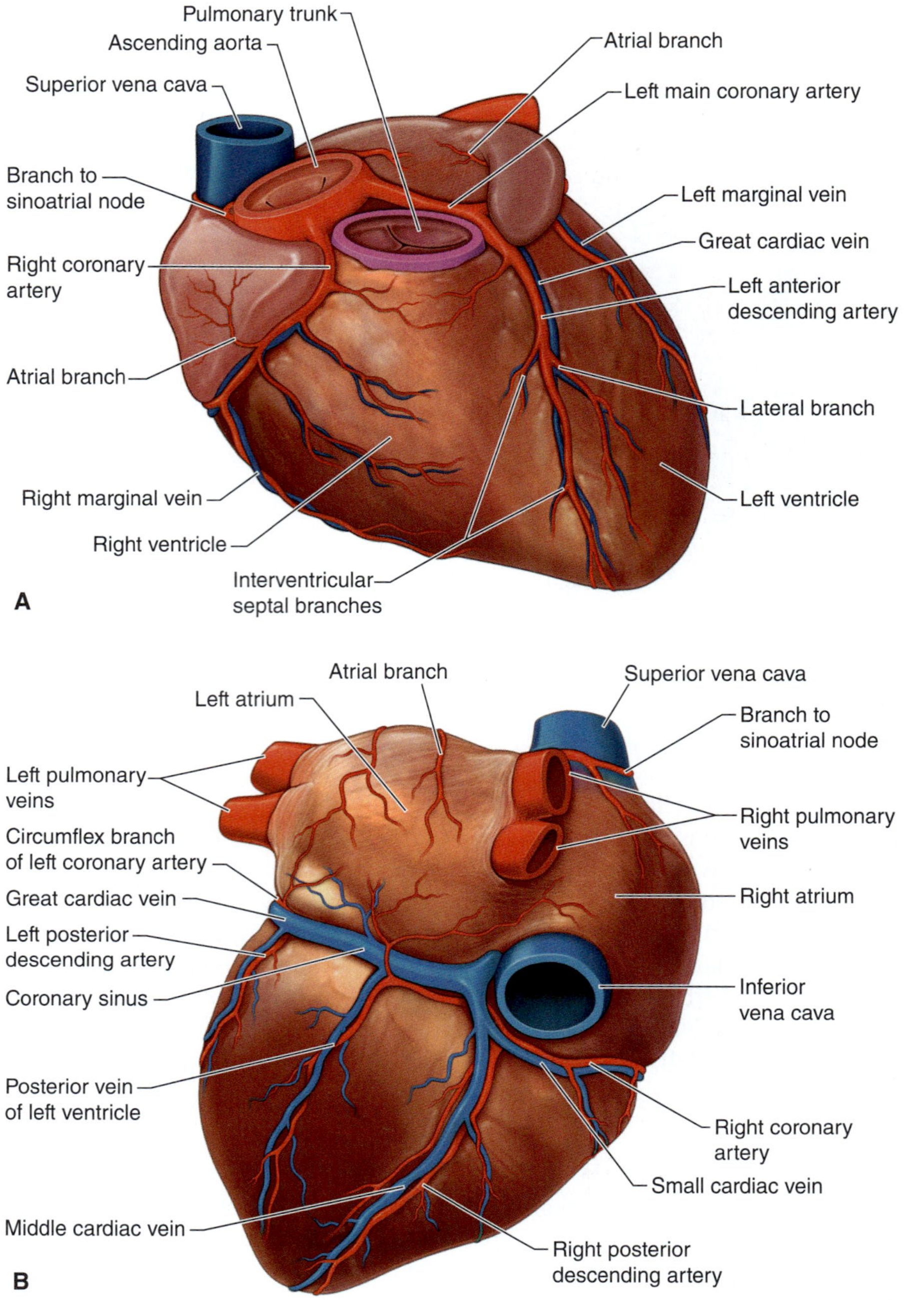

Figure 16-3 The coronary arteries and major veins of the heart. **A.** Anterior view. **B.** Posterior view.

blood to the entire left heart. A significant obstruction to blood flow through the left main coronary artery can be lethal.

The LAD supplies blood to the anterior wall and apex of the left ventricle as well as to the anterior portion of the interventricular septum. The smaller arterial branches that supply the septum also nourish the ventricular conduction system, including the bundle of His and the right and left bundle branches. The left circumflex (LCX) branch supplies arterial blood to the left atrium and the lateral and posterior portions of the left ventricle. In some individuals, the sinoatrial (S-A) node and the atrioventricular (A-V) node are also supplied by this branch. The LCX is usually the occluded vessel in a lateral wall infarction.

The right coronary artery (RCA) supplies nutrients and oxygen to the right atrium, the right ventricle, and the inferior wall of the left ventricle.

In most individuals, the RCA supplies the S-A and the A-V nodes as well as the posterior portion of the interventricular septum. With an inferior wall infarction, the RCA is most likely the vessel that has been occluded. With an anterior wall infarction, the LAD branch would be the most likely source of occlusion, with resulting complications in the ventricular conduction system (such as bundle branch blocks) or ventricular arrhythmias.

Venous drainage from the myocardium is carried by the coronary sinus, anterior cardiac veins, and thebesian veins. About 75% of the venous blood empties into the right atrium via the coronary sinus. The thebesian veins carry only a small portion of the unoxygenated blood that is emptied directly into all four chambers of the heart.

Cardiac Cycle

Figure 16-4 illustrates the electrical and mechanical events in the heart. Physical examination findings can be correlated with these electrophysiological mechanisms.

The cardiac cycle consists of two phases: systole and diastole. In **systole**, the myocardial fibers contract and tighten to eject blood from the ventricles (for this chapter, any mention of systole means ventricular systole, unless specifically called atrial systole). **Diastole** is a period of relaxation and reflects the pressure remaining in the blood vessels after the heart has pumped.

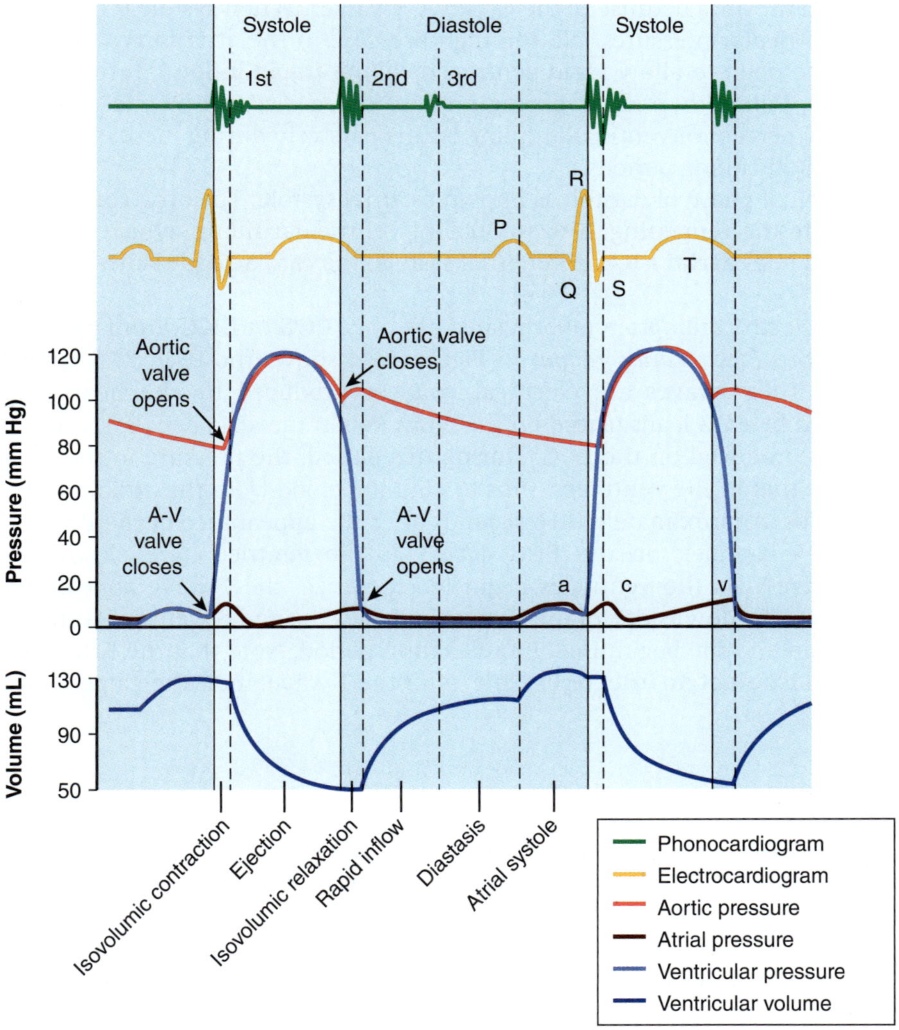

Figure 16-4 Events of the cardiac cycle.

> **NURSING TIP**
> **The American Heart Association's Recommendations for Exercise (2024)**
>
> For overall health benefits to the heart, lungs, and circulation, perform any moderate-to-vigorous-intensity aerobic activity using the following guidelines:
>
> - Avoid the risk of being sedentary. Spend less time sitting.
> - Get the equivalent of at least 150 minutes of moderate-intensity or 75 minutes of vigorous-intensity aerobic physical activity each week.
> - Increase your activity gradually over time.
> - More activity can lead to more benefit. Aim for 300 minutes or 5 hours of activity per week. Include muscle strengthening activity at least 2 days each week. This can include the use of weights or resistance bands.

> **NURSING TIP**
> **Calculating Target Heart Rate Zone**
>
> 1. Subtract the client's age in years from 220 to calculate the client's maximum heart rate.
> 2. The low end of the client's target heart rate (THR) zone is 50% of the value obtained in step 1. The high end of the client's THR zone is 85% of the value obtained in step 1. For example, a 48-year-old's THR zone would be calculated as follows:
> $(220 - 48) \times 0.50 = 86$ (low end)
> $(220 - 48) \times 0.85 = 146$ (high end)
>   Thus, the client's THR zone (range) would be 86 to 146 beats per minute.
> 3. If the client's goal is weight management and/or to burn fat, then the client should train to 50% to 65% of the maximum heart rate determined in step 1. If the client's goal is purely aerobic exercise, then the client should train to 65% to 85% of the maximum heart rate calculated in step 1.

Systole is divided into three phases, beginning with the isovolumic (or isometric) contraction phase, which marks the onset of a ventricular contraction. During this phase, the pressure is increasing but no blood is entering or leaving the ventricle. As the pressure rises in the left ventricle, the mitral valve closes (similar events occur in the right ventricle with the tricuspid valve). Closure of these A-V valves produces the first heart sound, known as S_1 (depicted as "1st" on the phonocardiogram [a recording of the heart sounds] curve in Figure 16-4).

Once the pressure in the left ventricle exceeds that in the aorta, and the pressure in the right ventricle exceeds that in the pulmonary artery, the semilunar (aortic and pulmonic) valves open and blood is rapidly ejected. This rapid ejection phase is also referred to as early systole. It is followed by a third phase of the reduced ejection, which is also known as late systole.

Ventricular diastole begins with the isovolumic, or isometric, relaxation phase. During this phase, ventricular ejection ceases and the pressure in the left ventricle is reduced to less than that in the aorta. This permits a backflow of blood from the aorta to the left ventricle, causing the aortic valve to close (similar events occur in the pulmonary artery to cause the pulmonic valve to close). The closure of the semilunar valves produces the second heart sound, known as S_2 (depicted as "2nd" on the phonocardiogram curve in Figure 16-4). When the A-V and semilunar valves are closed, the pressure in the left ventricle falls rapidly.

Atrial pressures then rise as a result of a large amount of blood accumulating in the atria because of the closed A-V valves. When systole is over and the ventricular pressures fall, the high pressure in the atria forces the A-V valves to open to allow rapid ventricular filling (rapid inflow) during early diastole. Filling then slows during a phase called diastasis or mid-diastole. Seventy percent of ventricular filling occurs passively during these early and middiastolic filling periods.

The final phase of diastole is known as atrial systole. The atria contract to complete the remaining 20% to 30% of ventricular filling, which is often referred to as **atrial kick**. After atrial systole, the cardiac cycle starts all over again.

The electrocardiogram (abbreviated as either **ECG** or **EKG**, from the German word *Elektrokardiogramm*) in Figure 16-4 shows the P, Q, R, S, and T waves. These waves are electrical voltages produced by the heart and recorded by ECG leads placed on the body. When the atria depolarize, the P wave is produced on the ECG. During this period, the pressure in the atria exceeds that in the ventricles, thus forcing the blood from the atria into the ventricles. Approximately 0.16 seconds after the appearance of the P wave, the QRS complex on the ECG occurs as the ventricles are electrically depolarized. As the ventricles begin to repolarize, the T-wave appears on the ECG. The downslope of the T wave indicates the end of ventricular repolarization and the beginning of a relaxation period. Note that the ECG contains an **isoelectric line**, or flat line, after the T wave, indicating a period of electrical rest.

Conduction System of the Heart

The **sinoatrial (S-A) node** is the normal pacemaker of the heart and is located about 1 mm below the right atrial epicardium at its junction with the superior vena cava. It initiates a rhythmic impulse approximately 60 times per minute. The infranodal atrial pathways conduct the impulse initiated in the S-A node to the **atrioventricular (A-V) node** via the myocardium of the right atrium. The three infranodal pathways are the anterior, middle, and posterior tracts. Meanwhile, the Bachmann bundle conducts the impulse from the S-A node to the left atrium. In the absence of a signal from the S-A node, the A-V node has its own intrinsic rate of 40 to 60 impulses per minute. The A-V node, also known as the A-V junction, delays the impulse received from the atria before transmitting it to the ventricles, to give them time to fill before the next systole. The impulse then travels very rapidly from the A-V node to the bundle branch system via the bundle of His. The bundle branch system is composed of the right bundle branch (RBB) and the left bundle branch (LBB). The RBB carries the impulse down the right side of the interventricular septum into the right ventricle. The LBB separates into three fascicles that relay the impulse to the left ventricle. Finally, the Purkinje fibers arising from the distal portions of the bundle branches transmit the impulse into the subendocardial layers of both ventricles. Barring interference with the connections described previously, the final transmission of the impulse allows depolarization of the ventricles to occur, followed by a normal systole. Figure 16-5 depicts the normal conduction pathways of the heart. If A-V node disease causes transmission of the electrical signal to be blocked, the intrinsic rate of the ventricles kicks in at a rate of fewer than 40 beats per minute. Normal conduction of the heart produces an ECG rhythm called normal sinus rhythm. An abnormal heart rhythm is called an **arrhythmia** or **dysrhythmia**.

NURSING TIP

Atrial Fibrillation

One of the most common arrhythmias seen on ECG is atrial fibrillation (AF). AF is a rhythm where the atria are quivering rather than contracting. There are multiple atrial depolarizations but the electrical activity is erratically conducted through the AV node resulting in an irregular, often rapid ventricular rate. The loss of atrial contraction leads to a decrease in up to 30% of the cardiac output and clients can experience hypotension, fatigue, diaphoresis, and palpitations. It also can cause stagnation of the blood and the formation of clots which can lead to stroke.

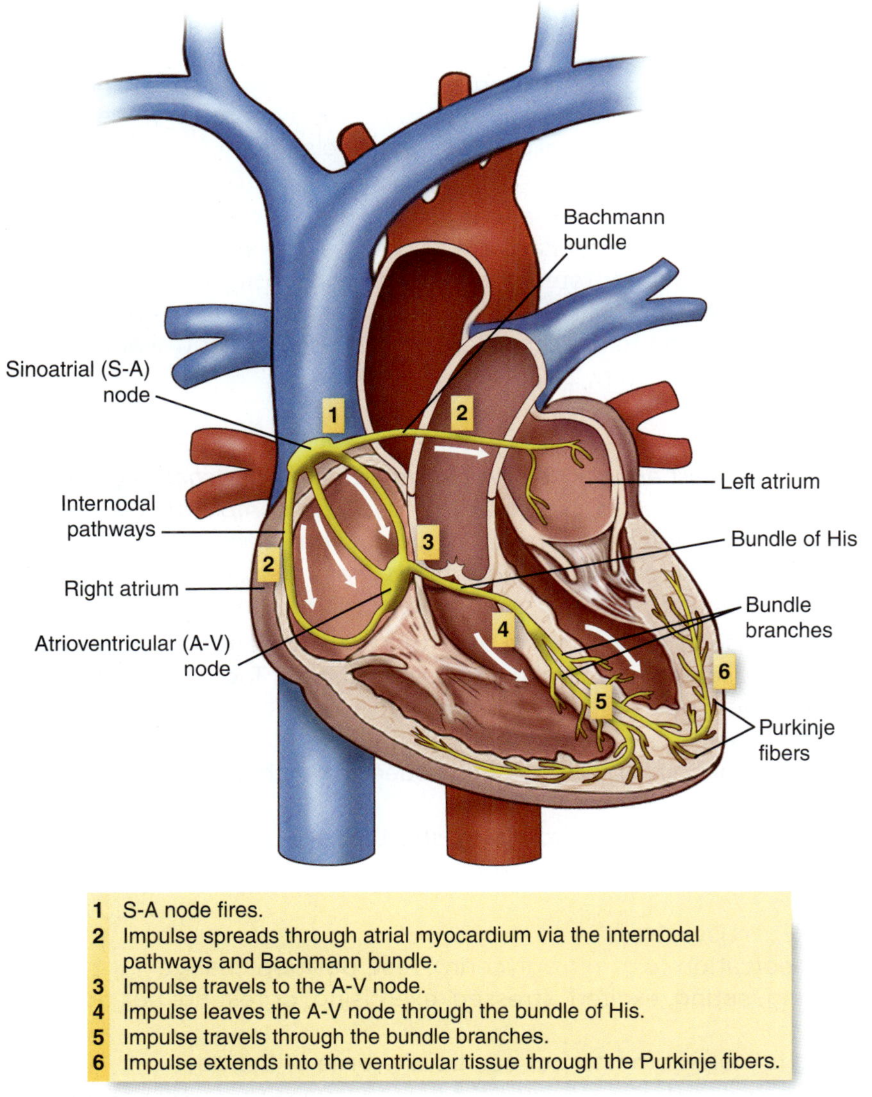

Figure 16-5 Conduction system of the heart.

HEALTH HISTORY

The heart health history provides insight into the link between a client's life/lifestyle and heart information and pathology.

CLIENT PROFILE

Diseases that are age-, sex-, and race-specific for the heart are listed. Table 16-1 differentiates the common cardiac disorders. Table 16-2 differentiates congenital cardiac defects.

Age Rheumatic fever (5–15)

Mitral valve prolapse (can develop at any age, serious symptoms occur in males >50)

Valve **stenosis** (narrowing or constriction of a diseased heart valve): mitral valve stenosis (15–40); aortic valve stenosis (older adults, symptoms generally don't appear until age 70–80)

Valve regurgitation (backward flow of blood through a heart valve). This can occur for many reasons, but older age is a risk factor.

Coronary artery disease (CAD) (40 to >80, risk increases with age)

Dilated or congestive cardiomyopathy (40–60)

Myocardial infarction (MI) (40 to >80, risk increases with age)

Sex

Female Higher mortality rate after a severe MI; marked rise in CAD after menopause; atrial septal defect (ASD).

Females experiencing a MI may not have the classic warning signs experienced by males. Instead, they may complain of unusual fatigue, sleep disturbance, and/or shortness of breath.

Combination hormone therapy is no longer used to prevent cardiac disease in healthy, postmenopausal females. If hormone therapy is used for the symptoms of menopause, it should be taken only in the smallest dose over the shortest feasible period.

Male Marked predisposition to CAD; ventricular septal defect (VSD)

Race Black, Indigenous, and people of color are at greater risk for complications from cardiovascular disease. Black Americans are at greatest risk for death from cardiovascular disease. They have higher rates of hypertension, obesity, and diabetes leading to higher rates of stroke and MI. This is related more to social determinants and disparities in health care than to biology (Centers for Disease Control and Prevention, 2023; Medical News Today, 2021).

CHIEF COMPLAINT

Common chief complaints for the heart are defined and information on the characteristics of each sign or symptom is provided. Keep in mind that the following complaints can also be signs of a potential cardiac problem: diaphoresis; dyspnea on exertion; change in color of lips, face, or nails; fatigue; feeling of doom; lightheadedness; peripheral edema; shortness of breath; syncope; extremity pain; and/or tingling/numbness in the extremities.

1. **Chest Pain** Subjective sense of discomfort in the thorax; also referred to as angina if it is caused by myocardial ischemia. Not all chest pain is angina. Table 16-3 differentiates different origins of chest pain.

   Radiation Arm, shoulder, neck, jaw, teeth

   Quality Crushing, heavy, tight, stabbing, burning, squeezing, aching, smothering, or perceived as indigestion

   Associated Manifestations Nausea and vomiting, shortness of breath (SOB), restlessness, anxiety, weakness, feeling of impending doom, diaphoresis, faintness, dizziness

   Aggravating Factors Exercise, stress

   Alleviating Factors Medication (e.g., nitroglycerin), rest, position change

   Setting While dreaming, eating, excited, stressed, exercising, or resting; hot or cold environment

   Timing Early morning is more common but can be any time of the day

2. **Palpitations** Irregular heartbeats; the sensation of a rapidly throbbing or fluttering heart

Quality Skipped heartbeats, throbbing, pounding, fluttering
Associated Manifestations Anxiety, weakness, nausea, SOB, chest pain, perspiration, fainting
Aggravating Factors Smoking, caffeine, exercise
Alleviating Factors Rest
Setting Resting, smoking, exercising, drinking, or eating food or beverages containing caffeine
Timing After exercise or at rest

PAST HEALTH HISTORY

The various components of the past health history are linked to heart pathology and heart-related information.

Medical History

Cardiac Specific Angina, cardiogenic shock, cardiomyopathy, chest trauma, congenital anomalies, congestive heart failure (CHF), CAD, endocarditis, hyperlipidemia, MI, myocarditis, pericarditis, cardiac tamponade, rheumatic fever, valvular disease, hypertension, arrhythmia, heart block

Noncardiac Specific Bleeding or blood disorder, diabetes mellitus, gout, Marfan syndrome, pheochromocytoma, primary aldosteronism, renal artery disease, CVA, thyroid disease, autoimmune disorders, cancers, history of chemotherapy or radiation treatment

Surgical History Ablation of accessory pathways, cardiac catheterization, chest surgery for trauma or pulmonary pathology, congenital heart defect repair, coronary artery bypass graft (CABG), coronary stents, directional coronary atherectomy (DCA), electrophysiology studies (EPS), heart transplant, implantable or internal cardioverter/defibrillator (ICD) placement, myotomy or myectomy, percutaneous laser myoplasty, pacemaker insertion, percutaneous transluminal coronary angioplasty (PTCA), pericardial window, pericardiectomy, pericardiotomy, valve replacement

Allergies Aspirin (most clients who are recovering from an MI receive aspirin), intravenous pyelogram (IVP) dye (injected during a cardiac catheterization) and seafood (both contain iodine compounds), latex (found in gloves used for procedures), betadine (used as a skin surface prep for cardiac and vascular procedures), heparin (used on cardiopulmonary bypass or for thromboprophylaxis)

Medications Antianginals, antiarrhythmics, anticoagulants, antihypertensives, antihyperlipidemics, diuretics, inotropics, thrombolytic enzymes, vasodilators, GLP-1

Communicable Diseases Rheumatic fever (valvular dysfunction), untreated syphilis (aortic regurgitation, aortitis, and aortic aneurysm), viral myocarditis (cardiomyopathy), COVID-19, (myocarditis, pericarditis, arrhythmias), tuberculosis (pericarditis, pericardial effusion, tamponade)

Injuries and Accidents Chest trauma (falls, motor vehicle accidents, blunt force)

Childhood Illnesses Rheumatic fever (valvular dysfunction)

FAMILY HEALTH HISTORY

Familial heart diseases are listed.

Aneurysm, CAD, hypertrophic cardiomyopathy, Marfan syndrome, mitral valve prolapse (MVP), MI, rheumatic fever, sudden cardiac death, long QT syndrome, congenital cardiac defects

SOCIAL HISTORY

The components of the social history are linked to heart factors and pathology.

Alcohol Use Prolonged use of alcohol can interfere with the normal pumping function and electrical activity of the heart, leading to **cardiomegaly** (enlargement of the heart), poor left ventricular contractility, ventricular dilation, palpitations, peripheral edema, fatigue, and SOB.

Thiamine deficiencies that usually occur concurrently with alcohol abuse may contribute to arrhythmias and heart failure.

Excessive alcohol intake may play a role in the pathogenesis of dilated cardiomyopathy, angina, CAD, arrhythmias, and beriberi heart disease. The use of alcohol in moderation, up to 2 ounces a day, has been associated with increased HDL cholesterol and lower rates of heart disease, but the American Heart Association (AHA) does not recommend drinking alcohol to gain health benefits (2019).

Tobacco Nicotine, inhaled through smoking tobacco and vaping, or chewing/dipping tobacco, increases catecholamine release, leading to elevated cardiac output, heart rate, and blood pressure. Nicotine also inhibits the development of collateral circulation, causes peripheral vasoconstriction, thickens cardiac arterioles, causes platelet aggregation, leads to arrhythmias, and neutralizes heparin, thus increasing the risk of thrombus formation. The nicotine and tobacco habit contribute to the pathogenesis of CAD, angina, and atherosclerosis. Exposure to other people's tobacco smoke increases the cardiac risk for nonsmokers.

Recreational Drug Use Injecting illegal drugs increases risk of vein collapse and contracting bacterial infections of the blood, heart valves, or blood vessels from the use of nonsterile needles and the embolization of localized infections from the injection site. IV drug use also carries the risk of oversedation and respiratory and cardiac arrest. Amphetamines, cocaine, and heroin affect the central nervous system and can cause altered consciousness, hyperthermia, hypertension, tachycardia, seizures, coronary vasospasm, myocardial infarction, arrhythmias, coronary artery dissection, and dilated cardiomyopathy.

Sexual Practice Sexual activity is generally safe for clients if their cardiovascular disease has been stabilized. Clients who have symptoms such as exertional chest pain or a vagal response should defer sexual activity until they have been assessed by a medical professional and stabilized. Clients who use nitrate drugs should never take phosphodiesterase type 5 inhibitors for erectile dysfunction. Postmenopausal females with heart disease can safely use topical or vaginal estrogen to treat painful intercourse and vaginal atrophy. Clients may avoid taking their cardiac medications because of the impact on sexual function. This should be discussed openly so the risk can be mitigated.

Travel History Chagas disease: Severe arrhythmias, mitral regurgitation or insufficiency, and cardiomegaly; caused by a protozoan parasite endemic to Central America, South America, and the Southwestern United States. Tuberculosis (TB): pericarditis and effusion can lead to constrictive pericarditis and cardiac tamponade in clients who have lived or traveled to areas with high TB rates.

Work Environment Exposure to toxic substances at the place of employment can cause cardiac pathology. Heavy metal exposure (e.g., arsenic, aluminum, lead, cadmium, mercury, nickel) can lead to heart ischemia, arrhythmia, and heart failure.

Home Environment A dirty fireplace may cause a smoky environment that leads to the worsening of chest pain.

Hobbies and Leisure Activities Clients with cardiac pathology may report a decline in the ability to participate in any activity that involves exertion. Understanding how clients spend their time helps determine functional status.

Stress Can cause tachycardia and arrhythmias, and lead to sudden death.

HEALTH MAINTENANCE ACTIVITIES

This information provides a bridge between health maintenance activities and heart function.

Sleep Dyspnea, orthopnea, or paroxysmal nocturnal dyspnea (PND)

Diet Eating disorders (e.g., bulimia) and liquid protein diets have been associated with sudden death due to electrolyte imbalances (e.g., hypokalemia).

Foods high in vitamin K may reduce the effectiveness of some anticoagulants.

Awareness of the sodium content of the tap water in your area (home water softeners often contain sodium).

Caffeine (in coffee, tea, soft drinks, chocolate, over-the-counter medications) is a sympathomimetic amine that increases the blood pressure and heart rate, elevates the serum catecholamine level, and can lead to arrhythmias (especially premature atrial contractions).

BMI score should be 18.5 to 24.9 kg/m² (see Chapter 7).

Socioeconomic factors and food insecurity are associated with poor nutrition quality and high chronic disease states. Food deserts, poor nutritional education, misinformation, and the use of federal food assistance programs may inhibit clients from choosing heart-healthy dietary options.

Exercise Physical exercise is essential to a healthy life. The body is made to be active and does not respond well to being sedentary for long periods. The aim of an individual's cardiovascular fitness program should be the attainment of the THR (see the Nursing Tip box titled "Calculating Target Heart Rate Zone" to determine THRs) to increase cardiovascular tone. In general, it is recommended that aerobic exercise or sustained physical activity for at least 20 to 30 minutes per day, 3 to 5 times per week, positively affects one's cardiovascular conditioning. It may be helpful to assess a client's activity status to determine cardiac risk. The Duke Activity Status Index is an activity scale that estimates functional status and capacity. This can be found at the website: *https://www.mdcalc.com/calc/3910/duke-activity-status-index-dasi*.

Stress Management Exercise, time management, pet therapy, reading, listening to music, eating, biofeedback, yoga, imagery, massages, transcendental meditation, participation in a variety of support groups; the AHA (2024) provides tips on managing stress.

Use of Safety Devices Clients with older pacemakers and implantable cardioverter defibrillators (ICDs) should avoid areas with magnetic fields (including MRI scanners). Keep microwaves, cellular phones (especially digital cellular phones), walkie-talkies, headphones, and earbuds at least 6 inches away from a pacemaker or ICD as they may cause interference. Electric fences or pet containment systems should also be avoided.

Health Checkups ECG, chest x-ray, heart rate, blood pressure, lipid profile, HbA1c if diabetic

NYHA CLIENT CLASSIFICATION

The New York Heart Association (NYHA) classification provides a template for classifying the degree of heart failure in clients. This standardization of functional status evaluates limitations during physical activity and anginal symptoms (e.g., fatigue, palpitations, dyspnea, angina).

- Class I - No limitation in ordinary physical activity such as walking, climbing stairs, etc. Ordinary physical activity does not cause angina, fatigue, or breathing problems such as shortness of breath. This client has no objective evidence of cardiovascular disease.
- Class II – Slight limitation of physical activity. Clients are comfortable at rest. Ordinary physical activity results in fatigue, palpitation, or dyspnea. This client has objective evidence of minimal cardiovascular disease.
- Class III - Marked limitation of physical activity. Clients are comfortable only at rest. Less than ordinary activity causes fatigue, palpitation, or dyspnea. This client has objective evidence of moderately severe cardiovascular disease.
- Class IV - Inability to carry on any physical activity without discomfort. Symptoms are present even at rest or with minimal exertion. If any physical activity is undertaken, discomfort is increased. This client has severe cardiovascular disease and has severe limitations on life's activities.

American Heart Association (2023)

Table 16-1 Cardiac Disorders

Disorder	Definition	Common Findings
Acute coronary syndrome (ACS)	An umbrella term used to describe a constellation of events associated with an acute myocardial ischemic episode, ranging from unstable angina to myocardial infarction	Chest pain that is similar to angina except that it is more intense and more persistent (>30 minutes), not fully relieved by rest or nitroglycerin, and accompanied by systemic symptoms (e.g., nausea, shortness of breath, sweating, or apprehension)
Aortic regurgitation or insufficiency	Backflow of blood from the aorta to the left ventricle during diastole because of an incompetent valve	Dyspnea, paroxysmal nocturnal dyspnea (PND), orthopnea, palpitations, angina, fatigue, syncope, diastolic murmur
Aortic stenosis	A narrowing or constriction of the aortic valve obstructing the ejection of blood from the left ventricle during systole	Syncope, fatigue, weakness, palpitations, angina, systolic murmur
Arrhythmia	A malfunction of the electrical conduction system of the heart leading to an irregular heart rhythm	Palpitations, chest pain, dizziness, syncope
Atherosclerosis (coronary artery disease)	A type of arteriosclerosis; localized accumulations of lipid-containing material within the blood vessels	Angina, MI, CHF, sudden cardiac death, arrhythmias
Cardiac tamponade	Compression of the heart resulting from the accumulation of excess fluid in the pericardium	Beck's triad (hypotension, distended neck veins, and distant heart sounds); pulsus paradoxus
Cardiogenic shock	A shock of cardiac origin caused by pump failure	Pulmonary congestion; peripheral edema; hypotension; tachycardia; decreased pulse pressure; cool, pale, and clammy skin
Cardiomyopathy • congestive or dilated • hypertrophic • restrictive	Heart muscle disease resulting in the heart having a diminished ability to pump	CHF-type symptoms, cardiomegaly with dilated or congestive form, familial history with hypertrophic form
Congestive heart failure (CHF)	A condition whereby pump failure makes the heart unable to maintain cardiac output sufficient to meet the metabolic needs of the body; the left ventricle, the right ventricle, or both may fail	Left-sided: anxiety, diaphoresis, rales, S_3, cough, PND, fatigue Right-sided: dependent pitting edema, hepatomegaly, weight gain, hepatojugular reflux
Endocarditis (bacterial)	Infection of the endocardial surface or the heart valves	Fever; chills; fatigue; anorexia; nausea and vomiting; arthralgia; back pain; dyspnea; splinter hemorrhages of the nails; petechiae, positive blood cultures
Marfan syndrome (annuloaortic ectasia)	A syndrome of congenital collagen deficiency affecting the connective tissues	Client may be tall and thin with hyperextensive joints and long arms, legs, and fingers; aortic dissection; aortic regurgitation; mitral regurgitation; arrhythmias

Table 16-1 Cardiac Disorders—cont'd

Disorder	Definition	Common Findings
Metabolic syndrome (insulin-resistance syndrome)	Characterized by a group of metabolic risk factors that place clients at greater risk for coronary artery disease, stroke, and/or peripheral vascular disease as well as type 2 diabetes	Abdominal obesity and insulin resistance or glucose intolerance are the predominant risk factors associated with this disorder. Others include hyperlipidemia, hypertension, a prothrombotic state, and/or a proinflammatory state.
Mitral regurgitation or insufficiency	The backflow of blood from the left ventricle to the left atrium during systole, resulting from an incompetent valve	CHF-type symptoms; history of rheumatic fever, infection, trauma, or mitral valve prolapse; systolic murmur
Mitral stenosis	A narrowing or constriction of the mitral valve obstructing blood flow from the left atrium to the left ventricle during diastole	CHF-type symptoms, history of rheumatic heart disease or congenital heart defect, diastolic murmur, thrill at apex
Myocardial infarction	Myocardial cell death due to prolonged ischemia	Nausea and vomiting, diaphoresis, shortness of breath, abnormal heart and lung sounds, angina, arrhythmias, CHF, cardiogenic shock
Myocarditis	Inflammation of the heart's muscular tissue	History of rheumatic fever, viral or parasitic infection, irregular pulse, tenderness over the pericardium, may lead to dilated cardiomyopathy
Pericarditis	An inflammation of the pericardium; origin may be viral, malignant, or autoimmune	Precordial pain that increases with inspiration or in the supine position; pain may be relieved by leaning forward; fever; fatigue; pulsus paradoxus; pericardial friction rub and possible pericardial effusion
Pulmonary regurgitation or insufficiency	The backflow of blood from the pulmonic valve to the right ventricle because of an incompetent valve	Dyspnea on exertion (DOE), fatigue, diastolic murmur
Pulmonary stenosis	A narrowing or constriction of the pulmonic valve causing an obstruction to the ejection of blood from the right ventricle	DOE, fatigue, right-sided heart failure symptoms, systolic murmur
Tricuspid regurgitation or insufficiency	The backflow of blood from the right ventricle to the right atrium because of an incompetent valve	Dyspnea, fatigue, systolic murmur
Tricuspid stenosis	A narrowing or constriction of the tricuspid valve obstructing blood flow from the right atrium to the right ventricle	Dyspnea, fatigue, diastolic murmur, right-sided CHF
Ventricular aneurysm	The dilation of a portion of necrosed ventricular wall after an MI	Tachyarrhythmias, CHF-type symptoms, clot formation, arterial emboli, rupture, cardiac tamponade, systolic murmur

Table 16-2 Congenital Cardiac Defects

A congenital cardiovascular defect (CCD), also known as a congenital heart defect (CHD), occurs when the heart or blood vessels near the heart do not develop normally before birth. CCDs occur in about 1% of live births (CDC, 2023). Treatment depends on the type and severity of the defect. Many children with CCDs survive into adulthood. Often the cause of the defect is unknown, but it may be related to teratogenic, genetic, or random factors. The majority of clients with CCDs require long-term follow-up for the management of persistent problems such as arrhythmias, myocardial changes, ventricular failure, prosthetic materials, or endocarditis.

Most CCDs either obstruct blood flow in the heart or vessels near the heart or cause blood to flow through the heart in an abnormal pattern. Another rare defect occurs when the right or left side of the heart is not completely formed. About 1 in 4 babies who have a critical CHD requires surgery or a procedure to correct/minimize the anomaly within the first year of life (CDC, 2023).

Classification	Disorder	Definition	Common Findings	Treatment Options	Special Considerations
Obstruction Defects	Pulmonary stenosis (PS)	Occurs when a defective pulmonary valve does not open properly. Thus, the right ventricle must pump harder than normal to overcome the obstruction.	If stenosis is severe, especially in babies, cyanosis may occur. Older children may not have symptoms. A pulmonic systolic ejection click, murmur, and/or a diminished S_2, possibly with a wide split, may be auscultated. Client may also have a thrill.	Required when the pressure in the right ventricle is higher than normal. Obstruction can be relieved by balloon valvuloplasty or open-heart surgery.	Most clients will need subacute bacterial endocarditis (SBE) prophylaxis. Before and after treatment for their CCD, clients need to take antibiotics before certain dental and surgical procedures to prevent endocarditis.
	Aortic stenosis (AS)	Occurs when the aortic valve is narrowed. This makes it hard for the heart to pump blood to the body.	Chest pain, DOE, unusual tiring, dizziness, or fainting may occur. A systolic ejection murmur may be auscultated. Client may also have a thrill.	The need for surgery depends on the severity of the stenosis. The stenosis may be relieved by enlarging the valve opening. Eventually, the valve may have to be replaced with an artificial valve.	• Most clients will need SBE prophylaxis. • Lifelong follow-up is required.
	Coarctation of the aorta (COA)	When the aorta is constricted, blood flow to the lower part of the body is obstructed. Also, the blood pressure above the obstruction is increased.	Symptoms of CHF and hypertension may develop in the week after birth. Blood pressure that is higher in the upper extremities than the lower extremities is suggestive of COA.	Balloon angioplasty or surgery, or both.	• Most clients will need SBE prophylaxis. • Defect may reoccur. • Hypertension may ensue even after repair. • Lifelong follow-up is required.

			A systolic murmur will often be present. Absent or weak femoral pulses are another hallmark sign. A heave over the left ventricle may be observed. In adulthood, the upper body may be more developed than the lower body.		
	Bicuspid aortic valve	Occurs when the aortic valve has only two cusps, rather than the normal three.	There may be no symptoms in childhood but by adulthood, the valve can become stenotic or regurgitant. Thus, a diastolic or systolic murmur may be auscultated depending on the condition of the valve.	Treatment depends on how well the valve functions.	Most clients will need SBE prophylaxis.
	Subaortic stenosis	Refers to a narrowing of the left ventricle just below the aortic valve. Thus, blood flowing out of the left ventricle is limited. This condition may be congenital or it may be the result of a type of cardiomyopathy known as idiopathic hypertrophic subaortic stenosis (IHSS).	Client may have an ejection murmur and thrill.	Treatment depends on the cause and severity of the narrowing; may include medications or surgery.	Most clients will need SBE prophylaxis.
	Ebstein anomaly	Occurs when the tricuspid valve is displaced downward into the right ventricle. Usually associated with an atrial septal defect (ASD).	In mild cases, there are no symptoms. Later, clients may complain of tiredness, palpitations, or an abnormal heartbeat. In severe cases, children may turn cyanotic and have CHF.	Medications for mild cases and surgery for severe cases.	Most clients will need SBE prophylaxis.

Continued

Table 16-2 Congenital Cardiac Defects—cont'd

Classification	Disorder	Definition	Common Findings	Treatment Options	Special Considerations
Septal Defects	Atrial septal defect (ASD); Patent foramen ovale (PFO)	Occurs when there is an opening between the heart's atria. In ASD, the septal tissue fails to develop in utero. In PFO, the foramen ovale fails to close when the newborn takes its initial breath at delivery. Thus, blood from the left atrium flows into the right atrium instead of flowing through the left ventricle, out of the aorta, and through the rest of the body.	Many children have few, if any, symptoms. A systolic ejection murmur, a diastolic murmur, a fixed widely split S_2, or a heave may be auscultated. Signs of CHF may occur in older clients.	Open-heart surgery in some cases.	None.
	Ventricular septal defect (VSD)	Occurs when there is an opening between the heart's lower chambers. Thus, blood that has returned from the lungs and has been pumped into the left ventricle flows into the right ventricle instead of being pumped directly through the aorta. The heart may enlarge because it has to pump extra blood to meet the oxygenation needs of the body and thus may become overworked.	Client may have high pulmonary pressures. A lift is often observed, a thrill may be palpated, and a harsh holosystolic murmur may be auscultated. Children with VSDs may have poor weight gain, slow growth, feeding difficulties, DOE, and failure to thrive (FTT).	Open-heart surgery for a large defect.	• Most clients will need SBE prophylaxis. • After a VSD has been successfully repaired with surgery, prophylactic antibiotics are usually not required. • Lifelong follow-up is required.

	Eisenmenger complex or syndrome	Consists of both a VSD and pulmonary hypertension. Therefore, blood shunts from the right side of the heart to the left, causing the right ventricle to enlarge. It may also include an overriding aorta whereby a malpositioned aorta receives ejected blood from both ventricles.	Severe CHF and cyanosis with a right-to-left shunt. Clients may have healthy childhoods but become progressively cyanotic in adulthood, with poor exercise tolerance. Syncope may occur. Problems might not arise until pregnancy or some other type of cardiovascular stress occurs.	Surgery followed by a possible heart or heart-lung transplant.	• Most clients will need SBE prophylaxis. • Lifelong follow-up is required.
	Atrioventricular canal defect (also known as endocardial cushion defect or atrioventricular septal defect)	Consists of both a large hole in the center of the heart plus a single, large valve (which is a combination of the tricuspid and mitral valves) that crosses the defect. Eventually, the heart may enlarge because it has to pump extra blood and thus may become overworked. The defect may be complete, intermediate, or partial (the most common form).	Babies may become undernourished because they do not grow normally. Pulmonary hypertension occurs because there is increased blood flowing to the lungs. Clients may present with CHF. S_2 may be widely split. Diastolic and systolic murmurs may be auscultated.	Surgery.	• Most clients will need SBE prophylaxis. • A reconstructed valve may not work normally. • About 40% to 50% of clients with this defect have Down syndrome.
Cyanotic Defects	Tetralogy of Fallot	Has four components: 1. VSD 2. Stenosis at or beneath the pulmonic valve 3. Right ventricular hypertrophy 4. Dextroposition of the aorta (the aorta now lies directly over the VSD)	Cyanosis may occur soon after birth or with rapid breathing. Older children may faint during exercise because not enough blood flows to the lungs to supply the body with oxygen. Subsequently, clubbing of the fingers and toes may occur. Clients may have a heave as well as a systolic ejection murmur, a loud S_2, and a thrill.	Surgery.	Most clients will need SBE prophylaxis.

Continued

Table 16-2 Congenital Cardiac Defects—cont'd

Classification	Disorder	Definition	Common Findings	Treatment Options	Special Considerations
	Transposition of the great arteries	Occurs when the positions of the pulmonary artery and the aorta are reversed. The aorta is connected to the right ventricle, so most of the blood returning to the heart from the body has not gone through the lungs to be oxygenated. The pulmonary artery is connected to the left ventricle, so most of the blood returning from the lungs goes back to the lungs again.	Cyanosis, tachypnea without respiratory distress, loud S_2, poor feeding in infants.	Surgery.	• Most clients will need SBE prophylaxis. • Lifelong follow-up is required. • This defect is rare (<1% of all congenital heart defects).
	Tricuspid atresia	There is no tricuspid valve in this defect; therefore, blood cannot flow from the right atrium to the right ventricle. Thus, the right ventricle is small and underdeveloped. The child's survival depends on whether there is both an ASD and a VSD.	Cyanosis.	If left untreated, clients will die. Thus, surgery is required.	• Most clients will need SBE prophylaxis. • Lifelong follow-up is required.
	Pulmonary atresia	With this defect, there is no pulmonary valve; therefore, blood cannot flow from the right ventricle into the pulmonary artery and the lungs. The right ventricle may be small and underdeveloped. The tricuspid valve may also be abnormal. An ASD allows blood to exit the right side of the heart. A coexisting PDA is the only source of lung blood flow.	Cyanosis, clubbing, dyspnea, or tachypnea.	Medications and surgery.	• Most clients will need SBE prophylaxis. • Lifelong follow-up is required.

Truncus arteriosus	Consists of only one artery, which arises from the heart and forms the aorta and the pulmonary artery. May also have a VSD. There are four types of this defect depending on how the pulmonary arteries originate from the single arterial vessel.	Cyanosis, CHF, tachypnea, or poor feeding. A systolic ejection click is often heard, as well as a harsh pansystolic murmur.	Medications and surgery.	• Most clients will need SBE prophylaxis. • Lifelong follow-up is required.
Total anomalous pulmonary venous connection	Occurs when the pulmonary veins do not connect to the left atrium. Instead, they drain through abnormal connections to the right atrium.	Cyanosis.	Surgery.	• Lifelong follow-up is required.
Hypoplastic left heart syndrome	Results in an underdeveloped left side of the heart. May also have an ASD, PDA, or both.	Babies become ashen within days of birth, sometimes cyanotic. They will also have rapid breathing and difficulty in feeding. CHF, shock, and multisystem organ failure may be present.	Compassionate care, medications, surgery, and/or possibly a heart transplant.	• This heart defect is usually fatal without treatment. • Most clients will need SBE prophylaxis. • Lifelong follow-up is required.
Patent ductus arteriosus (PDA)	Occurs when the ductus, which is patent in utero, fails to close after birth. This allows blood to mix between the pulmonary artery and aorta. Consequently, the right ventricle has to work harder and pulmonary hypertension may ensue.	If ductus is large, children may tire quickly, grow slowly, breathe rapidly, and catch pneumonia easily. A continuous, harsh, loud, and machine-like murmur is often heard throughout systole and diastole.	Surgery.	SBE prophylaxis is usually stopped 6 months after surgical repair unless there are concurrent cardiac defects.

Table 16-3 Differentiating Chest Pain

All of these conditions (excluding musculoskeletal) are life-threatening and require immediate attention.

Etiology	Pain	Related Factors
Cardiac Ischemia (also known as acute coronary syndrome)	Burning, squeezing or aching, heaviness, smothering	• Not reproducible by palpation of the chest wall, may be relieved with rest or oxygen, and may or may not be accompanied by ECG changes. • Myocardial ischemia may lead to myocardial infarction; when in doubt, assume a cardiac cause and follow your institution's chest pain protocol.
Aortic (Thoracic) Dissection	Sudden, sharp, and tearing; radiates to shoulders, neck, back, and abdomen	• Neurological complications: hemiplegia, sensory deficits secondary to carotid artery occlusion. • May present with a new murmur, bruits, or unequal blood pressure in upper extremities.
Pericarditis	Positional ache, dyspnea	• May also present with a pericardial friction rub or distended neck veins.
Pulmonary Embolus	Sudden onset, sharp or stabbing, varies with respiration	• May also present with dyspnea, tachypnea, fever, tachycardia, diaphoresis, or deep vein thrombosis (DVT).
Pneumothorax	Sudden onset, tearing, or pleuritic, worsened by breathing	• May also have dyspnea, tachycardia, decreased breath sounds, and a deviated trachea. Refer to Chapter 15 for further information.
Pneumonia	Stabbing that is exacerbated by coughing and deep breathing	• Presents with fever, chills, productive cough, tachypnea. Refer to Chapter 15 for further information.
Esophageal Rupture	Sudden onset upon swallowing or constant retrosternal, epigastric pain	• May mimic signs and symptoms of a pneumothorax. • Consider esophageal rupture when a client has experienced forceful vomiting, penetrating trauma, a severe epigastric blow, or a first or second rib fracture.
Miscellaneous: Musculoskeletal	Reproducible by chest wall palpation	• May be relieved by position changes.
Miscellaneous: Recreational Drug Use (cocaine, amphetamines, or stimulants)	Cardiac ischemia pain (as listed previously)	• May produce a direct, toxic effect on the myocardium.

Equipment

- Appropriate PPE
- Stethoscope
- Watch or smartphone that counts seconds

Examination of the Precordium

The cardiovascular physical examination has two major components:

1. Assessment of the **precordium** (the area on the anterior surface of the body overlying the heart, great vessels, pericardium, and some pulmonary tissue)
2. Assessment of the periphery (detailed in Chapter 17)

Assessment in Brief

Heart Examination

Assessment of the Precordium

- Inspection
  - Aortic area
  - Pulmonic area
  - Midprecordial area
  - Tricuspid area
  - Mitral area
- Palpation
  - Aortic area
  - Pulmonic area
  - Midprecordial area
  - Tricuspid area
  - Mitral area

Assessment of the Precordium (cont.)

- Auscultation
  - Aortic area
  - Pulmonic area
  - Midprecordial area
  - Tricuspid area
  - Mitral area
  - Mitral and tricuspid areas (S_3)
  - Mitral and tricuspid areas (S_4)
  - Murmurs
  - Pericardial friction rub
  - Prosthetic heart valves

Assistive Devices

- Artificial cardiac pacemakers
- Hemodynamic monitor
- Chest tubes
- ECG monitor

NURSING CHECKLIST

General Approach to Heart Examination

1. Observe standard precautions and don personal protective equipment (PPE) such as gloves, gown, face shield, goggles, N-95 respirator mask, or face mask if your client's status warrants these protective measures.
2. Explain to the client what you are going to do.
3. Ensure that the room is warm, quiet, and well-lit.
4. Expose the client's chest only as much as is needed for the examination.
5. Position the client in a supine or sitting position.
6. Stand to the client's right side. The light should come from the side opposite where you are standing so that shadows can be accentuated.

Inspection, palpation, and auscultation should be performed systematically, using cardiac landmarks. Percussion has limited usefulness in cardiac examination because x-rays and other diagnostic tests provide the same information in a much more accurate manner. The cardiac landmarks (Fig. 16-6) are defined as follows:

1. The aortic area is the second intercostal space (ICS) to the right of the sternum.
2. The pulmonic area is the second ICS to the left of the sternum.
3. The midprecordial area, Erb's point, is located in the third ICS to the left of the sternum.
4. The tricuspid area is the fifth ICS to the left of the sternum. Other terms for this area are the right ventricular area or the septal area.

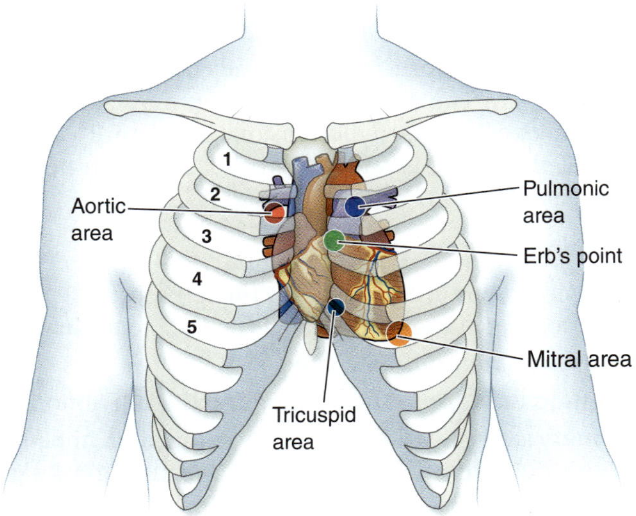

Figure 16-6 The cardiac landmarks. (The numbers between the ribs represent the intercostal spaces.)

5. The mitral area is the fifth ICS at the left midclavicular line. Other terms for this area are the left ventricular area or the apical area.

These cardiac landmarks are the locations where the heart sounds are heard best, not where the valves are actually located. The mitral area correlates anatomically with the apex of the heart; the aortic and pulmonic areas correlate anatomically with the base of the heart. Examination of the heart should proceed in an orderly fashion from the base of the heart to the apex, or from the apex of the heart to the base.

Risk Factors

Cardiac Disease

Fixed: Increasing age, sex (male), heredity (including race and family history).

Modifiable (client can modify, treat, or control by changing their lifestyle and/or taking medicine): Tobacco use, high blood cholesterol, high blood pressure, physical inactivity, obesity and overweight, and diabetes.

Other Factors That Contribute to Heart Disease: Stress, alcohol, diet/nutrition.

Clients can assess their risk of having a heart attack or dying from coronary heart disease in the next ten years by using the Heart Attack Risk Calculator found at *www.heart.org.*

Inspection

Once the chest is exposed, the examination begins with visually inspecting the chest. Skin color, evidence of scars indicating prior surgery or implanted device, symmetry, and movements such as heaves/lifts or pulsations are all observed. Heaves/lifts are discussed in the following section on palpation.

Aortic Area

E
1. Lightly place your index finger on the angle of Louis.
2. Move your finger laterally to the right of the sternum to the rib. This is the second rib.
3. Move your finger down beneath the second rib to the ICS. The aortic area is located in the second ICS to the right of the sternum.

N **No pulsations should be visible.**

A A pulsation in the aortic area is an abnormal finding.

P A pulsation in the aortic area may indicate the presence of an aortic root aneurysm. The aneurysm's dilation may become bigger when the client experiences hypertension. A rupture can occur at any time, but the risk is greater when the aneurysm becomes 5 cm or more in diameter.

Pulmonic Area

E
1. Lightly place your index finger on the left second ICS.
2. The pulmonic area is located at the second ICS to the left of the sternum.

N **No pulsations should be visible.**

A A pulsation or bulge in the pulmonic area is an abnormal finding.

P Pulmonary stenosis, which is usually congenital, impedes blood flow from the right ventricle into the lungs, causing a bulge. The right side of the heart then dilates and the right ventricle becomes hypertrophied to accommodate the load.

Midprecordial Area

E
1. Lightly place your index finger on the left second ICS.
2. Continue to move your finger down the left rib cage, counting the third rib and the third ICS.
3. The midprecordial area, or Erb's point, is located at the third ICS, left sternal border. Both aortic and pulmonic murmurs may be heard here.

N **No pulsations should be visible.**

A The presence of a pulsation or a systolic bulge in the midprecordial area is an abnormal finding.

P A left ventricular aneurysm can produce a midprecordial pulsation. Ventricular aneurysms can develop for several weeks following an acute MI. With an MI, the hydraulic stress on the infarcted area may cause the damaged ventricular wall to bulge and become extremely thin during systole.

A A retraction in the midprecordial area is an abnormal finding.

P Pericardial disease can produce retractions in this area (retractions occur when there is pulling in some of the tissues of the precordium, depending on the activities of the heart).

Tricuspid Area

E
1. Lightly place your index finger on the left third ICS.
2. Continue to move your finger down the left rib cage, counting the fourth rib, the fourth ICS, and the fifth rib followed by the fifth ICS.
3. The tricuspid area is located at the fifth ICS, left of the sternal border.

N **No pulsations should be visible.**

A A visible systolic pulsation in the tricuspid area is an abnormal finding.

P A visible systolic pulsation can result from right ventricular enlargement secondary to an increased stroke volume. Anxiety, hyperthyroidism, fever, and pregnancy are clinical situations that produce an increased stroke volume.

Mitral Area

E
1. Lightly place your index finger on the left fifth ICS.
2. Move your finger laterally to the midclavicular line. This is the mitral landmark. In a large-breasted client, have the client displace the left breast upward and to the left, so you can locate the mitral landmark.

N **Normally, there is no movement in the precordium except at the mitral area, where the left ventricle lies close enough to the skin's surface that it visibly pulsates during systole. The apical impulse at the mitral landmark is generally visible in about half of the adult population. This pulsation is also known as the point of maximal impulse (PMI) and occurs simultaneously with carotid pulsation.**

A **Hypokinetic** (decreased movement) pulsations at the mitral area are considered abnormal.

P Conditions that place more fluid between the left ventricle and the chest wall, such as pericardial effusion or cardiac tamponade, produce a hypokinetic or absent pulsation. In obese individuals, excess subcutaneous tissue dampens the apical impulse. Low-output states such as shock produce a less palpable apical impulse from the reduced

> **NURSING TIP**
> **PMI Versus Apical Impulse**
> The term *PMI* has fallen out of favor because it can be a misnomer if cardiac pathology causes a stronger impulse in a different region. Any movement other than the apical impulse is abnormal and should be described in terms of type, location, and timing in relation to the cardiac cycle.

blood volume and decreased myocardial contractility. Keep in mind that absent pulsations are normal in half of the adult population.

A **Hyperkinetic** (increased movement) pulsations are always abnormal when located at the mitral area.

P High-output states such as mitral regurgitation, thyrotoxicosis, severe anemia, and left-to-right heart shunts are potential causes of hyperkinetic pulsations.

Palpation

Inspection and palpation of the heart go hand in hand. Again, you must be systematic in this part of the examination and palpate the cardiac landmarks starting at either the base or the apex of the heart. During palpation, assess for the apical impulse, pulsations, **thrills** (vibrations that feel similar to what one feels when a hand is placed on a purring cat), and **heaves** (lifting of the cardiac area secondary to an increased workload and force of left ventricular contraction; also referred to as lift). The client should be in a supine position for this portion of the examination.

Palpate the cardiac landmarks for:

E
1. Pulsations: Using the finger pads, locate the cardiac landmark and palpate the area for pulsations (Fig. 16-7).
2. Thrills: Using the palmar surface of the hand at the base of the fingers (also known as the ball of the hand), locate the cardiac landmark and palpate the area for thrills (Fig. 16-8).
3. Heaves: Follow step 2 and palpate the area for heaves.

Aortic Area

E Palpate the aortic area for pulsations, thrills, and heaves.

N **No pulsations, thrills, or heaves should be palpated.**

A Palpation of a thrill in the aortic area is an abnormal finding.

P Aortic stenosis and aortic regurgitation create turbulent blood flow in the left ventricle, which may be palpated as a thrill.

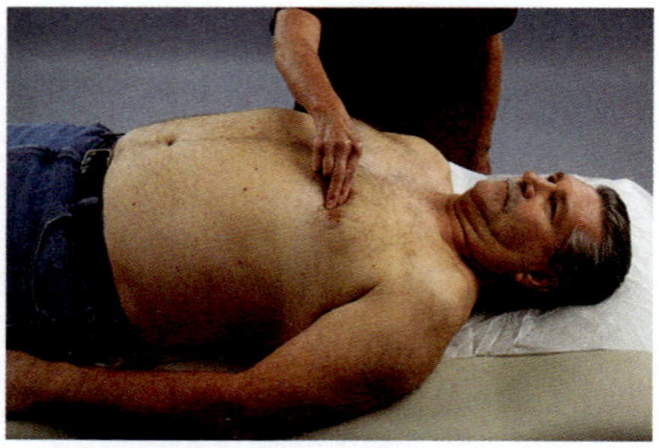

Figure 16-7 Palpating for pulsations.

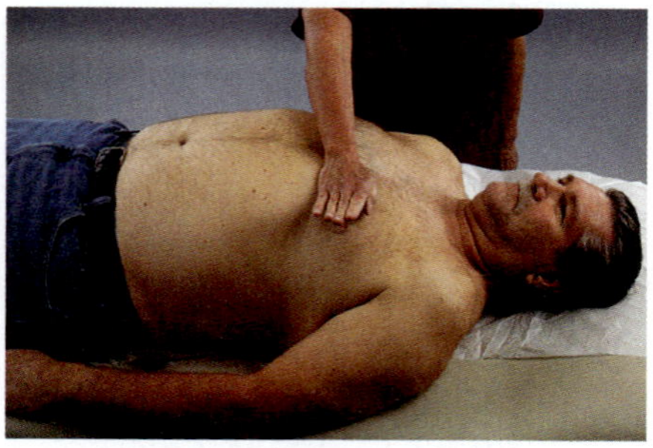

Figure 16-8 Palpating for thrills.

> **NURSING TIP**
> **Mechanical Circulatory Support Devices**
> Cardiogenic shock post-MI and cardiac surgery despite maximal medical therapy may be treated with a mechanical circulatory support device. These devices are used as a bridge to recovery or heart transplant based on whether the client's condition is reversible.
> - Intra-Aortic Balloon Pump: provides counterpulsation during diastole decreasing the oxygen demands of the heart and increasing coronary perfusion. Generally inserted in the femoral artery and advanced to sit in the thoracic aorta above the renal arteries and below the aortic knob.
> - TandemHeart Ventricular Assist Device: decreases the workload of the left ventricle by draining blood from the left atrium and infusing back into the systemic circulation via the femoral artery.
> - Impella®**:** a microaxial pump placed across the aortic valve that drains blood from the left ventricle and injects it into the aorta decreasing the work of the left ventricle.
> - Veno-Arterial Extracorporeal Membrane Oxygenator (V-A ECMO): cannulas are placed in the femoral or jugular vein and the femoral or axillary artery. Blood is aspirated by the venous catheter, directed through a membrane oxygenator outside the body, and returned to the arterial circulation via the arterial catheter bypassing the heart and lungs.

Pulmonic Area

E Palpate the pulmonic area for pulsations, thrills, and heaves.

N **No pulsations, thrills, or heaves should be palpated.**

A Palpation of a thrill in the pulmonic area is an abnormal finding.

P Pulmonic stenosis and pulmonic regurgitation create turbulent blood flow in the right ventricle, which may be palpated as a thrill.

Midprecordial Area

E Palpate the midprecordial area for pulsations, thrills, and heaves.

N **No pulsations, thrills, or heaves should be palpated.**

A Palpation of pulsations in the midprecordial area is an abnormal finding.

P Both a left ventricular aneurysm and an enlarged right ventricle can produce a pulsation in the midprecordial area.

Tricuspid Area

E Palpate the tricuspid area for pulsations, thrills, and heaves.

N **No pulsations, thrills, or heaves should be palpated.**

A Palpation of a thrill in the tricuspid area is an abnormal finding.

P Tricuspid stenosis and tricuspid regurgitation create turbulent blood flow in the right atrium, which may be palpated as a thrill.

A Palpation of a heave in the tricuspid area is an abnormal finding.

P Right ventricular enlargement may produce a heave in the tricuspid area secondary to an increased workload.

Mitral Area

E Palpate the mitral area for pulsations, thrills, and heaves. If a pulsation (apical impulse) is not palpable, turn the client to the left side and palpate in this position (Fig. 16-9). This position facilitates palpation because the heart shifts closer to the chest wall.

N **The apical impulse is palpable in approximately half of the adult population. It is felt as a light, localized tap that is 1 to 2 cm in diameter. The amplitude is small and it can be felt immediately after the first heart sound, lasting for about one-half of systole. This impulse may be exaggerated in young clients. A thrill is not found in the normal adult population. A heave is absent in the healthy adult.**

A A thrill palpated at the fifth ICS at the left midclavicular line is an abnormal finding.

P Mitral stenosis and mitral regurgitation may produce a thrill from the turbulent blood flow found in the left atrium.

A A visible heave, or sustained apex beat, displaced laterally to the left sixth ICS at the anterior axillary line is an abnormal finding. It is usually more than 3 cm in diameter and has a large amplitude.

P Left ventricular hypertrophy produces a laterally displaced apical impulse because of the increased size of the left ventricle in the thorax and the subsequent shifting of the heart. In addition, the hypertrophied muscle works harder during a contraction to produce a heave or sustained apex beat. This frequently occurs in conditions such as aortic stenosis, systemic hypertension, and idiopathic hypertrophic subaortic stenosis (which is a form of hypertrophic cardiomyopathy).

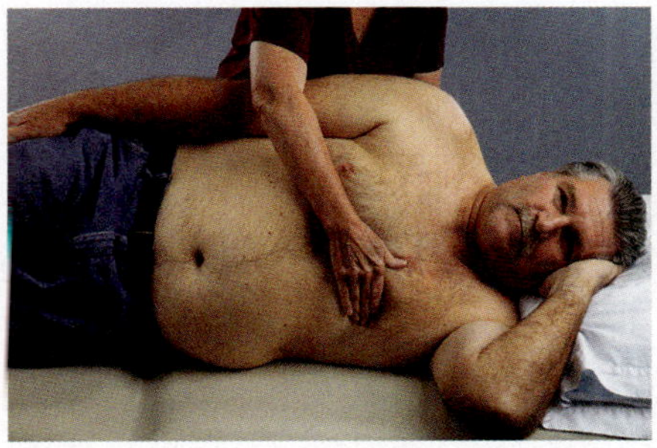

Figure 16-9 Palpating the apical impulse with the client on the left side.

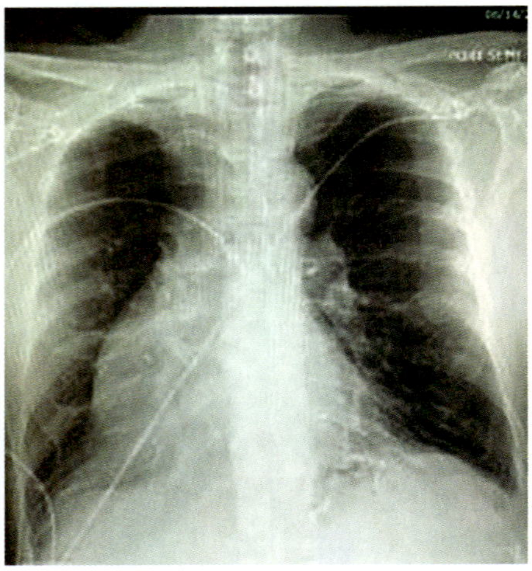

Figure 16-10 Dextrocardia.

A A hypokinetic pulsation, usually less than 1 to 2 cm in diameter and of small amplitude, is an abnormal finding.

P Conditions that place more fluid between the left ventricle and the chest wall, such as pericardial effusion or cardiac tamponade, produce a hypokinetic or absent pulsation. In obesity, the excess subcutaneous tissue dampens the apical impulse. Low-output states such as shock produce a less palpable apical impulse from the reduced blood volume and decreased myocardial contractility.

A A hyperkinetic pulsation, usually greater than 1 to 2 cm in diameter and of increased amplitude, is an abnormal finding.

P High-output states such as mitral regurgitation, thyrotoxicosis, severe anemia, and left-to-right heart shunts are potential causes of hyperkinetic pulsations.

NURSING TIP
Dextrocardia

Dextrocardia is the term for the rare condition where the heart is located on the right side of the chest with the axis positioned to the right (refer to Figure 16-10). *Situs solitis* is the term used when only the heart position is abnormal with the aorta and abdominal organs in normal position. *Situs inversus* describes the condition where all organs exist in mirror image of their normal position. ECG leads and defibrillator pads should be placed correctly to avoid errors or misinterpretation of data. Most of these clients have no symptoms and the condition is usually detected by imaging studies done for another reason. Educating clients about their condition is of the utmost importance so they can inform their providers of this condition.

NURSING CHECKLIST
General Approach to Heart Auscultation

1. Explain to the client what you are going to do.
2. Expose the client's chest only as much as is needed for the examination. Never auscultate through any type of clothing.
3. Position the client in a supine or sitting position. The left lateral position may be used for auscultation of the mitral and tricuspid areas. Also, the upright, leaning-forward position may be used for thorough auscultation of the aortic area (Fig. 16-11).
4. Stand to the client's right side.
5. Use the correct headpiece of the stethoscope. The diaphragm transmits high-frequency sounds, whereas the bell is used for low-pitched sounds. Keep in mind when using the bell that it should rest lightly on the skin. If too much pressure is applied, the bell will act like a diaphragm.
6. Warm the headpiece in your hands before touching it to the client.
7. Listen to all four of the valvular cardiac landmarks at least twice. During the first auscultation, identify S_1 and S_2, and then listen for a possible S_3 and S_4. During the second auscultation, listen for murmurs and friction rubs. As you gain expertise, you may be able to listen for S_1, S_2, S_3, S_4, murmurs, and friction rubs all at the same time.
8. Listen for at least a few cardiac cycles (10 to 15 seconds) in each area. It may be helpful to close your eyes when you auscultate heart sounds to facilitate increased auditory concentration.

NURSING TIP
Heart Auscultation Practice

In addition to practicing auscultation in the clinical setting, it is possible to refine auscultation skills on the Internet. Several of the websites listed online allow the listener to hear a variety of normal and pathological heart sounds.

Auscultation

Aortic Area

E Place the diaphragm of the stethoscope on the aortic landmark and listen for S_2.

N **S_2 is caused by the closure of the semilunar valves. S_2 corresponds to the "dub" sound in the phonetic "lub-dub" representation of heart sounds. S_2 heralds the onset of diastole. S_2 is louder than S_1 at this landmark (Fig. 16-12A).**

A The components of S_2 are A_2 (aortic) and P_2 (pulmonic). A greatly intensified or diminished A_2 is considered abnormal (Fig. 16-12B).

P Arterial hypertension, which increases the pressure in the aorta, may be suspected in the case of a greatly intensified A_2. Aortic stenosis, in which the aortic valve is calcified or thickened, may be the cause of a diminished A_2.

A An ejection **click** is an abnormal systolic sound that is high-pitched and can radiate in the chest wall. It is created by the opening of the damaged valve. An ejection click does not vary with the respiratory cycle. An ejection click follows S_1 (Fig. 16-12C).

P An ejection click can be auscultated in aortic stenosis, where the calcified valve produces this sound on opening.

Pulmonic Area

E Place the diaphragm of the stethoscope on the chest wall at the pulmonic landmark and listen for S_2.

N **S_2 is also heard in the pulmonic area. S_2 is louder than S_1 at this landmark, as depicted in Figure 16-12A. It is softer than the S_2 auscultated in the aortic area because the pressure on the left side of the heart is greater than that on the right. There is a normal physiological splitting of S_2 that is heard best in the pulmonic area. The components of a split S_2 are A_2 (aortic) and P_2 (pulmonic) (Fig. 16-12D). The aortic component occurs slightly before the pulmonic component during inspiration. The physiology of a split S_2 is that during inspiration, because of the more negative intrathoracic pressure, the venous return to the right side of the heart increases. Thus, pulmonic closure is delayed because of the extra time needed for the increased blood volume to pass through the valve. Normally, the A_2 component of the split S_2 is louder than the P_2 component because of the greater pressures in the left side of the heart.**

A When a split S_2 occurs that is abnormally wide, the aortic valve closes early and the pulmonic valve closes late. There is a split on both inspiration and expiration, but a wider split on inspiration, as shown in Figure 16-12E.

P Delayed closure of the pulmonic valve may be due to a delay in the electrical stimulation of the right ventricle, as seen with right bundle branch block.

A Fixed splitting, a wide splitting that does not change with inspiration or expiration, is abnormal (Fig. 16-12F). The pulmonic valve consistently closes later than the aortic valve. The right side of the heart is already ejecting a large volume, so filling cannot be increased during inspiration.

P Right ventricular failure that results in a prolonged right ventricular systole or a large atrial septal defect can lead to fixed splitting.

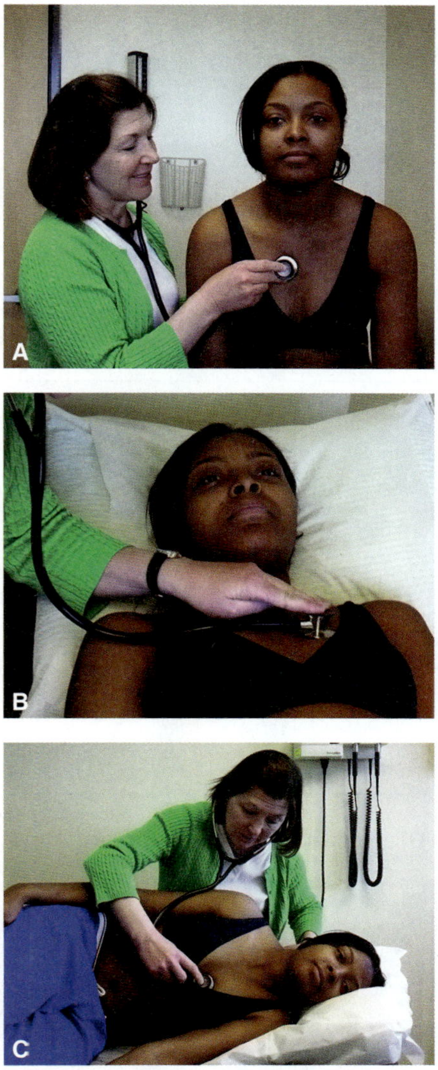

Figure 16-11 Auscultating the heart. **A.** At the aortic landmark in a client who is in a sitting position. **B.** At the pulmonic landmark in a client who is in a supine position. **C.** At the tricuspid landmark in a client who is in a left lateral position.

A In paradoxical splitting, the aortic valve closes after the pulmonic valve because of the delay in left ventricular systole. This occurs during expiration and disappears with inspiration. It is considered abnormal (Fig. 16-12G).

P Left bundle branch block, aortic stenosis, patent ductus arteriosus, severe hypertension, and left ventricular failure are conditions in which paradoxical splitting may be auscultated.

A A pulmonic ejection click always indicates an abnormality (Fig. 16-12H).

P A pulmonic ejection click is caused by the opening of a diseased pulmonic valve. It is heard loudest on expiration and is quieter on inspiration. It occurs early in systole and it does not radiate.

A A P_2 that is louder than or equal in volume to A_2 is abnormal, as is a greatly diminished P_2 (Fig. 16-12I).

P A loud P_2 is expected in pulmonary hypertension, where the pressures in the pulmonary artery are abnormally high. A diminished P_2 can occur in pulmonic stenosis, when the pulmonic valve is calcified or thickened.

Midprecordial Area

Erb's point is where both aortic and pulmonic murmurs may be auscultated. Refer to the discussion on murmurs later in this chapter for additional information.

Tricuspid Area

E Place the diaphragm of the stethoscope on the chest wall at the tricuspid landmark to listen for S_1.

N **S_1 in the tricuspid area is softer than the S_1 auscultated in the mitral area because the pressure in the left side of the heart is greater than that in the right. S_1 is louder than S_2 at this landmark (Fig. 16-12J). There is a normal physiological splitting of S_1 that is best heard in the tricuspid area (Fig. 16-12K). This split occurs because the mitral valve closes slightly before the tricuspid valve due to greater pressures in the left side of the heart. The components of a split S_1 are M_1 (mitral) and T_1 (tricuspid). Physiological splitting disappears when the client holds their breath.**

A A split S_1 with an abnormally wide split is pathological (Fig. 16-12L). The split is wider than usual during inspiration and is still heard on expiration.

P A split S_1 is usually due to electrical malfunctions such as right bundle branch block or mechanical problems such as mitral stenosis. In mitral

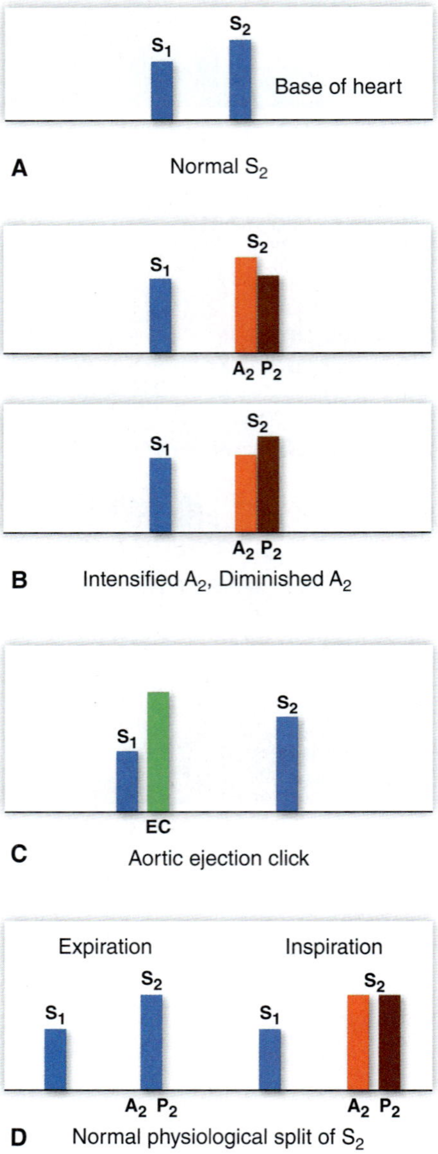

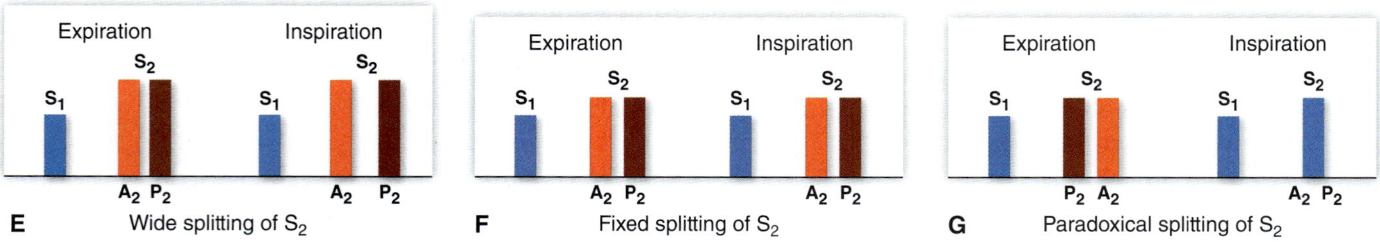

Figure 16-12 Summation of heart sounds. **A.** Normal S_2. **B.** Intensified A_2, diminished A_2. **C.** Aortic ejection click. **D.** Normal physiological split of S_2. **E.** Wide splitting of S_2. **F.** Fixed splitting of S_2. **G.** Paradoxical splitting of S_2.

stenosis, the tricuspid valve can close before the mitral valve closes because of calcification of the diseased mitral valve.

Mitral Area

E 1. Place the diaphragm of the stethoscope over the mitral area to identify S_1.
2. If you are unable to distinguish S_1 from S_2, palpate the carotid artery with the hand closest to the head while auscultating the mitral landmark. You will hear S_1 with each carotid pulse beat.

N **S_1 is heard the loudest in the mitral area. S_1 is caused by the closure of the mitral and tricuspid valves. S_1 corresponds to the "lub" sound in the phonetic "lub-dub" representation of heart sounds. S_1 is louder than S_2 at this landmark (Fig. 16-12J). S_1 also heralds the onset of systole. At normal or slow heart rates, systole (the time occurring between S_1 and S_2) is usually shorter than diastole. Diastole constitutes two-thirds of the cardiac cycle, with systole being the other third. The intensity of S_1 depends on:**

1. The adequacy of the A-V cusps in halting the ventricular blood flow

2. The mobility of the cusps

3. The position of the cusps and the rate of ventricular contraction

A An abnormally loud S_1 occurs when the mitral valve is wide open when systolic contraction begins, then slams shut (Fig. 16-12M).

P A loud S_1 occurs in mitral stenosis, short PR interval syndrome (0.11 to 0.13 seconds), or in high-output states such as tachycardia, hyperthyroidism, and exercise.

A A soft S_1 is abnormal (Fig. 16-12N).

P A soft S_1 can indicate mitral incompetence or regurgitation. This can be due to rheumatic fever, where the mitral valve has only limited motion.

A A variable abnormal S_1 occurs when diastolic filling time varies. Both a soft and a loud S_1 can be auscultated (Fig. 16-12O).

P A variable S_1 can occur with complete heart block, where the atria and the ventricles are beating independently, and in atrial fibrillation, where the ventricles are beating irregularly.

A An opening **snap** is an early diastolic sound that is high-pitched. It is abnormal (Fig. 16-12P).

P An opening snap is caused by the opening of a diseased valve and can be auscultated in mitral stenosis. The sound does not vary with respirations and can radiate throughout the chest. It follows S_2 and can be differentiated from an S_3 because it occurs earlier than an S_3.

A In tachycardia, the heart rate increases, diastole shortens, and systole and diastole become increasingly difficult to distinguish. Tachycardia is abnormal.

P Tachycardia can occur during exercise, fever, anxiety, pregnancy, and conditions that lead to hypertrophy, such as heart failure.

A A holosystolic (pansystolic murmur) that begins after S1 going into an S2 is abnormal.

P A holosystolic murmur is created with the incompetence or regurgitation of the mitral valve, which causes flow from the left ventricle into the left atria during systole. Acute mitral regurgitation (MR) is

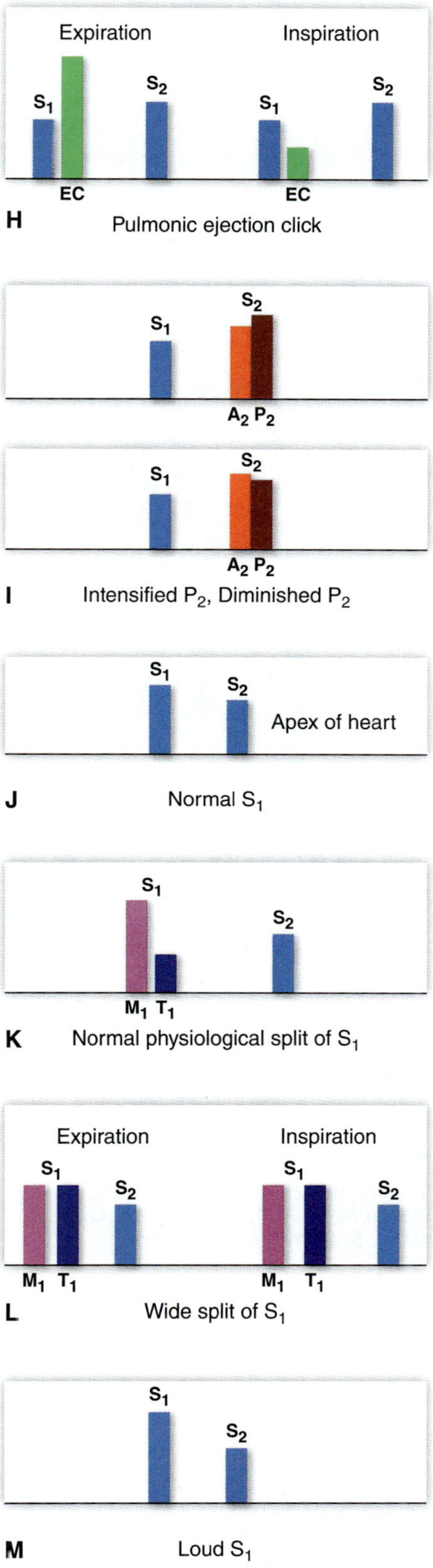

Figure 16-12—cont'd H. Pulmonic ejection click. **I.** Intensified P_2, diminished P_2. **J.** Normal S_1. **K.** Normal physiological split of S_1. **L.** Wide split of S_1. **M.** Loud S_1.

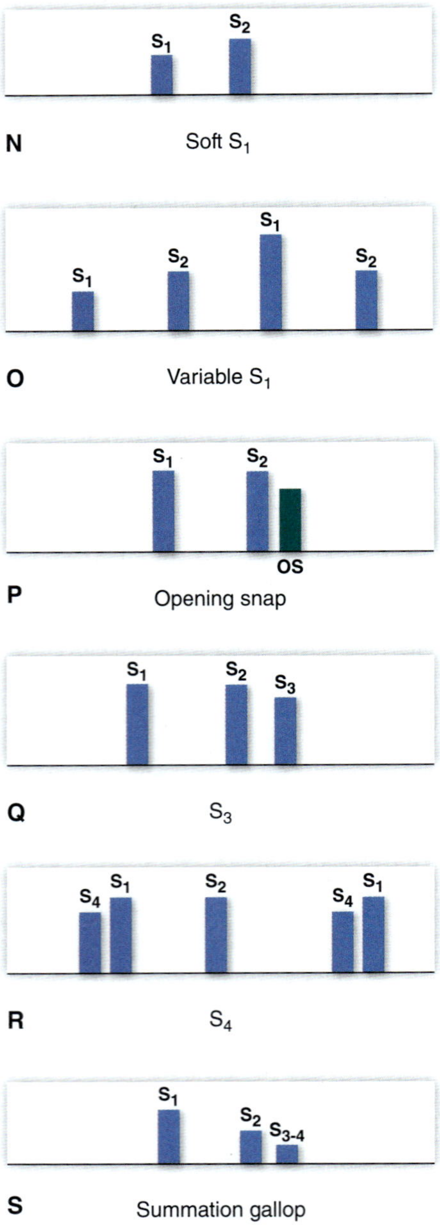

Figure 16-12—cont'd N. Soft S_1. **O.** Variable S_1. **P.** Opening snap. **Q.** S_3. **R.** S_4. **S.** Summation gallop.

caused by infective endocarditis, rheumatic fever, papillary muscle rupture, or ventricular ischemia during MI.

Mitral and Tricuspid Areas (S_3)

Auscultation of the mitral and tricuspid areas is repeated for low-pitched sounds, specifically an S_3 (otherwise known as a ventricular diastolic **gallop**, or extra heart sound). An S_3 is an early diastolic filling sound that originates in the ventricles and is therefore heard best at the apex of the heart. A right-sided S_3 (tricuspid area) is heard louder during inspiration because the venous return to the right side of the heart increases with more negative intrathoracic pressure. An S_3 sound occurs just after an S_2 (Fig. 16-12Q).

E
1. Place the bell of the stethoscope lightly over the mitral landmark. When the S_3 originates in the left ventricle, it is heard best with the client in a left lateral decubitus position and exhaling.
2. When originating in the right ventricle, an S_3 can best be heard by placing the bell of the stethoscope lightly over the third or fourth ICS at the left sternal border.
3. Auscultate for 10–15 seconds for a left- or right-sided S_3.

N **An S_3 heart sound can be a normal physiological sound in children and young adults. After the age of 30, a physiological S_3 is very infrequent. An S_3 can also be normal in high-output states such as the third trimester of pregnancy.**

A In an adult, an S_3 heart sound may be one of the earliest clinical findings of cardiac dysfunction. A loud, persistent S_3 can be an ominous sign. The average life expectancy after a persistent S_3 sound is detected is approximately 4 to 5 years.

P An S_3 is caused by rapid ventricular filling. An S_3 sound may occur with ventricular dysfunction, excessively rapid early diastolic ventricular filling, and restrictive myocardial or pericardial disease. It often indicates congestive heart failure and fluid overload.

Mitral and Tricuspid Areas (S_4)

An S_4 heart sound, or atrial diastolic gallop, is a late diastolic filling sound associated with atrial contraction. An S_4 can be either left- or right-sided and is therefore heard best in the mitral or tricuspid areas. An S_4 is a late diastolic filling sound that occurs just before S_1 (Fig. 16-12R).

Sometimes, the S_3 and the S_4 heart sounds can occur simultaneously in middiastole, thus creating one loud diastolic filling sound. This is known as a summation gallop (Fig. 16-12S).

E
1. Place the bell of the stethoscope lightly over the mitral area.
2. Place the bell of the stethoscope lightly over the tricuspid area.
3. Auscultate for 10 to 15 seconds for a left- or right-sided S_4 in each location.

N **An S_4 heart sound may occur with or without any evidence of cardiac decompensation. A left-sided S_4 is usually louder on expiration. A right-sided S_4 is usually louder on inspiration.**

A The presence of an S_4 can indicate cardiac decompensation.

P An S_4 heart sound can be auscultated in conditions that increase the resistance to filling because of a poorly compliant ventricle (e.g., MI, CAD, CHF, and cardiomyopathy) or in conditions that result in systolic overload (e.g., HTN, aortic stenosis, and hyperthyroidism).

NURSING TIP
S_3 Heart Sound

Phonetically, an S_3 heart sound is thought to resemble the pronunciation of the word *Kentucky:*

S_1	S_2	S_3
Ken	túc	ky

Murmurs

Murmurs are distinguished from heart sounds by their longer duration. Murmurs may be classified as innocent (which are always systolic and are not associated with any other abnormalities), functional (which are associated with high-output states), or pathological (which are related to structural abnormalities). Murmurs are produced by turbulent blood flow in the following situations:

1. Flow across a partial obstruction
2. Increased flow through normal structures
3. Flow into a dilated chamber
4. Backward or regurgitant flow across incompetent valves
5. Shunting of blood out of a high-pressure chamber or artery through an abnormal passageway

When assessing for a murmur, analyze the murmur according to the following seven characteristics:

1. Location: area where the murmur is heard the loudest (e.g., mitral, pulmonic, etc.).
2. Radiation: transmission of sounds from the specific valves to other adjacent anatomic areas. For example, mitral murmurs can often radiate to the axilla.
3. Timing: phase of the cardiac cycle in which the murmur is heard. Murmurs can be either systolic or diastolic. If the murmur occurs simultaneously with the pulse, it is a systolic murmur. If it does not, it is a diastolic murmur. Murmurs can further be characterized as **pansystolic** or **holosystolic**, meaning that the murmur is heard throughout all of systole. Murmurs can also be characterized as early, mid-, or late systolic or diastolic murmurs.
4. Intensity: Table 16-4 describes the six grades of loudness or intensity. The murmur is recorded with the grade over the Roman numeral "VI" to show the scale being used (e.g., III/VI).
5. Quality: harsh, rumbling, blowing, or musical.
6. Pitch: high, medium, or low. Low-pitched murmurs should be auscultated with the bell of the stethoscope; high-pitched murmurs should be auscultated with the diaphragm of the stethoscope.
7. Configuration: pattern that the murmur makes over time (Fig. 16-13). The configuration of a murmur can be described as **crescendo** (soft to loud), **decrescendo** (loud to soft), crescendo-decrescendo (soft to loud to soft), or plateau (sound is sustained).

E

1. The client should be in the same position for murmur auscultation as for the first auscultation (i.e., supine or sitting).
2. Auscultate each of the following cardiac landmarks for 10 to 15 seconds:
   a. Aortic and pulmonic areas, with the diaphragm of the stethoscope
   b. Mitral and tricuspid areas, with the diaphragm of the stethoscope
   c. Mitral and tricuspid areas, with the bell of the stethoscope
3. Label the murmur using the characteristics of location, radiation, timing, intensity, quality, pitch, and configuration. See Table 16-4 for information on grading heart murmurs.
4. You may also have the client sit up, lean forward, completely exhale, and hold their breath while you listen at the right and left second and third ICSs for aortic murmurs (especially aortic regurgitation).

N **No murmur should be heard; however, a physiological or functional murmur in children and adolescents may be innocent.**

> **NURSING TIP**
>
> **S_4 Heart Sound**
>
> Phonetically, an S_4 heart sound is thought to resemble the pronunciation of the word *Tennessee:*
>
> | S_4 | S_1 | S_2 |
> |---|---|---|
> | Ten | nes | sée |

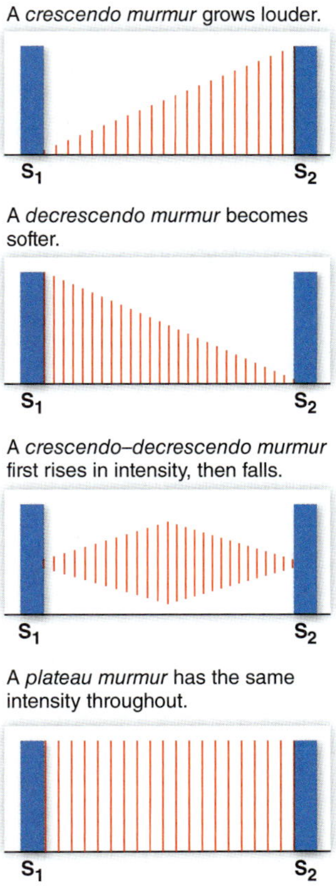

Figure 16-13 Characteristic patterns of murmurs.

Table 16-4 Grading Heart Murmurs

Grade	Characteristics
I	Very faint; heard only after a period of concentration
II	Faint; heard immediately
III	Moderate intensity
IV	Loud; may be associated with a thrill
V	Loud; stethoscope must remain in contact with the chest wall to hear; thrill palpable
VI	Very loud; heard with stethoscope off chest wall; thrill palpable

NURSING TIP

Pericardial Friction Rub Versus Pleural Friction Rub

- A pericardial friction rub produces a *high*-pitched, multiphasic, and scratchy (may be leathery or grating) sound that *does not* change with respiration. It is a sign of pericardial inflammation.
- A pleural friction rub produces a *low*-pitched, coarse, and grating sound that *does* change with respiration. When the client holds their breath, the sound disappears. The client may also complain of pain upon breathing. It is a sign of visceral and parietal pleurae inflammation.

These murmurs are usually systolic, short, grade I or II, vibratory, heard at the left sternal border, and nonradiating. No cardiac symptoms accompany the murmur.

A Abnormal murmurs of stenosis can be found in each of the four valvular cardiac landmarks.

P Stenosis occurs when a valve that should be open remains partially closed. It produces an increased **afterload** or pressure overload. Stenosis may develop from rheumatic fever, congenital defects of the valves, or calcification associated with the aging process.

A Abnormal murmurs of regurgitation or insufficiency can be auscultated in each of the four valvular cardiac landmarks.

P Regurgitation or insufficiency occurs when a valve that should be closed remains partially open. An insufficient valve causes volume overload, or increased **preload**. Regurgitation frequently results from the effects of rheumatic fever and congenital defects of the valves.

Pericardial Friction Rub

E
1. Position the client in a supine position, in the knee-chest position, or leaning forward.
2. Auscultate from the sternum (third to fifth ICS) to the apex (mitral area) with the diaphragm of the stethoscope for 10 to 15 seconds.
3. Characterize any sound according to its location, radiation, timing, quality, and pitch.

N **No pericardial friction rub should be auscultated.**

A A pericardial friction rub is always an abnormal finding. It is heard best during held inspiration or expiration. It does not change with the respiratory cycle. Table 16-5 gives additional information on pericardial friction rubs.

P Pericardial friction rubs are caused by the rubbing together of the inflamed visceral and parietal layers of the pericardium. They may be present in conditions such as **pericarditis** (inflammation of the pericardium) and renal failure.

Prosthetic Heart Valves

E N **Prosthetic heart valves can be located in any of the four heart valves, although mitral and aortic valve replacements are the most common. Refer to the aortic and mitral valve auscultation discussions.**

A Prosthetic heart valves produce abnormal heart sounds. Furthermore, mechanical prosthetic valve sounds can sometimes be heard without the use of a stethoscope.

P Mechanical prosthetic valves (e.g., caged-ball, tilting disk, and bileaflet valves) produce "clicky" opening and closing sounds. Homograft (human tissue) and heterograft (animal tissue) valves produce sounds that are like those of human valves; however, they usually produce a murmur.

Table 16-5 Murmurs and Pericardial Friction Rub

Heart Sound	Location/Radiation	Quality/Pitch	Configuration
Systolic Murmurs			
Aortic stenosis	Second right ICS; may radiate to neck or left sternal border	Harsh/medium	Crescendo/decrescendo
Pulmonic stenosis	Second or third left ICS; radiates toward shoulder and neck	Harsh/medium	Crescendo/decrescendo
Mitral regurgitation	Apex; fifth ICS, left midclavicular line; may radiate to left axilla and back	Blowing/high	Holosystolic/plateau
Tricuspid regurgitation	Lower left sternal border; may radiate to right sternum	Blowing/high	Holosystolic/plateau
Diastolic Murmurs			
Aortic regurgitation	Second right ICS and Erb's point; may radiate to left or right sternal border	Blowing/high	Decrescendo
Pulmonic regurgitation	Second left ICS; may radiate to left lower sternal border	Blowing/high	Decrescendo
Mitral stenosis	Apex; fifth ICS, left midclavicular line; may get louder with client on left side; does not radiate	Rumbling/low	Crescendo/decrescendo
Tricuspid stenosis	Fourth ICS, at sternal border	Rumbling/low	Crescendo/decrescendo
Pericardial Friction Rub	Third to fifth ICS, left of sternum; does not radiate	Leathery, scratchy, grating/high	Three components: 1. Ventricular systole 2. Ventricular diastole 3. Atrial systole

NURSING CHECKLIST

Assessing Clients With Cardiac Assistive Devices

The client with cardiac disease may need the assistance of special equipment to maintain optimal health. The presence of cardiac assistive devices must be noted during the inspection process. Consider the following to assist you in observing these devices:

1. Artificial cardiac pacemakers (e.g., temporary external chest pacing, temporary internal pacing, permanent pacemaker); implantable cardiac defibrillator (ICD)
   a. The pacemaker is on. Check the settings.
   b. The ICD is on. Check the settings. This information should be in the client's chart or EHR. The device manufacturer representative may have to be called to interrogate an internal device if there are any problems. Check your facility's policy for verifying and controlling the settings.

c. Observe the client's telemetry waveform to verify the device is functioning at the proper settings.
d. Check for external pacer wires. Wires should be protected from electrical hazards per your facility's policy.
e. The insertion site is free of infection.
f. The appropriate dressing is intact and in place.

2. Hemodynamic monitoring: Right atrial pressure (RAP) line; left atrial pressure (LAP) line; pulmonary artery (PA) catheter (Swan-Ganz)
   a. Check the goal of the line (e.g., fluid, monitoring).
   b. The monitor's alarms are on. The appropriate limits are set.
   c. The transducer level is at the client's right atrium (phlebostatic axis—fourth ICS, midaxillary line).
   d. The pressure bag(s) is pumped to 300 mm Hg.
   e. Change the flush bag(s) per your facility's policy.
   f. The line is safely secured to the client or the bed (it is not just dangling).
   g. The insertion site is free of infection.
3. Chest tubes
   a. Identify the location of the chest tube(s).
   b. Determine whether the chest tube is used to evacuate air or fluid.
   c. Ascertain if drainage system is wet suction or dry suction. In dry suction, there is water only in the water seal chamber and you cannot hear bubbling unless there is an air leak.
   d. Determine whether the chest tube is on wall suction or water seal.
   e. Confirm the amount of suction ordered and check the control dial (dry) or the water level (wet) to ensure the suction level is correct.
   f. The chest tube connections are secured.
   g. The chest tube is kink-free.
   h. The insertion site and surrounding chest are free from subcutaneous emphysema.
   i. The insertion site is free of infection.
4. ECG monitoring
   a. The client's skin is intact where the ECG pads are located.
   b. The ECG pads are placed on the correct anatomic locations.
   c. The monitor's alarms are on. The appropriate limits are set.

U.S. Preventive Services Task Force (USPSTF)

Grade B Recommendations:

- The USPSTF recommends offering or referring adults with cardiovascular disease risk factors to behavioral counseling interventions to promote a healthy diet and physical activity.
- The USPSTF recommends that clinicians prescribe a statin for the primary prevention of CVD for adults aged 40 to 75 years who have 1 or more CVD risk factors (i.e., dyslipidemia, diabetes, hypertension, or smoking) and an estimated 10-year risk of a cardiovascular event of 10% or greater.

Retrieved November 8, 2025, from *https://uspreventiveservicestaskforce.org/uspstf/recommendation-topics/uspstf-a-and-b-recommendations*

CASE STUDY

The Client With Cardiac Tamponade

This case study illustrates the application and objective documentation of the cardiac examination. Marques Jackson is a 44-year-old Black man who lives in a suburban area with his husband of 4 years. Marques was in his usual state of health until the spring when he contracted COVID-19. After recovery, Marques had persistent shortness of breath with activity and was found to have severe aortic stenosis on an echocardiogram. Marques underwent an elective mechanical aortic valve replacement (AVR) 3 weeks ago and was recovering well at home until 2 to 3 days ago. At that time Marques began experiencing sharp anterior chest pain and shortness of breath. Marques now presents to the emergency department with husband, Todd.

HEALTH HISTORY

CLIENT PROFILE

44-year-old Black man

CHIEF COMPLAINT

"Increasing chest pain and shortness of breath"

PRESENT HEALTH

Client is status post mechanical AVR 3 weeks ago for aortic stenosis secondary to a bicuspid aortic valve. Hospital course was significant for atrial fibrillation, which converted after 6 hours with IV amiodarone. Client was discharged on warfarin, amiodarone, oxycodone, and acetaminophen for pain. Was recovering well and stopped taking pain medication last week. Two days ago started feeling progressively shorter of breath and started having aching pain over his heart. Client noticed a racing heart and feeling dizzy when standing. Denies fever, chills, weight change, swelling in extremities, cough, muscle aches, or anxiety. This feels markedly different than incisional pain and has not been relieved with acetaminophen.

PAST HEALTH HISTORY

Medical History Heart murmur due to bicuspid aortic valve, diagnosed after having COVID-19
Hypertension for 12 years
Gastroesophageal reflux disease for 8 years

Surgical History AVR with mechanical valve 3 wks ago

Allergies No medications, latex, insects, foods, or environmental allergies

Medications Warfarin 5 mg orally daily
Amlodipine 5 mg orally daily
Amiodarone 200 mg orally daily
Acetaminophen 1,000 mg orally every 8 hours as needed for pain.
Pantoprazole 20 mg orally every morning

Communicable Diseases COVID-19 this year completed 5-day course of molnupiravir; was treated in college for a STI, not sure which

Injuries and Accidents None

Differing Abilities Admits to bilateral hearing loss (has history of playing loud music)

Blood Transfusions None

Childhood Illnesses None that he can recall

Immunizations Up to date as child; annual flu shot, tetanus booster before surgery
COVID-19 vaccine mRNA—2 initial vaccines and 1 booster; no HPV vaccine

FAMILY HEALTH HISTORY

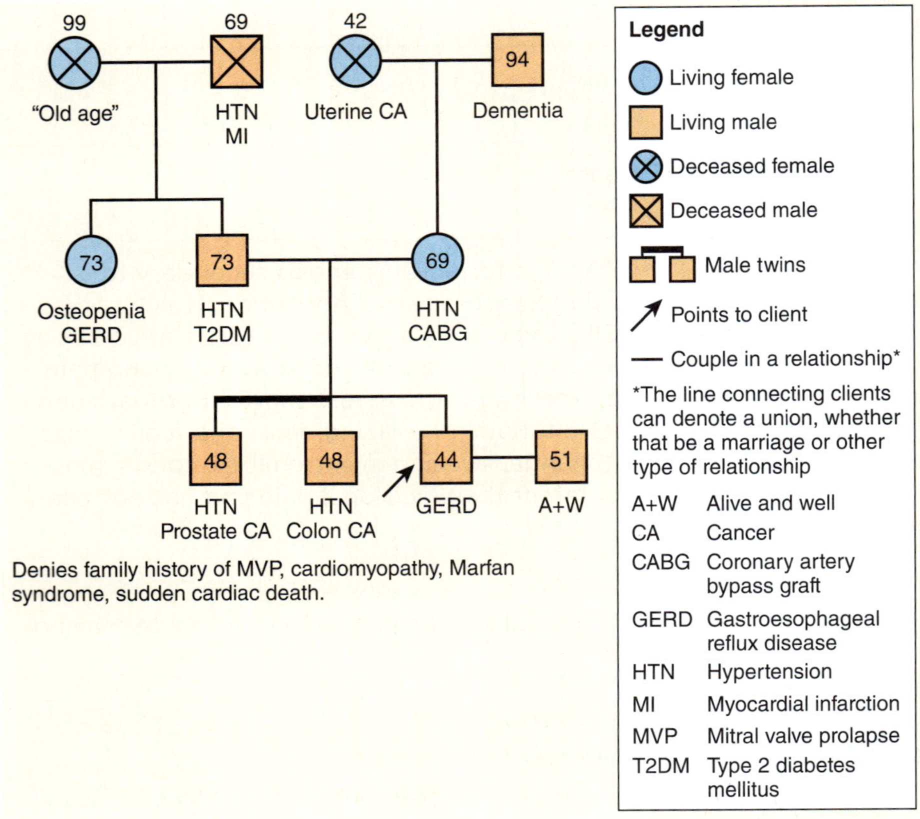

SOCIAL HISTORY

Alcohol Use 1-2 beers 3×/week, none since surgery

Tobacco Use Smoked in college, 4-year pack history, none since then

Recreational Drug Use Smoked marijuana in college, none since

Domestic and Intimate Partner Violence Denies

Sexual Practice Sexually active, monogamous with husband for 4 years; 5 lifetime partners

Travel History Has traveled only within the United States, no travel in last month

Work Environment Works in Information Technology for the city but has not returned to work since surgery

Home Environment Lives on the 18th floor of a high-rise condominium that was built in 2001. Has smoke and carbon monoxide detectors. No exposure to open fires, smoking, or chemicals. Lives with husband.

Hobbies and Leisure Activities Generally active, runs and hikes on the weekends. Home is located close to running/biking paths. Hikes are within a 1-hour drive. Likes to visit brew pub after hikes.

Stress Job has been stressful but he enjoys it. Gets along with work colleagues. He is due to return to work in 3 weeks.

Education Masters in Information Technology

Economic Status Relatively comfortable but worries about the economy. Health benefits are provided through his job.

Military Service None

Religion Does not practice any religion

Ethnic Background African American

Roles and Relationships Married to husband for 4 years

Husband works as a lawyer for the Department of Justice. Sees parents and brothers infrequently as they live 1,500 miles away.

Characteristic Patterns of Daily Living Has been getting up early and walking after breakfast. Normally would be at work from 7 a.m. to 4 p.m. but has spent his days reading and napping since surgery. Walks a second time before dinner. Has not been able to walk in past 2 days.

HEALTH MAINTENANCE ACTIVITIES

Sleep Was sleeping well, 7 to 8 hours nightly but pain kept him up last night, had to sit upright to breathe.

Diet Poor appetite. Usually eats "healthy."

Exercise Walking twice a day until 2 days ago.

Stress Management "I was not stressed until my pain started."

Use of Safety Devices Wears seat belt.

Health Checkups Followed up with Cardiac Surgery Nurse Practitioner last week and was told that his postoperative course was "right on target." "Everything looked good."

RISK FACTORS

Fixed Male
Heredity (paternal grandfather had a fatal MI at age 69)

Major Modifiable Hypertension

CLIENT CLASSIFICATION

NYHA I (until today)

PHYSICAL EXAMINATION

Examination of the Precordium

Inspection
Aortic area: No visible pulsation
Pulmonic area: No visible pulsation
Midprecordial area: No visible pulsation
Tricuspid area: No visible pulsation
Mitral area: No visible pulsation

Palpation
Aortic area: Thrill present; no pulsation or heave
Pulmonic area: No pulsation, thrill, or heave
Midprecordial area: No pulsation, thrill, or heave
Tricuspid area: No pulsation, thrill, or heave
Mitral area: No pulsation, thrill, or heave

Auscultation
Aortic area: Muffled S_2, I/VI systolic murmur; valve click present
Pulmonic area: Muffled S_2
Midprecordial area: Muffled S_1, no S_3 or S_4
Tricuspid area: Muffled S_1, no S_3 or S_4
Mitral area: Muffled S_1, no S_3 or S_4

Additional Significant Findings Vital signs: Blood pressure: 94/52 mm Hg, right arm, sitting; pulsus paradox auscultated with manual BP check
Pulse rate: 110/min and regular
Respirations: 24 breaths per minute
Oxygen saturation on room air: 92%
Temperature: 98.0°F
Additional findings: Jugular venous distention present in supine and semi-Fowler positions, cool extremities, weak pulses

DIAGNOSTIC DATA

Chest X-ray Enlarged cardiac silhouette

ECG Sinus tachycardia. Pulsus alternans in all leads.

Echocardiogram Pericardial effusion, diastolic right ventricular collapse, systolic right atrial collapse. Engorged inferior vena cava with minimal respiratory variation.

CLINICAL JUDGMENT IN ACTION

1. What cues indicate that the client is having cardiac distress?
2. What interventions have the highest priority?
3. What assessment findings indicate clinical improvement or decline in this client?

Review Questions

1. The heart receives oxygen via constant blood flow through the coronary arteries. What is the condition that results when coronary blood flow does not meet the needs of the heart such as during physical activity or stress?
   a. Ischemia
   b. Stenosis
   c. Pericarditis
   d. Arrhythmia

2. A client is admitted to the cardiac care unit with an acute inferior myocardial infarction and a new first-degree heart block. Which of the following coronary arteries is the most likely occluded vessel?
   a. Left anterior descending coronary artery (LAD)
   b. Left main coronary artery (LM)
   c. Right coronary artery (RCA)
   d. Left circumflex coronary artery (LCX)

3. Nurses can advise clients to mitigate their cardiac risk through lifestyle modification. Which of the following risk factors are clients unable to modify? Select all that apply.
   a. Smoking
   b. Family history
   c. Obesity
   d. Race
   e. Age
   f. Stress

4. A 68-year-old client is discharged after having a successful coronary artery bypass graft surgery. The client has a 48-pack-year history of cigarette smoking and expresses a desire to quit. The client asks the nurse about the effects smoking has on the body. The nurse informs the client that nicotine can lead to which of the following cardiac conditions? Select all that apply.
   a. Tachycardia
   b. Hypertension
   c. Cardiomyopathy
   d. Peripheral vasoconstriction
   e. Congestive heart failure

5. A 70-year-old male presents with 10/10 chest pain described as sharp, tearing, and radiating to the back. A physical examination reveals significantly lower blood pressure in the left arm than in the right arm. You immediately recognize that this may be which cardiac emergency?
   a. Acute coronary syndrome
   b. Acute aortic dissection
   c. Cardiac tamponade
   d. Pneumonia

6. A client is admitted with severe aortic stenosis for a transcatheter aortic valve replacement. What are the expected physical examination findings for this client?
   a. A loud systolic murmur in the second intercostal space to the right of the sternum that radiates to the neck
   b. A rumbling nonradiating diastolic murmur in the left midclavicular line
   c. A grating, nonradiating rub in the third to fifth intercostal space
   d. A very loud S_3 heard in the 3rd intercostal space to the left of the sternum

7. The nurse palpates the apical impulse and detects a hyperkinetic pulsation in the mitral area. Which conditions are associated with hyperkinetic pulsation? Select all that apply.
   a. Mitral regurgitation
   b. Thyrotoxicosis
   c. Severe anemia
   d. Left-to-right heart shunt
   e. Pericarditis

8. A client with a history of injecting heroin is admitted with a heart rate of 108, and an oral temperature of 100.2°F (37.9°C). Splinter hemorrhages of the nails are noted as well as scattered petechiae on the feet. What cardiac condition do you suspect this client is experiencing?
   a. Myocarditis
   b. Cardiogenic shock
   c. Ventricular aneurysm
   d. Infective endocarditis

9. A 34-year-old client wants to exercise to lose weight. Using the target heart rate calculation, what is the heart rate goal?
   a. 80 to 104 bpm
   b. 93 to 121 bpm
   c. 100 to 140 bpm
   d. 186 bpm

10. The nurse auscultates the client's chest and detects an S_4 heart sound. The nurse recalls that the sound produced by S_4 is thought to resemble the pronunciation of which of the following words?
   a. Kentucky
   b. New Jersey
   c. Tennessee
   d. Virginia

CHAPTER 17

Peripheral Vasculature System and Lymphatic System

Learning Outcomes

1. Identify the anatomy and physiology of the peripheral vasculature system and lymphatic system.
2. Conduct a complete health history on a client with a peripheral vascular system and lymphatic system condition.
3. Perform a physical examination on a healthy adult and an adult with peripheral vasculature system and lymphatic system pathology.
4. Differentiate between normal clinical findings from a client's physical examination and the pathophysiology of abnormal clinical findings.
5. Identify risk factors for peripheral artery disease.
6. Identify risk factors for chronic arterial insufficiency.
7. Assess if a client's peripheral vascular system's or lymphatic system's assistive devices are adversely affecting a client's health.
8. Identify risk factors for varicose veins.
9. Identify risk factors for lymphoma.
10. Identify the United States Preventive Services Task Force recommendations for the peripheral vasculature system and lymphatic system.
11. Document a complete history and physical examination of a client with peripheral vascular system and lymphatic system pathology.

The peripheral vasculature system and lymphatic system are primarily assessed in the four limbs and neck. Clinicians are familiar with the peripheral vasculature system assessment because pathology occurs frequently in this system. Conversely, lymphatic system pathology occurs less frequently and can be easily overlooked in the physical examination.

Anatomy and Physiology

Peripheral Vascular System

The circulatory system consists of arterial pathways, which are the distribution routes, and venous pathways, the collection system that returns the blood to the central pumping station, the heart. Figure 17-1 shows the journey of the blood through the systemic and pulmonary circuits.

Arterial walls are composed of three layers. The innermost layer is known as the tunica intima and is composed of the endothelium and some connective tissue. The tunica media is the middle layer and is composed of both smooth muscle and an elastic type of connective tissue. The outer layer, the tunica externa or adventitia, has a more fibrous connective tissue that is arranged longitudinally.

As the arterial system branches and subdivides on its way to the periphery, the diameters of the vessels decrease. Arterioles are the smallest group of

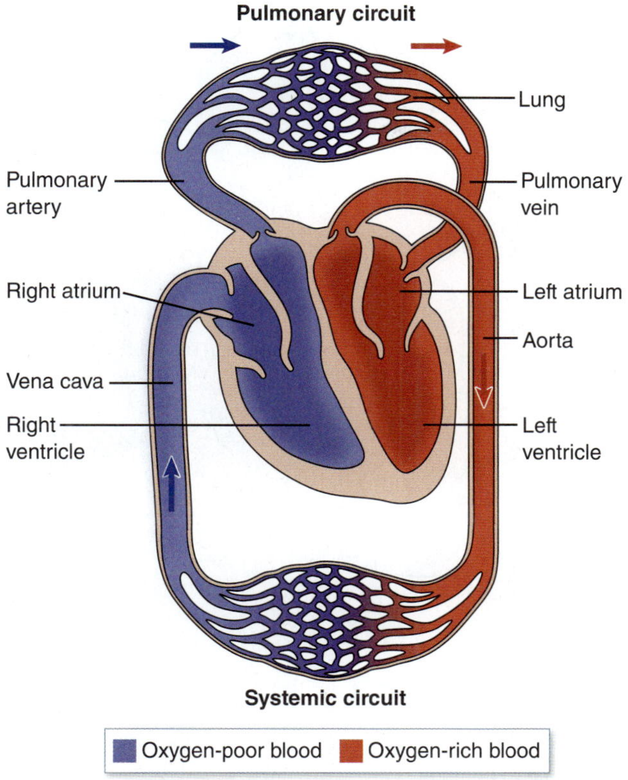

Figure 17-1 The systemic and pulmonary circuits. The systemic pump consists of the left side of the heart, and the pulmonary circuit pump consists of the right side of the heart.

arteries, with a diameter of less than 0.5 mm. It is here that the rapid velocity of blood flow found in the larger arteries begins to decrease. Blood flow becomes even slower in the capillaries arising from each arteriole. The walls of the capillaries are only one cell thick, which, coupled with the slow rate of blood flow, provides optimal conditions for the exchange of nutrients and wastes and the transfer of fluid volume between the plasma and the interstitium.

After leaving the capillaries, the blood flows into the low-pressure venous system beginning with vessels known as venules. Veins are similar in construction to arteries, but they have much less elasticity, thinner walls, and greater diameters. One-way valves are found in most veins where blood is carried against the force of gravity, such as in the lower extremities. Arteries do not have valves.

As blood passes from the arterial system through the capillaries, there is a change from the pulsatile character of arterial flow to a steady flow in the venous system. Arterial pulsations are caused by intermittent contractions of the left ventricle. Figures 17-2 and 17-3 illustrate the arterial and venous networks of blood flow.

Lymphatic System

The lymphatic (or lymphoid) system name is derived from its relationship to **lymphocytes**, the white blood cells that play a key role in the body's immune system. Lymphatics supplement the cardiovascular system—and help maintain fluid balance—by collecting interstitial (or extracellular) fluids that have leaked from surrounding tissues through the thin walls of the capillaries and returning them to circulating blood. This interstitial fluid is a component of blood plasma and contains nutrients that the tissue cells need. Also, the lymphatic system assists the digestive tract by absorbing lipids (or fats) and fat-soluble vitamins and transporting these elements to the venous

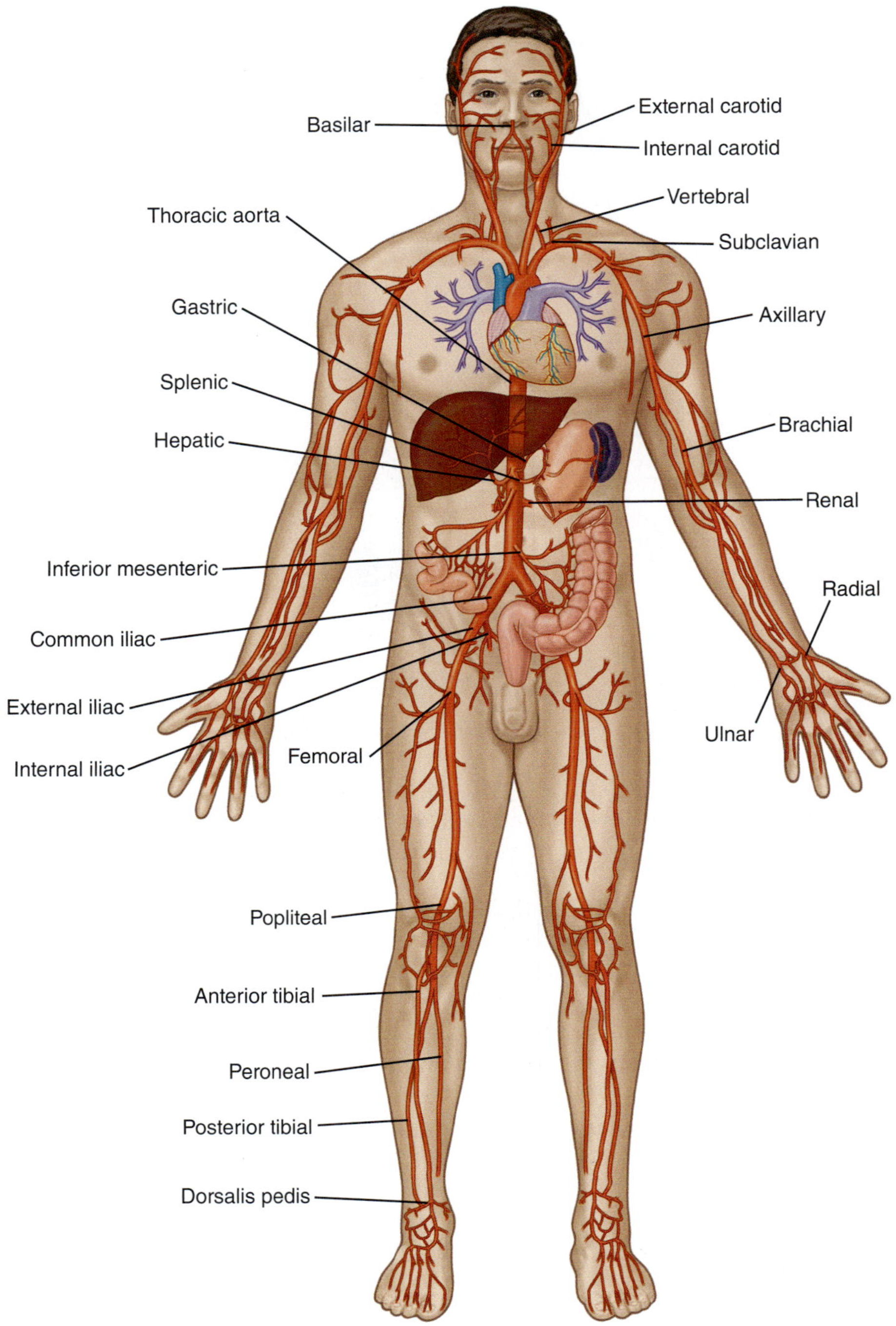

Figure 17-2 Arterial system anatomy.

circulation; it also supports the immune system by producing lymphocytes (disease-fighting white blood cells) that destroy bacteria, toxins, and particulate matter. The lymphatic system is composed of fluid (known as lymph), vessels that transport the lymph, and organs that contain lymphoid tissue.

Lymphatic Vessels

The transport of lymph through the lymphatic vessels (Fig. 17-4) moves in only one direction and is slow compared with cardiac circulation: 3 liters/day versus 4 to 5 liters/minute. Additionally, there are no lymphatic pumps. Instead, lymph moves through the lymphatic vessels with assistance from skeletal muscle action, smooth muscle contraction, and respiratory movement. Any backflow of lymph is prevented by valves within the vessels.

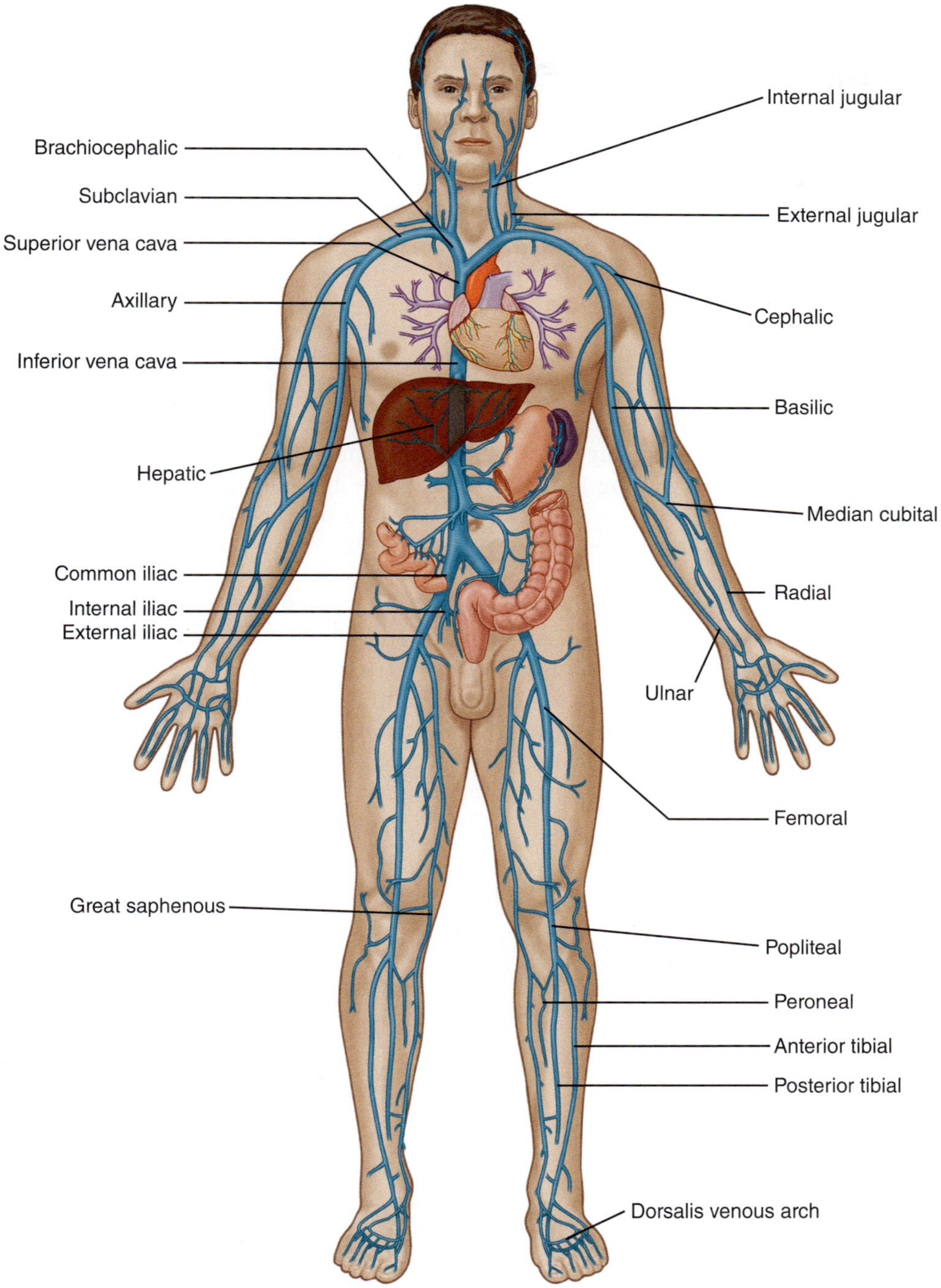

Figure 17-3 Venous system anatomy.

Lymphatic drainage occurs by way of lymphatic trunks, which are named after the areas of the body they supply. For example, lymph drains from the legs, abdominal wall, and pelvic organs via the lumbar trunk; the intestinal trunk drains organs of the abdominal cavity; the broncho-mediastinal and intercostal trunks serve the thorax; the arms are drained from the subclavian trunk; and parts of the head and neck are drained by the jugular trunk. The lymphatic trunks eventually join either the thoracic duct or the right lymphatic duct; however, most of the lymph in the body reaches the venous system via the thoracic duct. After leaving one of these collecting ducts, lymph becomes part of the plasma by entering the veins just before the blood returns to the right atrium of the heart.

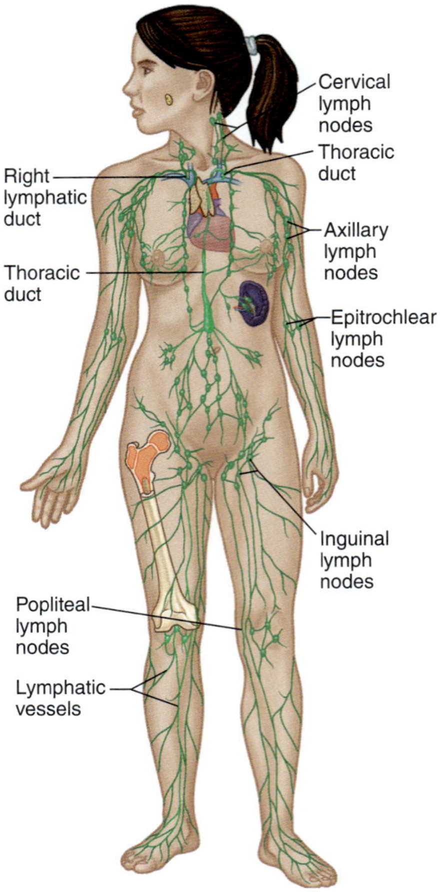

Figure 17-4 Lymphatic vessels.

Lymphatic Organs

Lymphatic organs (Fig. 17-5) are classified as either primary or secondary. The primary organs are the thymus gland and the bone marrow, which consist of sites where two types of immunoprotective cell lines originate and/or mature: T lymphocytes (or T-cells) and B lymphocytes (or B-cells). The secondary organs are the lymph nodes, spleen, and small masses of lymph tissue dispersed throughout the body (e.g., Peyer patches, the appendix, tonsils, and some regions of the body's mucosal surfaces). They contain the locations where lymphocytes continue to mature; they also trap antigens for exposure to T- and B-cells.

The thymus gland is located in the upper chest region, posterior to the sternum, and between the lungs. It grows until puberty but becomes less active and shrinks thereafter; this atrophy is thought to be the reason why T-cell production decreases as one grows older. For this reason, vaccines are given at a young age, so that they will have the most impact. The hollow shafts of the long bones contain bone marrow that produces T- and B-cells. Unlike the thymus gland, the bone marrow does not atrophy at puberty; therefore, the production of B-cells remains unchanged despite advancing age.

The **lymph nodes** or glands (Fig. 17-6) are small, bean-shaped structures that house T- and B-cells as well as other cells that can help the T-cells by filtering out antigens and presenting them to these immune cells. Thus, when aggravated, this combination of cells found in the lymph nodes can unite to present an immune response. Thousands of lymph nodes, each of which is supplied by an artery and a vein, are found along the lymphatic routes of the body. They are especially clustered around the axilla (axillary nodes), neck (cervical nodes), groin (inguinal nodes), and knees (popliteal nodes).

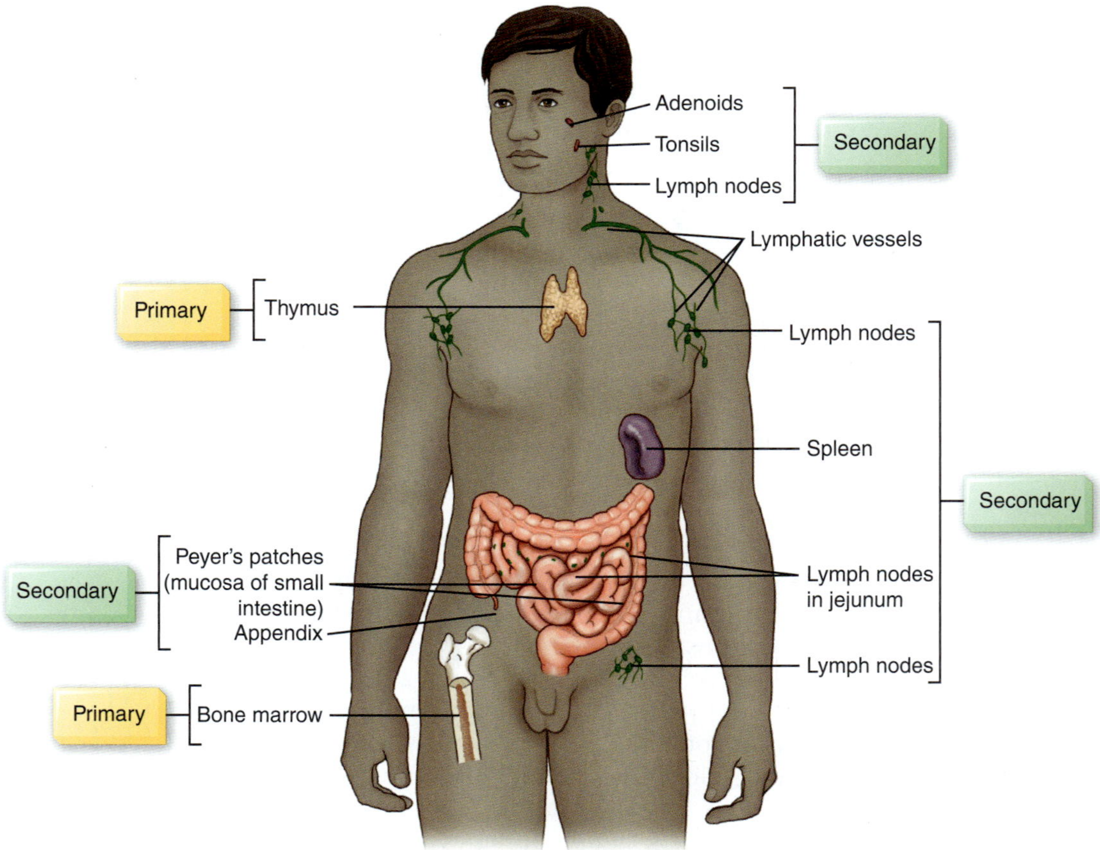

Figure 17-5 Lymphatic organs.

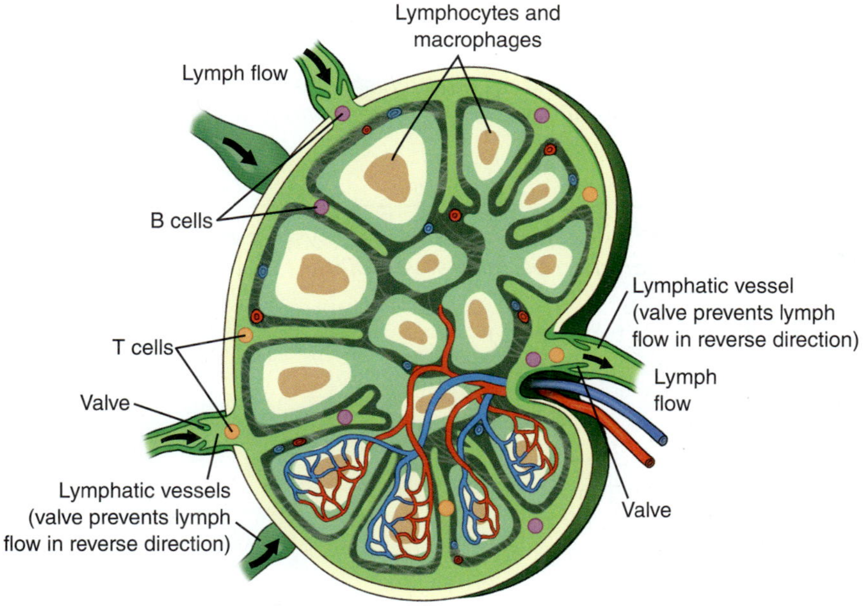

Figure 17-6 A lymph node.

Lymphocytes exit the lymph nodes in lymph through the lymphatic vessels. At some point, they cross back into the bloodstream and are transported to tissues throughout the body, whereupon they seek to react with foreign antigens. Eventually, they return to the lymphatic vessels, and the cycle begins again.

The spleen is a fist-sized organ located in the abdomen behind the stomach; it is the largest lymphatic organ. The spleen is similar in structure to a lymph node, but instead of filtering lymph, it filters blood. The spleen has two important types of tissue: the red pulp (which contains macrophage cells that engulf and then digest cellular debris and pathogens) and the white pulp (which holds a majority of lymphocyte cells that are the major cellular components of the adaptive immune response). Although humans can live without a spleen, those who have had it damaged or removed are highly susceptible to infection, because it can no longer fulfill its active role in immune responses.

Peyer patches are clusters of lymphatic nodules that line the ileum of the small intestine. The appendix is rich in lymphatic tissue, although its function remains unknown. Tonsils are lymphatic nodules found in the mucosa that line the throat. Actually, there are seven tonsils, but the single pharyngeal tonsil is the best known. Some regions of the body's mucosal surfaces (e.g., the gastrointestinal, respiratory, reproductive, and urinary tracts) have nodules known as mucosa-associated lymphoid tissue (or MALT) that contain lymphocytes and macrophages that protect against bacteria and other pathogens that enter the body via food, air, or urine.

Some lymphatic diseases are congenital, but others are the result of an illness or injury. In any case, most lymphatic disorders result in **lymphedema**, a condition whereby the lymphatic system is obstructed and localized swelling occurs, including the tissues. Tissues with unresolved lymphedema are susceptible to infection. Because the lymphatic system affects every body organ, its dysfunction also contributes to arthritis, autoimmune disorders, chronic infection, and peripheral vascular disease.

HEALTH HISTORY

The peripheral vasculature system and lymphatic system health history provide insight into the link between a client's life/lifestyle and peripheral vasculature system and lymphatic system information and pathology.

CLIENT PROFILE

Diseases that are age- and sex-specific for the peripheral vasculature system and lymphatic system are listed. Table 17-1 differentiates common peripheral vasculature system and lymphatic system disorders.

Age Hodgkin lymphoma (15 to 39; after age 75)
Non-Hodgkin lymphoma (risk increases with age)
Raynaud phenomenon (18 to 50)
Hypertension (HTN) (20 to 70)
Arteriosclerosis (50 to 70)
Peripheral artery disease (PAD) (>50)
Cerebrovascular accident (CVA) (50 to 70)
Abdominal aortic aneurysm (AAA) (60 to 70)
Chronic arterial insufficiency (>60)

Sex

Female Raynaud phenomenon, varicose veins.

Like heart disease, peripheral vasculature disease (PVD) has been understudied in females. However, some believe that its prevalence among females is now equal to that among males.

Male Peripheral artery disease, chronic arterial insufficiency; more likely to develop lymphoma of all types.

Race

Non-Hispanic White Non-Hodgkin lymphoma
Black CVA, HTN, PVD, peripheral artery disease (PAD)
Hispanic and Filipino HTN
Native American CVA

Although race is a social construct, the experience of racial bias can result in illness due to chronic inflammation, stress hormone release, metabolic disorders, endothelial damage, and thrombosis. All these factors increase the risk for vascular disease.

CHIEF COMPLAINT

Common chief complaints for the peripheral vascular system and lymphatic system are defined, and information on the characteristics of each sign or symptom is provided.

1. **Syncope** Fainting caused by a transient decrease in cerebral blood flow

   Associated Manifestations Weakness, dizziness, numbness and tingling of extremities, headache, facial droop, inability to speak or slurred speech, visual changes

   Aggravating Factors Exercise, medications, fever, decreased food intake, or food abstinence

   Alleviating Factors May be relieved with rest or may resolve spontaneously

   Setting Any setting. Syncope with the above-associated factors is a sign of a CVA or transient ischemic attack (TIA). (See Nursing Tip: What Is a TIA or Mini-Stroke?)

2. **Peripheral Edema** Swelling of the extremities, usually the feet and hands but can include the abdomen and thighs. May be unilateral such as in a deep venous thrombosis (DVT) and lymphedema, or bilateral such as in venous insufficiency; bilateral lymphedema can occur depending on the location of affected lymph nodes.

   Associated Manifestations Pain to the extremity, coolness or warmth, pallor, rubor or discoloration, numbness, weakness, and paresthesia

   Aggravating Factors Continuous standing, high salt intake

   Alleviating Factors Lying down or elevating the feet, wearing compression garment

3. **Extremity Pain** Sense of discomfort usually occurring in the legs or feet

   Quality Cramping or aching (PAD)

   Severe pain in calf or back of the leg (DVT)

Associated Manifestations Swelling in the affected extremity, discoloration of the skin, tenderness, change in skin temperature, hair loss, paresthesia, and weakness can occur, fatigue noted in the legs, discomfort in the muscles of the hip, leg, or buttocks. Wounds to the lower extremities that weep or are difficult to heal, abdominal pain

Aggravating Factors Continual standing, walking, exercise, cold weather, smoking, stress, and pain increase with dangling the extremity to a dependent position in venous insufficiency

Alleviating Factors Rest, elevation, (leg elevation in venous insufficiency, dangling the leg to a dependent position in arterial insufficiency)

Setting Walking, exercise

4. Lymphadenopathy An enlarged lymph node in the neck, axilla, or groin

Associated Manifestations Tenderness at the lymph node site, swelling of associated distal extremity, fever, fatigue, weight loss, cough, sore throat

Aggravating Factors Presence of recent illness, injury, or event

Alleviating Factors Acetaminophen, ibuprofen, heat or ice

Setting Recent COVID-19 infection, exposure to Mpox

PAST HEALTH HISTORY

The various components of the past health history are linked to peripheral vasculature system and lymphatic system pathology and peripheral vasculature system and lymphatic system-related information.

Medical History

Peripheral Vasculature System AAA, PVD, PAD, DVT, varicose veins, lower extremity edema, HTN, hyperlipidemia, May-Thurner syndrome

Lymphatic System Lymphedema, lymphadenopathy, lymphomas, autoimmune disorders, Epstein Barr virus, HIV

Surgical History Aneurysm repair, peripheral vascular stenting, bypass grafting, carotid endarterectomy or stent, coronary artery bypass graft (CABG), limb amputation

Allergies Intravenous pyelogram (IVP) dye (injected during diagnostic testing such as in a CT scan) and seafood (both contain iodine compounds), latex (found in gloves used for procedures), betadine (used as a skin surface prep for vascular procedures)

Medications

Peripheral Vasculature System Antiplatelet, anticoagulants, antiarrhythmics, hypoglycemic agents, insulin, antihypertensives, dyslipidemics, diuretics, vasodilators, GLP-1

Lymphatic System Phenytoin, carbamazepine, atenolol, cephalosporins, sulfa, and penicillin (can cause reversible adenopathy); monoclonal antibodies, immunosuppressants, chemotherapy agents, steroids

Communicable Diseases Untreated syphilis (aortitis, aortic aneurysm); HIV (lymphadenopathy), COVID-19 (lymphadenopathy), Mpox (lymphadenopathy)

Injuries and Accidents Trauma to limbs or abdomen (splenic rupture), crush or impingement injury

FAMILY HEALTH HISTORY

Familial peripheral vasculature system and lymphatic system diseases are listed.

Aneurysm, CVA, HTN, Raynaud phenomenon, lymphomas

SOCIAL HISTORY

The components of the social history are linked to the peripheral vasculature system and lymphatic system factors and pathology.

Alcohol Use Excessive alcohol intake may play a role in the pathogenesis of HTN, PVD, and CVA

Tobacco Use Nicotine increases catecholamine release, leading to elevated blood pressure. Nicotine also inhibits the development of collateral circulation and causes peripheral vasoconstriction, thus increasing the risk of thrombus formation and atherosclerosis. Tobacco use can be associated with aneurysms, CVA, HTN, Raynaud phenomenon, and lymphomas.

Recreational Drug Use Amphetamines, cocaine, and heroin: HTN, hypotension, aortic rupture/dissection, aneurysm, CVA, lymphoma, Raynaud phenomenon

Travel History Arsenic poisoning: Systemic arterial disease, including gangrene and PVD; can be traced to the elevated arsenic content in contaminated drinking water and soil in some geographic locations

Work Environment Exposure to high levels of ionizing radiation, pesticides, and herbicides increases the risk for lymphoma.

Stress Chronic stress, depression, anxiety, anger, and negativity are associated with arrhythmia and HTN

HEALTH MAINTENANCE ACTIVITIES

This information provides a bridge between health maintenance activities and peripheral vasculature system and/or lymphatic system function.

Diet Caffeine (found in coffee, tea, energy drinks, soft drinks, chocolate, over-the-counter medications) is a sympathomimetic amine that increases blood pressure.

Reduced sodium intake and a diet centered on fresh produce are two of the recommendations for the prevention of HTN. Additionally, the DASH (Dietary Approaches to Stop Hypertension) diet is a dietary pattern promoted by the National Heart, Lung, and Blood Institute. High-fat diets are associated with atherosclerosis.

Exercise Increased physical activity is an important recommendation for the prevention of HTN, PVD, CAD, and CVA.

Health Checkups HTN: Blood pressure, pulse, and serum lipid profile

PAD: Angiogram, Ankle-Brachial index (ABI), serum lipid profile, Doppler ultrasound flow studies, magnetic resonance angiography (MRA), treadmill exercise test, photoplethysmography (PPG), pulse volume recording (PVR) waveform analysis, reactive hyperemia test, segmental blood pressure measurements

Table 17-1 Peripheral Vasculature and Lymphatic Disorders

Disorder	Definition	Common Findings
Acute arterial occlusion	Thrombus or embolus blocks blood flow through an artery	Sudden severe pain to the affected limb, pulseless, pallor.
Aneurysm	Localized abnormal dilation of a blood vessel	Abdominal aortic aneurysm (AAA, sometimes referred to as a "triple-A"). Usually, asymptomatic but can cause abdominal fullness. Ruptured AAA—severe, sudden, and continuous abdominal pain that radiates to the back. Thoracic aneurysm may involve aortic root, ascending aorta, arch, or descending aorta. Usually asymptomatic, but if very large can cause compression on esophagus, larynx, or trachea.
Aortic dissection	A tear in the innermost layer of the aorta allows blood to flow between the aortic walls and forces them apart and possibly rupture. Frequently caused by an injury to the torso or abdomen	Sudden, tearing pain in chest (thoracic aortic dissection) radiating to shoulders, neck, and back or abdomen (abdominal aortic dissection) radiating to the back. Hypotension, skin mottling distal to the dissection.
Cerebrovascular accident (CVA)	Brain damage that results from lack of blood flow to the brain; a CVA can have an embolic, thrombotic, or hemorrhagic cause	Decreased neurological function; headaches; hemiparesis; inability to speak; coma; abnormal cranial nerve findings.

Table 17-1 Peripheral Vasculature and Lymphatic Disorders—cont'd

Disorder	Definition	Common Findings
Deep vein thrombosis (DVT)	The formation of a blood clot in a deep vein (most commonly in the leg or pelvis); inflammation of a vein due to a blood clot	Unilateral edema; calf pain or tenderness; temperature and color changes in the affected leg; cyanosis in the foot.
Hypertension	Elevated blood pressure	Systolic blood pressure (SBP) 130 to 139 mm Hg or diastolic blood pressure (DBP) 80 to 89 mm Hg; most often asymptomatic; headaches or epistaxis; see Chapter 9 for further information.
Peripheral artery disease (PAD)	Vascular disorder of the arteries that supply the extremities; also known as peripheral vascular disease (PVD) or peripheral artery occlusive disease (PAOD)	Changes in the skin, including decreased skin temperature, or thin, brittle, shiny skin on the legs and feet; diminished pulses in the legs and the feet; gangrene; hair loss on the legs; impotence; restricted mobility; nonhealing wounds over pressure points; numbness, weakness, or heaviness in muscles; pain at rest, commonly in the toes, and at night while lying flat; pallor with elevated legs; reddish-blue discoloration of the extremities; severe pain; thickened toenails.
Raynaud phenomenon	A condition caused by abnormal blood vessel spasms in the extremities, especially in response to cold temperatures	Finger or toe becomes pale, cold, and numb, then becomes red, hot, and tingling.
Thrombophlebitis	A blood clot in an inflamed vein; most common in the legs, but can also occur in the arms. It can result from pooling of the blood, venous wall injury, and/or altered blood coagulation	Swelling, pain, tenderness, redness, and/or warmth in the affected extremity; if a vein close to the surface of the skin is affected, the client may have a red, hard, and/or tender cord just under the surface of the skin.
Thrombus/ embolus	A blood vessel blockage caused by a thrombus (a blood clot) or an embolus (a tiny mass of debris that moves through the bloodstream)	Pain, tenderness, and/or swelling around the site where the obstruction occurs.
Transient ischemic attack (TIA)	A temporary blockage of blood flow to part of the brain lasting from a few minutes up to 24 hours. It is impossible to know if a client is having a TIA or CVA at the onset of symptoms	Limb weakness, numbness, paresthesia, slurred speech, facial droop, visual changes, dizziness
Vasculitis	A general term for a spectrum of disorders in which the inflammation of blood vessels leads to narrowing and/or blockage of vessels	Signs and symptoms depend on which vessel(s) are involved; can include fever, fatigue, loss of appetite, muscle and joint pain, nerve problems (e.g., numbness or weakness), weight loss.
Lymphedema	Occurs when lymph cannot be adequately drained from the lymphatic system, resulting in swelling. Primary lymphedema is an inherited condition whereby lymphatic vessels are impaired or missing; secondary lymphedema happens with insufficiency of the regional lymphatics as a result of infection, surgery, or trauma. It can also occur after lumpectomy or mastectomy, after sentinel node biopsy, and after axillary node dissection. Refer to Figure 17-7	Swelling in the extremities.
Lymphoma	A group of cancers that originate in the lymphatic system	Chronic fatigue, weak immune function, weight loss, night sweats.

Table 17-1 Peripheral Vasculature and Lymphatic Disorders—cont'd

Disorder	Definition	Common Findings
Lymphadenopathy	Swelling of a single or group of lymph nodes from bacterial, viral, or fungal infections, autoimmune diseases or malignancy	Enlarged or swollen lymph nodes, fatigue; fever may accompany swelling.
Lymphadenitis	An inflammation of the lymph node(s) related to a bacterial infection of the node tissue	Redness of skin, swelling, and/or tenderness over the affected node.

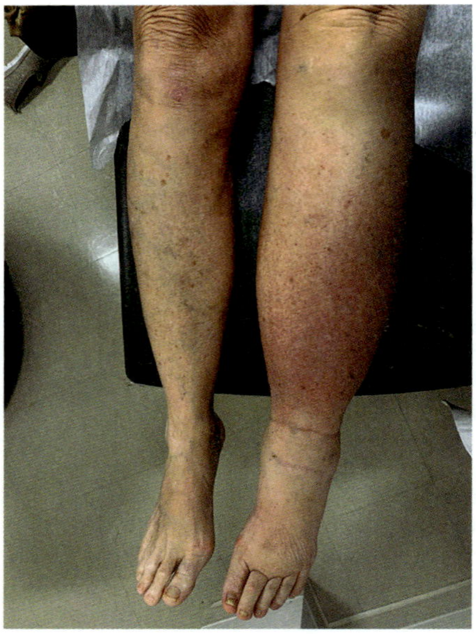

Figure 17-7 Note the lymphedema in the left lower leg. This client usually wears a compression bandage to promote lymphatic fluid drainage.

NURSING TIP

What is a TIA or Mini-stroke?

- A TIA (transient ischemic attack) is a medical emergency. Call 911 or a "CODE STROKE" (if in the hospital).
- A TIA is a transient lack of blood flow that completely resolves usually within minutes.
- Do not wait to see if symptoms resolve before calling for help.
- Blood clots cause TIAs just like strokes.
- A TIA is a warning. 10% to 15% of clients who have a TIA will have a CVA within 3 months, and if the TIA is untreated, 30% will have a stroke within 1 year.

(CDC, 2024)

Assessment in Brief

Peripheral Vasculature and Lymph Node Examinations

Examination of the Peripheral Vasculature

- Inspection of the jugular venous pressure
- Inspection of the hepatojugular reflux
- Palpation and auscultation of arterial pulses
- Inspection and palpation of peripheral perfusion
  - Color
  - Clubbing
  - Capillary refill
  - Skin temperature
  - Edema
  - Ulcerations
  - Skin texture
  - Hair distribution

Advanced Techniques

- Assessing for pulsus paradoxus
- Orthostatic hypotension assessment
- Assessing the venous system
  - Homan sign
  - Manual compression
  - Retrograde filling or Trendelenburg test
- Assessing the arterial system
  - Pallor
  - Color return and venous filling time
  - Allen test
  - ABI

Examining the Lymphatic System

- Inspection and palpation
  - Epitrochlear lymph nodes
  - Inguinal lymph nodes
  - Popliteal lymph nodes

Assistive Devices

- Hemodynamic monitoring
- Antiembolic stockings
- Intravenous catheters
- Pneumatic compression stockings
- Compression bandage for lymphedema
- Compression garment for lymphedema
- Intermittent pneumatic compression pump for lymphedema

Equipment

- Appropriate PPE
- Stethoscope
- Sphygmomanometer
- Watch or smartphone that counts seconds
- Tape measure
- Ruler

Examination of the Peripheral Vasculature

The components of the examination of the periphery include:

1. Inspection of the jugular venous pressure (JVP)
2. Inspection of the hepatojugular reflux
3. Palpation and auscultation of the arterial pulses
4. Inspection and palpation of peripheral perfusion

Inspection of the Jugular Venous Pressure

Identify the internal and external jugular veins (Fig. 17-8) with the client in a supine position with the head elevated to 30° or 45° so that the jugular veins are visible. Tangential lighting (lighting across the veins rather than on top of the veins) will facilitate the examination. Both sides of the neck should be examined. The external jugular veins are more superficial than the internal jugular (IJ) veins and traverse the neck diagonally from the center of the clavicle to the angle of the jaw. The IJ veins are larger and are located deep below the sternocleidomastoid muscle adjacent to the carotid arteries. The pulsations of the IJ veins can be difficult to identify visually because the veins are deep and their pulsations can be confused with those of the adjacent carotid arteries.

Jugular vein pulsations consist of two or three waves (Fig. 17-9). These waves are called the *a, c,* and *v* waves. The *a* wave, which is produced by the contraction of the right atrium, reflects the backflow of blood into the vena cava as the right atrium ejects blood into the right ventricle. The *a* wave occurs just before S_1.

The *c* wave occurs at the end of S_1 and is produced when the right ventricle begins to contract. The *c* wave is caused by both the slight backflow of blood into the right atrium when the ventricular contraction occurs and the bulging of the tricuspid valve backward toward the right atrium because of increased right ventricular pressure.

The *v* wave results from the slow buildup of blood in the right atrium during the ventricular contraction (when the tricuspid valve is closed) and occurs during late systole. The *v* wave disappears when the tricuspid valve opens and blood flows rapidly into the right ventricle.

Two negative slopes, the *x* and *y* descents, also occur in the jugular venous pulse. The *x* descent occurs after the *c* wave and reflects the fall of the right atrial pressure when the tricuspid valve closes and the right atrium relaxes.

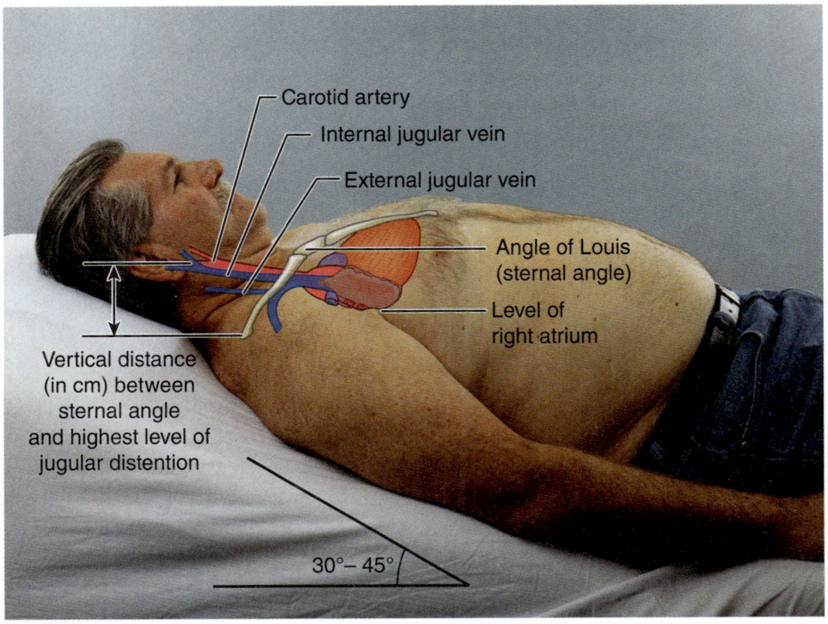

Figure 17-8 Inspection of jugular venous pressure.

NURSING CHECKLIST

General Approach to Peripheral Vasculature Examination

1. Observe standard precautions and don personal protective equipment (PPE) such as gloves, gown, face shield, goggles, N-95 respirator mask, or face mask if your client's status warrants these protective measures.
2. Explain to the client what you are going to do.
3. Ensure that the room is warm and well-lit.
4. Use a drape and uncover only those areas that are necessary as the examination is done.
5. Position the client in a supine or sitting position.

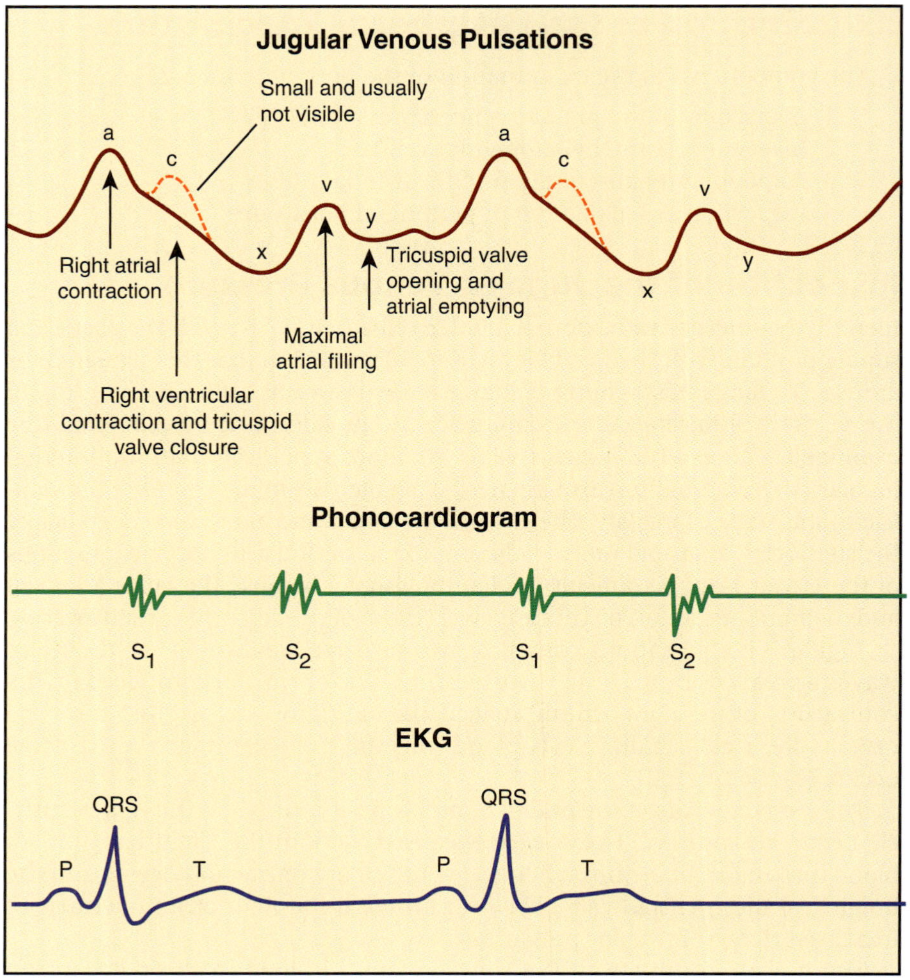

Figure 17-9 Jugular venous pulse waves in relation to the phonocardiogram and electrocardiogram (EKG).

The *y* descent follows the *v* wave and occurs when the tricuspid valve opens and blood flows rapidly from the right atrium into the right ventricle.

These waves and descents are clearly noted when the client has a direct central venous pressure (CVP) line and the right atrial pressure waves are depicted on an oscilloscope.

Information about the CVP can be obtained directly via a catheter inserted into one of the jugular veins (the IJ veins are the veins of choice for cannulation because they do not have valves and they provide a more direct route to the right atrium) or indirectly as discussed in the next section.

E 1. To indirectly estimate a client's CVP, first determine the JVP (Fig. 17-8):

a. Place the client at a 30° to 45° angle (the highest position where the neck veins remain visible).

b. Measure the vertical distance in centimeters from the client's sternal angle to the top of the distended neck vein. This will give you the JVP.

c. Knowing that the sternal angle is roughly 5 cm above the right atrium, take the JVP measurement obtained in the previous step and add 5 cm to get an estimate of the CVP. For example, a JVP of 2 cm at a 45° angle estimated on a client's right side is equivalent to a CVP of 5 + 2, or 7 cm.

2. Direct CVP measurements in the client with a central venous cannula should be obtained with the client in the supine position or reclining at no more than a 45° angle.
   a. Do not forget to level the transducer at the client's right atrium (phlebostatic axis—fourth ICS, midaxillary line) before obtaining any CVP reading.
   b. When recording CVP measurements, chart the angle of the client when the measurement was taken.

N **A JVP reading of less than 4 cm is considered normal. Normally, the jugular veins are:**
- **Most distended when the client is flat because gravity is eliminated and the jugular veins fill**
- **1 to 2 cm above the sternal angle when the head of the bed is elevated to a 45° angle**
- **Absent when the head of the bed is at a 90° angle**
- **Normal direct CVP readings are 3 to 8 cm H_2O or 0 to 8 mm Hg**

A A JVP greater than 4 cm is considered abnormal.

P An elevated JVP can be due to increased right ventricular pressure, increased blood volume, or an obstruction to right ventricular flow.

A Bilateral jugular venous distention (JVD) is abnormal.

P JVD indicates an increased JVP, which occurs in conditions such as congestive heart failure (CHF).

A Unilateral JVD is abnormal.

P Unilateral JVD indicates a local vein blockage.

A JVD with the head of the bed elevated up to a 90° angle is abnormal.

P JVD at a 45° to 90° angle (Fig. 17-10) indicates more serious pathology, such as severe right ventricular failure, constrictive pericarditis, or cardiac tamponade.

A An increased *a* wave is abnormal.

P An increased *a* wave can occur with stenosis of the tricuspid valve (because the right atrium has difficulty emptying the blood into the right ventricle) or when the right ventricle is enlarged and the right atrium must contract more forcefully to fill it. An increased *a* wave can also occur in complete heart block because the right atrium contracts at its own pace against a closed tricuspid valve.

A An enlarged *v* wave is abnormal.

P An enlarged *v* wave can occur with tricuspid regurgitation or insufficiency. It is exaggerated when the tricuspid valve allows blood to flow back from the right ventricle to the right atrium during systole, thus causing the *x* slope to be replaced by a large *c–v* wave. It can also occur with right-sided heart failure, where the right ventricle becomes so enlarged that it forces the tricuspid valve to stretch and allow blood back into the right atrium.

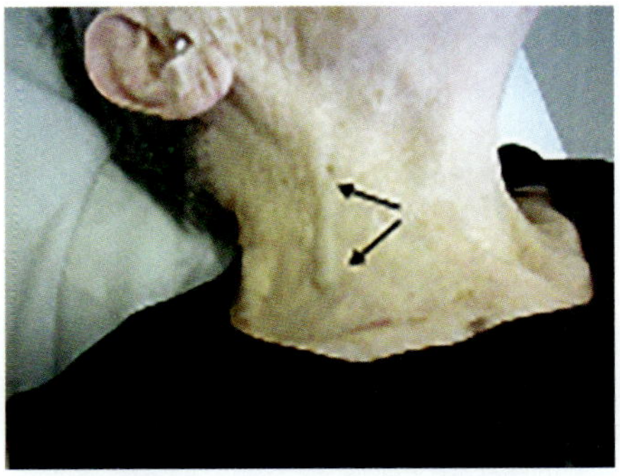

Figure 17-10 Positive JVD in client positioned at a 45° angle. This client had not taken their morning diuretic and was complaining of SOB.

Inspection of the Hepatojugular Reflux

Hepatojugular reflux is a test that is very sensitive in detecting right ventricular failure. This procedure is performed if the CVP is normal but right ventricular failure is suspected.

E 1. Place the client flat in bed, or elevated to a 30° angle if the jugular veins are visible. Remind the client to breathe normally.

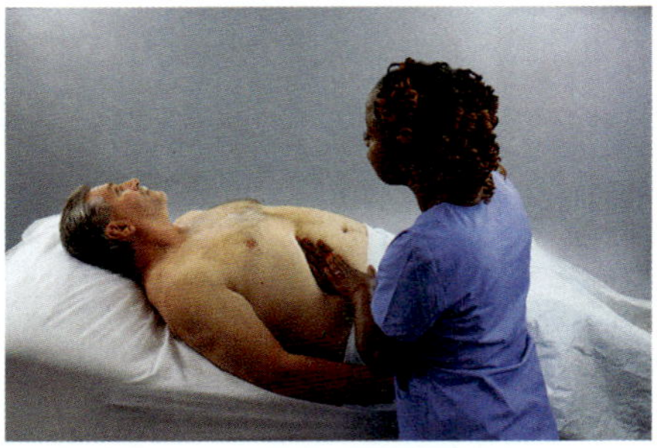

Figure 17-11 Hepatojugular reflux.

2. Using single or bimanual deep palpation, press firmly on the right upper quadrant of the abdomen for 30 to 60 seconds.
3. Observe the neck for an elevation in JVP (Fig. 17-11).

N **Normally, this maneuver should not elicit any change in the jugular veins.**

A A rise of more than 1 cm in JVP is abnormal.

P A rise in JVP that occurs with this maneuver is suggestive of right-sided congestive heart failure or fluid overload. The heart simply cannot accept the increase in venous return.

Palpation and Auscultation of Arterial Pulses

Information concerning the function of the right ventricle is gained via examination of the venous pulses; however, examination of the arterial pulses provides information about the left ventricle. The pulses to be evaluated are the temporal, carotid, brachial, radial, femoral, popliteal, posterior tibial, and dorsalis pedis. The radial arteries are most frequently examined, due to their easy accessibility. In a cardiac arrest situation, the carotid pulse is the artery of choice for palpation. The carotid pulses should not be palpated together because excessive stimulation can elicit a vagal response and slow the heart rate. Palpating both carotid pulses at the same time could also cut off circulation to the client's head and brain.

E

1. The arterial pulse examination is best facilitated with the client in a supine position with the head of the bed elevated at 30° to 45°. If the client cannot tolerate such a position, then the supine position alone is acceptable
2. Using your dominant hand, palpate the pulses with the pads of the index and middle fingers. The number of fingers used will be determined by the amount of space where the pulse is located.
3. Evaluate the pulse in terms of:
   a. Rate.
   b. Rhythm: If there is an irregularity in the pulse rate, then auscultate the heart.
   c. Amplitude: Refer to Chapter 9 for grading scales.
   d. Symmetry: Palpate the pulses on both sides of the body simultaneously (except the carotid pulses).
4. If a peripheral pulse cannot be palpated, an amplification device can be used to detect the presence, rate, and rhythm at that location (Fig. 17-12).
5. Assess the "5 Ps" when examining a client with a suspected arterial occlusion: pain, pallor, pulselessness, paresthesia, and paralysis.
6. Using the bell of the stethoscope, auscultate the temporal, carotid, and femoral pulses for **bruits**, which are blowing sounds heard when blood flow becomes turbulent as it rushes past an obstruction. Ask the client to hold their breath during auscultation of the carotid pulse, because respiratory sounds can interfere with auscultation.

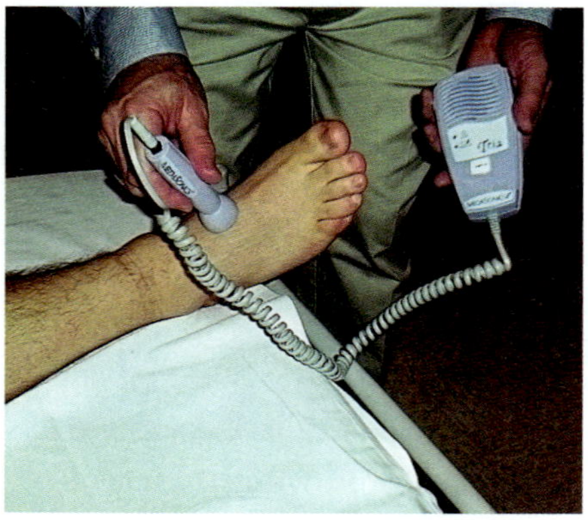

Figure 17-12 Use of a Doppler ultrasound to detect a dorsalis pedis pulse.

N **Refer to Chapter 9 for normal pulse rate, rhythm, and amplitude. When assessing symmetry, the pulses should be equal bilaterally. No bruits should be auscultated in the temporal, carotid, or femoral pulses.**

A P Figure 17-13 illustrates abnormal pulses with possible etiologies.

A Asymmetrical pulses are abnormal.

Normal

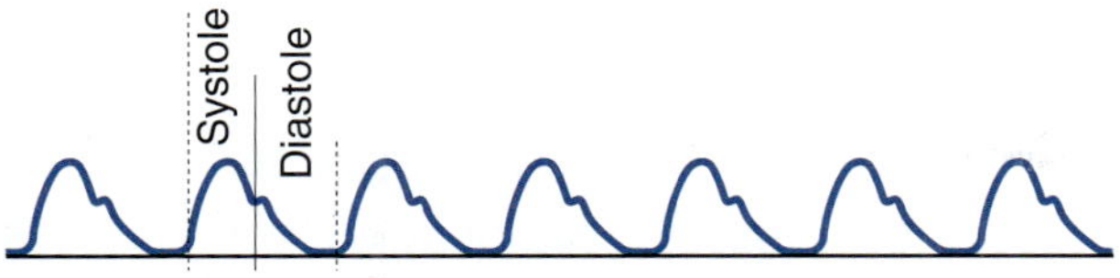

Hypokinetic/Weak Pulse

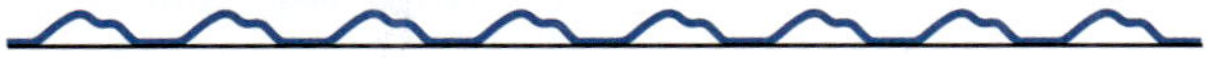

Characteristics:
a. Amplitude is decreased
b. Can be obliterated easily with palpation

Possible causes:
a. Decreased stroke volume
(1) Hypovolemia
(2) Congestive heart failure
(3) Cardiogenic shock
b. Increased peripheral vascular resistance
(1) Aortic stenosis
(2) Constrictive pericarditis

Hyperkinetic/Bounding Pulse

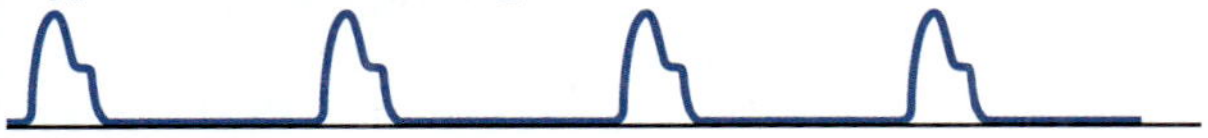

Characteristics:
a. Amplitude is increased
b. Easily palpable

Possible causes:
a. Hyperdynamic states
(1) Exercise
(2) Fever
(3) Hyperthyroidism
(4) Anxiety
(5) Septic shock
b. Rigid aorta
(1) Aging
(2) Atherosclerosis

Water-Hammer Pulse

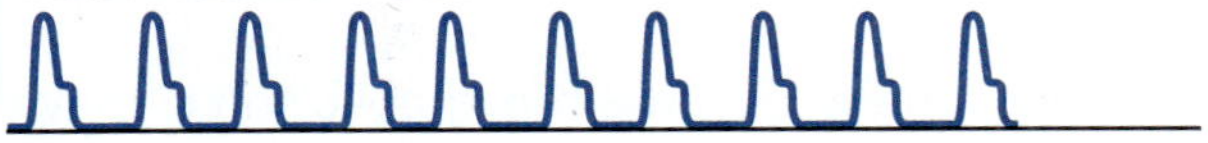

Characteristics:
a. Occurs when a high stroke volume results in an increased rate of ejection of blood flow from the left ventricle followed by a rapid fall in ejection
b. Also known as a collapsing pulse

Possible causes: Occurs when there is an abnormally rapid runoff of blood such as in patent ductus arteriosus and aortic regurgitation

Pulsus Alternans

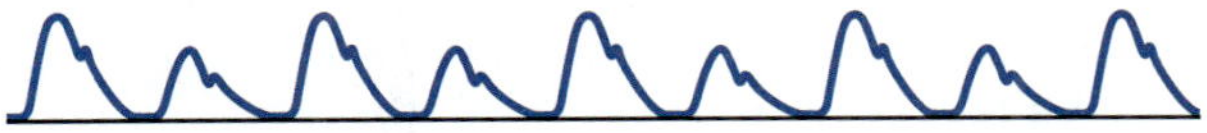

Characteristics: Rhythm is normal; however, alternates between increased amplitude and decreased amplitude

Possible causes:
a. Left ventricular failure
b. Cardiac tamponade

Bigeminal Pulse

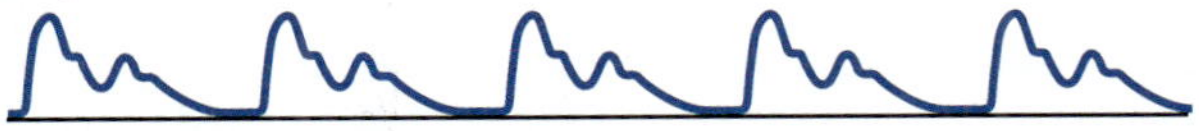

Characteristics: Rhythm is irregular (pulse with increased amplitude is followed by a pulse with decreased amplitude)

Possible causes: Dysrhythmias such as premature ventricular contractions, premature atrial contractions

Pulsus Paradoxus

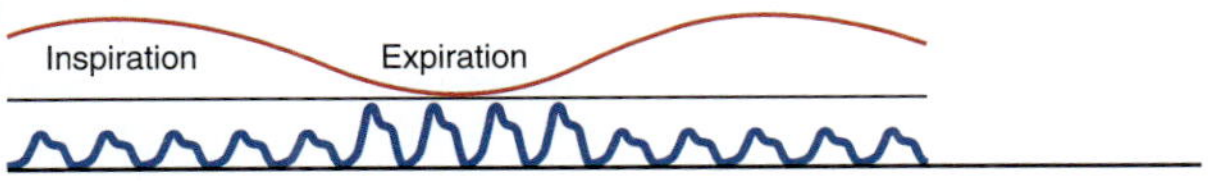

Characteristics: Marked decrease (10 mm Hg or more) in pulse amplitude during inspiration and increased amplitude during expiration

Possible causes:
a. Cardiac tamponade
b. Pericardial effusion
c. Constrictive pericarditis
d. Restrictive cardiomyopathy
e. Severe chronic obstructive lung disease
f. Superior vena cava obstruction

Pulsus Bisferiens

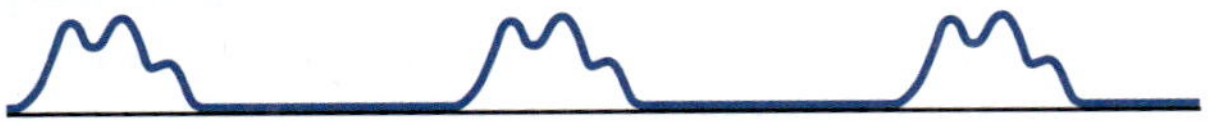

Characteristics: A pulse with a double peak. The first peak is believed to be the pulse pressure; the second peak is believed to be produced by reflected waves from the periphery

Possible causes:
a. Aortic regurgitation
b. Combined aortic stenosis and aortic regurgitation
c. Idiopathic hypertrophic subaortic stenosis (IHSS)

Figure 17-13 Alterations in arterial pulses.

P Variations in the symmetry of pulses can occur because of anatomic differences in the depths and locations of the arteries.

A Absent pulses are abnormal.

P An arterial occlusion may result in an absent pulse distal to the occlusion.

A Auscultation of bruits at the temporal, carotid, or femoral areas is abnormal.

P Bruits in these areas can be caused by an obstruction related to atherosclerotic plaque formation, a jugular vein-carotid artery fistula, or high-output states such as anemia or thyrotoxicosis.

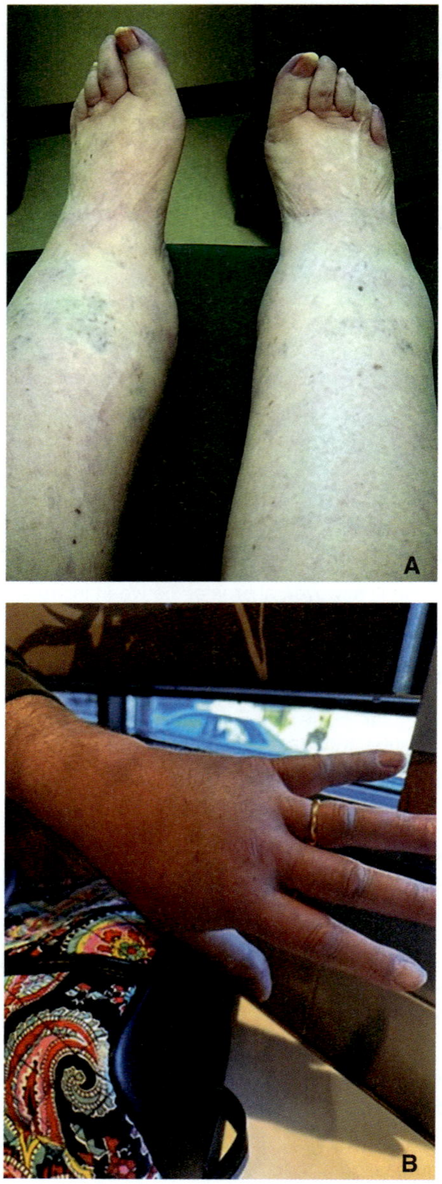

Figure 17-14 Edema. **A.** This client presented with lower extremity edema. The client stopped taking the prescribed diuretic the previous day. **B.** This client developed left hand edema after a fall. The client should remove the ring as soon as possible to prevent finger ischemia.

ADVANCED TECHNIQUE

Assessing for Pulsus Paradoxus

During inspiration, the blood flow into the right side of the heart is increased, the right ventricular output is enhanced, and pulmonary venous capacitance is increased, resulting in less blood reaching the left ventricle. These mechanisms account for a decrease in both the left ventricular stroke volume and arterial pressure. An exaggerated form of this mechanism is referred to as **pulsus paradoxus**.

E
1. Place the client in a supine position. Instruct them to breathe normally.
2. Apply the blood pressure cuff.
3. Inflate the cuff to 20 mm Hg above the client's last systolic blood pressure reading.
4. Slowly deflate the cuff until the first systolic sound is heard.
5. Observe the client's respirations, because the systolic sound may disappear during normal inspiration.
6. Slowly deflate the cuff again and note the point at which all of the systolic sounds are heard regardless of respirations.

N **The difference between the first systolic sound and the point at which all the systolic sounds are heard is the paradox. The paradox should be less than or equal to 10 mm Hg.**

A A paradox greater than 10 mm Hg is considered abnormal (refer to Figure 17-13).

P Pulsus paradoxus can occur in conditions such as cardiac tamponade, pericardial effusion, constrictive pericarditis, restrictive cardiomyopathy, severe chronic obstructive lung disease, and superior vena cava obstruction because all of these conditions can result in a decreased blood return to the left ventricle.

Inspection and Palpation of Peripheral Perfusion

Peripheral perfusion can be impaired with any pathological state that affects the flow of blood through the peripheral arteries and veins. Components of peripheral perfusion examination include peripheral pulse, color, clubbing, capillary refill, skin temperature, edema (Fig. 17-14), ulcerations, skin texture, hair distribution, and special techniques for the assessment of arterial and venous blood flow.

E
1. Inspect the fingers, toes, or points of trauma on the feet and legs for ulceration. Inspect the sides of the ankles for ulceration.
2. Advanced techniques for assessing the venous system (discussed in more detail later):
   a. **Homan sign**
   b. Manual compression
   c. Retrograde filling or Trendelenburg test

ADVANCED TECHNIQUE

Orthostatic Hypotension Examination

When an individual stands, blood pools in the lower part of the body and the blood pressure falls transiently. However, in the healthy individual, **baroreceptors** (receptors located in the walls of most of the great arteries) located in the carotid sinus area sense the decrease in blood pressure and initiate reflex vasoconstriction and increase the heart rate. These mechanisms bring the blood pressure back to normal. When this mechanism fails, **orthostatic hypotension** may ensue and an evaluation must be made. When assessing for orthostatic hypotension, take the client's blood pressure and heart rate with the client in supine and standing positions. If a client is unable to stand, vital signs may be taken in the sitting position with the legs dangling.

E 1. Have the client lie flat for 5 minutes. This time ensures that no reflex mechanisms from the upright position are influencing the blood pressure). Measure and record the blood pressure and the heart rate in this position.

2. Next, assist the client to a sitting position with the feet dangling. Wait 1 to 3 minutes. (There is no consensus in the literature regarding how long to wait after a position change before obtaining the next set of vital signs). Retake the blood pressure and heart rate. Record the blood pressure and the heart rate. Ask about any symptoms of weakness or dizziness related to the position change. If the client becomes weak or dizzy, or the blood pressure is <90/60 mm Hg, assist them back to a supine position.

3. Assist the client to a standing position. Measure the blood pressure and heart rate again after 1 minute and then at 3 minutes. Again, ask about any symptoms of weakness, dizziness, or visual changes related to the position change. Observe for diaphoresis or pallor. If the client becomes symptomatic or shows signs of syncope, assist them back to a supine position.

N **There is controversy as to whether orthostatic vital signs are useful for determining fluid status; however, as a low-cost, low-risk test, it continues to be utilized to make tentative diagnoses and assist in the management of syncope.**

A Subtract the 3-minute standing values from the supine position values. A decline of 20 mm Hg of systolic pressure or 10 mm Hg of diastolic pressure indicates orthostatic hypotension. A heart rate increase of 30 beats per minute after 3 minutes indicates hypovolemia. If the blood pressure drops upon standing but resolves at 3 minutes, this is not orthostatic hypotension; however, it indicates the need for education about changing positions slowly to prevent falls and injury.

P Orthostatic hypotension can occur in clients who are hypovolemic, have a neurogenic condition, or are experiencing side effects from prescribed medication.

3. Advanced techniques for examining the arterial system (discussed in more detail later):
   a. **Pallor**
   b. Color return (CR) and venous filling time (VFT)
   c. **Allen Test**

N **Ulcerations: No ulcerations should be noted.**

A Arterial ulcerations are abnormal. They usually occur at toes or points of trauma on the feet or legs (Fig. 17-15). Arterial ulcerations have well-defined edges, black or necrotic tissue with a deep, pale base without bleeding. The affected skin is hairless or disrupted. The skin is shiny, thick, and waxy. Arterial ulcerations are exceedingly painful with claudication. Pain is relieved by resting with limb dependency.

P The location and characteristics of ulceration are due to inadequate arterial flow, such as in peripheral artery disease (PAD) and diabetes mellitus. Most distal arterial beds are prone to ulceration. The pain is caused by ischemia.

P Arterial ulcers on the tips of the fingers, toes, or nose can be caused by Raynaud phenomenon (Fig. 17-16). Arteriolar spasms lead to pallor and pain in the affected area, followed by cyanosis, with numbness, tingling, and burning; rubor also develops. Over time,

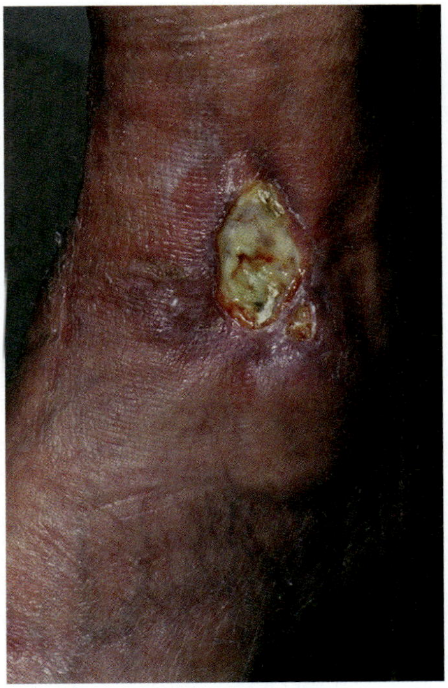

Figure 17-15 Arterial ulceration.

Risk Factors

Chronic Arterial Insufficiency

- Age (>60 years old)
- Smoking
- Sex (males > females)
- Hypertension
- Diabetes mellitus
- Hyperlipidemia

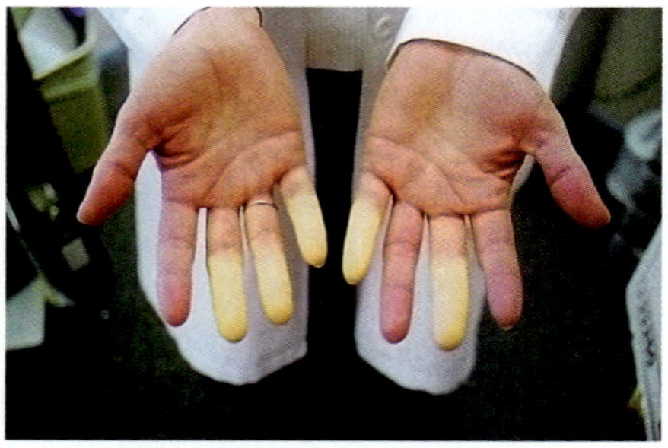

Figure 17-16 Early-stage Raynaud phenomenon. Note the pallor in the distal half of some of the fingers.

the affected area may develop an ulcer. Attacks occur bilaterally and last minutes to hours.

A Venous ulcerations are abnormal (Fig. 17-17). They usually occur at the sides of the ankle. Venous ulcerations have uneven edges and ruddy tissue with thin, shiny skin that lacks the support of subcutaneous tissue. The affected skin is hairless or disrupted. Venous ulcerations cause a deep muscular pain with aching and cramping relieved by leg elevation.

P Ulcers are due to inadequate venous flow that results when communication between the superficial and deep veins is compromised. Both the characteristics and the pain are related to inadequate venous blood flow. Table 17-2 compares features of arterial and venous insufficiency.

Risk Factors

Peripheral Artery Disease (PAD)

Fixed (client cannot alter): Age (especially over age 50), sex (male), ethnicity (Black), history of heart disease or cerebrovascular disease, diabetes mellitus and chronic kidney disease, postmenopausal females, family history of dyslipidemia/hypertension

Modifiable (client can reduce risk of PAD by controlling these factors): coronary artery disease and cerebrovascular disease, impaired glucose tolerance, dyslipidemia, hypertension, obesity (BMI >30 kg/m^2), physical inactivity, smoking or use of tobacco products

Warning: Those who smoke or have diabetes have the highest risk of complications from PAD because these risk factors also impair blood flow.

NURSING TIP

Peripheral Artery Disease (PAD)

Clients with PAD are encouraged to have the following: routine measurements of Ankle-Brachial index (ABI); high-dose statin therapy for lowering low-density lipoprotein cholesterol; antihypertensive therapy, smoking-cessation intervention; antiplatelet therapy with aspirin or clopidogrel; supervised exercise training for clients with intermittent claudication to reduce symptoms and improve function; and endovascular intervention if critical limb ischemia (CLI) is present or medical management and exercise is ineffective.
(Gerhard-Herman et al, 2017)

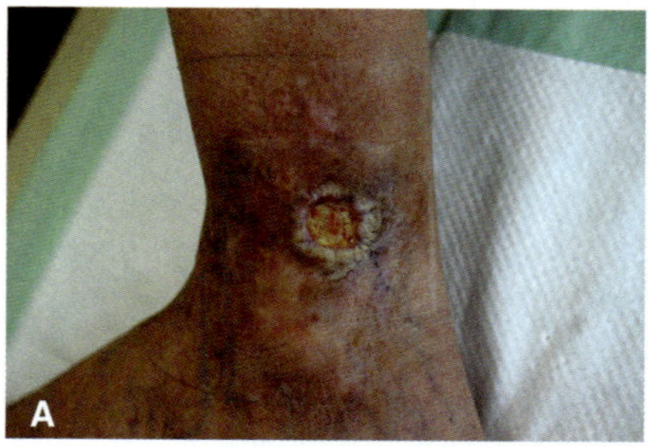

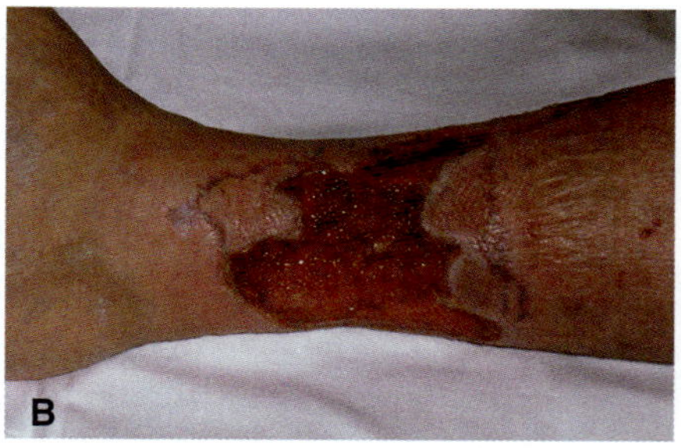

Figure 17-17 Venous ulcerations. **A.** Note the thin, shiny skin of this chronic venous stasis ulcer. **B.** Note the acute ulcerations at the side of the ankle.

Table 17-2 Arterial Versus Venous Insufficiency

	Arterial Insufficiency	Venous Insufficiency
Wounds	Occur as a result of ischemia from impaired circulation of oxygenated blood; wounds are deep, have smooth edges, and are well-defined	Occur because of inadequate functioning of the venous system; wounds are shallow and have irregular shapes
Pain	Severe; there may be pain with walking (claudication)	Mild to moderate
Pulses	Diminished or absent	Normal
Edema	Absent	Present
Skin temperature	Cold or cool	Warm
Skin	Thin and shiny; hair loss; rubor	Flaky/dry; may have a brownish color
Nails	Yellow	Normal
Leg elevation	Increases pain	Decreases pain
Related disorders	• Aneurysm • Aortic dissection • Arterial stasis ulcer • Buerger disease • Carotid artery stenosis • Chronic arterial insufficiency	• Chronic venous insufficiency • DVT • Thrombophlebitis (venous thrombus) • Varicose veins • Venous stasis ulcer

NURSING CHECKLIST

Assessing Clients With Peripheral Vascular System and Lymphatic System Assistive Devices

The client with peripheral vascular system and lymphatic system pathology may need the assistance of special equipment to maintain optimal status. The presence of these assistive devices must be noted and inspected as part of the examination. Consider the following to assist you in observing these devices:

1. Hemodynamic monitoring
   a. Check the goal of the line (e.g., fluid, monitoring).
   b. The monitor's alarms are on. The appropriate limits are set.
   c. The transducer level is at the client's right atrium (phlebostatic axis—fourth ICS, midaxillary line).
   d. The pressure bag(s) is pumped to 300 mm Hg.
   e. Change the flush bag(s) per your facility's policy.
   f. The line is safely secured to the client or the bed (it is not just dangling).
   g. The insertion site is free of infection.
2. Antiembolic stockings
   a. Identify if the stockings are knee-high or thigh-high.
   b. Ensure that they are the correct size (see the manufacturer's directions for correct sizing).
   c. The client has palpable or audible pulses in the lower extremities.
   d. The stockings have been removed at least once per day to assess the client's skin.
3. IV catheters
   a. Determine whether the catheter is inserted peripherally or centrally.
   b. The insertion site is free of infection, infiltration, or thrombophlebitis.
   c. Verify that the correct fluid is infusing.
   d. Verify that the correct additives are in the IV fluid.
   e. Determine the rate of the IV.
   f. Determine when the IV can be discontinued.
   g. Rotate IV site per your facility's policy.

4. Pneumatic compression stockings
   a. Ensure that the client has some sort of stocking between the legs and the plastic enclosures.
   b. The device is turned on.
   c. The stockings have been removed at least once per day to assess the client's skin.
5. Compression bandage for lymphedema (enhances lymphatic fluid drainage) (Fig. 17-18)
   a. Low stretch bandages that encircle the limb are applied by the client.
   b. Limb should maintain arterial pulse and skin temperature.
6. Compression garment for lymphedema (enhances lymphatic fluid drainage)
   a. Ensure proper size and pressure (determined by severity of lymphedema and body habitus).
   b. Limb should maintain arterial pulse and skin temperature.
7. Intermittent pneumatic compression pump (sleeve is worn on affected limb connected to a pump that sequentially inflates and deflates to enhance lymphatic fluid reabsorption)
   a. Use as prescribed for specified period.

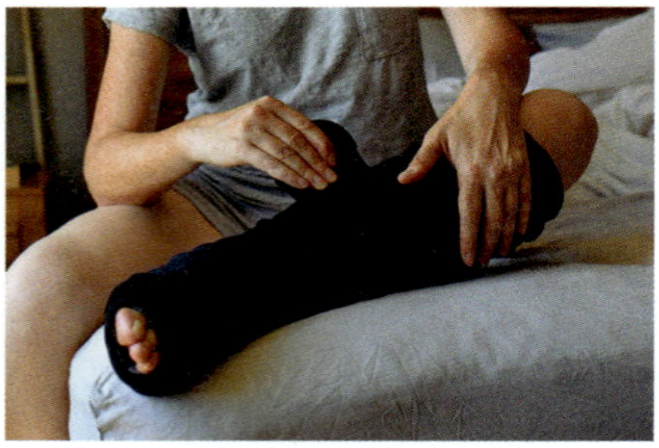

Figure 17-18 Compression bandage for leg lymphedema.

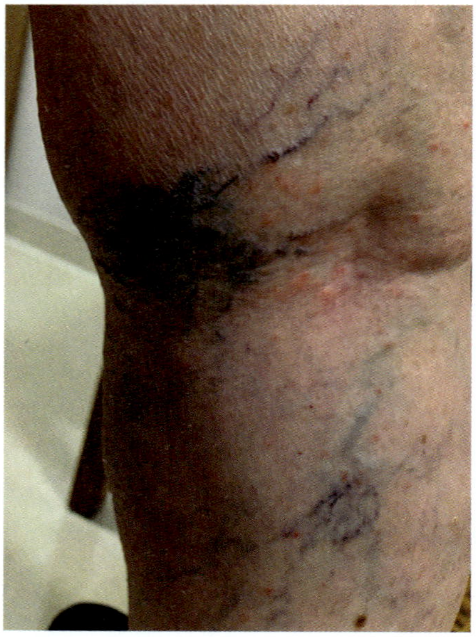

Figure 17-19 Varicose veins.

ADVANCED TECHNIQUE

Assessing the Venous System

Homan Sign

It is important to note that because a Homan sign has a low sensitivity (an indication of the frequency of a positive test result in a population with the disease) for thrombophlebitis, the use of this test has fallen out of favor with some health care providers. The Homan test is also controversial because there have been reports of the dislodging of deep vein thromboses (DVT) with the performance of the maneuver. In addition, conditions other than DVT could yield positive results from this test. A positive Homan sign is present in less than 20% of all DVT cases.

E 1. With the client's knee slightly bent, sharply dorsiflex the client's foot and ask the client if this maneuver elicits pain in the calf.
2. Repeat this technique with the other foot.

N **There should be no complaints of calf pain when this is evaluated.**

A A positive Homan sign may be abnormal.

P A positive Homan sign may indicate thrombophlebitis or DVT. Early detection of thrombophlebitis is essential because it can lead to life-threatening complications such as pulmonary embolism, which occurs when a thrombus breaks loose from the vein and travels to the lung. Three factors can disrupt the balance between blood-clotting activators and inhibitors. Known as Virchow triad, they are stasis of blood flow, an injured venous wall, and hypercoagulability. All three of these factors can predispose a client to thrombosis. Thrombosis can occur in either deep or superficial veins.

Manual Compression

Manual compression tests the competency of the saphenous vein's valves.

E 1. Palpate the dilated vein with one hand.
2. Use the other hand to compress the same vein 20 cm higher in the leg.
3. Note if an impulse is felt.

N **If the valves are competent, you will not feel the impulse because competent valves block the transmission of the impulse.**

A An impulse felt with manual compression is abnormal.

P Varicose veins are dilated, tortuous veins that are caused by incompetent valves (Fig. 17-19). They are most prevalent in the saphenous veins of the lower extremities.

E Examination **N** Normal Findings **A** Abnormal Findings **P** Pathophysiology

Retrograde Filling, or Trendelenburg Test

The retrograde filling, or Trendelenburg test, assesses the competency of the valves in the communicating and saphenous veins (evaluating varicose veins).

E
1. Raise the client's leg 90° to drain the venous blood.
2. Place a tourniquet or your hands around the upper thigh to occlude the saphenous vein.
3. Instruct the client to stand so that venous filling can be noted.
4. Release the compression and watch venous filling again.

N **Normal veins fill from below the occlusion and within 35 seconds as blood flows down from the arteries to the veins. Following the release of the hands or tourniquet, there should be no additional filling because competent valves prevent the backflow of blood.**

A A varicose vein that fills from above is abnormal.

P A varicose vein fills from above because of the backward flow of blood through incompetent valves. If sudden, additional filling occurs when the hands or tourniquet are removed, it is another indication that varicosities occur because of incompetent valves.

ADVANCED TECHNIQUE

Assessing the Arterial System

Pallor

E
1. Instruct the client to raise the extremities.
2. Note the time it takes for pallor, or lack of color, to develop.

N **Normally no pallor develops within 60 seconds.**

A Pallor that develops quickly in the extremities when the extremities are lifted is abnormal.

P Pallor that develops quickly is indicative of arterial insufficiency. The quicker the pallor develops, the more severe the disease.

Color Return and Venous Filling Time

E
1. To drain the feet of venous blood, elevate the supine client's legs approximately 12 inches and ask them to move their feet up and down at the ankles for approximately 1 minute.
2. Next, place the client in a sitting position on the edge of the bed, with the legs dangling over the side.
3. Note the time it takes for the color to return to the legs and for the superficial veins to refill.

N **Normal color return (CR) is 10 seconds and venous filling time (VFT) is 15 seconds.**

A A delayed CR of 15 to 25 seconds or a VFT of 20 to 30 seconds is abnormal.

P Moderate ischemia is defined as a delayed CR of 15 to 25 seconds or a VFT of 20 to 30 seconds.

A A delayed CR of 40 seconds or more or a VFT of 40 seconds or more is abnormal.

P Severe ischemia is defined as a delayed CR of 40 seconds or more or a VFT of 40 seconds or more.

Allen Test

The Allen test is used to assess the patency of the radial and ulnar arteries (Fig. 17-20). This test is usually performed before radial artery cannulation

Risk Factors

Varicose Veins

Varicose veins affect approximately 10% of the adult population and occur four times more often in females than in males. The pathogenesis of varicose veins remains unknown; however, it is not uncommon to find varicose veins in clients:

- Who have a family history of varicose veins
- Whose occupation requires long periods of standing
- Who have obesity
- Who are pregnant

NURSING TIP

Varicose Vein Prevention

Measures to prevent unnecessary pressure on the leg veins include:

- Avoid heavy lifting
- Avoid excessive weight gain
- Avoid crossing legs
- Wear support pantyhose or knee-high antiembolic stockings
- Stop smoking
- Elevate legs and feet while sitting
- Exercise

E Examination N Normal Findings A Abnormal Findings P Pathophysiology

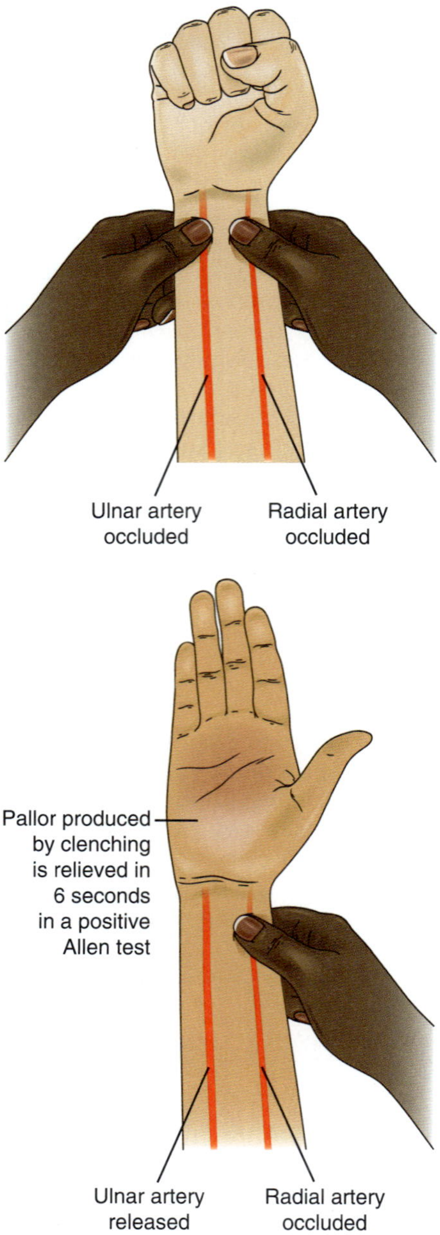

Figure 17-20 The Allen test.

because radial artery cannulation can be associated with radial artery thrombosis. If the radial artery becomes occluded with a thrombus, the continued viability of the hand depends on collateral blood flow from the ulnar artery.

E
1. Ask the client to make a tight fist. If the client is unresponsive, raise the arm above the heart for several seconds to force blood to leave the hand.
2. Apply direct pressure on the radial and ulnar arteries to obstruct blood flow to the hand as the client opens and closes the fist.
3. Instruct the client to open the hand, with the radial artery remaining compressed. If the client is unresponsive, keep the arm above the heart level.
4. Examine the palmar surface of the hand for a blush or pallor within 15 seconds.

N **If the radial artery is compressed, the blood flow through the ulnar artery should be sufficient to maintain the normal palm color after the client unclenches the fist. Also, if the ulnar artery is compressed, the blood flow through the radial artery should be sufficient to maintain the normal palm color. This is a positive Allen test.**

A If the color does not return to normal within 6 seconds after the client unclenches the fist, then obstruction of either the radial or the ulnar arteries may be present. This is a negative Allen test. Thus, the radial artery should not be punctured for an arterial blood gas or invasive arterial line.

P Atherosclerosis or a thrombus can cause either artery to not be patent.

ADVANCED TECHNIQUE

Ankle-Brachial Index (ABI)

The ABI is an easy, dependable, and inexpensive test used in the assessment of peripheral artery disease (PAD). Clients are evaluated annually, to note the progression of the disease as well as their response to treatment.

E
1. Have the client remove socks and shoes, as well as roll up sleeves and/or pant legs (but do not obstruct blood flow).
2. The client should rest in a supine position for 5 minutes before the readings are taken.
3. Place blood pressure (BP) cuffs snugly on the client's arms and above the ankles.
4. Apply a small amount of gel to the first brachial artery site and place the Doppler probe at the point with the loudest signal.
5. Inflate the BP cuff 20 mm Hg above the occlusion pressure.
6. Deflate the cuff at approximately 2 mm Hg per second, listening for the blood flow sound to return (this is the systolic pressure). Rapidly deflate the cuff after auscultating this systolic pressure and record the results.
7. Repeat this process for the other arm and record the results.
8. Use either the posterior tibial (PT) or dorsalis pedis (DP) for auscultation when obtaining ankle pressures. Again, apply a small amount of gel to the first site and place the Doppler probe at the point with the loudest signal.
9. Inflate the BP cuff 20 mm Hg above the occlusion pressure.
10. Deflate the cuff at approximately 2 mm Hg per second, listening for the blood flow sound to return. Rapidly deflate the cuff after auscultating the systolic pressure and record the results.
11. Repeat this process for the other ankle and record the results.

12. For the left-side ABI, divide the left ankle systolic pressure by the higher of the two brachial systolic pressures and record the results. Repeat this process for the right-side ABI, using the right ankle systolic pressure divided by the higher of the two brachial systolic pressures. For example, if the left ankle systolic pressure was 148 and the higher brachial systolic pressure was 152, then the ABI is 0.97 (148 ÷ 152).

N **An ABI range of 0.95 to 1.2 is considered normal.**

A An ABI of less than 0.90 is abnormal. An ABI greater than 0.60 but less than 0.90 indicates mild PAD. An ABI between 0.40 and 0.59 signals moderate PAD. An ABI less than 0.39 denotes severe PAD, with ischemia noted in an ABI less than 0.25.

P These abnormal values indicate PAD. Note that the ABI reading may not be accurate for clients who have diabetes, kidney disease, or some older adult clients, as they may have rigid blood vessels that make it difficult to compress the BP cuff to get accurate readings.

NURSING CHECKLIST

General Approach to Lymphatic System Examination

1. Observe standard precautions and don PPE such as gloves, gown, face shield, goggles, N-95 respirator mask, or face mask if the client's status warrants these protective measures.
2. Explain to the client what you are going to do.
3. Ensure that the room is warm and well-lit.

Inspection and Palpation of Lymph Nodes

Refer to Chapter 11 for examination techniques on the lymphatic vessels that drain the head and neck; Chapter 14 for the regional lymphatics of the breast, including axillary lymph nodes; and Chapter 18 on the lymphatic functions of the spleen and appendix. Examination of the thymus and bone marrow requires specialty diagnostic testing and is outside the scope of this discussion. Examination of epitrochlear, inguinal, and popliteal lymph nodes will be discussed here.

Inspection and Palpation of Epitrochlear Lymph Nodes

Epitrochlear lymph nodes are located approximately 3 cm proximal to the medial humeral epicondyle in the groove between the biceps and triceps muscles. They drain lymph afferently from the ulnar aspect of the forearm and hand, the little and ring fingers, and the ulnar part of the middle finger. These nodes are not routinely examined unless there is suspicion of infection distal to the elbow.

E
1. Place the client in a sitting position.
2. Support the client's hand with your hand.
3. Observe the epitrochlear area for lymphadenopathy.
4. With the other hand, reach behind the elbow and place your finger pads in the groove between the biceps and the triceps muscles (Fig. 17-21), superior to the medial condyle of the humerus (along the inside of the upper arm).
5. Palpate the epitrochlear nodes for size, shape, consistency, tenderness, and mobility.

N **Normally, epitrochlear lymph nodes are not visible or palpable.**

A An enlarged epitrochlear lymph node is abnormal.

P An infection (e.g., cat scratch disease, dog bite) in the forearm or hand can lead to palpable and tender epitrochlear nodes. Keep in mind that this enlargement might be a sign that the nodes are performing their job; when the infection subsides, the lymph node(s) should return to normal size.

P Malignancies can cause enlarged, hard, and nontender epitrochlear nodes.

Risk Factors

Lymphoma

Fixed (client cannot alter): Age (non-Hodgkin lymphoma risk increases with age), sex(male), race (non-Hispanic White), family history of lymphoma, history of HIV, human T-cell lymphotropic virus and Epstein Barr virus (EBV), exposure to high levels of ionizing radiation

Modifiable (client can reduce risk of lymphoma by controlling these factors): exposure to pesticides and herbicides

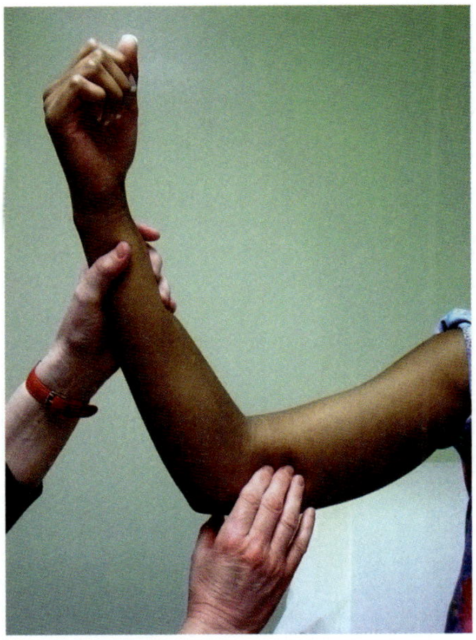

Figure 17-21 Palpation of epitrochlear lymph nodes.

E Examination N Normal Findings A Abnormal Findings P Pathophysiology

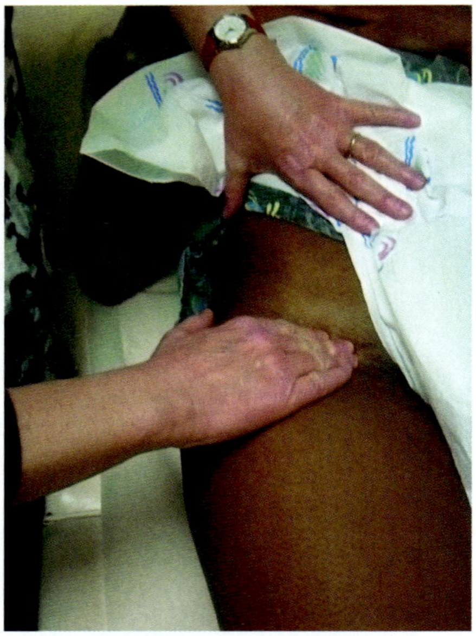

Figure 17-22 Palpation of inguinal lymph nodes.

Inspection and Palpation of Inguinal Lymph Nodes

The inguinal area contains both deep and superficial lymph nodes, but only the latter are palpable. These lymph nodes are grouped into superior and inferior chains. The superior chain is located horizontally near the inguinal ligament, and the inferior chain lies vertically below the junction of the saphenous and femoral veins.

E
1. Place the client in a supine position, with the knees slightly flexed.
2. Drape the genital area.
3. Inspect the groin for lymphadenopathy.
4. Using the finger pads of the second, third, and fourth fingers, apply firm pressure and palpate the inguinal area with a rolling motion (Fig. 17-22).
5. Palpate inguinal nodes for size, shape, consistency, tenderness, and mobility.
6. Repeat this process on the other side.

N **Inguinal lymph nodes should not be seen. It is normal to palpate small, soft, movable, and nontender nodes less than 1 cm in diameter.**

A The presence of inguinal lymph nodes greater than 1 cm in diameter or elicitation of nonmovable, tender lymph nodes is abnormal.

P Large, palpable nodes can be attributed to localized or systemic infections. Remember that this enlargement might be a sign that the nodes are performing their job; when the infection subsides, the lymph node(s) should return to normal size.

P More serious pathology associated with inguinal lymphadenopathy includes processes associated with cancer or lymphomas.

A The presence of swelling in the legs is abnormal.

P The inguinal nodes filter lymph from the legs before the lymph heads toward the thoracic duct, so swelling in the legs may indicate an obstruction. Use a tape measure to assess the client's calf circumference if any swelling is noted in the lower limbs.

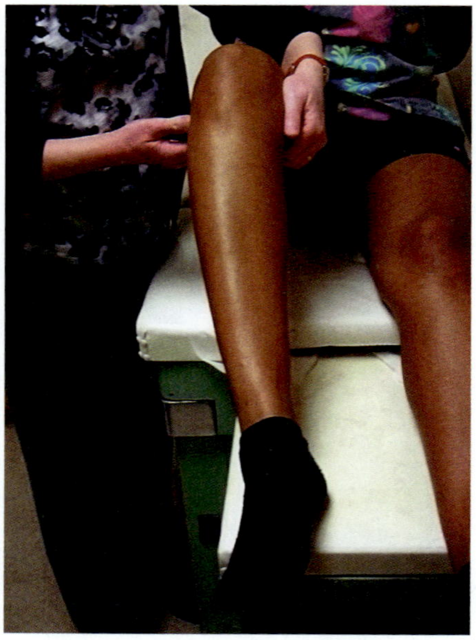

Figure 17-23 Palpation of popliteal lymph nodes.

Inspection and Palpation of Popliteal Lymph Nodes

Popliteal lymph nodes average five to seven per lower extremity and are embedded in the fat of the popliteal fossa.

E
1. Place the client in a supine position, with the knees slightly flexed.
2. Using the finger pads of the second, third, and fourth fingers of both hands, apply firm pressure and palpate the popliteal fossa of each leg (Fig. 17-23).
3. Palpate popliteal nodes for size, shape, consistency, tenderness, and mobility.
4. If an enlarged node is palpated, ask the client to assume a side-lying or prone position to inspect for visible lymphadenopathy.

N **Normally, popliteal lymph nodes are not visible or palpable.**

A An enlarged popliteal lymph node is abnormal.

P Enlarged popliteal nodes may result from foot injuries. Consider that this enlargement might be a sign that the nodes are performing their job; when the infection subsides, the lymph node(s) should return to normal size.

P A popliteal abscess may be mistaken for swollen nodes and occurs with inflammation of the knee joint, leg, or foot.

U.S. Preventive Services Task Force (USPSTF)

Grade A Recommendation:

- The USPSTF recommends screening for hypertension in adults 18 years or older with office blood pressure measurement (OBPM). The USPSTF recommends obtaining blood pressure measurements outside of the clinical setting for diagnostic confirmation before starting treatment.

Grade B Recommendations:

- The USPSTF recommends 1-time screening for abdominal aortic aneurysm (AAA) with ultrasonography in men aged 65 to 75 who have ever smoked.
- The USPSTF recommends offering or referring adults with cardiovascular disease risk factors to behavioral counseling interventions to promote a healthy diet and physical activity.
- The USPSTF recommends that clinicians prescribe a statin for the primary prevention of CVD for adults aged 40 to 75 years who have 1 or more CVD risk factors (i.e., dyslipidemia, diabetes, hypertension, or smoking) and an estimated 10-year risk of a cardiovascular event of 10% or greater.

Retrieved November 8, 2025, from *https://www.uspreventiveservicestaskforce.org/uspstf/recommendation-topics/uspstf-a-and-b-recommendations*

CASE STUDY
The Client With Leg Claudication

This case study illustrates the application and objective documentation of the peripheral vasculature system and lymphatic system examination. Ronan O'Malley is a 78-year-old Irish American retired attorney. Ronan has been having leg pain with walking for 6 months, and the pain is getting worse. Ronan recognizes that with a history of diabetes, hypertension, hyperlipidemia, and peripheral artery disease, exercise is important to maintaining health. Ronan feels frustrated that the pain is affecting quality of life. Ronan feels "old" because reliance on a cane to prevent falls has been necessary. Ronan worries about what will happen if his Parkinson disease progresses and what kind of help might be needed.

HEALTH HISTORY

CLIENT PROFILE

Ronan O'Malley is a 78-year-old Irish American male.

CHIEF COMPLAINT

"My left leg hurts when I walk."

HISTORY OF PRESENT ILLNESS

Ronan has a known history of bilateral peripheral artery disease and had a femoral-popliteal bypass on the right leg in 2015. Ronan has been experiencing increasing left lower extremity pain symptoms over the last 6 months. The pain usually occurs after walking approximately 100 yards and is relieved with rest. Client denies pain at rest, change in temperature, or color of the leg or foot; denies right leg pain. Has taken acetaminophen 500 mg every 4 hours for pain (usually 6 doses daily for the past month).

PAST HEALTH HISTORY

Medical History Hypertension, hyperlipidemia, type 2 diabetes, peripheral artery disease, bilateral carotid stenosis, Parkinson disease

Surgical History
- Cervical disc C2-4 fusion (10/2019)
- Femoral artery to popliteal artery bypass graft surgery on right leg (11/2015)
- Angioplasty of the right superficial femoral artery (6/2014)
- Bilateral cataract extraction (12/2013)
- Tonsillectomy as a child

Denies complications from all surgeries

Allergies No known drug allergies

Medications Atorvastatin 80 mg orally daily
Carbidopa-levodopa 25/100 mg orally three times daily
Clopidogrel 75 mg orally daily
Aspirin 81 mg orally daily
Lisinopril 40 mg orally daily
Hydrochlorothiazide 25 mg orally daily
Metformin 500 mg orally 2 times per day
Acetaminophen 500 to 1,000 mg orally as needed for pain

Communicable Diseases Denies recent COVID-19 exposure

Injuries and Accidents None that he can recall

Differing Abilities Denies

Blood Transfusions Unsure if any blood product was received with past surgeries

Childhood Illnesses Does not remember

Immunizations Initial COVID-19 vaccine completed and has had 7 boosters
PCV 13, PCV 20, and PPSV 23 completed
Zoster recombinant completed
Received RSV vaccine in 2024
Believes tetanus is current
Receives yearly flu shot

FAMILY HEALTH HISTORY

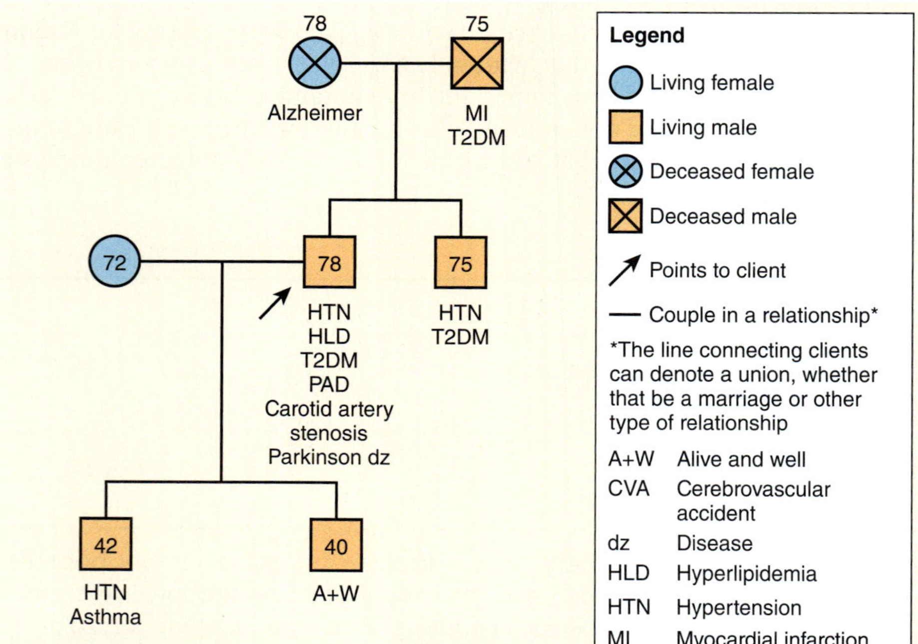

Denies family history of CVA, aneurysm, Raynaud dz, lymphoma.

SOCIAL HISTORY

Alcohol Use 1 glass of bourbon before dinner and 1 glass of wine with dinner

Tobacco Use 1 pack of cigarettes per day for 41 years, 41 pack year/history. Quit in 2013

Recreational Drug Use "Never"

Domestic and Intimate Partner Violence Denies

Sexual Practice Sexually active, one current partner. Married to female partner for 44 years. No other partners

Travel History No recent travel. Used to travel out of the country annually but has not done so for 10 years due to health

Work Environment Retired at age 70. Was a bankruptcy lawyer for the Department of Justice for 45 years

Home Environment Lives in a single-family home with 3 levels, with bedroom on second floor. Checks smoke/carbon monoxide detectors monthly. Has fire extinguisher in kitchen

Hobbies and Leisure Activities Likes to watch movies, read books, do puzzles.

Stress Denies stressors since retirement

Education Juris Doctor law degree

Economic Status No financial concerns

Military Service Was Army ROTC for 2 years in college, served one summer in Germany, and then left the service

Religion Nondenominational

Ethnic Background Irish American

Roles and Relationships Ronan's parents emigrated to the U.S. a few years before he was born. Ronan does not know any relatives in Ireland because his parents broke off all communication with them when they emigrated. Ronan's parents are now deceased. Client has an older brother, Liam, who is seen regularly. Ronan and Liam are planning to go to Ireland in 4 months to learn about their family heritage. Ronan has been married for 44 years and has 2 grown sons who live locally. Ronan's sons and their families come over once a month for a family dinner—they all get along. Client's wife, Susie, works part-time as a teaching aid in the public school system. Susie does the grocery shopping, cooking, and cleaning.

Characteristic Patterns of Daily Living "I can't sleep past 6 AM, but then I usually nap in my chair in the afternoon. I'm in bed at 11 pm after the news. I guess I'm pretty sedentary."

HEALTH MAINTENANCE ACTIVITIES

Sleep Sleeps 6-7 hours/night plus daytime napping

Diet Attempts healthy diet. "Mainly lean meat and fish with a salad. I have been trying to stay on my diabetic diet, counting carbs and checking my blood sugar."

Exercise Had been walking daily, but it has become increasingly difficult. Now uses a cane. Feels anxious about falling

Stress Management Listens to music and podcasts as well as audiobooks

Use of Safety Devices Always wears seat belt. Has a cane and now has to use it even in the house

Health Checkups Every 6 months sees primary care nurse practitioner. HbA1c checked every 6 months. Has remained in goal <7%. Has not seen vascular surgeon since 2015 surgery

PHYSICAL EXAMINATION

Examination of the Peripheral Vascular

Inspection of JVP (indirect) No distention

Inspection of Hepatojugular Reflux Negative, no change in jugular veins

Palpation and Auscultation of Arterial Pulses

- Rate: 72
- Rhythm: Regular

Pulses:

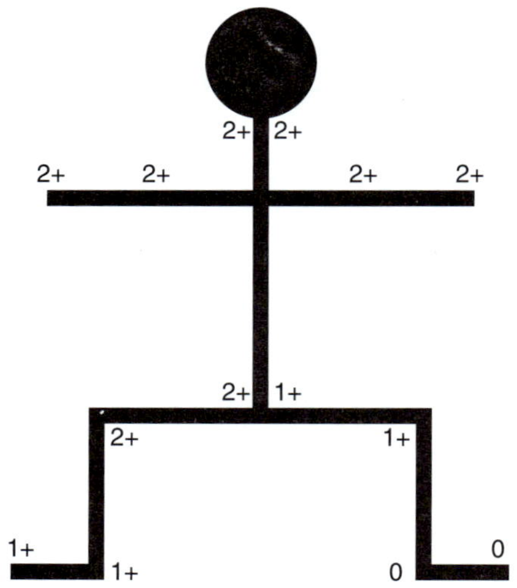

Dorsalis pedis: left pulse absent with no Doppler signal present
Posterior tibial: Doppler signal present on left
Bruits: Left femoral bruit auscultated. No right femoral bruit

Inspection and Palpation of Peripheral Perfusion

Color: Right leg warm to touch, color pink. Left leg cool from knee through toes, pale without cyanosis

Clubbing: None

Capillary refill: 3 seconds in all extremities except for the left foot, with greater than 5 seconds noted in that foot

Skin temperature: Warm throughout except cool from knee down on left leg

Edema: No pedal edema

Ulcerations: None

Skin texture: Smooth, even. No varicose veins noted

Hair distribution: Hair loss noted midcalf through ankles bilaterally

EXAMINATION OF THE LYMPHATIC SYSTEM

Inspection No swelling in epitrochlear, inguinal, or popliteal areas

Palpation

Epitrochlear: No palpable lymph nodes
Inguinal: No palpable lymph nodes
Popliteal: No palpable lymph nodes

CLINICAL JUDGMENT IN ACTION

1. What cues indicate the client is having a peripheral vasculature disorder?
2. What interventions have the highest priority?
3. What assessment findings indicate clinical improvement in this client?

Review Questions

1. What are the risk factors for lymphoma? Select all that apply.
   a. Female sex
   b. Exposure to pesticides
   c. HIV
   d. Diabetes mellitus
   e. Tobacco use
   f. Exposure to ionizing radiation
   g. Hispanic heritage

2. Which statement is true about the circulatory system?
   a. The circulatory system consists of arteries which are distribution pathways and veins that collect blood and return it to the heart
   b. The circulatory system consists of arteries that use valves to move blood against gravity and veins that move blood in a pulsatile manner
   c. The circulatory system consists of arteries that are larger and have thin walls and veins that are smaller and more elastic
   d. The circulatory system consists of the arterial low-pressure system and the venous high-pressure system

3. Vaccines are given at a young age when they will have the most impact because of what characteristic of a lymphatic organ?
   a. Bone marrow can produce B-cells throughout the aging process
   b. Tonsils trap antibodies to destroy T-and B-cells
   c. The thymus gland grows until puberty and then shrinks afterward
   d. Lymph nodes unite to present an immune response

4. Which of the following are important to remember about a TIA? Select all that apply.
   a. Waiting to see if symptoms resolve can save a client the inconvenience of a costly work-up.
   b. Blood clots cause TIAs just like strokes.
   c. A TIA is not dangerous because symptoms completely resolve.
   d. A TIA is a medical emergency.
   e. It is impossible to know if a client is experiencing a TIA or a stroke at the onset of symptoms.
   f. Weakness, facial droop, slurred speech, and paresthesia can be symptoms of both a stroke and a TIA.

5. The nurse observes right-sided JVD with a JVP of 6 in a client with chest pain. The left jugular vein has a JVP of 3. What conclusion can the nurse draw from this examination finding?
   a. The client has right-sided heart failure, but normal left heart function.
   b. This is a normal examination finding because the right heart pressure is always higher than the left.
   c. The client has a positive hepatojugular reflux.
   d. The client has a local vein blockage on the left.

6. What phenomenon occurs during inspiration that results in a decrease in filling of the left ventricle and can be observed in clients with cardiac tamponade and restrictive pericarditis?
   a. Homan test
   b. Pulsus paradoxus
   c. Ankle-Brachial index
   d. Orthostatic hypotension

7. Enlarged inguinal lymph nodes are noted on examination with tenderness to palpation. The nurse recognizes that this finding could be attributed to which of the following conditions? Select all that apply.
   a. Metastatic cancer
   b. Lymphoma
   c. Cat scratch fever of the lower extremity
   d. Systemic infection
   e. Seasonal allergies
   f. Ingestion of toxins

8. A bruit is a sign of turbulent blood flow. Nurses recognize this as a significant clinical finding because it indicates which condition?
   a. An obstruction in the blood vessel
   b. Adequate flow in a high-pressure blood vessel
   c. Hypertensive emergency
   d. Systemic fluid overload

9. A 30-year-old client experiences acute calf pain with erythema and swelling after returning to New York from a business trip to Japan. The nurse taking the health history in the emergency department recognizes that the client is most at risk for which vascular condition?
   a. Varicose veins
   b. Acute arterial occlusion
   c. Deep venous thrombosis
   d. Raynaud phenomena

10. Which of the following interventions help prevent varicose veins? Select all that apply.
    a. A low-fat diet
    b. Smoking cessation
    c. Wearing antiembolic stockings
    d. Crossing the legs frequently
    e. Elevating the legs when possible

CHAPTER

18 Abdomen

Learning Outcomes

1. Identify the anatomy and physiology of the abdomen.
2. Conduct a complete health history on a client with an abdominal condition.
3. Perform a physical examination on a healthy adult and an adult with abdominal pathology.
4. Differentiate between normal clinical findings from a client's physical examination of the abdomen and the pathophysiology of abnormal clinical findings.
5. Identify risk factors for abdominal cancers: esophageal, stomach, pancreatic, colorectal, liver, renal, and bladder.
6. Identify risk factors for hepatitis.
7. Identify risk factors for urinary tract infections.
8. Identify the United States Preventive Services Task Force recommendations for the abdomen.
9. Document a complete health history and physical examination of a client with abdominal pathology.

Assessing the abdomen requires a complete understanding of anatomical and abdominal examination norms. Examination of the abdomen provides significant information about the various functions of the gastrointestinal, cardiovascular, and genitourinary systems.

Anatomy and Physiology

Abdominal Cavity

The abdomen is the largest cavity of the body. It is located between the diaphragm and the symphysis pubis, is oval-shaped, and contains several vital organs. The posterior wall of the cavity includes the lumbar vertebrae, the sacrum, and the coccyx. The iliac bones and the lateral portion of the ribs shape the sides of the abdominal cavity (Figs. 18-1 and 18-2). These bony structures are held together by muscular tissue that surrounds the entire abdominal cavity. The muscles of the abdomen include the rectus abdominis, transversus abdominis, external oblique, and internal oblique. The **linea alba**, a tendinous tissue that extends from the sternum to the symphysis pubis in the midline of the abdomen, is situated between the rectus abdominis muscles (Fig. 18-3).

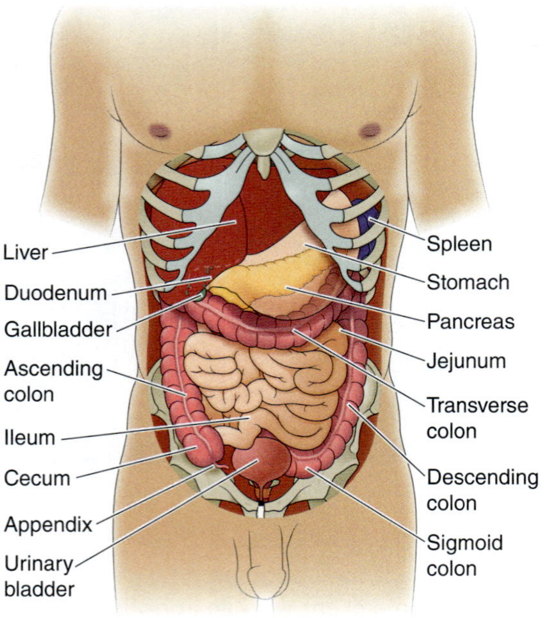

Figure 18-1 Structures of the abdomen: Anterior view.

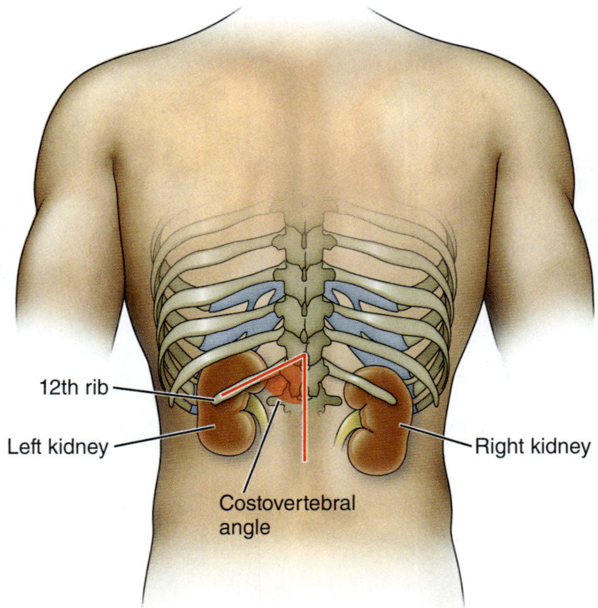

Figure 18-2 Structures of the abdomen: Posterior view.

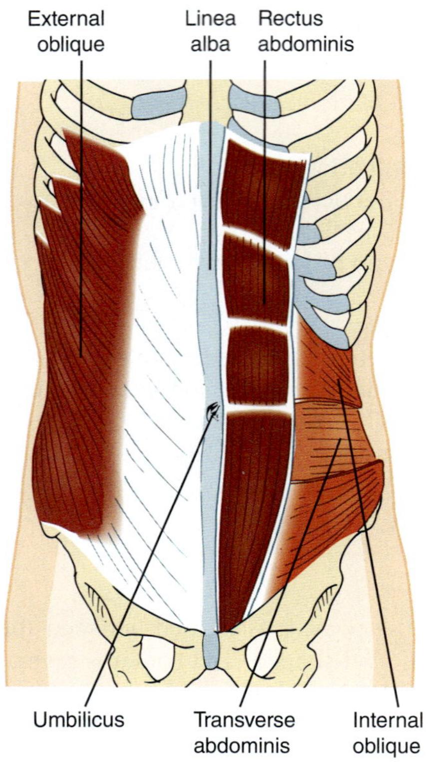

Figure 18-3 Abdominal musculature.

Peritoneum

The abdominal cavity's endothelial lining consists of peritoneal serous membranes. The serous layer that lines the walls of the cavity itself is called the parietal peritoneum and that which covers the organs is called the visceral peritoneum. The potential space between the two layers is referred to as the peritoneal cavity. This cavity is completely closed in the male, whereas openings exist for the fallopian tubes in the female.

The organs covered with peritoneum and held in place by mesentery are referred to as intraperitoneal organs. The intraperitoneal organs are the spleen, gallbladder, stomach, liver, bile duct, small intestine, and large intestine. In contrast, the organs situated behind the peritoneum and without mesenteric attachment are known as retroperitoneal organs. The retroperitoneal organs are the pancreas, kidneys, ureters, and bladder.

Abdominal Vasculature

The aorta is the largest artery in the body. Below the level of the diaphragm, the descending aorta becomes the abdominal aorta, giving rise to arterial vessels that supply the abdominal wall and gastrointestinal organs with blood (Fig. 18-4). At about the fourth lumbar vertebra, the aorta bifurcates to become the right and left common iliac arteries.

Anatomical Mapping

Anatomical maps serve as a frame of reference during examination of the abdomen. The abdominal cavity can be subdivided using two methods: quadrants or nine regions.

The four-quadrant technique is the most commonly used examination approach in clinical practice (Fig. 18-5). For accuracy in documentation, the abdominal surface is divided into four sections by imaginary vertical and horizontal lines intersecting at the umbilicus. Commit to memory the location of abdominal organs according to quadrants (Table 18-1). Table 18-2 lists pathologies by the quadrant or region where the pain is perceived.

Another strategy for pinpointing the location of abdominal examination findings is via nine abdominal anatomical regions (Fig. 18-6). You can also use the anatomical landmarks in Figure 18-7.

Abdominal Viscera (Organs)

Stomach

The stomach is a J-shaped, pouchlike organ located in the left upper quadrant of the abdomen beneath the diaphragm; it lies to the right of the spleen and is partially covered by the liver.

The stomach functions as a reservoir where the complex mechanical and chemical processes of digestion occur. Hydrochloric acid and digestive enzymes are secreted by the stomach to aid digestion. Little absorption of foodstuffs occurs in the stomach. Foodstuffs are liquified via gastric secretions into a semisolid substance called chyme. The usual capacity of the stomach is 1 to 1.5 L. In a regulated manner, chyme is released into the small intestine's duodenum for further digestion and absorption.

Small Intestine

The small intestine is a tubular-shaped organ extending from the pyloric sphincter to the ileocecal valve at the opening of the large intestine. The majority of foodstuffs are digested and absor bed in the small intestine. The convoluted loops of intestine are relatively mobile and can measure from 10 feet to 30 feet, depending on the degree of muscular relaxation of the intestinal wall and the size of the individual. Portions of the small intestine can be found in all four abdominal quadrants. The three segments of the small intestine are the duodenum, the jejunum, and the ileum. The duodenum is the first and shortest section. It plays a significant role in digestion because hormonal secretions are released and both the common bile and main pancreatic ducts open into the duodenum. The jejunum, the second component, is composed of circular mucosal folds that provide surface area for nutrient absorption. The ileum absorbs bile salts and vitamin B_{12}. The ileum terminates at the ileocecal valve.

Table 18-1 Four-Quadrant Anatomical Map

Right Upper Quadrant (RUQ)	Left Upper Quadrant (LUQ)
Liver	Left lobe of liver
Gallbladder	Stomach
Pylorus	Spleen
Duodenum	Pancreas (body)
Pancreas (head)	Portion of left kidney and adrenal gland
Portion of right kidney and adrenal gland	Splenic flexure of colon
Hepatic flexure of colon	Sections of transverse and descending colons
Section of ascending and transverse colons	
Right Lower Quadrant (RLQ)	**Left Lower Quadrant (LLQ)**
Appendix	Sigmoid colon
Cecum	Section of descending colon
Lower pole of right kidney	Lower pole of left kidney
Right ureter	Left ureter
Right ovary	Left ovary
Right spermatic cord	Left spermatic cord

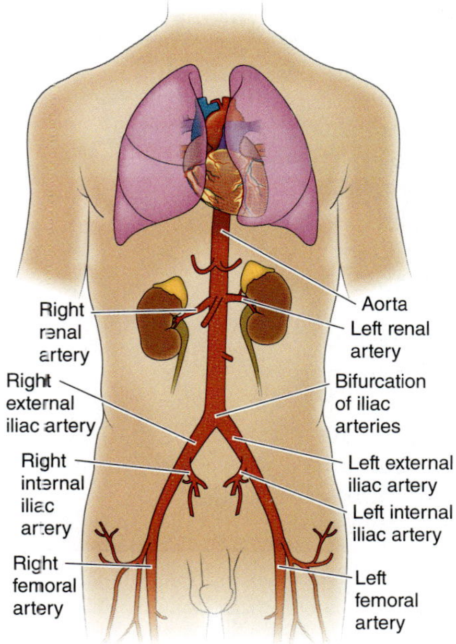

Figure 18-4 Abdominal vasculature.

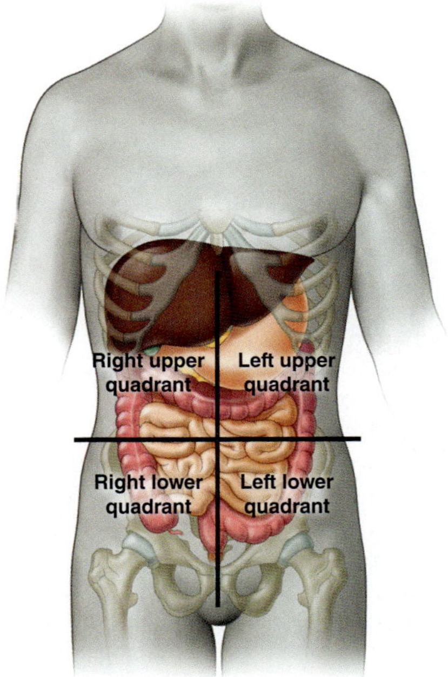

Figure 18-5 Abdominal quadrants.

Table 18-2 Etiologies of Abdominal Pain: Anatomical Regions Where They Are Perceived

Right Upper Quadrant	Epigastrium	Left Upper Quadrant
Biliary stone Cholecystitis Cholelithiasis Colitis Duodenal ulcer Gastric ulcer Hepatic abscess Hepatitis Hepatomegaly Nephrolithiasis Pancreatitis Pneumonia Pulmonary embolus Pyelonephritis	Abdominal aortic aneurysm Appendicitis (early) Biliary stone Cholecystitis Cholelithiasis Diverticulitis Gastroesophageal reflux disease/ gastritis Hiatal hernia Myocardial infarction Pancreatitis Peptic ulcer disease	Colitis Gastric ulcer Gastritis Myocardial infarction Nephrolithiasis Pneumonia Pulmonary embolus Pyelonephritis Splenic enlargement Splenic rupture
	Periumbilical	
	Abdominal aortic aneurysm and dissection Appendicitis (early) Diverticulitis Intestinal obstruction Irritable bowel syndrome Mesenteric ischemia Pancreatitis Peptic ulcer Recurrent abdominal pain (in children) Small bowel obstruction Volvulus	
Right Lower Quadrant		**Left Lower Quadrant**
Appendicitis Diverticulitis Ectopic pregnancy (ruptured) Endometriosis Hernia (strangulated) Inflammatory bowel disease Irritable bowel syndrome Mittelschmerz		Diverticulitis Ectopic pregnancy (ruptured) Endometriosis Hernia (strangulated) Inflammatory bowel disease Irritable bowel syndrome Mittelschmerz Ovarian cyst
Right Lower Quadrant		**Left Lower Quadrant**
Ovarian cyst Pelvic inflammatory disease Renal calculi Salpingitis Uterine fibroids		Pelvic inflammatory disease Renal calculi Salpingitis Uterine fibroids
	Diffuse	
	Gastroenteritis Herpes zoster Muscle strain Peritonitis	

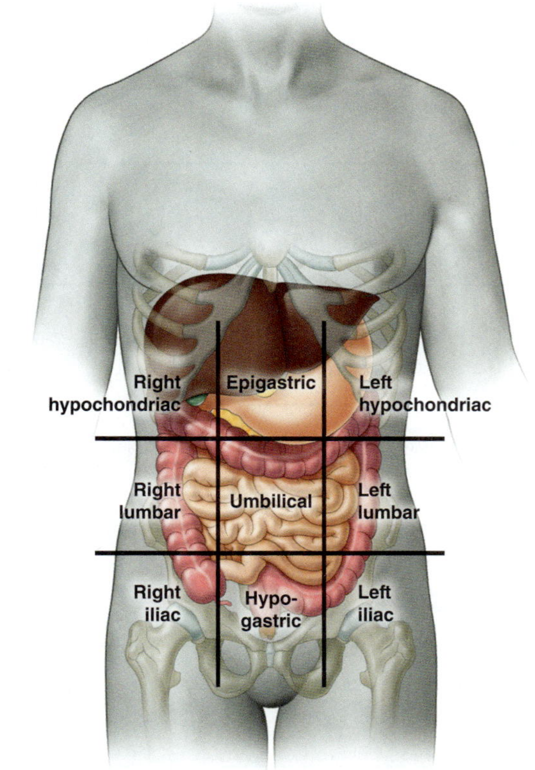

Figure 18-6 Nine abdominal anatomical regions.

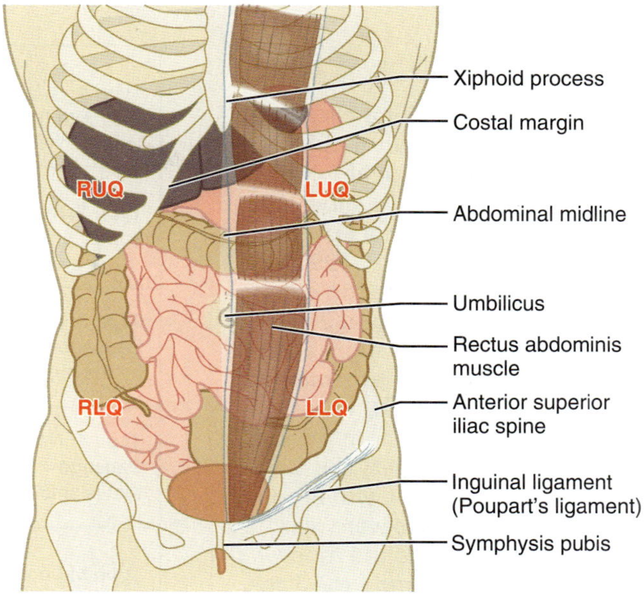

Figure 18-7 Abdominal examination landmarks. When describing the pathology of the abdomen, it is useful to use these anatomical landmarks: 1. xiphoid process; 2. costal margin; 3. abdominal midline; 4. umbilicus; 5. rectus abdominis muscle; 6. anterior superior iliac spine; 7. inguinal ligament (Poupart's ligament); 8. symphysis pubis. LLQ = left lower quadrant, LUQ = left upper quadrant, RLQ = right lower quadrant, RUQ = right upper quadrant.

Large Intestine

The large intestine is a tubular-shaped organ extending from the ileocecal valve to the anus. It has a greater diameter than the small intestine and can vary considerably in length, depending on the size of the individual, but generally is about 5 feet long.

The four segments of the large intestine are the ascending, transverse, descending, and sigmoid colons. The cecum is the blind pouch that is continuous with the ascending colon, the large intestine located in the lower right quadrant of the abdomen.

The work of the large intestine is to form stool from cellulose, indigestible fibers, fat, bacteria, cellular debris, and inorganic materials, and then carry these intestinal contents to the end of the gastrointestinal tract. An additional function of the large intestine is the absorption of water and electrolytes. Water absorption occurs primarily in the ascending colon, under the influence of the osmotic pressure gradient produced by sodium ions. The large intestine has limited digestive function.

> **NURSING TIP**
> **Cause of Flatulence**
> Most gases are nitrogen and oxygen derived from swallowing. Bacterial gas formation occurs in the large intestine and is expelled as flatus.

Liver

The liver is the largest solid organ in the body. It lies directly below the diaphragm. The liver is located in the right upper quadrant but extends across the midline into the left upper quadrant. In the right upper quadrant, the superior aspect of the liver is at the fifth rib, or at the nipples. The lower border does not extend more than 1 to 2 cm below the right costal margin.

The functions of the liver are complex and varied, and can be divided into:

- Storage (carbohydrates, amino acids, vitamins, minerals, and blood)
- Detoxification and filtration (drugs, hormones, and bacteria)
- Metabolism (carbohydrates, proteins, fat, ammonia to urea)
- Synthesis and secretion (bile production—600 to 1,000 mL/day, formation of lymph, bile salts, plasma proteins, fibrinogen, blood-clotting substances, and antibodies)

> **NURSING TIP**
>
> **Bristol Stool Form Scale**
>
> It can be difficult for a client to describe the exact nature of stools. To assist in identifying stool, it is practical to show the client the Bristol Stool Form Scale (Lewis & Heaton, 1997). This can provide clues on colon transit time. Types 1 and 2 can be classified as constipation, and the client usually needs to strain with defecation (Fig. 18-8). Types 3 and 4 are the most comfortable stools to pass. Stool types 5, 6, and 7 are associated with urgency, with 7 constituting severe diarrhea. Type 1 stool spends the most time in the colon and type 7 the least.

Bristol Stool Chart

Type 1: Severe constipation Separate hard lumps of stool	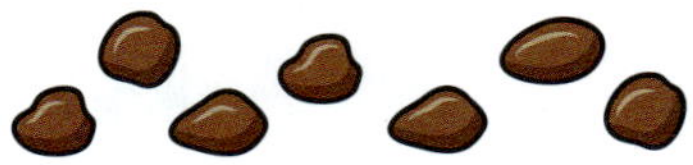
Type 2: Mild constipation Lumpy and sausage-shaped stool	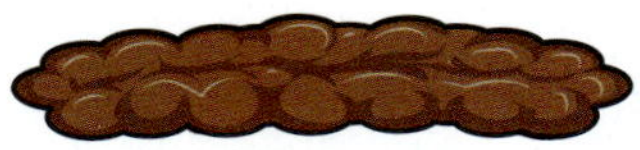
Type 3: Normal Sausage-shaped stool with cracks on the surface	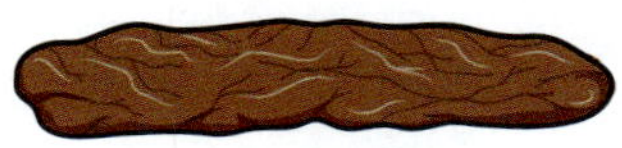
Type 4: Normal Sausage- or snake-shaped stool that is smooth and soft	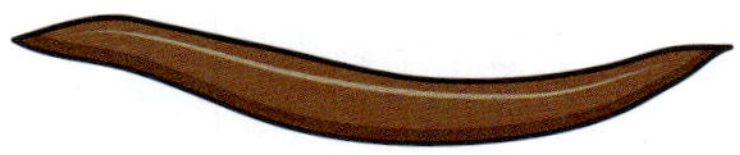
Type 5: Lacks fiber Soft blobs with clear edges	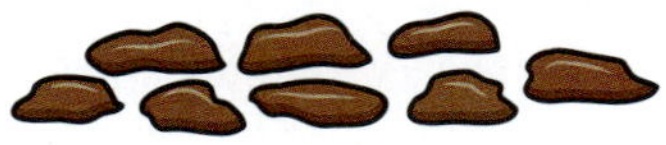
Type 6: Mild diarrhea Mushy stool with ragged edges	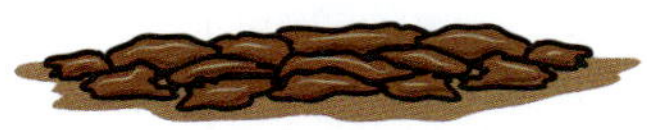
Type 7: Severe diarrhea Liquid stool with no solid pieces	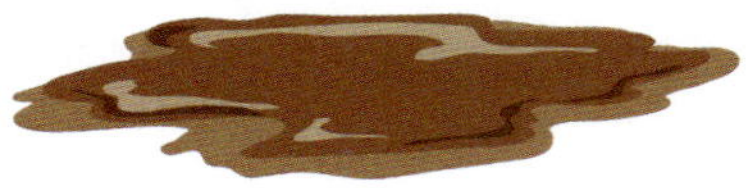

Figure 18-8 Bristol Stool Form Scale.

Gallbladder

The gallbladder is a pear-shaped sac located in the right upper quadrant of the abdomen. It is attached to the inferior surface of the liver.

The primary role of the gallbladder is to store and concentrate the bile produced by the liver. Bile contributes to fat digestion and absorption. The gallbladder stores approximately 30 to 50 mL of bile and releases bile in the presence of cholecystokinin, pancreozymin, and parasympathetic stimulation. As the gallbladder contracts, bile is released through the cystic duct into the common bile duct, which drains into the duodenum.

Pancreas

The pancreas is an elongated accessory organ of digestion. It lies in a transverse position along the posterior abdominal wall. It is located in the upper right and upper left quadrants of the abdomen. The pancreas is both an exocrine gland that secretes bicarbonate and pancreatic enzymes (which aid in digestion), and an endocrine gland that secretes the hormones insulin, glucagon, and gastrin.

Spleen

The spleen is the largest lymph organ in the body. It is oval-shaped and is composed of white, pulpy lymphoid tissue and red pulp containing capillaries and venous sinuses. It is located behind the fundus of the stomach, below the diaphragm, and above the left kidney and splenic flexure. The spleen is found in the left upper quadrant of the abdomen.

The spleen is part of the reticuloendothelial system and serves the body as a filter and a reservoir for red blood cell mass. During events that can cause vasoconstriction, such as hemorrhage or exercise, the spleen contributes needed blood to the general circulation. As a filter, the spleen rids the body of old or deformed red blood cells and platelets.

Vermiform Appendix

The vermiform appendix extends off the lower cecum in the right lower quadrant. This fingerlike appendage fills with digestive materials from the cecum. The vermiform appendix frequently does not empty completely, causing obstruction and subsequent infection.

Kidneys, Ureters, and Bladder

The kidneys are bean-shaped organs that lie tucked against the posterior abdominal wall. The left kidney is slightly larger in some individuals. Because of the superior placement of the liver over the right kidney, that kidney tends to hang about half an inch lower than the left, between T12 and L3.

The primary function of the kidneys is to rid the body of waste products and to maintain homeostasis through regulation of the acid-base balance, fluid and electrolyte balance, and arterial blood pressure.

Urine leaves the kidneys via the ureters. Peristaltic waves move the waste products to the bladder. The bladder stores urine. Normally the bladder holds 200 to 400 mL of urine, however, its capacity is greater.

HEALTH HISTORY

The abdominal health history provides insight into the link between a client's life/lifestyle and abdominal information and pathology.

CLIENT PROFILE

Diseases that are age- and sex-specific for the abdomen are listed.

Age Recurrent abdominal pain (2 to 15)
- Appendicitis (young child to 30)
- Peptic ulcer disease (>30, with an increased incidence in the older adult)
- Cholecystitis (40 to 50)
- Diabetes mellitus, type 2 (>45)
- Diverticulosis (>50)
- Esophageal cancer (>55)
- Stomach cancer (60 to 80)
- Pancreatic cancer (>65)
- Colorectal cancer (>50)
- Bladder cancer (>55)
- Pernicious anemia (older adult)
- Mesenteric arterial insufficiency or infarct (more prevalent in older adults, especially those with arteriosclerotic or atherosclerotic disease)

Sex
- **Female** Gallbladder disease, mittelschmerz (ovulatory pain), celiac disease
- **Male** Colorectal cancer, pancreatic cancer, esophageal cancer, liver cancer, stomach cancer, renal cancer, bladder cancer, cirrhosis, duodenal ulcer, diverticulosis

Race/Ethnicity Bladder cancer: White Americans
- Colorectal cancer: Native Americans, Alaska Natives, Black Americans, people of Ashkenazi Jewish descent
- Liver cancer: Asian Americans, Pacific Islanders
- Pancreatic cancer: Black Americans
- Renal cancer: Black Americans
- Stomach cancer: Black Americans, Hispanic Americans, Native Americans, Asian Americans, Pacific Islanders

CHIEF COMPLAINT

Common chief complaints for the abdomen are defined, and information on the characteristics of each sign or symptom is provided.

1. **Nausea** An uncomfortable sensation in the stomach and abdominal region
   Quality Retching (dry heaves)
   Associated Manifestations Vomiting, medication use, fever, chills, foods eaten, fluids consumed, diarrhea, pregnancy
   Aggravating Factors Noxious odors
   Alleviating Factors Flat soda, dry crackers, sleep, antiemetics
   Timing Early morning, bedtime, middle of the night, after eating, after missed menstrual period
2. **Vomiting** Expulsion of contents from the upper gastrointestinal tract via contraction of abdominal wall muscles and relaxation of the esophageal sphincter
   Quality Color (bright red: fresh blood; coffee-grounds appearance: "old" blood that has had time to mix with digestive juices; dark brown or black: bile; other colors may occur secondary to food intake), projectile
   Associated Manifestations Nausea, medications, fever, chills, abdominal pain, headache, foods eaten, fluids consumed, weight loss, diarrhea, pregnancy
   Aggravating Factors Noxious odors
   Alleviating Factors Flat soda, dry crackers, sleep, antiemetic medications
   Timing Early morning, bedtime, middle of the night, after eating, after missed menstrual period
3. **Diarrhea** Frequent watery stools resulting in the loss of essential electrolytes
   Quality Color; presence of blood or mucus, fatty or frothy appearance; presence of undigested food; unusual odor
   Associated Manifestations Abdominal cramping, pain, physical weakness, weight loss, fever, stress, consumption of sugar-free food/drink
   Aggravating Factors Food, medications, stress
   Alleviating Factors Diet (bananas, rice, apples, toast), medications, fluids with electrolyte supplement, physical rest
   Setting History of inflammatory bowel disease, irritable bowel diseases, celiac disease
   Timing Recent travel, especially areas with unpotable water; recent antibiotic use; laxative use; stool softener use; contaminated well water
4. **Constipation** Infrequent stools resulting in the passage of dry, hard fecal waste
   Quality Color, odor, appearance of blood
   Associated Manifestations Physical discomfort, rectal fullness, nausea, bloating, pain with defecation
   Aggravating Factors Food, medications (e.g., iron, narcotics), stress
   Alleviating Factors High-fiber diet, medications (e.g., laxatives, stool softeners, enemas), physical activity, increased fluid intake
   Setting Decreased fluid intake
5. **Abdominal Pain** Discomfort in the abdomen; may be visceral, parietal, or referred pain (Table 18-3 and Figure 18-9)
   Quality Dull, burning, sharp, gnawing, stabbing, cramping (severe cramping is referred to as colic pain), aching
   Associated Manifestations Bleeding, flank pain, weight loss, nausea and vomiting, jaundice, eructation, fever or chills, changes in bowel habits, flatus, prolonged immobility, menstrual cycle, cough/wheeze
   Aggravating Factors Position, stress, eating, smoking, medications (e.g., aspirin, steroids, NSAIDs), alcohol or drug use, caffeine, food (spicy, citrus, mint, chocolate)
   Alleviating Factors Antacids, proton pump inhibitors (PPI), histamine-2 antagonists, rest, diet, stress management, position change
   Setting Home environment, work environment, mealtimes, social occasions involving alcohol or drug use
   Timing Pre- or postprandial, nighttime, seasonal, stressful situations, menstruation, gradual, sudden

6. **Hoarseness** Husky or harsh quality of the voice due to gastroesophageal reflux disease (GERD) or other conditions
   - **Quality** Audible, inaudible
   - **Associated Manifestations** GERD, fever, sore throat, malaise, vocal cord mass
   - **Aggravating Factors** Inhalation of chemicals or noxious fumes, smoking, overuse of voice, alcohol use, recent upper respiratory infections (URIs), recent head and neck surgery, intubation, neck trauma, recumbent or supine position within 2 hours of eating
   - **Alleviating Factors** Medications, adequate hydration, voice rest
   - **Setting** Public speaking, singing, yelling, normal speech, after eating, reclining after eating especially if fatty foods were consumed
   - **Timing** Continuous, intermittent
7. **Increased Flatulence** Passage of excess gas via the rectum
   - **Quantity** Marked increase over client's normal status
   - **Associated Manifestations** Ingestion of certain foods (onions, cabbage, beans, cauliflower, corn, wheat, barley, rye)
   - **Aggravating Factors** Food or medications
   - **Alleviating Factors** Avoidance of particular foods that are fermentable
   - **Timing** Following meals
8. **Dysuria** Painful urination
   - **Location** Suprapubic, near urinary meatus, costovertebral angle
   - **Quality** Burning, stabbing
   - **Associated Manifestations** Abdominal/flank/testicular pain, fever, chills, current sexually transmitted infection (STI) or urinary tract infection (UTI), hematuria, dribbling, urethral discharge, decreased urinary flow, urgency, hesitancy, nocturia, recent sexual intercourse
   - **Aggravating Factors** Presence of prostatic stones or renal calculi, decreased oral intake
   - **Alleviating Factors** Medications (e.g., antibiotics, pyridium, analgesics, D-mannose), passage or surgical removal of stone, transurethral resection of the prostate, increased oral intake
   - **Setting** New sexual partner in the last 6 months, a sexual partner known to have other sexual partners, unprotected intercourse, vigorous intercourse, wiping genitalia back to front (female), recent explosive diarrhea
   - **Timing** At start of urination, midstream, throughout stream, sense of urgency, pregnancy
9. **Nocturia** Night arousal to void
   - **Associated Manifestations** Hesitancy, decrease in force of urinary stream, postvoid dribbling, urge incontinence
   - **Aggravating Factors** Enlarged prostate, diabetes mellitus, diuretics, UTI, alcohol ingestion, anticholinergic medications, diuretics, decongestants, cough medicines
   - **Alleviating Factors** Adrenergic antagonists, 5-alpha-reductase inhibitors, transurethral resection of prostate, elimination of causative medications
10. **Urinary Incontinence** Involuntary loss of urine
    - **Quality** Constant, intermittent, dribbling, large volumes, hesitancy
    - **Quantity** Frequency, urgency, number of pads used
    - **Associated Manifestations** Recent surgery, coughing, sneezing, crying, laughing, heavy lifting, activity, medications, UTI, constipation, spinal cord lesions, neurological disease
    - **Aggravating Factors** Medications, caffeine intake, alcohol intake
    - **Alleviating Factors** Pelvic floor muscle rehabilitation, bladder training, biofeedback, anti-incontinence devices, medications
    - **Setting** Accessibility of toilet, distance to toilet, adequate lighting to toilet, grab bars by toilet, height of toilet seat
    - **Timing** Nocturia, after childbirth, after menopause

PAST HEALTH HISTORY

The various components of the past health history are linked to abdominal pathology and abdomen-related information.

Medical History

Abdomen Specific Malignancies, peritonitis, cholecystitis, appendicitis, pancreatitis, small bowel obstruction, ulcerative colitis, Crohn disease, hepatitis, hiatal hernia, diverticulitis, diverticulosis, peptic ulcer disease, acute renal failure, chronic renal failure, gallstones, kidney stone, irritable bowel syndrome, gastroesophageal reflux disease, *Helicobacter pylori* infection *(H. pylori),* UTI, parasitic infections, food poisoning, cirrhosis, infectious mononucleosis, hyper- or hypoadrenalism, malabsorption syndromes (e.g., celiac disease), gut fermentation syndrome

Non-Abdomen Specific Pulmonary tuberculosis, malaria, heart disease, thyroid or parathyroid disease, pneumonia, URIs, allergies, postnasal discharge, sinusitis, stress, STI, puberty, menopause, diabetes, ketoacidosis, ectopic pregnancy, cystic fibrosis, endometriosis, lupus, sickle cell anemia

Surgical History

Abdomen Specific Cholecystectomy, gastrectomy, Billroth I or II, ileostomy, colostomy, appendectomy, colectomy, nephrectomy, pancreatectomy, ileal conduit, portal caval shunt, splenectomy, hiatal/umbilical/ventral/femoral/inguinal hernia, hernia repair, removal of renal calculi, liver transplant, renal transplant, bariatric surgery, Stretta procedure, esophageal dilation, PEG placement

Non-Abdomen Specific Hysterectomy with or without bilateral salpingo-oophorectomy

Allergies Ingestion of certain food types or medications may cause gastric irritation, nausea, and vomiting; lactose intolerance, celiac disease

Medications Histamine-2 antagonists, PPI, antibiotics, probiotics, gastrointestinal motility enhancer, lactulose, antacids, vitamins, antiparasitics, anticholinergics, steroids, antidiarrheals, electrolytes, laxatives, stool softeners, insulin, antiemetics, antiflatulents, tumor necrosis factor blocker, aminosalicylates, monoclonal antibody, 5-HT_3 receptor antagonist

Communicable Diseases Hepatitis A virus (HAV), hepatitis B virus (HBV), hepatitis C virus (HCV), hepatitis D virus (HDV), hepatitis E virus (HEV), STI, HIV, Mpox, tuberculosis, infectious mononucleosis, intestinal parasites

Injuries and Accidents Abdominal trauma such as ruptured or bruised organs, gunshot wounds, or knife stabbings; swallowing of foreign bodies

Blood Transfusions Since 1992 blood and blood products have been tested for HIV and other communicable diseases. There is still a risk of contracting a communicable disease, but it is very small.

Immunizations Hepatitis A and hepatitis B vaccines

FAMILY HEALTH HISTORY

Familial abdominal diseases and disorders are listed.

Malignancies of the stomach, liver, pancreas, colon, bladder; peptic ulcer disease, diabetes mellitus, familial adenomatous polyposis, inflammatory bowel disease, irritable bowel syndrome, polycystic kidney disease, colitis, malabsorption syndromes (e.g., celiac disease), cystic fibrosis

SOCIAL HISTORY

The components of the social history are linked to abdominal factors and pathology.

Alcohol Use Altered nutrition, impaired gastric absorption, increased risk for upper and lower gastrointestinal bleeding, cirrhosis of liver

Recreational Drug Use Opioids reduce peristalsis and are associated with the development of constipation. Injected drug use is a risk factor for HAV, HBV, HCV, HDV.

Sexual Practice Men who have sex with men (MSM) and individuals who have numerous sex partners increase their risk for HAV, HBV, HCV, HDV.

Travel History Infectious diarrhea may be caused by bacteria such as *Escherichia coli* and parasites in contaminated food or water.

Work Environment Hazardous chemical exposure can increase the risk for various cancers. Health-care workers, emergency medical and public safety workers, as well as day-care workers have a higher risk for hepatitis because of their exposure to blood and body fluids. Refer to Hepatitis Risk Factors for additional information.

Home Environment Living in an environment with poor sanitation and contaminated food and water are risk factors for HAV and HEV.

Hobbies and Leisure Activities Sports such as lacrosse, football, rugby, and boxing often associated with traumatic injuries

Economic Status Bacterial, viral, and parasitic diseases from poor sanitation

HEALTH MAINTENANCE ACTIVITIES

This information provides a bridge between health maintenance activities and abdominal function.

Sleep Nocturnal pain with peptic ulcer disease; hiatal hernia/GERD discomfort in recumbent position

Diet Healthy diet as a means of avoiding abdominal pathology; gallbladder attack after fatty meals; caffeinated beverages, coffee, tea, alcohol, tomatoes, citrus, onions, garlic, chocolate, spicy food, fatty food, and fried food exacerbate GERD; smoked foods, salted fish/meat, pickled vegetables, frequent consumption of processed, grilled, or charcoaled meats increase the risk for stomach cancer

Exercise Regular exercise facilitates gastrointestinal functioning.

Stress Management High stress levels are associated with stress ulcers.

Use of Safety Devices Shoulder and lap restraints in automobiles to prevent abdominal injuries; appropriate sports safety equipment to protect abdominal region

Health Checkups Blood chemistry: Elevated glucose and HbA1c might indicate onset of diabetes mellitus; elevated liver function tests may indicate liver or gallbladder pathology

Blood count: Anemia can indicate a silent gastrointestinal bleed

Urinalysis: Dark color may signify bilirubin in urine; urine culture may indicate a UTI

Stool guaiac: Positive results must be investigated for colorectal pathology

Colonoscopy: Screening (a preventive procedure to identify any pathology in a client who has no symptoms) versus diagnostic (procedure to identify probable pathology in a client with symptoms)

Esophageal manometry: May show slowed esophageal motility or increased contractions

Capsule endoscopy: May show tumors, ulcerations, or other disease of the small intestine

Fluoroscopy esophagram: May show reflux, polyps/tumors, strictures, swallowing/muscular disorder

H. pylori breath test: Positive result indicates *H. pylori* bacteria in the stomach which can lead to stomach ulceration

Small intestine bacterial overgrowth breath test: positive results may reveal cause of bloating, diarrhea, and digestive symptoms

Fecal microbiota transplant: Feces from a healthy person are inserted into a client with chronic infections such as *Clostridioides difficile (C. diff)*

Table 18-3 Differentiating Abdominal Pain

	Visceral Pain	Parietal Pain	Referred Pain
Origin	Originates in the abdominal organs	Originates in the parietal peritoneum	Originates from abdominal organs to non-abdominal locations (e.g., chest, spine, or pelvis). The sensory cortex perceives pain via nerve fibers where the internal abdominal organs were located in fetal development (Fig. 18-9)
Cause	Hollow structures become painful when they contract forcefully or when distended (e.g., intestines); solid organs become painful when stretched	Inflammation	Nerve innervation
Characteristics	Deep, dull, poorly localized; usually begins as dull pain, but when it becomes intense, is associated with nausea, vomiting, pallor, and diaphoresis	Sharp, precisely localized; usually severe from the onset and intensifies with movement	Well localized; pain is from a disorder in another site, for example: duodenal pain (back and right shoulder); pancreatic pain (back and left shoulder)

NURSING TIP

Bloody Vomitus

Hematemesis, or the vomiting of blood, may be attributed to gastrointestinal ulcers or esophageal varices. Active bleeding is a medical emergency, and the client should be promptly treated.

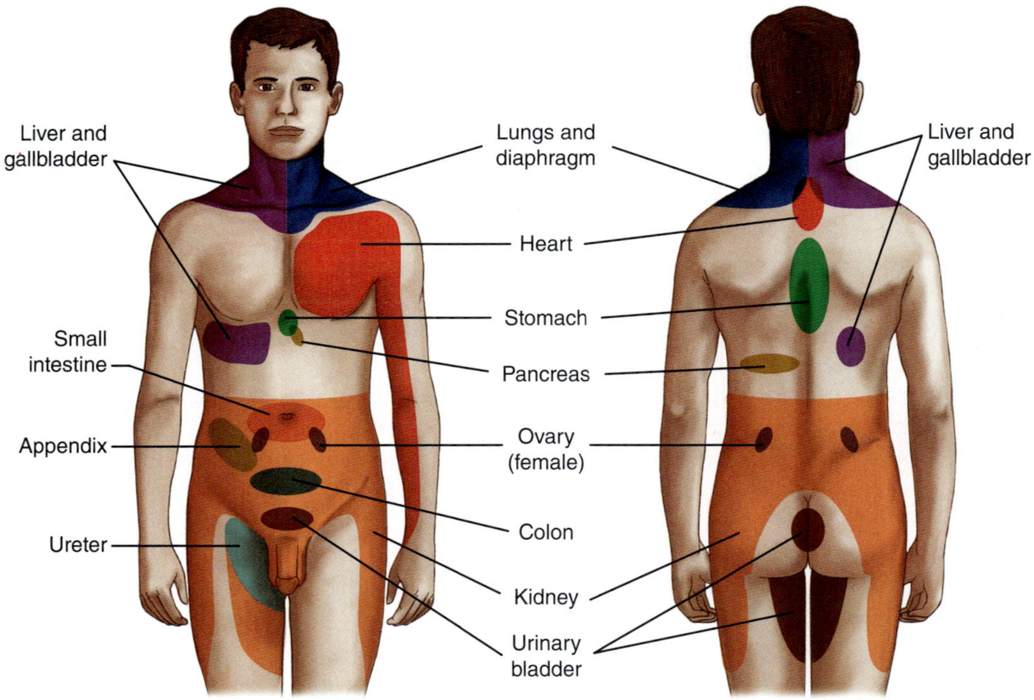

Figure 18-9 Areas of referred pain.

NURSING TIP

American Cancer Society Guidelines for the Early Detection of Colorectal Cancer and Polyps

Beginning at age 45, adults of average risk should be screened for colorectal cancer and polyps. Individuals who are in good health and with a life expectancy of more than 10 years should continue regular colorectal cancer screening through the age of 75. For individuals ages 76 through 85, the decision to be screened should be based on a person's preferences, life expectancy, overall health, and prior screening history. Individuals over age 85 should no longer get colorectal cancer screening.

For screening purposes, individuals are considered at average risk if they do not have:

- A personal history of colorectal cancer or certain types of polyps
- A family history of colorectal cancer
- A personal history of inflammatory bowel disease (ulcerative colitis or Crohn disease)
- A confirmed or suspected hereditary colorectal cancer syndrome, such as familial adenomatous polyposis (FAP) or Lynch syndrome (hereditary nonpolyposis colon cancer or HNPCC)
- A personal history of getting radiation to the abdomen or pelvic area to treat a prior cancer

Individuals of average risk should follow one of these testing schedules:

Tests that find polyps and cancer:

- Flexible sigmoidoscopy every 5 years*, or
- Colonoscopy every 10 years, or
- CT colonography (virtual colonoscopy) every 5 years*

Tests that primarily find cancer:

- Yearly guaiac-based fecal occult blood test (gFOBT)*, **, or
- Yearly fecal immunochemical test (FIT) every year*, **, or
- Multitargeted stool DNA test (mt-sDNA) every 3 years*

* If the test is positive, a colonoscopy should be done.

** The multiple stool take-home test should be used. One test done by a [health-care provider] is not adequate for testing.

Adapted from *https://www.cancer.org/cancer/colon-rectal-cancer/detection-diagnosis-staging/acs-recommendations.html* (retrieved December 17, 2025).

NURSING CHECKLIST

General Approach to Abdominal Examination

1. Observe Standard Precautions and don Personal Protective Equipment (PPE) such as gloves, gown, face shield, goggles, N-95 respirator mask, or face mask if the client's status warrants these protective measures.
2. Greet the client and explain the examination technique.
3. Ensure that the room is at a warm, comfortable temperature to prevent the client from chilling and shivering.
4. Use a quiet room that will be free from interruptions.
5. Utilize an adequate light source. This includes both a bright overhead light and a freestanding lamp for tangential lighting.
6. Ask the client to urinate before the examination. Save a urine sample for analysis if indicated.
7. Drape the client from the xiphoid process to the symphysis pubis, then expose the client's abdomen.
8. Position the client comfortably in a supine position with knees flexed over a pillow or position the client so that the arms are either folded across the chest or at the sides to ensure abdominal relaxation.
9. Stand to the right side of the client for the examination.
10. Visualize the underlying abdominal structures during the examination process so that you can accurately describe the location of any pathology.
11. Have the client point to tender areas; examine these last. Mark these and other significant findings (scars, dullness, and so on) on the body diagram in the client's chart.
12. Watch the client's face closely for signs of discomfort or pain.
13. Help the client relax by using an unhurried approach, diverting attention with questions, and so on.
14. Ensure that your hands and the stethoscope are warm to promote client comfort.

Assessment in Brief

Abdominal Examination

Inspection

- Contour
- Symmetry
- Rectus abdominis muscles
- Pigmentation and color
- Scars
- Striae
- Respiratory movement
- Masses and nodules
- Visible peristalsis
- Pulsation
- Umbilicus

Auscultation

- Bowel sounds
- Vascular sounds
- Venous hum
- Friction rub

Percussion

- General percussion
- Liver span
- Liver descent
- Spleen
- Stomach
- Fist percussion
    - Kidney
    - Liver
- Bladder

Palpation

- Light palpation
- Abdominal muscle guarding
- Deep palpation
- Liver
    - Bimanual method
    - Hook method
- Spleen
- Kidneys
- Aorta
- Bladder

Advanced Techniques

- Liver scratch test
- Assessing for ascites
    - Shifting dullness
    - Puddle sign
    - Fluid wave
- Murphy sign
- Rebound tenderness
- Rovsing sign
- Cutaneous hypersensitivity
- Iliopsoas muscle test
- Obturator muscle test
- Ballottement

Assistive Devices

- Tubes
    - Enteral tube
    - Nasogastric suction tube
    - Intestinal tube
    - Gastrostomy
    - Peritoneal dialysis catheter
- Drains
    - Abdominal cavity drain
    - Biliary drain
- Intestinal diversions
    - Colostomy
    - Ileostomy
- Urinary diversions
    - Ileal conduit
    - Ureteral stent
    - Indwelling catheter

Equipment

- Appropriate PPE
- Drapes
- Small pillow for under knees
- Tape measure or small ruler with centimeter markings
- Marking pencil
- Gooseneck lamp for tangential lighting
- Stethoscope
- Sterile safety pin or sterile needle

NURSING TIP

7 Fs of Abdominal Distention

Seven possible causes of abdominal distention are:

- Fat
- Fluid (ascites)
- Flatus
- Feces
- Fetus
- Fatal growth (malignancy)
- Fibroid tumor

Examination of the Abdomen

The order of abdominal examination is inspection, auscultation, percussion, and palpation. Auscultation is performed second because palpation and percussion can alter bowel sounds.

Inspection

Contour

E 1. View the contour of the client's abdomen from the costal margin to the symphysis pubis.

2. Position tangential light lengthwise across the client's abdomen at a right angle.
3. Position yourself on a horizontal plane looking at the client's abdomen and view the contour (Fig. 18-10).

N **In the normal adult, the abdominal contour is flat (straight horizontal line from the costal margin to symphysis pubis) or rounded (convexity of the abdomen from the costal margin to symphysis pubis).**

A Assessment reveals a large, convex, symmetrical profile from the costal margin to the symphysis pubis.

P A large convex abdomen can result from one of the 7 Fs (refer to the Nursing Tip on the 7Fs).

A A convex abdomen that has a marked increase at the height of the umbilicus is abnormal.

P A protuberant abdomen can result from a wide range of disorders. Taut stretching of the skin across the abdominal wall may occur (refer to the Nursing Tip on the 7Fs).

A A concave, symmetrical profile from the costal margin to the symphysis pubis is abnormal.

P A scaphoid abdomen reflects a decrease in fat deposits, a malnourished state, or flaccid muscle tone.

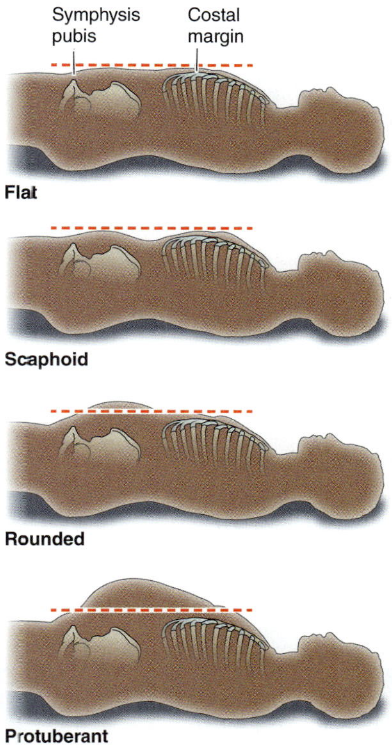

Figure 18-10 Abdominal contours.

Symmetry

E
1. View the symmetry of the client's abdomen from the costal margin to the symphysis pubis.
2. Move to the foot of the examination table and recheck the symmetry of the client's abdomen.

N **The abdomen should be symmetrical bilaterally.**

A Assessment reveals an asymmetrical abdomen.

P Asymmetry may be caused by a tumor, cysts, bowel obstruction, enlargement of abdominal organs, or scoliosis. Bulging at the umbilicus can indicate an umbilical hernia.

P If the abdomen is asymmetrical at the site of a surgical incision or scar, suspect an incisional hernia.

Rectus Abdominis Muscles

E
1. Instruct the client to raise the head and shoulders off the examination table.
2. Observe the rectus abdominis muscles for separation.

N **The symmetry of the abdomen remains uniform; no ridge is observed parallel to the umbilicus or between the rectus abdominis muscles.**

A A ridge between the rectus abdominis muscles is observed.

P A ridge between the rectus abdominis muscles is known as diastasis recti abdominis and is attributed to marked obesity or past pregnancy. The observed separation of rectus abdominis muscles is caused by increased intra-abdominal pressure and is not considered to be harmful or ominous.

Pigmentation and Color

E View the color of the client's abdomen from the costal margin to the symphysis pubis.

N **The abdomen should be uniform in color and pigmentation.**

A Uneven skin color or pigmentation is abnormal.

Risk Factors

Esophageal Cancer

- Age (risk increases after age 55)
- Gender (male)
- Gastroesophageal reflux disease
- Barrett esophagus
- Tobacco use
- Alcohol use
- Obesity
- Diet (a diet high in fruits/vegetables decreases the risk)
- Achalasia (esophageal sphincter disorder)
- History of other cancers (e.g., lung, mouth, throat)
- Rare conditions such as tylosis and Plummer-Vinson syndrome
- Chemical exposure (e.g., lye ingestion)
- Esophageal human papillomavirus

Adapted from *https://www.cancer.org/cancer/esophagus-cancer/causes-risks-prevention/risk-factors.html* (retrieved December 17, 2025).

E Examination **N** Normal Findings **A** Abnormal Findings **P** Pathophysiology

P The presence of jaundice suggests liver dysfunction. The yellow discoloration of the skin in light-skinned clients is due to the accumulation of bilirubin in the blood. The average level for visible jaundice is 2 mg/dL.

P In light-skinned individuals, the observation of a blue tint at the umbilicus suggests free blood in the peritoneal cavity, known as **Cullen sign**. Such bleeding can occur either following the rupture of a fallopian tube secondary to an ectopic pregnancy, or with acute hemorrhagic pancreatitis.

P Six or more café au lait spots that are more than 1.5 cm in diameter may be associated with neurofibromatosis type 1, also known as von Recklinghausen disease, a familial condition associated with the formation of neurofibromas.

A Engorged abdominal veins are abnormal.

P The appearance of engorged or dilated veins around the umbilicus is called **caput medusae**. It is associated with circulatory obstruction of the superior or the inferior vena cava. In some instances, this condition is related to obstruction of the portal vein or emaciation.

A A network of dilated veins on the abdomen is abnormal.

P A network of dilated veins on the abdomen occurs in portal hypertension, cirrhosis, and vena cava obstruction secondary to increased venous pressures.

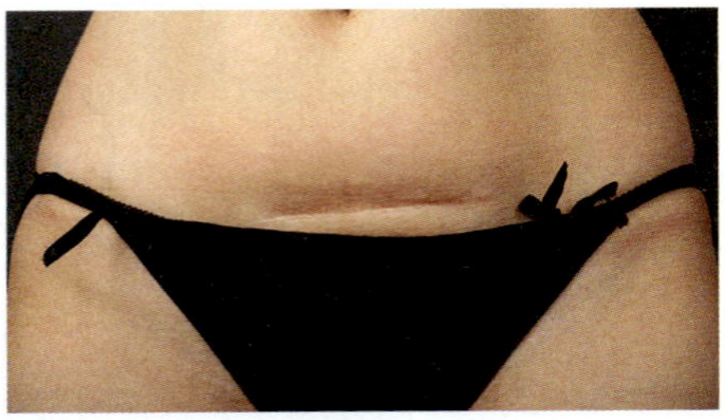

Figure 18-11 Abdominal scar from a Caesarean section.

Scars

E
1. Inspect the abdomen for scars from the costal margin to the symphysis pubis.
2. Note the location, size, and condition (old or new) of all scars.
3. Document the size, location, and condition in the client record.

N **There should be no abdominal scars.**

A Scars are present (Fig. 18-11).

P The location of scars discloses useful information about the client's surgical history. Dense, irregular, collagenous scars are keloids, which are more common in the higher-pigmented skin of persons of color and may be associated with traumatic injuries or burns. The presence of surgical scars may indicate internal adhesions.

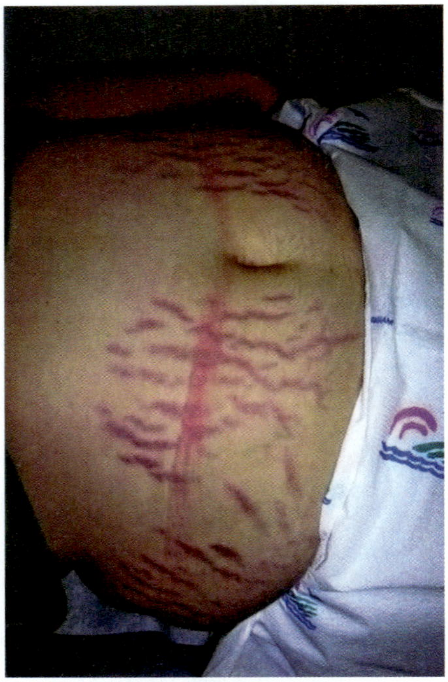

Figure 18-12 Abdominal striae.

Striae

E Observe the abdominal skin for **striae**, or abdominal atrophic lines or scars.

N **No evidence of striae is present.**

A Striae are present (Fig. 18-12).

P Striae, atrophic lines or streaks, occur when there has been rapid or prolonged stretching of the skin. Abdominal striae may be caused by Cushing syndrome, abdominal tumors, obesity, ascites, or pregnancy. Following pregnancy, striae are a normal finding.

Respiratory Movement

E Observe the abdomen for smooth, even respiratory movement.

N **There is no evidence of respiratory retractions. Normally, the abdomen rises with inspiration and falls with expiration.**

A Abnormal respiratory movements and retractions are observed.

P The origin of abnormal respirations due to an abdominal disorder may include appendicitis with local peritonitis, pancreatitis, biliary colic, or a perforated ulcer.

Masses and Nodules

E 1. Observe the abdominal skin for nodules and masses.
2. Have the client touch the chin to the chest.

N **No masses or nodules are present.**

A Abdominal masses or nodules are present.

P The presence of abdominal masses or nodules may indicate tumors, metastases of an internal malignancy, or pregnancy.

P Multiple small, soft, rubbery masses can be seen in neurofibromatosis. Refer to Figure 18-13.

P A bulge over an abdominal incision may indicate an incisional hernia. A ventral hernia can appear as a bulge in the abdominal wall.

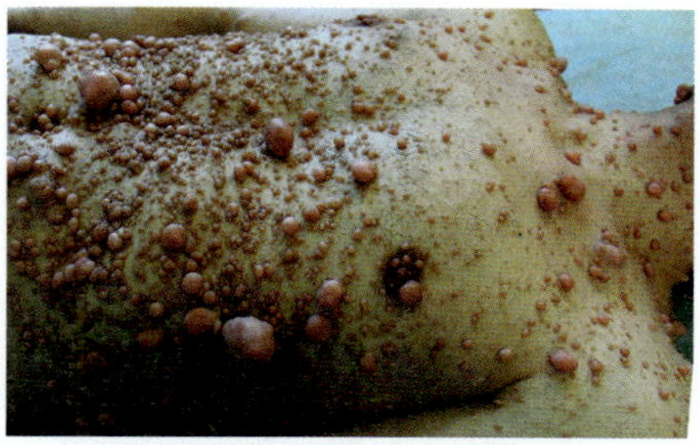

Figure 18-13 Neurofibromatosis.

Visible Peristalsis

E Observe the abdominal wall for surface motion.

N **Ripples of peristalsis may be observed in clients of thin body habitus. Peristaltic movement slowly traverses the abdomen in a slanting, downward direction.**

A Strong peristaltic contractions are observed.

P Strong peristaltic waves may indicate intestinal obstruction.

Pulsation

E Inspect the epigastric area for pulsations.

N **In the client with a normal build, a nonexaggerated pulsation of the abdominal aorta may be visible in the epigastric area. In clients with a heavy build, pulsations may not be visible.**

A Marked, strong abdominal pulsations are observed.

P Widened pulse pressure and strong epigastric pulsations may indicate an aortic aneurysm. An exaggerated pulsation can also occur in aortic regurgitation and right ventricular hypertrophy.

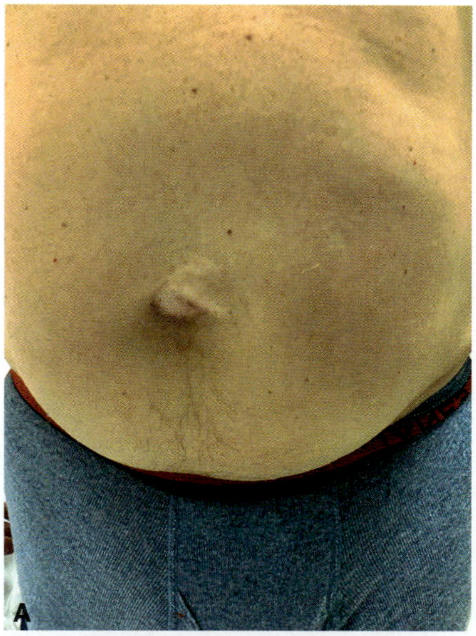

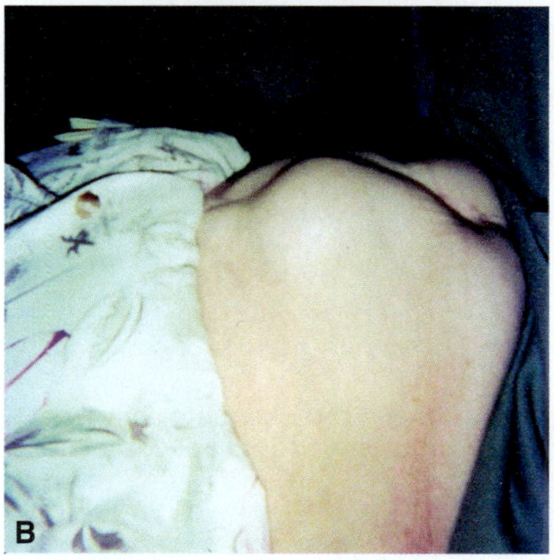

Figure 18-14 Hernias. **A.** Umbilical hernia. **B.** Ventral hernia.

Umbilicus

E 1. Observe the umbilicus in relation to the abdominal surface.
2. Ask the client to flex the neck and perform the Valsalva maneuver.
3. Observe for protrusion of the intestine through the umbilicus.

N **The umbilicus is depressed and beneath the abdominal surface.**

A The umbilicus protrudes above the abdominal surface.

P Umbilical hernia in the adult is the protrusion of part of the intestine through an incomplete umbilical ring (Fig. 18-14A). Umbilical hernia is confirmed by inserting the index finger into the navel and feeling an opening in the fascia. It can often be seen when the client's intra-abdominal pressure increases when coughing, sneezing, laughing, and straining occur.

A A singular protrusion in the abdominal wall is abnormal.

P A ventral hernia is a protrusion that occurs in an area other than the umbilicus or groin (Fig. 18-14B). It frequently occurs at postoperative sites.

P The umbilicus that appears as a nodule may be the manifestation of abdominal carcinoma with metastasis to the umbilicus. This physical finding is known as Sister Mary Joseph nodule.

P Intra-abdominal pressure from ascites, masses, or pregnancy can cause the umbilicus to protrude.

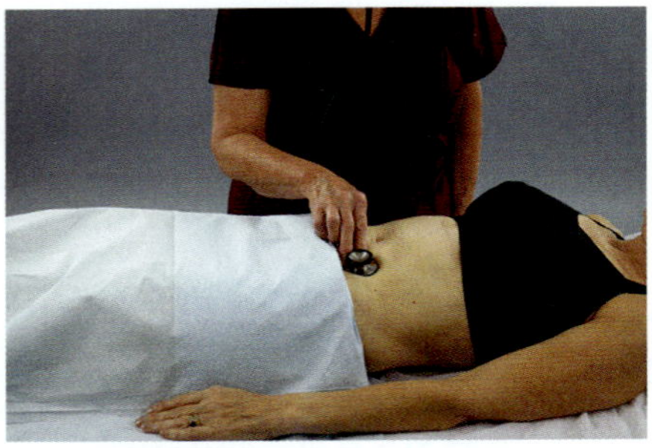

Figure 18-15 Technique of abdominal auscultation.

Auscultation

Before examining the abdomen, if the client has a nasogastric tube that is connected to suction, discontinue the suction to avoid interfering with auscultation findings. Remember to turn the suction back on after the examination.

Bowel Sounds

E

1. Place the diaphragm of the stethoscope lightly on the abdominal wall beginning at the RLQ.
2. Listen to the frequency and character of the bowel sounds. It is necessary to listen for at least 5 minutes in an abdominal quadrant before concluding that bowel sounds are absent.
3. Move the diaphragm to the RUQ, LUQ, and LLQ (Fig. 18-15).

N **Bowel sounds are heard as intermittent gurgling sounds throughout the abdominal quadrants. Usually, they are high-pitched sounds and occur 5 to 30 times per minute. Bowel sounds result from the movement of air through the gastrointestinal tract. Normally, bowel sounds are always present at the ileocecal valve area (RLQ).**

Normal hyperactive bowel sounds are called borborygmi. They are loud, audible, gurgling sounds. Borborygmi may be due to hyperperistalsis ("stomach growling") or the sound of flatus in the intestines.

A Absent bowel sounds are abnormal.

P Absent bowel sounds are indicative of late intestinal obstruction, both mechanical and nonmechanical in nature. Mechanical obstruction of the bowel may result from extraluminal lesions such as adhesions, hernias, and masses. In nonmechanical obstruction, the gastrointestinal lumen remains unobstructed, but the muscles of the intestinal wall cannot move its contents. This type of obstruction can be caused by physiological, neurogenic, or chemical imbalances that result in paralytic ileus.

A Hypoactive bowel sounds are abnormal.

P Hypoactive or diminished bowel sounds indicate decreased motility of the bowel and can occur with peritonitis and nonmechanical obstruction. Other causes include inflammation, gangrene, electrolyte imbalance, and intraoperative manipulation of the bowel.

A Hyperactive bowel sounds are abnormal.

P Hyperactive or increased bowel sounds signify increased motility of the bowel and can result from gastroenteritis, diarrhea, laxative use, and subsiding ileus.

P Auscultation of high-pitched, tinkling hyperactive bowel sounds is indicative of partial obstruction. These sounds are caused by the powerful peristaltic action of the bowel segment attempting to eject its contents through a narrow, constricted area. Frequently, clients complain of abdominal cramping.

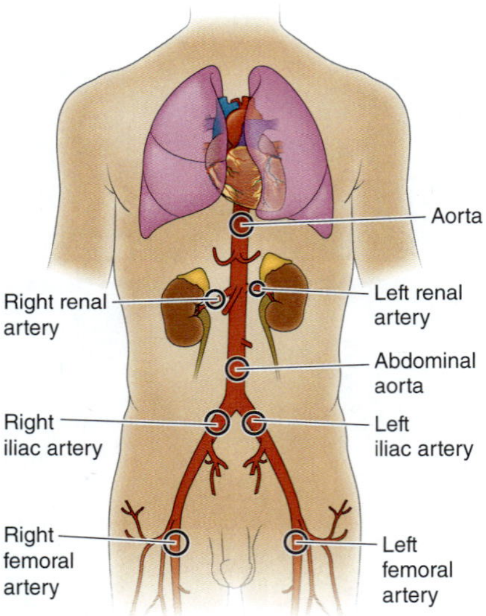

Figure 18-16 Stethoscope placement for auscultating abdominal vasculature.

Vascular Sounds

E

1. Place the bell of the stethoscope over the abdominal aorta, renal arteries, iliac arteries, and femoral arteries (Fig. 18-16).
2. Listen for bruits over each area (Fig. 18-17).

N **No audible bruits are auscultated.**

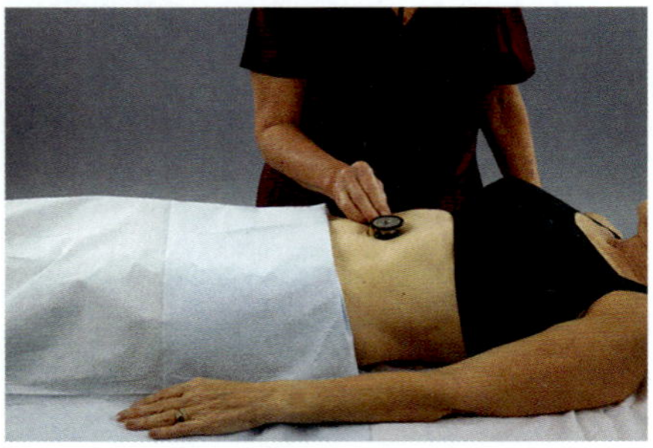

Figure 18-17 Auscultation for aortic bruits with bell of stethoscope.

NURSING CHECKLIST

General Approach to Abdominal Assistive Devices

For all tubes, drains, and intestinal and urinary diversions, note color, odor, amount, consistency, and the presence of blood in any drainage. Check for an obstruction if there is no drainage. The skin around the device should be intact without excoriation.

Tubes

1. Enteral Tubes
   a. Nasogastric, nasoduodenal, or nasojejunal.
   b. Check the residual amount frequently.
2. Nasogastric Suction Tubes
   a. Levin or Salem sump.
   b. Ensure that the suction setting (intermittent or continuous) is set at the appropriate suction level.
3. Intestinal Tubes
   a. Miller-Abbott, Cantor, Johnston, or Baker.
   b. Ensure that the tube is advancing with peristalsis as expected.
   c. Ensure that the suction setting is at the appropriate suction level.
4. Gastrostomy
   a. Continuous versus intermittent feeding.
   b. With intermittent feedings, a clamp is applied when not in use.
   c. Tube should be secured to the abdomen.
   d. Check that dressing is applied.
5. Peritoneal Dialysis Catheter
   a. Continuous ambulatory versus automated peritoneal dialysis.
   b. Catheter is capped when not in use.
   c. Catheter should be secured to the abdomen.

Drains

1. Abdominal cavity drain (e.g., Jackson-Pratt, Hemovac)
   a. To self-suction or wall suction; if wall suction, ensure that it is set at the appropriate level.
2. Biliary drain (T-tube)
   a. Tube is below insertion site.

Intestinal Diversions

1. Colostomy
   a. Stoma is pink.
   b. Skin barrier should be used around stoma if appliance is worn.
   c. Evacuation method: natural or irrigation.
2. Ileostomy
   a. Stoma is pink.
   b. Skin barrier is used and appliance is worn.
   c. If client has Kock pouch, nipple valve is pink; frequency of drainage.

Urinary Diversions

1. Ileal conduit
   a. Stoma is pink.
   b. Skin barrier is used with appliance.
2. Ureteral stents
   a. Stent is secured to collection bag.
   b. No bleeding from insertion site.
3. Indwelling catheter
   a. Balloon inflated.
   b. Catheter secured to client to prevent dislodgement.
   c. Urinary collecting bag is closed.
   d. Drainage tube is below level of bladder and without kinks.

A Audible bruits are auscultated.

P A bruit over an abdominal vessel indicates turbulence of blood flow and suggests a partial obstruction. Bruits can occur with abdominal aortic aneurysm, renal artery stenosis, and femoral artery stenosis.

Venous Hum

E Using the bell of the stethoscope, listen for a **venous hum**, or a continuous, medium-pitched sound, in all four quadrants.

N Venous hums are normally not present in adults.

A A continuous pulsing or fibrillary sound is auscultated.

P A venous hum in the periumbilical area is usually due to obstructed portal circulation. Portal hypertension caused by cirrhosis of the liver impedes portal circulation.

Friction Rubs

E
1. Using the diaphragm of the stethoscope, listen for a friction rub over the right and left costal margins, the liver, and the spleen.
2. Listen for a friction rub in all four quadrants.

N **No friction rubs should be present.**

A Friction rubs are high-pitched sounds that resemble the sound produced by two pieces of sandpaper being rubbed together. The sound increases with inspiration.

P Friction rubs occur when tumors, inflammation, or infarct cause the visceral layers of the peritoneum to rub together over the liver and the spleen.

Percussion

General Percussion

E
1. Systematically percuss all four quadrants. Begin percussion in the RUQ and proceed to the LUQ, then move down to the LLQ and cross to the RLQ (Fig. 18-18).
2. Visualize each organ in the corresponding quadrant; note when tympany changes to dullness.

N **Tympany is the predominant sound heard because air is present in the stomach and the intestines. It is a high-pitched sound of long duration. In clients with obesity, it may be difficult to elicit tympany due to the quantity of adipose tissue. Dullness is normally heard over organs such as the liver or a distended bladder. Dull sounds are high-pitched and of moderate duration.**

A Dullness over areas where tympany normally occurs, such as over the stomach and intestines, is considered abnormal.

P Dullness may be caused by a mass or tumor, pregnancy, ascites, or a full intestine.

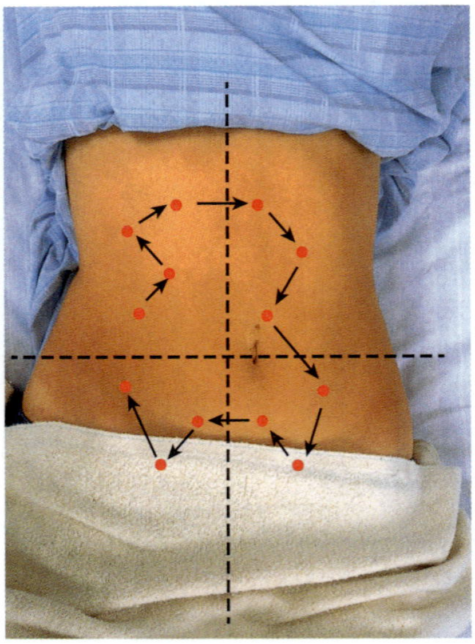

Figure 18-18 Direction of pattern of abdominal percussion.

Liver Span

E
1. Stand to the right side of the client.
2. Begin at the right midclavicular line below the umbilicus and percuss upward to determine the lower border of the liver (Fig. 18-19A).
3. With a marking pen, mark where the sound changes from tympany to dullness.
4. Then, at the right midclavicular line, percuss downward from an area of lung resonance to one of dullness.

5. With a tape measure or ruler, measure the two marks in centimeters (Fig. 18-19B).

N **Normally, the distance between the two marks is 6 to 12 cm in the midclavicular line. There is a direct correlation between body size and the size of the liver. The mean span for a man is 10.5 cm and for a woman is 7.0 cm.**

A A liver span greater than 12 cm or less than 6 cm is considered abnormal.

P The liver span is increased when the liver becomes enlarged. Hepatomegaly can occur with various liver diseases such as hepatitis, cirrhosis, cardiac or renal congestion, cysts, or metastatic tumors.

P The liver span can be falsely increased when the upper border is obscured by the dullness of lung consolidation with pneumonia or pleural effusion.

P The liver span can be decreased in the later stages of cirrhosis when the disease causes liver atrophy.

P The liver span can be falsely decreased when gas in the colon, tumors, or pregnancy pushes the lower border of the liver upward.

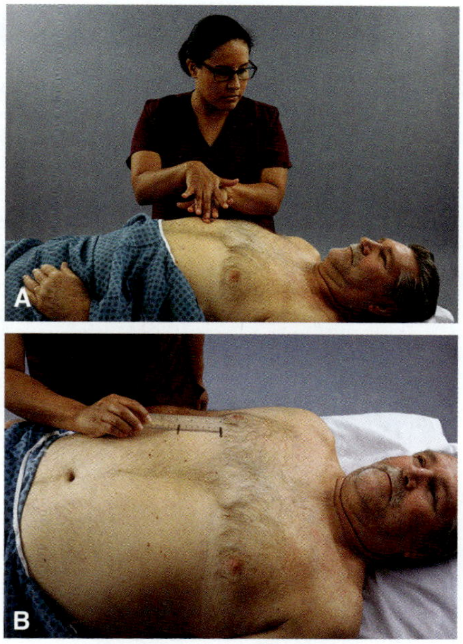

Figure 18-19 Percussing liver span. **A.** Determining lower liver border. **B.** Measuring liver span.

Liver Descent

E
1. Percuss the liver descent by asking the client to take a deep breath and hold it (because on inspiration, the diaphragm moves downward).
2. Again, percuss the lower border of the liver at the right midclavicular line by percussing from tympany to dullness. Have the client exhale.
3. Repercuss the liver-lung border.
4. Mark where the change in sound takes place.
5. Measure the difference in centimeters between the two lower borders of the liver.

N **Normally, the area of lower border dullness descends 2 to 3 cm.**

A The liver descent is considered abnormal if it is greater or less than 2 to 3 cm.

P A liver descent greater than 2 to 3 cm can be due to hepatomegaly, as in cirrhosis.

P A liver descent of less than 2 cm can be due to abdominal tumors, pregnancy, or ascites.

ADVANCED TECHNIQUE

Assessing the Liver Border: Liver Scratch Test

It can be difficult to palpate the liver border if a client's abdomen is distended or if the muscles are tense. An alternative method to determine the lower edge of the liver is the liver scratch test.

E
1. Place your stethoscope in the right midclavicular line at the lower rib cage.
2. With your other hand, scratch short strokes in the right midclavicular line starting in the right lower quadrant of the abdomen (Fig. 18-20).
3. Continue to scratch with short strokes every 1 to 2 cm toward the stethoscope.
4. The scratching sound will be louder when you reach the lower liver border.

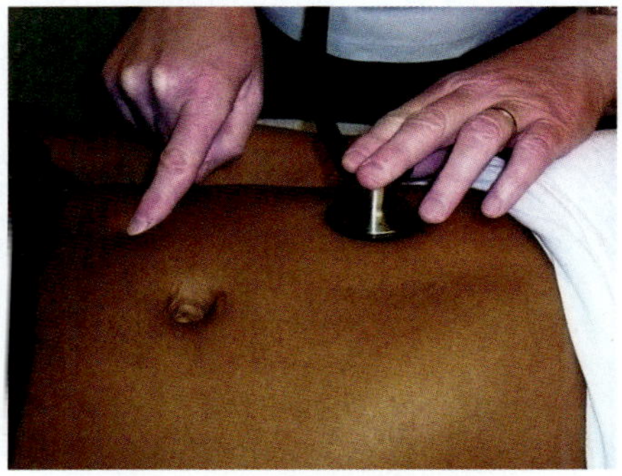

Figure 18-20 Performing the liver scratch test.

Risk Factors

Hepatitis A Virus (HAV) Risk Factors

- Food and water contamination
- Poor sanitation (sewage disposal)
- Poor personal hygiene (poor hand washing, especially after defecation)
- People experiencing homelessness
- International travel, especially in less developed countries or endemic areas
- People with close personal contact with an international adoptee
- Sexual contact with an infected person
- Males who have sex with males
- People who use or inject drugs
- Chronic liver disease including other types of hepatitis
- HIV Infection
- People with occupational risk exposure (e.g., working in a day-care center where diapers are changed)

Hepatitis B Virus (HBV) Risk Factors

- Injection drug use with shared needles
- Frequent contact with blood/body fluids and exposure to contaminated needles or other sharp instruments (e.g., health-care workers)
- HIV infection
- Hepatitis C infection
- High-risk sexual activity (multiple partners)
- Sex partners of people with HBV infection
- Males who have sex with males
- Living with HBV-infected person
- Household contacts of people with known HBV infection (sharing personal care items such as a razor or toothbrush, or exposure to an open skin lesion)
- Perinatal transmission
- People born in regions of the world where HBV infection is common
- U.S.- born people not vaccinated as infants whose parents were born in regions with high rates of HBV infection
- Incarceration in a jail, prison, or other detention setting
- Home hemodialysis/peritoneal dialysis or in-center hemodialysis
- Chronic liver disease/damage/inflammation

Hepatitis C Virus (HCV) Risk Factors

- Injection drug use
- HIV infection
- Infant born to HCV-infected mother
- Sex with an HCV-infected person
- Males who have sex with males
- Sharing personal care items with HCV-infected persons (e.g., razor, toothbrush)
- Health-care, emergency medical, and public safety personnel after needle sticks, sharps, or mucosal exposures to HCV-positive blood
- Maintenance hemodialysis
- Chronic ALT elevation
- People who received blood, blood products, and organs before 1992

Hepatitis D Virus (HDV) Risk Factors

Hepatitis D Virus (HDV) is rare in the United States. HDV only occurs in persons who also have HBV.

- People chronically infected with HBV
- Infants born to mothers infected with HDV
- Sex partners of persons infected with HBV and HDV
- Coinfection with HIV and HBV
- Males who have sex with males
- Injection drug use
- Household contacts of people with HDV infection
- Health-care and public safety workers at risk for occupational exposure to blood or blood-contaminated body fluids
- Hemodialysis clients

Hepatitis E Virus (HEV) Risk Factors

Hepatitis E Virus (HEV) occurs rarely in the United States. Primarily it is spread by the fecal-oral route.

- Contaminated water supply
- Areas with poor sanitation
- Infected foods (e.g., uncooked/undercooked pork, shellfish)

Adapted from *https://www.cdc/gov/hepatitis-a/hcp/clinical-overview/index.html* (Retrieved December 17, 2025).
Adapted from *https://www.cdc/gov/hepatitis-b/hcp/clinical-overview/index.html* (Retrieved December 17, 2025).
Adapted from *https://www.cdc.gov/hepatitis-c/hcp/clinical-overview/index.html* (Retrieved December 17, 2025)
Adapted from *https://www.cdc/gov/hepatitis-d/about/index.html* (Retrieved December 17, 2025).
Adapted from *https://www.cdc/gov/hepatitis-e/about/index.html* (Retrieved December 17, 2025).

Risk Factors

Stomach Cancer

- *Helicobacter pylori (H. pylori)* infection
- Age (60 to 80)
- Sex (male)
- Race/Ethnicity (Black Americans, Hispanic Americans, Native Americans, Asian Americans, and Pacific Islanders)
- Diet (smoked foods, salted fish/meat, pickled vegetables; frequent consumption of processed, grilled, or charcoaled meats)
- Tobacco use
- Alcohol use (3 or more drinks per day)
- Overweight/obese
- Occupation (e.g., coal, metal, and rubber industries)
- Previous stomach surgery (partial gastrectomy)
- Adenomatous stomach polyps
- Pernicious anemia
- Type A blood
- Family history of stomach cancer
- Inherited cancer syndromes (e.g., hereditary diffuse gastric cancer, Lynch syndrome, familial adenomatous polyposis, gastric adenoma and proximal polyposis of the stomach, Li-Fraumeni syndrome, Peutz-Jeghers syndrome)
- Common variable immune deficiency

Adapted from *https://www.cancer.org/cancer/types/stomach-cancer/causes-risks-prevention/risk-factors.html* (retrieved December 17, 2025).

Risk Factors

Pancreatic Cancer

- Age >45 but majority are >65
- Sex (male)
- Race (Black)
- Family history of pancreatic cancer
- Tobacco use
- Overweight/obese
- Diabetes mellitus
- History of chronic pancreatitis
- Exposure to chemicals (e.g., used in dry cleaning and metal working)
- Inherited genetic syndromes (e.g., hereditary breast and ovarian cancer syndrome, hereditary breast cancer, ataxia telangiectasia, familial atypical multiple mole melanoma syndrome, hereditary pancreatitis, Lynch syndrome, and Peutz-Jeghers syndrome)

Adapted from *https://www.cancer.org/cancer/types/pancreatic-cancer/causes-risks-prevention/risk-factors.html* (retrieved December 17, 2025).

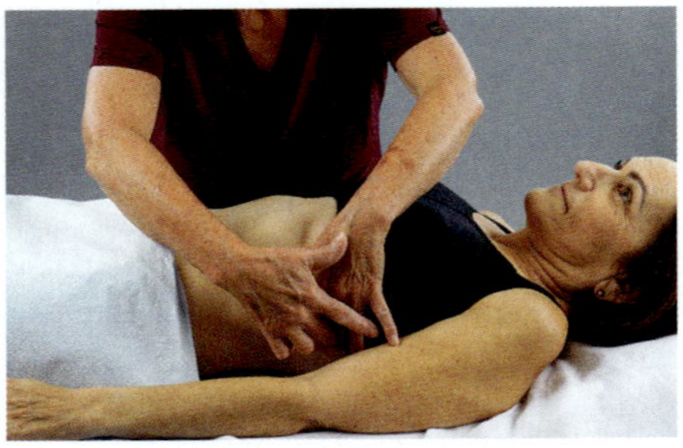

Figure 18-21 Percussion of the spleen.

Spleen

E
1. Percuss the lower level of the left lung slightly posterior to the midaxillary line and continue downward (Fig. 18-21).
2. Percuss downward until dullness is ascertained. In some individuals, the spleen is positioned too deeply to be discernable by percussion.

N **Normally, the upper border of dullness is found 6 to 8 cm above the left costal margin. Splenic dullness may be heard from the 6th to the 10th rib.**

A Dullness beyond the 8 cm line is indicative of splenic enlargement. However, a full stomach or a feces-filled intestine may mimic the dullness of splenic enlargement. Moreover, gastric or colonic air may obscure the dullness of the spleen.

P Splenic enlargement can be due to portal hypertension resulting from liver disease; other potential causes are mononucleosis, thrombosis, stenosis, atresia, angiomatous deformities of the portal or splenic vein, cysts, or aneurysm of the splenic artery.

Stomach

E Percuss for a gastric air bubble in the LUQ at the left lower anterior rib cage and left epigastric region.

N **The tympany of the gastric air bubble is lower in pitch than the tympany of the intestine.**

A An increase in size of the gastric air bubble is abnormal.

P An increase in size of the gastric air bubble accompanied by gastric distention can suggest gastric dilation.

Bladder

E
1. Percuss upward from the symphysis pubis to the umbilicus.
2. Note where the sound changes from dullness to tympany.

N **A urine-filled bladder is dull to percussion. A recently emptied bladder should not be percussible above the symphysis pubis.**

A It is abnormal to percuss a bladder that has recently been emptied. The urine that remains in the bladder after urination is called residual urine. A bladder may also be dull to percussion when the client has difficulty voiding.

P The inability to completely empty the bladder occurs in older adults; in postoperative, bedridden, and acutely ill clients; and in clients with neurogenic bladder dysfunction.

P Difficulty voiding can occur in conjunction with benign prostatic hypertrophy (see Chapter 23 for additional information), urethral pathology, and some medications (e.g., antipsychotics: phenothiazine; anticholinergics: atropine; antihypertensives: hydralazine).

Fist Percussion

Fist percussion is performed over the kidneys and liver to assess for tenderness.

Kidney

E
1. Place the client in a sitting position.

ADVANCED TECHNIQUE

Assessing for Ascites: Shifting Dullness, Puddle Sign, and Fluid Wave

Assess the client for **ascites** (Fig. 18-22), or excess accumulation of fluid in the abdominal cavity. There are three methods to evaluate for ascites: **shifting dullness**, **puddle sign**, and **fluid wave**.

Shifting Dullness

E
1. Standing to the right, with the client supine, percuss over the top of the abdomen, beginning at the midline.
2. Percuss outward toward the right side of the client, following a downward direction (Fig. 18-23A).
3. Mark on the abdomen where percussion changes from tympany to dullness, because this change is indicative of settled fluid in the flanks of the abdominal cavity.
4. Turn the client onto the right side.
5. Repercuss the upper side of the abdomen, moving downward.
6. If the percussion sound changes from tympany to dullness above the prior-marked fluid line, this shifting dullness test is positive for ascites.
7. Repeat the same technique on the client's left side. Change the client's position from the right to the left side (Fig. 18-23B).
8. Mark where the percussion changes from tympany to dullness.

N **There should be no change from tympany to dullness.**

A There is a marked change from tympany to dullness as you percuss outward and downward. Ascites is present in the abdominal cavity.

P Ascitic fluid sinks with gravity, which accounts for the dullness in dependent areas. Ascites is found in cirrhosis and other liver diseases.

Puddle Sign

E
1. Ask the client to kneel and assume the knee-chest position for several minutes.
2. Percuss the umbilical area (Fig. 18-24).

N **The umbilical area should remain tympanic.**

A The umbilical area percusses dull.

P The ascitic fluid pools in the dependent area of the umbilicus because of gravity.

Fluid Wave

E
1. With the client in a supine position, stand on the client's right side.
2. Have the client or a second nurse firmly place the ulnar side of the right-hand midline on the abdomen to prevent displacement of fat.
3. Place your right hand on the client's right hip or flank area. Reach across the client with your left hand and deliver a blow to the client's left hip or flank area (Fig. 18-25).
4. Assess if a fluid wave is felt on your right hand or the second nurse's hand.

N **No fluid wave should be felt.**

A A fluid wave is easily felt if a large amount of ascites is present. This sign is often negative until the ascites is obvious. In addition, the fluid wave is sometimes positive in people without ascites.

P The factors that contribute to the development of ascites are increased vascular resistance to hepatic outflow, increased hepatic lymph flow and extravasation of fluid into the peritoneal cavity, portal hypertension and increased capillary filtration pressure, hypoalbuminemia and decreased colloid osmotic serum pressure, disordered kidney function, and excessive secretion of antidiuretic hormone.

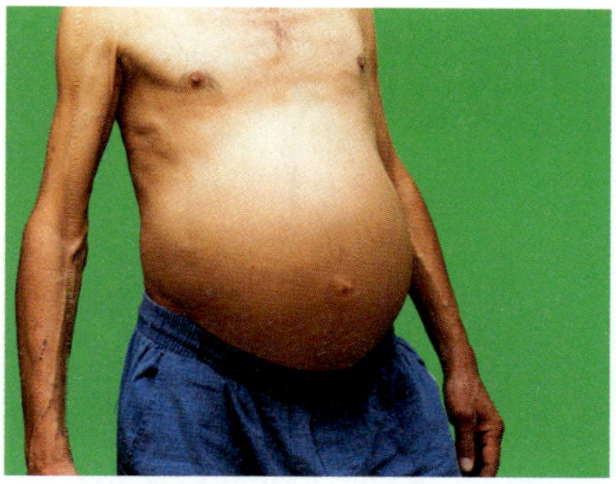

Figure 18-22 Ascites.

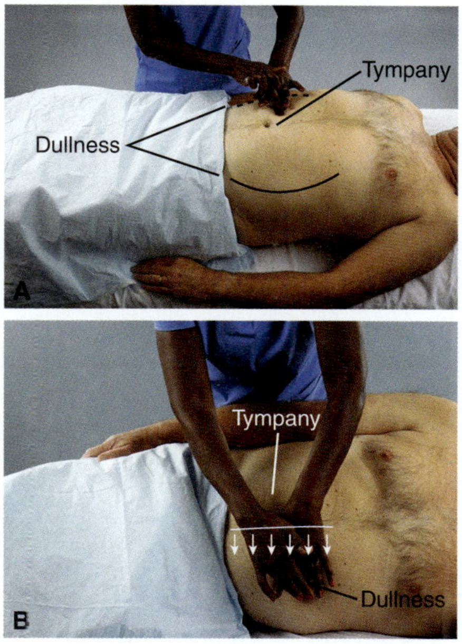

Figure 18-23 Percussion for ascites: Shifting dullness. **A.** Client supine. **B.** Client on left side.

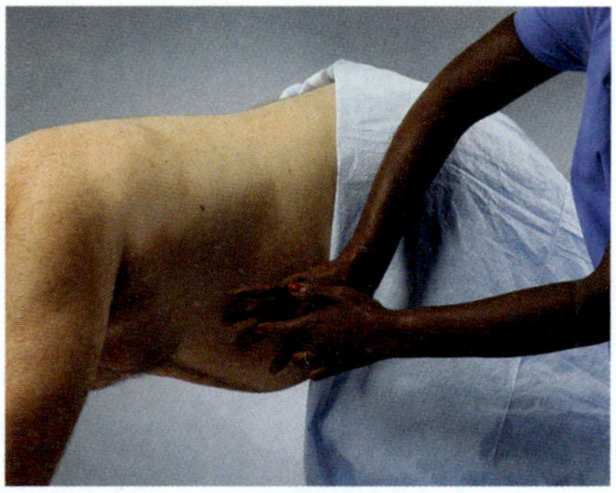

Figure 18-24 Percussion for ascites: Puddle sign.

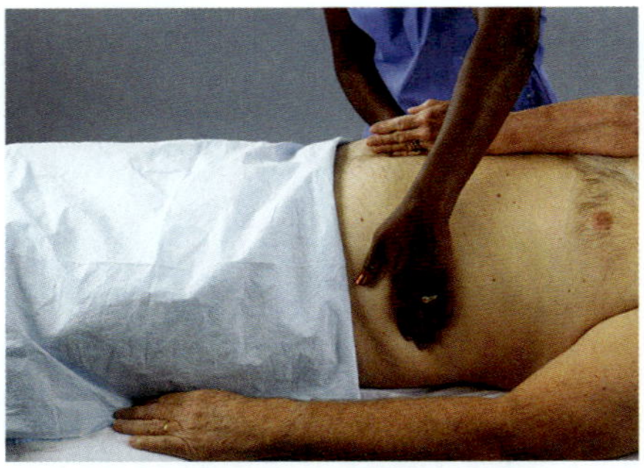

Figure 18-25 Palpation for ascites: Fluid wave.

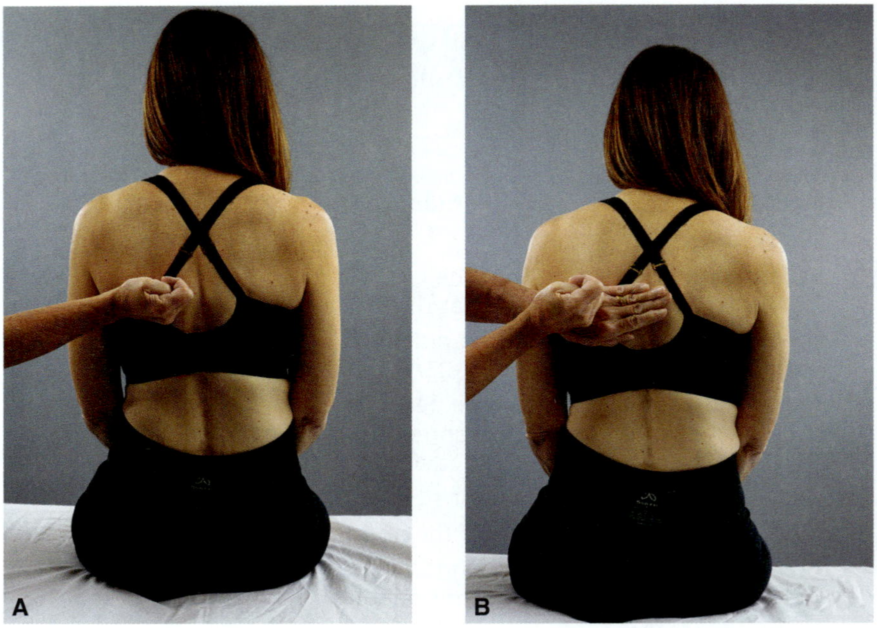

Figure 18-26 Fist percussion of the left kidney. **A.** Direct fist percussion. **B.** Indirect fist percussion.

> **NURSING TIP**
> **Monitoring Ascites**
> It is often helpful to monitor ascites by measuring the client's abdomen at its largest diameter. To promote consistency among nurses, it is advised that marks be drawn on the client's abdomen showing the placement of the tape measure. An increase in abdominal circumference indicates an ascites that is increasing in size.

2. Strike the costovertebral angle with a closed fist (direct fist percussion, Figure 18-26A) or
   Place the palmar surface of one hand over the costovertebral angle (CVA). Strike that hand with the ulnar surface of the fist of the other hand (indirect fist percussion, Figure 18-26B).
3. Ask the client what was felt. Observe the client's reaction.
4. Repeat on the other side.

N **No tenderness should be elicited.**

A Tenderness or pain over the costovertebral angle is abnormal.

P Costovertebral angle tenderness can occur in pyelonephritis.

Liver

E
1. Place the client in a supine position.
2. Place the palmar surface of one hand over the lower right rib cage (where the liver was percussed).
3. Strike that hand with the ulnar surface of the fist of the other hand (indirect fist percussion, Figure 18-27).
4. Ask the client what was felt. Observe the client's reaction.

N **No tenderness should be elicited.**

A Tenderness or pain that can be elicited over the liver is abnormal.

P Liver tenderness can occur in conjunction with cholecystitis or hepatitis.

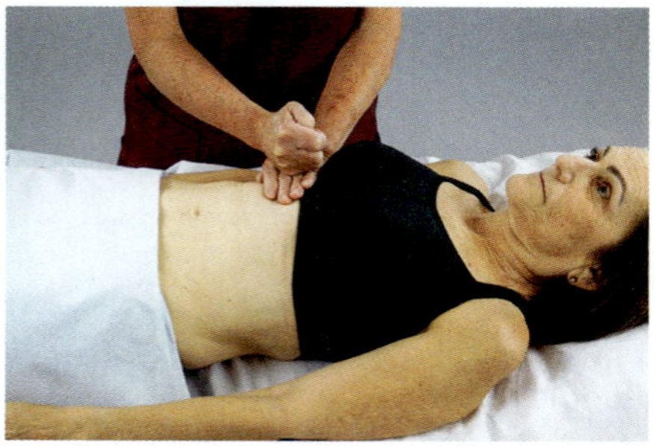

Figure 18-27 Indirect fist percussion of the liver.

Palpation

Light Palpation

E
1. With your hands and forearm on a horizontal plane, use the pads of the approximated fingers to depress the abdominal wall 1 cm (Fig. 18-28).
2. Avoid short, quick jabs.
3. Lightly palpate all four quadrants in a systematic manner.

4. Never palpate over areas where bruits are auscultated, as palpation may cause rupture.

N **The abdomen should feel smooth with consistent softness.**

A Light palpation reveals changes in skin temperature, tenderness, or large masses.

P Tenderness and elevated skin temperature can be due to inflammation. Large masses can be due to tumors, feces, or enlarged organs.

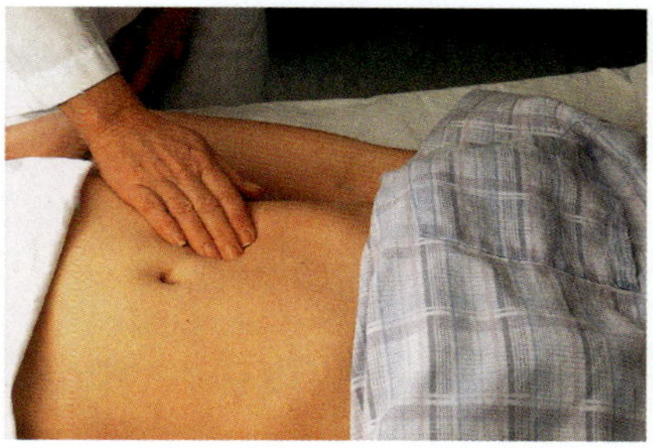

Figure 18-28 Light palpation of the abdomen.

Abdominal Muscle Guarding

To determine whether muscle guarding is involuntary:

E 1. Perform light palpation of the rectus muscles during expiration.
2. Note muscle tensing.

N **Muscle guarding, or tensing of the abdominal musculature, is absent during expiration. The abdomen is soft. Normally, the client cannot exercise voluntary muscle tensing during expiration.**

A Muscle guarding of the rectus muscles occurs during expiration.

P Involuntary muscle guarding suggests irritation of the peritoneum, as in peritonitis.

Deep Palpation

In performing deep palpation of all four quadrants, you can use either a one-handed or a two-handed method.

E 1. With the one-handed method, use the palmar surface of the extended fingers to depress the skin approximately 5 to 8 cm (2 to 3 inches) in the RLQ (Fig. 18-29A).
2. A two-handed approach is used when palpation is difficult because of obesity or muscular resistance. With the bimanual technique, the nondominant hand is placed on top of the dominant hand. The bottom hand is used for sensation, and the top hand is used to apply pressure (Fig. 18-29B).
3. Identify any masses and note location, size, shape, consistency, tenderness, pulsation, and degree of mobility.
4. Continue palpation of the RUQ, LUQ, and LLQ.

N **There should be no abnormal masses, bulges, or swelling. Normally, only the aorta and the edge of the liver are palpable. When the large colon or the bladder is full, palpation is possible.**

A The gallbladder, liver, spleen, fecal-filled colon, or flatus-filled cecum should not be palpable. Masses, bulges, and swellings are also considered abnormal.

P Organomegaly can be caused by many pathological states, such as cholecystitis, hepatitis, or cirrhosis; masses, bulges, or swelling can be due to tumors, fluids, feces, flatus, or fat.

> **NURSING TIP**
> **Abdominal Palpation**
> - Ensure that your hands are warm, to promote client comfort and prevent muscle guarding.
> - Before beginning the palpation, ask the client to cough. Coughing can elicit a sharp twinge of pain if peritoneal irritation is present. Palpate this area and other known areas of pain or tenderness last.
> - Instruct the client to take slow, deep breaths through the mouth.
> - Begin with gentle pressure and gradually increase it.
> - If the client is very ticklish, have the client perform self-palpation with your hand over the client's hand. Gradually remove the client's hand when the ticklishness is gone.
> - Observe the client's face while performing abdominal palpation for changes in expression that can indicate pain or discomfort.

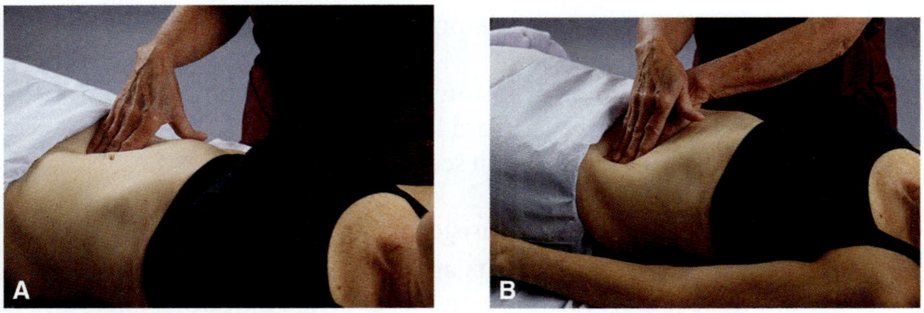

Figure 18-29 Deep palpation. **A.** One-handed method. **B.** Bimanual method.

Liver

Liver palpation can be performed by one of two methods: the bimanual method or the hook method.

Bimanual Method

E
1. Stand on the client's right side, facing the client's head.
2. Place the left hand under the client's right flank at about the 11th or 12th rib.
3. Press upward with the left hand to elevate the liver toward the abdominal wall.
4. Place the right hand parallel to the midline at the right midclavicular line below the right costal margin or below the level of liver dullness.
5. Instruct the client to take a deep breath.
6. Push down deeply and under the costal margin with your right fingers. On inspiration, the liver will descend and contact the hand (Fig. 18-30A).
7. Note the level of the liver.
8. Note the size, shape, and consistency. Note any masses.

Hook Method

E
1. Stand on the client's right side, facing the client's feet.
2. Place both hands side by side on the right costal margin below the border of liver dullness.
3. Hook the fingers in and up toward the costal margin and ask the client to take a deep breath and hold it.
4. Palpate the liver's edge as it descends (Fig. 18-30B).
5. Note the level of the liver.
6. Note the size, shape, and consistency. Note any masses.

N **A normal liver edge presents as a firm, sharp, regular ridge with a smooth surface. Normally, the liver is not palpable, although it may be felt in extremely thin adults.**

Risk Factors

Colorectal Cancer

- Age >50
- Male
- Race/ethnicity (American Indian, Alaska Native, Black American, Ashkenazi Jewish descent)
- Personal history of adenomatous polyps or colorectal cancer
- Personal history of chronic inflammatory bowel disease (ulcerative colitis, Crohn disease)
- Personal history of radiation to the abdomen or pelvis
- History of cholecystectomy
- Family history of colorectal cancer or adenomatous polyps
- Family history of a hereditary colorectal cancer syndrome (Lynch syndrome, Turcot syndrome, Gardner syndrome, attenuated familial adenomatous polyposis, Peutz-Jeghers syndrome, MUTYH-associated polyposis, cystic fibrosis)
- Lack of physical activity
- Diet: Low fruit and vegetable consumption, high-fat diet, diet high in red meats
- Overweight/obese
- Alcohol use (moderate to heavy)
- Tobacco use
- Type 2 diabetes

Adapted from *https://www.cancer.org/cancer/types/colon-rectal-cancer/causes-risks-prevention/risk-factors.htm* (retrieved December 17, 2025).

Risk Factors

Liver Cancer

- Male
- Race/ethnicity (Asian Americans, Pacific Islanders)
- Chronic hepatitis B or C virus
- Alcohol abuse
- Tobacco use
- Cirrhosis
- Metabolic dysfunction-associated steatotic liver disease (MASLD)
- Primary biliary cirrhosis
- Type 2 diabetes
- Obesity
- Inherited metabolic disease (e.g., hereditary hemochromatosis)
- Rare diseases (e.g., Wilson disease, alpha1-antitrypsin deficiency, acute intermittent porphyria, tyrosinemia, glycogen storage diseases, porphyria cutanea tarda)
- Aflatoxin exposure (fungus that can contaminate food)
- Vinyl chloride and thorium dioxide exposure
- Anabolic steroids

Adapted from *https://www.cancer.org/cancer/types/liver-cancer/causes-risks-prevention/risk-factors.html* (retrieved December 17, 2025).

A If the liver is palpable below the costal margin both medially and laterally, it is abnormal.

P An enlarged liver can be due to congestive heart failure, hepatitis, encephalopathy, cirrhosis, nonalcoholic fatty liver disease, cysts, or cancer.

A A liver that is enlarged, has an irregular border and nodules, and is hard is abnormal.

P These findings suggest liver malignancy. Tenderness may or may not be present.

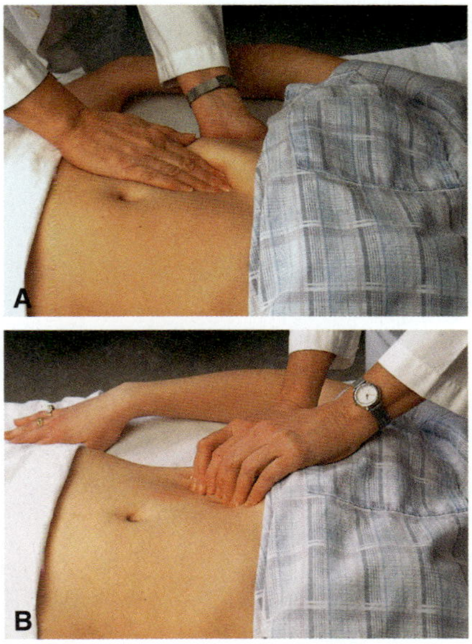

Figure 18-30 Palpation of the liver. **A.** Bimanual method. **B.** Hook method.

Spleen

Use the bimanual technique to palpate the spleen.

E
1. Stand on the client's right side.
2. Reach across and place the left hand beneath the client and over the left costovertebral angle. Press upward to lift the spleen anteriorly toward the abdominal wall.
3. With the right hand, press inward along the left costal margin while asking the client to take a deep breath (Fig. 18-31). Palpate the spleen gently, because an enlarged spleen will be very tender and may rupture.
4. The procedure can be repeated with the client lying on the right side, with the hips and knees flexed. This position will facilitate the spleen coming forward and to the right because the spleen is located retroperitoneally.
5. Note the size, shape, and consistency. Note any masses.

N **The spleen should not be palpable.**

A Because of its retroperitoneal position in the body, the spleen becomes palpable only when it has become enlarged to three times its normal size. An enlarged spleen is usually very tender.

P Splenomegaly can be due to inflammation, congestive heart failure, cancer, cirrhosis, or mononucleosis.

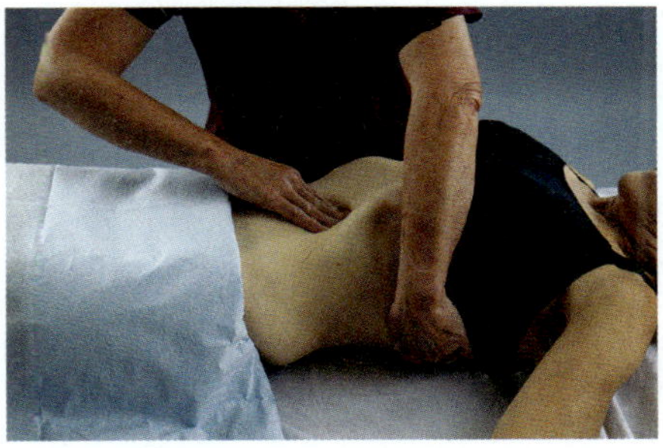

Figure 18-31 Palpation of the spleen.

ADVANCED TECHNIQUE

Assessing for Cholecystitis: Murphy Sign

E
1. With the client supine, stand on the client's right side.
2. Palpate below the liver margin at the lateral border of the rectus muscle.
3. Have the client take a deep breath.

N **No pain is elicited.**

A Pain is present with palpation. The client may stop inhaling to guard against the pain. This is known as Murphy sign.

P Murphy sign is positive in inflammatory processes of the gallbladder, such as cholecystitis.

Kidneys

E
1. Stand on the client's right side.
2. Place one hand on the right costovertebral angle on the client's back.
3. Place the other hand below and parallel to the costal margin.
4. As the client takes a deep breath, press hands firmly together and try to feel the lower pole of the kidney (Fig. 18-32).

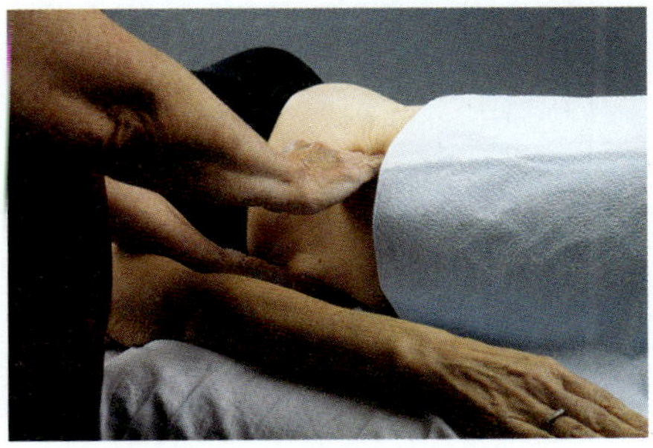

Figure 18-32 Palpation of the right kidney.

Risk Factors

Renal Cancer

- Male
- Race/Ethnicity (Native American, Alaska Native, Black)
- Hypertension (whether it is treated or not)
- Smoking
- Overweight/obese
- Occupational exposure (e.g., trichloroethylene, cadmium)
- Family history of renal cancer
- Genetics (von Hippel-Lindau disease, hereditary papillary renal cell carcinoma, hereditary leiomyomatosis and renal cell cancer, Birt-Hogg-Dubé syndrome, hereditary paraganglioma-pheochromocytoma syndromes, familial renal cancer, Cowden syndrome, tuberous sclerosis, BAP1 tumor predisposition syndrome, sickle cell trait and disease)
- Advanced renal disease especially those requiring dialysis

Adapted from *https://www.cancer.org/cancer/types/kidney-cancer/causes-risks-prevention/risk-factors.html* (retrieved December 17, 2025).

5. At the peak of inspiration, press the fingers together with greater pressure from above than from below.
6. Ask the client to exhale and to hold the breath briefly.
7. Release the pressure of your fingers.
8. If the kidney has been "captured," it can be felt as it slips back into place.
9. Note the size, shape, and consistency. Note any masses.
10. For the left kidney, reach across the client and place the left hand under the client's left flank.
11. Apply downward pressure with the right hand below the left costal margin and repeat steps 4 through 9.

N **The kidneys should not be palpable in a normal adult. However, the lower pole of the right kidney may be felt in very thin individuals. Kidneys are more readily palpable in older adults due to loss of muscle tone and muscle bulk.**

A Enlarged kidneys are abnormal. The right kidney may be difficult to distinguish from an enlarged liver. Left kidney enlargement may be difficult to distinguish from an enlarged spleen.

P Enlarged, palpable kidneys can be caused by hydronephrosis, neoplasms, or polycystic kidney disease.

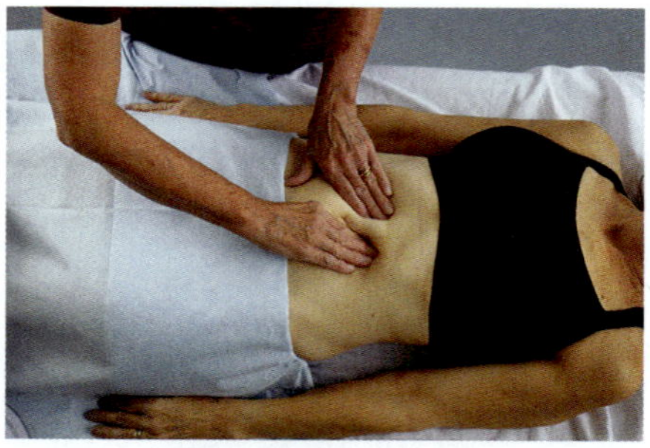

Figure 18-33 Palpation of the aorta.

Aorta

Do not palpate a client's aorta if an aneurysm is suspected, as it may dissect and lead to renal failure, loss of limb, or death.

E
1. Press the upper abdomen with one hand on each side of the abdominal aorta, slightly to the left of the midline.
2. Assess the width of the aorta and the direction of its pulsation (Fig. 18-33).

N **The aorta width is 2.5 to 4.0 cm, and the aorta pulsates in an anterior direction.**

A Aorta width greater than 4.0 cm is abnormal. Lateral pulsation of the aorta is also abnormal.

P A widened aorta and lateral pulsations suggest an abdominal aortic aneurysm.

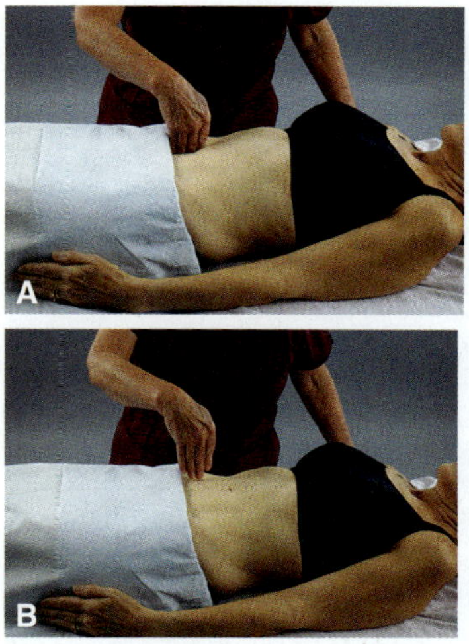

Figure 18-34 Rebound tenderness. **A.** Apply firm pressure to the abdomen. **B.** Quickly release the pressure.

ADVANCED TECHNIQUE

Assessing for Abdominal Inflammation: Rebound Tenderness

Rebound tenderness is assessed if pain has been elicited during palpation or if the client has reported pain. Rebound tenderness is an abnormal finding frequently associated with peritoneal inflammation or appendicitis. Be prepared to recognize that rebound tenderness assessment could elicit a strong pain response from the client. It is imperative to test for rebound tenderness away from the site where the pain is initially determined and to conclude abdominal examination with this test. If other tests are positive, omit this assessment.

E
1. Apply several seconds of firm pressure to the abdomen, with the hand at a 90° angle (perpendicular to the abdomen) and the fingers extended (Fig. 18-34A).
2. Quickly release the pressure (Fig. 18-34B).

N **Pain is not elicited.**

A As the abdominal wall returns to its normal position, the client complains of pain at the pressure site (direct rebound tenderness) or at another site (referred rebound tenderness).

P Rebound tenderness may indicate peritoneal irritation. The rebound effect of the internal structures indented by this technique causes sharp pain in the area of inflammation.

P Pain in the RLQ can indicate appendicitis. This location is known as **McBurney point**.

ADVANCED TECHNIQUE

Assessing for Appendicitis: Rovsing Sign

Rovsing sign is a differential technique to elicit referred pain, reflective of peritoneal inflammation secondary to appendicitis.

E
1. Press deeply and evenly in the LLQ for 5 seconds.
2. Note the client's response.

N **No pain should be elicited.**

A Abdominal pain felt in the RLQ is abnormal and is a positive Rovsing sign.

P Rovsing sign is based on the concept that changes in intraluminal pressure will be transmitted through the intestine when the ileocecal valve is competent. Pressing the LLQ traps air within the large intestine and increases the pressure in the cecum. When the appendix is inflamed, this increase in pressure causes pain.

NURSING TIP

Differentiating Kidney Palpation

Features distinguishing an enlarged liver and an enlarged kidney include:

1. The edge of the liver tends to be sharper and to extend medially and laterally, whereas the pole of the kidney is more rounded.
2. In addition, the edge of the liver cannot be "captured," whereas an enlarged kidney can be.

Features distinguishing an enlarged left kidney from an enlarged spleen include:

1. A palpable notch on the medial edge of the organ favors the spleen.
2. Percussion of the spleen produces dullness because the bowel is displaced downward; however, resonance is heard over the left kidney because of the intervening bowel.

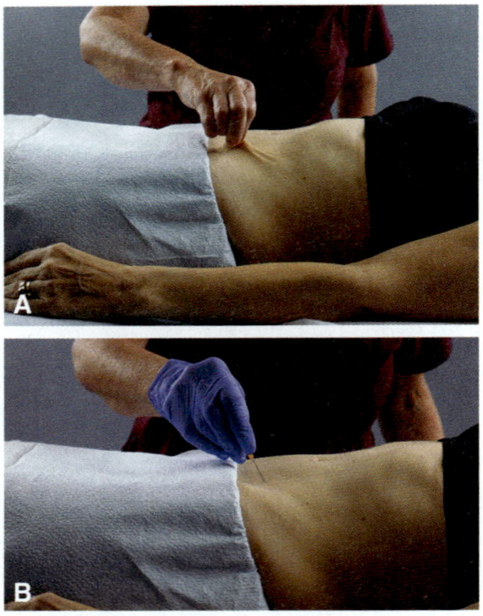

Figure 18-35 Assessment of cutaneous hypersensitivity. **A.** Lift a fold of skin away from the underlying muscle. **B.** Stimulate the skin with a sterile needle.

ADVANCED TECHNIQUE

Assessing for Abdominal Inflammation: Cutaneous Hypersensitivity

On stimulation with a sterile pin or by lifting a fold of skin away from the musculature, **cutaneous hypersensitivity** zones of sensory nerves initiate a painful response. The irritative stimulus detects specific zones of peritoneal irritation.

E 1. Lift a fold of skin away from the underlying muscle (Fig. 18-35A) or stimulate the skin by gently jabbing the abdominal surface with a sterile pin (Fig. 18-35B).
2. Observe for pain response.

N **No adverse reaction should be noted.**

A The client experiences an exaggerated sense of pain.

P Cutaneous hypersensitivity indicates a zone of peritoneal irritation.

P Localized pain in all or part of the RLQ may accompany appendicitis.

P Midepigastrium pain could signal a peptic ulcer.

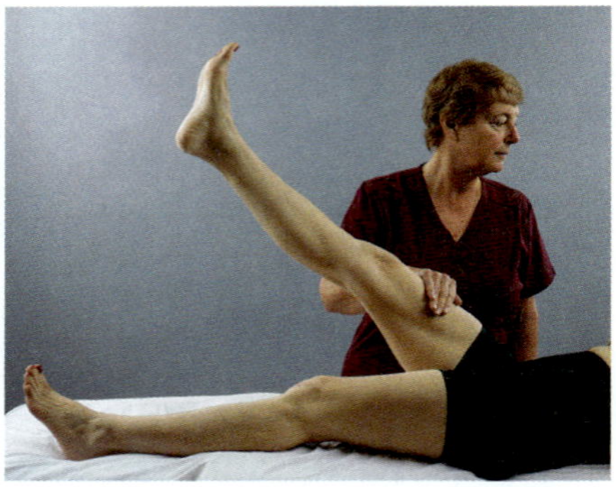

Figure 18-36 Iliopsoas muscle test.

ADVANCED TECHNIQUE

Assessing for Appendicitis: Iliopsoas Muscle Test

When a client presents with acute abdominal pain, an inflamed or perforated appendix may be distinguished via irritation of the lateral iliopsoas muscle.

E 1. Place your hand over the right thigh and push downward as the client raises the leg, flexing at the hip (Fig. 18-36).
2. Observe for pain response in the RLQ as described by the client.

N **Normally, the client should experience no pain.**

A The client experiences pain in the RLQ.

P This pain indicates an inflammation of the iliopsoas muscle in the groin and is caused by an inflamed appendix.

ADVANCED TECHNIQUE

Assessing for Appendicitis or Pelvic Abscess: Obturator Muscle Test

Another differential technique used to help determine whether the client is experiencing appendicitis is eliciting the **obturator sign**. This test can be used when a pelvic abscess is suspected. Both conditions may irritate the obturator internus muscle.

E 1. Flex the right leg at the hip and knee at a right angle.
2. Rotate the leg both internally and externally (Fig. 18-37).
3. Observe for pain response.

N **No pain is elicited with this maneuver.**

A Pain is elicited in the hypogastric area.

P This pain indicates irritation of the obturator muscle and can be caused by a ruptured appendix or pelvic abscess.

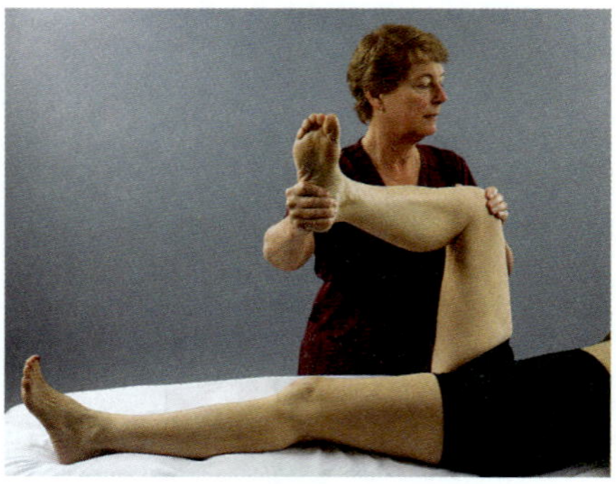

Figure 18-37 Obturator muscle test.

E Examination N Normal Findings A Abnormal Findings P Pathophysiology

> ## ADVANCED TECHNIQUE
> ### Assessing for Abdominal Mass: Ballottement
> **Ballottement** is a palpation technique used to displace excess fluid in the abdominal cavity to locate an organ or mass.
>
> **E** 1. Extend the fingers of the right hand in a straight line, perpendicular to the abdominal surface.
> 2. Stiffen the fingers.
> 3. Jab the abdominal surface in the desired area (Fig. 18-38).
> 4. Determine whether the intended organ is felt at the fingertips.
>
> **N** **Excluding during pregnancy, internal organs are not felt during this assessment technique.**
>
> **A** Internal masses, or organs such as the liver or spleen, are palpated.
>
> **P** The presence of ascites transmits external pressure to an internal organ or mass. The resulting impact felt on palpation is known as ballottement. It determines the presence of a free-floating abdominal mass, which can indicate a cancerous process in the abdominal cavity. Pain should not be elicited. A painful response would indicate inflammation and require further investigation.

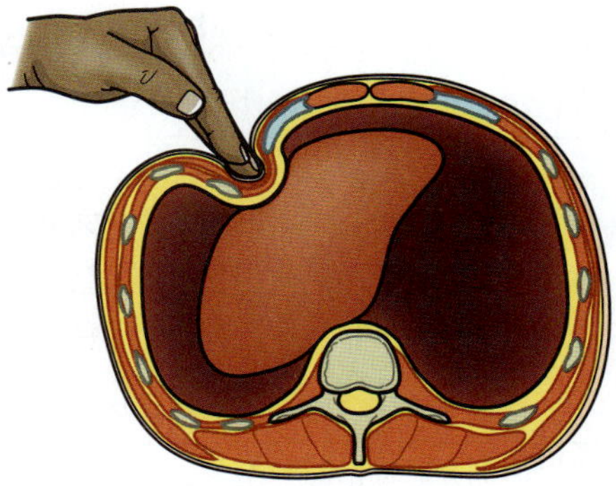

Figure 18-38 Abdominal ballottement.

Bladder

E 1. Using deep palpation, palpate the abdomen at the midline, starting at the symphysis pubis and progressing upward to the umbilicus (Fig. 18-39).
2. If the bladder is located, palpate the shape, size, and consistency.

N **An empty bladder is not usually palpable. A moderately full bladder is smooth and round, and it is palpable above the symphysis pubis. A full bladder is palpated above the symphysis pubis, and it may be close to the umbilicus.**

A A bladder that is nodular or asymmetrical is abnormal.

P A nodular bladder may indicate malignancy. An asymmetrical bladder may result from a tumor in the bladder or an abdominal tumor that is compressing the bladder.

A It is abnormal to palpate a bladder that has recently been emptied.

P Men with benign prostatic hypertrophy may be unable to completely empty the bladder because of the pressure that the enlarged prostate places on the bladder.

P Various types of urinary incontinence, due to altered mental status, muscle function, medications, and other factors, can lead to incomplete bladder emptying. Table 18-4 gives additional information on urinary incontinence.

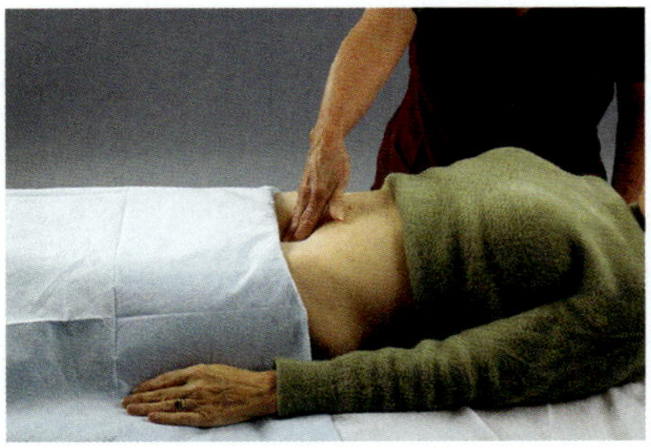

Figure 18-39 Palpation of the bladder.

> ## NURSING TIP
> ### Urinary Incontinence
> Use the acronym "DIAPPERS" to guide your thought processes when considering nonbladder etiologies of urinary incontinence, especially in the older adult:
>
> **D** = delirium
> **I** = infection
> **A** = atrophic vaginitis
> **P** = pharmacological agents: diuretics, alcohol, benzodiazepines, anticholinergics, calcium channel blockers, alpha-adrenergics, caffeine
> **P** = psychological disorder: depression, Parkinson disease
> **E** = endocrine disorder: diabetes mellitus, diabetes insipidus; excessive urinary output, heart failure
> **R** = restricted mobility
> **S** = stool impaction; stroke
>
> Adapted from Resnick, N. M. (1984). Urinary incontinence in the elderly. *Medical Grand Rounds, 3,* 281–290.

Table 18-4 Types of Urinary Incontinence

Type	Definition	Etiology
Stress	Involuntary loss of urine with activities that increase abdominal pressure (e.g., sneezing, coughing, laughing, heavy lifting, physical activity)	Childbirth, pregnancy, previous abdominal surgery, prostate surgery, radiation therapy
Urge	Involuntary loss of urine due to detrusor muscle hyperactivity; usually associated with a strong desire to void with a larger volume of urine	Stroke, dementia, multiple sclerosis, Parkinson disease, brain tumor, urinary tract tumors, urinary tract infection
Overflow	Involuntary loss of urine due to an overextended bladder; incontinence occurs when bladder pressure exceeds urethral pressure; usually small amount of urine occurs during dribbling; may be some hesitancy and frequency	Fecal impaction, diabetic neuropathy, obstruction of the bladder or urethra (due to prostate cancer, benign prostatic hypertrophy)
Functional	Involuntary loss of urine due to the inability to reach the toilet because of physical, cognitive, or environmental impairments	Immobility, dementia, inaccessible toilet, inappropriate lighting, physical restraints

Risk Factors

Bladder Cancer

- Race (White)
- Age >55
- Male
- Smoking
- Occupational chemical exposure (e.g., rubber/textile/leather/paint plant workers, hairdressers, printers)
- Personal history of bladder cancer or other urothelial cancers
- Family history of bladder cancer
- Pelvic radiation therapy
- Bladder birth defects
- Chronic bladder inflammation (e.g., UTIs, nephrolithiasis, schistosomiasis, bladder stones, chronic indwelling urinary catheter use)
- Medications (e.g., cyclophosphamide and pioglitazone)
- Dietary supplements containing aristolochic acid
- Arsenic ingestion (in contaminated drinking water)

Adapted from *https://www.cancer.org/cancer/types/bladder-cancer/causes-risks-prevention/risk-factors.html* (retrieved December 17, 2025).

Risk Factors

Urinary Tract Infection (UTI)

General Risk Factors

- History of childhood UTI
- History of recent UTI
- Decreased fluid intake
- Decreased frequency of voiding
- Incomplete bladder emptying
- Known structural abnormality
- Nephrolithiasis
- Neurogenic bladder dysfunction (e.g., spinal cord injury, multiple sclerosis)
- Indwelling urinary catheter
- Urinary instrumentation
- Sexually transmitted infections
- Diabetes
- Bowel incontinence
- Inadequate personal hygiene in genitalia
- Medications (e.g., canagliflozin, dapagliflozin, empagliflozin)
- Immunosuppression
- HIV with a CD4 + T-lymphocyte cell count <200 uL

Female Risk Factors

- Diaphragm use
- Spermicide use
- Postmenopausal
- Increased sexual activity
- Failure to void after sex
- Pregnancy
- Oral contraceptive use
- Cystocele

Male Risk Factors

- Age >50
- Benign prostatic hypertrophy
- Uncircumcised
- Sexual intercourse with persons of the same sex
- Anal sex

U.S. Preventive Services Task Force (USPSTF)

Grade A Recommendation:

- The USPSTF recommends screening for colorectal cancer in all adults aged 50 to 75 years with either a guaiac fecal occult blood test (gFOBT), fecal immunochemical test (FIT), stool DNA test (sDNA-FIT), colonoscopy, CT colonography, or flexible sigmoidoscopy in adults. Recommended intervals for colorectal cancer screening tests include:

High-sensitivity gFOBT or FIT every year
sDNA-FIT every 1 to 3 years
CT colonography every 5 years
Flexible sigmoidoscopy every 5 years
Flexible sigmoidoscopy every 10 years + FIT every year
Colonoscopy screening every 10 years

Grade B Recommendations

- The USPSTF recommends one-time screening for abdominal aortic aneurysm (AAA) with ultrasonography in men aged 65 to 75 years who have ever smoked.
- The USPSTF recommends screening for colorectal cancer in adults aged 45 to 49 years with either a guaiac fecal occult blood test (gFOBT), fecal immunochemical test (FIT), stool DNA test (sDNA-FIT), colonoscopy, CT colonography, or flexible sigmoidoscopy. Recommended intervals for colorectal cancer screening tests include:

High-sensitivity gFOBT or FIT every year
sDNA-FIT every 1 to 3 years
CT colonography every 5 years
Flexible sigmoidoscopy every 5 years
Flexible sigmoidoscopy every 10 years + FIT every year
Colonoscopy screening every 10 years

- The USPSTF recommends screening for hepatitis B virus (HBV) infection in adolescents and adults at increased risk for infection.
- The USPSTF recommends screening for hepatitis C virus (HCV) infection in adults aged 18 to 79 years.

Retrieved December 17, 2025, from *https://www.uspreventiveservicestaskforce.org/uspstf/recommendation-topics/uspstf-a-and-b-recommendations*

CASE STUDY

The Client With Pancreatitis

This case study illustrates the application and objective documentation of the abdominal examination. Andrew Miller is a 62-year-old White male. He has had many different jobs over the years in roofing and "odd jobs" as a daily worker. In the past few years, Mr. Miller has developed a worsening alcohol addiction that has left him homeless and without work. The drinking increased when the client's girlfriend moved out of the apartment. He remains estranged from his girlfriend but sees his son, Blake, regularly. Blake occasionally houses the client for short periods of time, but Mr. Miller frequently sleeps in a car. Mr. Miller has been to the emergency department four times in the past 5 months for alcohol intoxication. Over the past 3 days, Mr. Miller has developed increasing left upper quadrant abdominal pain and nausea. Blake brings Andrew in today for evaluation.

HEALTH HISTORY

CLIENT PROFILE

62-year-old White male

CHIEF COMPLAINT

"My stomach up here is hurting, and I've been feeling nauseated."

HISTORY OF PRESENT ILLNESS

Mr. Miller's symptoms started 3 days ago around the midafternoon with increasing pain in his left upper abdomen, sometimes also having pain in the epigastric area that radiates to the back. The abdominal pain is a constant "sharp and stabbing" pain. Mr. Miller tried taking "a few" acetaminophen and bismuth subsalicylate to try and alleviate the pain, but neither helped. The abdominal pain worsens after eating or drinking although he has felt less hungry with the pain. He rates the pain as 9/10. Client then developed persistent nausea and has vomited a few times over the last 2 days. Denies hematemesis. Client does not have a thermometer so has been unable to measure his temperature and admits to feeling "shaky" and "hot." Client denies chest pain, palpitations, dyspnea, urinary frequency, pain with urination, diarrhea, melena, or hematochezia. Client reports abdominal bloating.

PAST HEALTH HISTORY

Medical History Hypertension diagnosed age 51
Hyperlipidemia diagnosed age 58

Surgical History Cholecystectomy age 40 without complications

Allergies Sulfa antibiotic caused rash

Medications Lisinopril 20 mg daily prescribed but has not taken in months
Simvastatin 40 mg daily prescribed but has not taken in months

Communicable Diseases Denies

Injuries and Accidents Closed right ankle fracture age 31 after fall from ladder, denies sequelae

Differing Abilities Denies

Blood Transfusions Denies

Childhood Illnesses Had chickenpox as child

Immunizations Client does not know vaccine status except receiving one COVID-19 "shot" sometime in 2021

FAMILY HEALTH HISTORY

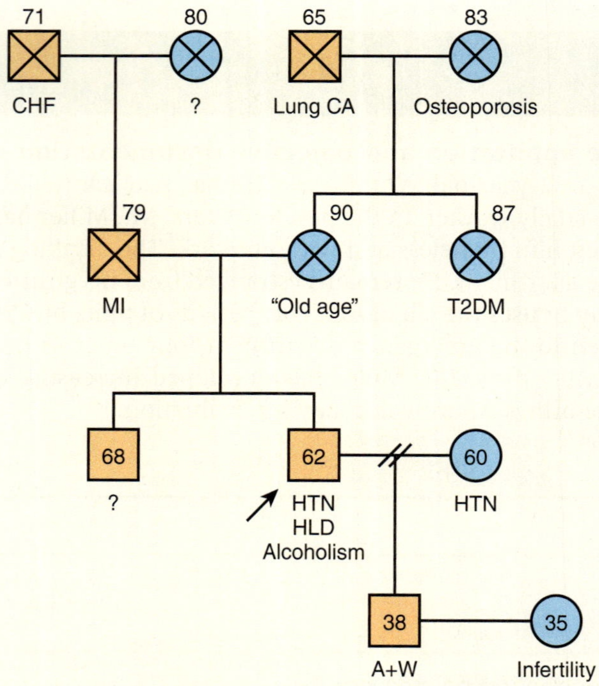

Legend

- Living female
- Living male
- Deceased female
- Deceased male
- Points to client
- Couple in a relationship*
- Divorced/No relationship

*The line connecting clients can denote a union, whether that be a marriage or other type of relationship

?	Unknown
A+W	Alive and well
CA	Cancer
CHF	Congestive heart failure
HLD	Hyperlipidemia
HTN	Hypertension
MI	Myocardial infarction
T2DM	Type 2 diabetes mellitus

Denies family history of gastrointestinal cancers, Crohn disease, ulcerative colitis, kidney disease, or malabsorption syndromes.
Above information was provided by client's son due to the client's pain status.

SOCIAL HISTORY

Alcohol Use "About a liter of whiskey" daily for "a long time"

Tobacco Use Smokes 1 PPD since age 18

Recreational Drug Use Denies

Domestic and Intimate Partner Violence Denies

Sexual Practice Estranged from girlfriend, heterosexual, no current partner

Travel History None in past several years, has never traveled internationally

Work Environment Unemployed

Home Environment Sleeps in an inoperable car most nights, in warmer weather may sleep on a park bench; does not like to go to local housing shelter to sleep

Hobbies and Leisure Activities Seeing friends around the library, goes to library in warm weather to cool off in air conditioning

Stress Unemployment, lack of adequate nighttime residence, no insurance, unable to pay for recent emergency room visits

Education High school diploma

Economic Status "I have nothing, my son, Blake, supports me a little."

Military Service Denies

Religion Nonpracticing Presbyterian

Ethnic Background No affiliation

Roles and Relationships Has son Blake who helps him when possible. Blake's wife does not get along with client and gets "mad" when client spends the night at their house. Blake states it is getting increasingly hard to help his father with worsening alcohol abuse.

Characteristic Patterns of Daily Living Sleeps in late most days, visits a food kitchen for lunch, some days looks for work, usually drinking by the afternoon, visits with friends who are also unhoused

HEALTH MAINTENANCE ACTIVITIES

Sleep 10 to 12 hours nightly

Diet Eats what is being served at food kitchen

Exercise None

Stress Management Drinking alcohol

Use of Safety Devices None

Health Checkups Does not routinely visit the doctor, only when client is feeling ill. Uses emergency department for health care. Never had a colonoscopy. No lung cancer screening

PHYSICAL EXAMINATION

Inspection

Contour Distended

Symmetry Symmetrical bilaterally

Rectus Abdominis Muscles Intact, no separation

Pigmentation and Color Uniform color/pigmentation

Scars Four faded 1 cm laparoscopic scars in the right upper abdomen

Striae None

Respiratory Movement No retractions

Masses and Nodules None

Visible Peristalsis None

Pulsation None

Umbilicus No hernias

Auscultation

Bowel Sounds Normoactive
Vascular Sounds No bruit
Venous Hum None
Friction Rub None

Percussion

General Percussion Tympany
Liver Span 8 cm in the right MCL
Liver Descent Unable to hold breath
Spleen Unable to detect
Stomach Tympany
Fist Percussion No costovertebral angle tenderness, no liver tenderness
Bladder Not detected

Palpation

Light Palpation Soft, tenderness in the left upper quadrant
Abdominal Muscle Guarding Guarding in the upper abdomen
Deep Palpation Severe tenderness in the epigastrium and LUQ, no masses

Liver No hepatomegaly

Spleen No splenomegaly

Kidneys Nonpalpable

Aorta 2 cm with anterior pulsation

Bladder Nonpalpable

Laboratory Data	Client's Values	Normal Values
WBC	16 k/mm^3	4–11 k/mm^3
HGB	13.3 g/dL	12–16 g/dL
HCT	38.7%	38–45%
PLT	384 k/mm^3	140–344 k/mm^3
BUN	18 mg/dL	8–21 mg/dL
Creatinine	1.1 mg/dL	0.8–1.3 mg/dL
Total Bilirubin	1.0 mg/dL	<1.2 mg/dL
Alkaline phosphatase	129 units/L	44–147 units/L
AST	50 units/L	10–40 units/L
ALT	65 units/L	10–55 units/L
Lipase	1100 units/L	10–150 units/L
Amylase	220 units/L	30- 125 units/L

CT Abdomen and Pelvis with Oral and IV Contrast

Impression: Liver is normal in size without masses or lesions. Mild hepatic steatosis is present. The gallbladder is absent. No intestinal colitis, obstruction, or masses seen. The pancreas is diffusely enlarged with homogeneous enhancement and stranding of the peripancreatic fat.

CLINICAL JUDGMENT IN ACTION

1. What cues indicate that the client is having a disorder of the abdomen?
2. What interventions have the highest priority?
3. What assessment findings indicate clinical improvement or decline in this client?

Review Questions

1. Which organ is oval-shaped, located behind the fundus of the stomach, and is responsible for providing needed blood to general circulation during hemorrhage and filtering old red blood cells and platelets from the body?
   a. Liver
   b. Spleen
   c. Gallbladder
   d. Kidney

2. A 45-year-old male presents to the emergency room with complaints of RUQ abdominal pain, bloating, nausea, and vomiting. The nurse notes the client's abdomen is distended and is unable to percuss the lower edge of the liver. Which advanced technique should the nurse use to measure the lower edge of the liver to assess for hepatomegaly?
   a. Fluid wave
   b. Obturator test
   c. Shifting dullness
   d. Liver scratch test

3. An urgent care clinic nurse examines a client with right lower quadrant pain. Visualizing the abdominal organs and using the four-quadrant technique, which of the following anatomical structures is located in this abdominal quadrant? Select all that apply.
   a. Appendix
   b. Pancreas
   c. Cecum
   d. Right ovary
   e. Liver
   f. Section of the descending colon

4. Which type of pain originates in the abdominal organs, is caused by contraction or distention of hollow structures, is dull and poorly localized, and can be associated with nausea and vomiting when it becomes intense?
   a. Visceral pain
   b. Referred pain
   c. Nociceptive pain
   d. Parietal pain

5. Which of the following individuals is at the highest risk for developing renal cancer?
   a. A 63-year-old Korean female with a history of gastroesophageal reflux disease
   b. A 70-year-old Black male who smokes and had asbestos exposure in the workplace
   c. A 54-year-old Native American female with a history of hepatitis C
   d. A 67-year-old Hispanic male with a history of ulcerative colitis

6. A 58-year-old female presents to the primary care clinic with complaints of constipation for the last 4 days. When obtaining the health history, the nurse determines which of the client's medications may be contributing factor(s) to constipation? Select all that apply.
   a. Lisinopril
   b. Metformin
   c. Ferrous sulfate
   d. Magnesium
   e. Oxycodone

7. While performing an abdominal examination on a client, the nurse notes that the abdomen is rounded, symmetrical, and without visible masses. The nurse also notes several atrophic lines and streaks across the abdomen. In which conditions can striae be found? Select all that apply.
   a. Cushing syndrome
   b. Gastric ulcer
   c. Cholecystitis
   d. Ascites
   e. Pregnancy

8. A 70-year-old male is being treated for a small bowel obstruction and has a nasogastric tube set to low intermittent suction. After the nurse completes the inspection of the abdomen, what should be the next action?
   a. Reposition the client to the left lateral recumbent position.
   b. Auscultate the abdomen by placing the diaphragm of the stethoscope lightly on the abdominal wall starting in the RLQ.
   c. Turn off the low intermittent suction.
   d. Beginning in the RLQ, percuss all four quadrants noting areas of tympany and dullness.

9. While using the fist percussion technique, the nurse notes the client experienced tenderness over the right costovertebral angle. What conclusion does the nurse make?
   a. This is an abnormal finding and present in a client with pyelonephritis.
   b. This is a normal finding and present in a client with Crohn disease.
   c. This is an abnormal finding and present in a client with appendicitis.
   d. This is a normal finding.

10. Which of the following individuals is at the highest risk for contracting hepatitis C?
    a. A 21-year-old female traveling in Southeast Asia eating local street food
    b. A 49-year-old male who received a kidney transplant in 2015
    c. A 37-year-old male with a history of chronic pancreatitis
    d. A 65-year-old female who shared a razor with a HCV-infected roommate

CHAPTER

19 Musculoskeletal System

Learning Outcomes

1. Identify the anatomy and physiology of the musculoskeletal system.
2. Conduct a complete health history on a client with a musculoskeletal system condition.
3. Perform a physical examination on a healthy adult and an adult with musculoskeletal system pathology.
4. Differentiate between normal clinical findings from a client's physical examination of the musculoskeletal system and the pathophysiology of abnormal clinical findings.
5. Identify risk factors for sports injuries.
6. Identify risk factors for osteoporosis.
7. Identify risk factors for osteoarthritis.
8. Assess if musculoskeletal system assistive devices are adversely affecting a client's health.
9. Identify the United States Preventive Services Task Force recommendations for the musculoskeletal system.
10. Document a complete health history and physical examination of a client with musculoskeletal system pathology.

The musculoskeletal system provides the ability to maintain and change body position in response to both internal and external stimuli. Muscles and bones allow a person to maintain an upright position and erect posture. Muscle contraction and joint movement allow an individual to move. Alterations in the musculoskeletal system will affect an individual's ability to complete activities of daily living and engage in occupational or recreational activities. The human body systems interact with and are dependent on each other for proper function. The musculoskeletal system is no exception. The musculoskeletal system is dependent on the neurological system for muscle tone and contraction. The cardiac, respiratory, and hematological systems provide oxygenated red blood cells to support muscle function and aerobic respiration while the bone marrow of the skeletal system provides new red blood cells, white blood cells, and platelets for the hematological and immune systems. Our internal organs and central nervous system depend on the skeleton for physical protection. The skeleton is dependent on the dermatological and endocrine systems to maintain calcium in the bone and the blood. A disturbance in one system affects the other systems to varying degrees.

Anatomy and Physiology

The musculoskeletal system consists of an intricate framework of bones, joints, skeletal muscles, and supportive connective tissue (cartilage,

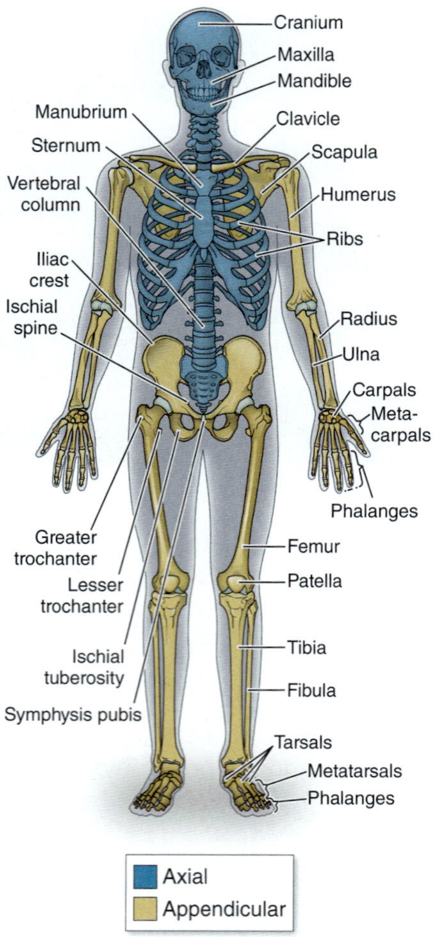

Figure 19-1 Adult skeleton: Anterior view.

tendons, and ligaments). Although the primary purpose of the musculoskeletal system is to support body position and enable mobility, it also protects underlying soft organs and stores minerals. In addition, it produces platelets, red blood cells, and white blood cells. Only those aspects of the musculoskeletal system that are responsible for body position and mobility are discussed in this chapter.

Bones

The adult human skeleton is composed of 206 bones (Fig. 19-1). Bone is ossified connective tissue. The skeleton is divided into the central **axial skeleton** (facial bones, skull, auditory ossicles, hyoid bone, ribs, sternum, and vertebrae) and the peripheral **appendicular skeleton** (limbs, pelvis, scapula, and clavicle). A bone's size and shape are directly related to the range of motion (ROM), directional movement, and weight-bearing function and capacity of that bone. In some cases, bone size, shape, and location are also related to the protection of underlying internal organs and tissues (e.g., the ribs in relation to the lungs, heart, and brain).

Shape and Structure

Bones have long, short, flat, rounded, or irregular shapes. A long bone consists of a shaft (**diaphysis**) with two large ends (**epiphyses**). The end of the epiphysis articulates with the epiphysis of another bone to form a joint. A 2- to 4-mm layer of articular cartilage covers the end of each epiphysis to minimize stress and friction on the bone ends during movement and weight-bearing. The thickness of the cartilage layer varies, depending on the amount of stress placed on that joint. The interior of the diaphysis is the **medullary cavity**. Red and yellow marrow exist within the medullary cavity. Red marrow is a primary site for blood cell production. Yellow marrow provides energy storage in the form of lipid reserves.

Short bones are found in the hands (carpals) and feet (tarsals). Flat bones, such as the skull, sternum, ribs, and parts of the pelvic girdle, are associated with the protection of underlying organs or soft tissues. Rounded, or sesamoid, bones are often encased in the fascia or a tendon near a joint; an example is the patella. Irregular bones include the mandible, vertebrae, and the auditory ossicles of the inner ear.

Muscles

There are more than 600 muscles in the human body. They can be classified as either cardiac, smooth, or skeletal muscles. Cardiac and smooth muscles are involuntary, meaning that the individual has no conscious control over the initiation and termination of the muscle contraction. Skeletal muscle is the largest type of muscle and the only type of voluntary muscle. Skeletal muscle enables mobility by exerting a pull on the bones near a joint. In addition, skeletal muscle creates the body contour and contributes to overall body weight. Fig. 19-2 illustrates the major muscles. It is estimated that 40% to 50% of adult body weight is due to the weight of the skeletal muscles. Muscles vary in size and strength in every person and are affected by age, sex, genetics, exercise, and nutrition.

Tendons

A strong connective tissue sheath (**epimysium**) acts as the outer covering of the muscle belly. The ends of the epimysium extend beyond the muscle belly to form the **tendons** of the muscle. The tendon attaches the muscle to a bone.

Cartilage

Hyaline cartilage is an avascular, dense, connective tissue. Articular cartilage is an example of hyaline cartilage that covers the ends of opposing bones. Its

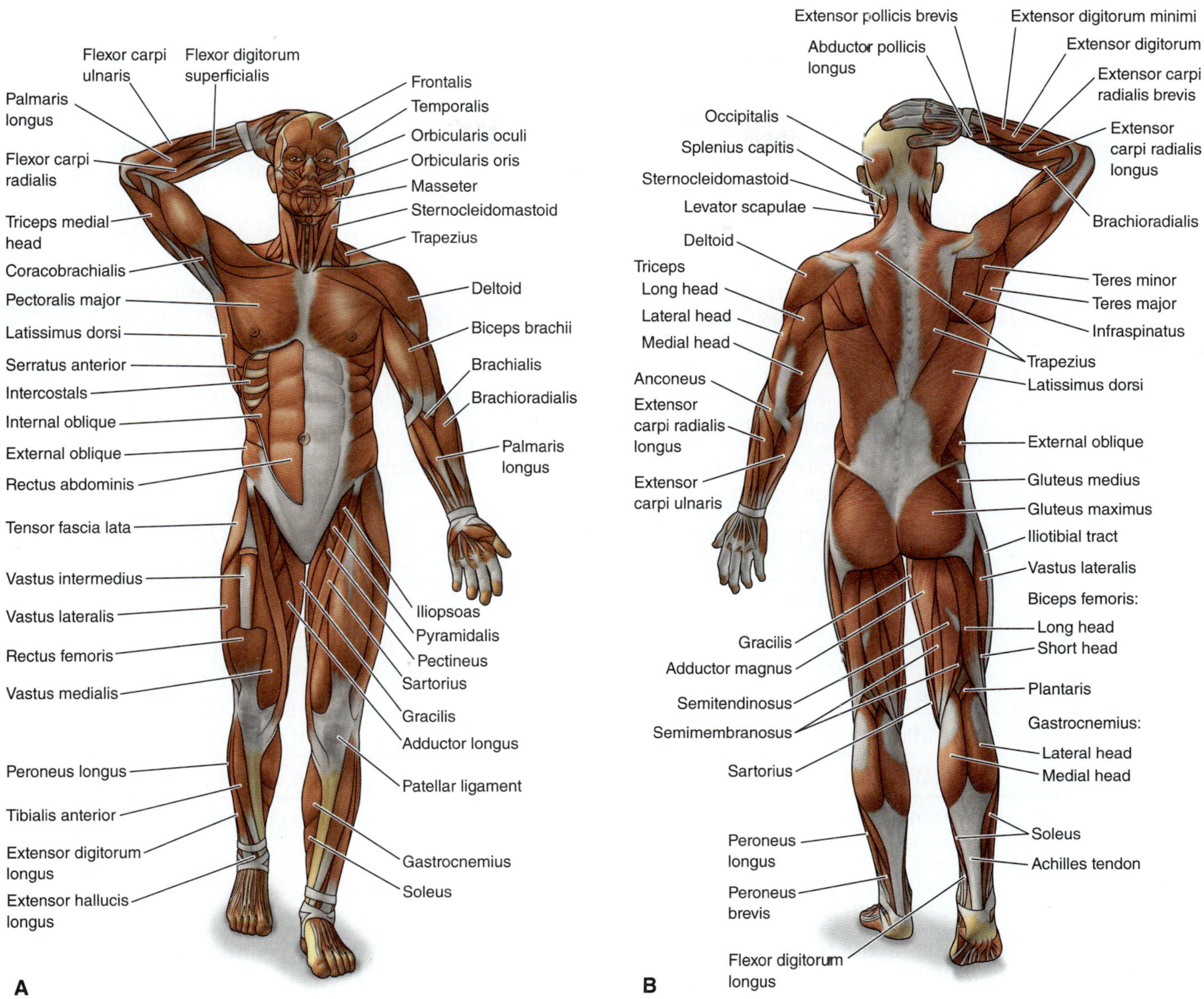

Figure 19-2 Muscles of the body. **A.** Anterior view. **B.** Posterior view.

resilience allows it to withstand increased pressure and tension. A second type of cartilage is fibrocartilage. The menisci within the knee joint are a good example of this type of cartilage. A third type of cartilage is elastic cartilage, a flexible cartilage with a large elastic fiber content. Two examples of this flexible type of cartilage are the tip of the nose and the pinna of the ear.

Ligaments

Ligaments are composed of strong, fibrous, connective tissue. They connect bones to each other at the joint level and encase the joint capsule. Ligaments may be seen as oblique to or parallel to a joint (e.g., knee) or encircling the joint (e.g., hip). Ligaments support purposeful anatomically normal joint movement and prevent abnormal or excessive joint movement that could result in injury to that type of joint.

Bursae

Bursae are sacs filled with fluid that act as cushions between two nearby structures (e.g., between tendon and bone or between skin and bony prominence) to reduce friction with tissue movement. They can also develop in response to prolonged friction or pressure over tissues.

Joints

A **joint** is a union between two bones. Many of the structures that a joint is composed of help to secure the bones firmly together but allow for varying degrees of movement between the two bones. Contraction of overlying skeletal muscle will act to alter the angle of the two bones by pulling the distal bone toward or away from the proximal bone. Terms used for joint ROM are described in Table 19-1.

Table 19-1 Descriptive Terms for Joint Range of Motion

Term	Description	Change in Joint Angle
Flexion	Bending of a joint so that the articulating bones on either side of the joints are moved closer together	Decreased
Extension	Bending the joint so that the articulating bones on either side of the joint are moved farther apart	Increased
Hyperextension	Extension beyond the neutral position	Increased beyond the angle of extension
Adduction	Moving the extremity medially and toward the midline of the body	Decreased
Abduction	Moving the extremity laterally and away from the midline of the body	Increased
Internal rotation	Rotating the extremity medially along its own axis	No change
External rotation	Rotating the extremity laterally along its own axis	No change
Circumduction	Moving the extremity in a conical fashion so that the distal aspect of the extremity moves in a circle	No change
Supination	Rotating the forearm laterally at the elbow so that the palm of the hand turns laterally to face upward	No change
Pronation	Rotating the forearm medially at the elbow so that the palm of the hand turns medially to face downward	No change
Opposition	Moving the thumb to touch the little finger of the same hand	No change
Eversion	Tilting the foot inward, with the medial side of the foot lowered	No change
Inversion	Tilting the foot outward, with the lateral side of the foot lowered	No change
Dorsiflexion	Flexing the foot at the ankle so that the toes move toward the chest	Decreased
Plantar flexion	Moving the foot at the ankle so that the toes move away from the chest	Increased
Elevation	Raising a body part in an upward direction	No change
Depression	Lowering a body part	No change
Protraction	Moving a body part anteriorly along its own axis (parallel to the ground)	No change
Retraction	Moving a body part posteriorly along its own axis (parallel to the ground)	No change
Gliding	One joint surface moves over another joint surface in a circular or angular nature	No change

Of the three classifications of skeletal joints found in the adult human skeleton (synarthroses, amphiarthroses, and diarthroses), only the synovial joint (diarthroses) is considered freely movable. Examples of each joint are provided in Table 19-2. Table 19-3 shows categories of the major synovial joints. The synovial joint allows body movement.

A synovial membrane lines a large portion of the interior lining of the joint space (Fig. 19-3). The primary purpose of the synovial membrane is to secrete fluid for joint lubrication, nourishment, and waste removal. Normally, the joint space contains only 1 to 3 mL of synovial fluid. Excessive synovial joint fluid is called a **synovial effusion**. The joint space is enclosed by a capsule, a fibrous connective tissue layer, which helps to contain synovial fluid in the joint, adds some physical stability, and contributes to proprioception.

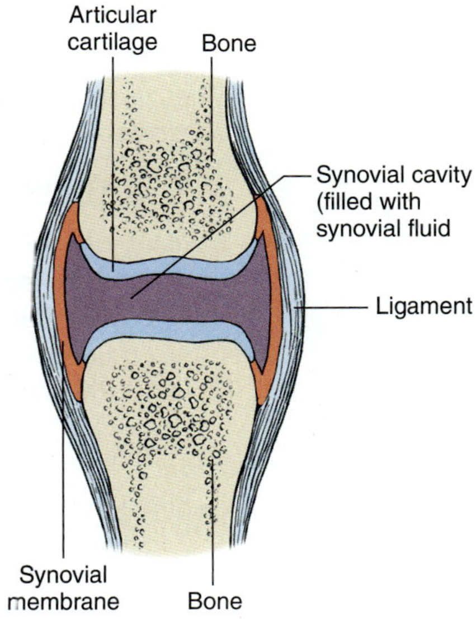

Figure 19-3 Synovial joint.

Table 19-2 Categories of Skeletal Joints

Category	Degree of Movement	Examples
Diarthroses (synovial)	Freely movable	Shoulder, elbow, wrist, thumb, hip, knee, ankle, and joint between first and second cervical vertebrae
Amphiarthroses	Slightly movable	Intervertebral joints (disc spaces), manubriosternal joint, radioulnar joint, and symphysis pubis
Synarthroses	Immovable	Epiphyseal growth plate (adult), skull sutures (child), between the distal ends of the radius and ulna, between the distal ends of the tibia and fibula, and the attachment of the root of a tooth to the alveolar process of the maxilla or mandible

Table 19-3 Categories of Synovial Joints

Category	Description	Example
	Uniaxial Joints	
Hinge joint	Angular movement in one axis and in one plane	Elbow, fingers, knee
Pivot joint (trochoid)	Rotary movement in one axis; a ring rotates around a pivot, or a pivotlike process rotates within a ring	Radioulnar joint, atlanto-axial joint of the first and second cervical vertebrae
	Biaxial Joints	
Saddle joint (sellar)	Articulating surface of one bone is convex and articulating surface of second bone is concave	Metacarpal bone of thumb, trapezium bone of carpus
Condyloid joint	Angular motion in two planes without axial rotation	Wrist between the distal radius and the carpals
	Multiaxial Joints	
Ball and socket joint (spheroidal)	Round end of bone fits into cuplike cavity of another bone; provides movement around three or more axes, or in three or more planes	Shoulder, hip
Gliding joint	Gliding movement	Vertebrae, tarsal bones of ankle

HEALTH HISTORY

The musculoskeletal health history provides insight into the link between a client's life/lifestyle, and musculoskeletal information and pathology.

CLIENT PROFILE

Diseases that are age-, sex-, and race-specific for the musculoskeletal system are listed.

Age Osteosarcoma (10 to 20 and 50 to 60)
Ankylosing spondylitis (20 to 40)
Bursitis (20 to 40)
Rheumatoid arthritis (onset 20 to 40 unless juvenile form of the disease)
Systemic lupus erythematosus (SLE) (25 to 35)
Low back pain (LBP) (30 to 50)
Gout (onset over 30, postmenopausal female)
Osteoporosis (menopausal female)
Carpal tunnel syndrome (pregnant or menopausal female)
Degenerative joint disease or osteoarthritis (onset after age 55 in females and before age 45 in males)
Multiple myeloma (50 to 70)
Paget disease (50 to 70)
Fibromyalgia (40 to 75)
Polymyalgia rheumatica (>50)

Sex

Female Osteoporosis, rheumatoid arthritis, scoliosis, carpal tunnel syndrome, SLE, postmenopausal gout, scleroderma, myasthenia gravis, multiple sclerosis (MS), senile kyphosis, fibromyalgia, polymyalgia rheumatica

Male Ankylosing spondylitis, gout, Paget disease, Reiter syndrome, Dupuytren contracture, psoriatic arthritis, muscular dystrophy (MD), amyotrophic lateral sclerosis (ALS), LBP

Race

White Rheumatoid arthritis, osteoarthritis, polymyalgia rheumatica, osteoporosis, Paget disease, Dupuytren contracture, ALS, ankylosing spondylitis

Black SLE, rheumatoid arthritis

CHIEF COMPLAINT

Common chief complaints for the musculoskeletal system are defined, and information on the characteristics of each sign or symptom is provided.

1. Pain The subjective sense of discomfort in the axial or appendicular skeleton

Location Muscle, bone, tendon, ligament, or joint; monoarticular or polyarticular; symmetrical or asymmetrical

Quantity Degree of interruption in the client's usual activities of daily living (ADL) (e.g., changes in ambulation, bathing, dressing, food preparation, working, sitting, transfer to a sitting or standing position, climbing stairs, lifting, pushing, and pulling)

Associated Manifestations Inflammation, skin abrasion, laceration, bruising, hematoma, stiffness, deformity, muscle spasm, paresthesia, decreased joint mobility, restriction of weight-bearing and movement, excessive weakness or fatigue, mental depression, insomnia, guarding of the painful area, crying, moaning, facial grimacing, anxiety, social withdrawal, agitation, restlessness, diaphoresis, tachycardia, elevated blood pressure, tachypnea

Aggravating Factors Muscle contraction, muscle spasm, joint movement, partial or full weight-bearing, obesity, dependent position, cold and damp weather, noncompliance with physical or occupational therapy guidelines

Alleviating Factors Restriction of movement, position change, non-weight-bearing, limb elevation and rest, ice, heat, analgesics, anti-inflammatory agents, steroids, muscle relaxants, local anesthetic agents, whirlpool therapy, transcutaneous electrical nerve stimulation (TENS), acupuncture, acupressure, assistive devices for use during weight-bearing and mobility, splints

Setting Recent untreated streptococcal infection; after COVID-19 infection; recent injury

Timing Sudden, insidious, intermittent, continuous, improving, or worsening. Musculoskeletal pain may be of an acute or chronic nature. Acute pain is associated with a recent onset and a short duration. Chronic pain has a malignant or nonmalignant etiology and lasts longer than 6 months.

2. **Weakness** The subjective sense of an overall decrease in strength and endurance

Location Local or diffuse, central or peripheral

Quantity Effect on ADLs

Associated Manifestations Fatigue, muscle atrophy, decreased sensation, decreased joint mobility, decreased muscle strength, discomfort, decreased ability to do ADLs

Aggravating Factors Overexertion, fatigue, immobility, noncompliance with physical or occupational therapy guidelines, physical or emotional stress

Alleviating Factors Rest, adequate nutrition and hydration, electrolyte replacement therapy, physical and occupational therapy geared toward muscle-strengthening exercises and adaptive techniques

Setting Neuromuscular conditions, after injury/illness

3. **Limited Movement** Decrease in mobility caused by a problem with impulse transmission to the muscle, stimulation of a muscle, the ability of that muscle to contract sufficiently to move the joint, or bone stability

Location Diffuse, or localized to a specific joint or muscle group

Quantity Range of joint motion compared with maximum potential or previous measurement

Associated Manifestations Pain, inflammation, stiffness, muscle atrophy, weakness, deformity, crepitus, joint effusion

Aggravating Factors Overexertion, immobility, excessive weight gain, noncompliance with medication regime (e.g., anti-inflammatory agents), noncompliance with physical and occupational therapy guidelines

Alleviating Factors Physical and occupational therapy, anti-inflammatory agents, analgesics, ice, heat, rest, reduction of fractures, correction of dislocation or subluxation

4. **Stiffness** The subjective sense of inflexibility

Location Diffuse, or localized to a specific joint

Quantity Effect on ADLs

Associated Manifestations Joint inflammation, muscle atrophy, deformity, contracture, immobility, pain, palpable joint crepitus, limited range of joint motion

Aggravating Factors Immobility, aging, overexertion (especially without adequate warming-up and cooling-down sessions during exercise), noncompliance with medication regime (e.g., anti-inflammatory agents), noncompliance with physical and occupational therapy guidelines

Alleviating Factors Physical and occupational therapy, exercise, anti-inflammatory agents, analgesics, heat, rest, massage, muscle relaxants

Setting Cold and damp environment

Timing Sudden or insidious, time of day (e.g., morning stiffness for more than 30 minutes is associated with rheumatoid arthritis), in relation to vigorous or excessive physical exercise

5. **Deformity** The congenital or acquired alteration in the configuration of the axial or appendicular skeleton

Location General (e.g., decreased overall body size) or localized (e.g., disruption in limb length and alignment due to a fracture)

Quality Degree of cosmetic alteration, inability to perform ADLs, degree of musculoskeletal dysfunction (adverse changes in mobility, weight-bearing, and the ability to maintain body posture and position)

Associated Manifestations Enlarged skull, jaw protrusion, forehead protrusion, abnormal joint angle, limb malalignment, missing or extra digits, missing limb, discrepancy in limb length or width, abnormal posture, muscle atrophy, joint contractures

Aggravating Factors Certain body positions or movements

Alleviating Factors Surgery, skeletal or skin traction, manual reduction of a fracture or dislocation, limb elevation, ice, physical therapy, splint, cast, brace

Timing Sudden or insidious, temporary or permanent

PAST HEALTH HISTORY

The various components of the past health history are linked to musculoskeletal pathology and musculoskeletal-related information.

Medical History

Musculoskeletal Specific Rheumatoid arthritis, osteoarthritis, osteoporosis, Paget disease, gout, ankylosing spondylitis, osteogenesis imperfecta, loosening or malfunction of joint prosthesis, aseptic necrosis, chronic LBP, herniated nucleus pulposus, chronic muscle spasms or cramps, scoliosis, poliomyelitis, polymyalgia rheumatica, osteomalacia, rickets, Marfan syndrome, scleroderma, spina bifida, congenital deformity, MD, MS, myasthenia gravis, ALS, Guillain-Barré syndrome, Reiter syndrome, carpal tunnel syndrome, paralysis, Ehler-Danlos syndrome

Non-Musculoskeletal Specific Immunosuppression, necrotizing fasciitis, gas gangrene, tetanus, sickle cell anemia, SLE, Lyme disease, blood dyscrasias (including hemophilia), multiple myeloma, diabetes mellitus with or without peripheral neuropathy, hypocalcemia, hypercalcemia, hypopituitarism, hyperpituitarism, hyperparathyroidism, hypoparathyroidism, hyperthyroidism, hypothyroidism, peripheral vascular disease with or without claudication, malnutrition, obesity, menopause

Surgical History Joint aspiration, therapeutic joint arthroscopy, joint replacement, synovectomy, meniscectomy, arthrodesis, open reduction and internal fixation (ORIF), discectomy, laminectomy, spinal fusion, spinal instrumentation, repair of torn rotator cuff, debridement, limb or digit amputation, reattachment of a limb or digit

Medications Narcotic or nonnarcotic analgesics, anti-inflammatory agents, antigout agents, muscle relaxants, steroids, calcitonin, calcium and vitamin D supplements, intra-articular injections, bisphosphonates, RANK Ligand inhibitor, sclerostin inhibitor, selective estrogen receptor modulator, human parathyroid hormone

Communicable Diseases Poliomyelitis

Injuries and Accidents Fracture, dislocation, subluxation, tendon tear, tendonitis, muscle contusion, joint strain or sprain, spinal cord injury, torn rotator cuff, traumatic amputation of a digit or limb, crush injury, back injury (including herniated vertebral disc), sports-related injury (e.g., golf elbow, tennis elbow, pitcher's shoulder), cartilage damage

Differing Abilities Amputation, hemiplegia, paraplegia, quadriplegia, need for brace or splint, limb in a cast, need for supportive devices, muscle atrophy

Childhood Illnesses Poliomyelitis, juvenile arthritis

FAMILY HEALTH HISTORY

Familial musculoskeletal diseases are listed.

Rheumatoid arthritis, osteoporosis, ankylosing spondylitis, gout, Paget disease, Dupuytren contracture, SLE, Marfan syndrome, osteomalacia, congenital defect

SOCIAL HISTORY

The components of the social history are linked to musculoskeletal factors and pathology.

Alcohol Use Increased use associated with increased risk of osteoporosis

Tobacco Use Increased use associated with increased risk of osteoporosis

Recreational Drug Use The use of recreational drugs can impair cognitive ability leading to musculoskeletal injury and accidents

Work Environment Manual movement of heavy objects (lifting, pushing, pulling), duties requiring repetitive motions (e.g., keyboard use, hammering), duties requiring prolonged standing or ambulation, use of hazardous equipment, availability and use of safety equipment (e.g., lifting equipment, availability of back support vest or brace)

Home Environment Design of home (e.g., number of floors, width of doorways, stairs, location of bedroom and bathroom), elevated toilet seat, bar in bathtub or shower, access ramp

Hobbies and Leisure Activities Basketball, wrestling, gymnastics, hockey, ballet, aerobics, use of free weights and exercise machines, baseball, football, lacrosse, rugby, cycling, running, horseback riding, skiing, hiking, tennis, pickleball, racquetball, swimming, camping, gardening, painting, needlepoint, carpentry, rollerblading, skateboarding, reading, watching sports, etc.

Stress Stress can be deleterious to clients with autoimmune chronic diseases affecting the musculoskeletal system, such as multiple sclerosis, systemic lupus erythematosus, and rheumatoid arthritis. During times of stress, these clients may experience additional discomfort, stiffness, loss of mobility, and fatigue.

Roles and Relationships Decreased self-esteem, decreased independence, or isolation secondary to immobility or pain

HEALTH MAINTENANCE ACTIVITIES

This information provides a bridge between health maintenance activities and musculoskeletal function.

Sleep Sleeping positions that may cause pain, need for pillow support, need for firm mattress

Diet Intake of dairy products and protein, use of dietary supplements or vitamins (especially calcium and vitamin D)

Exercise Prevents disuse atrophy, promotes bone growth (especially weight-bearing exercise), can aggravate existing musculoskeletal conditions, and cause musculoskeletal trauma

Use of Safety Devices Use of back support vest or lifting equipment for movement of heavy objects (e.g., Hoyer lift, forklift), safety shields when using hazardous equipment, protective padding (wrist or knee guards), helmet, use of gait belt for adult assistance/moving

Health Checkups Immunizations up to date, especially polio and tetanus, DEXA scan

NURSING TIP

Ensuring Home Safety

To ensure a safe home environment, encourage clients (especially those who have an increased risk for injury in the home) to avoid:

- Loose or unsecured rugs (e.g., scatter rugs, rugs on stairways)
- Stairways without banisters or stairways with loose banisters
- Stairs with a slippery surface
- Dim lighting, especially near stairways or steps
- Ill-fitting shoes; loose, unlaced shoes; shoes with high heels; or shoes with slippery soles
- Household clutter beneath waist level
- Electrical or phone cords that are too long and fall on the floor
- Wet or waxed floors
- Unrestrained small pets
- Bathtubs or shower stalls without a nonskid surface
- Lack of grab bars in the bathroom near the toilet and tub or shower stall
- Objects that are not within easy reach
- Wet or icy outdoor steps and sidewalks

NURSING CHECKLIST

General Approach to Musculoskeletal Examination

1. Observe Standard Precautions and don personal protective equipment (PPE) such as gloves, gown, face shield, goggles, N-95 respirator mask, or face mask if your client's status warrants these protective measures.
2. Assist the client to a comfortable position.
3. Offer pillows or folded blankets to support a painful body part.
4. If necessary, because of a painful body part or limited mobility, help the client with disrobing. Allow the client extra time to remove clothing.
5. To maximize client comfort during the physical examination, maintain a warm temperature in the examination room.
6. Be clear in your instructions to the client if you are asking the client to perform a certain body movement or to assume a certain position. Demonstrate the desired movement if necessary.
7. Notify the client before touching or manipulating a painful body part.
8. Inspection, palpation, range of motion, and muscle testing are performed on the major skeletal muscles and joints of the body in a cephalocaudal, proximal-to-distal manner. Always compare paired muscles and joints.
9. Examine nonaffected body parts before examining affected body parts.
10. Avoid unnecessary or excessive manipulation of a painful or injured body part.
11. If necessary, because of a painful body part or limited mobility, assist the client with dressing after the physical examination. Allow the client extra time to get dressed.
12. Some musculoskeletal disorders may affect the client more during certain parts of the day. Arrange for the follow-up appointment to be during the client's time of optimal function.

Assessment in Brief

Musculoskeletal Examination

General Assessment

- Overall appearance
- Posture
- Gait and mobility

Range of Motion

- Active and passive ROM
- Use of goniometer

Muscle Strength

- Muscle strength grading scale

Advanced Techniques

- Measuring limb circumference
- Using a goniometer
- Chvostek sign (assessing for neuroexcitability)
- Drop arm test (assessing for rotator cuff damage)
- Neer impingement sign (assessing for rotator cuff inflammation or injury)
- Hawkins impingement sign (assessing for rotator cuff inflammation or injury)
- Trousseau sign (assessing for neuroexcitability)
- Assessing grip strength using a blood pressure cuff
- Tinel sign (assessing for carpal tunnel syndrome)
- Phalen sign (assessing for carpal tunnel syndrome)
- Finklestein test (assessing for de Quervain tenosynovitis)
- Trendelenburg test (assessing for hip dislocation)
- Measuring limb length
- Bulge sign (assessing for small effusions)
- Patellar ballottement (assessing for large effusions)
- Apley grinding sign (assessing for meniscal tears)
- McMurray sign (assessing for meniscal tears)
- Drawer test (assessing the cruciate ligaments)
- Lachman test (assessing the anterior cruciate ligament)
- Varus stress test (assessing the lateral collateral ligament)
- Valgus stress test (assessing the medial collateral ligament)
- Anterior drawer test (assessing for ankle sprain)

- Talar tilt test (assessing for ankle sprain)
- Assessing status of distal limbs and digits
- Thompson squeeze test (assessing for ruptured Achilles tendon)
- Adams forward bend test (assessing for scoliosis) and use of the scoliometer
- Straight leg raising test (Lasègue test) (assessing for herniated disc)
- Milgram test (assessing for herniated disc)

Inspection

- Muscle size and shape
- Joint contour and periarticular tissue

Palpation

- Muscle tone
- Joints

Examination of Joints

- Temporomandibular joint
- Cervical spine
- Shoulders
- Elbows
- Wrists and hands
- Hips
- Knees
- Ankles and feet
- Spine

Assistive Devices

- Crutches
- Cane
- Walker
- Brace, splint, immobilizer
- Cast
- Motorized scooter
- Wheelchair

Equipment

- Appropriate PPE
- Measuring tape: cloth tape measure that will not stretch
- **Goniometer**: protractor-type instrument with two movable arms to measure the angle of a skeletal joint during ROM
- Sphygmomanometer and blood pressure cuff
- Felt-tip marker

Examination of the Musculoskeletal System

The complete musculoskeletal examination described in this chapter is designed for clients who have musculoskeletal complaints or disease or who have difficulty with ADLs. The screening, or musculoskeletal miniexamination, is conducted on all other clients and should include only general assessment: inspection and palpation of major muscles and joints, inspection of ROM as the client moves through the examination, and muscle strength of the arms and legs.

General Assessment

Overall Appearance

E

1. Obtain height and weight. Refer to Chapter 7.
2. Observe the client's ability to bear weight on the lower extremities during standing and ambulation. Assess the amount of weight-bearing placed on each of the lower extremities. See Table 19-4 for a description of terms defining weight-bearing status.
3. Identify obvious structural abnormalities. Obvious structural deformities can be acute or chronic in nature. Acute obvious structural abnormalities are time limited and short in duration such as days, or weeks (Fig. 19-4). Chronic obvious deformities result from congenital or acquired conditions that can last for a long period of time or for the client's lifetime (Fig. 19-5).

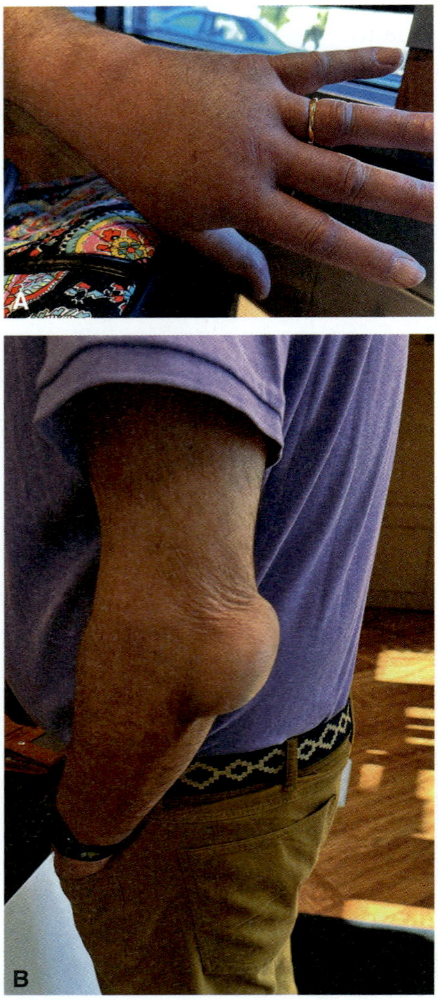

Figure 19-4 Acute obvious structural abnormalities. **A.** Hand edema caused by a fall. The ring needs to be removed before circulation is cut off to the digit. **B.** Elbow hematoma caused by falling on ice.

Table 19-4 Weight-Bearing Status

Status	Charting Abbreviation	Limits
Full weight-bearing	FWB	Full body weight may be placed upon the affected limb with standing or ambulating. Frequently no ambulation aid is utilized.
Weight-bearing as tolerated or to tolerance	WBAT or WBTT	A client may bear as much weight on the affected leg as is comfortable. The client shifts more weight or less weight to the affected leg using pain as the guide.
Partial weight-bearing	PWB	A percentage of the client's body weight or specific weight amount may be supported by the affected leg. The client can stand with the affected leg on a scale and adjust the amount of force placed on the leg to appreciate what that percentage of body weight feels like. Client may use crutches, a walker, or a cane.
Toe-touch or touch-down weight-bearing	TTWB or TDWB	No body weight may be placed on the affected leg. The foot of the affected leg may touch the floor for balance only while standing or ambulating. Clients usually use crutches to ambulate.
Non-weight-bearing	NWB	No body weight may be placed on the affected leg. The leg does not touch the floor and is held off the floor while standing or ambulating. Clients usually use crutches to ambulate.

4. Note nonverbal indications of discomfort (e.g., restricted weight-bearing or movement, frequent shifting of position, facial grimacing, excessive fatigue).

N **Body height and weight should be appropriate for age and sex. See Chapter 7. The client should be able to enter the assessment area via independent ambulation. Structural defects should be absent. There should be no outward indications of discomfort during rest, weight-bearing, or joint movement. There should be a distinct and symmetrical relationship among the limbs, torso, and pelvis.**

A An excessively tall, short, overweight, or underweight client is abnormal.

P Marfan syndrome affects multiple systems. The musculoskeletal changes are increased height for age due to an increased length of the distal limbs, extra digits, joint instability, pectus excavatum, and kyphosis.

P Dwarfism, a congenital disorder, is manifested by a decrease in body size. It is regarded as proportionate if both limb and trunk size are smaller than average. The decrease in size may affect only the limbs, which then appear out of proportion to the torso size.

P Severe osteoporosis and ankylosing spondylitis can result in height loss due to vertebral compression fractures and thoracic kyphosis.

P Obesity is considered to be a contributing factor in the development of both degenerative joint disease and low back pain. The stress of bearing excess body weight in the standing and ambulating positions can lead to loss of protective joint cartilage and joint pain in the hips and knees.

A Any weight-bearing status other tha n full weight-bearing is abnormal.

P Pain from an injury or arthritis may lead to an inability to fully bear weight.

A Structural defects are abnormal.

P **Acromegaly**, due to hyperpituitary function, may result in an enlarged skull with jaw protrusion and in an increase in the size of the hands, feet, and long bones (see Chapter 11 for additional information). The increased length of the long bones can contribute to increased height.

P A missing limb can be due to a congenital defect, surgery, or trauma (see Figs. 19-5 C and D).

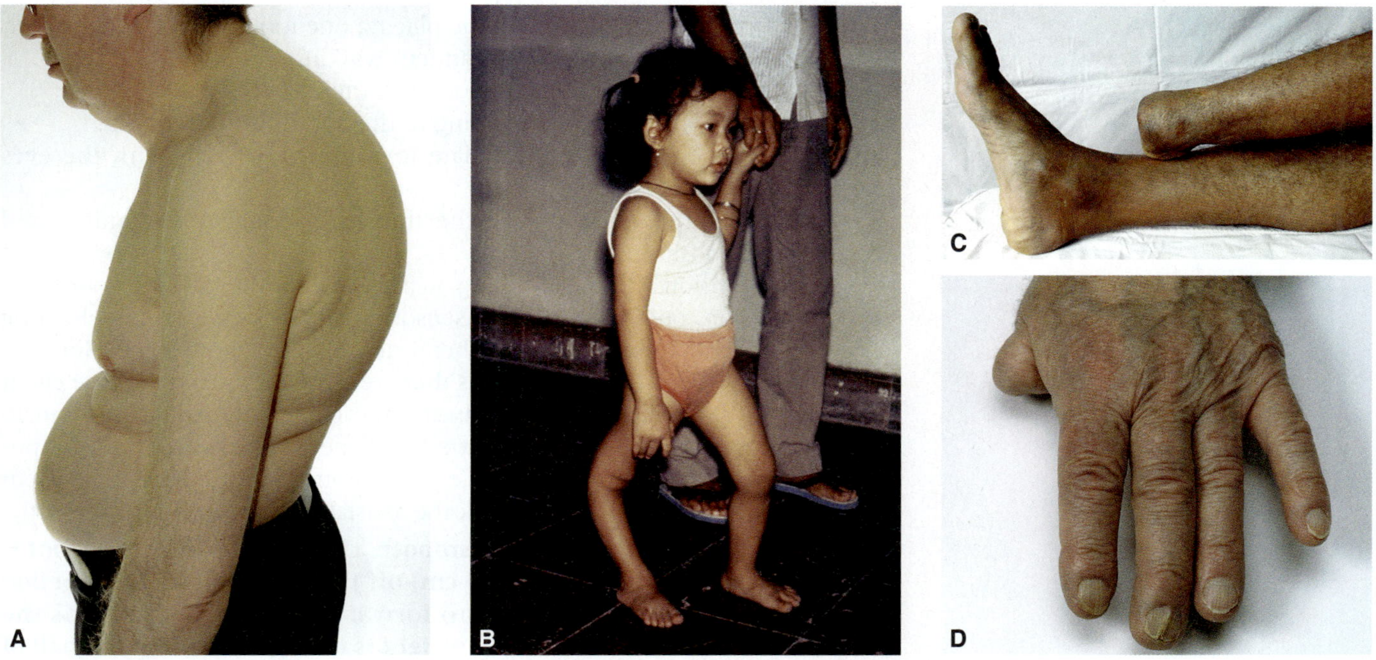

Figure 19-5 Chronic obvious structural abnormalities. **A.** Kyphosis. **B.** A leg deformity resulting from polio. **C.** An amputated left foot due to complications of diabetes. **D.** Loss of left thumb from a workplace injury.

P Pectus excavatum and pectus carinatum are abnormal findings. See Chapter 15 for additional information.

P Scoliosis and kyphosis are abnormal findings. They are discussed later in this chapter in the "Spine" section.

Posture

E

1. Instruct the client to stand upright with the feet together.
2. Observe the client while standing in front, then behind.
3. Observe the structural and spatial relationship of the head, torso, spine, pelvis, and limbs. Assess for symmetry of the shoulders, scapulae, and iliac crests.
4. Ask the client to sit; observe posture.

N **In the standing position, the torso and head are upright. The head is midline and perpendicular to the horizontal line of the shoulders and pelvis. The shoulders and hips are level, with symmetry of the scapulae and iliac crests. The arms hang freely from the shoulders. The feet are aligned, and the toes point forward. The extremities are proportional to the overall body size and shape, and the limbs are also symmetrical with each other. The knees face forward, with symmetry of the level of the knees. There is usually less than a 2 inches (5 cm) interval between the knees when the client stands with the feet together, facing forward. When full growth is reached, the arm span is equal to the height. In the sitting position, both feet should be placed firmly on the floor surface, with toes pointing forward.**

A Forward slouching of the shoulders produces a false thoracic kyphosis.

P These findings can be caused by poor posture habits.

Gait and Mobility

E

1. Observe the client walking normally across the examination room.
2. Observe the client walking on the toes and then on the heels of the feet.
3. Observe the client walking by placing one foot in front of the other, in a "heel-to-toe" fashion (tandem walking).
4. Observe the client walking forward, then backward.
5. Observe the client sidestepping to the left, then to the right.
6. Instruct the client to ambulate forward a few steps with the eyes closed.
7. Observe the client during the transfer between the standing and sitting positions.
8. Use caution when examining a client with limited ability, poor coordination, poor balance, or a sensory deficit (e.g., visual loss, hearing loss, limb amputation, peripheral neuropathy, hemiplegia). Some of the positions and movements that are necessary may place the client at increased risk of falling during the examination. Be prepared to support the client to prevent a fall. If necessary, omit those components of the musculoskeletal examination that would place the client at high risk for injury, or seek the assistance of a second nurse.

N **Walking is initiated in one smooth, rhythmic fashion. The foot is lifted 1 to 2 inches (2.5 to 5 cm) off the floor and then propelled 12 to 18 inches (30 to 45 cm) forward in a straight path. As the heel strikes the floor, body weight is then shifted onto the ball of that foot. The heel of the foot is then elevated off the floor before the next step forward. The client remains erect and balanced**

during all stages of gait. Step height and length are symmetrical for each foot. The arms swing freely at the side of the torso but in opposite direction to the movement of the legs. The lower limbs can bear full body weight during standing and ambulation. Before turning, the head and neck turn toward the intended direction, followed by the rest of the body. The client should be able to transfer easily to various positions.

A Indications of gait disturbance include hesitancy or multiple attempts to initiate ambulation, unsteadiness, staggering, grasping for external support, high stepping, foot scraping due to inability to raise the foot completely off the floor, persistent toe or heel walking, excessive pointing of the toes inward or outward, asymmetry of step height or length, limping, stooping during walking, wavering gait, shuffling gait, waddling gait, excessive swinging of the shoulders or pelvis, and slow or rapid step speed. See Table 19-5 for examples of abnormal gait patterns.

P Causes of abnormal gait include muscle weakness, joint deterioration, malalignment of the lower limbs, paralysis, lack of coordination or balance, fatigue, and pain.

P Limited mobility due to stiffness is associated with degenerative joint disease, rheumatoid arthritis, Paget disease, and Parkinson disease.

P Severe thoracic kyphosis will alter the body's center of gravity and affect balance during both standing and ambulation.

P Pathological fracture of the femoral shaft during the stress of weight-bearing may occur during standing or ambulation. Pathological fracture can occur if the bone has been significantly weakened by malignancy, osteoporosis, Paget disease, or osteomalacia.

P Fragility fracture refers to a fracture following a fall from standing height or less and in the absence of other trauma. Bone weakened by osteoporosis has a low bone mineral density and is vulnerable to breakage during what is otherwise considered to be a minor trauma. Fragility fractures are common among older adults and often affect the wrist, vertebrae, and hip. These clients are at risk for more fragility fractures in the future. Fall precautions, physical therapy, proper use of assistive devices, medications to strengthen bone, and avoidance of medications that can induce postural hypotension can reduce the risk of fragility fractures.

A When rising from or sitting in a chair, the client may have to lean on the armrest for external support. The client may also tend to rock forward and push off from the armrest for propulsion upward into the standing position. Discomfort felt while bearing the body's weight in the standing position may be reduced in the sitting position.

P Because of stiffness and discomfort, the client with a degenerative joint disease of the hip joint often has difficulty rising from a sitting position without assistance.

Inspection

Muscle Size and Shape

E

1. Survey the overall appearance and symmetry of the muscle mass.
2. Ask the client to contract the muscle without inducing movement (isometric muscle contraction), relax the muscle, and then repeat the muscle contraction.
3. Look for any obvious muscle contraction.

Table 19-5 Abnormal Gait Patterns

Gait Type	Gait Description	Possible Pathology
Antalgic	Shortened period of weight-bearing on the affected leg during ambulation; usually due to pain.	Arthritis or injury of the lower extremity, discomfort or pain with bearing weight
Apraxic	A client with an apraxic gait will have difficulty initiating or carrying out movements of ambulation. When initiated, walking appears to be slow and have a shuffling pattern.	Frontal lobe disorders, Alzheimer disease, or multiinfarct dementia
Cerebellar ataxia	When walking, the client appears to stagger. The gait is uncoordinated with a wide base. Clients typically have trouble executing turns. These clients frequently have an associated positive Romberg test.	Multiple sclerosis, cerebellar dysfunction leading to incoordination of muscle movements
Sensory ataxia	The client will ambulate with an excessively high stepping gait. The feet are typically slapped hard against the ground while walking. Because of the lack of proprioception and sensory input, clients will frequently actively watch where they are walking.	Loss of sensory input, including proprioception, leading to incoordination of movement Spinal-cord dysfunction involving the dorsal columns and peripheral sensory neuropathy
Festinating	The client experiences difficulty in both starting and stopping ambulation. As clients ambulate, they will have short, shuffling steps. The body is flexed at the hips, elbow, and knees. Clients appear somewhat rigid with the neck and trunk flexed forward.	Parkinson disease
Foot drop or steppage	The client's knee and foot are lifted markedly high while ambulating, as if walking up stairs. When the leg is brought down, the foot slaps onto the floor due to absence of ankle dorsiflexors.	Peroneal nerve injury, dysfunction of the tibialis anterior or peroneal muscles, polio, and lumbar disc herniation
Scissors	The knees are adducted or crossed. The client ambulates with short, uncoordinated, stiff steps. The lower leg appears to move forward in a semicircular arc of motion as the body sways sideways.	Upper motor neuron disorders, multiple sclerosis
Short leg	The client ambulates with a clear limp. This is usually noted if the client has a leg-length discrepancy greater than 1 inch (2.5 cm).	Congenital or traumatic limb length discrepancy, congenital hip dislocation, hip or knee flexion contracture
Spastic hemiplegia	While ambulating, the client's affected lower extremity is held extended at the hip, knee, and ankle. The foot is held in an inverted position. The affected leg is swung forward in a semicircular, lateral arc of motion. The affected arm is held firmly against the body with the elbow, hand, and wrist flexed while the shoulder is adducted.	Corticospinal tract lesion, cerebral palsy
Trendelenburg	Weak abductor muscles allow the pelvis to tilt down to the nonaffected side while bearing weight on the affected leg. To compensate for the pelvis tilt while ambulating, a client may tilt the torso toward the affected side to counterbalance the pelvic tilt and attempt to maintain a level pelvis.	Muscular dystrophy, polio, superior gluteal nerve injury, hip abductor weakness, lumbar radiculopathy involving L5 nerve root

N **Muscle contour will be affected by the individual's genetics, nutrition, exercise, and activity patterns. Muscle shape may be accentuated in certain body areas (e.g., the limbs and upper torso) but should be symmetrical. There may be hypertrophy in the dominant hand. During muscle contraction, you should be able to visualize sudden tautness of the muscle area. Muscle relaxation will be associated with termination of muscle tautness. There is no involuntary movement.**

Hypertrophy refers to an increase in muscle size and shape due to an increase in the muscle fibers (Fig. 19-6). Hypertrophy is detected as a unilateral or bilateral increase in the contour of the muscle. During contraction, the borders of the muscle will become accentuated. An increase in muscle strength will accompany the increase in muscle size. Bilateral hypertrophy is common among athletes involved in weightlifting or other activities that require repetitive motion against opposing resistance. Hypertrophy of the proximal arms is often seen in clients who are dependent on a wheelchair for mobility yet can propel the wheelchair manually.

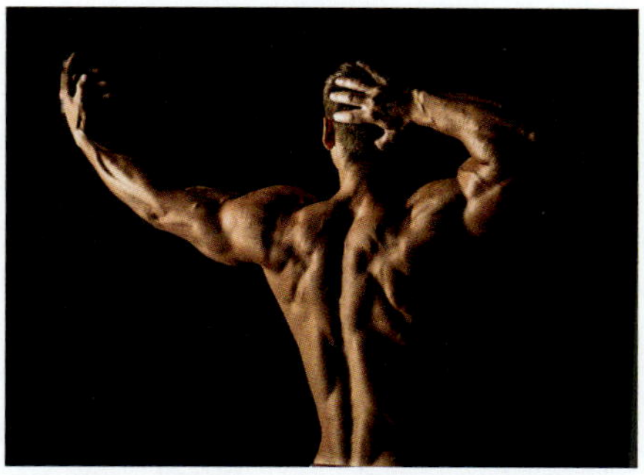

Figure 19-6 Muscle hypertrophy from weight-lifting.

A **Atrophy** describes a reduction in muscle size and shape. The contour of the skeletal muscle is less distinct than usual (Fig. 19-7). Atrophy may be local or diffuse.

P Generalized atrophy is directly related to prolonged immobility of the body as a whole unless isometric exercises were routinely performed during the period of immobility. It is accentuated by poor nutrition.

P Generalized atrophy may also be noted in grossly obese clients who lead sedentary lifestyles.

P Local atrophy is often detected in the limb or limbs affected by hemiparesis, paraplegia, or quadriplegia. It is also seen following the removal of a limb cast or splint (disuse atrophy).

A There is involuntary muscle movement.

P See Table 19-6.

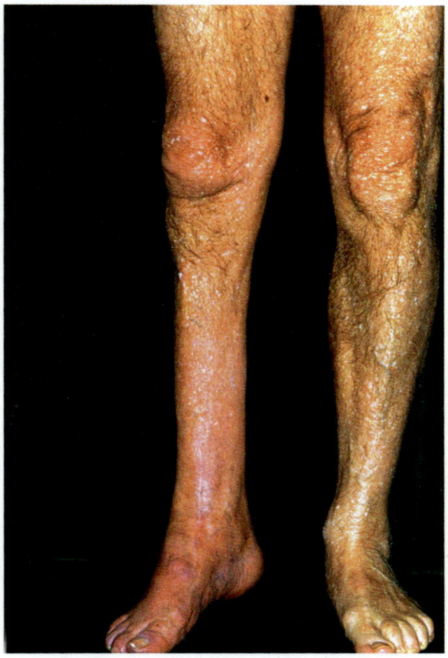

Figure 19-7 Atrophy of the right calf muscle.

Joint Contour and Periarticular Tissue

E
1. Observe the shape of the joint while the joint is in its neutral anatomical position.
2. Visually inspect the area of skin and subcutaneous tissue surrounding that joint. Assess the periarticular area for erythema, swelling, bruising, nodules, deformities, masses, skin atrophy, or skin breakdown.

N **Joint contour should be somewhat flat in extension, and smooth and rounded in flexion. You should be unable to detect any difference between periarticular tissue, the skin, and subcutaneous tissue. Bilateral joints should be symmetrical in position and appearance. There should be no observable erythema, swelling, bruising, nodules, deformities, masses, skin atrophy, or skin breakdown.**

A Enlargement of the joint is an abnormal finding.

P Joint inflammation can result from inflammatory disorders such as rheumatoid arthritis and gout (Fig. 19-8). Periarticular nodules may also be seen in the client with gout.

P Trauma to the joint and its extra-articular structures will also result in joint inflammation.

A Deformity of the joint capsule is an abnormal finding.

P Immobility results in joint contractures, which cause the joint to be permanently fixed in one position. The acquired joint position may be one within its normal range of joint motion or an abnormal joint position.

P Joint destruction from rheumatoid arthritis may result in a joint becoming fixed in one position.

Table 19-6 Involuntary Muscle Movements

Type	Description
Fasciculation	Visible twitching of a group of muscle fibers that may be stimulated by the tapping of a muscle.
Fibrillation	Ineffective, uncoordinated muscle contraction that resembles quivering.
Spasm	Sudden muscle contraction. A cramp is a muscle spasm that is strong and painful. Clonic muscle spasms are contractions that alternate with a period of muscle relaxation. A tonic muscle spasm is a sustained contraction with a period of relaxation.
Tetany	Paroxysmal tonic muscle spasms, usually of the extremities. The face and jaw may also be affected by spasm. Tetany may be associated with discomfort.
Chorea	Rapid, irregular, and jerky muscle contractions of random muscle groups. It is unpredictable and without purpose. It can involve the face, upper trunk, and limbs. Sometimes the client tries to incorporate the movement into voluntary movement, which may appear grotesque and exaggerated. The client may have difficulty with chewing, speaking, and swallowing.
Tremors	A period of continuous shaking due to muscle contractions. Although the quality of the tremors will be influenced by the cause, the amplitude and the frequency should remain the same. Tremors may be fine or coarse, rapid or slow, continuous or intermittent. They may be exacerbated during rest and attempts at purposeful movements, or by certain body positions.
Tic	Sudden, rapid muscle spasms of the upper trunk, face, or shoulders. The action is often repetitive and may decrease during purposeful movement. It can be persistent or limited in nature.
Ballism	Jerky, twisting movements due to strong muscle contraction.
Athetosis	Slow, writhing, twisting type of movement. The client is unable to sustain any part of the body in one position. The movements are most often in the fingers, hands, face, throat, and tongue, although any part of the body can be affected. The movements are generally slower than in chorea.
Dystonia	Similar to athetosis, but differing in the duration of the postural abnormality, and involving large muscles such as the trunk. The client may present with an overflexed or overextended posture of the hand, pulling of the head to one side, torsion of the spine, inversion of the foot, or closure of the eyes along with a fixed grimace.
Myoclonus	A rapid, irregular contraction of a muscle or group of muscles, such as the type of jerking movement that occurs when drifting off to sleep.
Tremors at rest	Asymmetrical and coarse movements that disappear or diminish with action. They tend to diminish or cease with purposeful movement.
Action tremors	Symmetrical or asymmetrical movements that increase in states of fatigue, weakness, drug withdrawal, hypocalcemia, uremia, or hepatic disease. This type of tremor may be induced in a normal individual when required to maintain a posture that demands extremes of power or precision. Action tremors are also called postural tremors.
Intention tremors	These tremors may appear only on voluntary movement of a limb and may intensify on termination of movement.
Asterixis	This is a variant of a tremor. The rate of limb flexion and extension is irregular, slow, and of wide amplitude. The outstretched limb temporarily loses muscle tone.

P Joint dislocation or subluxation will alter the normal contour of a joint. **Dislocation** refers to a complete dislodgment of one bone out of the joint space. **Subluxation** is a partial dislodgment of a bone from its position in the joint space.

A Alteration in periarticular skin and subcutaneous tissue is an abnormal finding.

P Trauma to the joint results in inflammation and bruising of the periarticular tissue. Joint trauma may include strain, sprain, contusion, dislocation, subluxation, or fracture within or near the joint capsule.

P The client with rheumatoid arthritis often presents with periarticular skin atrophy and subcutaneous nodules near a joint (e.g., elbow).

P Synovial effusion within the joint capsule may cause a bulging appearance that extends into the periarticular area.

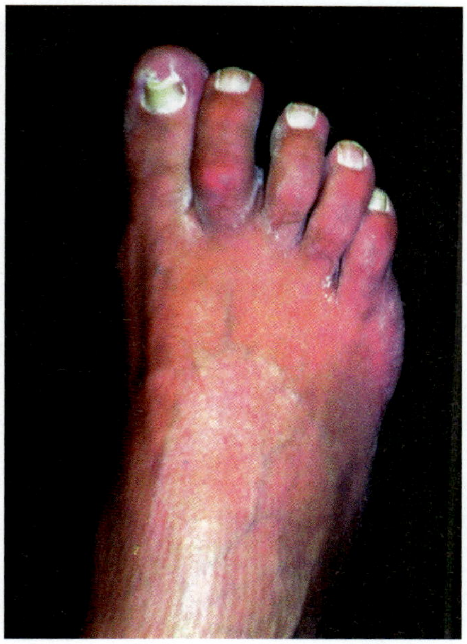

Figure 19-8 Joint inflammation of gout. Note the erythema and edema of the right second metatarsal interphalangeal joint.

ADVANCED TECHNIQUE

Measuring Limb Circumference

Limb circumference is measured when a limb looks larger or smaller than its counterpart during inspection.

E During muscle relaxation, measure the limbs at exactly the same distance from a nearby joint (e.g., the knee or elbow) at the site of maximal limb diameter (Fig. 19-9).

N **Bilateral measurements should be within ⅜ to 1¼ inches (1 to 3 cm) of each other. A slight increase in the circumference of the dominant arm is normal.**

A A discrepancy in limb circumference of 1 ¼ inches (3 cm) or more is abnormal.

P Atrophy results from disuse of a limb, as may occur following a stroke (see Fig. 19-7).

P Swelling following trauma to soft tissue or bone (e.g., crush injury or fracture) results in an increased limb circumference.

P Unilateral hypertrophy can result from selected activities that use one side of the body more than the other (e.g., tennis arm).

P Unilateral hypertrophy may also be the result of compensating for a deficit in the corresponding limb. For example, a client with hemiparesis of a limb will present with some degree of hypertrophy of the nonaffected arm muscles.

P A unilateral increase in calf circumference may accompany a deep vein thrombosis. In addition to increased calf circumference, a client may develop a positive Homan sign.

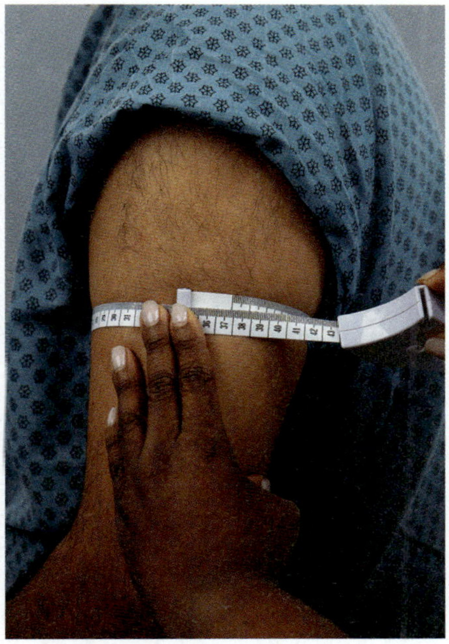

Figure 19-9 Measuring limb circumference.

Palpation

Muscle Tone

E

1. Palpate the muscle by applying light pressure with the finger pads of the dominant hand. Note any tenderness.
2. Note the change in muscle shape as the muscle belly (wide central aspect of the muscle) tapers off to become a tendon.
3. Ask the client to alternately perform muscle relaxation and isometric muscle contraction. Note the change in palpable muscle tone between relaxation and isometric contraction.
4. Palpate the muscle belly during contraction induced by voluntary movement of a nearby joint.

5. Perform a passive ROM to all extremities and note whether these movements are smooth and sustained.

N **Muscle tone refers to the partial muscle contraction state that is maintained for the muscle to respond quickly to the next stimulus. On palpation, the muscle should feel smooth and firm, even during the phase of muscle relaxation. There should be no pain. Normal muscle tone provides light resistance to passive stretch. During muscle contraction, especially against moderate external resistance to nearby joint movement, you will be able to palpate a significant overall increase in the firmness of the muscle belly. Muscle tone increases during anxiety or excitable states. Tone decreases during rest and sleep. You will be able to palpate the muscle belly and detect a change in its shape as it tapers down to become a tendon. The hypertrophied muscle will have an enlarged shape. You will detect muscle tautness even during the phase of relaxation.**

A **Hypotonicity** (flaccidity) is a decrease in muscle tone. When the muscle is palpated, it feels flabby and soft to the touch. When a flaccid limb is held away from the body and then released, it falls quickly with gravity.

P Etiology of flaccidity may include diseases involving the muscles, anterior horn cells, or peripheral nerves.

A **Spasticity** refers to an increase in muscle tension on passive stretching (especially rapid or forced stretching of the muscle). It is often noted with extreme flexion or extension.

P Upper motor neuron dysfunction is associated with spasticity.

A The atrophied muscle will feel small and flabby, even during the phase of muscle contraction.

P Refer to the description of atrophy in the "Muscle Size and Shape" section.

A A muscle spasm represents persistent muscle contraction without relaxation. The muscle belly will feel taut and the client may complain of discomfort over the muscle area. The spasm may also result in involuntary joint movement or a change in body position.

P Spasm follows fracture and may alter the distance between the bone fragments. Spasm is also common in the affected limbs of clients with paralysis, electrolyte imbalance, peripheral vascular disease, and cerebral palsy.

A Muscle pain may occur with or without palpation.

P Moderate to severe muscle pain of the neck, shoulders, or proximal thigh is associated with fibromyalgia. Pain or tenderness upon palpation of at least 11 out of 18 trigger points located on the back of the neck, upper chest, trunk, low back, and lower extremities is consistent with fibromyalgia. Palpation will often result in burning and gnawing pain (Fig. 19-10).

P Polymyalgia rheumatica involves stiffness and pain of the muscles. Symptoms of this inflammatory syndrome are located primarily in the shoulders, hips, and neck.

A Crepitus refers to a grating sensation or sound caused by two rough musculoskeletal surfaces rubbing together. Crepitus is more commonly detected with joint movement than it is with muscle contraction.

P Crepitus detected during palpation of muscle contraction, especially in a nonarticulating area, may indicate shaft fracture due to trauma

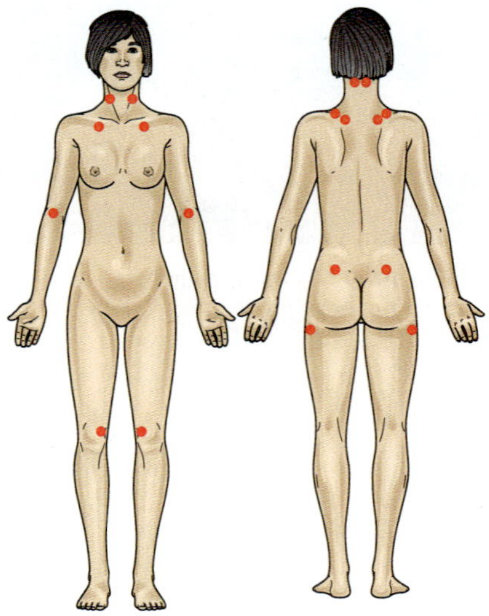

Figure 19-10 Fibromyalgia trigger points.

or loss of bone density. Muscle spasm following fracture may bring bone fragments in contact with each other, resulting in crepitus.

P Crepitus may result from the movement of an inflamed tendon and its covering sheath.

P Clients with osteoarthritis may have crepitus present with joint movement.

A Muscle masses detected on palpation are an abnormal finding.

P Muscle or tendon rupture will present as an inappropriate muscle mass above the joint due to retraction of the muscle. The muscle mass may be accentuated by muscle contraction. An example is a complete rupture of the Achilles tendon, resulting in a mass noted in the calf area.

P Displaced fracture (e.g., of the femoral shaft near the hip joint) will often result in palpation of the displaced bone near or into a muscle.

P Dislocation of a joint will also result in the palpation of the displaced bone in an abnormal position in relation to the surrounding musculature.

Joints

E

1. With the joint in its neutral anatomical position, begin palpating the joint by applying light pressure with the finger pads of the dominant hand 2 to 3 inches (5 to 7 cm) away from the center of the joint.
2. Palpate from the periphery inward to the center of the joint. Identify the soft tissue and bony landmarks while palpating the joint.
3. Note any swelling, pain, tenderness, warmth, or nodules.
4. Use a gentle approach when examining the client with severe osteoporosis or bone metastasis, because pathological fracture can occur with minor stress.

N **When the major skeletal joints are palpated in their neutral anatomical positions, the external joint contour will feel smooth, strong, and firm. The shape of the joint corresponds to that specific joint type. The area surrounding the joint (periarticular tissue) is free from swelling, pain, tenderness, warmth, and nodules. As the joint is moved through its normal ROM, it should be able to articulate in proper alignment without any visible or palpable deformity. Palpation of joint movement produces a smooth sensation, without tactile detection of crepitus, locking, or popping. A synovial membrane is not palpable under normal circumstances.**

A Bony enlargement or bony deformities of the joint are considered abnormal findings. Refer to Table 19-7, which provides a tool for grading joint swelling, tenderness, and limitations.

P Urate deposits associated with gout will result in a reactive synovitis, producing joint inflammation and enlargement (Fig. 19-11). Urate crystals accumulate in the joint as a result of a prolonged elevation of serum uric acid and create a mass called tophus. The affected joint will be extremely warm and tender to the touch. Although the great toe is most commonly affected, gout can also affect other joints, such as the hands.

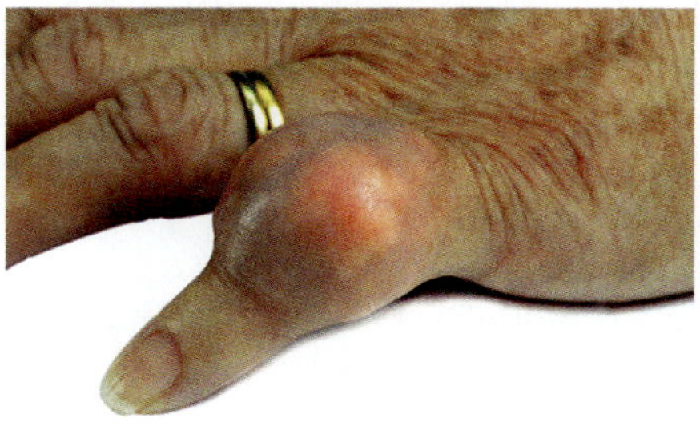

Figure 19-11 Gout tophus.

A Subcutaneous nodules detected in the periarticular area are abnormal.

P Rheumatoid arthritis is associated with subcutaneous nodules over the bony prominences and extensor joint surfaces (e.g., olecranon process of the elbow). These nodules are painless, firm but movable, and of normal skin color. They are more of a cosmetic concern than a threat to nearby joint function, although the overlying skin is at risk for breakdown due to irritation or pressure.

Table 19-7 Grading of Joint Swelling, Tenderness, and Limitation

Grade	Swelling (S)	Tenderness (T)	Limitation (L)
0	None	None	None
1	Mild	Mild, but tolerable tenderness upon palpation	25% decrease in joint range of motion
2	Moderate	Moderate tenderness upon palpation (which the client can tolerate but prefers not to)	50% decrease in joint range of motion
3	Marked	Light pressure or palpation induces an intolerable tenderness	75% decrease in joint range of motion
4	Maximum	Slight skin motion or sensation induces an intolerable tenderness	Complete loss of joint range of motion

0 = normal *1 = mild abnormality* *2 = moderate abnormality* *3 = marked abnormality* *4 = maximum abnormality*

Example: S3/T3/L4 = marked joint swelling with intolerable joint tenderness upon light pressure and with complete loss of joint range of motion.

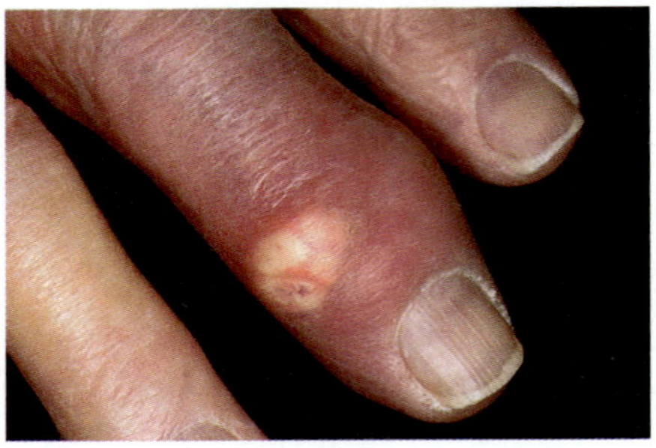

Figure 19-12 Tophi.

P Tophi nodules may be detected in the client with chronic gout, and they represent soft tissue reaction to uric acid crystal deposition (Fig. 19-12). They are often found on the great toes.

A Palpable, audible, severe crepitus that presents as more of a coarse than a fine sensation is abnormal.

P Crepitus is often palpated in joints affected by acute rheumatoid arthritis and degenerative joint disease due to a loss of articular cartilage and contact with bone surfaces.

P Bony overgrowth, muscle contracture, dislocation, and subluxation are associated with joint crepitus.

A Any tenderness felt on light touch or joint palpation is considered abnormal. You must differentiate between tenderness on palpation of the joint at rest versus tenderness during joint movement.

P Joint pain due to septic arthritis can occur 10 to 14 days after untreated streptococcal pharyngitis or tonsillitis.

P Increased joint capsule pressure with a significant joint effusion may induce discomfort with light touch or pressure to the joint in the neutral position.

P Localized joint tenderness may be detected in the presence of joint contusion, infection, or synovitis.

A Periarticular warmth, with temperature exceeding overall body temperature, indicates an underlying problem.

P Joint inflammation (e.g., due to acute rheumatoid arthritis or recent trauma) and gout produce significant joint warmth because of the increased localized perfusion associated with the inflammatory process.

Range of Motion (ROM)

E
1. Ask the client to move the joint through each of its various ROM movements.
2. Note the angle of each joint movement.
3. Note any pain, tenderness, or crepitus.
4. If the client is unable to perform full active ROM, then passively move each joint through its ROM.

ADVANCED TECHNIQUE

Assessing Joint ROM: Using a Goniometer

E

1. With the joint in its neutral position, place the center of the goniometer over the joint so that the two distal arms of the goniometer are in alignment with the proximal and distal bones adjacent to that joint.
2. Move the joint through its ROM and note the degree of the joint angle visible on the center of the goniometer (Fig. 19-13).

N **Refer to the specific sections on joints for the ROM for each joint movement.**

A Abnormalities of joint function are indicated by the client's inability to voluntarily and comfortably move a joint in the directions and to the degrees that are considered the norms for that joint.

P Degenerative joint disease, rheumatoid arthritis, and joint trauma are some of the many musculoskeletal disorders that prevent the affected joint from moving through its normal ROM.

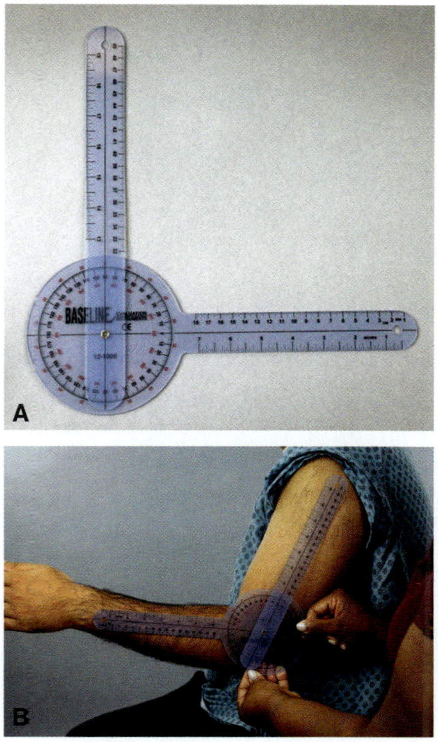

Figure 19-13 Assessing joint ROM with a goniometer. **A.** Goniometer. **B.** Goniometer measuring ROM of the left elbow joint.

5. Always stop if the client complains of pain, and never push a joint beyond its anatomical angle.
6. Use a goniometer to determine the exact ROM in joints with limited ROM. Refer to the Advanced Technique for using a goniometer.

Muscle Strength

Each muscle group is assessed for strength via the same movements as are performed in ROM. Muscle strength can be assessed indirectly by reviewing the client's ability to perform daily activities that involve lifting, pushing, pulling, grasping, walking, climbing stairs, and transferring to a sitting position. Muscle strength can be assessed directly using the Muscle Strength Grading Scale (Table 19-8).

E

1. Note whether muscle groups are strong and equal.
2. Always compare the right and left sides of paired muscle groups.
3. Note involuntary movements.

Table 19-8 Muscle Strength Grading Scale

Functional Ability Description	Scale (%)	0–5/5 Scale
Complete range of joint motion against both gravity and full manual resistance from the nurse.	100%	5/5 Normal (N)
Complete range of joint motion against both gravity and moderate manual resistance from the nurse.	75%	4/5 Good (G)
Complete range of joint motion possible only without manual resistance from the nurse.	50%	3/5 Fair (F)
Complete range of joint motion possible only with the joint supported by the nurse to eliminate the force of gravity and without any manual resistance from the nurse.	25%	2/5 Poor (P)
Muscle contraction detectable but insufficient to move the joint even when the forces of both gravity and manual resistance have been eliminated.	10%	1/5 Trace (Tr)
Complete absence of visible and palpable muscle contraction.	0%	0/5 None (O)

N **Normal muscle strength allows for a complete voluntary range of joint motion against both gravity and moderate to full resistance. Muscle strength is equal bilaterally. There is no observed involuntary muscle movement.**

A A decrease in skeletal muscle strength is significant if the complete range of joint motion is either impossible or possible only without resistance or gravity. A neurological consultation and diagnostic work-up are advised if there is a drastic reduction in muscle strength that results in a muscle strength grading value of 3 or less (corresponding to 50% or less of normal muscle strength). Further evaluation is also warranted if external support is needed to move a joint through its normal range of joint motion.

P Local decrease in muscle strength will accompany muscle atrophy of the limbs secondary to disuse.

P Diffuse reduction in muscle strength is associated with general atrophy, severe fatigue, malnutrition, muscle relaxant medications, long-term steroid use, and deteriorating neuromuscular disorders. These deteriorating neuromuscular diseases include, but are not limited to, ALS, MD, MS, myasthenia gravis, and Guillain-Barré syndrome.

A One-sided muscle weakness or paralysis is considered abnormal.

P Unilateral weakness or paralysis is indicative of **hemiparesis** (**hemiplegia**) from a cerebrovascular accident, brain tumor, or head trauma.

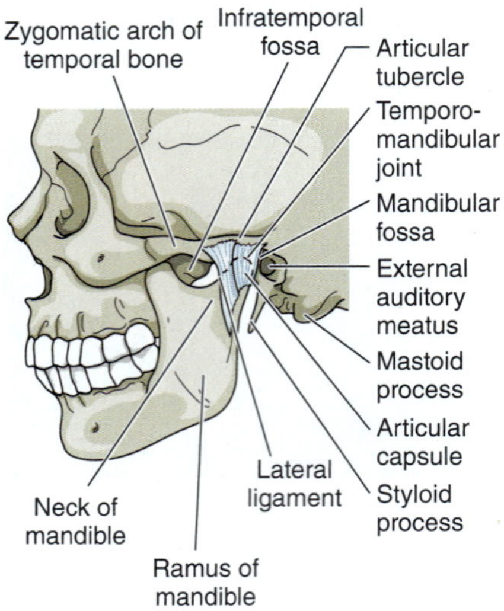

Figure 19-14 Anatomy of the temporomandibular joint (sagittal section).

Examination of Joints

Temporomandibular Joint

E
1. Stand in front of the client.
2. Inspect the right and left temporomandibular joints (Fig. 19-14).
3. Palpate the temporomandibular joints (Fig. 19-15).
   a. Place your index and middle fingers over the joint.
   b. Ask the client to open and close the mouth.
   c. Feel the depression into which your fingers move with an open mouth.
   d. Note the smoothness with which the mandible moves.
   e. Note any audible or palpable click as the mouth opens.
4. Assess ROM (Fig. 19-16). Ask the client to:
   a. Open the mouth as wide as possible.
   b. Push out the lower jaw.
   c. Move the jaw from side to side.
5. Palpate the strength of the masseter and temporalis muscles as the client clenches the teeth. This assesses cranial nerve V.

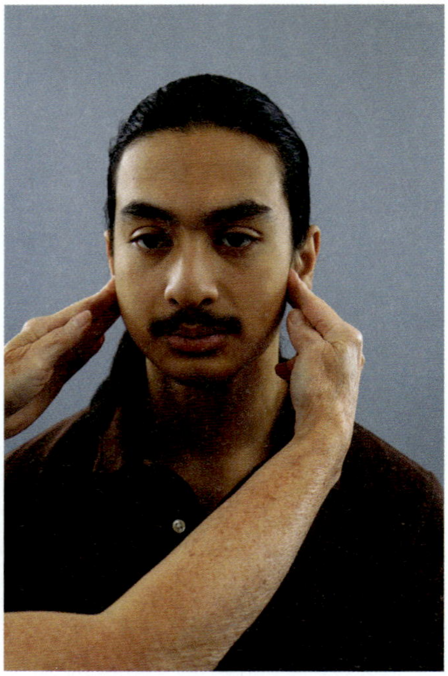

Figure 19-15 Palpation of the temporomandibular joint.

N **It is normal to hear or palpate a click when the mouth opens. The mouth can normally open 1¼ to 2¼ inches (3 to 6 cm) with ease. The lower jaw protrudes without deviating to the side and moves ⅜ to ½ inches (1 to 2 cm) with lateral movement.**

A Pain, limited ROM, and crepitus can occur in temporomandibular joint dysfunction.

P Temporomandibular joint dysfunction can occur secondary to malocclusion, arthritis, dislocation, poorly fitting dentures, myofascial dysfunction, and trauma.

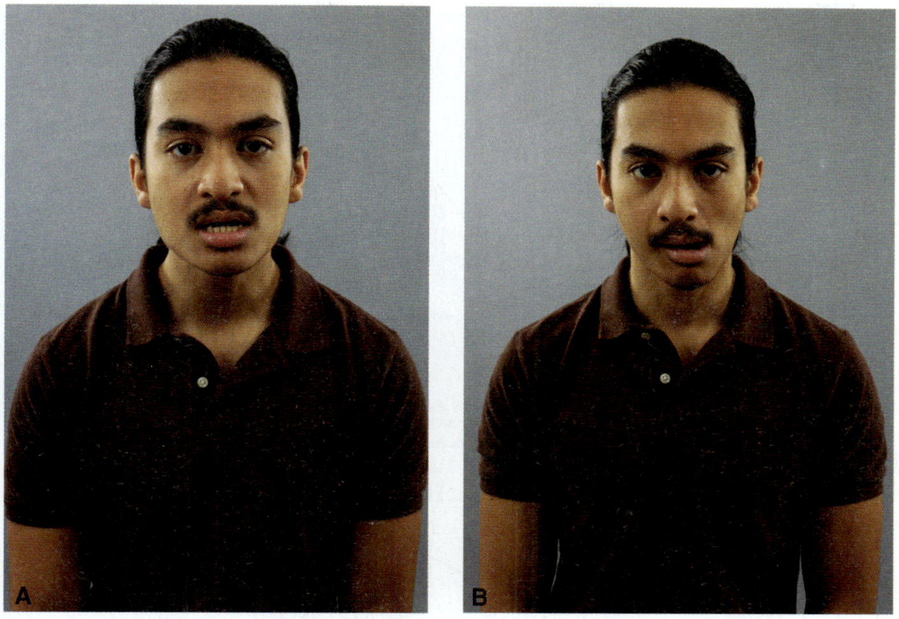

Figure 19-16 Range of motion of the temporomandibular joint. **A.** Pushing out the lower jaw. **B.** Moving the jaw from side to side.

P Osteonecrosis of the jaw may present as swelling, pain, or loosening of the teeth. This may be associated with the use of osteoporosis medications such as bisphosphonates.

ADVANCED TECHNIQUE

Assessing for Neuroexcitability: Chvostek Sign

E
1. The client can be assessed in the standing, sitting, or supine position.
2. While the client is facing forward, tap the side of the face just below the temple area anterior to the ear, using the middle or index finger (Fig. 19-17).
3. Observe for ipsilateral changes in facial expression immediately after tapping the face.
4. Repeat the procedure on the other side of the face.

N **There will be no change in the client's facial expression when the temple area is stimulated.**

A A positive Chvostek sign, indicated by an ipsilateral muscle spasm of the mouth and cheek, is abnormal. The muscle spasm will occur in an upward direction, toward the temple.

P A positive Chvostek sign is suggestive of neuroexcitability associated with hypocalcemia and tetanus infection.

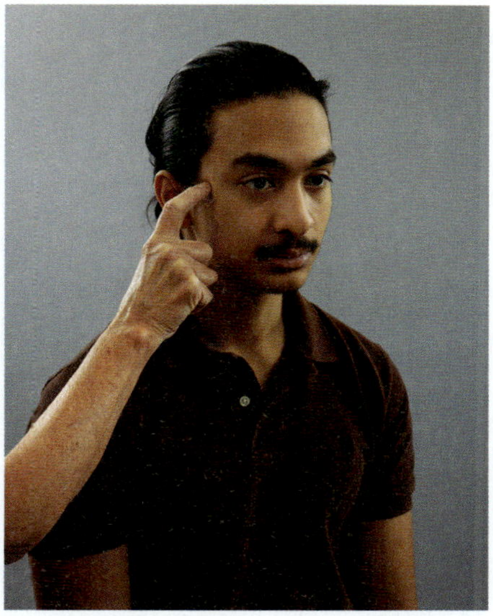

Figure 19-17 Assessing for Chvostek sign.

Cervical Spine

E
1. Stand behind the client.
2. Inspect the position of the cervical spine.
3. Palpate the spinous processes (Fig. 19-18) of the cervical spine and the muscles of the neck.

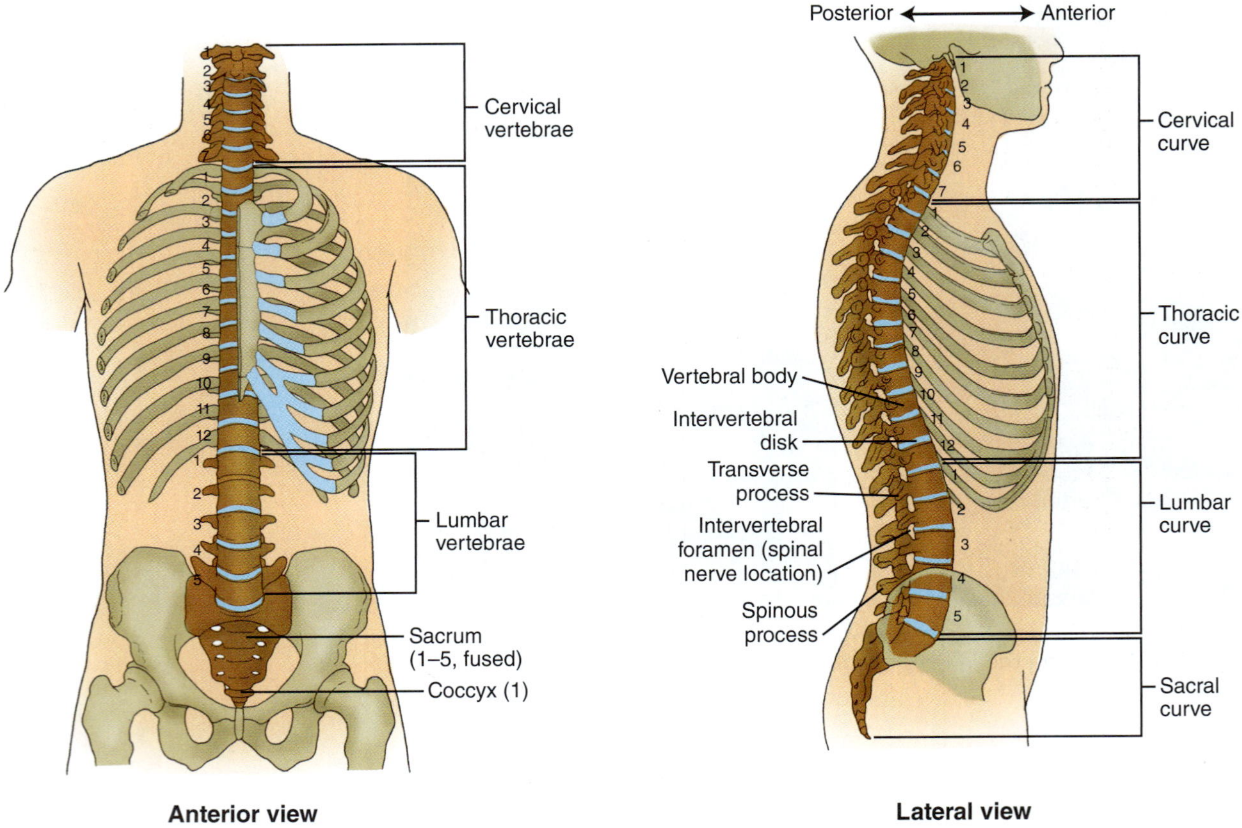

Figure 19-18 Anatomy of the spine.

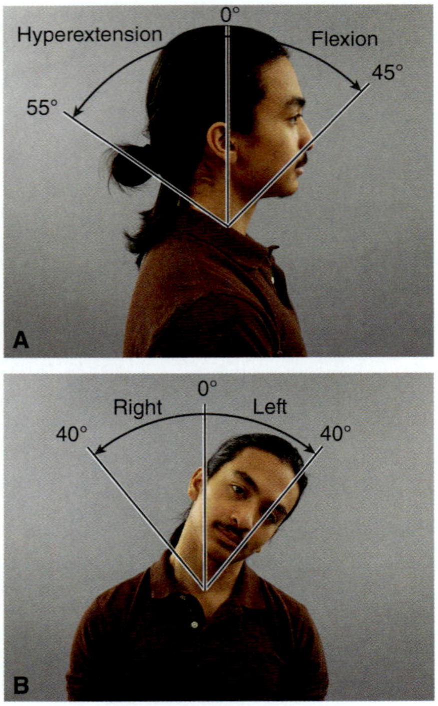

Figure 19-19 Range of motion of the cervical spine. **A.** Flexion, hyperextension. **B.** Lateral bending.

4. Stand in front of the client.
5. Assess the ROM of the cervical spine (Fig. 19-19). Ask the client to:
   a. Touch the chin to the chest (flexion).
   b. Look up at the ceiling (hyperextension).
   c. Move each ear to the shoulder on its respective side without elevating the shoulder (lateral bending).
   d. Turn the head to each side to look at the shoulder (rotation).
6. Assess the strength of the cervical spine by repeating the movements in step 5d while applying opposing force. This also assesses the function of cranial nerve XI.
7. Never move the head and neck of a client with a suspected neck injury. Movement can result in permanent spinal cord injury. Refer the client to an orthopedist or a neurosurgeon immediately. Use caution when applying mild to moderate resistance during neck examination, especially when the client has a known musculoskeletal disorder.

N **The cervical spine's alignment is straight with a gentle concave curvature, and the head is held erect. The normal ROM for the cervical spine is flexion—45°, hyperextension—55°, lateral bending—40° to each side, rotation—70° to each side. Hypertrophy of the neck muscles due to weight-lifting exercises will produce the appearance of a thick neck.**

A A neck that is not erect and has a loss of or excessive cervical curve is abnormal.

P Degenerative joint disease of the cervical vertebrae may result in lateral tilting of the head and neck.

P Muscle spasm of the cervical muscles can result in a flattening of the cervical curve.

P Torticollis is discussed in Chapter 11.

A A change in the size of the neck is abnormal.

P Klippel-Feil syndrome is the congenital absence of one or more cervical vertebrae along with fusion of the upper cervical vertebrae and bilateral elevation of the scapulae, resulting in a shortened neck appearance. It may be accompanied by a low hairline, webbing of the neck, and decreased neck mobility.

A Inability of the client to perform ROM and pain and tenderness on palpation are abnormal.

P Osteoarthritis, neck injury, disc degeneration (among older adult clients or from occupational stress), and spondylosis can manifest as an inability to perform some degree of ROM. Pain and tenderness to palpation may also be present.

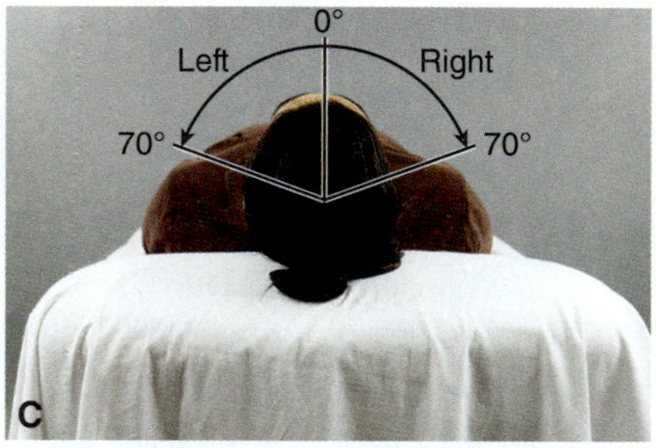

Figure 19-19—cont'd C. Rotation.

Shoulders

E
1. Stand in front of the client.
2. Inspect the size, shape, and symmetry of the shoulders (Fig. 19-20).
3. Move behind the client and inspect the scapula for size, shape, and symmetry.
4. Palpate the bony structures of the shoulders and surrounding muscles of the shoulder girdle.
   a. Palpate from the sternoclavicular joint along the clavicle to the acromioclavicular joint.
   b. Palpate the acromion, subacromial area, scapula, the proximal humerus, the anterior aspect of the glenohumeral joint, and the biceps groove.

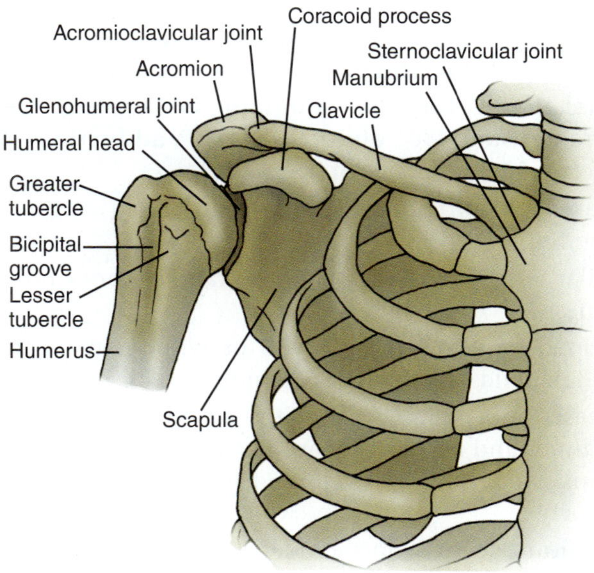

Figure 19-20 Anatomy of the shoulder joint.

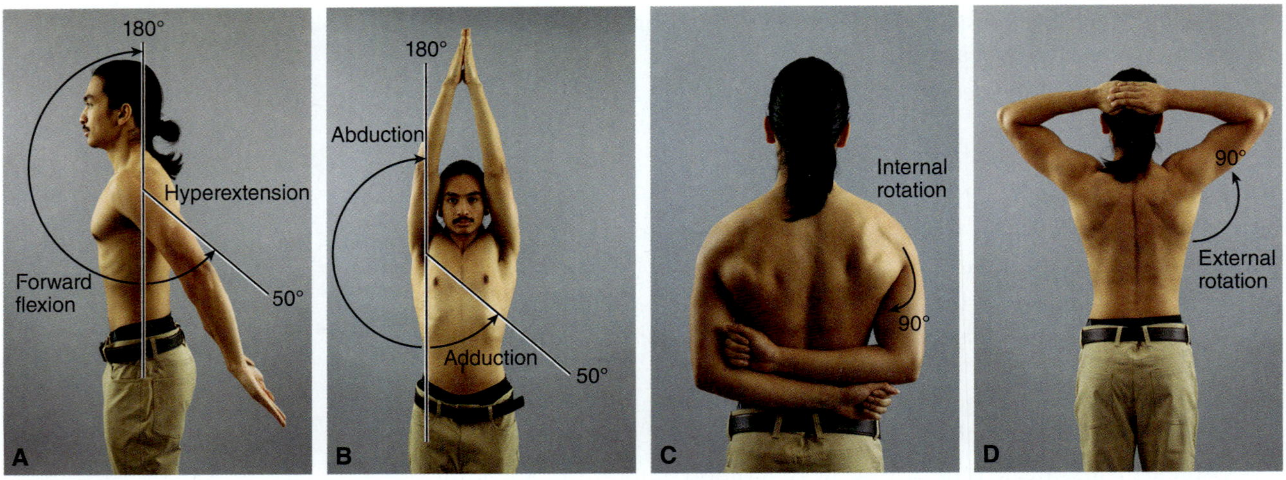

Figure 19-21 Range of motion of the shoulder joint. **A.** Forward flexion, hyperextension. **B.** Abduction, adduction. **C.** Internal rotation. **D.** External rotation.

5. Assess ROM of the shoulders (Fig. 19-21). Ask the client to:
   a. Place arms at the side, elbows extended, and move the arms forward in an arc (forward flexion).
   b. Move the arms backward in an arc as far as possible (hyperextension).
   c. Place arms at side, elbows extended, and move both arms out to the sides in an arc until the palms touch together overhead (abduction).
   d. Move one arm at a time in an arc toward the midline and cross it as far as possible (adduction).
   e. Place hands behind the back and reach up, trying to touch the scapula (internal rotation).
   f. Place both hands behind the head with elbows flexed (external rotation).
   g. Shrug the shoulders. This assesses cranial nerve XI function.
6. Assess the strength of the shoulders by applying opposing force to the ROM movement in step 5g.

N **The shoulders are equal in height. There is no fluid or edema palpable in the shoulder girdle. Crepitus is absent. The normal ROM for the shoulder is forward flexion—180°, hyperextension—50°, abduction—180°, adduction—50°, internal rotation—90°, external rotation—90°.**

A Increased outward prominence of the scapula (winging) is an abnormal finding.

P Scapular winging is indicative of serratus anterior muscle injury or weakness.

A Decreased movement, pain with or without movement, swelling from fluid, and asymmetry are abnormal.

P Decreased movement, pain with or without movement, swelling from fluid, and asymmetry are associated with immobility, osteoarthritis, and injury. Swelling from fluid is usually best seen anteriorly.

P A significant decrease in shoulder ROM is seen in a frozen shoulder (adhesive capsulitis). In a frozen shoulder, the glenohumeral joint gradually loses active and passive ROM, especially abduction and external rotation. The joint capsule becomes fibrotic and stiff. Stroke with loss of shoulder movement and rotator cuff pathology are common etiologies. There tends to be a greater incidence of adhesive capsulitis in people with diabetes.

P Subacromial bursitis of the shoulder can result from overuse of the shoulder in repetitive activity such as swimming.

P An acromioclavicular joint separation (separated shoulder) causes pain in the acromioclavicular joint. Swelling and deformity frequently occur at the distal end of the clavicle. A separated shoulder can occur with a fall directly on the shoulder joint or blunt trauma to the shoulder.

P Shoulder subluxation and dislocation are common athletic injuries. Clients with recurrent subluxations may feel the glenohumeral joint partially pop out of the socket and pop back in without medical intervention. The shoulder may lose its usual rounded contour with a sustained dislocation. With an anterior dislocation, fluid is usually seen anteriorly, whereas, with a posterior dislocation, fluid is usually best seen posteriorly.

P In biceps tendinitis, the client is tender with palpation of the biceps tendon in the bicipital groove. Excessive straining, as with lifting heavy objects, can rupture an inflamed biceps tendon. This can lead to a bulge and deformity of the biceps muscle.

P Shoulder pain that is not induced by palpation and ROM often occurs in clients experiencing cardiac dysfunction such as a myocardial infarction (MI). Be alert to other signs and symptoms of an MI, such as chest pain, nausea, vomiting, indigestion, shortness of breath, and diaphoresis. If the client complains of any of these symptoms, immediately refer the client to an appropriate healthcare facility.

ADVANCED TECHNIQUE

Assessing for Rotator Cuff Damage: Drop Arm Test

The rotator cuff is composed of four muscles (supraspinatus, infraspinatus, teres minor, and subscapularis) and their tendons. The tendons insert into the proximal humerus at the tuberosities. The rotator cuff stabilizes the glenohumeral joint.

The drop arm test assesses for rotator cuff damage.

E
1. Manually abduct the client's affected arm.
2. Ask the client to slowly lower the raised arm to the side while maintaining extension of the elbow (Fig. 19-22).
3. Observe the speed at which the client lowers the arm.

N **The client will be able to slowly lower the arm to the side while maintaining the elbow in extension.**

A An abnormal (positive) drop arm test is manifested by the client's inability to slowly lower the arm to the side (e.g., the arm quickly falls to the side of the torso), or by severe pain occurring in the shoulder while the arm is slowly lowered to the side.

P An abnormal drop arm test is indicative of a rotator cuff tear. It is caused by trauma to the shoulder.

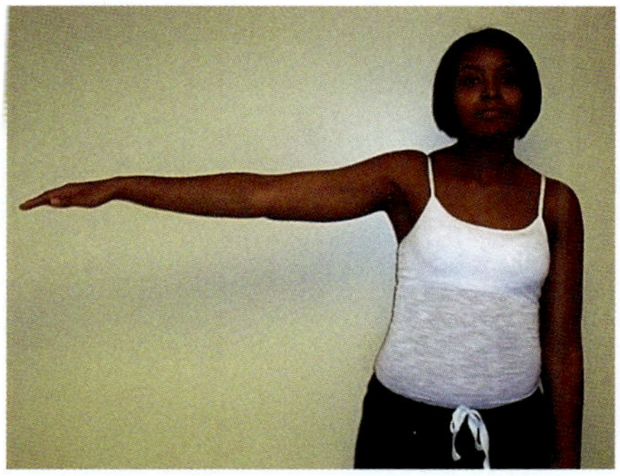

Figure 19-22 Drop arm test.

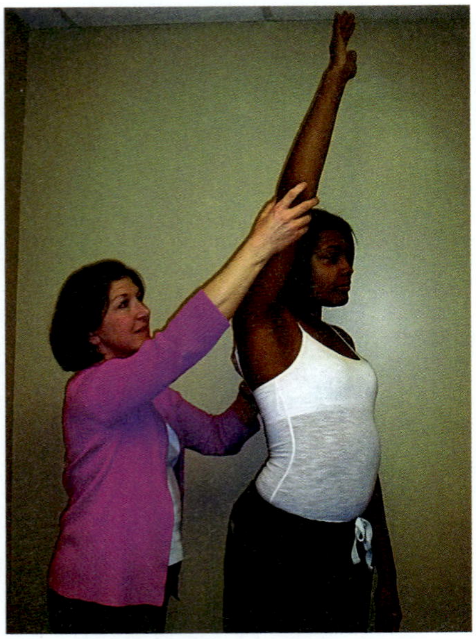

Figure 19-23 Neer impingement sign.

ADVANCED TECHNIQUE

Assessing for Impingement Syndrome and Rotator Cuff Tear: Neer Impingement Sign

E
1. The client can be in either a seated or a standing position.
2. Stand behind the client.
3. Stabilize the shoulder girdle by placing one hand over the scapula and trapezius of the arm to be tested.
4. With the other hand, grasp the client's arm posteriorly slightly proximal to the elbow.
5. While holding the elbow, flex the client's shoulder until the arm is in a flexed and abducted position with the arm at the side of the client's head (Fig. 19-23).

N **The client will be able to fully flex/abduct the shoulder. There will be no pain, crepitus, or instability while the examiner is raising the client's arm.**

A A positive Neer impingement sign is abnormal. The client will have pain while the arm is being raised and the shoulder girdle is being stabilized.

P As the client's arm is raised with this test, the greater tuberosity of the humerus and the acromion are being compressed. A client with injured or inflamed soft tissue (i.e., rotator cuff or bursa) at the shoulder, which gets compressed with this maneuver, will have pain.

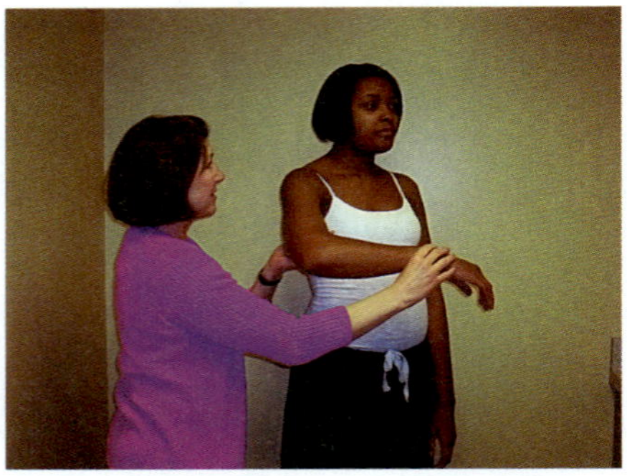

Figure 19-24 Hawkins impingement sign.

ADVANCED TECHNIQUE

Assessing for Impingement Syndrome and Rotator Cuff Tear: Hawkins Impingement Sign

E
1. Have the client in a seated or standing position.
2. Stand next to the client on the same side as the shoulder to be examined.
3. Support the client's elbow and hold the wrist of the arm to be examined (Fig. 19-24).
4. Place the client's arm in position with the shoulder at 90° of flexion, the elbow flexed to 90°, and the forearm in pronation.
5. While supporting the arm, internally rotate the client's shoulder.

N **The client will be able to flex the shoulder and elbow to 90° with the forearm in a pronated position. There will be no pain, crepitus, or instability while internally rotating the client's shoulder.**

A A positive Hawkins impingement sign is abnormal. The client will have pain at the shoulder with internal rotation during this test.

P As the client's shoulder is internally rotated with this test, the greater tuberosity of the humerus and the acromion are being compressed. A client with injured or inflamed soft tissue (i.e., rotator cuff or bursa) at the shoulder, which gets compressed with this maneuver, will have pain.

Elbows

E
1. Stand to the side of the elbow being examined.
2. Support the client's forearm on the side that is being examined (approximately 70°).

3. Inspect the elbow in flexed and extended positions. Note the olecranon process and the grooves on each side of the olecranon process (Fig. 19-25).
4. Using your thumb and middle fingers, palpate the elbow. Note the olecranon process, the olecranon bursa, the groove on each side of the olecranon process, the radial head, and the medial and lateral epicondyles of the humerus.
5. Assess ROM of the elbows (Fig. 19-26). Ask the client to:
   a. Bend the elbow (flexion).
   b. Straighten the elbow (extension).
   c. Hold the arm straight out, bent 90° at the elbow, and turn the palm upward toward the ceiling (supination).
   d. Turn the palm down toward the floor (pronation).
6. Assess the strength of the elbow:
   a. Stabilize the client's arm at the elbow with your nondominant hand. With your dominant hand, grasp the client's wrist.
   b. Ask the client to flex the elbow (pulling it toward the chest) while you apply opposing resistance (Fig. 19-27).
   c. Ask the client to extend the elbow (pushing it away from the chest) while you apply opposing resistance.

N **The elbows are at the same height and are symmetrical in appearance. The normal ROM for the elbow is flexion—160°, extension—0°, supination—90°, pronation—90°.**

A Elbows that are not symmetrical are abnormal. The forearm is not in its usual alignment. Pain is present.

P Elbow asymmetry and forearm malignment occur in a dislocation or a subluxation of the elbow. They usually occur from sports-related injuries, falls, or motor vehicle crashes.

A Localized tenderness and pain with palpation or elbow flexion and extension are abnormal.

P Epicondylitis occurs from repetitive motions of the forearm, such as hammering, using a screwdriver, or tight gripping. Lateral epicondylitis (tennis elbow) is caused by injury and inflammation to the extensor tendon at the lateral epicondyle, and medial epicondylitis (golfer's

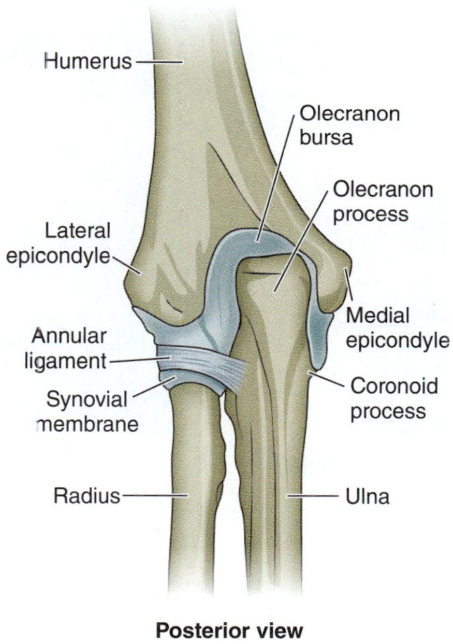

Figure 19-25 Anatomy of the elbow joint (posterior view, left elbow).

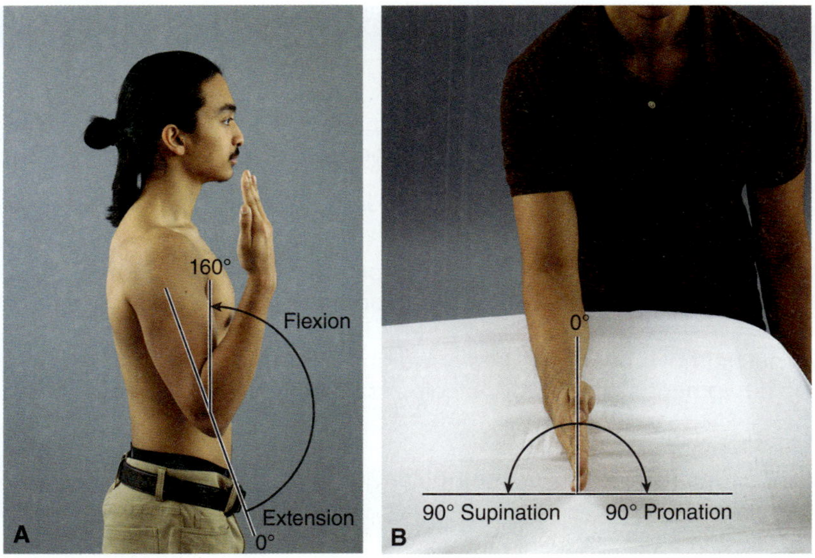

Figure 19-26 Range of motion of the elbow joint. **A.** Flexion, extension. **B.** Supination, pronation.

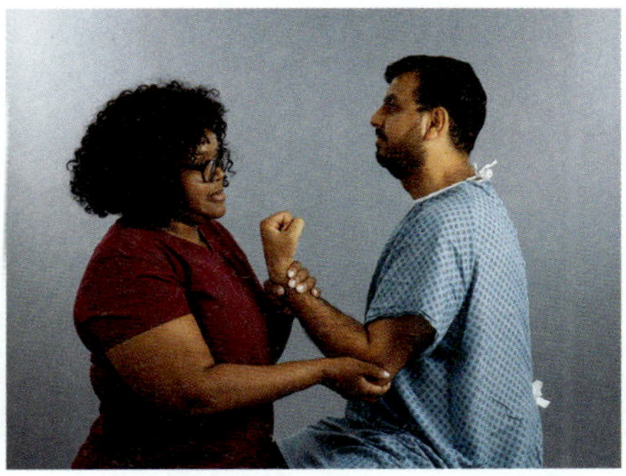

Figure 19-27 Assessing strength of the elbow.

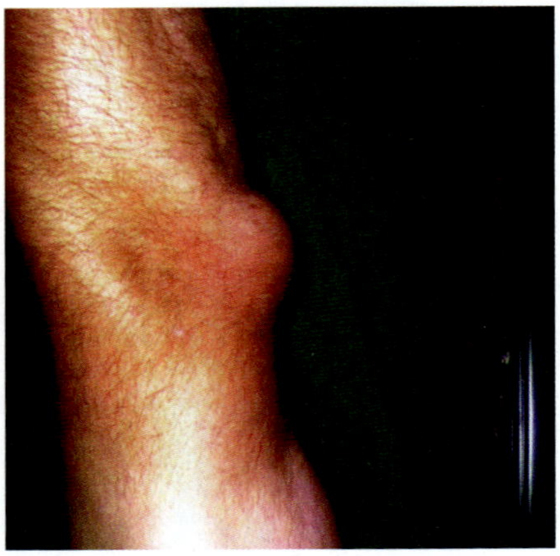

Figure 19-28 Olecranon bursitis.

elbow) is caused by injury and inflammation to the flexor tendon at the medial epicondyle.

P Radial head fractures usually result from falls. Frequently, the elbow is flexed in a 90° position. Any client, particularly an older adult, who complains of elbow pain after suffering a fall must be carefully examined for a radial head fracture.

P A flexion contracture of the elbow may be seen in a client with hemiparesis following a cerebrovascular accident.

A Red, warm, swollen, and tender areas in the grooves beside the olecranon process are abnormal. Synovial fluid may be palpable and is soft or boggy.

P Inflammatory processes such as gouty arthritis, rheumatoid arthritis, and SLE can cause these clinical manifestations.

P Olecranon bursitis (Fig. 19-28) usually results from repetitive motions but can also be caused by infection or an acute injury. ROM is usually not affected.

NURSING TIP

Comprehensive Musculoskeletal Assessment

A comprehensive musculoskeletal examination encompasses the elements described in this chapter as well as an assessment of the skin (refer to Chapter 10), peripheral vasculature (refer to Chapter 17), sensation, and deep tendon reflexes (refer to Chapter 20).

ADVANCED TECHNIQUE

Assessing for Neuroexcitability: Trousseau Sign

E
1. Place the client in a sitting or a supine position.
2. Apply a blood pressure cuff to the client's upper arm.
3. Inflate the blood pressure cuff to 10 mm Hg above the client's systolic blood pressure for 1 to 3 minutes.
4. Observe for twitching of the hand and fingers or a carpopedal spasm on the side being tested.

N **There will be no visible twitching or spasm of the hand and fingers during cuff inflation.**

A A positive Trousseau sign, indicated by visible ipsilateral twitching of the hand and fingers or a carpopedal spasm during cuff inflation, is abnormal. A carpopedal spasm occurs with flexion of the wrist, metacarpophalangeal joints, a nd thumb with hyperextension of the fingers.

P A positive Trousseau sign is suggestive of neuroexcitability associated with hypocalcemia and tetanus infection.

Risk Factors

Sports Injuries

Although exercise has been proven beneficial for good health and mobility, noncompliance with recommended guidelines can increase the risk of injury during exercise. Identification of risk factors for sports injury should be a part of the nursing assessment. These factors include, but are not limited to:

- The lack of medical clearance before the initiation of any aggressive exercise program following a period of prolonged sedentary activity
- Aggressive cardiovascular activity not accompanied by adequate warm-up (before) or cool-down (after) periods
- The lack of adequate and appropriate instruction on the use of exercise equipment (such as treadmills and weight machines)
- Not using a "spotter" assistant during gymnastic movements and heavy weightlifting
- Improperly fitting and unsecured protective equipment such as bicycle helmets, equestrian helmets, a mouthpiece, eye goggles, and shin pads
- Improperly fitting and unsupportive running shoes
- The lack of "rest days" between long-distance runs (e.g., 20 miles during marathon training)
- Obesity
- Lack of conditioning
- Prior heat-related injury
- Insufficient rehabilitation from a prior sport injury

E Examination **N** Normal Findings **A** Abnormal Findings **P** Pathophysiology

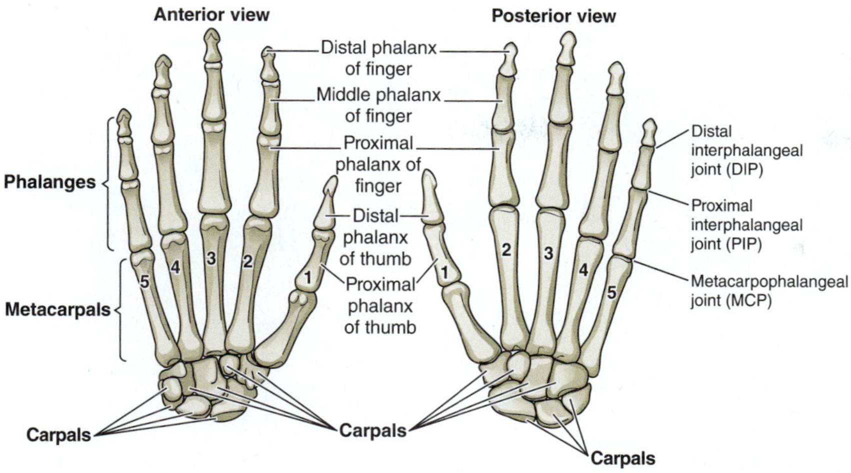

Figure 19-29 Anatomy of the wrist and hand.

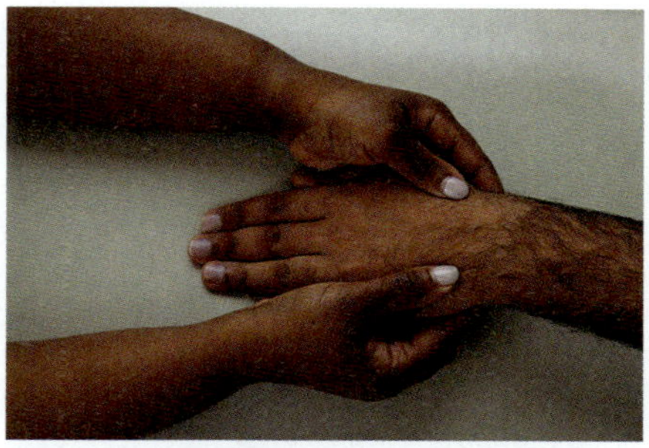

Figure 19-30 Palpating the wrist joint.

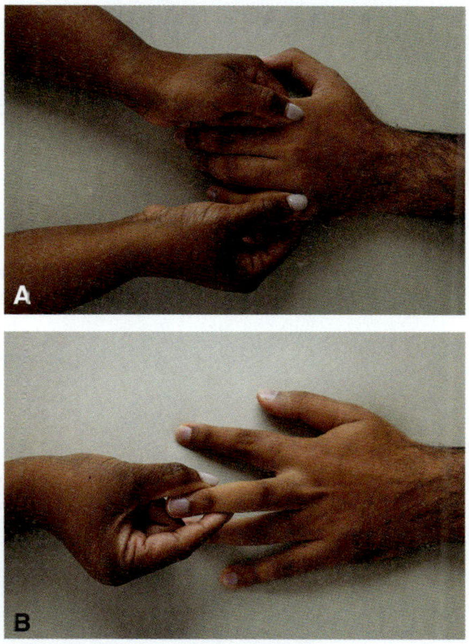

Figure 19-31 Palpating the hand joints. **A.** Metacarpophalangeal joints. **B.** Distal interphalangeal joint.

Wrists and Hands

E

1. Stand in front of the client.
2. Inspect the wrists and the palmar and dorsal aspects of the hands. Note the shape, position, contour, and number of fingers (Fig. 19-29).
3. Inspect the **thenar eminence** (the rounded prominence at the base of the thumb).
4. Support the client's hand in your two hands, with your fingers underneath the client's hand and your thumbs on the dorsum of the client's hand.
5. Palpate the joints of the wrist by moving your thumbs from side to side (Fig. 19-30). Feel the natural indentations. Palpate the indentation at the wrist along the radial border of the wrist just distal to the radius. This space is called the "anatomical snuff box."
6. Palpate the joints of the hand:
   a. Use your thumbs to palpate the metacarpophalangeal joints, which are immediately distal to and on each side of the knuckle (Fig. 19-31A).
   b. Between your thumb and index finger, gently squeeze the sides of the proximal and distal interphalangeal joints (Fig. 19-31B).
7. Assess the ROM of the wrists and hands (Fig. 19-32). Ask the client to:
   a. With the palm down, straighten the hand and wrist (extension), then bend it up at the wrist toward the ceiling (hyperextension).
   b. Bend the hand down at the wrist toward the floor (flexion).
   c. Bend the fingers up at the metacarpophalangeal joint toward the ceiling (hyperextension).
   d. Bend the fingers down at the metacarpophalangeal joint toward the floor (flexion).
   e. With the hand and wrist straight, deviate the hand from side to side at the wrist. (Radial deviation is movement toward the thumb, and ulnar deviation is movement toward the little finger).
   f. Make a fist with the thumb on the outside of the clenched fingers.
   g. Spread the fingers apart (abduction).
   h. Touch the thumb to each fingertip. Touch the thumb to the base of the little finger.

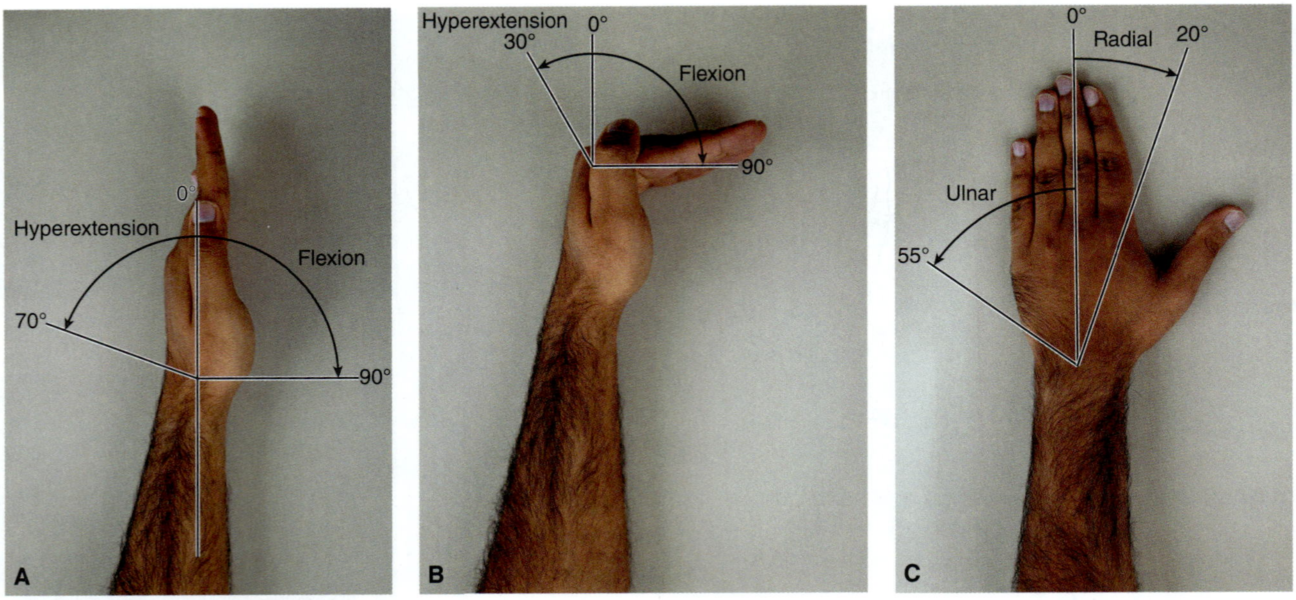

Figure 19-32 Range of motion of the wrist and hand joints. **A.** Hyperextension, flexion of the wrist. **B.** Flexion, hyperextension of the fingers. **C.** Radial, ulnar deviation of the wrist.

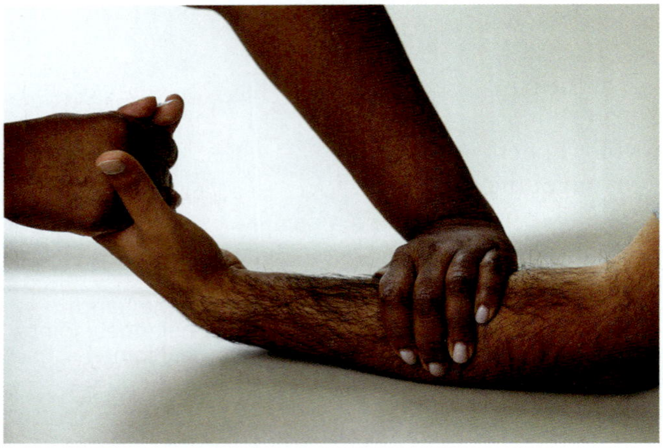

Figure 19-33 Assessing strength of the wrist.

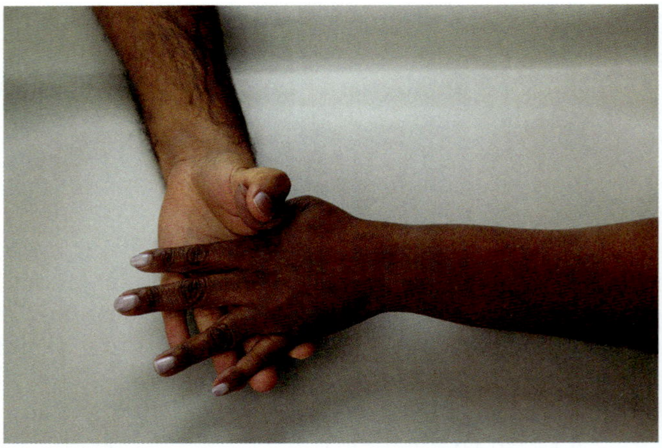

Figure 19-34 Assessing strength of the fingers.

8. Assess the strength of the wrists. Ask the client to:
   a. Place the arm on a table with the forearm supinated. Stabilize the forearm by placing your nondominant hand on it.
   b. Flex the wrist while you apply resistance with your dominant hand (Fig. 19-33).
   c. Place the arm in a pronated position. Stabilize the forearm, and extend the wrist while you apply resistance.
9. Assess the strength of the fingers. Ask the client to:
   a. Spread the fingers apart (abduct) while you apply resistance (Fig. 19-34).
   b. Push the fingers together (adduct) while you apply resistance.
10. Assess the strength of the hand grasp. Ask the client to:
   a. Grasp your dominant index and middle fingers in the client's dominant hand and your nondominant index and middle fingers in the client's nondominant hand (Fig. 19-35).
   b. Squeeze your fingers as hard as possible.
   c. Release the grasp.

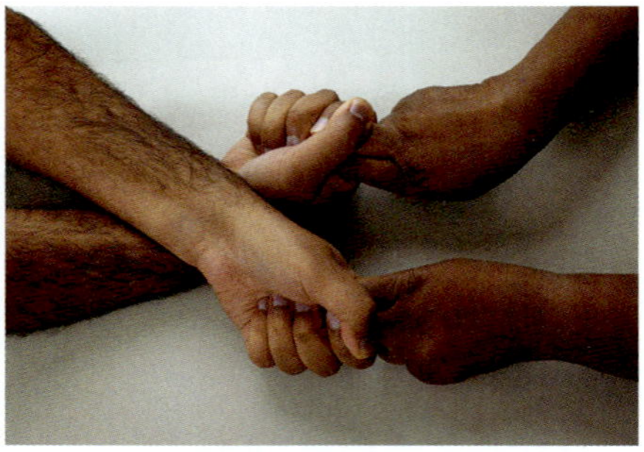

Figure 19-35 Assessing strength of the hand grasp.

N **There are five fingers on each hand. The normal ROM for the wrists is extension—0°, hyperextension—70°, flexion—90°, radial deviation—20°, ulnar deviation—55°. The normal ROM for the metacarpophalangeal joints is hyperextension—30° and flexion—90°.**

A Extra fingers, loss of fingers, or webbing between fingers is abnormal.

P **Polydactyly** is the congenital presence of extra digits. **Syndactyly** is the congenital webbing or fusion of fingers or toes (Fig. 19-36).

A Bony enlargement or bony deformities of the joints of the hand are abnormal.

P Osteoarthritis is associated with bony enlargement of the proximal interphalangeal joint (**Bouchard node**) and the distal interphalangeal joint (**Heberden node**) of the finger. These enlargements are hard and nontender. Bony enlargement may be masked by subcutaneous swelling. Bony enlargement is usually symmetrical (Fig. 19-37).

P Rheumatoid arthritis results in ulnar deviation (Fig. 19-38), swan-neck deformity, and boutonnière deformities of the fingers. In ulnar deviation, the fingers deviate to the ulnar side of the body. In swan-neck deformity, there is flexion of the metacarpophalangeal joint, hyperextension of the proximal interphalangeal joint, and flexion of the distal interphalangeal joint. In other words, the finger appears to go up, down, and up again. In boutonnière deformity, there is flexion of the proximal interphalangeal joint with hyperextension of the distal interphalangeal joint. The client frequently complains of pain, especially early in the morning. The joints may feel boggy on palpation. ROM may be restricted.

A A round, cystic growth near the tendons of the wrist or joint capsule is abnormal.

P A **ganglion cyst** is a benign growth that is frequently nontender and more prominent on the dorsum of the hand and wrist (Fig. 19-39).

A Flexion contracture of the fingers is abnormal.

P Dupuytren contracture is a flexion contracture that frequently affects the little finger, ring finger, and middle finger. Pain does not normally accompany this disorder. It is caused by the progressive contracture of the palmar fascia from an unknown etiology (Fig. 19-40).

A Muscular atrophy of the thenar eminence is abnormal.

P Muscular atrophy of the thenar eminence occurs as a result of median nerve compression, such as in carpal tunnel syndrome.

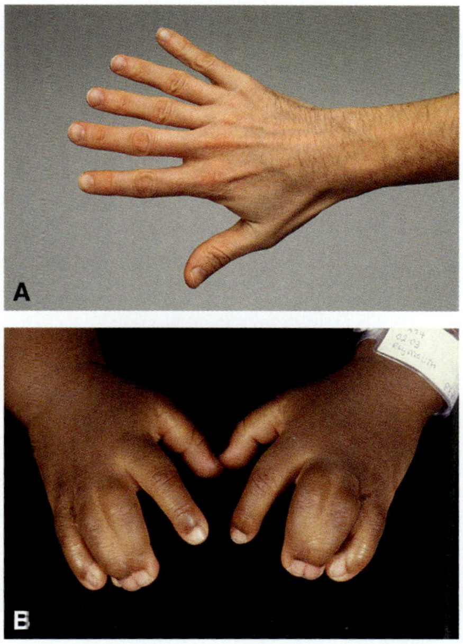

Figure 19-36 Finger anomalies. **A.** Polydactyly. **B.** Syndactyly.

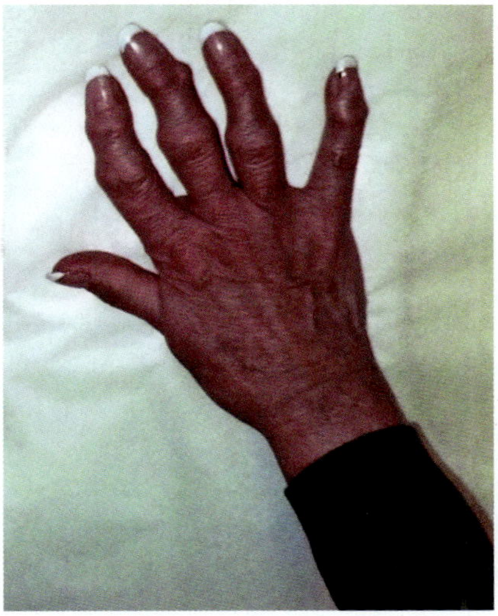

Figure 19-37 Bouchard nodes and Heberden nodes.

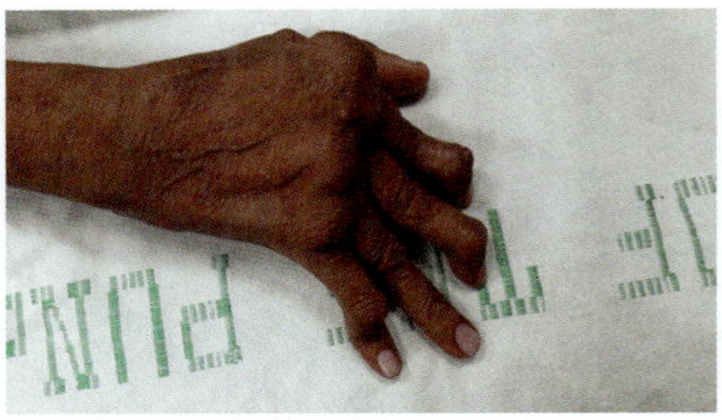

Figure 19-38 Ulnar deviation with swan neck and boutonnierre deformities.

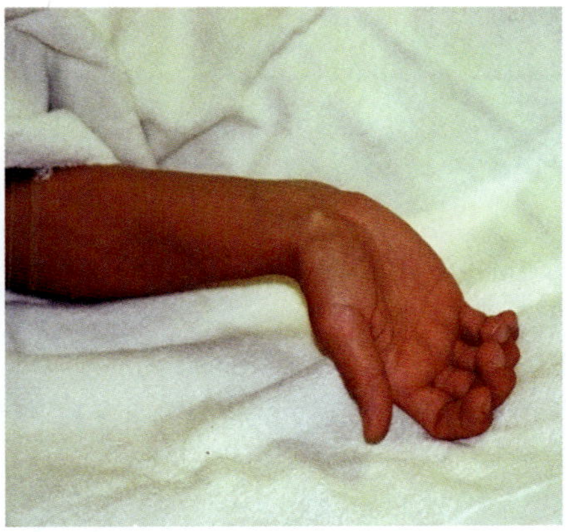

Figure 19-39 Ganglion cyst.

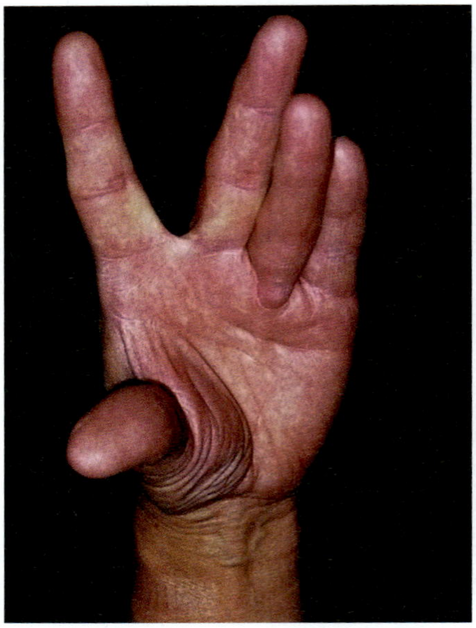

Figure 19-40 Dupuytren contracture.

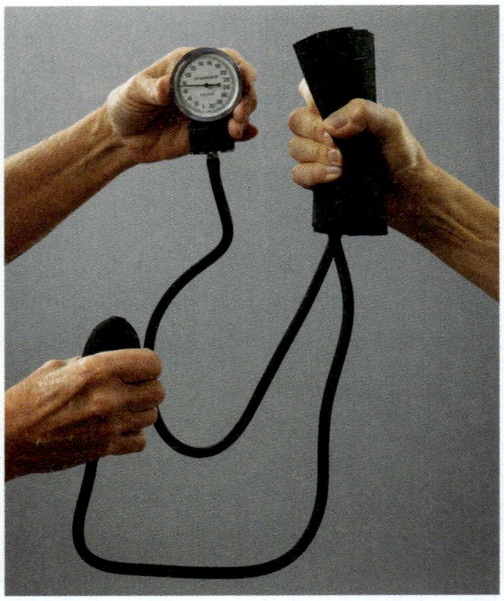

Figure 19-41 Assessing grip strength using a blood pressure cuff.

A Severe flexion ankylosis of the wrist is abnormal.

P Ankylosis can be caused by rheumatoid arthritis or severe disuse.

A Tenderness over the distal radius is abnormal.

P Tenderness over the distal radius can occur with a fracture of the distal radius.

P Pain slightly distal to the radius in the anatomical snuff box may represent a fracture of the scaphoid bone. This carpal bone has a high potential to not heal following a fracture.

A Wrist drop, demonstrated by the client's inability to extend the hand at the wrist, is abnormal.

P Radial nerve injury may cause wrist drop.

A Weak abduction of the fingers is abnormal.

P Ulnar nerve injury causes weakness in the fingers.

A Weakness of opposition of the thumb and ipsilateral finger against resistance is abnormal.

P Median nerve disorders, such as carpal tunnel syndrome, affect thumb opposition. Weak thumb opposition usually occurs from injuries where the hand is outstretched during a fall or from a twisting motion.

ADVANCED TECHNIQUE

Assessing Grip Strength Using a Blood Pressure Cuff

E

1. Roll up a blood pressure cuff into a ball and inflate the cuff to 20 mm Hg.
2. Ask the client to squeeze the inflated cuff (to determine the strength of the hand grasp action).
3. Note the increase in mm Hg during the grasp (Fig. 19-41).
4. Assess the strength of the other hand.

N **A healthy individual can usually achieve 150 mm Hg during a strong hand grasp action.**

A A hand grasp that measures below 150 mm Hg is abnormal.

P Neurological pathology, such as in stroke and myasthenia gravis, as well as musculoskeletal diseases such as MS and rheumatoid arthritis, can lead to decreased grip strength.

ADVANCED TECHNIQUE

Assessing for Carpal Tunnel Syndrome: Tinel Sign

The median nerve lies within the carpal tunnel of the wrist (Fig. 19-42A). Compression of the tunnel leads to median nerve neuropathy. The client may complain of paresthesias and burning, especially in the first three fingers, pain in the wrist and forearm, and a decreased ability to grasp objects due to a weak grip.

E
1. Place the client in a sitting position with the arm flexed at the elbow and the palm facing up.
2. Using the index or middle finger of the dominant hand, briskly tap the center of the client's wrist (median nerve) (Fig. 19-43).
3. Ask the client to describe the sensations that occur in the forearm, hands, thumb, or fingers.
4. Repeat the technique on the other wrist.
5. The pattern of pain, numbness, tingling, or sensory loss frequently corresponds with a specific nerve being irritated at the wrist or arm, including the radial, ulnar, or median nerve (Fig. 19-42B).

N **No tingling or burning will be noted in the hand, thumb, or fingers.**

A A positive Tinel test, indicated by pain, burning, or a tingling or pricking sensation that occurs in the hand, thumb, or index and middle fingers when the median nerve is tapped, is abnormal.

P A positive Tinel test is indicative of median nerve compression (carpal tunnel syndrome).

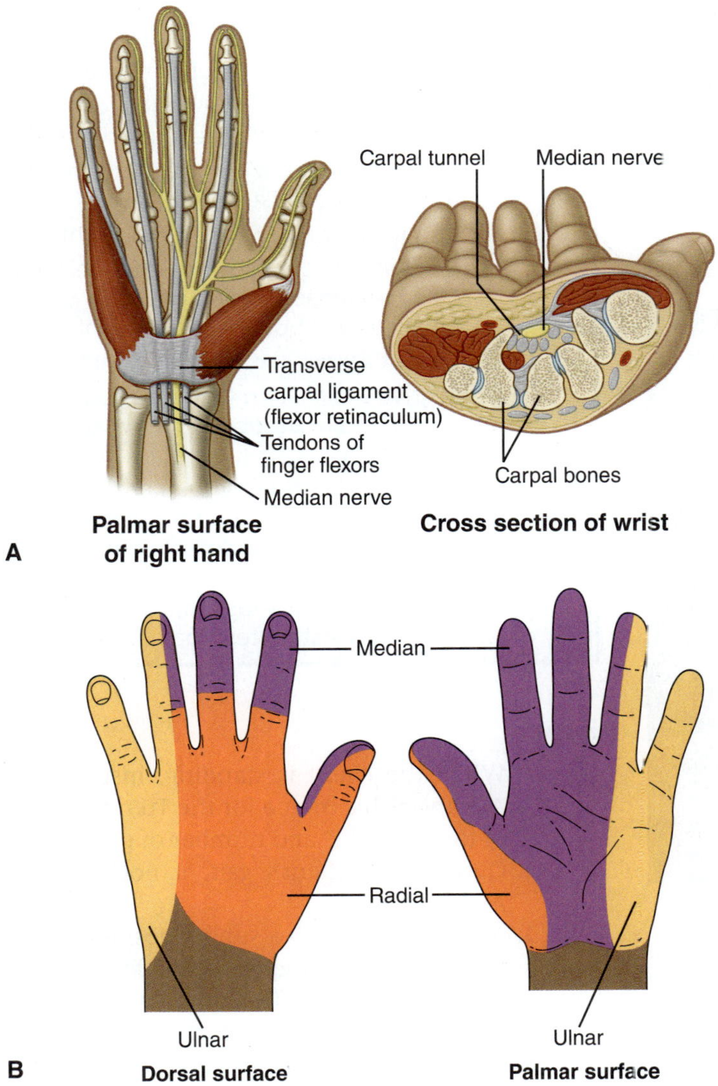

Figure 19-42 Carpal tunnel anatomy and nerve distribution. **A.** Anatomy of the carpal tunnel. **B.** Distribution of the ulnar, radial, and median nerves in the left hand.

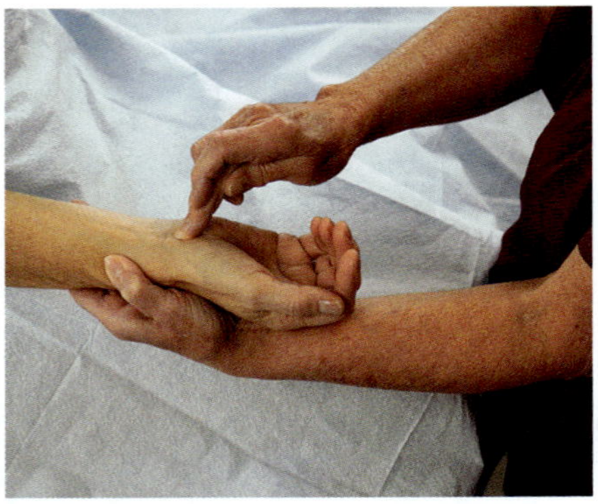

Figure 19-43 Assessing for Tinel sign.

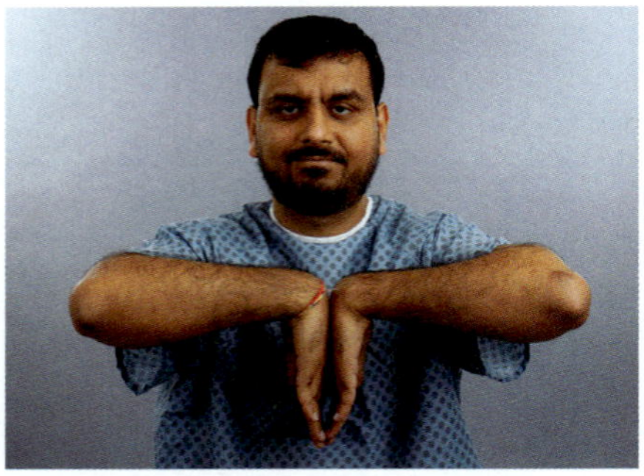

Figure 19-44 Assessing for Phalen sign.

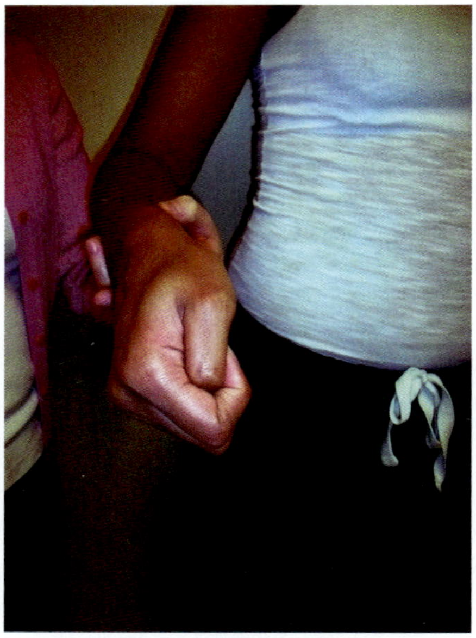

Figure 19-45 Finklestein test.

ADVANCED TECHNIQUE

Assessing for Carpal Tunnel Syndrome: Phalen Sign

E
1. Place the client in a sitting position with the arms flexed at the elbow and the backs of the hands pressed together (Fig. 19-44).
2. Ask the client to maintain the wrist flexion of 90° for at least 1 minute.
3. Ask the client to describe the sensations that occur in the hands and fingers.

N **There will be no change in the sensation of the hands and fingers.**

A A positive Phalen test, indicated by sensations of pain, burning, numbness, or paresthesia in the palmar aspect of the hand and the fingers (especially the first three fingers), is abnormal. These sensations disappear when the wrist joint is returned to its neutral anatomical position.

P A positive Phalen test is indicative of carpal tunnel syndrome.

ADVANCED TECHNIQUE

Assessing for De Quervain Tenosynovitis: Finklestein Test

E
1. Instruct the client to flex the thumb into the palm.
2. Ask the client to curl the fingers over the thumb, making a fist with the thumb inside the curved fingers.
3. With one hand, hold and stabilize the client's forearm just proximal to the wrist (Fig. 19-45).
4. With the other hand, grasp the client's fist.
5. Ulnarly deviate the client's wrist. This movement stretches the tendons (extensor pollicis brevis and abductor pollicis longus) along the radial border of the client's wrist.

N **The client's wrist can be moved into ulnar deviation without pain.**

A A positive Finklestein test is abnormal. The client will have pain along the radial border of the wrist while the wrist is deviated in an ulnar direction.

P De Quervain tenosynovitis is an inflammation of the extensor pollicis brevis and abductor pollicis longus. These tendons are positioned in the first dorsal compartment of the wrist along the radial border. These tendons can become irritated, painful, and inflamed due to overuse injuries. When the tendons are stretched with the Finklestein test, pain is elicited.

Hips

E
1. While the client is standing, inspect the iliac crests (refer to the Advanced Technique for the Trendelenburg test), size and symmetry of the buttocks, and number of gluteal folds (Fig. 19-46).
2. Observe the client's gait, if not previously assessed (see General Assessment).
3. Assist the client to a supine position on the examination table with the legs straight and the feet pointing toward the ceiling.
4. Palpate the anatomical landmarks at the hips and pelvis. Palpate the iliac spine, the greater trochanter, and hip joint.
5. Assess ROM of the hips (Fig. 19-47). Ask the client to:
   a. Raise the leg straight off the examination table with the knee extended (hip flexion with knee straight). The other leg should remain on the table.

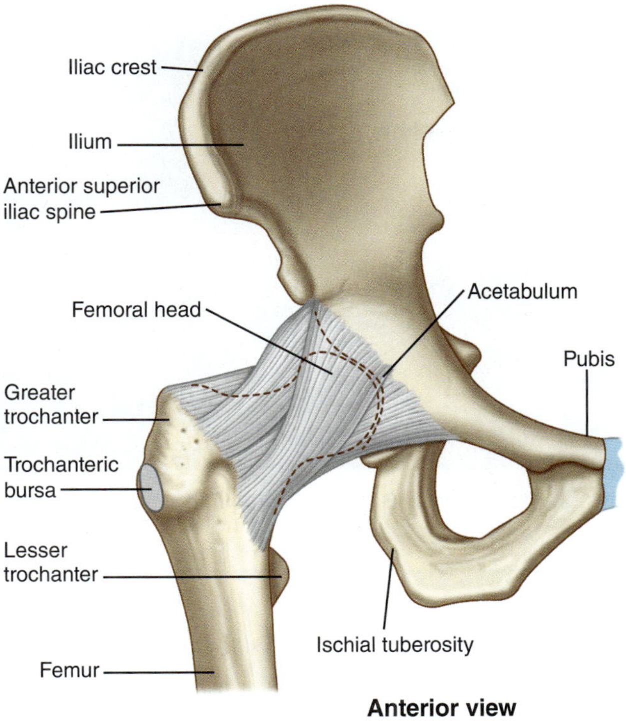

Figure 19-46 Anatomy of the hip joint.

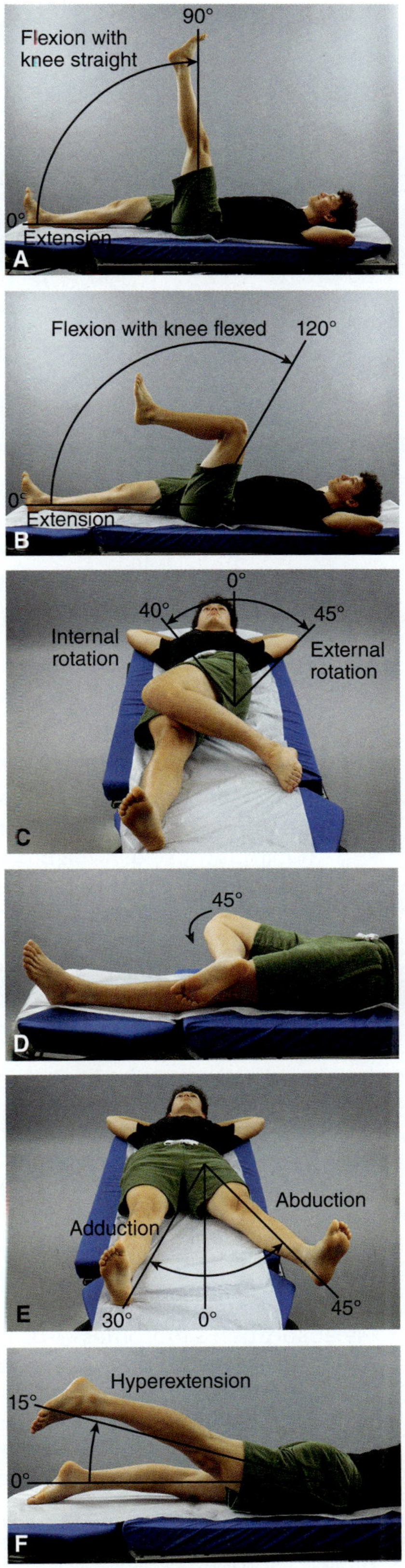

Figure 19-47 Range of motion of the hip joint. **A.** Flexion with knee straight. **B.** Flexion with knee flexed. **C.** Internal and external rotation. **D.** Position of the leg for full external rotation. **E.** Abduction and adduction. **F.** Hyperextension.

b. With the knee flexed, raise the leg off the examination table toward the chest as far as possible (hip flexion with knee flexed). The other leg should remain on the table. This is called the Thomas test.
c. Flex the hip and knee. Move the flexed leg medially as the foot moves outward (internal rotation).
d. Flex the hip and knee. Move the flexed leg laterally as the foot moves medially (external rotation).
e. With the knee straight, swing the leg away from the midline (abduction).
f. With the knee straight, swing the leg toward the midline (adduction).
g. Have the client roll over onto the abdomen and assume a prone position.
h. From the hip, move the leg back as far as possible while maintaining the pelvis on the table (hyperextension). This can also be performed while the client is standing.

6. Assist the client back to a supine position.
7. Assess the strength of the hips.
   a. Place the palm of your hand on the anterior thigh, above the knee. Instruct the client to raise the leg against your resistance (Fig. 19-48A). Assess the client's strength. Repeat on the other leg.
   b. Place the palm of your hand posteriorly above and behind the knee. Instruct the client to lower the leg against your resistance. Assess the client's strength. Repeat on the other leg.
   c. Place your hands on the lateral aspects of the client's legs at the level of the knee. Instruct the client to move the legs apart against your resistance; assess the strength of these muscles during the maneuver (Fig. 19-48B).
   d. Place your hands on the medial aspects of the client's legs just above the knee. Instruct the client to move the legs together against your resistance; assess the strength of these muscles during the maneuver.

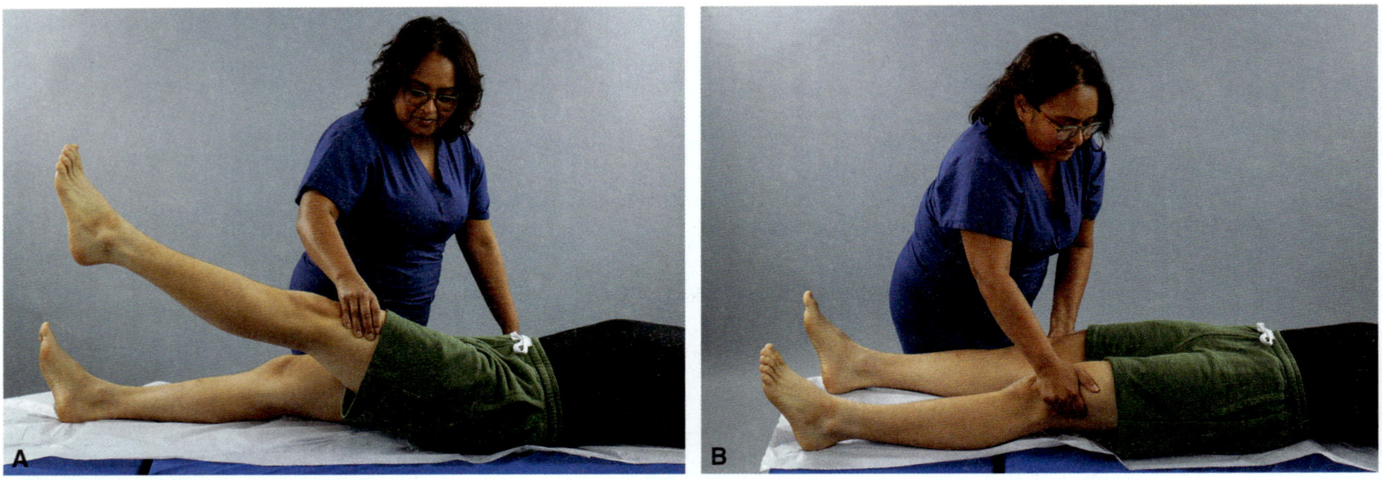

Figure 19-48 Assessing strength of the hip. **A.** Flexion with opposing force. **B.** Abduction with opposing force.

ADVANCED TECHNIQUE

Assessing for Hip Stabilization: Trendelenburg Test

E
1. Ask the client to stand on one foot, with the knee of the non-weight-bearing leg flexed to raise the foot off the floor.
2. Assess the symmetry of the iliac crests while the client is standing on one leg.
3. Repeat this technique on the other leg.

N **The iliac crest on the side opposite the weight-bearing leg elevates slightly.**

A It is abnormal for the iliac crest on the non-weight-bearing leg to drop.

P This finding is a positive Trendelenburg test; it indicates weakness of the gluteus medius and gluteus minimus muscles, which causes the hip on the unaffected side to drop. This finding can be attributed to muscle tear or nerve injury.

Risk Factors

Osteoporosis

- Increased age (>50), especially postmenopausal females
- Asians
- Whites
- Slender body build
- Smoking history
- Family history of osteoporosis
- Decreased physical activity
- Increased alcohol intake
- High caffeine intake
- Malabsorption syndromes (e.g., celiac disease)
- Malnutrition, including decreased calcium and vitamin D intake
- Increased stress
- Male gonadal insufficiency
- Rheumatoid arthritis
- Relative Energy Deficiency in Sports (RED-S); additional information on this condition is discussed in the Nursing Tip on RED-S
- Diabetes mellitus
- Blood disorders
- Anorexia and bulimia
- Surgical removal of ovaries
- Hyperparathyroidism
- Medications (e.g., steroids, anticonvulsants, lithium, tamoxifen, thyroxine, thiazide diuretics)

N **The normal ROM for the hips is flexion with knee straight—90°, flexion with knee flexed—120°, internal rotation—40°, external rotation—45°, abduction—45°, adduction—30°, hyperextension—15°.**

A A leg that is externally rotated and painful on movement is abnormal.

P These findings occur in hip fractures, which usually result from falls (especially in older adults). Hip fracture is the most serious fall-related fracture, often resulting in disability and death. This injury is often the pivotal event in an older adult's inability to remain independent in the home. Clinical manifestations of hip fracture include pain, inability to move the affected leg, inability to walk, and shortening of the affected leg with possible external rotation. The affected leg may also be shorter. See the Advanced Technique for guidelines on measuring limb length.

ADVANCED TECHNIQUE

Measuring Limb Length

E

1. Place the client in a supine position on the examination table with the legs extended.
2. Measure the leg from the anterior superior iliac spine to the medial malleolus (Fig. 19-49).
3. Repeat on the other limb.
4. Compare measurements.

N **Limb length measurements should be within ⅜ to 1¼ inches (1 to 3 cm) of each other.**

A A more than 1¼ inches (3 cm) difference in the length of limbs is abnormal.

P Asymmetry in lower limb length may be a congenital defect.

P Sudden unilateral decrease in limb length associated with pain occurs with fracture and dislocation of the hip and leg.

P A displaced proximal femoral shaft fracture (hip fracture) can result in limb shortening and internal or external rotation. Internal rotation is common if the client fell forward during the fall, and external rotation is common if the client fell onto the buttocks. The client is unable to straighten the leg into its neutral anatomical position.

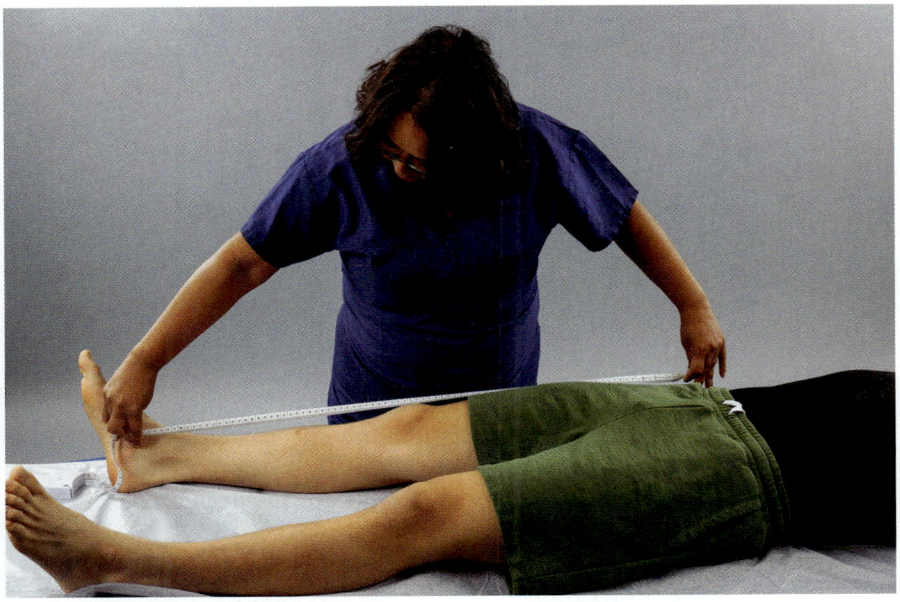

Figure 19-49 Measuring limb length.

NURSING TIP

DEXA Screening

Dual-energy X-ray absorptiometry (DEXA or DXA) screening is a painless procedure for measuring bone mineral density and for detecting bone density loss. Results can quantify bone as normal, osteopenic, or osteoporotic. Using a low level of radiation (or ultrasound waves in portable DEXA screening), the bones of the lower spine, hip, wrist, fingers, or heel can be scanned. The International Society for Clinical Densitometry (2015) recommends screening the following individuals:

- Females aged 65 or older
- Postmenopausal females under 65 years of age with risk factors for low bone mass
- Females during the menopausal transition with clinical risk factors for fracture, such as low body weight, prior fracture, or high-risk medication use
- Males age 70 years or older
- Males under 70 years of age with clinical risk factors for low bone mass
- Adults with a fragility fracture
- Adults with a disease or condition associated with low bone mass or bone loss
- Adults taking medications associated with low bone mass or bone loss
- Anyone being considered for pharmacological therapy for osteoporosis
- Anyone being treated for osteoporosis to monitor treatment effect
- Anyone not receiving therapy in whom evidence of bone loss would lead to treatment
- Females discontinuing estrogen should be considered for bone density testing according to the indications listed above

DEXA scans are usually repeated no more than every 2 years, as treatment protocols do not have short-term results.

E Examination N Normal Findings A Abnormal Findings P Pathophysiology

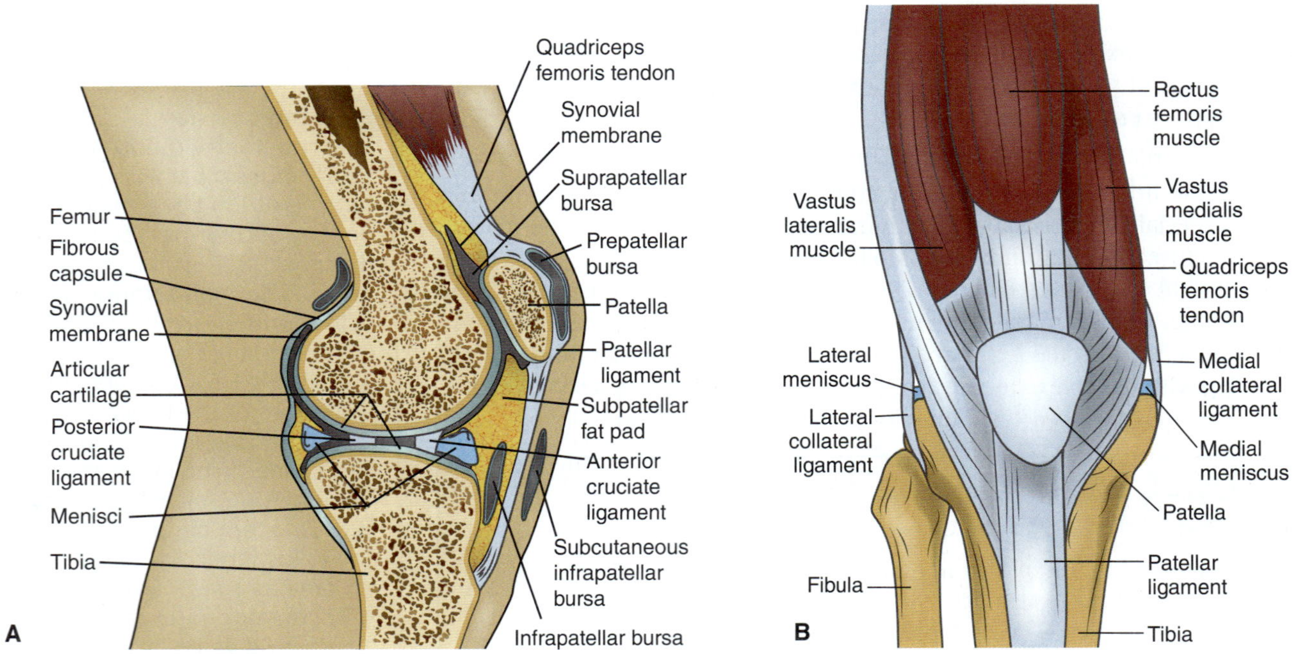

Figure 19-50 Anatomy of the right knee joint. **A.** Sagittal view. **B.** Anterior view.

A A positive Thomas test, when the client is unable to flex one knee and hip while simultaneously maintaining the other leg in full extension, is abnormal. There may be slight to moderate hip and knee flexion of the extended leg.

P Flexion contractures of the hip joint, such as in long-term degenerative joint diseases, will result in a positive Thomas test. This test will identify hip flexion contractures that are masked by lumbar lordosis.

Knees

E

1. With the client standing, note the position of the knees in relation to each other and in relation to the hips, thighs, ankles, and feet.
2. Ask the client to sit on the examination table with the knees flexed and resting at the edge of the table.
3. Inspect the contour of the knees. Note the normal depressions around the patella (Fig. 19-50).
4. Inspect the suprapatellar pouch and the prepatellar bursa.
5. Note the quadriceps muscle, located on the anterior thigh.
6. Palpate the knees, including the bony and muscular landmarks. The client may assume a supine position if this is more comfortable.
   a. Grasp the anterior thigh approximately 4 inches (10 cm) above the patella, with your thumb on one side of the knee and the other four fingers on the other side of the knee (Fig. 19-51).
   b. As you palpate, gradually move your hand down the suprapatellar pouch. Palpate the distal femur, medial and lateral femoral condyles, the patella, proximal tibia, and fibula. Be sure to palpate the quadriceps, patella tendon, hamstrings, popliteal fossa, and calf musculature.
7. Palpate the tibiofemoral joints. It is best to have the knee flexed to 90° when performing this assessment.
   a. Place both thumbs on the knee, with the fingers wrapped around the knee posteriorly.

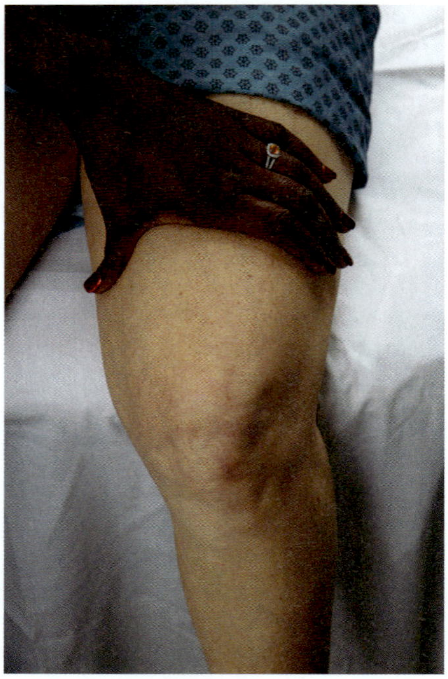

Figure 19-51 Palpating the knee.

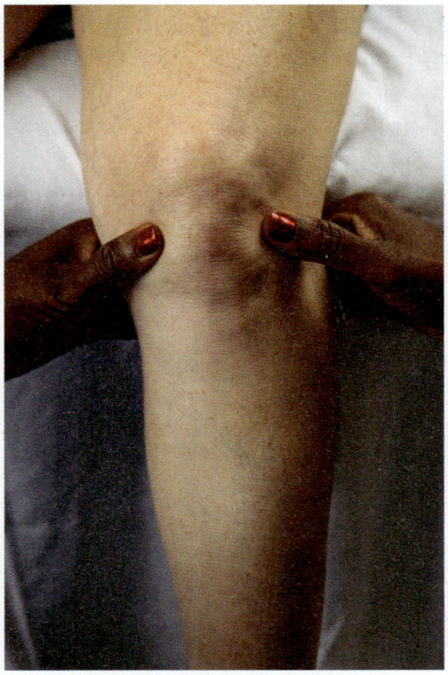

Figure 19-52 Palpating the tibiofemoral joint.

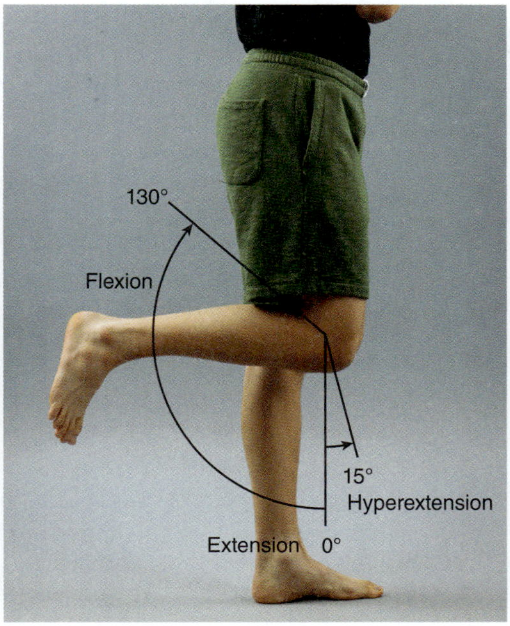

Figure 19-53 Range of motion of the knee joint: Flexion, extension, hyperextension.

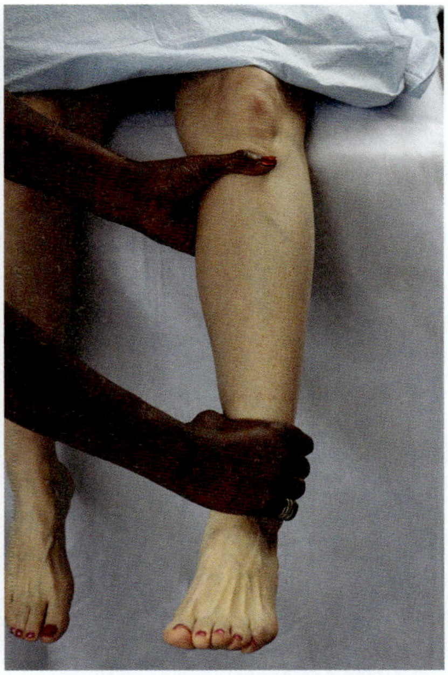

Figure 19-54 Assessing strength of knee joint.

   b. Press in with the thumbs as you palpate the tibial margins (Fig. 19-52).
   c. Palpate the medial and lateral collateral ligaments.
8. If knee fluid is suspected, test for the bulge sign and ballottement. See the Advanced Techniques on bulge sign and patellar ballottement.
9. Assess the ROM of the knees (Fig. 19-53). Ask the client to stand and:
   a. Bend the knee (flexion).
   b. Straighten the knee (extension). The client may also be able to hyperextend the knee during this movement.
10. Assess the strength of the knees with the client seated and the legs hanging off the table.
   a. Ask the client to bend the knee. Place your nondominant hand under the knee and place your other hand over the ankle.
   b. Instruct the client to straighten the leg against your resistance (Fig. 19-54).
   c. Ask the client to place the foot on the bed and the knee at approximately 45° of flexion. Place one hand under the knee and place the other hand over the ankle.
   d. Instruct the client to maintain the foot on the table despite your attempts to straighten the leg.

N **The knees are in alignment bilaterally and do not deviate medially or laterally. The normal ROM for the knees is flexion—130°, extension—0°; in some cases, hyperextension is possible up to 15°.**

A Alteration in lower limb alignment is considered an abnormal finding.

P **Genu valgum** (knock knees) is deviation toward the midline at the level of the knees (Fig. 19-55). Both legs are usually affected by the disorder. It is detected as an increased distance between the medial malleoli when the femoral condyles are close together and the patellae are facing forward. The knees appear closer together than is normal. Genu valgum can be congenital or acquired (rickets).

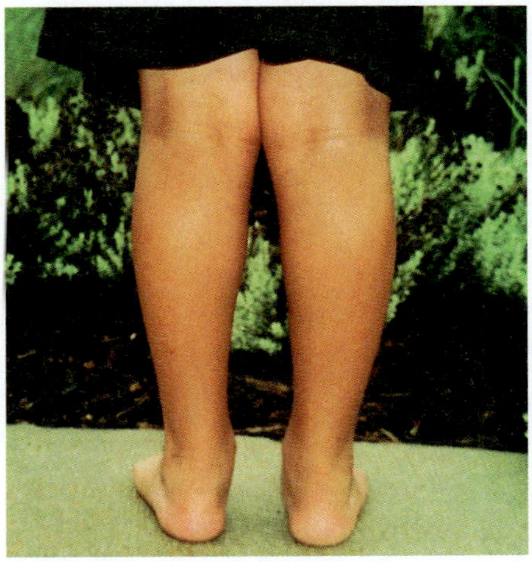

Figure 19-55 Genu valgum.

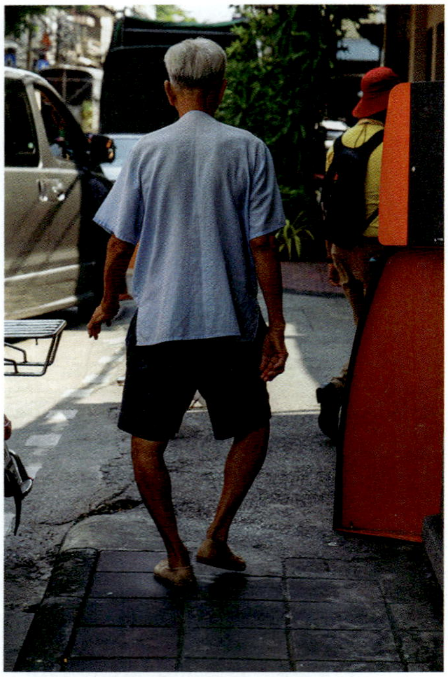

Figure 19-56 Genu varum.

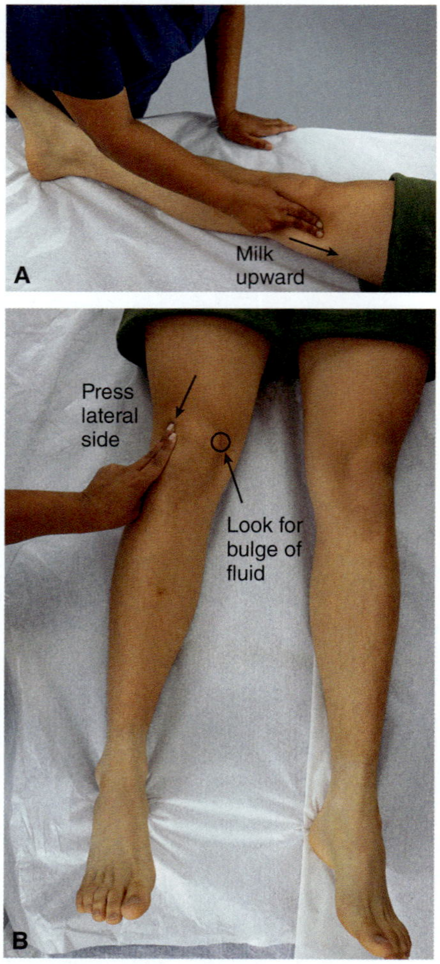

Figure 19-57 Assessing for bulge sign. **A.** Milking the patella. **B.** Observing for fluid.

P **Genu varum** (bow legs) is deviation away from the midline at the level of the knees (Fig. 19-56). Both legs are usually affected by the disorder. It is detected as an increased distance between the femoral condyles when the medial malleoli are close together and the patellae are facing forward. The knees appear farther apart than is normal. Genu varum can be congenital or acquired. This syndrome is common in horse jockeys due to the stretching of the nearby ligaments. It may also be seen in rickets, rheumatoid arthritis, and osteomalacia, due to the body's attempt to create a bone shape to tolerate the weight of the upper body.

NURSING TIP

Remembering Genu Valgum vs. Genu Varum

Genu Va**R**um: Let the "**R**" remind you that there is **R**oom between the client's knees, or that the knees are apa**R**t.
Genu Val**G**um: Let the "**G**" remind you that the client's knees are to**G**ether, or that they are stuck together like **G**lue.

A A knee effusion is present.

P A knee effusion can be associated with inflammation of the synovial lining of the knee, injury, or infection.

A A fullness or swelling in the popliteal fossa is abnormal.

P Fullness in the popliteal fossa can be associated with a Baker cyst (Fig. 19-58). A Baker cyst is a cystic mass in the medial popliteal fossa. If large enough, it can decrease the anatomical ROM of the knee. It is often detected in clients with rheumatoid arthritis.

ADVANCED TECHNIQUE

Assessing for Small Effusions: Bulge Sign

The bulge sign tests for small effusions (4 to 8 mL) in the knee.

E
1. Place the client in a supine position with the legs extended.
2. Firmly milk upward the medial aspect of the patella several times. This displaces any fluid (Fig. 19-57A).
3. Press or tap the lateral aspect of the knee.
4. Observe the hollow on the medial aspect of the knee for a bulge of fluid (Fig. 19-57B).

N **Normally there is no fluid return to the knee. This is a negative bulge sign.**

A The return of fluid to the medial aspect of the patella is abnormal.

P A positive bulge sign is present in joint effusion.

ADVANCED TECHNIQUE

Assessing for Large Effusions: Patellar Ballottement

Ballottement is performed to detect large effusions in the knee.

E
1. Place the client in a supine position with the knees extended.

2. Firmly grasp the thigh (with your thumb on one side and the four fingers on the other side) just above the patella. This compresses fluid out of the suprapatellar pouch and causes the patella to be slightly displaced out of the groove where it sits in the distal femur.
3. With your other hand, push the patella vertically back down toward the femur (Fig. 19-59).
4. Feel for a click as the patella is pushed through the fluid and then taps into the femur.

N **There is no palpable click. Normally, the patella is close to the femur because there is no excess fluid.**

A A palpable click is abnormal.

P When fluid is present between the femur and the patella, the patella "floats" on top of the femur. As the patella is pushed back, fluid is displaced and a palpable click is felt when the patella hits the femur.

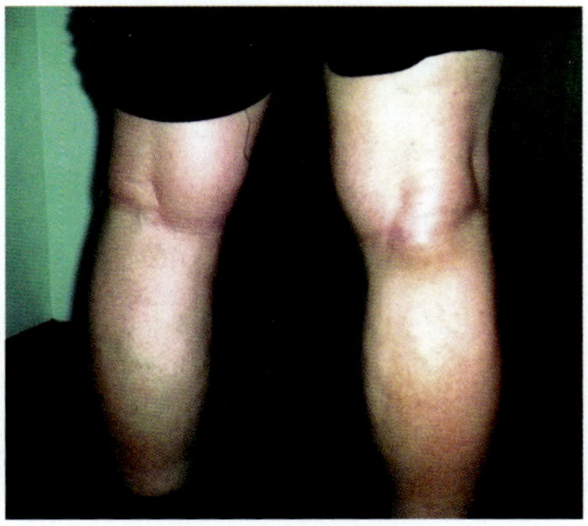

Figure 19-58 Baker cyst in the right popliteal fossa.

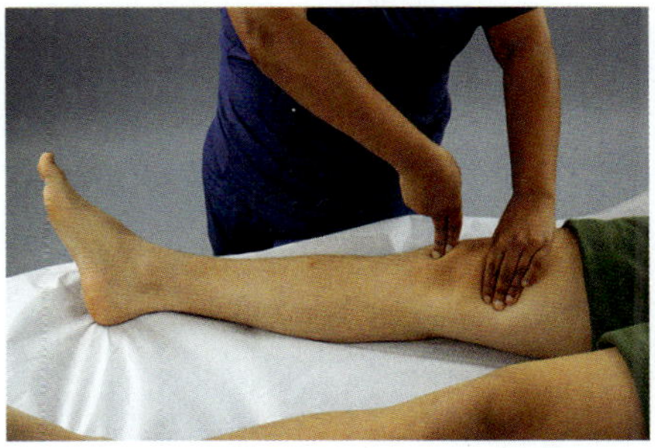

Figure 19-59 Patellar ballottement.

ADVANCED TECHNIQUE

Assessing for Meniscal Tears: Apley Grinding Sign

This test is performed to identify meniscal tears.

E
1. Place the client in a prone position on the examination table.
2. Manually flex the affected knee to a 90° angle so that the lower leg is perpendicular to the table.
3. With the dominant hand, apply firm downward pressure on the foot while simultaneously rotating the lower leg inward and then outward (Fig. 19-60).
4. Assess for pain, limited knee joint movement, or audible clicks during knee joint movement.

N **The client will be able to flex the knee joint to a 90° angle, no pain will be elicited, and no audible clicks will be heard during joint movement.**

A A positive Apley sign of the knee joint is indicated by knee pain, limited movement of the knee joint (locking of the knee joint), or audible clicks.

P A positive Apley sign is suggestive of torn meniscal cartilage within the knee joint.

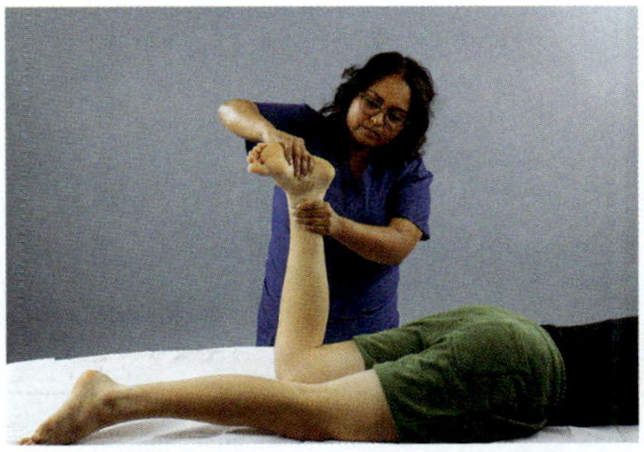

Figure 19-60 Assessing for Apley grinding sign.

ADVANCED TECHNIQUE

Assessing for Meniscal Tears: McMurray Sign

This test is performed to assess the integrity of the meniscus of the knee.

E
1. Place the client in a supine position on the examination table and stand on the affected side.
2. Manually flex the hip and knee. Hold the client's heel with one hand and stabilize the knee with the other hand (Fig. 19-61).
3. Using the hand that is holding the heel, internally rotate the leg while applying resistance to the medial aspect of the knee joint. This assesses the medial meniscus.

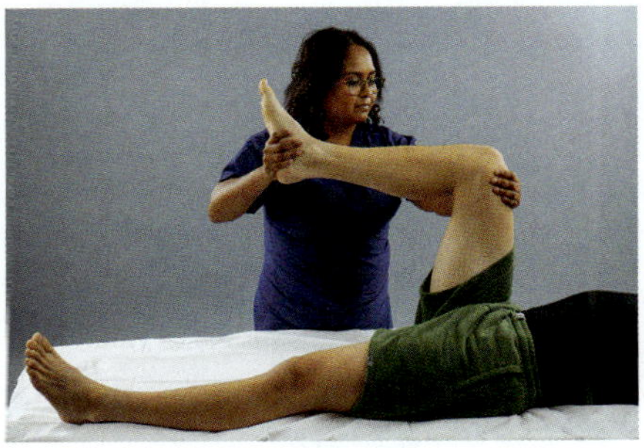

Figure 19-61 Assessing for McMurray sign.

4. Move the knee to a position of full extension. Note if full extension of the knee joint can be achieved or tolerated by the client.
5. Flex the hip and knee and externally rotate the leg. While stabilizing the knee joint, apply resistance to the lateral aspect of the knee joint. This assesses the lateral meniscus.
6. Assess for pain or an audible or palpable click of the knee joint.

N **The client will be able to extend the leg at the knee joint, and no pain or audible or palpable click will be detected.**

A A positive McMurray sign is indicated when the client is unable to extend the leg at the knee joint, when pain is present with the maneuver, or when an audible or palpable click is detected.

P A positive McMurray sign is suggestive of torn meniscus cartilage of the knee. The client may also state that full extension of the knee joint is impossible, that the knee joint "locks into place," or that "it feels like something is in the knee joint." If the torn meniscus cartilage is obstructing the articulating function of the joint, knee joint extension will be limited.

ADVANCED TECHNIQUE

Assessing the Cruciate Ligaments: Drawer Test

This test is performed to assess the stability of the anterior and posterior cruciate ligaments of the knee.

E
1. Assist the client to a supine position on the examination table.
2. Instruct the client to flex the right knee to 90° and to flex the right hip joint to 45°, placing the right foot flat on the examination table.
3. Sit on the client's right foot to stabilize it in place.
4. Observe for "sagging" of the tibia resulting in visible concavity below the patella ("sag" sign).
5. Place both hands on the client's right tibia, with the thumb of the right hand slightly medial to the patellar tendon and the left thumb slightly lateral to the patellar tendon (Fig. 19-62).
6. Attempt to move the tibia forward (anterior drawer test) and then backward (posterior drawer test).
7. Repeat on the left leg. Compare results.

N **You will not be able to pull the tibia forward more than 6 mm or to move the tibia backward at all. A firm endpoint should be noted with the drawer test. Concavity should not be detected distal to the patella.**

A An abnormal result is indicated by the ability to move the tibia forward more than ¼ inch (6 mm) or to move the tibia backward.

P Forward movement of the tibia more than ¼ inch (6 mm) indicates a tear in the anterior cruciate ligament of the knee. A false positive result may occur if the client has instability of the posterior cruciate ligament of the knee.

P Sagging of the tibia or backward movement of the tibia indicates a tear in the posterior cruciate ligament of the knee.

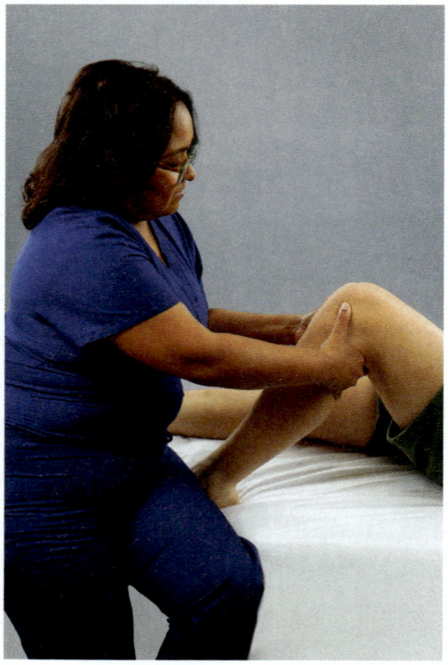

Figure 19-62 Drawer test.

ADVANCED TECHNIQUE

Assessing the Anterior Cruciate Ligament: Lachman Test

This test is performed to assess the stability of the anterior cruciate ligament of the knee. It is considered the most reliable assessment technique for detecting instability of the anterior cruciate ligament.

E
1. Place the client in a supine position on the examination table with the affected knee flexed to approximately 30°. The unaffected leg should be fully extended and in contact with the examination table.
2. Stabilize the femur of the affected leg by holding the leg above the knee joint with one hand.
3. Grasp the affected lower leg beneath the knee with the other hand and attempt to move the tibia anteriorly.
4. Note any movement or changes in the infrapatellar slope.

N **When the tibia is moved forward, the infrapatellar tendon slope should still be noticeable.**

A It is abnormal for the infrapatellar tendon slope to no longer be noticeable when the tibia is moved forward.

P A positive Lachman test is indicative of damage to the anterior cruciate ligament of the knee.

NURSING TIP

Relative Energy Deficiency in Sport (RED-S)

In the past, female athletes who experienced irregular menstrual periods, low bone mineral density, and disordered eating were diagnosed with a condition known as the female athlete triad. A better understanding of the complexity and imbalance of athletes and the complexity of energy needs and expenditure has given rise to a condition known as relative energy deficiency in sport (RED-S).

Low energy availability lies at the center of RED-S, and it is directly related to a whole host of complications that can result when athletes aren't adequately fueled, not only for their athletic performance but to sufficiently meet their body's physiological needs to support healthy functioning.

Energy availability is the difference between energy intake (food) and energy expenditure (exercise). There are two key factors to consider when interpreting this calculation; one, energy expenditure refers to that which is in excess of the energy required for activities of daily living, and two, that the result must be interpreted in relation to fat-free mass or muscle mass.

Research has shown that optimal energy availability is achieved around 45 kcal/kg of fat free mass. Low energy availability occurs when energy availability approaches 30 kcal/kg of fat free mass or lower. This is the point at which an athlete is considered to be impacted by RED-S.

Where the Female Athlete Triad represented the interrelationship between low energy availability, menstrual function, and bone health, RED-S recognizes that the complications of low energy availability are more extensive and that these complications are not just limited to female bodies.

RED-S reestablishes athlete health as the primary focus when it comes to fueling for optimal sport performance. Athletes and their coaches can become so focused on fueling for sport performance with pre-, intra-, and postworkout nutrition that fueling to maintain optimal health in the time between training and competition gets neglected. RED-S highlights the importance of fueling to support the functions required for optimal health first since efforts to fuel specifically for sport performance will be counterproductive without having the body's basic needs met.

When an athlete doesn't have adequate energy availability in the context of sport performance, the body is forced to adjust by reducing the energy allotted to support vital body systems and processes. This ultimately leads to a disruption in numerous hormonal, metabolic, and functional processes. As a result of low energy availability, metabolic rate, menstrual function, bone health, immunity, protein synthesis, cardiovascular, and psychological health can suffer.

Research shows that a decline in the above-mentioned body systems and processes can result in the following performance-related consequences for the athlete:

- Decreased endurance performance
- Increased injury risk
- Decreased training response
- Impaired judgment
- Decreased coordination
- Decreased glycogen stores
- Decreased muscle strength

In addition, athletes who are affected by low energy availability may develop nutrient deficiencies including anemia, chronic fatigue, and increased risk of infections and illnesses, all of which have the potential to harm health and performance.

With the new focus on energy availability that RED-S brings to the forefront, it is now easier to see how this syndrome can be just as present in male athletes as it is in females, bringing new awareness to the hormonal health of males as well as the prevalence of disordered eating in this population that can lead to low energy availability.

Research shows that low energy availability occurs at a comparable rate in males and females. Not surprisingly, it seems that athletes competing in weight-sensitive sports, regardless of sex, experience low energy availability at an increased rate compared with those who compete in sports where leanness is not as important for performance, appearance, or requirement to meet a competition weight category (Bentall, 2020).

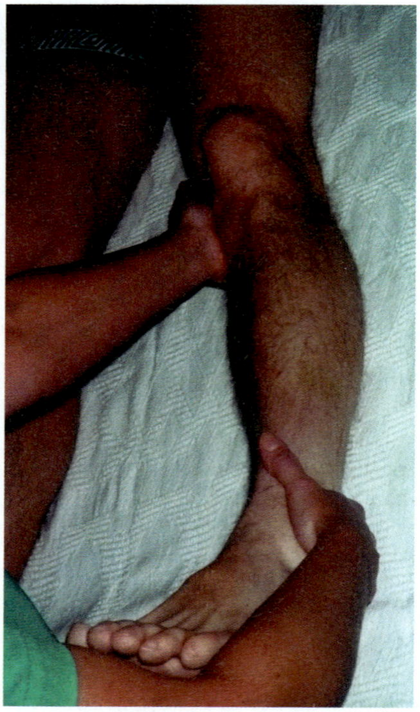

Figure 19-63 Varus stress test.

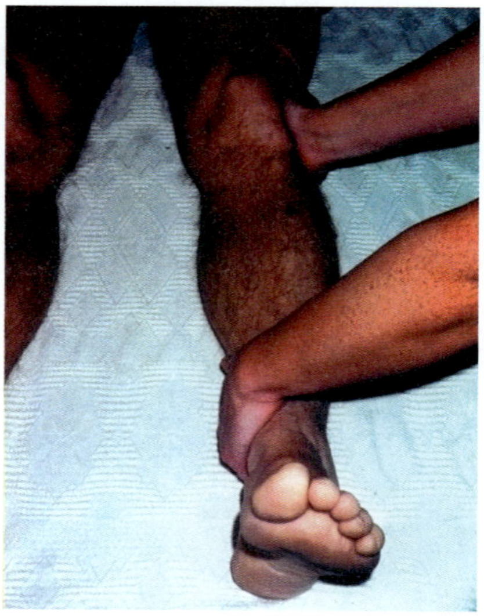

Figure 19-64 Valgus stress test.

ADVANCED TECHNIQUE

Assessing the Lateral Collateral Ligament: Varus Stress Test

E
1. Place the client in a supine position on the examination table.
2. Slightly abduct and slightly flex the affected leg.
3. Place one hand on the medial aspect of the affected knee.
4. Place your other hand on the lateral aspect of the same ankle.
5. Apply varus stress (lateral movement) to the knee and attempt to move the ankle medially (Fig. 19-63).
6. Note pain or laxity with movement.

N **There should be no pain or laxity when varus stress is applied.**

A Pain or laxity with varus stress is abnormal.

P Pain or laxity with varus stress may indicate a tear in the lateral collateral ligament.

ADVANCED TECHNIQUE

Assessing the Medial Collateral Ligament: Valgus Stress Test

E
1. Place the client in a supine position on the examination table.
2. Slightly abduct the affected leg.
3. Place one hand on the lateral aspect of the affected knee.
4. Place your other hand on the medial aspect of the same ankle.
5. Apply valgus stress (medial movement) to the knee and attempt to move the ankle laterally (Fig. 19-64).
6. Note pain or laxity with movement.

N **There should be no pain or laxity when valgus stress is applied.**

A Pain or laxity with valgus stress is abnormal.

P Pain or laxity with valgus stress may indicate a tear in the medial collateral ligament.

Ankles and Feet

E
1. Inspect the ankles and feet (Fig. 19-65) as the client stands, walks, and sits (bearing no weight).
2. Inspect the alignment of the feet and toes with the lower leg.
3. Inspect the shape and position of the toes.

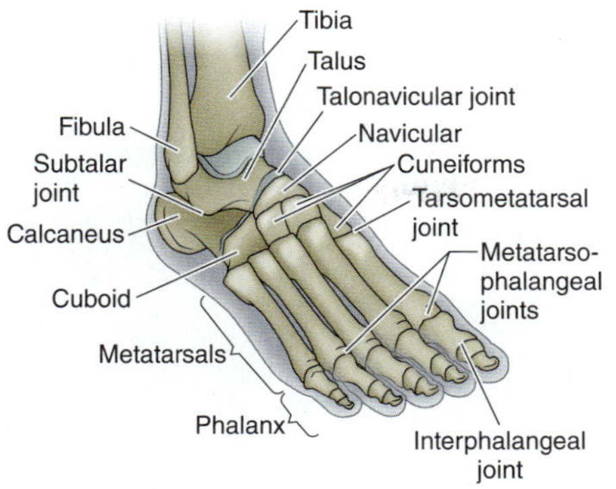

Figure 19-65 Anatomy of the ankle and foot.

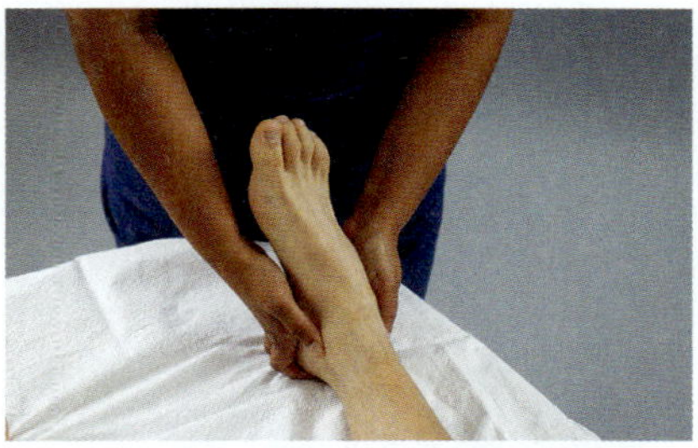

Figure 19-66 Palpation of the ankle.

4. Assist the client to a supine position on the examination table.
5. Stand by the client's feet.
6. Palpate the ankle and foot (Fig. 19-66).
   a. Grasp the heel with the fingers of both hands. Palpate the posterior aspect of the heel at the calcaneus.
   b. Use your thumbs to palpate the medial malleolus (bony prominence on the distal medial aspect of the tibia) and the lateral malleolus (bony prominence on the distal lateral aspect of the fibula).
   c. Move your hands forward and palpate the anterior aspects of the ankle and foot, particularly at the joints.
   d. Palpate the inferior aspect of the foot over the plantar fascia.
   e. Use your finger pads to palpate the Achilles tendon, as well as the tendons and ligaments on the medial and lateral ankle joint.
   f. Using your thumb and index finger, palpate each metatarsophalangeal joint.
   g. Between your thumb and index finger, palpate the medial and lateral surfaces of each interphalangeal joint.
7. Assess ROM of the ankles and feet (Fig. 19-67). Ask the client to:
   a. Point the toes toward the chest by moving the ankle (dorsiflexion).
   b. Point the toes toward the floor by moving the ankle (plantar flexion).
   c. Turn the soles of the feet outward (eversion).
   d. Turn the soles of the feet inward (inversion).
   e. Curl the toes toward the floor (flexion).
   f. Spread the toes apart (abduction).
   g. Move the toes together (adduction).
8. Assess the strength of the ankles and feet.
   a. Assist the client to a supine position on the examination table with the legs extended and the feet slightly apart.
   b. Stand at the foot of the examination table.
   c. Place one hand on top of the client's right foot and place your other hand on top of the client's left foot.
   d. Ask the client to attempt to point the toes toward the chest (dorsiflexion) against your resistance.
   e. Place one hand on the sole of the client's right foot and place your other hand on the sole of the client's left foot.
   f. Ask the client to attempt to point the toes down (plantar flexion) against your resistance. This technique can also be performed one foot at a time, as shown in Fig. 19-68.

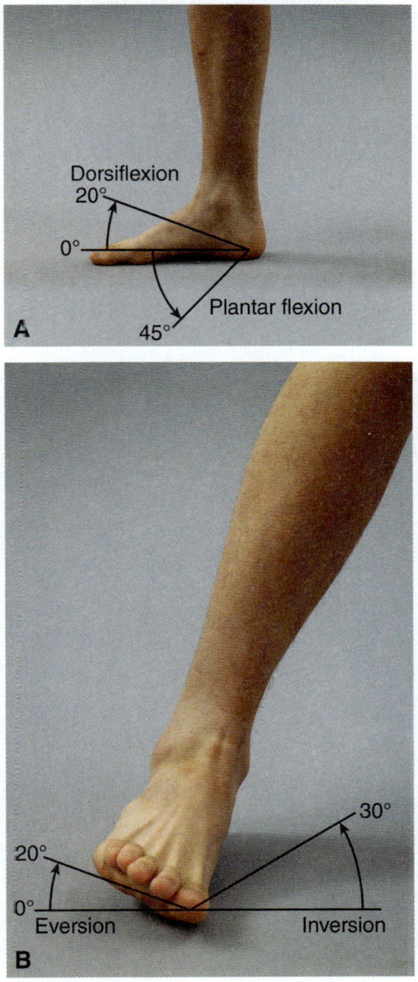

Figure 19-67 Range of motion of the ankle and foot. **A.** Plantar flexion, dorsiflexion. **B.** Eversion, inversion.

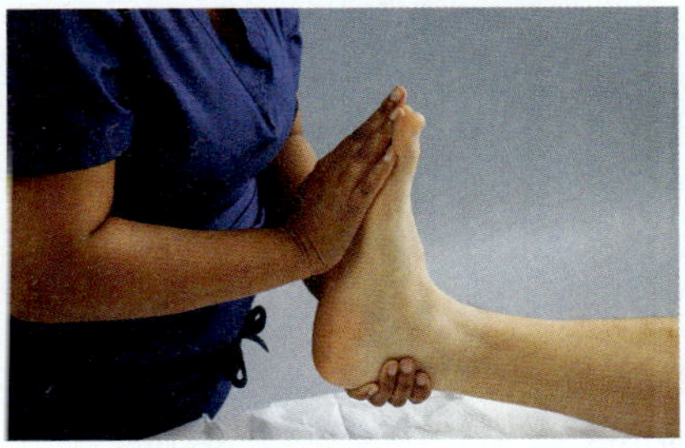

Figure 19-68 Strength of the ankle and foot.

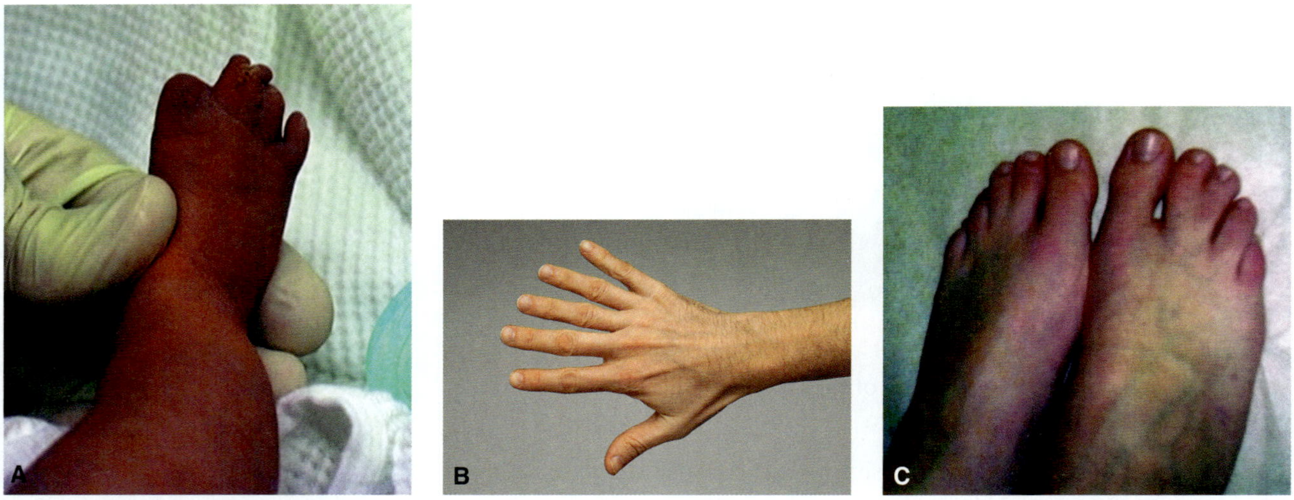

Figure 19-69 Toe abnormalities. **A.** Congenital loss of the right big toe. Also note the syndactyly in the second and third digits. **B.** Polydactyly. **C.** Syndactyly in the 2nd and 3rd metatarsals of the right foot.

9. Examine the client's shoes and observe for wear in unusual areas. This provides information on the client's weight-bearing. Keep this in mind as you watch the client stand and walk.

N **The foot is in alignment with the lower leg. The foot has a longitudinal arch. There is no pain over the plantar fascia upon palpation. The normal ROM for the ankles and feet is dorsiflexion—20°, plantar flexion—45°, eversion—20°, inversion—30°, abduction—30°, and adduction—10°.**

A Extra toes or webbing between the toes is congenital; loss of toes can be congenital or acquired (Fig. 19-69A).

P Polydactyly is the presence of extra digits (Fig. 19-69B). Syndactyly is the congenital webbing or fusion of toes (Fig. 19-69C).

A An alteration in the shape and position of the foot is considered abnormal.

P **Pes varus** describes a foot that is turned inward toward the midline.

P **Pes valgus** occurs when the foot is turned laterally away from the midline.

P **Pes planus** (flat foot) refers to a foot with a low longitudinal arch.

P **Pes cavus** refers to a foot with an exaggerated arch height.

P In **hallux valgus** (bunion), the big toe deviates laterally while the first metatarsal is deviated medially (Fig. 19-70). The metatarsophalangeal joint enlarges and becomes inflamed from the pressure. A bursa may form at this point. Hallux valgus can be congenital or caused by narrow shoes and arthritis.

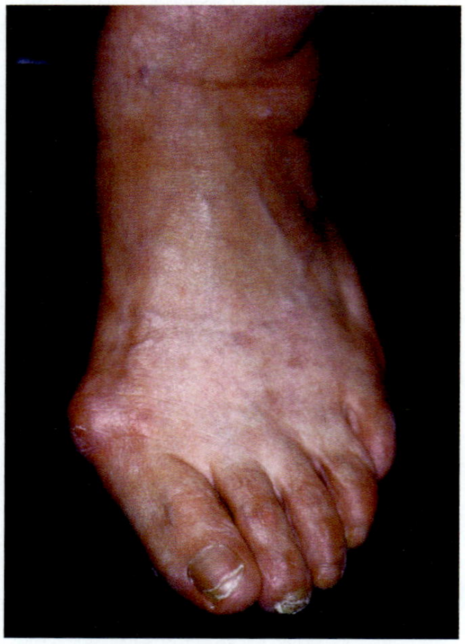

Figure 19-70 Hallux valgus.

P Tight shoes can also cause **hammertoe**. In hammertoe, there is a flexion of the proximal interphalangeal joint and hyperextension of the metatarsophalangeal joint. A corn or callus can develop from undue pressure at the point of flexion (Fig. 19-71).

P A **corn** is a conical area of thickened skin. It extends into the dermis and can be painful. Corns are caused by pressure on the affected area, particularly over bony prominences. Tight shoes and hammertoe can cause corns.

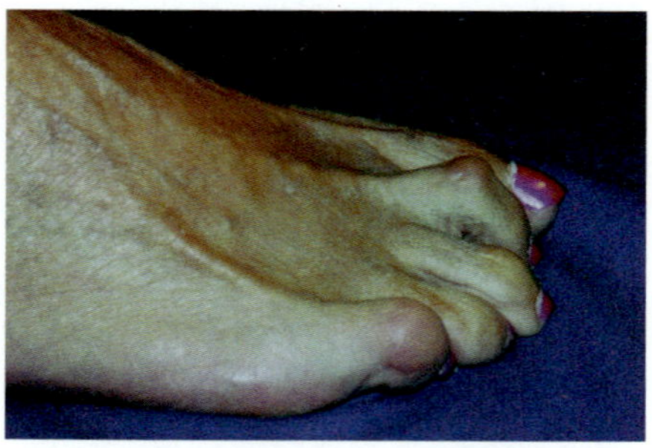

Figure 19-71 Hammertoe on the 2nd digit and corn on the 2nd and 5th digits.

P A **callus** is a thickening of the skin due to prolonged pressure (Fig. 19-72). It usually occurs on the sole of the foot and is not painful.

A Pain over the plantar fascia is abnormal.

P Plantar fasciitis is an inflammation of the plantar fascia where it attaches to the calcaneus. The pain tends to be worst first thing in the morning and with prolonged standing, sitting, or walking.

A A swollen, red, warm, and painful metatarsophalangeal joint is abnormal.

P The first metatarsophalangeal joint is usually affected in acute gouty arthritis.

A Decreased ROM of the ankle is abnormal.

P The client with an ankle sprain or fracture secondary to injury or trauma complains of pain on palpation and ROM. Crepitus may be present in an ankle fracture. Ankle sprain cannot always be differentiated from an ankle fracture without the use of X-rays.

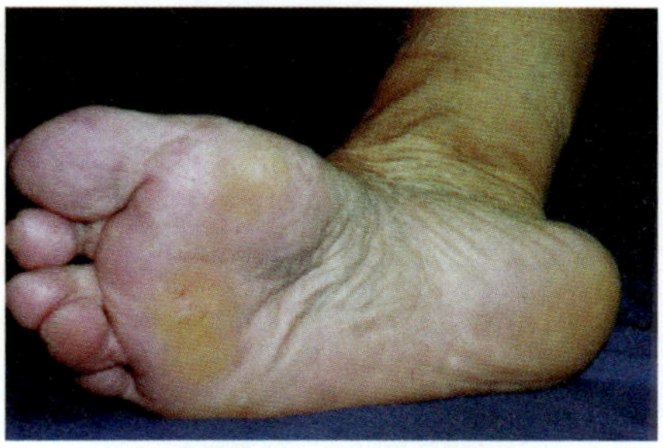

Figure 19-72 Callus.

ADVANCED TECHNIQUE

Assessing for Ankle Sprain: Anterior Drawer Test

E

1. Have the client sit with the feet hanging freely.
2. Grasp the heel of the foot with the injured ankle with one hand.
3. Place the other hand over the anterior aspect of the tibia on the affected side and firmly grasp the leg about 2¼ inches (6 cm) above the joint line (Fig. 19-73).
4. Firmly hold and stabilize the tibia as you apply an anterior forward motion with the hand holding the heel.
5. Note any pain or movement of the ankle and compare with the unaffected ankle.

N **There should be no pain or forward movement of the ankle.**

A It is abnormal to have pain or anterior movement of the ankle.

P Anterior movement and pain of the ankle indicate a possible tear in the anterior talofibular ligament (Fig. 19-74).

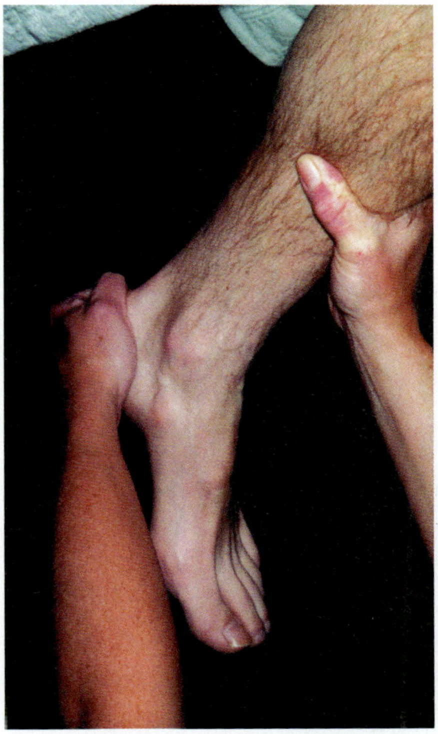

Figure 19-73 Anterior drawer test of the ankle.

ADVANCED TECHNIQUE

Assessing for Ankle Sprain: Talar Tilt Test

E

1. Have the client sit with the feet hanging freely.
2. Place your hands around the ankle of the affected leg so that the thumbs are inferior to the malleoli.
3. Passively invert and evert the ankle through ROM (Fig. 19-75).
4. Note the movement of the ankle.
5. Compare with the unaffected ankle.

N **Normally, there should be an equal talar tilt, or ROM, through inversion and eversion of both ankles.**

A It is abnormal if the injured ankle has pain and a talar tilt that is more than 5° to 10° than the unaffected ankle.

P A talar tilt greater than 5° to 10° and pain may indicate a tear in the calcaneofibular ligament.

E Examination **N** Normal Findings **A** Abnormal Findings **P** Pathophysiology

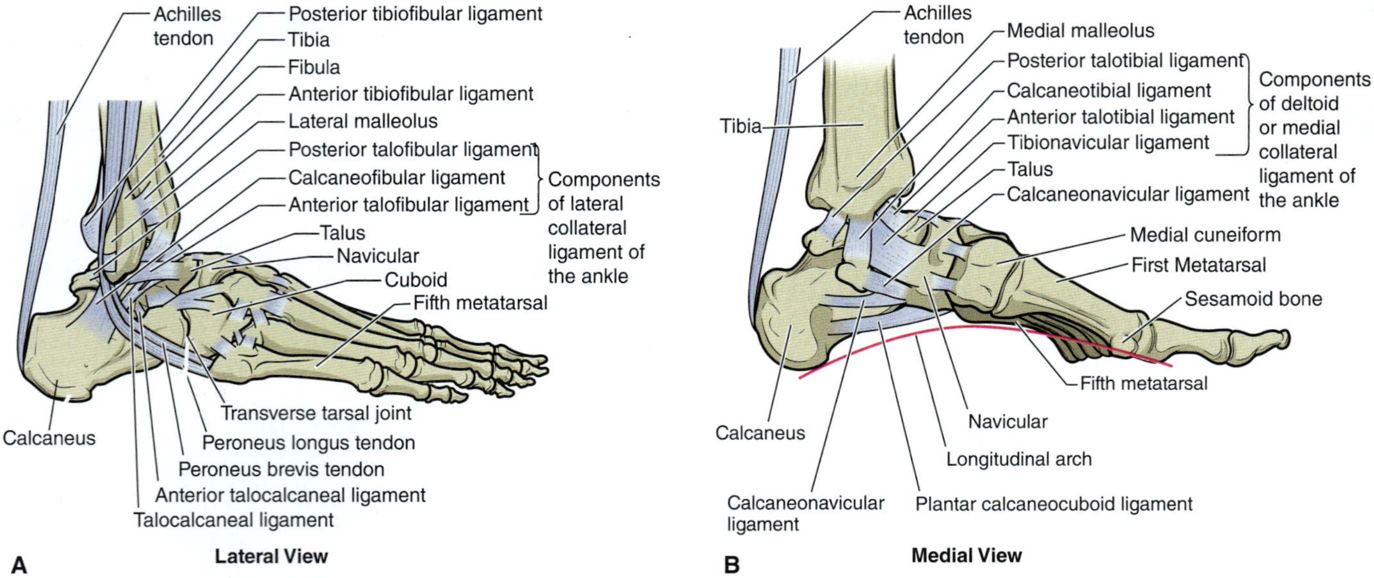

Figure 19-74 Ligaments of the ankle. **A.** Lateral view. **B.** Medial view.

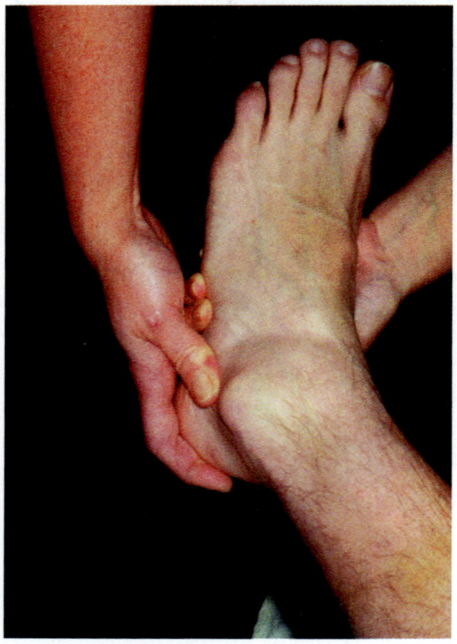

Figure 19-75 Talar tilt test.

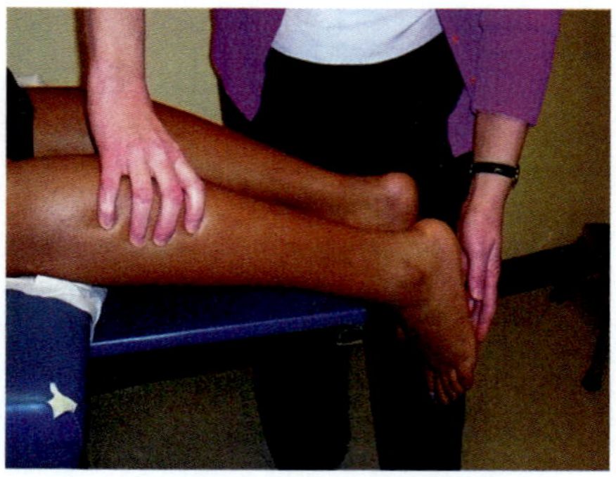

Figure 19-76 Thompson squeeze test.

NURSING TIP

Diet and Vitamin D

Calcium and phosphorus are the primary components of healthy bone. Vitamin D is essential for promoting the absorption of both of these elements from the gastrointestinal tract. Protein is essential for healthy muscle. A diet that is lacking in calcium, phosphorus, vitamin D, and/or protein can promote adverse changes in the musculoskeletal system, such as osteoporosis and osteomalacia. Exposure to sunlight helps to promote vitamin D production in the body. Supplemental vitamins and minerals may be necessary for the client with lactose intolerance who cannot consume these essential elements easily through the dietary intake of dairy products. Fortunately, calcium is also available in dark green, leafy vegetables.

ADVANCED TECHNIQUE

Assessing for Ruptured Achilles Tendon: Thompson Squeeze Test

E
1. Assist the client to a prone position with the feet hanging over the edge of the examination table.
2. Manually squeeze the calf muscles of the leg (Fig. 19-76).
3. Observe for plantar flexion of the foot being examined.

N **When the calf muscles are squeezed, you should be able to visualize plantar flexion of the foot on the leg being examined.**

P A positive Thompson test is manifested by the absence of plantar flexion when the calf muscles are squeezed.

P A positive Thompson test is suggestive of a ruptured Achilles tendon.

ADVANCED TECHNIQUE

Assessing Status of Distal Limbs and Digits

When you suspect distal limb or digit hypoperfusion due to trauma, injury, or pathology, conduct the following assessment:

E

1. Uncover the distal aspects of both limbs being assessed. A bilateral assessment permits comparison of the affected and unaffected limbs. When assessing an injured limb, assess the limb areas proximal and distal to the site of injury.
2. Assess for swelling.
3. Assess the vascular status of the distal limb and its digits (peripheral pulses, skin color, skin temperature, and capillary refill).
4. Ask the client to perform specific movements of the distal limb on command.
   a. To assess the ulnar nerve, ask the client to perform abduction of the fingers.
   b. To assess the radial nerve, ask the client to perform hyperextension of the thumb or wrist.
   c. To assess the median nerve, ask the client to perform opposition of the thumb to the little finger of the same hand.
   d. To assess the peroneal nerve, ask the client to perform dorsiflexion of the toes and ankle.
   e. To assess the tibial nerve, ask the client to perform plantar flexion of the toes and ankle.
5. When assessing sensation, instruct the client to close their eyes to prevent biased results. Use the thumb and index finger of the dominant hand to pinch certain areas of the distal limb.
   a. To assess the ulnar nerve, pinch the finger pad of the little finger.
   b. To assess the radial nerve, pinch the web space between the thumb and the index finger.
   c. To assess the median nerve, pinch the distal aspect of the index finger.
   d. To assess the peroneal nerve, pinch the lateral aspect of the great toe and the medial surface of the second toe.
   e. To assess the tibial nerve, pinch the medial and lateral surfaces of the sole of the foot.

N **The individual with normal perfusion to the limbs and digits will appear comfortable during rest and muscle contraction. Pain will not occur with movement of the distal limb or digits. Limb perfusion will be manifested by strong peripheral pulses, warm skin temperature, and a brisk capillary refill. There will be complete motor and sensory function of the distal limb and digits. The client will not experience any numbness or tingling.**

A Neurovascular deterioration, manifested by the "5 Ps" (pain, pallor, decreased perfusion, paresthesia, and paralysis) is abnormal.

P Neurovascular deterioration can occur in compartment syndrome. It is a severe complication of musculoskeletal trauma in which swelling is limited due to a confined space. As compartment syndrome worsens, clients will experience the "5Ps"; however, they may not be present at the same time. Pain is the most significant and the earliest clinical manifestation of acute compartment syndrome. It occurs distal to the site of injury and is induced by the contraction of the muscle compartment being compressed. Pain results from stretching of a muscle that is experiencing vascular compromise. Pain will be present at rest, can be worsened with passive stretch of the affected muscles, may seem out of proportion to the actual injury, and can be unimproved even with increasing dosages or frequency of pain medication.

P Inadequate arterial flow is a complication of digit or limb replantation following traumatic amputation.

P Arterial occlusion may also be detected as a complication of fracture or dislocation.

A Inadequate venous flow from the distal limb or digits, manifested by cyanosis, mottling, skin temperature that is warmer than usual, immediate capillary refill, and a distended or tense tissue turgor, is abnormal.

P Inadequate venous flow is a complication of digit or limb replantation following traumatic amputation.

Spine

E

1. Ask the client to stand and to leave the back of the gown open.
2. Stand behind the client so that you can visualize the posterior anatomy.
3. Inspect the position and alignment of the spine from a posterior and a lateral position.
4. Draw an imaginary line:
   a. From the head down through the spinous processes (Fig. 19-77).
   b. Across the top of the scapula.
   c. Across the top of the iliac crests.
   d. Across the bottom of the gluteal folds.
5. Palpate the spinous processes with your thumb.
6. Palpate the paravertebral muscles.
7. Assess ROM of the spine (Fig. 19-78). Ask the client to bend forward from the waist and touch the toes (flexion).
8. If necessary, stabilize the client's pelvis with your hands during the ROM assessment. Ask the client to:
   a. Bend to each side (lateral bending).
   b. Bend backward (hyperextension).
   c. Twist the shoulders to each side (rotation).

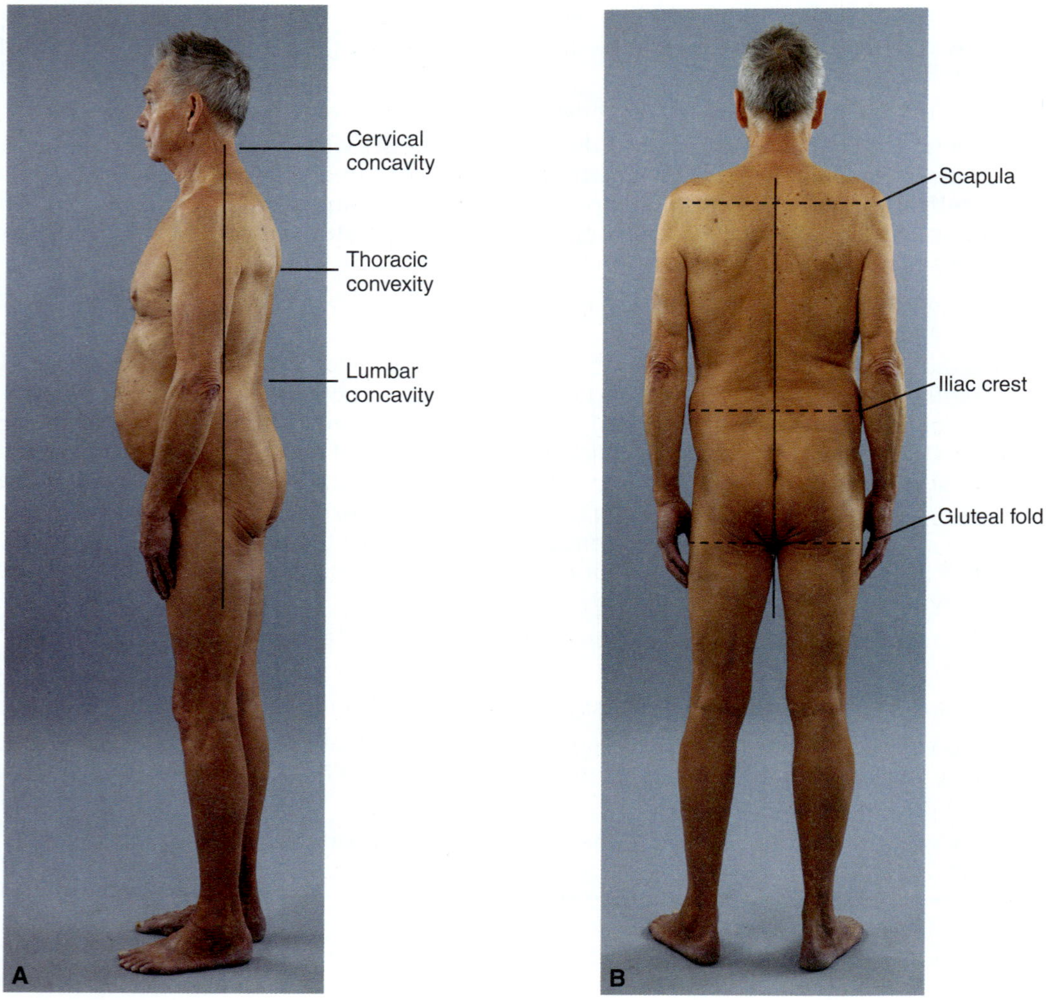

Figure 19-77 Alignment of spinal landmarks. **A.** Lateral view. **B.** Posterior view.

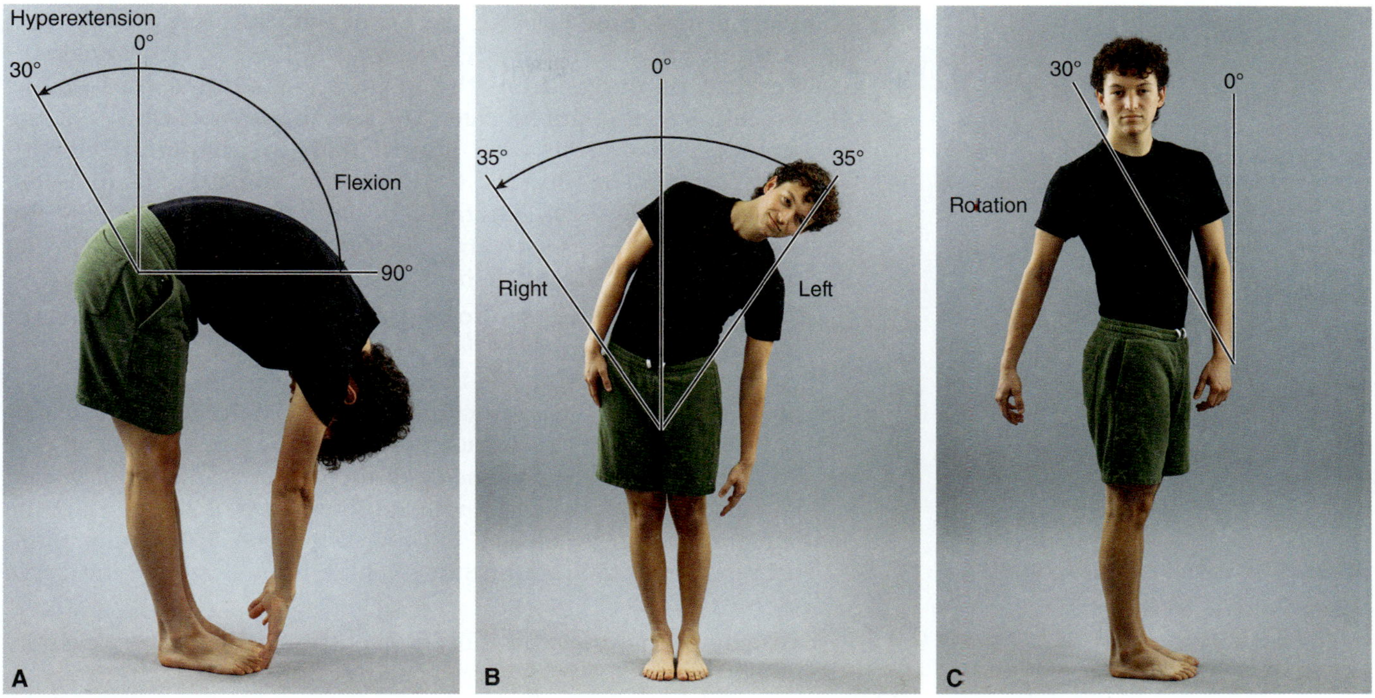

Figure 19-78 Range of motion of the spine. **A.** Flexion, hyperextension. **B.** Lateral bending. **C.** Rotation.

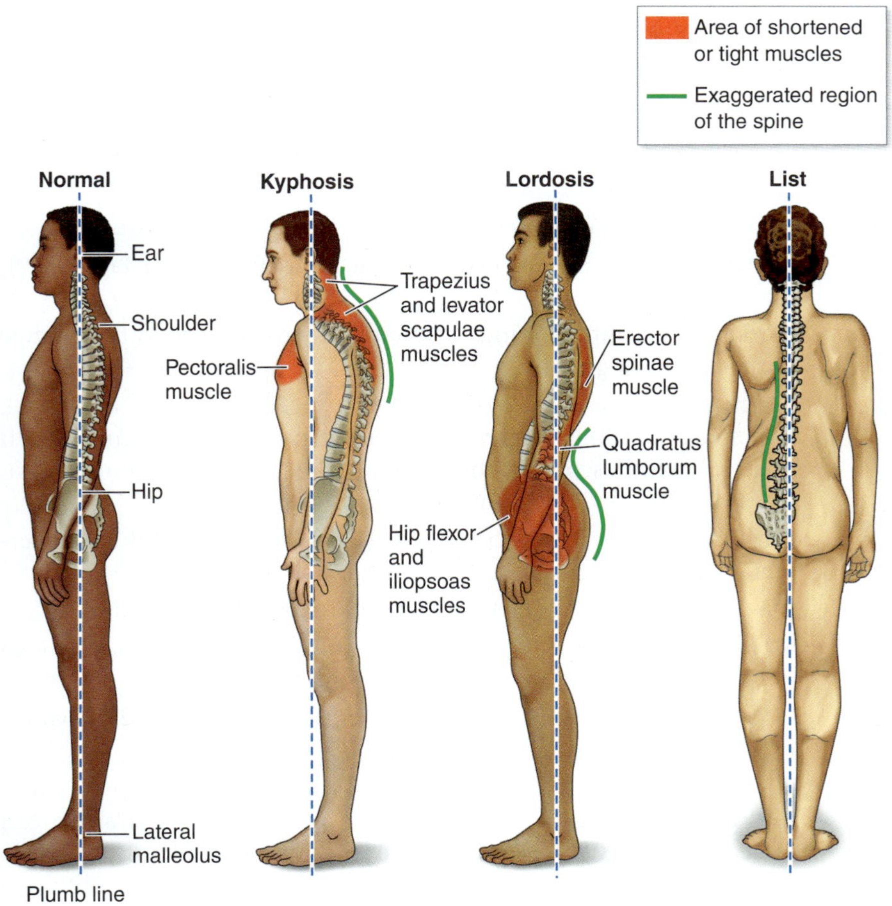

Figure 19-79 Normal spine and abnormalities of the spine.

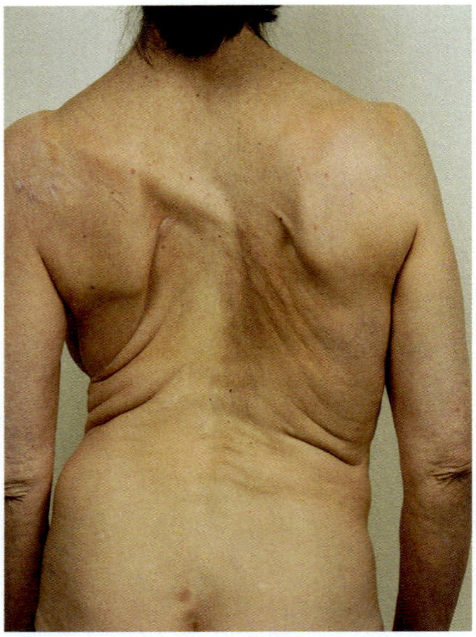

Figure 19-80 Scoliosis.

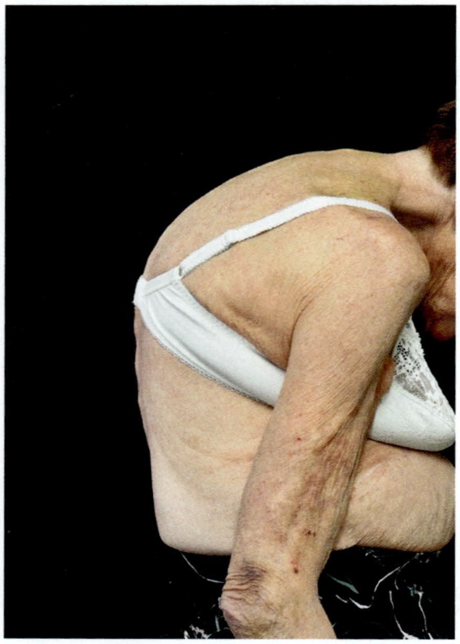

Figure 19-81 Kyphosis.

N **The normal spine has a cervical concavity, a thoracic convexity, and a lumbar concavity (Figs. 19-77 and 19-79). An imaginary line can be drawn from the head straight down the spinous processes to the gluteal cleft. The imaginary lines drawn at the scapulae, iliac crests, and gluteal folds are symmetrical with each other. The normal ROM of the spine is flexion—90°, hyperextension—30°, lateral bending—35°, and rotation—30°. As the client flexes forward, the concavity of the lumbar spine disappears and the entire back assumes a convex C shape.**

A From a posterior view, **scoliosis** (lateral curvature of the thoracic or lumbar vertebrae) may be detectable (Fig. 19-80) and is an abnormal finding. The curvature is visible despite voluntary attempts at proper posture. This is structural scoliosis. The curvature becomes accentuated on forward flexion from the waist. Scoliosis may also be accompanied by the asymmetry of the clavicles, uneven shoulder, and iliac crest levels, and a visible prominence of a scapula. If the lateral curvature is allowed to progress beyond 55°, cardiopulmonary problems can occur. Surgery may be indicated if the curve exceeds 40°.

P Structural scoliosis occurs most frequently in adolescence, especially in females.

A Functional scoliosis, which manifests itself only in a standing position, is abnormal.

P Functional scoliosis is due to unequal leg length or poor posture. Limb length should be measured.

A **Kyphosis**, an excessive convexity of the thoracic spine (Figs. 19-79 and 19-81), is abnormal. The client with kyphosis presents with the chin tilted downward onto the chest and with abdominal protrusion. There is also a decrease in the interval between the lower rib cage and the iliac crests. This appearance is due to forward and downward hunching of the head, neck, shoulders, and upper back.

P Kyphosis is frequently seen in older adults with osteoporosis.

A **Lordosis**, an excessive concavity of the lumbar spine (see Fig. 19-79), is abnormal.

P Lordosis is accentuated in obesity and pregnancy due to the change in the center of gravity.

A A **list**, which is a leaning of the spine (see Fig. 19-79), is abnormal. If an imaginary line is drawn straight down from T1, the gluteal cleft is lateral to it. In scoliosis, the imaginary line rests in the gluteal cleft, and the spine deviates from this straight line.

P A list can result from a herniated vertebral disc and painful paravertebral muscle spasms.

A It is abnormal to have iliac crests that are unequal in height.

P Scoliosis and congenital or acquired limb length discrepancies lead to iliac crests that are not equal in height.

A Decreased ROM is abnormal. This is usually accompanied by pain.

P Decreased ROM usually accompanied by pain can occur in back injury, osteoarthritis, and ankylosing spondylitis. Keep in mind that low back pain or tenderness of the costovertebral angle can indicate a musculoskeletal problem, a kidney problem, or a wide variety of other pathologies. Integrate the information obtained during the health history with clinical findings to guide your nursing interventions.

ADVANCED TECHNIQUE

Assessing for Scoliosis: Adams Forward Bend Test and Use of the Scoliometer

E
1. Instruct the client to disrobe to the underclothing.
2. Have the client stand upright with their feet together.
3. Stand behind the client.
4. Ask the client to bend forward from the waist with the hands held downward toward the feet and palms together (similar to a diving position). The head should be down, with the client looking at the floor.
5. Inspect and palpate the progression of the spinous processes, starting at the cervical spine and progressing in an inferior direction to the sacral area.
6. Draw an imaginary line through the spinous processes (or use a felt-tip marker to connect the spinous processes).
7. Place the scoliometer on the thoracic vertebrae in the midspinal line. Measure the angle of trunk rotation on the scoliometer.
8. Place the scoliometer on the lumbar vertebrae (Fig. 19-82) in the midspinal line and measure the angle of trunk rotation.

N **The imaginary (or real) line drawn through the spinous processes should be straight or with minimal deviation. The angle of trunk rotation reading on the scoliometer should be less than 7°.**

A It is abnormal to have moderate to severe lateral deviation of the spine. An angle of trunk rotation reading greater than 7° indicates scoliosis.

P Structural scoliosis usually develops in adolescence.

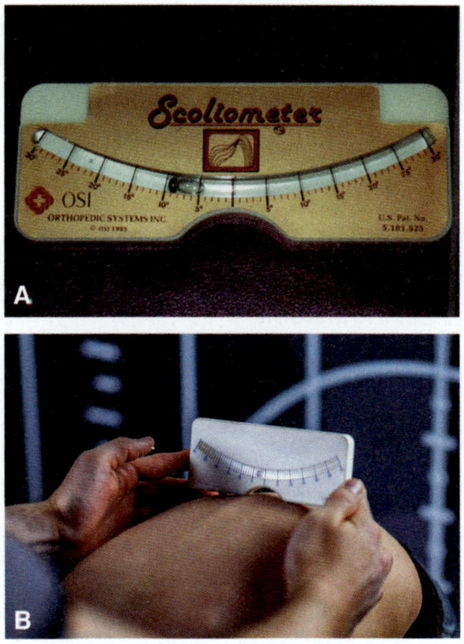

Figure 19-82 Scoliometer and its use. **A.** Scoliometer. **B.** Use of scoliometer.

ADVANCED TECHNIQUE

Assessing for Herniated Disc: Straight Leg Raising Test (Lasègue Test)

E
1. Assist the client to a supine position on the examination table.
2. Place one hand on the heel of the right foot and place the other hand behind the upper calf area of the same leg.
3. Maintain the foot in its neutral anatomical position.
4. Raise the leg to the angle at which leg pain occurs if present.
5. With the extended leg still raised to its maximum height, manually dorsiflex the foot (Fig. 19-83).
6. Repeat the technique on the left leg.

N **The client will be able to flex the hip joint and raise the straight leg to a hip flexion angle of 90°. There will be no leg pain with lifting of the extended leg or with dorsiflexion of the foot while the leg is raised.**

A A positive straight leg raising test is abnormal. The client will be unable to raise the extended leg to a 90° angle of hip joint flexion. Leg pain may occur with any lifting of the straight leg, and this discomfort will increase when the foot is dorsiflexed while the leg is in the raised position.

P Irritation of the lumbar nerve roots causes pain in the affected leg. Pain at less than 40° of elevation generally means an irritated nerve root caused by a herniated lumbar vertebral disc. Pain may also occur in the opposite leg.

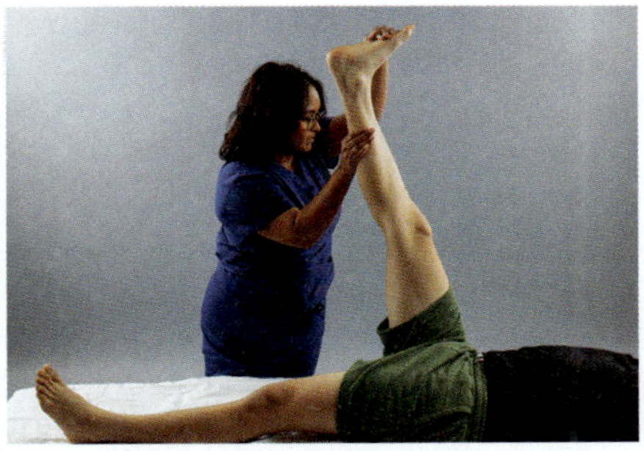

Figure 19-83 Straight leg raising test.

E Examination **N** Normal Findings **A** Abnormal Findings **P** Pathophysiology

Risk Factors

Osteoarthritis

- Obesity
- Family history of osteoarthritis
- Age >40–50
- Joint deformity
- Overuse of joint
- History of joint trauma
- Joint instability
- Diabetic neuropathy
- Joint infection or inflammation

ADVANCED TECHNIQUE

Assessing for Herniated Disc: Milgram Test

E 1. Place the client in a supine position on the examination table with both legs fully extended and resting on the table.

2. Instruct the client to raise both legs at least 2 inches (5 cm) off the examination table while maintaining the legs in extension for at least 30 seconds.

N **The client will be able to hold the extended legs in the raised position for at least 30 seconds.**

A The inability to maintain straight legs in the raised position for at least 30 seconds is suggestive of pressure on the spinal nerves and is abnormal.

P A positive Milgram test is often indicative of a herniated intervertebral disc.

NURSING CHECKLIST

Musculoskeletal Assistive Devices

Assistive devices may be necessary to support musculoskeletal structure and function. The need for such devices automatically indicates an underlying musculoskeletal disorder. For each assistive device, determine the reason for its use.

Crutches

Determine the following:

1. Amount of weight-bearing allowed on affected lower limb
2. Appropriate crutch height
3. Type of crutch gait and appropriateness for the amount of weight-bearing on affected leg: two-point crutch gait (partial weight-bearing); three-point crutch gait (partial or non-weight-bearing); four-point alternate crutch gait (partial or full weight-bearing); swing gait (non-weight-bearing)
4. Condition of crutches (padded handles, rubber tips)
5. Ease of transfer into and out of a chair
6. Ease of stair climbing with the crutches
7. Client wearing flat, properly fitted shoes with nonskid surfaces
8. Signs or symptoms of skin breakdown or distal limb hypoperfusion

Cane

Determine the following:

1. Shape of handle (C or T)
2. Number of points on contact surface
3. Appropriateness for client's height
4. Cane used on unaffected side
5. Refer to numbers 4–8 in the section on crutches

Walker

Determine the following:

1. Amount of weight-bearing allowed on the lower limb
2. Type of walker (e.g., rolling or pickup walker)
3. Appropriateness for client's height
4. Client's ability to grip and propel the walker forward with rolling walker; client's ability to grip, lift, and propel the walker forward with pickup walker (Fig. 19-84)
5. Refer to numbers 4–8 in the section on crutches

Brace, Splint, Immobilizer

Determine the following:

1. Location of device (e.g., limb, neck, torso, lower back, or pelvis)
2. Joint position maintained by device (e.g., extension, flexion, or abduction)
3. Joint motion allowed by device
4. If a movable device is used, whether the hinge joint of the device is aligned with the skeletal joint

5. Padding under pressure points of device
6. Amount of weight-bearing allowed on the affected leg (lower leg device)
7. Client wearing flat, properly fitted shoes with nonskid surfaces
8. Signs or symptoms of skin breakdown or distal limb hypoperfusion

Cast

Determine the following:

1. Plaster or fiberglass
2. Location of cast
3. Joint position maintained (e.g., extension, flexion, or abduction)
4. Joint motion allowed
5. Edges of the cast covered with tape to prevent skin irritation
6. Amount of weight-bearing allowed (lower leg cast)
7. Damage to cast (e.g., cracked, flaking or crumbling, dented, wet, softening)
8. Visible discoloration on the cast (e.g., from underlying wound drainage or bleeding)
9. Significant odor around the cast (e.g., a musty or foul smell)
10. Signs or symptoms of skin breakdown or distal limb hypoperfusion

Motorized Scooters

Determine the following:

1. Ease and ability to safely transfer to and from a scooter
2. Physical and cognitive ability to safely operate the steering system
3. Ability to maintain posture and position while operating the scooter
4. Condition of the scooter (seating, wheels, steering system, etc.)
5. Location for scooter use (indoor, outdoor, both)
6. Weight capacity of scooter adequate
7. Adequate access between rooms, maneuvering space, ramps, and surfaces for operating scooter
8. Does scooter meet mobility and ADL needs
9. Vehicle transportation needs
10. Appropriate size of scooter for client body size and habitus
11. Additional medical device needs on scooter (e.g., oxygen)

Wheelchair

Determine the following:

1. Condition of wheelchair (seating, secondary supports, padding, wheels, etc.)
2. Ease of transfer into and out of the wheelchair
3. Signs or symptoms of skin breakdown or distal limb hypoperfusion
4. Pressure relieving seating system or cushions
5. Adequate chair stability while client seated
6. Seating system provides sufficient support for seated client allowing normal anatomical alignment for the client
7. Condition of head, pelvic, or trunk supports
8. Type of wheelchair safe and appropriateness for client's condition, needs, abilities, and functional impairments (cognition, comorbidities, strength, and sensory-motor function, vision, hearing, postural control, occupation, social and transportation needs, home and occupational environment)
9. Appropriate size of a wheelchair for client's body size and habitus

U.S. Preventive Services Task Force (USPSTF)

Grade B Recommendations:

- The USPSTF recommends screening for osteoporosis to prevent osteoporotic fractures in postmenopausal women younger than 65 years who are at increased risk for an osteoporotic fracture as estimated by clinical risk assessment.
- The USPSTF recommends screening for osteoporosis to prevent osteoporotic fractures in women 65 years or older.

Retrieved December 17, 2025, from *https://www.uspreventiveservicestaskforce.org/uspstf/recommendation-topics/uspstf-a-and-b-recommendations*

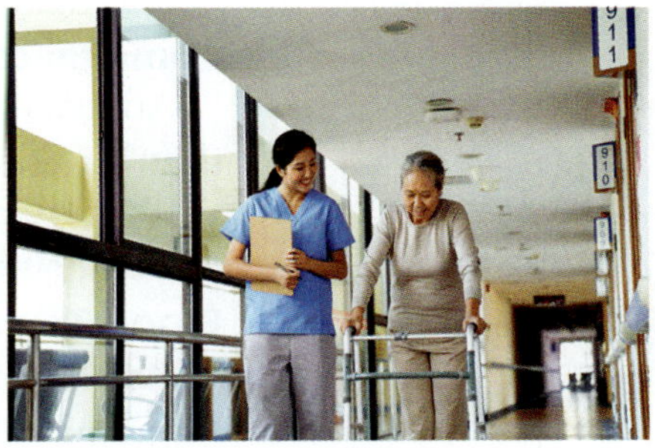

Figure 19-84 The nurse assesses the client's ability to use the walker correctly.

CASE STUDY
The Client With Acute Shoulder Pain

This case study illustrates the application and objective documentation of the musculoskeletal examination. Alex Chun was working at a construction site when a sudden onset of shoulder pain occurred after lifting a heavy object. Alex presents to the urgent care clinic for evaluation and treatment.

HEALTH HISTORY

CLIENT PROFILE

48-year-old Asian male

CHIEF COMPLAINT

"My right shoulder hurts."

HISTORY OF PRESENT ILLNESS

48-year-old client brought to the urgent care clinic. While at work 2 days ago client attempted to lift a heavy object and felt a sudden onset of sharp pain in the right shoulder with an immediate loss of strength. The shoulder pain is constant with 8/10 intensity. Right arm is immobilized in a sling, which seems to help reduce the pain to 6/10. Ice applied to the shoulder is not helping with the pain. Any movement with the shoulder worsens the pain. Reports taking "a lot" of hydrocodone that was obtained from a friend for the shoulder injury and pain, but it is only helping a little. This is in addition to the prescribed oxycodone taken twice daily since the accident.

PAST HEALTH HISTORY

Medical History Hypertension well controlled on meds since age 33

Chronic low back pain (LBP) and headaches for 20 years that started with his military deployments. Sees pain management provider at the Veterans Affairs (VA) clinic every month. Current treatment effective

Post-traumatic stress disorder (PTSD) and mild traumatic brain injury (TBI) following a blast injury while in combat in Afghanistan 15 years ago

Bilateral knee osteoarthritis

Surgical History Right wrist surgery after fall at age 16, no complications

Vasectomy at age 40

Allergies No known medication allergies. Denies environmental allergies

Medications

Lisinopril 10 mg daily

Hydrochlorothiazide 50 mg daily

Oxycodone-controlled release 10 mg every 12 hours prn

MVI daily

Communicable Diseases Denies

Annual PPD was negative 6 months ago.

Injuries and Accidents Right wrist fracture at age 16 after falling from a ladder.

TBI 15 years ago—no further information available at this time

Special Needs Denies

Blood Transfusions None

Childhood Illnesses Chickenpox at 9 years of age

Immunizations Fully immunized against childhood illnesses

COVID-19 vaccination "up to date"

Received annual flu shot in October of this year. Last tetanus shot was 3 years ago

FAMILY HEALTH HISTORY

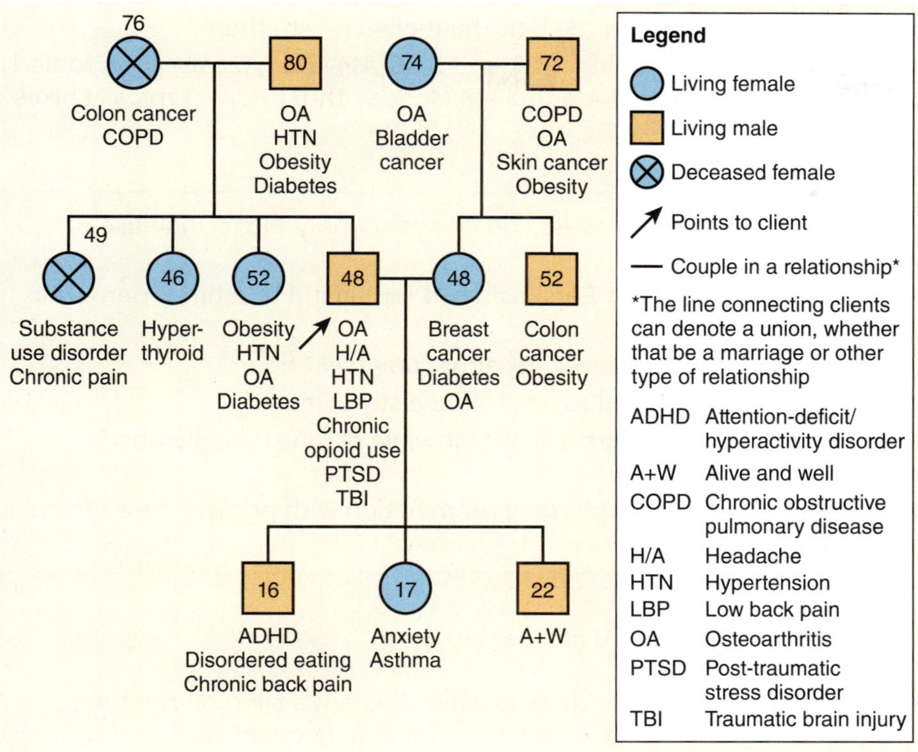

SOCIAL HISTORY

Alcohol Use Drinks 2 to 3 beers daily after work, admits up to 6 drinks daily on the weekends

Tobacco Use Denies

Recreational Drug Use Denies "illegal" drug use (i.e., cocaine or heroin) or diagnosis of substance use disorder; occasional marijuana joint

Domestic and Intimate Partner Violence Denies

Sexual Practice Married to wife of 28 years. In a monogamous heterosexual relationship. No history of STIs

Travel History No recent history of travel, none outside the country since leaving the military

Work Environment Employed with same company for past 10 years. Travels to wherever the construction site is located. Usually within 45 minutes of home. This is the first work-related injury at this company.

Home Environment Lives with wife and 2 teenage children. Smoke detectors in home. All guns in home have gun locks and are in a safe. Has one indoor/outdoor cat at home

Hobbies and Leisure Activities Enjoys bike riding and woodworking

Stress Reports no major stressors. Regularly visits with a pain management clinic and mental health nurse practitioner (NP) at the VA primarily for PTSD, TBI, and chronic LBP

Education Has a high school education; attended trade school after high school

Economic Status Middle-class family

Military Service Served for 6 years in the Marine Corps. Three combat deployments to Afghanistan and Iraq. Honorably discharged

Religion Baptist, attends church service regularly

Ethnic Background Chinese descent, second generation American

Roles and Relationships Married to wife for 28 years. Describes relationship as stable. Father to two teenage children who live at home and one son who is away at Marine boot camp. Reports having a "decent" relationship with them

Characteristic Patterns of Daily Living Wakes at 5:30 AM and typically goes to bed at 10 PM. Works full time between 7 AM to 3 PM Monday thru Friday. Typically bikes after work

HEALTH MAINTENANCE ACTIVITIES

Sleep 7–8 hours per night, feels well rested and sleeps soundly. No routine use of sedative/hypnotic agents to induce sleep

Diet Tries to maintain a balanced diet. Eats fast food for lunch 1 to 2 times per week. Doesn't snack in the evening

Exercise Bike riding 3 to 5 times per week for approximately 1 hour

Stress Management Exercise is useful to help reduce stress in life

Use of Safety Devices Routinely wears a seat belt while driving. Usually obeys traffic guidelines

Health Checkups Has routine annual physical examination with primary care provider

PHYSICAL EXAMINATION

General Assessment

Overall Appearance Height: 5 feet 11 inches (180 cm)
Weight: 175 lbs (79.5 kg)
No obvious deformities. Uses no assistive devices. Wearing a sling on right arm. No open wounds or lesions noted. Client is alert and fully oriented.

Posture Seated on examination table with an erect posture

Gait and Mobility Normal gait noted with ambulation

Inspection

Muscle Size and Shape Well-developed and contoured limb musculature. No muscle hypertrophy or atrophy noted. No obvious involuntary muscle movement or deformities noted.

Joint Contour and Periarticular Tissue Edema and mild ecchymosis of the right shoulder. No joint angulation or deformity. Remaining joint contours appear normal.

Palpation

Muscle Tone Normal muscle tone associated with muscle contraction in all extremities. No muscle spasm or soft tissue masses palpated in the extremities.

Joints Diffuse pain with palpation of the right shoulder. No specific point tenderness noted on palpation over the bicep tendon or deltoid muscle. No pain over the clavicle, acromioclavicular (AC) joint, acromion, or scapula.

Range of Motion Intact but pain-limited active motion at the right shoulder with flexion, extension, internal and external rotation. Unable to perform active abduction with right arm. Full, smooth, painless ROM of left shoulder in all planes. Passive shoulder motion is full bilaterally with discomfort at the right shoulder.

Muscle Strength Muscle strength 3/5 at the right shoulder with flexion, extension, internal and external rotation but 0/5 with attempted abduction. Strength is 5/5 with the left shoulder in all directions.

Sensation* Sensation is grossly intact in the upper extremities bilaterally to light touch.

Reflexes* Biceps, triceps, and brachioradialis deep tendon reflexes (DTR) bilaterally 2+/4+

Skin/Vascular* Skin is warm, dry, and intact. Radial pulses bilaterally 2+/4+. Brisk capillary refill

Advanced Techniques Positive drop arm test and Neer impingement sign of the right shoulder

*included in a comprehensive musculoskeletal examination

CLINICAL JUDGMENT IN ACTION

1. What cues indicate that the client is having a musculoskeletal disorder?
2. What interventions have the highest priority?
3. What assessment findings indicate clinical improvement or decline in this client?

Review Questions

1. Which of the following are considered freely movable joints?
   a. Synarthroses
   b. Amphiarthroses
   c. Diarthroses
   d. Semiarthrosis
2. Which of the following range of motion maneuvers is described as *moving the extremity laterally and away from the midline of the body*?
   a. Eversion
   b. Flexion
   c. Abduction
   d. Elevation
3. Which of the following best describes a Trendelenburg gait?
   a. The client ambulates with short, uncoordinated, stiff steps with the knees adducted or crossed and the lower leg appearing to move forward in a semicircular arc of motion as the body sways sideways.
   b. Difficulty initiating ambulation but, when initiated, walking appears to be slow and have a shuffling pattern.
   c. An excessively high stepping gait with the feet slapped hard against the ground while walking.
   d. The pelvis tilts down to the nonaffected side while bearing weight on the affected leg. A client may tilt the torso toward the affected side.
4. During the examination of a client with an acute painful injury to the shoulder, the nurse notes that the client is unable to slowly lower the arm after the nurse passively brings the arm into an abducted position. What test was conducted on this client?
   a. Drop arm
   b. Impingement
   c. Drawer
   d. Finklestein
5. While practicing in the outpatient surgery center, the nurse is preparing a client for carpal tunnel surgery to release compression of the median nerve. What history or physical examination finding is consistent with carpal tunnel syndrome?
   a. The client has complaints of pain and tingling in the fourth and fifth fingers of the hand with repeated grasping activities.
   b. When the nurse taps over the wrist, the client experiences a muscle spasm of the entire hand.
   c. After 45 seconds with the wrist of the affected limb flexed, the client experiences pain, numbness, and tingling in the first, second, and third fingers.
   d. When inspecting the palm of the affected hand the nurse notes hypertrophy of the thenar eminence.
6. The nurse is evaluating hip range of motion in a client who had a recent fall at a skilled nursing facility. The nurse assesses passive external rotation of the hip by doing which of the following maneuvers?
   a. Raise the leg straight off the examination table with the knee extended.
   b. With the knee flexed, raise the leg off the examination table, bringing the flexed knee toward the chest as far as possible.
   c. Flex the hip and knee. Move the flexed leg laterally as the foot moves medially.
   d. With the knee and hip in extension, slide the leg laterally.

7. While examining a client with an acute onset of knee pain, the nurse notices the client has a positive ballottement test and bulge sign. What is the likely cause for this?
   a. Joint effusion
   b. Referred pain
   c. A prior knee surgery
   d. Quadriceps weakness

8. A medical surgical nurse is caring for a client who experienced trauma to the forearm. The nurse should be aware that compartment syndrome, a surgical emergency, can occur. Of the "5 P" signs and symptoms, what is the earliest and most significant finding this client might exhibit that would alert the nurse to potential compartment syndrome?
   a. Paresthesia of the fingers
   b. Pallor of the arm and hand
   c. Pulselessness at the radial artery
   d. Pain not controlled with medication

9. A registered nurse at a nursing home responds to a client who has fallen. The nurse suspects a hip fracture based on the physical examination findings. What examination finding would lead the nurse to consider a potential fractured hip has occurred?
   a. The affected leg is visibly shorter that the opposite side.
   b. The client walks with a limp.
   c. The leg is held in a position of internal rotation.
   d. There is decreased sensation to the leg with a light touch.

10. What are some of the risk factors for osteoporosis? Select all that apply.
    a. Muscular body build
    b. Smoking history
    c. Celiac disease
    d. Bulimia
    e. Frequent steroid use

CHAPTER

20 Mental Status and Neurological System

Learning Outcomes

1. Identify the anatomy and physiology of the central nervous system, the peripheral nervous system, and the autonomic nervous system.
2. Conduct a complete health history on a client with a mental status or neurological system condition.
3. Perform a physical examination on a healthy adult and an adult with a mental status and neurological system pathology.
4. Differentiate between normal clinical findings from a client's mental status and neurological system physical examination and the pathophysiology of abnormal clinical findings.
5. Identify risk factors for a cerebrovascular accident.
6. Identify risk factors for suicide.
7. Identify the United States Preventive Services Task Force recommendations for mental status and the neurological system.
8. Document a complete health history and physical examination of a client with a mental status and neurological system pathology.

The nervous system controls all body functions and thought processes. The complex interrelationships among the various divisions of the nervous system permit the body to maintain homeostasis; receive, interpret, and react to stimuli; and control voluntary and involuntary processes, including cognition.

Anatomy and Physiology

The structure and function of the central nervous system and the peripheral nervous system are discussed.

Macrostructure

The scalp and skull are two protective layers covering the brain. The scalp performs a unique function in that it moves freely, helping to protect and cushion the head from traumatic injury. The skull is a rigid, bony cavity that has a fixed volume of approximately 1,500 mL.

Meninges

There are three layers of meninges (protective membranes), known as the dura mater, arachnoid mater, and pia mater, located between the brain and the skull (Fig. 20-1). The dura mater is the thick, tough, outermost layer. Below the dura mater is a small serous space known as the subdural space.

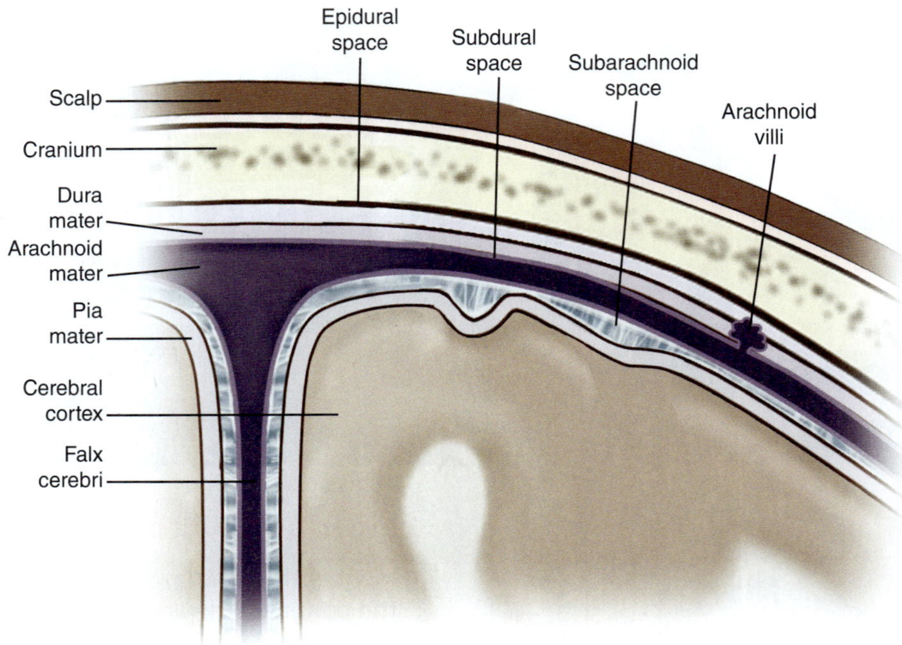

Figure 20-1 The meninges.

The arachnoid mater lies between the dura mater and the pia mater. Below the arachnoid mater is the subarachnoid space, where cerebrospinal fluid (CSF) is circulated. Portions of the arachnoid mater, called arachnoid villi, project into the subarachnoid space (also shown in Fig. 20-1). These absorb CSF.

The pia mater is thin and vascular. It is the innermost layer of the meninges. The pia mater helps form the choroid plexuses, which are vascular structures located in the ventricles of the brain that form CSF.

Central Nervous System

The brain and the spinal cord make up the central nervous system (CNS). The brain is divided into four main components: the cerebrum, the diencephalon, the cerebellum, and the brainstem. Each of these areas is subdivided into various anatomical areas.

Cerebrum

The cerebrum is the largest portion of the brain. It is incompletely divided into the right and left hemispheres by the longitudinal fissure. The two hemispheres are connected by the corpus callosum, which serves as a communication link between the left and right hemispheres.

The cerebral cortex, or the outermost layer of the cerebrum, contains gray matter. Higher cognitive functioning is dependent on the cerebral cortex and its interaction with other parts of the nervous system. The cerebral cortex is involved in memory storage and recall, conscious understanding of sensation, vision, hearing, and motor function. The basal ganglia are located deep within the cerebral hemispheres and function intricately with the cerebral cortex and the cerebellum in regulating motor activity.

Each cerebral hemisphere is divided into four lobes: the frontal, parietal, temporal, and occipital lobes. The locations and functions of each of the cerebral lobes are illustrated in Figure 20-2. A fifth lobe, called the limbic lobe, is anatomically part of the temporal lobe and is involved in emotional behavior and self-preservation.

Diencephalon

The diencephalon, a relay center for the brain, is composed of the thalamic structures: the thalamus, the epithalamus, and the hypothalamus. The

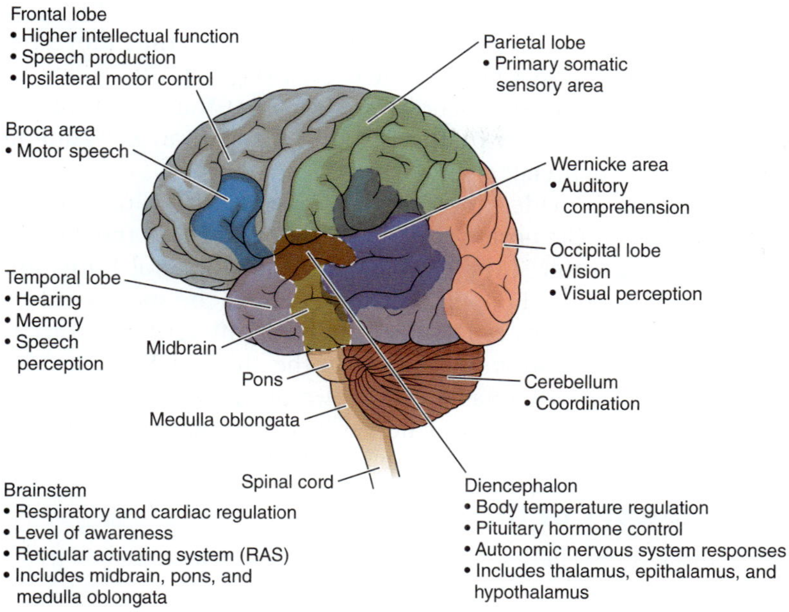

Figure 20-2 The locations and functions of the cerebral lobes, diencephalon, cerebellum, and brainstem.

hypothalamus is important in body temperature regulation, pituitary hormone control, and autonomic nervous system responses. It also plays a role in behavior via its connections with the limbic system.

Cerebellum

The cerebellum lies inferior to the occipital lobe and behind the brainstem. It is divided into two lateral lobes and a medial part called the vermis. The vermis is the part of the cerebellum concerned primarily with the maintenance of posture and equilibrium. Each cerebellar hemisphere is responsible for the coordination of movement of the ipsilateral (same) side of the body.

Brainstem

The brainstem is located immediately below the diencephalon and is divided into the midbrain, the pons, and the medulla oblongata. The reticular formation, a complex network of sensory fibers in the brainstem, contains centers that control respiratory, cardiovascular, and other maintenance of life functions. The ascending reticular activating system (RAS) is located in the brainstem and extends to the cerebral cortex. The RAS is mostly excitatory and is essential for arousal from sleep, maintaining attention, and perception of sensory input.

The midbrain contains the nuclei of cranial nerves III (oculomotor) and IV (trochlear), which are associated with the control of eye movements. The pons is located between the midbrain and the medulla oblongata. Sensory and motor nuclei of cranial nerves V (trigeminal), VI (abducens), VII (facial), and VIII (acoustic) are located in the pons. The medulla oblongata is located between the pons and the spinal cord. It contains the nuclei of cranial nerves IX (glossopharyngeal), X (vagus), XI (spinal accessory), and XII (hypoglossal). Also located in the medulla oblongata are the centers for reflexes such as sneezing, swallowing, coughing, and vomiting, as well as the centers regulating the respiratory and cardiovascular systems.

Spinal Cord

The spinal cord is a continuation of the medulla oblongata. It exits the skull at the foramen magnum and begins at the upper border of the atlas (C1), continuing downward to the conus medullaris, a tapered ending of the cord at about the level of the first or second lumbar vertebra (Fig. 20-3A). From the conus medullaris, a connective tissue filament called the filum terminale continues down to its attachment at the coccyx (Fig. 20-3B).

A cross section of the spinal cord will show that the central part of the cord is gray matter. The gray matter is in the shape of an H. White matter surrounds the gray matter.

The gray matter is made up of nerve cell bodies and short segments of unmyelinated fibers. The posterior portion of the H is called the dorsal horn, and the anterior portion is the ventral horn. Small lateral horns are also present in the thoracic and upper lumbar sections of the spinal cord.

The dorsal horn contains cell bodies of sensory (afferent) neurons, which receive and transmit sensory messages from the afferent fibers in the spinal nerve. The ventral horn contains cell bodies of motor (efferent) neurons, which send axons into the spinal nerves and innervate skeletal muscles, carrying signals from the brain and the spinal cord.

Motor Pathways of the CNS

There are three motor pathways in the CNS: the corticospinal or pyramidal tract, the extrapyramidal tract, and the cerebellum.

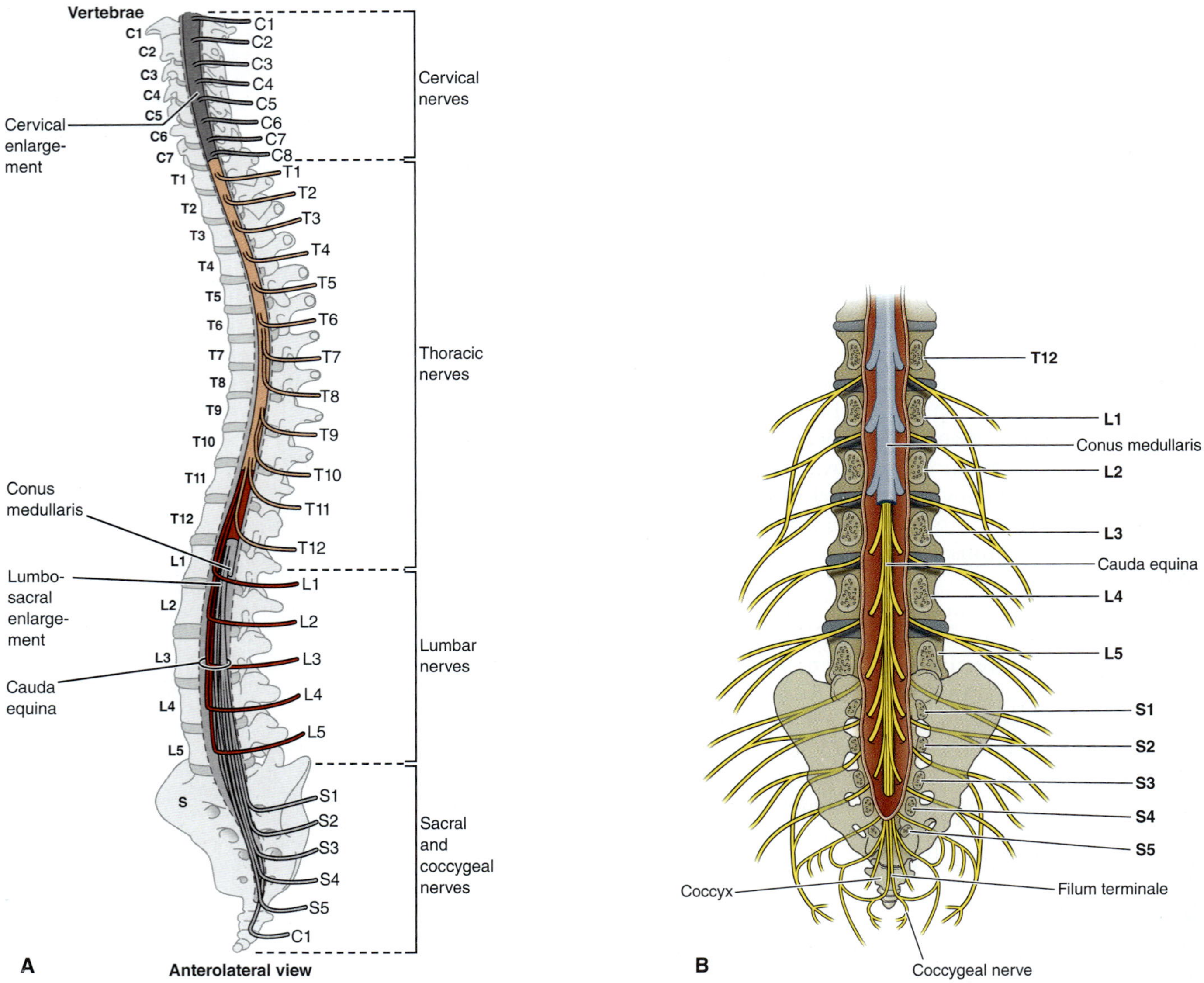

Figure 20-3 The spinal cord. **A.** The spinal cord and spinal nerves. **B.** Close-up of the caudal region of the spinal nerves.

Pyramidal Tract

The corticospinal pathway descends from the motor area of the cerebral cortex, through the midbrain, the pons, and the medulla. At the level of the medulla, 90% of the fibers of the corticospinal tract decussate (cross) to travel down the opposite side of the spinal cord, becoming the lateral corticospinal tract. The remaining fibers travel down the spinal cord in a tract known as the anterior corticospinal tract. Fibers of the lateral corticospinal tract synapse in the anterior horn (gray matter) at all levels of the cord just before they leave the cord (Fig. 20-4). The motor neurons above this synapse in the anterior horn are known as upper motor neurons. Upper motor neurons connect the cerebral cortex with the anterior horn and are entirely contained within the CNS. Lower motor neurons are motor neurons below the level of the upper motor neurons. Lower motor neuron cell bodies are located in the anterior horn, where they connect with the corticospinal tract. Lower motor neurons innervate skeletal muscle at the myoneural junction. They are responsible for purposeful, voluntary movement.

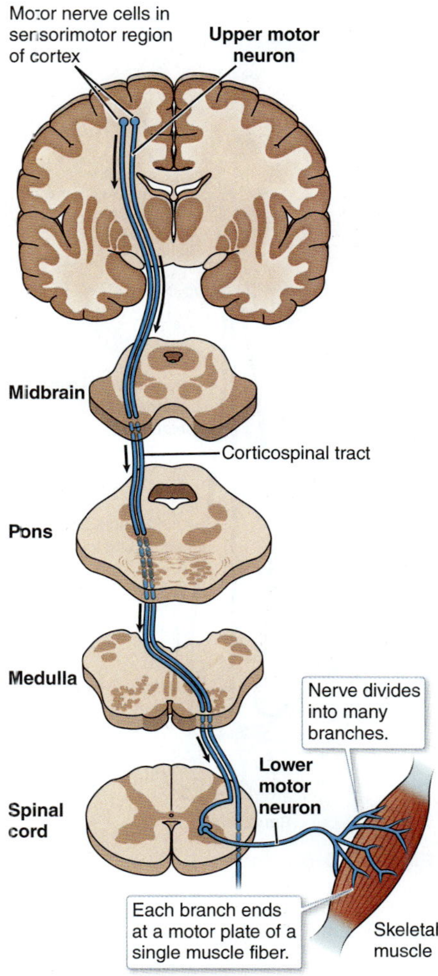

Figure 20-4 Motor pathways of the CNS.

Extrapyramidal Tract

The extrapyramidal tract includes all motor neurons in the motor cortex, basal ganglia, brainstem, and spinal cord that are outside the corticospinal, or pyramidal, tract (hence the name "extrapyramidal"). The extrapyramidal tract is responsible for controlling body movement, particularly gross automatic movements (e.g., walking), and for controlling muscle tone.

Sensory Pathways of the CNS

The sensory portion of the peripheral nervous system consists of afferent neurons divided into somatic afferent and visceral afferent neurons. Somatic afferent fibers originate in skeletal muscles, joints, tendons, and skin. Visceral fibers originate in the viscera. Both types of afferent fibers carry impulses from both the external and the internal environments to the CNS.

Afferent fibers containing impulses, or messages, enter the spinal cord through the dorsal roots. From the spinal cord, the message travels via the spinothalamic tracts or the posterior column to the thalamus and sensory cortex. The thalamus receives the message and interprets a general sensation. The impulse synapses with another sensory neuron to the sensory cortex, where the message is fully interpreted (Fig. 20-5).

Spinothalamic Tracts

In the spinal cord, the spinothalamic tracts synapse with a second sensory neuron and then decussate to the opposite side. The message is then carried up the tract. The lateral spinothalamic tract carries pain and temperature sensations, and the anterior spinothalamic tract carries the sensations of crude or light touch.

Posterior Column

The posterior column carries position, vibration, and fine-touch sensations. The nerve impulse enters the spinal cord and travels upward to the medulla, where a synapse with a second sensory neuron occurs. The neuron decussates to the opposite side of the medulla and continues to the thalamus and sensory cortex.

Blood Supply

Blood is supplied to the brain by two pairs of arteries, the internal carotid arteries (anterior circulation) and the vertebral arteries (posterior circulation). At the base of the brain lies the circle of Willis, an arterial anastomosis that links the anterior and posterior blood supplies (Fig. 20-6). The functional areas supplied by each of the main cerebral arteries are listed in Table 20-1.

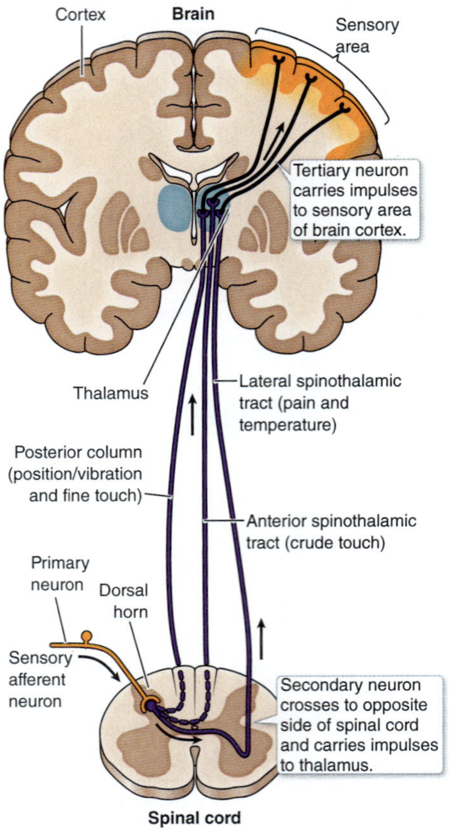

Figure 20-5 Sensory pathways of the CNS.

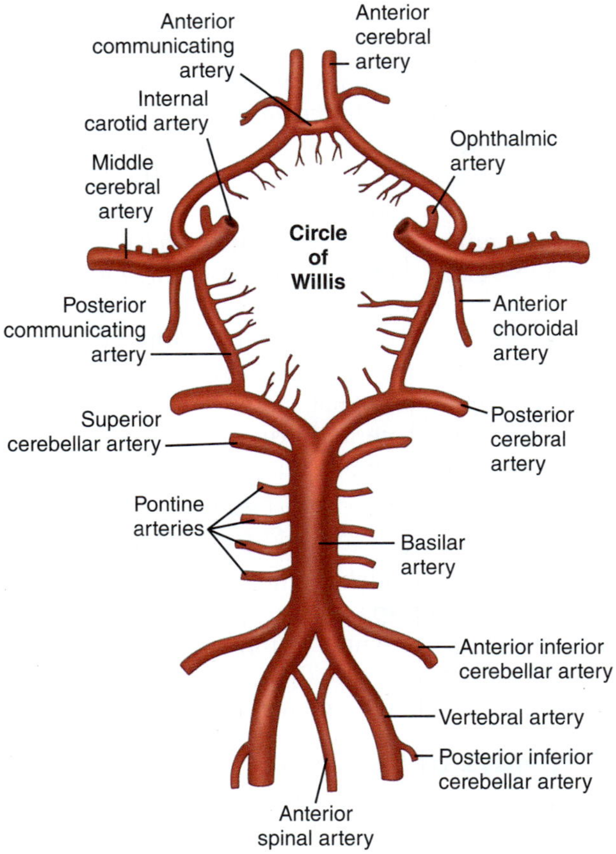

Figure 20-6 Major arteries of the brain.

Table 20-1 Cerebral Blood Supply

Artery	Functional Area
Anterior cerebral artery	Medial and inferior surfaces of each hemisphere: • Frontal lobe • Parietal lobe
Middle cerebral artery	Lateral surface of each hemisphere: • Frontal lobe • Temporal lobe • Parietal lobe • Occipital lobe
Posterior cerebral artery	Medial and inferior surfaces of each hemisphere: • Temporal lobe • Medial occipital lobe • Midbrain
Basilar artery	• Midbrain • Upper brainstem • Medulla oblongata
Cerebellar arteries	• Pons • Midbrain • Cerebellum

Peripheral Nervous System

The peripheral nervous system consists of nervous tissue found outside the CNS, including the spinal nerves, cranial nerves, and the autonomic nervous system.

Spinal Nerves

The 31 pairs of spinal nerves include 8 cervical, 12 thoracic, 5 lumbar, 5 sacral, and 1 coccygeal. Each spinal nerve is made up of a dorsal (afferent) root and a ventral (efferent) root. Each afferent spinal nerve root innervates a specific area of the skin, called a **dermatome**, for superficial cutaneous sensations. Figure 20-7 illustrates both the anterior and the posterior dermatomal distributions. Spinal nerves leaving the right side of the cord supply the right side of the body, and those leaving the left side supply the left side of the body.

Each of the eight cervical nerves exits above its corresponding vertebra. Each of the spinal nerves below the cervical portion exits below its corresponding vertebra. The spinal cord is not as long as the vertebral column, so the lumbar and sacral nerves are comparatively long. These longer roots are called the cauda equina, meaning "horse's tail" (Fig. 20-3B).

Cranial Nerves

There are 12 pairs of cranial nerves. They are designated in the order of their position with Roman numerals I through XII. Some cranial nerves have purely motor functions, and some have only sensory functions. Others have mixed sensory and motor functions. Table 20-2 summarizes the functions of the cranial nerves.

Autonomic Nervous System

The autonomic nervous system (ANS) is divided into two functionally different subdivisions: the sympathetic and the parasympathetic nervous systems.

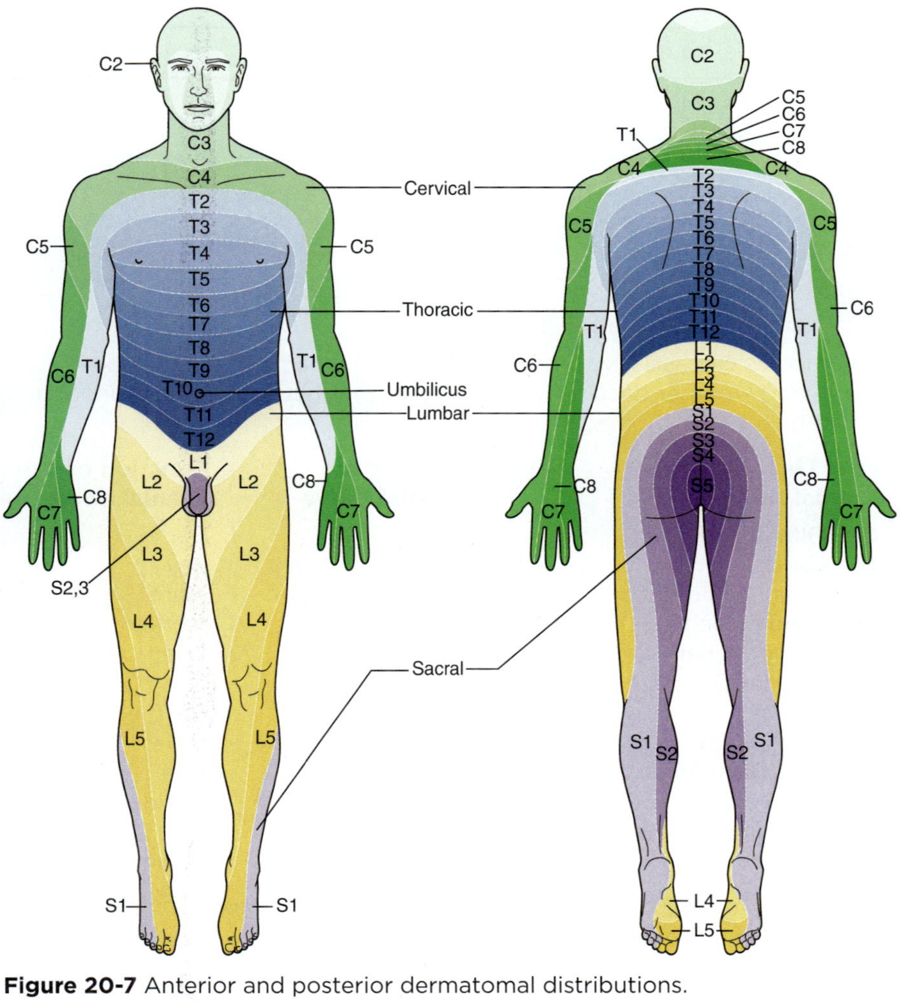

Figure 20-7 Anterior and posterior dermatomal distributions.

Table 20-2 The 12 Cranial Nerves and Their Functions

Name and Number	Function
Olfactory (I)	Smell
Optic (II)	Visual acuity, visual fields, funduscopic examination
Oculomotor (III)	Cardinal fields of gaze (EOM movement), eyelid elevation, pupil reaction, doll's eyes phenomenon
Trochlear (IV)	EOM movement
Trigeminal (V)	Motor: strength of temporalis and masseter muscles Sensory: light touch, superficial pain and temperature to face, corneal reflex
Abducens (VI)	EOM movement
Facial (VII)	Motor: facial movements Sensory: taste anterior two-thirds of tongue Parasympathetic: tears and saliva secretion*
Acoustic (VIII)	Cochlear: gross hearing, Weber and Rinne tests Vestibular: vertigo, equilibrium, nystagmus
Glossopharyngeal (IX)	Motor: soft palate and uvula movement, gag reflex, swallowing, guttural and palatal sounds Sensory: taste posterior one-third of tongue Parasympathetic: carotid reflex, chemoreceptors*
Vagus (X)	Motor and Sensory: same as CN IX Parasympathetic: carotid reflex, stomach and intestinal secretions, peristalsis, involuntary control of bronchi, heart innervation*
Spinal accessory (XI)	Sternocleidomastoid and trapezius muscle movements
Hypoglossal (XII)	Tongue movement, lingual sounds

*Cannot be directly assessed.
EOM = extraocular muscle; CN = cranial nerve.

NURSING TIP

Cranial Nerve Mnemonics

Mnemonics can assist you in remembering the name of each cranial nerve and whether each nerve has a sensory function, a motor function, or both.

First Letter of Cranial Nerve	Number of Cranial Nerve	Function of Cranial Nerve
On (Olfactory)	I	**S**ome
Old (Optic)	II	**S**ay
Olympus (Oculomotor)	III	**M**arry
Towering (Trochlear)	IV	**M**oney
Tops (Trigeminal)	V	**B**ut
A (Abducens)	VI	**M**y
Finn (Facial)	VII	**B**rother
And (Acoustic)	VIII	**S**ays
German (Glossopharyngeal)	IX	**B**ad
Viewed (Vagus)	X	**B**usiness
Some (Spinal Accessory)	XI	**M**arry
Hops (Hypoglossal)	XII	**M**oney

For cranial nerve function: **S** = sensory nerve, **M** = motor nerve, **B** = both sensory and motor nerves.

Table 20-3 Sympathetic Versus Parasympathetic Response

System	Sympathetic Response	Parasympathetic Response
Neurological	Pupils dilated Heightened awareness	Pupils normal size
Cardiovascular	Increased heart rate Increased myocardial contractility Increased blood pressure	Decreased heart rate Decreased myocardial contractility
Respiratory	Increased respiratory rate Increased respiratory depth Bronchial dilation	Bronchial constriction
Gastrointestinal	Decreased gastric motility Decreased gastric secretions Increased glycogenolysis Decreased insulin production Sphincter contraction	Increased gastric motility Increased gastric secretions Sphincter dilation
Genitourinary	Decreased urine output Decreased renal blood flow	Normal urine output

The ANS functions without voluntary control to maintain the body in a state of homeostasis. Most organs that are under the influence of the ANS have dual innervation of both the sympathetic and parasympathetic systems.

The sympathetic nervous system, sometimes called the thoracolumbar system, controls "fight or flight" actions. The parasympathetic nervous system (craniosacral) is responsible for the "general housekeeping" of the body. See Table 20-3 for specific system responses to autonomic stimulation.

Reflexes

A reflex action—a specific response to an adequate stimulus—occurs without conscious control. The stimulus can occur in a joint, muscle, or the skin and is transmitted to the CNS by one or more afferent, or sensory, neurons. The impulse enters the spinal cord through the dorsal root of a spinal nerve, where it synapses. Following synapse in the cord, the anterior motor neurons send an impulse via efferent neurons to the endplates of the skeletal muscle, causing the effector muscle to react (Fig. 20-8).

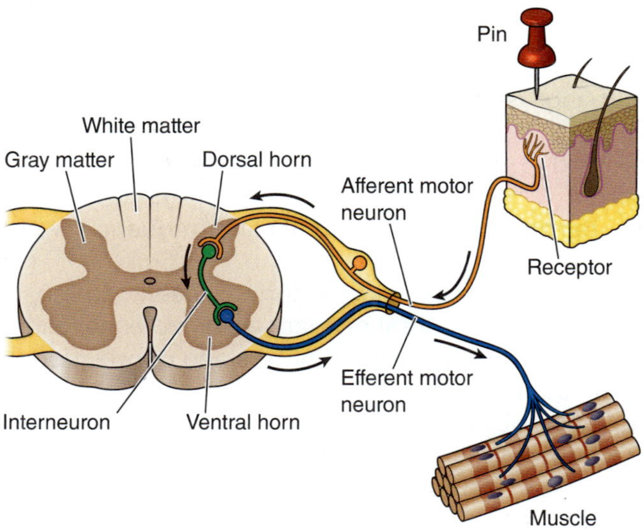

Figure 20-8 Monosynaptic reflex arc.

NURSING TIP
Preventing Traumatic Neurological Injuries

Teach your clients the importance of reducing the risk of traumatic injury:

- Always wear a helmet when riding a motorcycle or bicycle, rollerblading, skateboarding, horseback riding, skiing, snowboarding, or other high-risk activities.
- Buckle your seat belt whenever you are in the car, even if you have airbags. All children younger than 13 years should be restrained in the rear seat of vehicles for optimal protection (Durbin et al, 2018).
- When diving into the water, look for signs indicating water depth and observe "No Diving" signs. Jump feet first into the water to determine the depth of the water before diving head-first if you are unsure of the water's depth.

A monosynaptic reflex, such as the patellar reflex, involves two neurons: one afferent and one efferent. Polysynaptic reflexes involve many neurons in addition to the afferent and efferent limbs of the reflex arc. Reflexes are classified into three main categories: muscle stretch, or deep tendon reflexes (DTRs); superficial reflexes; and pathological reflexes.

HEALTH HISTORY

The neurological health history provides insight into the link between a client's life/lifestyle and mental status and neurological information and pathology.

CLIENT PROFILE

Diseases that are age-, sex-, and race-specific for mental status and neurological system are listed.

Age Panic disorder (adolescence to middle adulthood)
Anxiety disorder (adolescence to middle adulthood)
Phobias (mid-20s)
Schizophrenia (young adulthood)
Multiple sclerosis (MS) (20 to 40)
Myasthenia gravis (20 to 30)
Fibromyalgia (25 to 50)
Syringomyelia (30)
Huntington chorea (30 to 40)
Parkinson disease (>50)
Cerebrovascular accident (CVA) (>55)
Alzheimer disease (middle adult to older adult)

Sex

Female Panic disorder, generalized anxiety disorder, acute and posttraumatic stress disorders, mood disorders, postpartum depression, myasthenia gravis, MS, meningiomas, pseudotumor cerebri, migraine headaches, fibromyalgia

Male Cervical spine injuries, CVA, cluster headache, dyslexia

Race

Black Intracerebral hemorrhage (due to increased incidence of hypertension); CVA
Asian or Pacific Islander Intracranial hemorrhage
Hispanic Intracranial hemorrhage
White Multiple sclerosis

CHIEF COMPLAINT

Common chief complaints for mental status and neurological system are defined, and information on the characteristics of each sign or symptom is provided.

1. Headache See Chapter 11

2. Seizure A transient disturbance of cerebral function caused by an excessive discharge of neurons

Location Body parts involved
Quality General or localized
Quantity Number of minutes or seconds (per event) and frequency (weekly, monthly, every few months)
Associated Manifestations Incontinence, injury (tongue, cheeks, limbs), memory loss, cyanosis, respiratory arrest; postictal headache, somnolence, confusion, rash
Aggravating Factors Television viewing, bright lights, sleep deprivation, stress, flashing lights, hyperventilation, fever in children or infants, alcohol (use or withdrawal), hyperglycemia, hypoglycemia
Alleviating Factors Medications, time
Setting Sequence of events: warning (aura) such as headache, abdominal discomfort, euphoria or depression, visual hallucination; phases: tonic, clonic, postictal, fugue states, tick bite

Timing First occurrence, age at onset of seizures, associated trauma or presumed cause, sleeping hours, first awakening, menses

3. **Syncope** Abrupt loss of consciousness of brief duration due to decreased oxygen or glucose supply to the brain
   Quality Total versus partial loss of consciousness
   Quantity Duration of seconds, minutes, or hours; frequency (daily, monthly)
   Associated Manifestations Nausea, diaphoresis, dimmed vision, increased salivation, gastrointestinal bleeding, dyspnea, chest pain, palpitations, hemiparesis, transient focal deficits, seizures, migraine headache, associated illness (e.g., myocardial infarction, diabetes mellitus type 1)
   Aggravating Factors Injury, intense emotion, carotid occlusion, cardiovascular disorders, exertion, anemia, hypoglycemia, insulin peak, crowded space, decreased atmospheric oxygen
   Alleviating Factors Cool air, change in position, oxygen, glucose, medication, volume infusions
   Setting Hot, stuffy room; standing still for long periods, after COVID-19 infection
4. **Tremor** Repetitive, often regular, oscillatory movements of a body part caused by contraction of opposing muscle groups; usually voluntary muscles
   Location Voice, face, arms, hands, trunk
   Quality Postural, intention/essential, rest
   Aggravating Factors Fatigue, anxiety, caffeine, movement; hyperthyroidism, cerebellar disease, MS, Parkinson disease; medications (e.g., lithium, tricyclic antidepressants)
   Alleviating Factors Rest, propranolol, benzodiazepines, L-dopa, primidone, alcohol intake
   Setting Head or hands outstretched against gravity; with tasks requiring precision or fine motor grasp
   Timing Age of onset; intermittent, constant
5. **Pain** A sensation of discomfort, distress, or suffering
   Location Anatomical location (e.g., lower back, head)
   Quality Aching, stabbing, pounding, throbbing, burning, crushing, cramping
   Associated Manifestations Crying, muscular tenseness, depression, shortness of breath, diaphoresis, splinting or protective behaviors, focal deficits, limited range of motion, activity impairment, sleep disturbance, loss of bowel or bladder control
   Aggravating Factors Stress, excessive exercise, lifting, coughing or sneezing, posture changes, trauma, illness, extreme temperatures, humidity
   Alleviating Factors Medications, heat, cold, distraction, physical therapy, massage, exercise (e.g., physical therapy, stretching)
   Setting After accident or trauma
   Timing Minutes to constant; early morning, late day; daily, monthly
6. **Paresthesia** Abnormal sensations such as numbness, pricking, tingling
   Location Anatomical location (e.g., arms, hands, legs, feet)
   Quality Aching, stabbing, pins and needles, numbness
   Associated Manifestations Pain, stiffness, changes in gait, pulseless extremities, pallor, injury, ulcers, muscle wasting, traumatic injury, weakness, rash
   Aggravating Factors Activity, extreme cold, diabetes mellitus
   Alleviating Factors Medication, warmth, position changes
   Setting Tick bite, vitamin B_{12} or folate deficiency, diabetes, hypothyroidism, medications (e.g., metformin, proton pump inhibitors), injury, post COVID
7. **Disturbances in Gait** Abnormal way of moving on foot, walking, or running
   Quality Ataxic, spastic hemiplegia, hemiplegic, scissors, festinating, steppage, antalgic, apraxic, Trendelenburg
   Associated Manifestations Vertigo, visual impairments, blackouts, stroke, focal weakness, muscle wasting, abnormal movements or posture, spasticity, falling
   Aggravating Factors Fatigue, alcohol ingestion, vitamin D deficiency
   Alleviating Factors Rest, assistive devices
   Setting Level ground versus uneven terrain, CVA, neuromuscular pathology, neurosyphilis

8. Visual Changes Changes in visual acuity, visual fields, color perception, depth perception

Quality Blindness in particular field of vision; scotoma; perception of flashing, bright lights; blurriness

Associated Manifestations Vertigo, dizziness, nausea, weakness, headache

Aggravating Factors Darkness, fatigue, bright lights, reading, alcohol ingestion, medication

Alleviating Factors Rest, medications, glasses

Timing Abrupt, gradual, constant, intermittent, morning, evening

9. Vertigo The sensation of moving in space or objects moving around the person; also may be referred to as dizziness, lightheadedness

Quality Spinning sensations, dizziness, lightheadedness

Associated Manifestations Nausea, vomiting, headache, tinnitus, deafness, discharge from ear, cranial nerve palsies, hemiparesis, seizure, loss of consciousness, chest pain, palpitations, falling, rash

Aggravating Factors Motion, movement of head, changes in atmospheric pressure (weather), heights, amusement rides, anxiety, alcohol ingestion, pain, medications

Alleviating Factors Medications, lying down, maintaining a still posture

Setting Amusement rides, glassed-in elevators, rising from a seated or supine position, tick bite, after COVID-19 infection

Timing Sudden, gradual; seconds, minutes, days, months; constant, intermittent

10. Memory Disorders Change in ability to remember events or facts

Quality Recent or remote memory loss

Associated Manifestations Irritability, anxiety, agitation, confabulation, associated trauma, depression, fearfulness

Aggravating Factors Distraction, anxiety, medications, alcohol ingestion, drug abuse, unfamiliar environment, sleep deprivation, anesthesia, hypoxia, electrolyte imbalance, high altitude

Alleviating Factors Visual or auditory cues, familiarity with environment, oxygen, electrolyte replacement, narcotic reversal, detoxification

Setting Unfamiliar environment, neurosyphilis, after COVID-19 infection

Timing Nighttime, upon awakening, after general anesthesia in some older adults

11. Difficulty With Swallowing or Speech Inability to swallow food or drink, choking, or aspiration; changes in enunciation of words, volume of speech, content of speech, or comprehension of written or verbal language

Associated Manifestations Excessive drooling and saliva, paresis, dysarthria, weight loss, dehydration, irritability, depression, disease or damage to the CNS such as stroke or cerebral palsy

Aggravating Factors Fatigue, position, prolonged tracheal intubation, alcohol intake

Alleviating Factors Rest, quiet environment, thickened liquids, soft foods, varied communication tools

Setting Loud, chaotic environment; after prolonged intubation

PAST HEALTH HISTORY

The various components of the past health history are linked to mental status and neurological pathology and mental status and neurological-related information.

Medical History

Neurological Specific Headache, migraine, amyotrophic lateral sclerosis (ALS), MS, tumors, Guillain-Barré syndrome, cerebral aneurysm, arteriovenous malformations (AVM), CVA, migraines, Alzheimer disease, dementia, myasthenia gravis, congenital defects, seizures, head trauma, neuropathies, Parkinson disease, Tourette syndrome, Lyme disease

Mental health illness: anxiety disorders (generalized anxiety disorder, panic disorder, phobia, obsessive-compulsive disorder, posttraumatic stress disorder), mood disorder (major depressive disorder, dysthymia, bipolar disorder, cyclothymia), schizophrenia, postpartum depression, transient global amnesia

Non-Neurological Specific Hypertension, heart disease, cardiac surgery, peripheral vascular disease, invasive procedures, diabetes mellitus, leukemia, hypoglycemia, metabolic disorders, recent viral illness, chemotherapy, or other cancer treatment, COVID-19 infection

Surgical History Craniotomy, laminectomy, microdiscectomy, carotid endarterectomy, transsphenoidal hypophysectomy, cordotomy, lumbar puncture, epilepsy surgery, spinal fusion, ventriculoperitoneal shunt, ventriculostomy, aneurysmectomy or repair

Medications Antidepressants, antiseizure medications, narcotics, antianxiolytics, antipsychotics, mood stabilizers; medications to treat: insomnia, dementia, Parkinson disease, restless legs syndrome, narcolepsy, ADHD, nerve pain, headaches, migraines, sleep/wake disorders

Communicable Diseases COVID-19 infection, encephalitis, meningitis, poliomyelitis, HIV, dementia (neurosyphilis), botulism, cat scratch disease, rickettsial infections, toxoplasmosis, Mpox

Injuries and Accidents Closed head injury, acute subdural hematoma, chronic subdural hematoma, traumatic brain injury, concussion, postconcussion syndrome, spinal cord injury, quadriplegia, paraplegia, peripheral nerve damage

FAMILY HEALTH HISTORY

Familial neurological diseases are listed.

Congenital defects such as neural tube defects, hydrocephalus, AVM, headaches, epilepsy, Alzheimer disease, Huntington chorea, muscular dystrophies, lipid storage diseases, Gaucher disease, Niemann-Pick disease, mental health disorders

SOCIAL HISTORY

The components of the social history are linked to neurological factors and pathology.

Alcohol Use Clients suffering from chronic alcoholism may exhibit the following abnormal findings: Korsakoff psychosis, polyneuropathy, Wernicke encephalopathy, tremor

Tobacco Use Increased risk of stroke

Recreational Drug Use Neurological signs of drug use are listed in Table 20-4; seizures can occur with the ingestion of some illicit drugs

Sexual Practice HIV: headaches, memory and concentration impairment, mood disorders, movement disorders, seizure, CVA; neurosyphilis: impotence secondary to neuropathies, lower motor neuron lesions; Mpox: encephalitis, seizures

Travel History Tickborne illnesses in various locations in the United States (Lyme disease, Rocky Mountain spotted fever, anaplasmosis, babesia, ehrlichiosis, rickettsia, tularemia, Colorado tick fever, Heartland and Bourbon virus diseases, Powassan virus disease), malaria (many areas in Africa, India and other Asian countries, South America), Chagas disease (rural areas of Mexico, Central America, and South America)

Work Environment Exposure to continuous loud noise, performing repetitive-motion tasks, toxic chemical exposure (e.g., carbon dioxide, insecticides)

Home Environment Exposure to toxic substances (e.g., carbon monoxide, carbon dioxide, insecticides), lead paint

Hobbies and Leisure Activities Use of protective equipment; participation in contact sports or high-risk activities such as football, soccer, hockey, boxing, race car driving, motorcycling; hobbies involving repetitive motion (needlework), hiking/camping (at risk for Lyme disease and other tickborne illnesses)

Stress Headaches, migraines, fibromyalgia flares, and MS can be exacerbated by stress

Military Service Exposure to explosions can lead to traumatic brain injury

Ethnic Background

Jewish Tay-Sachs disease

Northern European MS

HEALTH MAINTENANCE ACTIVITIES

This information provides a bridge between health maintenance activities and mental status and neurological function.

Sleep Narcolepsy, insomnia

Diet Vitamin deficiencies can lead to neurological symptoms/conditions

Exercise Increases muscle strength, increases coordination

Use of Safety Devices Helmet, seat belt, eye shields, carbon monoxide detectors

Health Checkups Developmental milestones; neurological testing (e.g., electroencephalogram [EEG], electromyogram [EMG], sleep study, CT scan, MRI, lumbar puncture)

Table 20-4 Neurological Signs of Drug Ingestion

Examination Parameter	Hallucinogens	Cannabis (Marijuana)	Narcotics	Sedative-Hypnotics	CNS Stimulants
Pupils	Dilated React to light	Normal	Pinpoint Fixed	Normal	Dilated React to light
Deep tendon reflexes	Hyperactive	Normal	Normal	Hypoactive	Hyperactive
Speech	Normal	Often normal	Normal or dulled	Slurred	N/A
Coordination	Normal	Normal	Normal or unsteady	Ataxia	N/A
Sensorium	Often clear	Usually clear	Dulled	Confusion	May be confused
Sensory perception	Distorted	Distorted	Dulled	Dulled	Heightened
Memory	Unchanged	Transient loss	Unchanged	Impaired	Unchanged
Hallucinations	Any type	Rare	Rare	N/A	N/A
Delusions	Variable	Paranoid	N/A	N/A	Paranoid

CNS = central nervous system, N/A = not applicable.

NURSING CHECKLIST

General Approach to Mental Status and Neurological System Examination

1. Observe Standard Precautions and don personal protective equipment (PPE) such as gloves, gown, face shield, goggles, N-95 respirator mask or face mask if the client's status warrants these protective measures.
2. Greet the client and explain the examination techniques that you will be using.
3. Maintain a quiet, unhurried, self-confident demeanor to help relieve any feelings of anxiety or discomfort and to help the client relax during the examination.
4. Provide a warm, quiet, and well-lit environment.
5. After the mental status assessment, instruct the client to remove clothes, and provide an examination gown for the client to put on. Return to the room once the client is ready.
6. Begin the examination with the client in a comfortable, upright sitting position; or, for the client on bedrest, position the client comfortably, preferably with the head of the bed elevated, or flat, whichever is tolerated best or is within activity orders for the client.

Assessment in Brief

Mental Status and Neurological System Examination

Mental Status

- Physical appearance and behavior
  - Posture and movements
  - Dress, grooming, and personal hygiene
  - Facial expression
  - Affect
- Communication
- Level of consciousness
- Cognitive abilities and mentation
  - Attention
  - Memory
  - Judgment
  - Insight
  - Spatial perception
  - Calculation
  - Abstract reasoning
  - Thought process and content
  - Suicidal ideation

Motor System

- Muscle size
- Muscle tone
- Muscle strength
- Involuntary movements
- Pronator drift

Reflexes

- Deep tendon reflexes
  - Brachioradialis
  - Biceps
  - Triceps
  - Patellar
  - Achilles
- Superficial reflexes
  - Abdominal
  - Plantar
  - Anal
  - Cremasteric
  - Bulbocavernosus
- Pathological reflexes
  - Glabellar
  - Clonus
  - Babinski

Sensory

- Exteroceptive sensation
  - Light touch
  - Superficial pain
  - Temperature
- Proprioceptive sensation
  - Motion and position
  - Vibration sense
- Cortical sensation
  - Stereognosis
  - Graphesthesia
  - Two-point discrimination
  - Extinction

Cerebellar Function

- Coordination
- Station
- Gait

Advanced Techniques

- Doll's eyes phenomenon
- Romberg test
- Meningeal irritation
  - Nuchal rigidity
  - Kernig sign
  - Brudzinski sign
- Assessing for diabetic peripheral neuropathy

Cranial Nerves

- Olfactory nerve (CN I)
- Optic nerve (CN II)
  - Visual acuity
  - Visual fields
  - Funduscopic examination
- Oculomotor nerve (CN III)
  - Cardinal fields of gaze
  - Eyelid elevation
  - Pupil reactions
- Trochlear nerve (CN IV)
  - Cardinal fields of gaze
- Trigeminal nerve (CN V)
  - Motor component
  - Sensory component
- Abducens nerve (CN VI)
  - Cardinal fields of gaze
- Facial nerve (CN VII)
  - Motor component
  - Sensory component
- Acoustic nerve (CN VIII)
  - Cochlear division
    - Hearing
    - Weber test
    - Rinne test
  - Vestibular division
- Glossopharyngeal nerve (CN IX)
- Vagus nerve (CN X)
- Spinal accessory nerve (CN XI)
- Hypoglossal nerve (CN XII)

Equipment

- Appropriate PPE
- Pencil and paper
- Cotton wisp
- Cotton-tipped swab
- Penlight
- Tongue blade

- Tuning fork: 128 Hz or 256 Hz
- Reflex hammer
- Sterile needle or a sterile safety pin
- Familiar small objects (coins, key, paper clip)
- Vials containing odorous materials (coffee, orange extract, vinegar)
- Vials containing hot and cold water
- Vials with solutions for tasting: quinine (bitter), glucose solution (sweet), lemon or vinegar (sour), saline (salty)
- Snellen chart or Rosenbaum pocket screener
- Pupil gauge in millimeters
- Single-fiber monofilament

Examination of the Neurological System

A complete neurological examination includes an assessment of mental status, sensation, cranial nerves, motor function, cerebellar function, and reflexes. For clients with minor or intermittent symptoms, a rapid screening neurological examination may be used, as outlined in Table 20-5.

Mental Status

Much of the mental status assessment should be conducted during the interview, with the client comfortably positioned facing you. Mental status may also be assessed throughout the neurological examination. Assess physical appearance and behavior, communication, level of consciousness, cognitive abilities, and mentation while conversing with the client. The Mini-Cog is a screening tool that assesses cognition in older adults. This is discussed in Chapter 26.

Physical Appearance and Behavior

Posture and Movements

E 1. Note if the client's posture is relaxed, slumped, or stiff.
2. Observe the client's movements for control and symmetry.
3. Observe the client's gait (see Chapter 19).

N **The client should appear relaxed. The client should exhibit an erect posture, a smooth gait, and symmetrical body movements.**

A Restlessness, tenseness, and pacing can be abnormal.

P Restlessness, tenseness, and pacing may be signs of anxiety or metabolic disorders, which should alert you to further investigate these problems.

A Slumped posture, slow gait, poor eye contact, blank facies, and slow responses can be abnormal findings.

P Slumped posture, slow gait, poor eye contact, blank facies, and slow responses may be signs of depression.

A Stooped, flexed, or rigid posture; drooping neck; deformities of the spine; and tics are abnormal findings.

P Clients with kyphosis, scoliosis, Parkinson disease, cerebral palsy, osteoporosis, schizophrenia, muscular atrophy, myasthenia gravis, or stroke may exhibit these signs.

> **NURSING TIP**
>
> **Focusing on the Mental Status Assessment**
>
> In most cases, the information obtained during the health history is sufficient to assess mental status. A more specific mental status assessment should be performed if the following are noted:
>
> - Known brain lesion (e.g., stroke, tumors, trauma)
> - Suspected brain lesion (e.g., new seizures, headaches, behavioral changes)
> - Memory deficits
> - Confusion
> - Vague behavioral complaints (by significant others if client is unaware of or denies behavioral changes)
> - Aphasia
> - Irritability
> - Emotional lability/depression

Dress, Grooming, and Personal Hygiene

E 1. Note the appearance of the client's clothing, specifically:
a. Cleanliness
b. Condition
c. Age appropriateness
d. Weather appropriateness
e. Appropriateness for the client's socioeconomic group

Table 20-5 Neurological Screening Examination

Examination Parameter	Examination Skill	Comments
Mental status	Note general appearance, affect, speech content, memory, logic, judgment, and speech patterns during the history. Perform Glasgow Coma Scale (GCS) with motor examination component and pupil examination.	If any abnormalities or inconsistencies are evident, perform full mental status assessment. If GCS < 15, perform full assessment of mental status and consciousness. If motor examination is abnormal or asymmetrical, perform complete motor and sensory examinations.
Sensation	Assess pain and vibration in the hands and feet, light touch on the limbs.	If deficits are identified, perform a complete sensory assessment.
Cranial nerves	Assess CN II, III, IV, VI: visual acuity, gross visual fields, funduscopic examination, pupillary reactions, and extraocular movements. Assess CN VII, VIII, IX, X, XII: facial expression, gross hearing, voice, and tongue.	If any abnormalities exist, perform complete assessment of all 12 cranial nerves.
Motor system	Muscle tone and strength; abnormal movements; hand grasp.	If deficits are noted, perform a complete motor system examination.
Cerebellar function	Observe the client's: 1. Gait on arrival. 2. Ability to: a. Walk heel to toe b. Walk on toes c. Walk on heels d. Hop in place e. Perform shallow knee bends 3. Check Romberg test. 4. Finger to nose test. 5. Fine repetitive movements with hands.	If any abnormalities exist, perform complete cerebellar examination.
Reflexes	Assess the deep tendon reflexes and the plantar reflex.	If an abnormal response is elicited, perform a complete reflex assessment.

2. Observe the client's personal grooming (hair, skin, nails, teeth) for:
   a. Adequacy
   b. Symmetry
   c. Odor

N **The client should be clean and well-groomed and should wear clothing appropriate for age, weather, and socioeconomic status.**

A Poor personal hygiene, such as uncombed hair, body odor, or unkempt clothing, is abnormal.

P Poor personal hygiene and unkempt appearance may be indications of depression, schizophrenia, or dementia.

A Excessive, meticulous care and attention to clothing and grooming can be abnormal behaviors.

> **NURSING TIP**
> **Client History and Mental Status Assessment**
>
> 1. Begin the assessment as the client approaches you. Observe gait, posture, mode of dress, involuntary movements, voice, and other features that will help guide and refine your assessment priorities. Dress and grooming can be influenced by the client's economic status, age, home situation, and ethnic background. Information obtained during the health history will assist in determining appropriate dress and grooming for an individual client. It is helpful to directly ask the client about grooming routines and clothing choices if there is a question as to appropriateness.
> 2. The history should be comprehensive because neurological disorders can affect all body systems.
> 3. The history should be age-sensitive:
>   a. Utilize other family members when appropriate.
>   b. Acknowledge adolescents' ability to speak for themselves.
>   c. Do not make assumptions regarding older adult clients' ability to relate their own health histories.
> 4. Allow the client to remain clothed during the history and mental status assessment.
> 5. Consider language and cultural norms when obtaining the history and performing the mental status assessment.

P Excessive, meticulous care and attention to clothing and grooming may indicate obsessive-compulsive behavior.

A Obvious one-sided differences in grooming and dressing or the use of only one side of the body are abnormal.

P Stroke in the parietal lobe may cause the client to be aware of only one side of the body, which is termed one-sided neglect.

Facial Expression

E Observe for appropriateness of, variations in, and symmetry of facial expressions.

N **Facial expressions should be appropriate to the content of the conversation and should be symmetrical.**

A Extreme, inappropriate, or unchanging facial expressions or asymmetrical facial movements are abnormal.

P Abnormal facial expressions can occur in anxiety and depression. An unchanging facial expression can occur in a client with Parkinson disease. An unchanging facial expression may also indicate a lesion in the facial nerve (CN VII).

Affect

E
1. Observe the client's interaction with you, paying particular attention to both verbal and nonverbal behaviors.
2. Note if the client's affect appears labile, blunted, or flat.
3. Note the variations in the client's effect with a variety of topics.
4. Note any extreme emotional responses during the interview.

N **The appropriateness and degree of affect should vary with the topics and the client's cultural norms and be reasonable or eurhythmic (normal).**

A Blunted affect, manifested by the client shuffling into the examination room, slumping into a chair, moving slowly, and not making eye contact, is abnormal.

P A blunted effect may indicate depression.

A Unresponsive, inappropriate affect is abnormal.

P A flat, unresponsive affect may indicate depression or schizophrenia.

A Anger, hostility, and paranoia are abnormal responses in most clinical situations.

P Anger, hostility, and paranoia may be the responses of a paranoid schizophrenic individual.

A Euphoric, dramatic, disruptive, irrational, or elated behaviors are abnormal in most clinical situations.

P A manic-depressive client might display euphoria, dramatic, disruptive, irrational, or elated behaviors in the manic phase.

Communication

Communication skills should be assessed throughout the entire interview and physical examination.

E
1. Note voice quality, which includes voice volume and pitch.
2. Assess articulation, fluency, and rate of speech by engaging the client in normal conversation. Ask the client to repeat words and sentences after you or to name objects you point out.

3. Note the client's ability to carry out requests during the assessment, such as pointing to objects within the room as requested. Ask questions that require "yes" and "no" responses.
4. Write simple commands for the client to read and perform, for example, "point to your nose" or "tap your right foot." Reading ability may be influenced by the client's educational level or visual impairment.
5. Ask the client to write their name, birthday, a sentence the client composes, or a sentence that you dictate. Note the client's spelling, grammatical accuracy, and logical thought process.

N **The client should be able to produce spontaneous, coherent speech. The speech should have an effortless flow with normal inflections, volume, pitch, articulation, rate, and rhythm. The content of the message should make sense. Comprehension of language should be intact. The client's ability to read and write should match the client's educational level. Nonnative speakers may exhibit some hesitancy or inaccuracy in written and spoken language.**

A **Aphasia**, an impairment of language functioning, is abnormal.

P Aphasias are classified by the anatomy involved, behavioral speech manifestations, fluency of speech (fluent: rhythm, grammar, and articulation are normal; nonfluent: speech production is limited and speech is poorly articulated), and comprehension (receptive) versus expression (expressive) deficits. Other categories include amnesic, the inability to recall specific types of words; and central, a deficit in the coordination among the speech areas. See Table 20-6 for a summary of the characteristics and pathophysiology of specific aphasias. Most clients with aphasia will have some components of several aphasia classifications (e.g., a client with transcortical motor aphasia will usually have some degree of transcortical sensory aphasia as well).

A **Dysarthria**, a disturbance in muscular control of speech, is abnormal.

P Dysarthria is due to ischemia affecting motor nuclei of CN X and CN XII; defects in the premotor or motor cortex that provide motor input for the face, throat, and mouth; or cerebellar disease.

A **Dysphonia**, difficulty making laryngeal sounds, is abnormal and can progress to **aphonia** (total loss of voice).

P Dysphonia is usually caused by lesions of CN X or swelling and inflammation of the larynx. Gastroesophageal reflux can also cause dysphonia.

A **Apraxia**, the inability to convert the intended speech into the motor act of speech, is abnormal.

P Apraxia is due to dysfunction in the precentral gyrus of the frontal lobe.

A **Agraphia**, the loss of the ability to write, is abnormal.

P Agraphia is caused by lesions of Broca and Wernicke areas in the dominant side of the brain.

A **Alexia**, the inability to grasp the meaning of written words and sentences (word blindness), is abnormal.

P Alexia is usually due to a lesion of the angular gyrus and the occipital lobe.

NURSING TIP
Handedness

Note the dominant side/hand before conducting language testing. Handedness and cerebral dominance for language are closely allied. Clients with dominant-hemisphere lesions will frequently show communication abnormalities; for example, aphasia in the right-handed individual almost always indicates left-hemisphere disease.

NURSING TIP
The Client With Dysphonia

Clients with signs of dysphonia (impaired laryngeal speech) are at high risk for dysphagia (difficulty with swallowing) and therefore aspiration. A thorough assessment of swallowing is warranted before the client tries to eat unassisted.

Table 20-6 Classification of Aphasias

Aphasia	Pathophysiology	Expression	Characteristics
Broca aphasia	Motor cortex lesion in Broca area	Expressive Nonfluent	Speech slow and hesitant, the client has difficulty in selecting and organizing words. Naming, word and phrase repetition, and writing impaired. Subtle defects in comprehension.
Wernicke aphasia	Left hemisphere lesion in Wernicke area	Receptive Fluent	Auditory comprehension impaired, as is content of speech. Client unaware of deficits. Naming severely impaired.
Anomic aphasia	Left hemisphere lesion in Wernicke area	Amnesic Fluent	Client unable to name objects or places. Comprehension and repetition of words and phrases intact.
Conduction aphasia	Lesion in the arcuate fasciculus, which connects and transports messages between Broca and Wernicke areas	Central Fluent	Client has difficulty repeating words, substitutes incorrect sounds for another sound (e.g., *ping for ring*).
Global aphasia	Lesions in the frontal-temporal area	Mixed Fluent	Both oral and written comprehension severely impaired; naming, repetition of words and phrases, ability to write impaired.
Transcortical sensory aphasia	Lesion in the periphery of Broca and Wernicke areas (watershed zone)	Fluent	Impairment in comprehension, naming, and writing. Word and phrase repetition intact.
Transcortical motor aphasia	Lesion anterior, superior, or lateral to Broca area	Nonfluent	Comprehension intact. Naming and ability to write impaired. Word and phrase repetition intact.

Level of Consciousness (LOC)

Consciousness is the level of awareness of the self and the environment. Conscious behavior requires arousal, or wakefulness, and awareness, or cognition and affect. Arousal is controlled by the reticular activating system (RAS). The RAS activates the cortex after receiving stimuli from the somatic and special sensory pathways. Awareness is a higher-level function of the cerebral cortex, which interprets incoming sensory stimuli. Aspects of awareness at a higher level include judgment and thinking, which are generally evaluated as part of the cognitive assessment. Orientation is awareness of self and environment.

E

1. Observe the client's eyes when entering the room (environmental stimuli). Note whether the client's eyes are open or whether they open when you enter the room (before any verbalization). Note the client's response to any general environmental stimuli, such as noises or lights.
2. If the client's eyes are closed, call out the client's name (verbal stimuli). Observe whether the client's eyes are open, whether the client responds verbally and appropriately, and whether verbal commands are followed.
3. If the client does not respond to verbal stimuli, lightly touch the client's hand or gently shake the client awake.

> **NURSING TIP**
> **The Confused Client**
> The confused client should be thoroughly assessed for aphasia. A missed diagnosis because of "confusion" can be fatal if aphasia is present and due to a subdural hematoma. Check for other signs associated with a subdural hematoma, including headache, slow cerebration, decreasing level of consciousness, and ipsilateral pupil dilation with a sluggish response to light.

NURSING TIP

FAST and BE FAST Acronyms

The American Stroke Association recommends learning and sharing the warning signs of stroke to identify and reduce or reverse long-term complications. The FAST and BE FAST acronyms are used:

B = **Balance:** Is there a sudden loss or change in balance or coordination?

E = **Eyes:** Is there a sudden change or loss in vision in one or both eyes without pain? double vision?

F = **Face Drooping**: Does one side of the face droop, or is it numb? Ask the person to smile. Is the person's smile uneven?

A = **Arm Weakness**: Is one arm weak or numb? Ask the person to raise both arms. Does one arm drift downward?

S = **Speech Difficulty**: Is speech slurred? Or does the person have difficulty speaking/forming words?

T = **Time to call 911:** If tissue plasminogen activator (tPA) can be administered within 3 hours (FDA approved), it can restore blood flow to brain areas affected by a stroke and limit the risk of functional impairment.

Other symptoms to watch for include numbness of face/arm/leg, confusion, altered gait, vision changes, and severe headache.

*Information summarized from the following sources: National Institute of Neurological Disorders and Stroke (n.d.). *Tissue Plasminogen Activator for Acute Ischemic Stroke (Alteplase, Activase®).* NINDS Contributions to Approved Therapies. *https://www.ninds.nih.gov/about-ninds/impact/ninds-contributions-approved-therapies/tissue-plasminogen-activator-acute-ischemic-stroke-alteplase-activaser* When administered quickly after stroke, of damage and functional impairment; American Stroke Association. (2025). *Stroke Symptoms.* About Stroke. *https://www.stroke.org/en/about-stroke/stroke-symptoms;* Know the signs of stroke: BE FAST. *https://www.dukehealth.org/blog/know-signs-of-stroke-be-fast*

Risk Factors

Cerebrovascular Accident (CVA)—Stroke

- Age >55
- Male
- Black
- Hypertension
- Diabetes mellitus
- Cocaine use
- Cigarette smoking
- Hyperlipidemia
- Carotid artery disease
- Peripheral artery disease
- Atherosclerosis
- Atrial fibrillation and flutter
- History of cerebral aneurysm
- Family history of stroke
- Sickle cell disease
- Severe anemia
- IV drug abuse
- Alcohol abuse
- Physical inactivity
- Obesity
- Oral contraceptive use, especially in women over age 35 who smoke and have hypertension
- Patent foramen ovale
- Previous stroke, TIA (transient ischemic attack)
- Previous myocardial infarction

4. If the client is not responding to environmental, verbal, or light touch stimuli, proceed to the application of a painful stimulus.
   a. Apply pressure with a pen to the nailbed of each extremity, or
   b. Firmly pinch the trapezius muscle, or
   c. Apply pressure to the supraorbital ridge or the manubrium.
5. Observe the client's reaction to the painful stimulus. Note whether the client's eyes are open.
6. Observe whether the client can localize the painful stimulus by reaching for the area being stimulated. The strength of the client's extremities can be assessed by the strength and distance of movement during the attempt to reach the painful stimulus. Note any abnormal motor responses.
7. Compare the motor responses and strength of the responses of the right versus left sides of the client.
8. Note whether the client responds verbally to the painful stimulus.
9. Assess orientation by asking questions related to person, place, and time:
   a. Person: name of the client, name of spouse or significant other
   b. Place: where the client is now (what town, what state), where the client lives
   c. Time: the time of day, month, year, season
10. Determine the **Glasgow Coma Scale** (GCS) (Fig. 20-9) score, an international method for grading neurological responses of the injured or severely ill client. It is monitored in clients who have

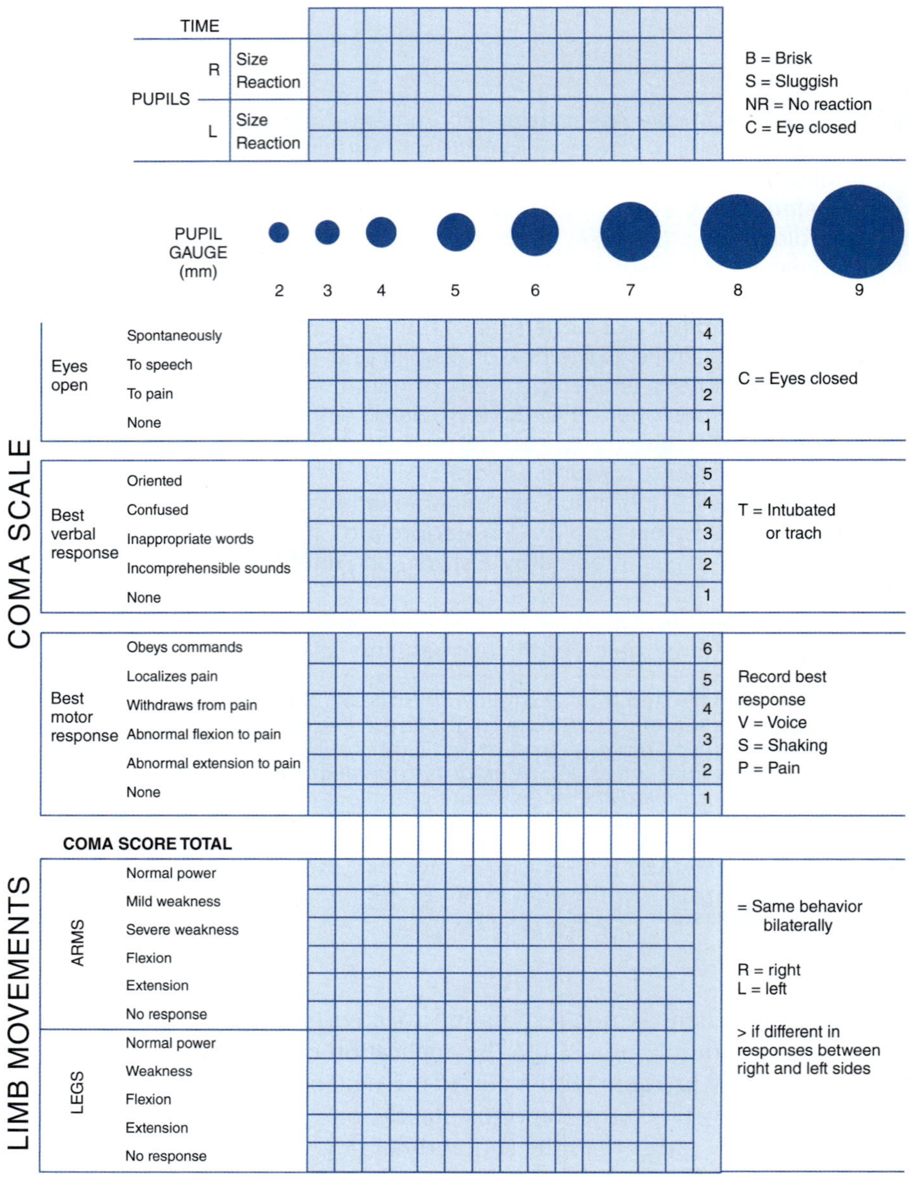

Figure 20-9 Neurological flow sheet, including Glasgow Coma Scale.

> ## NURSING TIP
> ### Application of Painful Stimuli
> 1. Application of painful stimuli is extremely upsetting to family members and therefore should not be performed in their presence or without a comprehensive explanation.
> 2. Apply only the amount of pressure needed to elicit a response.
> 3. If painful stimuli must be repeated, alternate sites when possible.
> 4. Pain applied centrally (e.g., trapezius muscle squeeze) that results in a response always indicates involvement of the cerebrum. Pain applied to an extremity (e.g., pen pressure on a nailbed) may elicit a reflex response or cerebral response, or both. Great care is needed when interpreting the significance of the response to pain from a client in a profound coma.

the potential for rapid deterioration in their level of consciousness. The GCS assesses three parameters of consciousness: eye opening (1–4 points), verbal response (1–5 points), and motor response (1–6 points). Most often, the Glasgow Coma Scale (GCS) is included in a neurological observation sheet, which also includes vital signs, motor movement and strength, and pupillary size and reactions, to give a more in-depth evaluation of the client's neurological status.

N **The client's best response to each of these categories (eye movement, verbal response, motor response) is recorded. The sum of the three categories is the total GCS score. The highest score of responsiveness is 15, and the lowest is 3. A score of 15 indicates a fully alert, oriented individual.**

A **P** See Table 20-7.

TABLE 20-7 Levels of Consciousness: Abnormalities and Pathophysiology

LOC	GCS	Response to Stimuli	Pupil Response	Pathophysiology	Prognosis
Confusion	14	Spontaneous but may be inappropriate Memory faulty Reflexes intact	Normal	Metabolic derangements Diffuse brain dysfunction	Good chance of recovery Must treat primary cause
Lethargy	13–14	Requires stimulus to respond (verbal, touch) Reflexes intact	Normal to unequal	Metabolic derangements Medications Increased ICP	Good chance of recovery Must treat primary cause
Stupor	12–13	Requires vigorous, continuous stimuli to respond Reflexes intact	Normal, unequal, or sluggish	Metabolic derangements Medications Increased ICP	Good chance of recovery Must treat primary cause
Permanent vegetative state	8–10	Responds to pain No cognitive response Reflexes abnormal	Normal	Anoxic ischemic insults	Irreversible
Locked-in syndrome	6	Awake and aware	Normal	Lesion in ventral pons All four extremities and lower cranial nerves paralyzed Myasthenia gravis Acute polyneuritis	Poor prognosis
Coma	3–6	Abnormal Varied response to pain Reflexes abnormal or absent	Abnormal Dilated or pinpoint	Anoxia Traumatic injury Space-occupying lesion Cerebral edema	Prognosis dependent on length of time in coma
Brain death	3	No response Reflexes abnormal or absent	Abnormal Dilated or pinpoint	Anoxia Structural damage	Irreversible

LOC = level of consciousness; GCS = Glasgow Coma Scale; ICP = intracranial pressure.

Cognitive Abilities and Mentation

Assessment of cognitive function includes testing for attention, memory, judgment, insight, spatial perception, calculation, abstraction, thought processes, and thought content. You will need:

- Preprinted lists of objects, phrases, and numbers for client recall and explanation
- Answers to long-term memory questions to accurately assess recall
- Alternate tests prepared for clients with language barriers, aphasia, deafness, blindness, and other conditions

Attention

E 1. Pronounce a list of numbers slowly (approximately 1 second apart), starting with a list of two numbers and progressing to a series of five or six numbers. For example, 2, 5; then 3, 7, 8; then 1, 9, 4, 3; and 1, 5, 4, 9, 0.

2. Ask the client to repeat the numbers in the correct order, both forward and backward.
3. Give the client a different series of the same number of digits if the client is unable to repeat the first series correctly. Stop after two misses of any length series.
4. Serial 7s is another method of assessing attention and concentration. Instruct the client to begin with the number 100 and to count backward by subtracting 7 each time: 100, 93, 86, 79, 72, 65, etc.
5. The client may also try serial 3s (counting backward from 100 by 3s) if unable to perform serial 7s.

N **The client should be able to correctly repeat the series of numbers up to a series of five numbers. The client should be able to recite serial 7s or serial 3s accurately to at least the 40s or 50s from 100 within 1 minute.**

A If the client has a short attention span, the client will not be able to repeat the numbers in sequence or perform serial 7s or 3s.

P Dementia, neurological injury or disease, and mental disabilities may impair attention.

P Some people who had a COVID-19 infection may report a shortened attention span and difficulty concentrating.

NURSING TIP

Cognitive Mental Status Screening

The Mini-Mental State Examination (MMSE) and the Montreal Cognitive Assessment (MoCA) are widely used tools for assessing cognitive mental status, detecting impairment following the course of an illness, and monitoring response to treatment. Both tools are useful in screening for the cognitive deficits seen in syndromes of dementia and delirium, but the MoCA is a better tool for identifying mild cognitive impairment (Pinto et al, 2019). The MMSE is the most frequently utilized short-screening tool for measuring clinical impairment in research and clinical settings (Arevalo-Rodriguez et al, 2021).

The MMSE contains 11 cognitive tasks and takes 10 to 15 minutes to administer. Time orientation, place orientation, immediate recall, short-term memory recall, serial 7s, reading, writing, drawing, and verbal/motor comprehension compose the bulk of the examination. The maximum score on the MMSE is 30, and scores greater than 24 are considered within the normal range. Clients who have scores lower than 24 should receive a more detailed neuropsychological evaluation.

The MMSE is a copyrighted screening tool that can be purchased from Psychological Assessment Resources, Inc. at: 16204 North Florida Avenue, Lutz, Florida 33549; phone: 1-800-331-8378; *www.parinc.com*

Memory

E
1. Assess immediate recall in conjunction with an attention span as discussed previously.
2. Give a list of three items that the client is to remember and repeat in 5 minutes. Have the client repeat the items to check initial understanding. During the 5 minutes, carry on a conversation as usual. Ask the client to repeat the items after the 5-minute time has elapsed.
3. If the client is unable to remember one or more of the objects, show a list containing the objects along with others, and check recognition.
4. Record the number of objects remembered over the number of objects given.
5. Long-term memory is memory that is retained for at least 24 hours. Commonly asked questions for testing long-term memory include the name of the partner, partner's birthday, mother's maiden name, name of the president, or client's birthday.

N **The client should be able to correctly respond to questions and identify all the objects as requested.**

A Memory loss is abnormal.

P Memory loss may be caused by pathologies such as neurological system infection, trauma, stroke, tumors, Alzheimer disease, seizure disorders, alcohol, and drug toxicity. Memory centers are located in the temporal lobe and the hippocampus. Damage to these areas, in the form of hemorrhage, ischemia, compression, or herniation, will cause memory impairment.

P Some people who had a COVID-19 infection may report memory difficulties. This is often referred to as "COVID brain fog." Ongoing research into long-term effects of COVID continues and no known etiology explains the cognitive changes.

Judgment

E
1. During the interview, assess whether the client is responding appropriately to social, family, and work situations that are discussed.

2. Note whether the client's decisions are based on sound reasoning and decision making.
3. Present hypothetical situations and ask the client to make decisions as to what their responses would be. For example: "What would you do if you saw a house burning?" or "What would you do if someone was choking?"
4. Interview the client's family or directly observe the client to assess judgment more carefully.

N **The client should be able to evaluate and act appropriately in situations requiring judgment.**

A Impaired judgment, the inability to act appropriately in situations, is abnormal.

P Frontal lobe damage, dementia, psychotic states, and mental disability may cause the client to exhibit a lack of appropriate judgment.

Insight

Insight is the ability to realistically understand oneself.

E 1. Ask the client to describe personal health status, reason for seeking health care, symptoms, current life situation, and general coping behaviors.
2. If the client describes symptoms, ask what life was like before the appearance of the symptoms, what life changes the illness has introduced, and whether the client feels a need for help.
3. Ask the client to draw a self-portrait; note the emphasis put on specific body parts, the client's ability to reproduce figures on paper, and the representation of any part of the self-portrait. Note the facial features and the feelings portrayed by the picture.

N **The client should demonstrate a realistic awareness and understanding of self.**

A Unrealistic perceptions of self are abnormal.

P Lack of insight may occur in the euphoric stages of bipolar affective disorders, endogenous anxiety states, or depressed states.

Spatial Perception

Spatial perception is the ability to recognize the relationships of objects in space.

E 1. Ask the client to copy figures that you have previously drawn, such as a circle, triangle, square, cross, and a three-dimensional cube.
2. Ask the client to draw the face of a clock, including the numbers around the dial.
3. Ask the client to identify a familiar sound while keeping the eyes closed, for example, a closing door, running water, or a finger snap.
4. Have the client identify right from left body parts.

N **The client should be able to draw the objects without difficulty and as closely as possible to the original drawing, and to identify familiar sounds and left and right body parts.**

A **Agnosia**, the inability to recognize the form and nature of objects or persons, is abnormal. It may be visual, auditory, or somatosensory. For example, the client may be unable to name or recognize objects, faces, or familiar objects by touch, or to identify the meaning of nonverbal sounds.

P Lesions in the nondominant parietal lobe impair the client's ability to appreciate self in relation to the environment and to conceive

NURSING TIP

Traumatic Brain Injury

The public health issue of traumatic brain injury (TBI) has grown in awareness, recognition, reporting, and surveillance; TBI is caused by a sudden insult to the brain from an external force, which may create temporary or permanent impairment (Capizzi et al, 2020). The injury can be a penetrating piercing of the skull and brain or a closed head injury in which the skull and brain remain intact. The person having the TBI may or may not lose consciousness. The most common causes of TBI are unintentional and include falls, being struck by an object, and motor vehicle crashes; other causes are assault, no mechanism specified, and intentional self-harm (Capizzi et al, 2020), The severity of the TBI can range from mild to severe and can even lead to death. Prompt identification and treatment can prevent serious long-term disability and death. Symptoms of TBI include headache, nausea, vomiting, confusion, fatigue, dizziness, lightheadedness, blurred vision, diplopia, tinnitus, photophobia, phonophobia, fatigue, memory deficits, impaired attention and concentration, change in sleep patterns, altered school or work performance, and behavioral or mood changes. These symptoms can last days, weeks, or months after the initial insult and are referred to as postconcussive syndrome. The postconcussive syndrome necessitates periodic neurological evaluation.

The effects of TBI are warranting changes in approaches to sports at all levels of play. Professional sports teams, as well as high school and college-level sports teams, have instituted programs to establish baseline neurological function preseason, midseason, and postseason. Research demonstrates that successive concussions, especially in a relatively short period, can lead to permanent neurological abnormalities that can affect quality of life. Many professional organizations publish concussion evaluation tools that are easily administered on the playing field. These tools include assessments of orientation, concentration, and memory. The CDC publishes concussion guidelines, screening/symptom tools, and other provider resources (*https://www.cdc.gov/heads-up/?CDC_AAref_Val=https://cdc.gov/headsup/providerd/index.html*).

Another focus on TBI comes from the U.S. military. Soldiers stationed in conflict areas are susceptible to blast explosions, such as from improvised explosive devices. Early diagnosis and treatment are essential for returning soldiers as they reintegrate into American society. Left untreated, increased cases of depression and posttraumatic stress disorder can result.

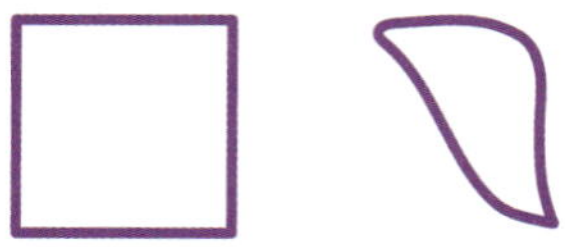

Figure 20-10 Constructional apraxia.

three-dimensional objects. Lesions in the occipital lobe will cause visual agnosia, and temporal lesions will cause auditory agnosia.

A Apraxia, the inability to perform purposeful movements despite the preservation of motor ability and sensation, is abnormal. **Constructional apraxia** is the inability to reproduce figures on paper (Fig. 20-10).

P Apraxia is usually associated with lesions of the precentral gyrus of the frontal lobe.

Calculation

The client's ability to perform serial 7s was discussed in the section on attention and is also an assessment of calculation.

E
1. Ask the client to add 3 to 100, then 3 to that number, until numbers greater than 150 are reached.
2. Note the amount of time needed for the calculations and any difficulty with them.

N **The client should be able to calculate the correct numbers upon subtraction or addition within educational abilities and with fewer than four errors in less than 1½ minutes.**

A **Dyscalculia**, the inability to perform calculations, is abnormal. Significant dyscalculia often accompanies aphasia. If dyscalculia is noted, a reassessment of speech and language ability should be performed.

P Dyscalculia may be caused by depression or anxiety, dementia, or mental disabilities. The most common cause of dyscalculia is a focal lesion in the dominant parietal lobe; however, calculation deficits have also been ascribed to focal lesions in the frontal, temporal, and occipital lobes.

Abstract Reasoning

E 1. Ask the client to describe the meaning of a familiar fable, proverb, or metaphor. Use examples that are meaningful within the context of the client's culture and language. Some examples from American culture are:
   a. The squeaky wheel gets the grease.
   b. A rolling stone gathers no moss.
   c. A stitch in time saves nine.
   d. People who live in glass houses shouldn't throw stones.
   e. Don't count your chickens before they hatch.
2. Note the degree of concreteness versus abstraction in the answers.

N **Clients should be able to give abstract meanings of proverbs, fables, or metaphors within their cultural understanding.**

A Conceptual concreteness—the inability to describe in abstractions, to generalize from specifics, and to apply general principles—is abnormal.

P Alterations of cognitive processes causing concreteness in thought may occur in clients with dementia, frontal tumors, or schizophrenia. Concreteness in thought processes may also indicate low intelligence.

Thought Process and Content

E 1. Observe the client's pattern of thought for relevance, consistency, coherence, logic, and organization.
2. Listen throughout the interview for flaws in the content of the conversation.

N **Thought processes should be logical, coherent, and goal oriented. Thought content should be based on reality.**

A Unrealistic, illogical thought processes and interruptions of the thinking processes, such as blocking, are abnormal. Blocking is demonstrated when an extended pause occurs during a sentence due to a repressed or painful subject matter. Sometimes, the thoughts following are unrelated to what the client was discussing.

P Abnormal thought processes are often due to schizophrenia.

A Flight of ideas, demonstrated when the client changes from subject to subject within a sentence, is abnormal. This is frequently due to distractions or word associations with a resultant lack of sense of purpose in the conversation.

P Clients experiencing manic episodes of bipolar affective disorder often demonstrate a flight of ideas.

A **Confabulation**, the making up of answers unrelated to facts, is abnormal.

P Confabulation is often related to aging, memory loss, disorientation, Korsakoff psychosis, and psychopathic disorders.

A **Echolalia**, the involuntary repetition of a word or sentence that was uttered by another person, is abnormal.

P Clients with schizophrenia and dementia can exhibit echolalia. Echolalia can also occur in clients with anxiety, amnesia, and after head injuries.

A **Neologism**, a word coined by the client that is meaningful only to the client, is an abnormal finding.

P Clients who are delirious or have schizophrenia may use neologisms.

A Delusions of persecution, grandiose delusions, hallucinations, illusions, obsessive-compulsiveness, and paranoia are examples of abnormal thoughts.

NURSING TIP

Depression Acronym

An easy way to remember the symptoms of clinical depression is to use the acronym "IN SAD CAGES."

IN Interest (loss of pleasure)
S Sleep disturbance
A Appetite change (increases or decreases)
D Depressed mood
C Concentration difficulties
A Activity level (retardation or agitation)
G Guilt feelings (low self-esteem)
E Energy loss (fatigue)
S Suicidal ideation

P Abnormal thought content is demonstrated in clients suffering from schizophrenia or dementia and in clients who use recreational drugs.

Table 20-8 compares and contrasts the various clinical parameters that distinguish dementia, depression, delirium, and acute confusion.

Table 20-8 Distinguishing Dementia, Depression, Delirium, and Acute Confusion

Parameter	Dementia	Depression	Delirium	Acute Confusion
Definition	Deterioration of all cognitive function with little or no disturbance of consciousness or perception Onset: gradual	An abnormal emotional state characterized by feelings of sadness, despair, and discouragement Onset: variable	A disorder of perception with heightened awareness, hallucinations, vivid dreams, and intense emotional disturbances Onset: sudden	An inability to think with customary clarity, and coherence Onset: variable
Pathophysiology	Alzheimer disease Metabolic disorders CVA Head injury	Inherited: neurochemical abnormalities Situational: acute loss of significant person CVA Parkinson disease Alzheimer disease Medications (e.g., steroids)	Withdrawal from alcohol and other drugs Drug intoxication Encephalitis Traumatic injury Febrile states Hypoxia Fluid and electrolyte imbalance	Metabolic disorders Drug intoxication Traumatic injury Febrile states
Attention	Impaired	Intact	Impaired: heightened or dulled	Impaired: dulled
Memory	Short term: impaired first Long term: intact for a while	Intact	Short term: impaired Long term: intact	Short term: impaired Long term: may be intact
Judgment	Impaired	Intact	Grossly impaired Impulsive Volatile	Impaired
Insight	Impaired	Impaired if in manic phase	Impaired	Impaired
Spatial perception	Impaired	Intact	Intact	May be impaired
Calculation	Impaired	May be intact	May be intact	Impaired
Abstract reasoning	Impaired	Intact	Impaired	Impaired
Thought process and content	Impaired	Intact but may demonstrate flight of ideas	Impaired, hallucinations present	Impaired, incoherent

CVA = cerebrovascular accident (stroke).

Suicidal Ideation

If the client has expressed feelings of sadness, hopelessness, despair, worthlessness, or grief, explore these feelings further with more specific questions, such as:

E 1. Have you ever felt so bad that you wanted to hurt yourself?
2. Do you feel like hurting yourself now?

N **The client should provide a negative response and be able to verbalize self-worth.**

A An affirmative response is abnormal and requires probing, such as:

Do you have a plan to hurt yourself?

Have you ever acted on this plan?

What would happen if you were dead?

Continued affirmative responses and expressions of worthlessness and hopelessness should be interpreted as suicidal ideation, a psychiatric emergency that requires immediate referral to a specialist.

P Suicidal ideation is associated with mental disorders, particularly depression, substance abuse, and schizophrenia.

Mental Health

Findings during the cognitive functioning examination may indicate the need for further mental health screening. Table 20-9 summarizes findings common to mental illness that may lead the practitioner to refer the client for further diagnostic study.

Risk Factors

Suicide

- Prior suicide attempts
- Mental illness, particularly with hopelessness
- Female (more suicide attempts)
- Male (more successful suicides)
- Family member with attempt history
- Substance abuse
- Alcohol abuse
- Trauma early in life
- History of physical/sexual abuse
- Unwillingness to seek help because of stigma
- Barriers to accessing mental health treatment
- Stressful life events or loss
- Easy access to lethal methods such as guns
- Suicidal ideation with or without a plan
- Posttraumatic stress (PTS)

(Park et al, 2020)

Table 20-9 Mental Illnesses

Disorder	Defining Characteristics	Population Characteristics
Anxiety Disorders	A group of conditions (panic, phobias, generalized anxiety disorder, obsessive-compulsive disorder, acute and posttraumatic stress disorders) that share extreme or pathological anxiety as the principal disturbance of mood or emotional tone	• Common across cultures • Early age onset • Relapsing or recurrent episodes • Periods of disability • Significant overlap with mood and substance abuse disorders
Panic Disorder • Panic attack • Panic disorder	The client has experienced at least two unexpected panic attacks and develops persistent concern over having recurring attacks or changes behavior to avoid or minimize such attacks	• Twice as common in females as males • Onset most common between adolescence and midadult life • Significant overlap with mood, substance abuse, and panic disorders
Phobias • Agoraphobia • Social phobia • Specific phobias	Marked fear of specific objects or situations	• Experienced by approximately 8% of the population • Typically begin in childhood • There is a second peak in the middle 20s of adulthood
Generalized anxiety disorder	Protracted period of anxiety and worry accompanied by multiple associated physical and cognitive symptoms	• Twice as common in females as males • Half of cases begin in childhood or adolescence • Symptoms increase with life stress or difficulties

Continued

Table 20-9 Mental Illnesses—cont'd

Disorder	Defining Characteristics	Population Characteristics
Obsessive-compulsive disorder	Obsessions are recurrent, intrusive thoughts, impulses, or images that are perceived as inappropriate, grotesque, or forbidden. Compulsions are repetitive behaviors or mental acts that reduce the anxiety that accompanies an obsession	• Equally common among the sexes • Begins in adolescence to young adult life in males • Female onset typically is young adult life • Familial pattern • Strongly associated with Tourette syndrome • Significant overlap with other anxiety disorders and major depressive disorder
Acute and posttraumatic stress disorders	Acute: The anxiety and behavioral disturbances that develop within the first month after exposure to an extreme trauma. If the symptoms persist for more than 1 month and are associated with functional impairment, the diagnosis is changed to posttraumatic stress disorder.	• Twice as prevalent in females as males • Develop in approximately 9% of those exposed to extreme trauma a. Rape b. Physical assault c. Near-death experience d. Witnessing murder and combat
Mood Disorders	A cluster of mental disorders (major depressive disorder, dysthymia, bipolar disorder, cyclothymia) best recognized by depression or mania.	• Rank among the top 10 causes of worldwide disability • More prevalent in females • Leading cause of absenteeism and diminished productivity at work • Common comorbidities include anxiety disorder, personality disorders, and chronic medical conditions • May be caused by: a. Dominant hemispheric strokes b. Hyperthyroidism c. Antihypertensives d. Cushing disease e. Oral contraceptives f. Pancreatic cancer g. Alcohol withdrawal
Major depressive disorder	• Five or more of the following symptoms have been present in the same 2-week period and represent a change from previous functioning; at least one symptom is either depressed mood or loss of interest or pleasure: • Depressed mood • Loss of interest or pleasure • Significant weight loss when not dieting • Insomnia or hypersomnia • Psychomotor agitation or retardation • Fatigue or loss of energy • Feeling of worthlessness • Diminished ability to think or concentrate; indecisiveness • Recurrent thoughts of death or suicidal ideation	• Leading cause of disability worldwide (Greenburg et al, 2021) • Two to three times more common among females (Thom et al, 2019) • Lifetime prevalence is 16.5% • Up to 85% of postpartum females experience transient mood disturbance; 7% to 13% of these females develop disabling or persistent depression • Most severe depressions more common among older adults • At least 50% will recur

Table 20-9 Mental Illnesses—cont'd

Disorder	Defining Characteristics	Population Characteristics
Dysthymia	A chronic form of depression, symptoms are constant for 2 years (1 year for children)	• Twice as many females as males are diagnosed • Affects about 1.5% of adults each year • If onset in childhood, associated strongly with subsequent substance abuse • Susceptible to major depression episode superimposed on dysthymia
Bipolar disorder • Type I (prior mania) • Type II (prior hypomanic episodes only)	Recurrent mood disorder featuring one or more episodes of mania or mixed episodes of mania and depression	• Equally common in males and females • Affects about 2% of adult population
Cyclothymia	Manic and depressive states of insufficient intensity or duration to merit a diagnosis of bipolar disorder or major depressive disorder	33% higher risk than general population to develop bipolar disorder
Schizophrenia	Profound disruption in cognition and emotion. Two or more of the following symptoms persist for a significant portion of time for 1 month: • Delusions • Hallucinations • Disorganized speech • Grossly disorganized or catatonic behavior • Negative symptoms: affective flattening, alogia (inability to express oneself through speech), or avolition (lack of motivation for work or other goal-directed activity)	• Onset during young adulthood • Females experience later onset than males; males and females are equally affected • One-year prevalence in adults is estimated to be 1.1% • Associated with significantly higher mortality rate than the general population • Suicide • Comorbid medical illness: visual and dental problems, hypertension, diabetes, and sexually transmitted infections

Information condensed from the following sources: Department of Health and Human Services, Office of the Surgeon General (US). (1999) Mental health: A report of the Surgeon General. *https://profiles.nlm.nih.gov/spotlight/nn/catalog/nlm:nlmuid-101584932X120-doc*; National Institute of Mental Health (n.d.). Accessed December 17, 2025. Health topics. Mental health information (n.d.). *https://www.nimh.nih.gov/health/topics*

NURSING TIP

Suicide and Crisis Lifeline

Starting in July 2022, the 988 Suicide and Crisis Lifeline started using a new three-digit dialing code that routes callers to the National Suicide Prevention, much like 911 routes callers to aid in a medical emergency. When people call, text, or chat 988, they will be connected to trained counselors. These trained counselors will listen, understand how the clients' problems are affecting them, provide support, and connect them to resources if necessary. The original phone number (1-800-273-TALK) will remain available to people in emotional distress or suicidal crisis.

Source: *https://988lifeline.org*

NURSING CHECKLIST

Assessing Sensation

1. Explain the procedure to the client before starting the examination.
2. The entire sensory examination is carried out with the client's eyes closed.
3. For a thorough sensory examination, the client should be in a supine position.
4. The client should be cooperative and reliable, although the pain examination may be performed on comatose clients.
5. Note the client's ability to perceive the sensation.
6. Much of the sensory component of the neurological examination is subjective; observe the client's reactions by watching the face for grimacing, or withdrawal of the stimulated extremity.
7. Compare the client's sensation on the corresponding areas bilaterally.
8. Note whether any sensory deficits follow a dermatome distribution.
9. The borders of any area exhibiting changes in sensation should be mapped by dermatomes (Fig. 20-7).

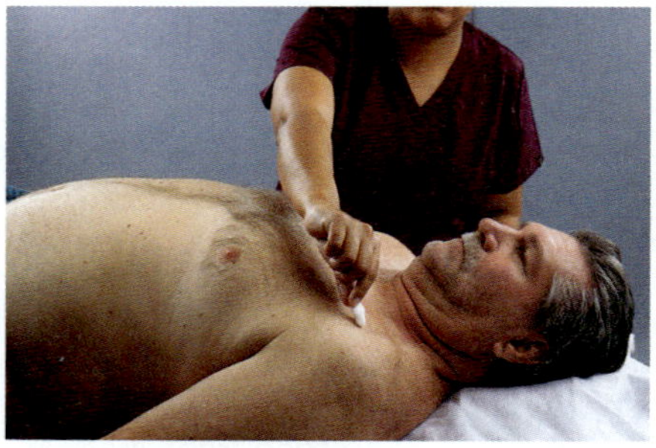

Figure 20-11 Assessment of light touch.

Sensory Examination

Sensation should be tested early in the neurological examination because of the detail involved and because the client's cooperation is required. The conclusions of the examination may be unreliable if the client becomes fatigued.

The sensory examination is divided into three sections. First, the exteroceptive sensations (superficial sensations that originate in the sensory receptors in the skin and mucous membranes) are tested. These are the sensations of light touch, superficial pain, and temperature.

Second, the proprioceptive sensations (deep sensations, with sensory receptors in the muscles, joints, tendons, and ligaments) are assessed. **Proprioception** is tested with the modalities of motion and position and vibration sense.

Finally, the cortical sensations (those that require cerebral integrative and discriminative abilities) are assessed. Stereognosis, graphesthesia, two-point discrimination, and extinction are tested.

Exteroceptive Sensation

For the entire exteroceptive sensation examination, expose the client's legs, arms, and abdomen.

Light Touch

E
1. Use a wisp of cotton and apply the stimulus with very light strokes (Fig. 20-11). If the skin is calloused, or for the thicker skin on the hands and soles, the stimulus may have to be intensified, although care must be taken not to stimulate subcutaneous tissues.
2. Begin with distal areas of the client's limbs and move proximally.
3. Test the hand, lower arm, abdomen, foot, and leg. Examination of sensation of the face is discussed in the Cranial Nerve section later in this chapter.
4. To prevent the client from being able to predict the next touch, alter the rate and rhythm of stimulation. Also, vary the sites of stimulation, keeping in mind that the right and left sides must be compared.
5. Instruct the client to respond by saying "now" or "yes" when the stimulus is felt, and to identify the area that was stimulated either verbally or by pointing to it.

N A P Refer to the Temperature section.

Superficial Pain

E
1. Use a sharp object (a sterile needle or sterile safety pin).
2. Establish that the client can identify sharp and dull sensations by touching the client with each stimulus and asking the client to describe what is felt. This will help alleviate some of the fears the client may have about being touched by a sharp object.
3. Hold the object loosely between the thumb and first finger to allow the sharp point to slide if too much pressure is applied.
4. Begin peripherally, moving in a distal to proximal direction and following the dermatomal distribution. If the impaired sensation is identified, move from impaired sensation to normal sensation for comparison. Attempt to define the area of impaired sensation (mapping) by proceeding from the analgesic area to the unaffected area.
5. Alternate the sharp point with the dull end to test the client's accuracy of shear sensation.

6. Instruct the client to reply "sharp," "dull," or "I don't know" as soon as the stimulus is felt and to indicate areas of the skin that perceive differences in pain sensation.
7. Compare the two sides, taking care not to proceed too fast or to cue the client with regularity in the stimulus presentation.

N A P Refer to the Temperature section.

Temperature

Assess temperature sensation only if abnormalities in superficial pain sensation are noted.

E
1. Use glass vials containing warm water (40°C to 45°C or 104°F to 113°F) and cold water (5°C to 10°C or 41°F to 50°F). Hotter or colder temperatures will stimulate pain receptors.
2. Touch the warm or cold test tubes on the skin, distal to proximal and following dermatome distribution.
3. Instruct the client to respond "hot," "cold," or "I can't tell" and to indicate where the sensation is felt.
4. As an alternative, other warm or cold items such as a cold tuning fork and a chemical disposable heat pack may be utilized.

N **The client should be able to perceive light touch, superficial pain, and temperature accurately, and be able to correctly perceive the location of the stimulus.**

A **Anesthesia** refers to an absence of touch sensation. **Hypesthesia** is a diminished sense of touch; this may also be called **hypoesthesia**. **Hyperesthesia** is marked acuteness to the sensitivity of touch. **Paresthesia** is numbness, tingling, or a pricking sensation. **Dysesthesia** is an abnormal interpretation of a stimulus, such as burning or tingling perceived from a stimulus such as touch or superficial pain. All of these findings are abnormal.

P Peripheral nerve lesions may cause anesthesia, hypesthesia, or hyperesthesia, which may be mapped out in the specific sensory distribution of the affected nerve. Lesions of the nerve roots produce areas of anesthesia and hypesthesia limited to the segmental distribution of the roots involved. Lesions in the brainstem or spinal cord can cause anesthesia, paresthesia, or dysesthesia.

A **Analgesia** refers to insensitivity to pain. **Hypalgesia** refers to diminished sensitivity to pain. **Hyperalgesia** is increased sensitivity to pain. These findings are abnormal.

P Lesions of the thalamus and the peripheral nerves and nerve roots can cause analgesia, hypalgesia, and hyperalgesia.

A Total unilateral loss of all forms of sensation is an abnormal finding.

P Total unilateral loss of all forms of sensation can occur due to an extensive lesion in the thalamus and results in gross disability.

A A "saddle" pattern of sensation loss is abnormal.

P A lesion of the cauda equina produces the "saddle" pattern of sensation loss, the loss of leg reflexes, and the loss of bowel and/or bladder sphincter control. If touch is preserved, the lesion is in or near the conus medullaris.

A The loss of touch sensation in the hands and lower legs (glove and stocking anesthesia) is abnormal.

P Glove and stocking anesthesia is common in polyneuritis of any cause.

A Unilateral loss of all exteroceptive sensation is abnormal.

P Unilateral loss of all exteroceptive sensation is abnormal and can be caused by a partial lesion in the thalamus or a lesion laterally situated in the upper brainstem. Hysteria can also lead to a unilateral loss of exteroceptive sensation.

Proprioceptive Sensation

Motion and Position

E
1. Grasp the client's index finger with your thumb and index finger. Hold the finger at the sides (parallel to the plane of movement) so as not to exert upward or downward pressure with your fingers and thus give the client any clues as to which direction the finger is moving. The client's fingers should be relaxed.
2. Have the client shut their eyes, and show the client what "up" and "down" feel like by moving the finger in those directions.
3. Use gentle, slow, and deliberate movements. Begin with larger movements that become smaller and less perceptible.
4. Instruct the client to respond "up," "down," or "I can't tell" after each time you raise or lower the finger.
5. Repeat this several times. Vary the motion to avoid establishing a predictable pattern.
6. Repeat steps 2 through 5 with the finger of the client's opposite hand, and then with the great toes.
7. If there appears to be a deficit in motion sense, proceed to the proximal joints such as wrists or ankles, and repeat the test.

N **The client should be able to correctly identify the changes in the position of the body parts.**

A Inability to perceive the direction of movement is abnormal.

P Peripheral neuropathies will interfere with position sense. A lesion of the posterior column will cause an ipsilateral loss of position sense. Lesions of the sensory cortex, the thalamus, or the connections between them (thalamocortical connections) may also disrupt position sense.

Vibration Sense

E
1. Strike the prongs of a low-pitch tuning fork (128 or 256 Hz) against the ulnar surface of your hand or your knuckles, and place the base of the fork firmly on the client's skin over bony prominences (Fig. 20-12). Be sure that your fingers touch only the stem of the fork, not the tines.
2. Begin with distal prominences such as a toe or finger, testing each extremity.
3. Instruct the client to say "now" when the buzzing, vibrating tuning fork is felt, and to report immediately when the vibrations are no longer felt.
4. Be sure that the client is reporting the vibration sense rather than hearing a humming sound or just feeling pressure from the tuning fork.
5. After the client can no longer feel the vibrations, determine whether the vibrations can, in fact, still be felt by holding the prongs while the tuning fork is left on the client.
6. If you detect a deficit in the vibratory sense in the peripheral bony prominences, progress toward the trunk by testing ankles, knees, wrists, elbows, anterior superior iliac crests, ribs, sternum, and spinous processes of the vertebrae.

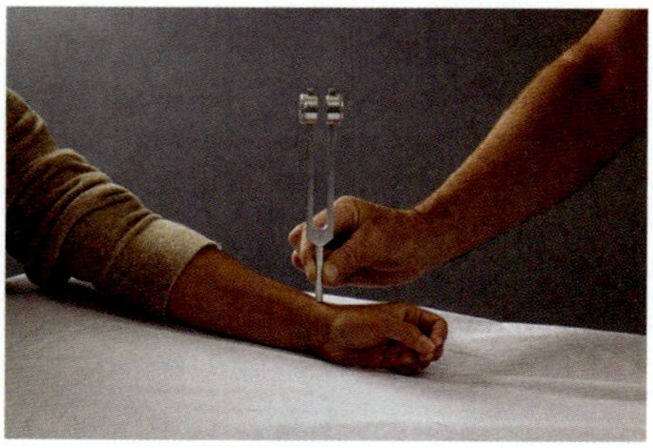

Figure 20-12 Assessment of vibration.

N **Normally, the client should be able to perceive vibration over all bony prominences.**

A The inability to perceive vibration sense is abnormal.

P Vibratory sense may be lost as a result of polyneuropathies (e.g., diabetic) or spinal cord lesions involving the posterior columns. The vibratory sensation may be perceived less in clients over age 65.

Cortical Sensation

Stereognosis

Stereognosis is the ability to identify objects by manipulating and touching them.

E
1. Place a familiar object (e.g., coin, button, closed safety pin, key) into the client's hand (Fig. 20-13).
2. Ask the client to manipulate the object, appreciating size and form.
3. Ask the client to name the object.
4. Repeat in the opposite hand with a different object.

N **The client should be able to identify the objects by holding them.**

A The inability to recognize the nature of objects by touch manipulation, termed **astereognosis**, is abnormal.

P Astereognosis is related to dysfunction of the parietal lobe, where the sensory cortex is located.

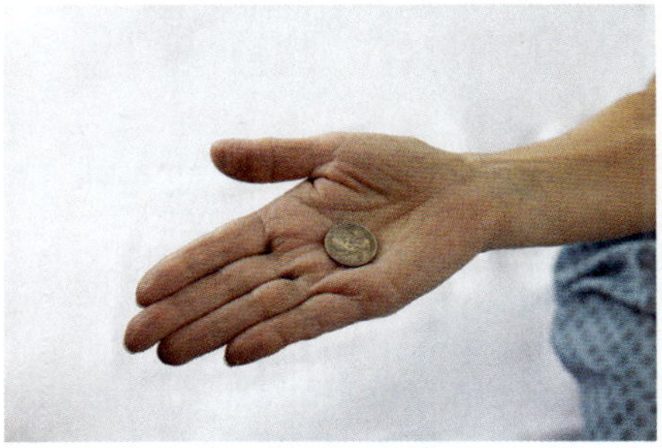

Figure 20-13 Assessment of stereognosis.

Graphesthesia

The ability to identify numbers, letters, or shapes drawn on the skin is termed **graphesthesia**.

E
1. Draw a number or letter with a blunt object (such as a closed pen or the stick of a cotton-tipped swab) on the client's outstretched palm. Make sure the number or letter is facing the client's direction (Fig. 20-14).
2. Ask the client to identify what has been written.
3. Repeat on the opposite side.

N **The client should be able to identify what number or letter has been written on the palm.**

A **Graphanesthesia** is the inability to recognize a number or letter drawn on the skin and is abnormal.

P Graphanesthesia, in the presence of intact peripheral sensation, indicates parietal lobe dysfunction.

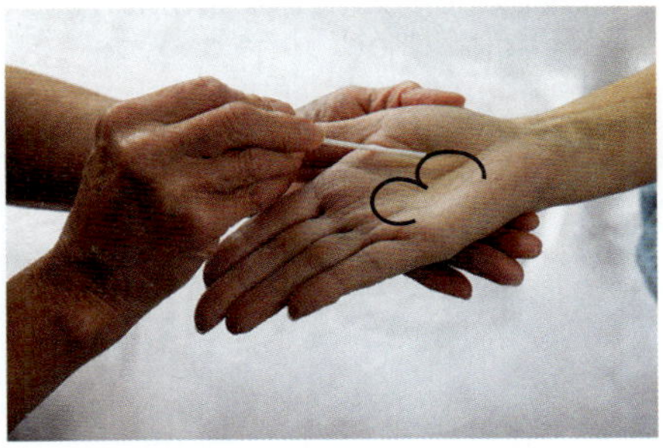

Figure 20-14 Assessment of graphesthesia.

Two-Point Discrimination

Two-point discrimination is tested by simultaneously and closely touching various parts of the body with two identical, sharp objects.

E
1. With two sterile pins or broken cotton-tipped swabs, simultaneously touch the tip of one of the client's fingers, starting with the objects far apart (Fig. 20-15).
2. Ask the client whether one or two points are felt.
3. Continue to move the two points closer together until the client is unable to distinguish two points. Note the minimum distance between the two points at which the client reports feeling the objects separately.
4. Irregularly alternate, using one or two pins throughout the test, to verify that the client is feeling two points.
5. Repeats steps 1–4 with the fingers of the opposite hand.
6. Other areas of the body that may be tested include the dorsum of the hand, the tongue, the lips, the feet, or the trunk.

N **The client should be able to identify two points at 5 mm apart on the fingertips. Other parts of the body vary widely in the normal distance of discrimination, such as the dorsum of the hand or feet, where a separation of as much as 20 mm may be necessary for discrimination. The client may be able to detect two points as close as 2 to 3 mm on the tip of the tongue.**

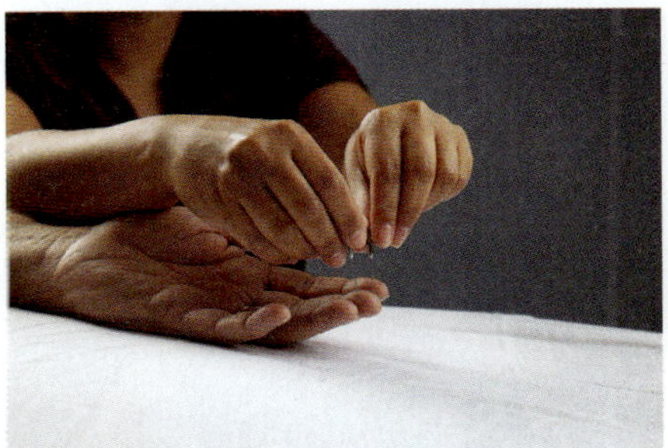

Figure 20-15 Assessing two-point discrimination.

NURSING TIP
Olfactory Examination

- Determine whether the nasal passages are patent by asking the client to breathe through first one nostril and then through the other while occluding the opposing nostril by pressing against it with a finger. Examination of the olfactory nerve may be delayed if the client has a severe cold, allergic rhinitis, nasal packing, had recent oral surgery, or if nasal steroids have been used for a prolonged period.
- Keep aromatic substances such as cloves, coffee, orange, or chocolate in closed glass vials until they are presented to the client.
- Avoid using noxious odors such as alcohol, camphor, ammonia, acetic acid, or formaldehyde, which may stimulate the trigeminal nerve endings in the nasal mucosa.

A Distances greater than those described previously that are required to identify two points are abnormal.

P Lesions in the parietal lobe impair two-point discrimination (with intact tactile sensation).

Extinction

Extinction (sensory inattention) is tested by simultaneously touching opposite sides of the body at an identical site. Use cotton-tipped swabs or your fingers.

E
1. Ask the client if one or two points are felt and where they are felt.
2. Remove the stimulus from one side while maintaining the stimulus on the opposite side.
3. Ask the client if one or two points are felt and where the sensations are felt.

N **The client should be able to feel both stimuli.**

A The inability to feel the two points simultaneously and to discriminate that one point has been removed is abnormal.

P A lesion in one parietal lobe may prevent the client from feeling the stimulus on the opposite side of the body even if sensation is intact on that side during a routine examination.

Cranial Nerves

A complete examination of the 12 cranial nerves is necessary when a baseline assessment is desired, if a tumor of a specific cranial nerve is suspected, or if periodic assessment is needed after surgery or radiation treatments. An abbreviated cranial nerve examination is an integral part of a neurological screening examination. The screening examination would include cranial nerves II, III, IV, and VI: visual acuity and gross visual fields, funduscopic examination, pupillary reactions, and extraocular movements; cranial nerves VII, VIII, IX, X, and XII: facial musculature and expression, gross hearing, voice, and inspection of the tongue.

Olfactory Nerve (CN I)

E
1. Ask the client to close their eyes.
2. Test each side separately by asking the client to occlude one nostril by pressing against it with a finger.
3. Ask the client to inhale deeply to cause the odor to surround the mucous membranes and adequately stimulate the olfactory nerve (Fig. 20-16).
4. Ask the client to identify the contents of each vial.
5. Present one odor at a time and alternate them from nostril to nostril.
6. Allow enough time to pass between the presentation of vials to prevent confusion of the olfactory system.
7. Record the number of substances tested and the number of times the client was able to correctly identify the contents.
8. Note whether a difference between the right and the left sides was apparent.

N **The client should be able to distinguish and identify the odors with each nostril.**

A **Anosmia,** the loss of the sense of smell, is abnormal.

P Total loss of the sense of smell may be caused by trauma to the cribriform plate, sinusitis, colds, or heavy smoking. Unilateral anosmia may be the result of an intracranial neoplasm, such as a meningioma of the sphenoid ridge compressing the olfactory tract or bulb.

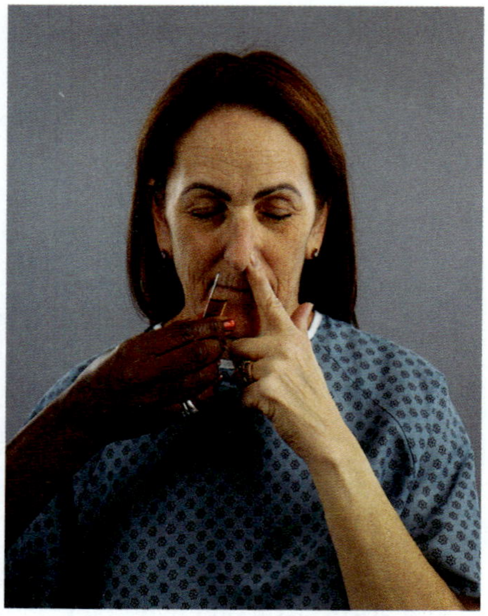

Figure 20-16 Assessment of CN I.

P Anosmia can develop with COVID-19 infection. It can take days or months to regain the sense of smell. Some people have not regained their sense of smell even years later. The etiology is unknown.

Optic Nerve (CN II)

Visual Acuity

(ENAP: See Chapter 12.)

Visual Fields

(ENAP: See Chapter 12.)

Funduscopic Examination

(ENAP: See Chapter 12.)

Oculomotor Nerve (CN III)

Cardinal Fields of Gaze

(ENAP: See Chapter 12.)

Eyelid Elevation

(ENAP: See Chapter 12.)

Pupil Reactions (Direct, Consensual, Accommodation)

(ENAP: See Chapter 12.)

> **ADVANCED TECHNIQUE**
>
> **Doll's Eyes Phenomenon**
>
> Assess the doll's eye phenomenon (oculocephalic reflex) (CN III) in the unconscious client. This tests the intactness of the vestibular and oculomotor pathways. The doll's eyes phenomenon should not be tested in a client with a suspected neck injury.
>
> **E**
> 1. Hold the client's eyelids open and rotate the client's head from the center to one side and then to the opposite side, holding briefly at the endpoints.
> 2. Watch for eye movement.
> 3. Further evaluate the oculocephalic reflex by alternately flexing and extending the head with the eyelids held as before.
>
> **N** **Normally, the eyes should deviate in the direction opposite the head (e.g., head up, eyes look down; head turned to the right, eyes look left) (Fig. 20-17).**
>
> **A** The client with an abnormal response will have eyes that appear to be painted onto a doll's head, hence the term doll's eyes phenomenon. Loss of the doll's eyes phenomenon is abnormal and is demonstrated when the eyes remain fixed with neither lateral nor vertical deviation in response to head movement.
>
> **P** Clients with low brainstem lesions will exhibit abnormal doll's eyes phenomenon.

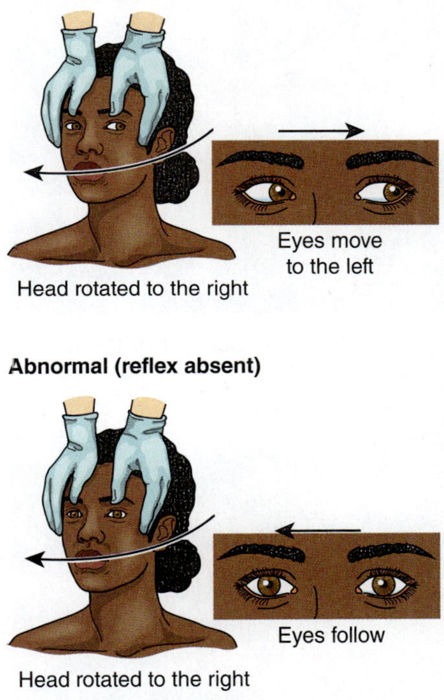

Figure 20-17 Assessing the oculocephalic reflex.

Trochlear Nerve (CN IV)

Cardinal Fields of Gaze

(ENAP: See Chapter 12.)

Trigeminal Nerve (CN V)

Motor Component

E 1. Instruct the client to clench the jaw.

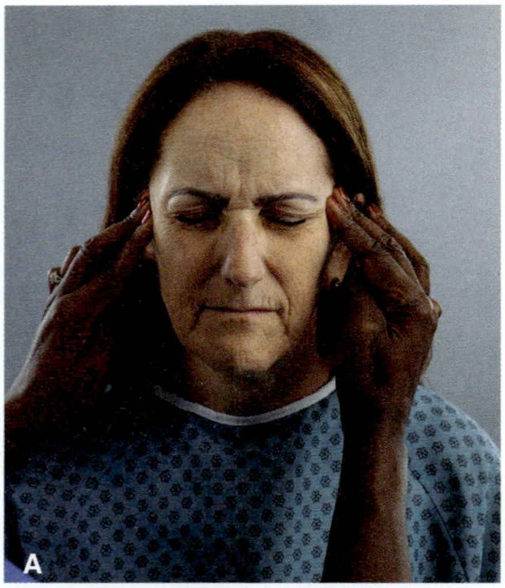

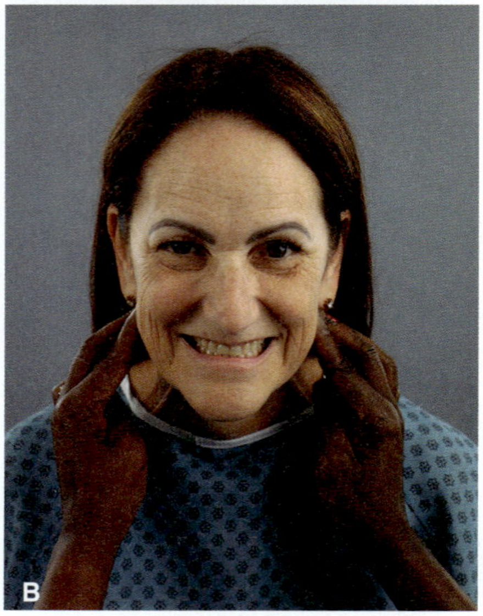

Figure 20-18 Assessment of the motor component of CN V. **A.** Temporalis muscles. **B.** Masseter muscles.

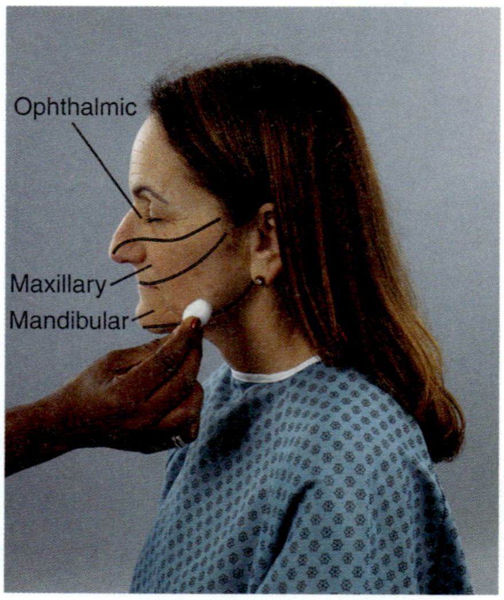

Figure 20-19 Assessment of the sensory component of CN V: Light touch.

2. Palpate the contraction of the temporalis (Fig. 20-18A) and masseter (Fig. 20-18B) muscles on each side of the face by feeling for contraction of the muscles with the finger pads of the first three fingers.
3. Ask the client to move the jaw from side to side against resistance from your hand. Feel for weakness on one side or the other as the client pushes against resistance.
4. Test the muscles of mastication by having the client bite down with the molars on each side of a tongue blade and comparing the depth of the impressions made by the teeth. If you can pull the tongue blade out while the client is biting on it, there is weakness in the muscles of mastication.
5. Observe for fasciculation and note the bulk, contour, and tone of the muscles of mastication.

Sensory Component

E

1. Instruct the client to close their eyes.
2. Test light touch by using a cotton wisp to lightly stroke the client's face in each area of the sensory distribution of the trigeminal nerve (Fig. 20-19).
3. Instruct the client to respond by saying "now" each time the touch of the cotton wisp is felt.
4. Test and compare both sides of the face.
5. To assess superficial pain sensation, use a sterile needle or a sterile safety pin. Before testing, show the client how the sharpness of the needle feels compared with the dullness of the opposite, blunt end. Testing with the blunt end will give some reliability to the assessment.
   a. Instruct the client to respond by saying "sharp" or "dull" when each sensation is felt.
   b. Irregularly alternate the sharp and dull ends, and again test each distribution area of the trigeminal nerve on both sides of the face.
6. Test temperature sensation if other abnormalities have been detected. Use vials of hot and cold water.
   a. Touch the vials to each dermatomal distribution area, alternating hot and cold.
   b. The client should respond by saying "hot" or "cold."
7. Because sensation to the cornea is supplied by the trigeminal nerve, test the corneal reflex (the motor component is CN VII). The corneal reflex should not be routinely assessed in conscious clients unless there is a clinical suspicion of trauma to CN V or CN VII.
   a. Ask the client to open their eyes and look away from you.
   b. Approach the client out of the line of vision to eliminate the blink reflex. You can stabilize the client's chin with your hand if it is moving.
   c. Lightly stroke the cornea with a slightly moistened cotton wisp (to avoid irritating the cornea) (Fig. 20-20). Avoid stroking just the sclera or the lashes of the eye. An alternative technique is to instill normal saline eye drops instead of a light stroke of a cotton wisp.
   d. Observe for bilateral blinking of the eyes.
   e. Repeat on the opposite eye.

N

The temporalis and masseter muscles should be equally strong on palpation. The jaw should not deviate and should be equally strong during side-to-side movement against resistance. The volume and bulk of the muscles should be bilaterally equal. Sensation to light touch, superficial pain, and temperature

should be present in the sensory distribution areas of the trigeminal nerve. The corneal reflex should cause bilateral blinking of the eyes.

A Lesions of the trigeminal nerve may give rise to either reduced sensory perception or to facial pain, both of which are abnormal.

P Aneurysms of the internal carotid artery next to the cavernous sinus may give rise to severe pain in the ophthalmic or mandibular distribution of the trigeminal nerve due to the pressure of the aneurysm on the nerve. Neoplasms that compress the Gasserian ganglion or root, such as meningiomas, pituitary adenomas, and malignant tumors of the nasopharynx, may cause facial pain and impairment of sensation. Head injuries, especially basilar skull fractures, may give rise to facial anesthesia and paralysis of the muscles of mastication.

A Trigeminal neuralgia (tic douloureux), characterized by brief, paroxysmal, unilateral facial pain along the distribution of the trigeminal nerve, is abnormal. The pain can be provoked by touch or movement of the face, such as in tooth brushing, yawning, chewing, or talking. There is no associated motor weakness.

P Trigeminal neuralgia may occur in clients with multiple sclerosis due to demyelinization of the CN V root. The client with a posterior fossa tumor may have trigeminal neuralgia. In most cases, no etiology is found.

A Continuous facial pain that is constant, burning, and stabbing is abnormal. The pain may be provoked by touch.

P Continuous facial pain that is constant, burning, and stabbing occurs in herpes zoster (shingles). The pain is unilateral and tends to follow the distribution of the ophthalmic distribution of the trigeminal nerve. Inflammatory lesions are found throughout the trigeminal pathways.

A Tetanus is characterized by tonic spasms interfering with the muscles that open the jaw (trismus), and it is abnormal. Dysphagia and spasms of the pharyngeal muscles are also observed in tetanus.

P Motor root involvement of the trigeminal nerve causes the spasm of the masseter muscles.

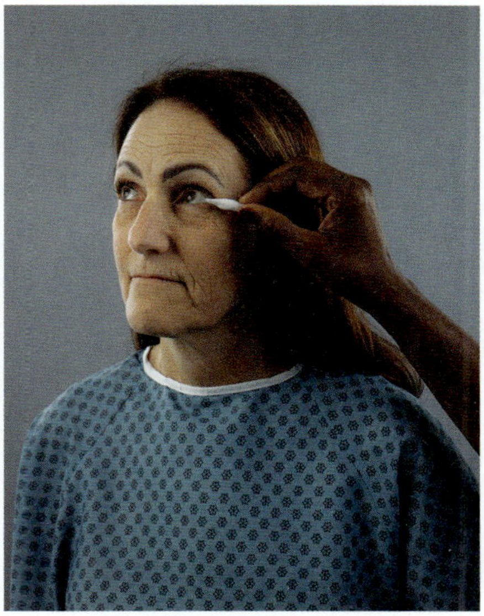

Figure 20-20 Assessment of the sensory component of CN V and motor component of CN VII: Corneal reflex.

Abducens Nerve (CN VI)

Cardinal Fields of Gaze

(ENAP: See Chapter 12.)

Facial Nerve (CN VII)

Motor Component

E
1. Observe the client's facial expressions for symmetry and mobility throughout the examination.
2. Note any asymmetry of the face, such as wrinkles or lack of wrinkles on one side of the face or one-sided blinking.
3. Test muscle contraction by asking the client to:
   a. Frown
   b. Raise the eyebrows
   c. Wrinkle the forehead while looking up
   d. Close the eyes lightly and then keep them closed against your resistance (Fig. 20-21)
   e. Smile, show teeth, purse lips, and whistle
   f. Puff out the cheeks against the resistance of your hands
4. Observe for symmetry of facial muscles and for weakness during the maneuvers in steps 3a–f.

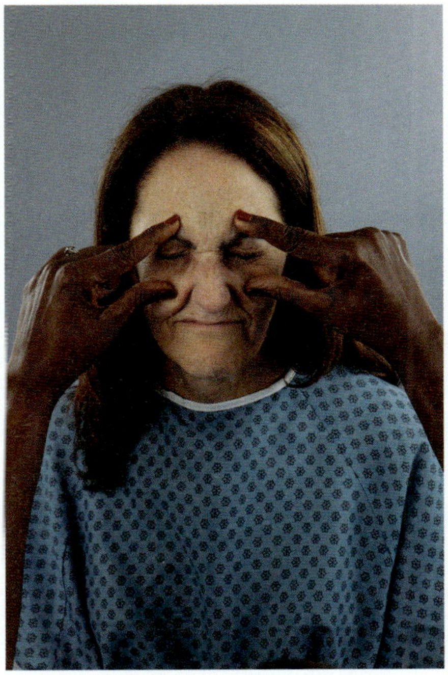

Figure 20-21 Assessment of the motor component of CN VII: Opening the client's eyes against resistance.

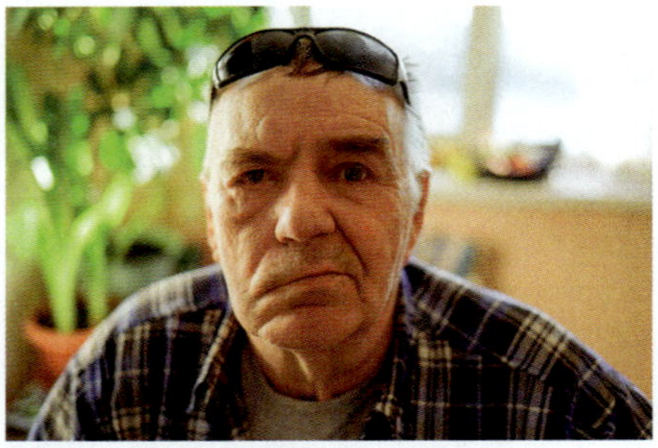

Figure 20-22 Bell palsy.

5. Note any abnormal movements such as tremors, tics, grimaces, or immobility.

N **Normal findings of the motor portion of the facial nerve include symmetry between the right and the left sides of the face, as well as between the upper and lower portions of the face at rest and while executing facial movements. There should be an absence of abnormal muscle movement.**

A **Bell palsy** (idiopathic facial palsy), characterized by complete flaccid paralysis of the facial muscles on the involved side, is abnormal. The affected side of the face is smooth, the eye cannot close, the eyebrow droops, the labiofacial fold is gone, and the mouth may droop (Fig. 20-22). Loss of the sensation of taste in the anterior two-thirds of the tongue may occur.

P Bell palsy is a lower motor neuron paralysis. Damage occurs along the facial nerve from its origin to its periphery. The etiology of Bell palsy is not entirely clear, and the diagnosis is one of exclusion. Diagnosis often includes consideration of five factors, including anatomical structure, viral infection, ischemia, inflammation, and cold stimulation responsivity. Bell palsy usually resolves within 2 weeks, but if prolonged can cause permanent damage and asymmetry (Zhang et al, 2019).

A Supranuclear facial palsy is characterized by paralysis in the lower one-third to two-thirds of the face; the upper portion of the face is spared. The nasolabial fold is flat, and the eye on the affected side can close, although more weakly. The client may be unable to keep the eye closed against resistance applied by the nurse. The muscles of the upper portion of the face remain intact. Supranuclear facial palsy is abnormal.

P Supranuclear facial palsy is due to an upper motor neuron lesion of the facial nerve.

Sensory Component

E

1. Sensory examination of the facial nerve is limited to testing taste. The portions of the tongue that are tested are:
   a. The tip of the tongue for sweet and salty tastes
   b. Along the borders and at the tip for sour taste
   c. The back of the tongue and the soft palate for bitter taste
2. Test both sides of the tongue with each solution.
3. The client's tongue should protrude during the entire assessment of taste, and talking is not allowed. For the client to identify the substance, the words sweet, salty, bitter, and sour should be written on a card so that the client can point to what is tasted. Be sure the client does not see which solution is being tested.
4. Cotton swabs may be used as applicators, using a different one for each solution.
5. Dip the cotton swab into the solution being tested and place it on the appropriate part of the tongue.
6. Instruct the client to point to the word that best describes the taste perception.
7. Instruct the client to rinse the mouth with water before the next solution is tested.
8. Repeat steps 5, 6, and 7 until each solution has been tested on both sides of the tongue.

N **Normal sensation is an accurate perception of sweet, sour, salty, and bitter tastes.**

A **Ageusia** (loss of taste) and **hypogeusia** (diminution of taste) are abnormal.

P Age, excessive smoking, extreme dryness of the oral mucosa, viral colds, medications, lesions of the medulla oblongata, and lesions of the parietal lobe may cause alterations in the sense of taste.

P Many people who had COVID-19 had ageusia and hypogeusia. Some people do not return to their baseline sense of taste even years after their COVID-19 infection.

Acoustic Nerve (CN VIII)

Cochlear Division

Hearing. (ENAP: See Chapter 13.)

Weber and Rinne Tests. (ENAP: See Chapter 13.)

Vestibular Division

The vestibular division of CN VIII assesses for vertigo.

E
1. During the history, ask the client if vertigo is experienced.
2. Note any evidence of equilibrium disturbances. Refer to the section on cerebellar examination.
3. Note the presence of nystagmus.

N **Vertigo is not normally present.**

A Vertigo describes an uncomfortable sensation of movement of the environment or the movement of self within a stationary environment; it is often accompanied by nausea, vomiting, and nystagmus.

P Vertigo is caused by a disorder of the labyrinth or the vestibular nerve. Causative factors may include migraine headache, which disrupts the supply of the internal auditory artery. Tumors of the cerebellopontine angle may cause vertigo by compressing the vestibular nerve. Head injuries that involve the labyrinth may cause vertigo. Blockage of the eustachian tube during ascent in an airplane may lead to vertigo.

A Ménière disease, characterized by vertigo that lasts for minutes or hours, low-pitched roaring tinnitus, progressive hearing loss, nausea, and vomiting, is abnormal. The client may also experience pressure in the ear.

P The main pathological finding is distention of the endolymphatic system, with degenerative changes in the organ of Corti.

Glossopharyngeal and Vagus Nerves (CN IX and CN X)

The glossopharyngeal and vagus nerves are tested together because of their overlap in function.

E
1. Examine soft palate and uvula movement and gag reflex as described in Chapter 13.
2. Assess the client's quality of speech for a nasal quality or hoarseness. Ask the client to produce guttural and palatal sounds, such as *k, q, ch, b,* and *d.*
3. Assess the client's ability to swallow a small amount of water. Observe for regurgitation of fluids through the nose. If the client is unable to swallow, observe how oral secretions are handled.
4. The sensory examination of the glossopharyngeal and vagus nerves is limited to taste on the posterior one-third of the tongue. This examination was previously discussed in the section on CN VII.

N **Refer to Chapter 13 for normal soft palate and uvula movement and gag reflex findings. The speech is clear, without hoarseness or a nasal quality. The client can swallow water or oral secretions**

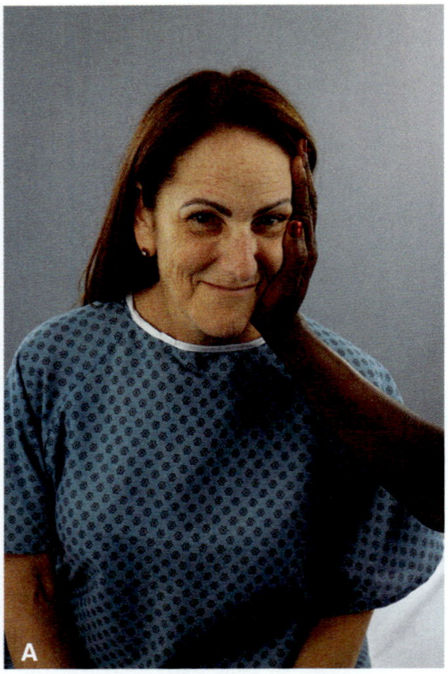

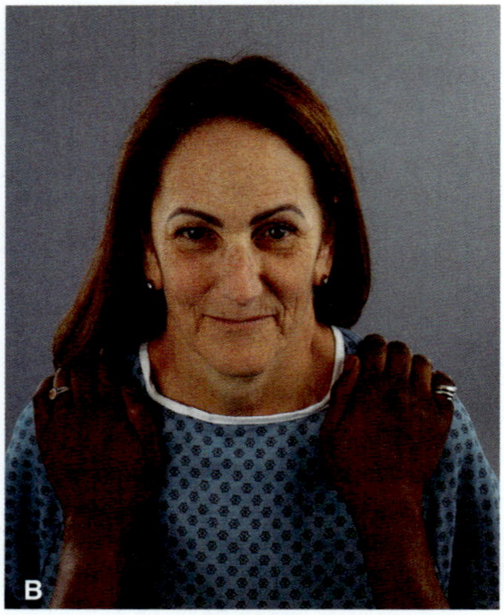

Figure 20-23 Assessment of CN XI. **A.** Strength of sternocleidomastoid muscle. **B.** Strength of trapezius muscles.

easily. Taste (sweet, salty, sour, and bitter) is intact in the posterior one-third of the tongue.

A Unilateral lowering and flattening of the palatine arch; weakness of the soft palate; deviation of the uvula to the normal side; mild dysphagia, regurgitation of fluids, and nasal quality of the voice; loss of taste in the posterior one-third of the tongue; and hemianesthesia of the palate and pharynx are abnormal.

P Unilateral glossopharyngeal and vagal paralysis, such as with trauma or skull fractures at the base of the skull, will cause these symptoms.

A Marked nasal quality of the voice, difficulty with guttural and palatal sounds, severe dysphagia with liquids, and the inability of the palate to elevate on phonation are abnormal.

P Bilateral vagus nerve paralysis will cause these more marked symptoms and often occurs simultaneously with signs and symptoms of other lower brainstem cranial nerve dysfunctions such as in progressive bulbar palsy in amyotrophic lateral sclerosis (ALS).

Spinal Accessory Nerve (CN XI)

E

1. Place the client in a seated or supine position. Inspect the sternocleidomastoid muscles for contour, volume, and fasciculation.
2. Place your right hand on the left side of the client's face. Instruct the client to turn the head sideways against the resistance of your hand (Fig. 20-23A).
3. Use the other hand to palpate the sternocleidomastoid muscle for the strength of contraction. Inspect the muscle for contraction.
4. Repeat steps 2 and 3 in the opposite direction. Compare the strength of the two sides.
5. To assess the function of the trapezius muscle, stand behind the client and inspect the shoulders and scapula for symmetry of contour. Note any atrophy or fasciculation.
6. Place your hands on top of the client's shoulders and instruct the client to raise the shoulders against the downward resistance of your hands (Fig. 20-23B). This can be performed in front of or behind the client.
7. Observe the movements and palpate the contraction of the trapezius muscles. Compare the strength of the two sides.

N **The client should be able to turn the head against resistance with a smooth, strong, and symmetrical motion. The client should also demonstrate the ability to shrug the shoulders against resistance with a strong, symmetrical movement of the trapezius muscles.**

A Inability to turn the head toward the paralyzed side, and a flat, noncontracting muscle on that side are abnormal findings. The contralateral sternocleidomastoid muscle may be contracted.

P These findings are the result of unilateral paralysis of the sternocleidomastoid muscle due to trauma, tumors, or infection affecting the spinal accessory nerve.

A The client's inability to elevate one shoulder, asymmetrical drooping of the shoulder and scapula, and a depressed outline of the neck are abnormal findings. The involved shoulder may also show atrophy and fasciculation of the muscles.

P Unilateral paralysis of the trapezius muscle may be suspected, usually due to trauma, tumors, or infection.

A P For information on torticollis, see Chapter 11.

Hypoglossal Nerve (CN XII)

E 1. See Chapter 13 for an assessment of tongue movement.
2. Assess lingual sounds by asking the client to say "la la la."

N **See Chapter 13 for normal tongue movements. Lingual speech is clear.**

A Inability or difficulty in producing lingual sounds is abnormal. The speech sounds lispy and clumsy.

P Lesions of the hypoglossal nerve will cause difficulty in the pronunciation of lingual sounds.

Motor System

For ENAP on muscle size, tone, strength, and involuntary movements, see Chapter 19. Additional abnormal findings and pathophysiology are:

A Extrapyramidal rigidity is evident when resistance is present during passive movement of the muscles in all directions and lasts throughout the entire range of motion. It may involve both flexor and extensor muscles and is abnormal.

P Extrapyramidal rigidity is due to lesions located in the basal ganglia.

A **Decerebrate rigidity** (decerebration) is characterized by rigidity and sustained contraction of the extensor muscles and is abnormal. The arms are adducted, extended, and hyperpronated. The legs are stiffly extended and the feet are plantar flexed (Fig. 20-24A). The back and neck may be arched and the teeth clenched (opisthotonos).

P Decerebration may be found in unconscious clients with a deep, bilateral diencephalic injury that progresses to midbrain dysfunction. Decerebrate rigidity may also occur due to midbrain and pontine damage, which occurs with compression of these structures due to expanding cerebellar or posterior fossa lesions. Severe metabolic disorders that depress diencephalic and forebrain function may also cause decerebration.

A **Decorticate rigidity** (decortication) is characterized by hyperflexion of the arms (flexion of the arms, wrists, and fingers; adduction of the arms), hyperextension and internal rotation of the legs, and plantar flexion (Fig. 20-24B). It is abnormal.

P Decorticate rigidity is found in unconscious clients with cerebral hemisphere lesions that interfere with the corticospinal tract.

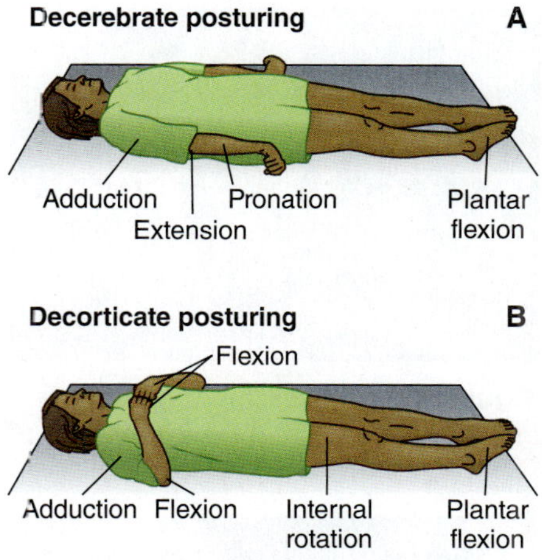

Figure 20-24 Motor system dysfunction. **A.** Decerebrate rigidity (abnormal extension). **B.** Decorticate rigidity (abnormal flexion).

Pronator Drift

E 1. Have the client extend the arms out in front with palms up for 20 seconds.
2. Observe for downward drifting of an arm.

N **There should be no downward drifting of an arm.**

A Downward drifting of an arm is abnormal.

P Downward drifting of an arm may indicate hemiparesis, such as in a stroke.

Cerebellar Function (Coordination, Station, and Gait)

Motor coordination refers to smooth, precise, and harmonious muscular activity. Movement requires the coordination of many muscle groups. Coordination is a complex process involving complicated neural integration of the

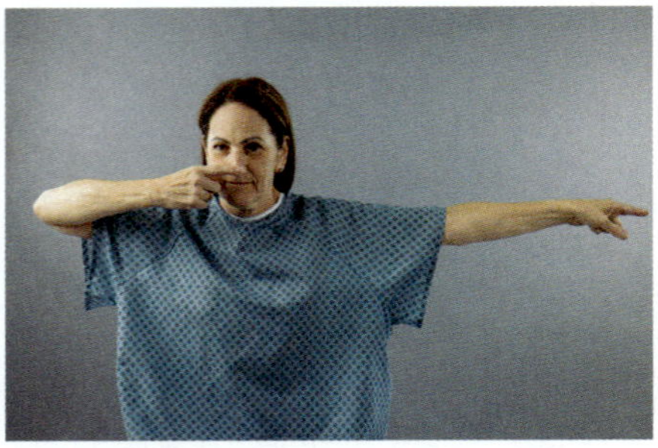

Figure 20-25 Assessment of coordination: Fingertip to nose touch.

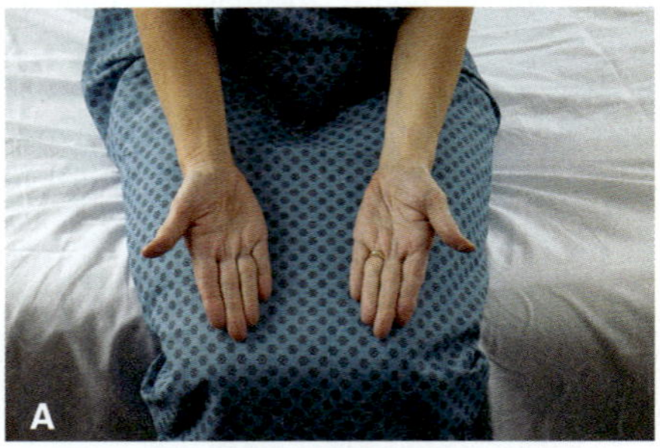

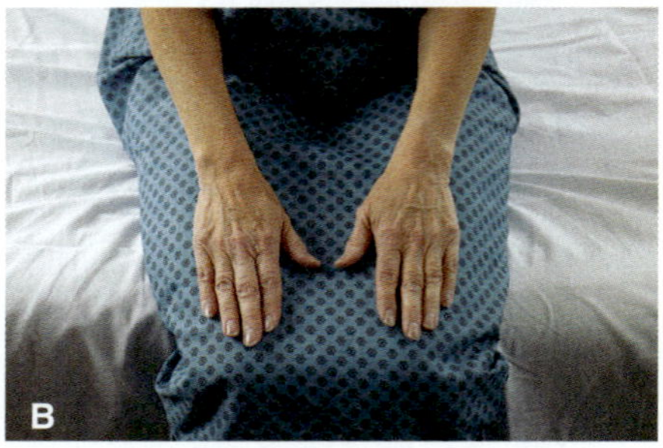

Figure 20-26 Assessment of coordination: Rapid alternating hand movements. **A.** Supination. **B.** Pronation.

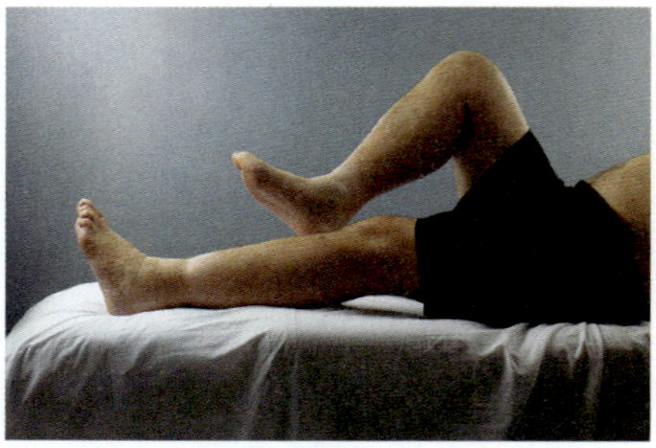

Figure 20-27 Assessment of coordination: Heel slide.

motor and premotor cortex, basal ganglia, cerebellum, vestibular system, posterior columns, and peripheral nerves.

Equilibratory coordination refers to the maintenance of an upright stance and depends on the vestibular, cerebellar, and proprioceptive systems. Nonequilibratory coordination refers to smaller movements of the extremities and involves the cerebellar and proprioceptive mechanisms.

Incoordination is categorized into three different types of syndromes: cerebellar, vestibular, and posterior column syndromes. Incoordination is not considered to be secondary to involuntary movements, paresis, or alterations of muscle tone.

Station refers to the client's posture, and gait refers to the client's manner of walking.

Coordination

E

1. Instruct the client to sit comfortably facing you, with eyes open and arms outstretched. Ensure that clients who wear corrective lenses (eyeglasses or contacts) are wearing them before assessing their coordination.
2. Ask the client to first touch the index finger to the nose, then alternate rapidly with the index finger of the opposite hand.
3. With the client's eyes closed, have the client continue to rapidly touch the nose with alternate index fingers (Fig. 20-25).
4. With the client's eyes open, ask the client to again touch a finger to their nose. Next, ask the client to touch your index finger, which is held about 18 inches (45 cm) away from the client.
5. Change the position of your finger as the client rapidly repeats the maneuver with one finger.
6. Repeat steps 4 and 5 with the other hand.
7. Observe for intention tremor or overshoot or undershoot of the client's finger.
8. To assess rapid alternating movements, ask the client to rapidly alternate patting the knees, first with the palms and then alternating palms with the backs of the hands (rapid supinating [Fig. 20-26A] and pronating [Fig. 20-26B] of the hands).
9. Ask the client to repeatedly touch the thumb to each of the fingers of the hand in rapid succession from the index to the fifth finger, and back.
10. Repeat step 9 with the other hand.
11. Observe coordination and the client's ability to perform these movements in rapid sequence.
12. With the client in a seated or supine position, ask the client to place the heel just below the knee on the shin of the opposite leg and to slide it down to the foot (Figs. 20 to 27).
13. Repeat with the opposite foot.
14. Observe coordination of the two legs.
15. Ask the client to draw a circle or a figure 8 with a foot, either on the ground or in the air (Figs. 20 to 28).
16. Repeat with the other foot.
17. Observe for coordination and regularity of the figure.
18. Test the lower extremities for rapid alternating movement by asking the client to rapidly extend the ankle ("tap your foot") or to rapidly flex and extend the toes of one foot.
19. Repeat with the opposite foot.
20. Note the rate, rhythm, smoothness, and accuracy of the movements.

N **The client can rapidly alternate touching finger to nose and moving finger from nose to your finger in a coordinated fashion.**

The client can perform alternating movements in a purposeful, rapid, and coordinated manner. The client demonstrates the ability to purposefully and smoothly run heel down shin with equal coordination in both feet and to draw a figure 8 or circles with the foot.

A **Dyssynergy**, the lack of coordinated action of the muscle groups, is abnormal. The client is unable to carry out smooth, coordinated movements. The client's movements appear jerky, irregular, and uncoordinated.

A **Dysmetria**, the impaired judgment of distance, range, speed, and force of movement, is abnormal. The client misjudges distance and overshoots.

A **Dysdiadochokinesia**, the inability to perform rapid alternating movements, is abnormal. The client is unable to abruptly stop one movement and begin another opposite movement.

P Cerebellar disease can lead to dyssynergy, dysmetria, or dysdiadochokinesia.

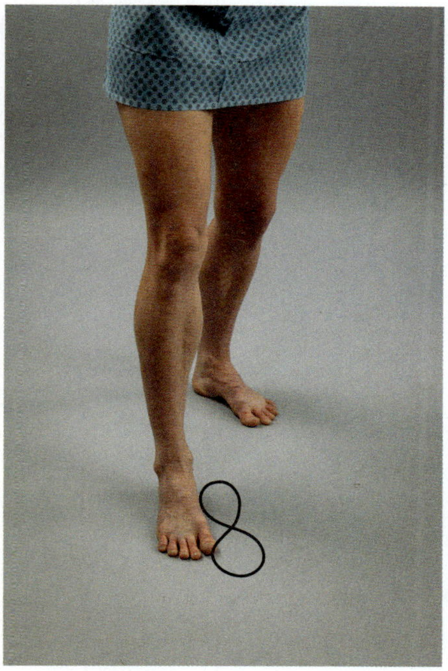

Figure 20-28 Assessment of coordination: Figure 8.

Station

(ENAP: See Chapter 19.)

Gait

E
1. See Chapter 19 for the gait assessment technique.
2. Ask the client to walk on tiptoes, then on heels.
3. Ask the client to walk in a straight line, touching heel to toe (tandem walking). The arms should be held at the side and the eyes should be open.
4. Note the client's ability to maintain balance.
5. Ask the client to hop in place, first on one foot and then on the other.

N **See Chapter 19 for normal gait findings. The client should be able to walk unaided on tiptoes and heels and walk heel to toe in a straight line without losing balance. The client should also be able to maintain balance while hopping on one foot, with bilateral equal strength.**

A P See Chapter 19.

ADVANCED TECHNIQUE

Romberg Test

E
1. Ask the client to stand erect, feet together and arms at side, first with eyes open, then closed.
2. Note the client's ability to maintain balance with eyes first open, then closed. Stand close to the client during this test to catch the client if they begin to fall.

N **The client should be able to maintain balance with eyes open or closed for 20 seconds and with minimal swaying.**

A The Romberg test is positive if the client becomes unsteady and tends to fall when the eyes are closed.

P In cerebellar disease, the client remains unsteady with the eyes open and closed. In posterior column disease with proprioceptive loss, the client becomes appreciably more unsteady with eye closure.

NURSING CHECKLIST
Assessing Reflexes

1. When testing reflexes, the client should be relaxed and comfortable.
2. Position the client so the extremities are symmetrical.
3. To elicit true reflexes, distract the client by talking about another topic.
4. Hold the reflex hammer loosely between the thumb and index finger and strike the tendon with a brisk motion from the wrist. The reflex hammer should make contact with the correct point on the tendon in a quick, direct manner.

   Even when the deep tendon reflex (DTR) is stimulated correctly, the client may not exhibit a DTR because of conscious thought. If this occurs, reinforcement may be necessary. Reinforcement is a technique used to distract the conscious thought of the DTR by concentrating on another action. Examples include the client clenching the teeth, grasping the thigh with the hand not being assessed, and grasping and pulling the wrists with the contralateral hands.
5. Observe the degree and speed of response of the muscles after the reflex hammer makes contact. Grading of DTR is as follows:
   0: absent
   + (1+): present but diminished
   ++ (2+): normal
   +++ (3+): mildly increased but not pathological
   ++++ (4+): markedly hyperactive repeating reflex (clonus)
6. Compare reflex responses of the right and the left sides. The normal response to taps in the correct area should elicit a brisk (++ or +++) contraction of the muscles involved.
7. When documenting the DTRs, you can use a stick figure as illustrated in the Case Study at the end of this chapter.

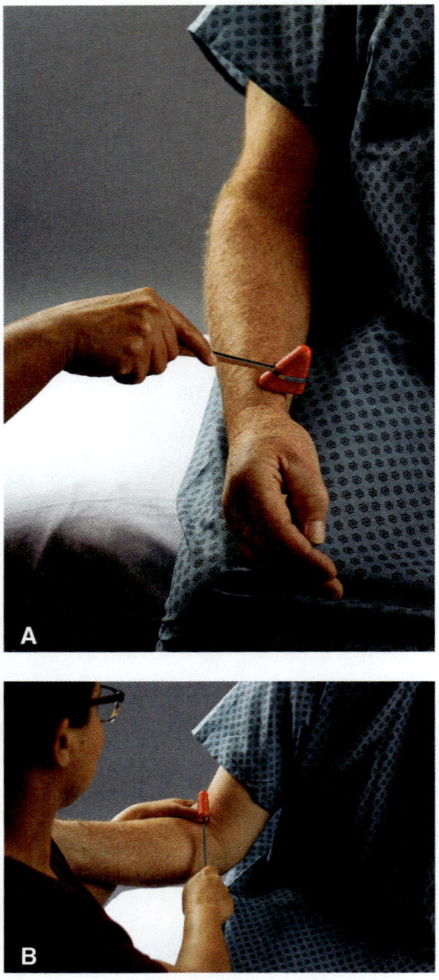

Figure 20-29 Assessment of deep tendon reflexes. **A.** Brachioradialis. **B.** Biceps.

Reflexes
Deep Tendon Reflexes
Brachioradialis

E
1. Flex the client's arm to 45°.
2. Support the client's relaxed arm either on the lap or semipronated on your forearm.
3. With the blunt end of the reflex hammer, strike the tendon of the brachioradialis above the styloid process of the radius (a few centimeters above the wrist on the thumb side) (Fig. 20-29A).
4. Observe for flexion and supination of the forearm.

N **Flexion and supination of the forearm are normal. An exaggerated reflex may also show flexion of the wrist and fingers and adduction of the forearm. Innervation of this reflex is through the radial nerve, with segmental innervation of C5 and C6.**

A P See the Achilles section.

Biceps

E
1. Flex the client's arm to between 45° and 90°.
2. Support the client's forearm on your forearm.
3. Place your thumb firmly on the biceps tendon just above the crease of the antecubital fossa (Fig. 20-29B).
4. Wrap your fingers around the client's arm and rest them on the biceps muscle to feel it contract.
5. Tap your thumb briskly with the pointed end of the reflex hammer.

6. Observe for contraction of the biceps muscle and flexion of the elbow.

N **Contraction of the biceps muscle and elbow flexion is normal. Innervation of the biceps reflex is through the musculocutaneous nerve with segmental innervation of C5 and C6.**

A P See the Achilles section.

Triceps

E
1. Flex the client's arm to between 45° and 90°.
2. Support the client's arm either on the lap or on your hand as shown in Figure 20-29C.
3. With the pointed end of the reflex hammer, tap the triceps tendon just above its insertion above the olecranon process of the elbow.
4. Observe for contraction of the triceps muscle and extension of the arm.

N **Contraction of the triceps muscle and arm extension is normal. Innervation of the triceps reflex is through the radial nerve, with segmental innervation of C7 and C8.**

A P See the Achilles section.

Patellar

E
1. Ask the client to sit in a chair or at the edge of the examination table.
2. Place your hand over the quadriceps femoris muscle to feel contraction.
3. With the other hand, tap the patellar tendon just below the patella with the blunt end of the reflex hammer (Fig. 20-29D).
4. If the client cannot tolerate a sitting position, support the flexed knee with your hand under it so the foot is hanging freely.
5. Observe for contraction of the quadriceps muscle and extension of the leg.

N **Contraction of the quadriceps muscle and leg extension is normal. Innervation of the patellar reflex is through the femoral nerve, with segmental innervation of L2, L3, and L4.**

A P See the Achilles section.

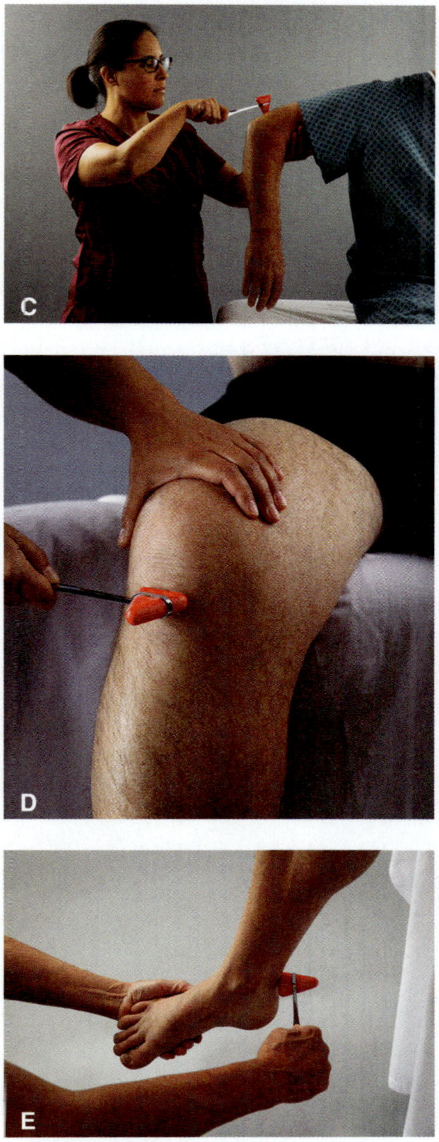

Figure 20-29—cont'd C. Triceps. **D.** Patellar. **E.** Achilles.

Achilles

E
1. Ask the client to sit with the feet dangling.
2. Slightly dorsiflex the client's foot.
3. With the blunt end of the reflex hammer, tap the Achilles tendon just above its insertion in the heel (Fig. 20-29E).
4. If the client is lying down, flex the leg at the knee and externally rotate the thigh. Place your nondominant hand under the foot to produce dorsiflexion. Apply the stimulus as described in step 3.
5. Observe for contraction of the muscles of the calf (gastrocnemius, soleus, and plantaris) and plantar flexion of the foot.

N **Contraction of the calf muscles and plantar flexion is normal. Innervation of the Achilles reflex is through the tibial nerve, with segmental innervation of L5, S1, and S2.**

A Absent or decreased deep tendon reflexes are abnormal.

P Diminished deep tendon reflexes usually result from interference in the reflex arc, and an absence may indicate a break in the reflex arc. Deep tendon reflexes are lost in deep coma, narcosis, deep sedation, and in magnesium sulfate toxicity. Hypothyroidism, sedative or hypnotic drugs, and infectious diseases may also diminish reflexes.

Clients with increased intracranial pressure frequently show decreased or absent deep tendon reflexes. Spinal shock also causes loss of these reflexes.

A Hyperactive deep tendon reflexes are abnormal. Hyperactive deep tendon reflexes are characterized by an increase in the speed of response and enhancement of the vigor of movement. The muscle contraction is sustained, with a minimal stimulus needed to elicit the response. Sometimes the adjacent muscles may also contract. Clonus may be present.

P Hyperactivity is associated with a loss of inhibition of the higher centers in the cortex and reticular formation and in lesions of the pyramidal system. Muscle stretch reflexes are also exaggerated in a light coma, tetany, tetanus, preeclampsia, and exlampsia. Clonus can occur in upper motor neuron lesions (e.g., CVA, brain tumor, MS, ALS, cerebral palsy, spinal cord injury, and TBI).

Superficial Reflexes

Abdominal

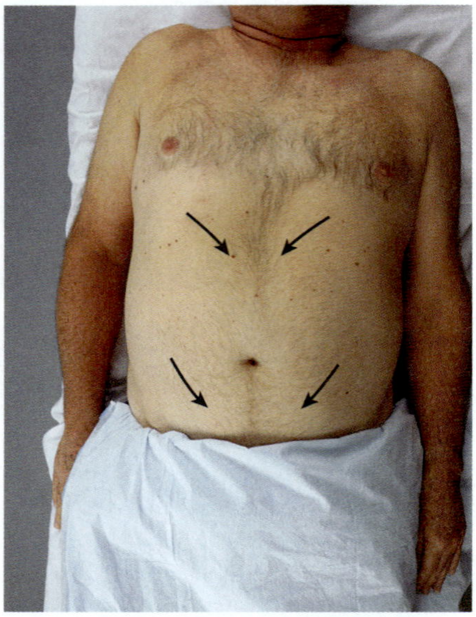

Figure 20-30 Assessment of superficial reflexes: Direction of stimulus for abdominal reflexes.

E

1. Drape and place the client in a recumbent position, arms at the sides, and knees slightly flexed. Stand to the right of the client.
2. Use a moderately sharp object to stroke the skin, such as the wooden tip of a cotton-tipped swab or a split tongue blade.
3. To elicit the upper abdominal reflex, stimulate the skin of the upper abdominal quadrants. From the tip of the sternum, stroke in a diagonal (downward and inward) fashion (Fig. 20-30).
4. Observe for contraction of the upper abdominal muscles and umbilical movement.
5. Repeat step 3 on the opposite side.
6. To elicit the lower abdominal reflex, stimulate the skin of the lower abdominal quadrants. From the area below the umbilicus, stroke in a diagonal (downward and inward) fashion to the symphysis pubis.
7. Observe for contraction of the lower abdominal muscles and umbilical movement.
8. Repeat step 6 on the opposite side.

N **It is normal for the upper abdominal muscles to contract upward and outward with a deviation of the umbilicus toward the stimulus. The upper abdominal reflex is innervated by the thoracic nerves with segmental innervation of T7, T8, and T9. It is normal for the lower abdominal muscles and the umbilicus to contract toward the stimulus. The lower abdominal reflex is innervated by the lower intercostal, iliohypogastric, and ilioinguinal nerves through segments T10, T11, and T12.**

A P See the Bulbocavernosus section.

Plantar

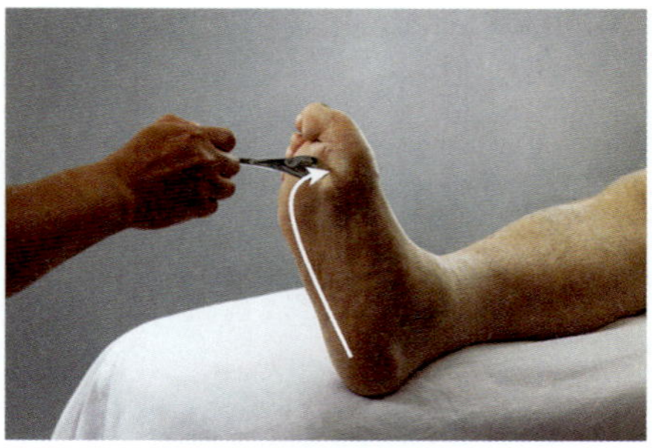

Figure 20-31 Assessment of superficial reflex: Plantar.

E

1. With the handle of the reflex hammer, stroke the outer aspect of the sole of the foot from the heel across the ball of the foot to just below the great toe (Fig. 20-31).
2. Observe for plantar flexion of the toes.
3. Repeat on the opposite foot.

N **It is normal to see plantar flexion of the toes. The plantar reflex is innervated by the tibial nerve with segmental innervation of L5, S1, and S2.**

A P See the Bulbocavernosus section.

Anal Reflex

E 1. The client should be in the lithotomy or supported side-lying position.
2. Using a gloved finger or a cotton-tipped swab, stroke the skin in the client's perianal region at the 3 o'clock position.
3. Observe for a contraction of the external anal sphincter.
4. Repeat step 2 on the opposite side at the 9 o'clock position.

N **There should be a contraction of the external anal sphincter toward the stimulus. This is sometimes called a positive "anal wink." Innervation of the anal reflex is primarily through the pudendal nerve with segmental innervation of S2, S3, and S4.**

A A decreased or absent anal reflex is abnormal.

P Spinal cord injury and tumors involving the S2–S4 nerve root can result in an absent anal reflex.

P A decreased anal reflex may also be present in clients who engage in anal sex or are abused with anal penetration.

Cremasteric

E 1. The client with male genitalia should be lying down with the thighs exposed and the testicles visible.
2. Stroke the skin of the inner aspect of the thigh near the groin from above downward (Fig. 20-32).
3. Observe for contraction of the cremasteric muscle and testicle movement.
4. Repeat step 2 on the opposite side.

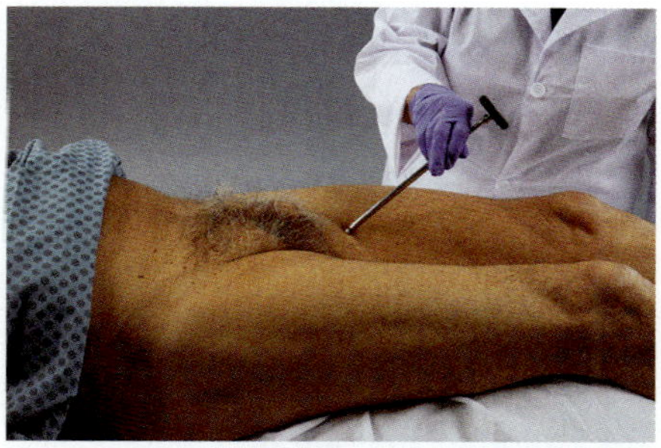

Figure 20-32 Assessment of superficial reflex: Cremasteric.

N **Contraction of the cremasteric muscle with the corresponding elevation of the ipsilateral testicle is normal. Innervation of the cremasteric reflex is through the ilioinguinal and genitofemoral nerves with segmental innervation of T12, L1, and L2.**

A **P** See the Bulbocavernosus section.

Bulbocavernosus

E 1. Pinch the skin of the foreskin or the glans penis.
2. Observe for a contraction of the bulbocavernosus muscle in the perineum at the base of the penis.

N **It is normal to see contraction of the bulbocavernosus muscle. The presence of this reflex in a paraplegic client after acute spinal cord injury indicates that the initial stage of spinal shock is past. Innervation of the bulbocavernosus muscle is primarily through the pudendal nerve with segmental innervation at segments S3 and S4.**

A Decreased or absent superficial reflexes are abnormal.

P Superficial reflexes are diminished or absent with dysfunction of the reflex arc, as with the muscle stretch reflexes. Superficial reflexes are complex because they involve the parietal areas and the motor centers of the premotor area and the pyramidal system. Lesions in the pyramidal tracts will cause a decrease or absence of superficial reflexes. These reflexes may also be lost in deep sleep and coma.

Pathological Reflexes

All of the reflexes described in this section are abnormal findings in adults and are not usually assessed unless the client's clinical presentation warrants it.

Glabellar

E 1. With your finger, tap the client on the forehead between the eyebrows.
2. Observe for a hyperactive blinking response.

A The presence of this reflex is abnormal.

P Clients with lesions of the corticobulbar pathways from the cortex to the pons, clients with Parkinson disease, and clients with glioblastoma of the corpus callosum will have a glabellar reflex.

Clonus

E 1. Have the client assume a recumbent position. Stand to the side.
2. Support the client's knee in a slightly flexed position.
3. Quickly dorsiflex the foot and maintain it in that position.
4. Observe for **clonus** (a rhythmic oscillation of involuntary muscle contraction).

A Sustained clonus is an abnormal finding.

P Sustained clonus indicates upper motor neuron disease (e.g., CVA, brain tumor, MS, ALS, cerebral palsy, spinal cord injury, and TBI). Table 20-10 summarizes the findings associated with upper and lower motor neuron dysfunction.

P Females with pre-eclampsia and eclampsia may also demonstrate clonus.

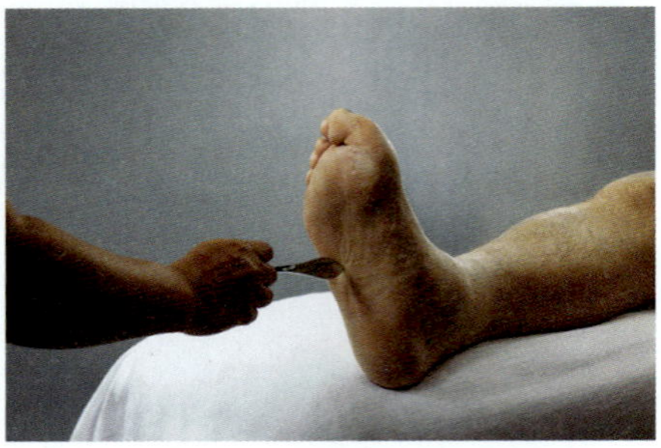

Figure 20-33 Assessment of pathological reflex: Babinski.

Babinski

E With the handle of the reflex hammer, stroke the client's sole as you did for the plantar reflex (Fig. 20-33). Use a slow and deliberate motion.

N **A Babinski reflex is normal in infants and toddlers until 15–18 months of age.**

A A positive Babinski reflex is noted when the client's toes abduct (fan) and the great toe dorsiflexes.

P Clients with lesions in the pyramidal system, such as in stroke or trauma, display a positive Babinski reflex.

Table 20-10 Comparison of Upper Motor Neuron and Lower Motor Neuron Lesions

Parameter	Upper Motor Neuron	Lower Motor Neuron
Muscle tone	Spasticity	Flaccidity
Muscle bulk	Late atrophy from disease; no fasciculations	Atrophy; fasciculations
Pronator drift	Positive	Absent
Deep tendon reflexes	Hyperreflexia	Hyporeflexia or absent
Babinski reflex	Positive	Absent
Clonus	Present	Absent

ADVANCED TECHNIQUE

Assessing for Diabetic Peripheral Neuropathy

Peripheral neuropathy is the diminished or absent perception of protective sensation on the plantar surfaces of the feet. The presence of peripheral neuropathy can be painful for the client and can lead to ulceration and foot injury.

E 1. The client may sit or lie down with legs extended and bare feet exposed.

2. Holding a single-fiber monofilament perpendicular to the plantar surface of the client's foot, apply just enough contact pressure to bend the monofilament fiber (Fig. 20-34). Testing must be done on sites without ulceration or calluses for accurate assessment.

3. Ask the client to tell you when the sensation is felt.

4. Test various locations on the foot.

N **It is normal to have intact sensation at all sites tested.**

A The client does not feel contact with the monofilament fiber.

P Lack of sensitivity indicates nerve damage caused by diabetes mellitus, viruses, toxins, trauma, tumors, vitamin deficiencies, or other sensory conditions.

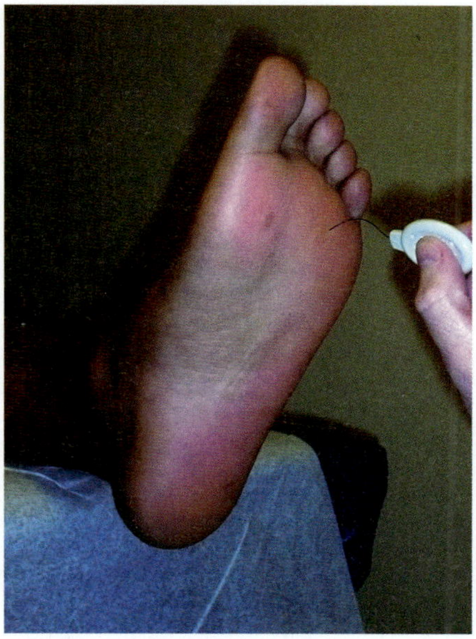

Figure 20-34 Testing for peripheral neuropathy with a monofilament fiber.

ADVANCED TECHNIQUE

Assessing for Meningitis

Meningeal Irritation

To assess the client for signs of meningeal irritation, look for nuchal rigidity, Kernig sign, and Brudzinski sign, all of which are abnormal findings. Other signs and symptoms include violent headache, photophobia, fever, nausea and vomiting, decreasing level of consciousness, and seizures. Definitive diagnosis is obtained through cultures of cerebrospinal fluid.

Nuchal Rigidity

Nuchal rigidity is the tendency of the client to maintain the head in an immobile, extended position. The client resists movement of the neck. Severe pain and spasms occur with movement.

E 1. Place the client in a supine position.

2. Flex the client's neck.

A The client resists the movement.

P Nuchal rigidity can be caused by meningeal irritation such as in meningitis. Meningitis is an infectious process of the meninges caused by bacteria, viruses, mycobacteria, fungi, or spirochetes. The organisms enter the subarachnoid space, causing an acute inflammatory response.

P Irritation of the subarachnoid space due to subarachnoid hemorrhage may cause meningeal irritation.

Kernig Sign

E 1. Place the client in a recumbent position.

2. Lift the client's leg and flex the knee at a right angle.

3. Attempt to extend the client's knee by pushing down on it.

A A positive Kernig sign is resistance to extension and pain (due to spasm of the hamstring), preventing extension of the leg.

P Kernig sign is caused by the stretching of irritated nerve roots and meninges.

NURSING TIP

Signs/Symptoms of Lyme Disease

- Erythema migrans (EM) lesion (refer to Chapter 10)
- EM rash on other parts of the body
- Headache
- Dizziness
- Fever/chills
- Lymphadenopathy
- Neck stiffness or painful neck flexion
- Malaise, fatigue, lethargy
- Arthralgias, myalgias
- Paresthesia
- Palpitations
- Shortness of breath

Brudzinski Sign

E 1. Place one hand under the client's neck and the other hand on top of the client's chest to prevent elevation of the body.

2. Flex the client's neck with a deliberate motion.

A Brudzinski sign is positive if the client responds with flexion of one or both legs up to the pelvis. The arms may also flex.

P A positive Brudzinski sign can be caused by meningeal irritation such as in meningitis. Meningitis is an infectious process of the meninges caused by bacteria, viruses, mycobacteria, fungi, or spirochetes. Organisms enter the subarachnoid space, causing an acute inflammatory response.

NURSING TIP

Meningococcal Meningitis

The Meningococcal (A, C, W, Y) and Meningococcal B meningitis vaccines are recommended by the CDC (2025) for adolescents and young adults. The CDC advises that the first dose of Meningococcal (serogroup A, C, W, Y) vaccination be administered at 11 to 12 years of age and a second dose be given at 16 years for all adolescents. Meningococcal B vaccination is recommended for low risk adolescents (age 16 to 23 with preferred dosing at 16 to 18 years old) using a shared decision-making model which includes a discussion of high risk for college students who attend a 4-year university, live in on-campus housing, or participate in sororities and fraternities.

For adults ages 19 and older both Meningococcal (A, C, W, Y) and Meningococcal B meningitis vaccines may be administered in special situations such as anatomical or functional asplenia (including sickle cell disease), HIV infection, persistent complement component deficiency, complement inhibitor use, travel to countries with hyperendemic or epidemic meningococcal disease, microbiologists routinely exposed to *Neisseria meningitidis,* and military recruits living in communal residences. Clinical shared decision-making with the client is used to discuss the advantages, disadvantages of the vaccines, while providing the client an opportunity to have questions answered.

Accessed December 17, 2025, from *https://www.cdc.gov/vaccines/hcp/imz-schedules/child-adolescent-notes.html#note-mening; https://www.cdc.gov/vaccines/hcp/imz-schedules/adult-notes.html#note-mening*

U.S. Preventive Services Task Force (USPSTF)

Grade B Recommendations:

- The USPSTF recommends screening for anxiety disorders in adults, including pregnant and postpartum persons.
- The USPSTF recommends screening for depression in the adult population, including pregnant and postpartum persons, as well as older adults.

Retrieved December 17, 2025, *https://www.uspreventiveservicestaskforce.org/uspstf/recommendation-topics/uspstf-a-and-b-recommendations#more*

CASE STUDY

The Client With Numbness in the Hands and Feet

This case study illustrates the application and objective documentation of mental status and neurological examination. Alicia Bennett is a 60-year-old high school math teacher with new onset numbness and weakness in the hands and feet. The client is concerned about this recent change in health status and what it means for their job and life.

HEALTH HISTORY

CLIENT PROFILE

60-year-old, left-handed, married White female

CHIEF COMPLAINT

"I have numbness and tingling in both hands and feet."

HISTORY OF PRESENT ILLNESS

Client reports symptoms began 3 to 4 days ago, "but they are getting worse fast. I am weak, tired, and afraid to walk because I might fall." Reports that it's "like I have gloves and socks on my hands and feet." Reports that the sensation is "moving up my legs and arms." Admits to not being able to hold on to things, dropping items, and not being able to support self out of chairs. "I can't get out of the car. I can't grade papers for my math students because I can't hold the pen. What is happening to me?" Reports 5/10 pain in bilateral upper and lower extremities that is characterized as dull and aching. Reports disruption of sleep and severely limited activities of daily living.

Associated symptoms include blurry vision, urinary retention (feeling like bladder not emptying), and imbalance. Denies fever, chills, headache, diplopia, tinnitus, shortness of breath, dyspnea on exertion, cough, orthopnea, chest pain, palpitations, paroxysmal nocturnal dyspnea, abdominal pain, nausea/vomiting, diarrhea/constipation, stool incontinence, hematuria, dysuria, urinary incontinence. Client has taken melatonin 5 mg to help sleep. No other self-treatment.

PAST HEALTH HISTORY

Medical History Hypertension, diagnosed 2010—well controlled
Generalized anxiety disorder (mild), diagnosed 2000—well controlled

Surgical History Wisdom teeth extraction (age 16)

Allergies No known drug allergies (NKDA)

Medications Lisinopril 10 mg daily
Escitalopram 10 mg daily
Melatonin 5 mg nightly for 3 days
Multivitamin daily
Calcium with Vitamin D3 daily (unknown dose)

Communicable Diseases Denies—but notes that she had a pretty bad "Flu with upper respiratory and gastrointestinal symptoms about a month ago." No residual symptoms at present

Injuries and Accidents Denies: falls, head injuries, loss of consciousness (LOC), motor vehicle accident (MVA)

Differing Abilities Denies

Blood Transfusions Denies

Childhood Illnesses Chickenpox at age 10

Immunizations Tetanus booster 2018, herpes zoster vaccine completed two-shot series in 2020, annual influenza vaccine, COVID-19 mRNA (Moderna) vaccine x2 with two boosters (last in fall 2022—was bivalent, none since)

FAMILY HEALTH HISTORY

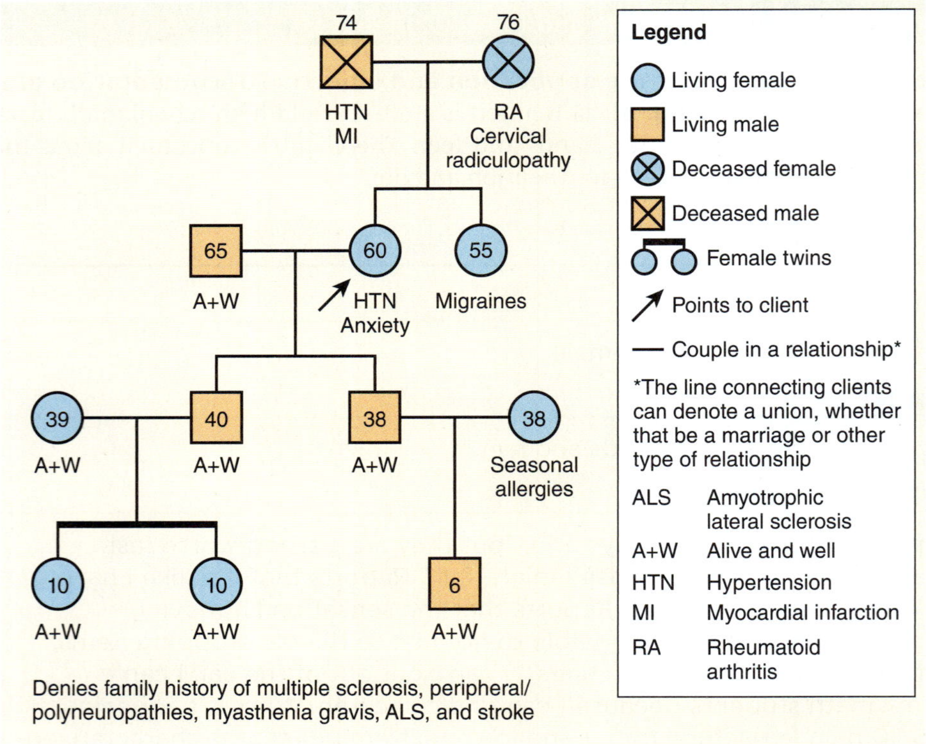

SOCIAL HISTORY

Alcohol Use Usually 0 to 1 servings a week, some weeks none. No drinking and driving, no binge drinking

Tobacco Use Denies current or prior use

Recreational Drug Use Denies

Domestic and Intimate Partner Violence Denies

Sexual Practice Heterosexual: One lifetime partner, in a monogamous relationship with husband. Denies history of sexually transmitted infections (STIs)

Travel History International travel to Europe and Caribbean for 7 days or less every other year; last trip was December 2019 before COVID

Work Environment 10th-grade honors precalculus and geometry teacher at local parochial school. There is currently no renovation occurring at the school. There has been a "bug" going around the school. Has friends/colleagues on faculty with whom client has positive relationship. No known contacts with similar symptoms

Home Environment Lives with 65 yo husband. Has comfortable home with air conditioning, security alarm system, modern appliances

Hobbies and Leisure Activities Reading, volunteers at pet shelter, plays tennis, participates in many church activities and committees

Stress Minimal—Happy at home and work. Children and grandchildren live close and visit often.

Education Master's Degree in Education

Economic Status Middle class

Military Status Denies

Religion Practicing Roman Catholic. Attends weekly Mass at local church. Client's faith is an important component of personal and family life.

Ethnic Background Identifies with Polish Catholic heritage

Roles and Relationships Wife, mother, grandmother, and sister. Many close family relationships and many friendships

Characteristic Patterns of Daily Living Works 40 hours per week at school and many hours at home grading students' papers. Socializes with friends on weekends.

HEALTH MAINTENANCE ACTIVITIES

Sleep 6 to 8 hours per night, restful and restorative; no sleep aids used until this illness

Diet Healthy, mostly whole foods, DASH/low-salt diet, avoids fast foods and sugar

Exercise Tennis 1 to 2 hours twice a week. Brisk walk 30 to 45 minutes 3 to 4 days/week

Stress Management Reading the Bible, praying, exercise, socializing, family time

Use of Safety Devices Wears seat belts, home has smoke/carbon monoxide detectors

Health Checkups Primary care every 6 months for hypertension and anxiety management

Colonoscopy (negative lesions/abnormalities, no polyps—2021)

Pap (negative for intraepithelial lesions or malignancy, negative HPV—2024),

Mammogram (gets annual mammogram, last result was in 2025; no suspicious masses or calcifications or areas of architectural distortion)

PHYSICAL EXAMINATION

Mental Status

1. Physical appearance and behavior:
   a. Posture and movements: Sitting on examination table, no demonstrated deficits
   b. Dress, grooming, and personal hygiene: Business casual clothes, clean and well-groomed
   c. Facial expression: Anxious facies
   d. Affect: Appropriate, maintains eye contact
2. Communication: Clear, fluent speech; follows instructions during examination
3. Level of consciousness: Awake, alert, and oriented; Glasgow Coma Scale score = 15
4. Cognitive abilities and mentation:
   a. Attention: Focused, on-task, interactive. Recites serial 7s accurately
   b. Memory: Intact short and longterm
   c. Judgment: Intact
   d. Insight: Appropriate, realistic
   e. Spatial perception: Intact
   f. Calculation: Intact
   g. Abstract reasoning: Intact
   h. Thought process and content: Coherent, logical
   i. Suicidal ideation: Denies

Sensory

1. Exteroceptive sensation:
   a. Light touch: Bilateral hyposensation to hands and wrists; bilateral hyposensation to legs below the knees
   b. Superficial pain: Equal and intact bilaterally
   c. Temperature: Equal and intact bilaterally
2. Proprioceptive sensation:
   a. Motion and position: Equal and intact bilaterally
   b. Vibration sense: Equal and intact bilaterally
3. Cortical sensation:
   a. Stereognosis: Absent/abnormal bilaterally
   b. Graphesthesia: Absent/abnormal bilaterally
   c. Two-point discrimination: Absent/abnormal bilateral fingers; intact bilaterally to torso
   d. Extinction: Absent/abnormal bilateral fingers; intact bilaterally to torso

Cranial Nerves

I: Smells oranges bilaterally
II: Visual acuity 20/20, visual fields by confrontation intact, no papilledema
III, IV, VI: Extraocular movements intact (EOM), pupils equally round, reactive to light and accommodation (PERRLA)
V: Temporalis and masseter muscles strong, corneal reflex intact, superficial pain and light touch present all facial areas
VII: Intact without facial asymmetry or palsy; taste deferred
VIII: No nystagmus; gross hearing intact; Weber: no lateralization; Rinne: air conduction > bone conduction (AC > BC)
IX and X: Intact gag reflex, clear speech, uvula midline; taste deferred
XI: Sternocleidomastoid and trapezius muscles strong and equal bilaterally
XII: Tongue midline, speech clear

Motor

1. Size: No muscle hypertrophy or atrophy; no involuntary movements
2. Tone: Firm and supple bilaterally
3. Strength: Bilateral upper extremities (UE) 5-/5, bilateral lower extremities (LE) 4/5
4. Involuntary movements: None
5. Pronator drift: None

Cerebellar Function

1. Coordination:
   a. Finger to nose: Intact bilaterally with eyes open and closed
   b. Rapid alternating movements: Rapid supination and pronation of the hands: intact bilaterally; heel slide: intact bilaterally
2. Station: Posture erect
3. Gait: Ambulates without assistive devices, ataxic gait, reaching for hand-holds (chair, furniture, hallway rail)
   a. Tiptoes and heel walking: Deferred
   b. Heel to toe in a straight line: Deferred
   c. Hopping on one leg: Deferred

Reflexes

Deep Tendon

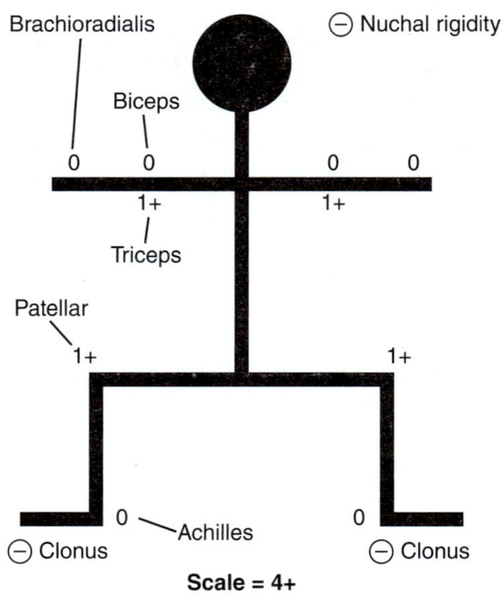

Superficial Deferred
Pathological Babinski: Absent

Advanced Technique

Romberg test: Positive with eyes open and closed
Nuchal rigidity: Absent
Brudzinski sign: Absent

LABORATORY DATA

Complete blood cell count (CBC), comprehensive metabolic panel (CMP), anc urinalysis (UA): within normal limits (WNL)

Heavy metal—negative for lead and mercury (normal results)

DIAGNOSTIC DATA

- Plain spinal X-ray imaging: Cervical, thoracic, and lumbar spines showed unremarkable alignment.
- Cervical and Lumbar MRI: Discogenic degenerative joint disease without focal spinal lesions. No foraminal or cord impingement noted.
- Lumbar Puncture for cerebrospinal fluid (CSF):
  Total protein: 180 mg/dL (normal 15 to 60 mg/dL)
  Glucose 53 mg/dL (normal: 40 to 85 mg/dL)
  Cell count 2 lymphocytes/mcL (normal: 0 to 5 lymphocytes/mcL
  RBC 0 (normal: 0)
- Electromyography (EMG) of upper extremities: Normal insertional activity with normal CMAP amplitude, mildly prolonged terminal latency, absent F-wave response. Conclusion: abnormal EMG

CLINICAL JUDGMENT IN ACTION

1. What cues indicate that the client is having a neurological disorder?
2. What interventions have the highest priority?
3. What assessment findings indicate clinical improvement or decline in this client?

Review Questions

1. A police officer and Army veteran presents for an annual physical examination. Which of the following risk factors indicate a need for specific screening for suicide risk? Select all that apply.
   a. Job/employment
   b. Healthy, low-salt diet
   c. Family history of suicide
   d. Alcohol misuse/abuse
   e. Posttraumatic stress (PTS) history

2. A 75-year-old client is brought in by a relative to discuss concerns about forgetfulness, confusion, and cognitive ability. The relative is concerned about the client losing car keys frequently and forgetting to turn off the stove. The family history includes multiple family members with dementia. Which of the following screening tools for cognition can be used to assess this client? Select all that apply.
   a. Mini-Mental State Examination (MMSE)
   b. Mini-Cog
   c. Montreal Cognitive Assessment (MoCA)
   d. Electroencephalogram (EEG)
   e. Electromyography (EMG)

3. The nurse preceptor in the Emergency Department asks the student nurse to record the Glasgow Coma Score (GCS) for a client who is evaluated following a motor vehicle accident. The student knows that the GCS score for a fully alert, oriented individual is which of the following?
   a. 18
   b. 15
   c. 12
   d. 3

4. A 54-year-old client with a history of postpartum depression should be regularly screened for what condition?
   a. Major depressive disorder
   b. Bipolar disorder
   c. Anxiety
   d. Agoraphobia

5. Which of the following clinical findings would be seen in a client experiencing a sympathetic nervous system response? Select all that apply.
   a. Pupil dilation
   b. Decreased heart rate
   c. Decreased gastric motility
   d. Bronchial constriction
   e. Decreased urine output

6. An intensive care unit (ICU) nurse is assessing the motor function of an unconscious client. The nurse should use which mechanism to test for peripheral pain response?
   a. Pressure on maxillary sinus
   b. Xiphoid process rub
   c. Squeezing the sternocleidomastoid muscle
   d. Pressure to the nailbed

7. An 87-year-old client, whose family has concerns about dementia, has difficulty identifying a familiar object (quarter) that has been placed in the hand to manipulate and handle while keeping their eyes closed. What is this abnormal finding called?
   a. Astereognosis
   b. Graphanesthesia
   c. Hypalgesia
   d. Dysesthesia

8. An 18-year-old client can frown, raise their eyebrows, and wrinkle their forehead while looking up. Which cranial nerve (CN) has the nurse evaluated?
   a. CN III
   b. CN IV
   c. CN VI
   d. CN VII

9. A 67-year-old client who takes metformin for type 2 diabetes mellitus complains of numbness and tingling on the bottom of the right foot. What is the best mechanism for the nurse to assess for nerve sensitivity and nerve damage?
   a. Babinski reflex
   b. Monofilament test
   c. Achilles reflex
   d. Romberg test

10. A 19-year-old college student lives in a dormitory with two roommates and has just completed the first semester. The client has been admitted to the hospital unit with fever, nuchal rigidity, and changes in mental status. Which meningeal assessments should the nurse conduct? Select all that apply.
    a. Kernig sign
    b. Romberg sign
    c. Tinel sign
    d. Brudzinski sign
    e. Phalen sign

CHAPTER

21 Female Genitalia

Learning Outcomes

1. Identify the anatomy and physiology of the female genitalia.
2. Describe the physiology of the female reproductive cycle.
3. Conduct a complete health history on a client with a female genitalia condition.
4. Perform a physical examination on a healthy adult client with female genitalia and on a client with female genitalia pathology.
5. Differentiate between normal clinical findings from a client's physical examination of the female genitalia and the pathophysiology of abnormal clinical findings.
6. Identify risk factors for vaginal infections.
7. Identify risk factors for female genitalia cancers.
8. Identify the Unites States Preventive Services Task Force recommendations for female genitalia.
9. Document a complete health history and physical examination on a client with a female genitalia pathology.

Assessment of the genitalia is often the last phase of a female's physical examination. The mortality rate due to cervical cancer has decreased substantially and continues to decline, from 2.8 per 100,000 females in 2000 to 2.2 per 100,000 females in 2022 (National Cancer Institute [NCI], n.d.). This decline can be attributed to early detection by physical examination and Papanicolaou tests (Pap smears) and, to a lesser extent, increased client knowledge of routine screening techniques. However, previous experiences of painful or embarrassing examinations may contribute to a client's apprehension about the examination process. By using a few commonsense techniques to diminish client discomfort and by empowering the client through education and participation in the examination, you can encourage the client in the management of their own health care. The female reproductive system is an area in which you can have a major impact on client health through routine screening, education, and integrating the client into the process of self-care.

Anatomy and Physiology

External Female Genitalia

The components of the external female genitalia are collectively referred to as the vulva. They consist of the mons pubis, labia majora, labia minora, clitoris, vulval vestibule and its glands, urethral meatus, and vaginal introitus (Fig. 21-1).

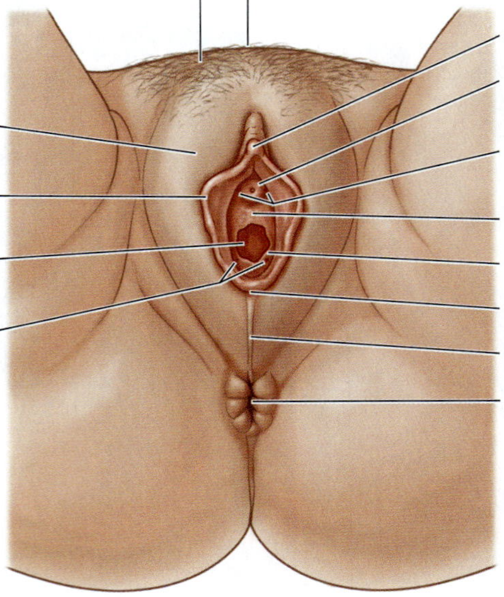

Figure 21-1 External female genitalia.

The **mons pubis** is a pad of subcutaneous fatty tissue lying over the anterior symphysis pubis. At puberty, a characteristic triangular pattern of coarse, curly hair known as the **escutcheon** develops over the mons pubis. The function of the mons pubis is to protect the pelvic bones, especially during coitus.

The **labia majora** are two longitudinal folds of adipose and connective tissue. They extend from the clitoris anteriorly and gradually narrow to merge and form the posterior commissure of the perineum. The outer surface of the labia majora becomes pigmented, wrinkled, and hairy at puberty. The inner surface is smoother, softer, and contains sebaceous glands. The function of the labia majora is to protect the vulval components that it surrounds.

Tucked within the labia majora are the **labia minora**, which enclose the vestibule. They are two thin folds of skin that extend to form the prepuce, or hood, of the clitoris anteriorly and a transverse fold of skin forming the **fourchette**, or frenulum, posteriorly. The labia minora contain sebaceous glands, erectile tissue, blood vessels, and involuntary muscle tissue, but no adipose tissue or hair follicles. The secretions of the sebaceous glands are bactericidal and aid in lubricating the vulval skin and protecting the skin from urine. Both the labia majora and the labia minora contain genital corpuscles that transmit erotic sensation.

The **clitoris** is a cylinder-shaped erectile body approximately 1 inch (2.5 cm) in length and ¼ inch (0.5 cm) in diameter, but normally less than ¾ inch (2 cm) of the body is visible on inspection. It is located at the superior aspect of the vulva and between the labia minora. The clitoris contains erectile tissue and has a significant supply of nerve endings.

The **vestibule** is the area between the two skinfolds of the labia minora. The vestibule is a boat-shaped area that contains the urethral meatus, openings of the Skene glands, hymen, openings of the Bartholin glands, and vaginal introitus.

The external urethral meatus is located in the superior aspect of the vestibule, approximately 1 inch (2.5 cm) inferior to the clitoris. It is characterized as an elongated dimple or slit. Surrounding the urethral meatus are **Skene glands**, also known as paraurethral glands, which provide lubrication to protect the skin. These tiny glands open in a posterolateral position to the urethral meatus, but they are not readily visible.

The **vaginal introitus** or orifice is situated at the inferior aspect of the vulval vestibule and is the entrance to the vagina. The size and shape of the vaginal introitus may vary. Surrounding the vaginal introitus is the **hymen**, an avascular, thin fold of connective tissue. It may be annular or crescentic in shape. The hymen may be broken by first-time sexual intercourse, strenuous physical activity, the use of tampons, masturbation, or menstruation, or it may be congenitally absent. Once the hymenal ring is perforated, small, irregular tags of tissue may be visible at the vaginal opening.

In the cleft between the labia minora and the hymenal ring lie the **Bartholin glands**, also known as the greater vestibular glands. Bartholin glands are small, pea-shaped glands located deep in the perineal structures. The ductal openings are not usually visible. The glands secrete a clear, viscid, odorless, alkaline mucus that improves the viability and motility of sperm along the female reproductive tract.

The **perineum** is located between the fourchette and the anus. Its composition of muscle, elastic fibers, fascia, and connective tissue gives it an exceptional capacity for stretching during childbirth. The **anal orifice** is located at the seam of the gluteal folds, and it serves as the exit of the gastrointestinal tract.

Internal Female Genitalia

The components of the internal female genitalia are the vagina, uterus, uterine tubes (also referred to as fallopian tubes), and ovaries (Fig. 21-2).

The **vagina** is a pink, hollow, muscular tube extending from the cervix to the vulva. It is located posterior to the bladder and anterior to the rectum, and it slopes backward at an angle of approximately 45° with the vertical plane of the body. The cervix projects into the vagina. This projection creates pouch-like recesses around the cervix. These recesses are divided into anterior, posterior, and lateral **fornices**. Abdominal organs such as the uterus, ovaries, appendix, cecum, colon, ureters, and distended bladder can be palpated through the thin walls of these fornices.

The vaginal walls consist of an outer layer of longitudinal and circular muscle fibers and a stratified squamous epithelium arranged in folds called rugae. Lactic acid is formed by the normal vaginal flora in conjunction with glycogen, which is contained in the superficial cells of the vagina. This maintains the vaginal pH and assists in the prevention of vaginal infections.

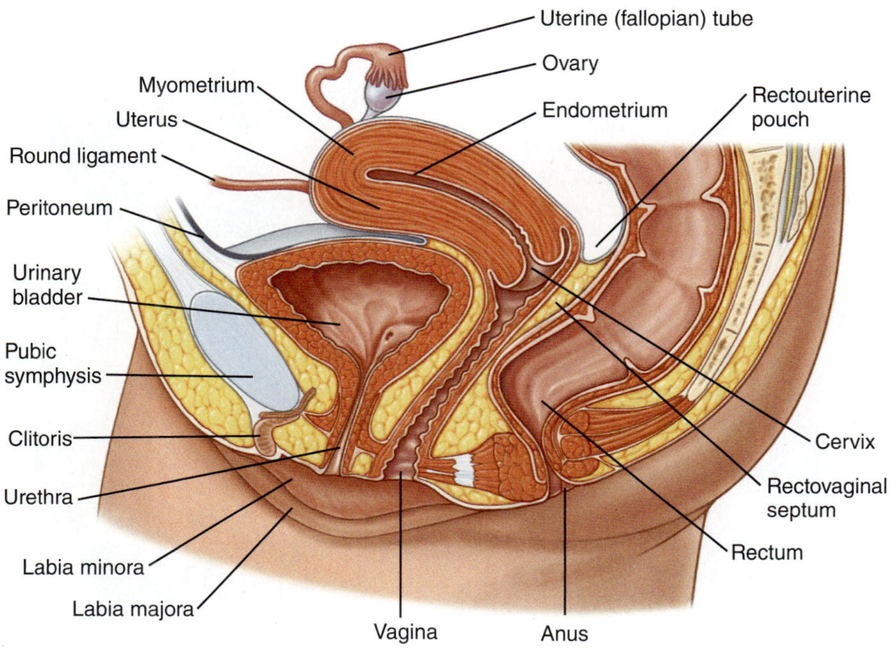

Figure 21-2 Right-sided sagittal section at the midline of internal pelvic organs.

The **uterus** is an inverted, pear-shaped, hollow, muscular organ in which an impregnated ovum develops into a fetus. The inferior aspect is the **cervix**; the superior aspect is the **fundus**. The most common position of the uterus is anteverted, but it may also be anteflexed, retroverted, retroflexed, or in a midplane position (Fig. 21-3). The mature, nonpregnant uterus weighs about 60 gm and is approximately 2¼ to 3¼ inches (5.5 to 8.0 cm) long, 1⅜ to 1⅝ inches (3.5 to 4.0 cm) wide, and ¾ to 1 inch (2.0 to 2.5 cm) thick. The uterus of a parous client, or one who has given birth, may be enlarged by ¾ to 1¼ inches (2 to 3 cm) in any of these dimensions.

Anatomically, the uterus can be divided into three parts: the body, the isthmus, and the cervix (Fig. 21-4). The body consists of the fundus, a raised, dome-shaped area on the superior portion of the uterus, and the cornu, the points of insertion of the uterine tubes. The uterine body has three layers: an outer layer of the peritoneum; a middle layer of muscle, called the myometrium; and an inner layer of columnar epithelium, mucous glands, and stroma, called the endometrium. It is this innermost layer that is shed and regenerated under normal hormonal influence during the menstrual cycle. The outer layer of the peritoneum forms a deep recess called the **rectouterine pouch**, or pouch of Douglas. It is the lowest point in the pelvic cavity and encompasses the lower posterior wall of the uterus, the upper portion of the vagina, and the intestinal surface of the rectum.

The **isthmus** is a constricted area between the body of the uterus and the cervix. The cervix is an open-ended canal approximately ¾ to 1¼ inches

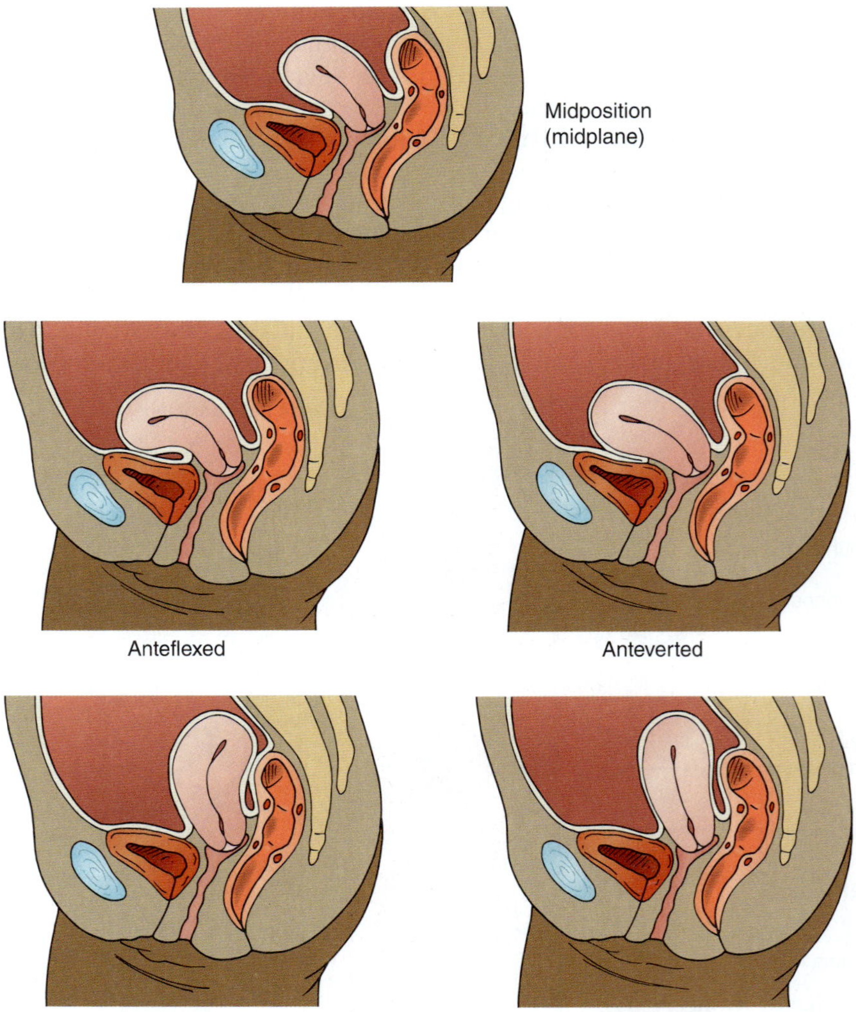

Figure 21-3 Positions of the uterus.

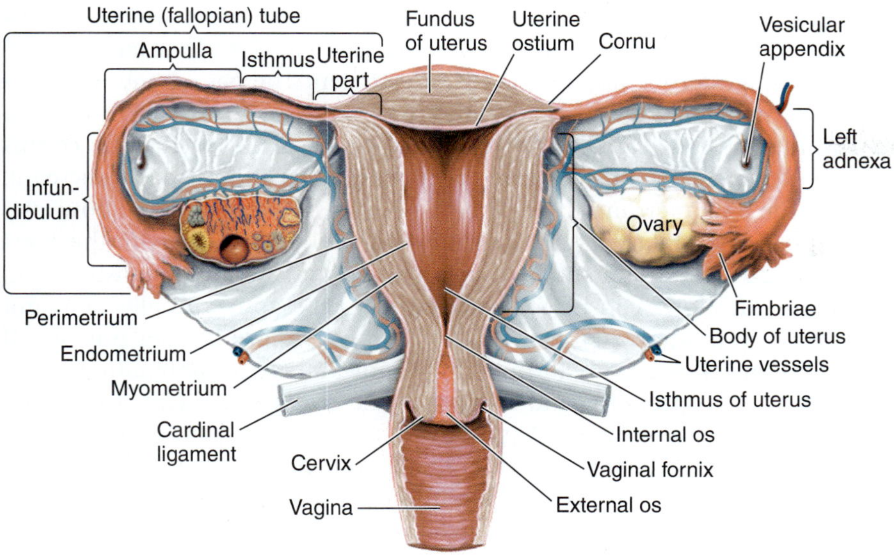

Figure 21-4 Coronal section of uterus and adnexal structures.

(2 to 3 cm) in length and diameter. Its internal os (opening) is at the isthmus and its external os extends into the vagina. The os of the **nulliparous** female, one who has not given birth, will be closed and tight. The os of a **parous** female, one who has given birth to one or more neonates, may be open by ⅜ inch (1 cm), and the orifice may be elongated and irregular. The endocervical canal is lined with mucus-secreting columnar epithelium. The ectocervix, which protrudes into the vagina, is covered with the same squamous epithelial cells that line the vagina. The point at which the two types of cells merge is the **squamocolumnar junction**. Its exact location varies with age but is clinically important because it is the point at which most cervical cancer originates.

The **adnexa** of the uterus consists of the uterine tubes, the ovaries, and their supporting ligaments. The **uterine tubes** extend from the cornu of the uterus to the ovaries and are supported by the broad ligaments. The tubes are approximately 3¼ to 5½ inches (8 to 14 cm) long. The distal, funnel-shaped end of the uterine tube is called the infundibulum. It has moving, fingerlike projections called fimbriae, which help direct ova from the ovary into the tube, where fertilization takes place. The uterine tubes are lined with ciliated squamous epithelium. The movement of the cilia and the peristaltic waves of the muscular layer of the tube propel the ovum toward the uterus, where implantation occurs.

The **ovaries** are a pair of almond-shaped glands, approximately 1¼ to 1⅝ inches (3 to 4 cm) in length, in the upper pelvic cavity. **Oogenesis**, the development and formation of an ovum, and hormonal production are the principal functions of the ovaries. The rectovaginal septum separates the rectum from the posterior aspect of the vagina.

The Female Reproductive Cycle

The female reproductive cycle consists of two interrelated cycles called the ovarian and the menstrual cycles. These cycles occur synchronously under neurohormonal control from the hypothalamus and the anterior pituitary gland.

The ovarian cycle consists of two phases: the follicular phase and the luteal phase. During the follicular phase, the actions of the follicle-stimulating hormone (FSH) and the luteinizing hormone (LH) from the anterior pituitary gland stimulate the ripening of one ovarian follicle called the Graafian follicle. The remaining follicles are suppressed by LH. Ovulation occurs when high levels of LH cause the release of the ovum from the Graafian follicle.

NURSING TIP

Client Education on the Reproductive Cycle

Educating the client about the reproductive cycle and its effects on the body will help the client to better understand the body's functioning and will assist the client in planning for gynecological examinations and birth control measures. The cervical mucus becomes clearer, thinner, and threadlike, indicating the onset of ovulation. The client can perform a **spinnbarkeit** test, the point at which the mucus can be drawn to a maximal length, by stretching vaginal mucus between the thumb and index finger. Tell the client it is normal to feel low abdominal or flank pain when the ovum is released during ovulation. A rise in basal body temperature indicates that ovulation has occurred. Spotting may also be present after ovulation.

During the luteal phase, LH stimulates the development of the corpus luteum. This yellow pigment that fills the Graafian follicle produces high levels of progesterone and low levels of estrogen. The basal body temperature rises, indicating that ovulation has occurred.

The menstrual cycle begins if implantation does not occur. The corpus luteum degenerates and the levels of progesterone and estrogen decrease, causing the endometrium to degenerate and shed. The menstrual flow lasts from 2 to 7 days and the cycles continue every 25 to 34 days, with the average being 28 days. The first day of the cycle is the first day of menstruation. The menstrual flow consists of blood and mucus and normally does not exceed 150 mL. Menstrual blood lacks fibrin; therefore, it does not clot. If clots do occur, they usually form in the vagina and are a combination of red blood cells, glycoproteins, and mucus. Cyclic changes associated with the menstrual cycle are shown in Figure 21-5.

The proliferative phase of the menstrual cycle occurs when the endometrial lining begins to regenerate under the influence of estrogen. Changes in the cervical mucosa also occur during this phase. The cervical mucus becomes clearer, thinner, and threadlike.

If conception and implantation of the fertilized ovum occur, the corpus luteum is maintained by the presence of human chorionic gonadotropin (HCG), which is secreted by the implanting blastocyst. HCG is the hormone tested in at-home pregnancy kits.

The female reproductive cycle begins at **menarche**, the onset of menstruation, which occurs between 9 and 16 years of age and ends at menopause, which occurs between 45 and 55 years of age. The onset of puberty, which

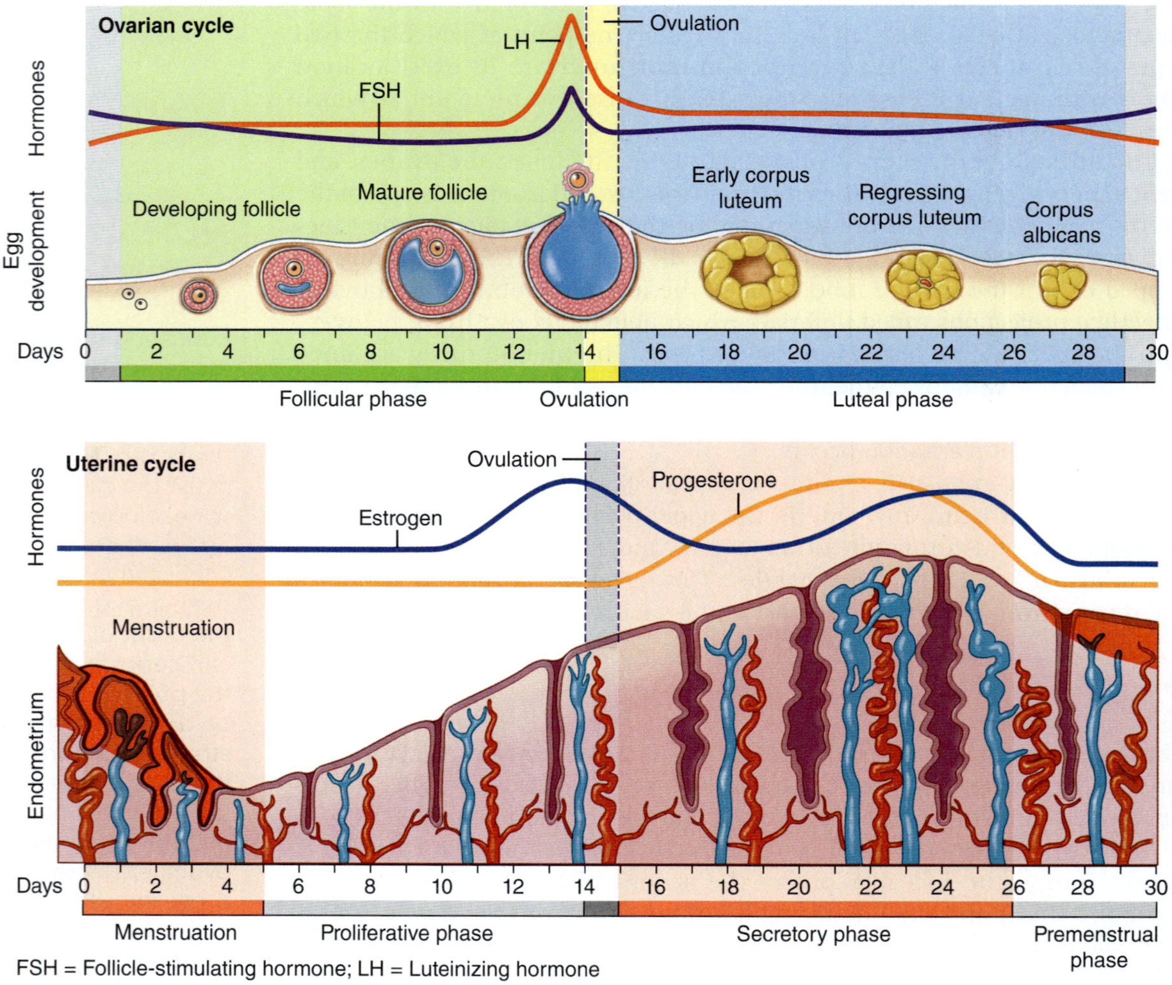

Figure 21-5 Cyclic changes associated with the menstrual cycle.

occurs between the ages of 8 and 9, is marked by significant increases in estrogen production and the development of secondary sex characteristics such as breast enlargement, hair distribution on the mons pubis, and contour changes of the hips and abdomen. Tanner stages of pubic hair development provide objective criteria for the evaluation of developmental changes in the appearance of female genitalia (Table 21-1).

Table 21-1 Sexual Maturity Rating (SMR) for Female Genitalia

Developmental Stage	Description
Stage 1 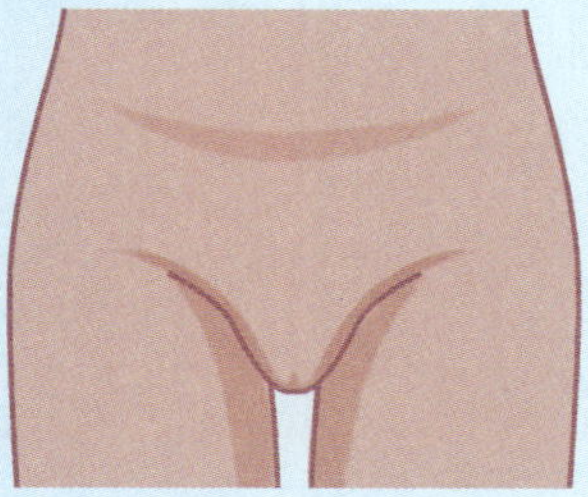	**Preadolescent Stage** (before age 8) No pubic hair, only body hair (vellus hair)
Stage 2 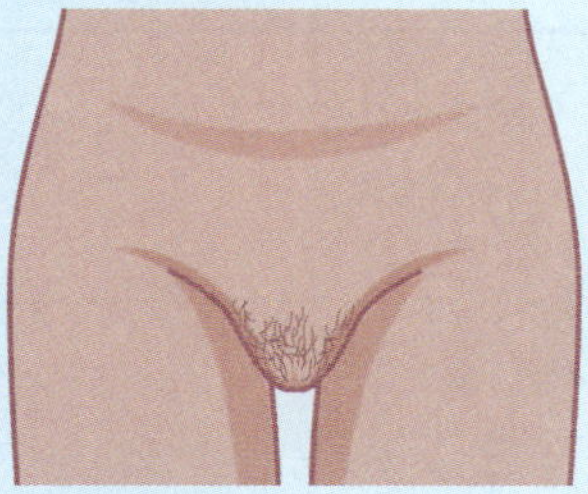	**Early Adolescent Stage** (ages 8 to 12) Sparse growth of long, slightly dark, fine pubic hair, slightly curly and located along the labia
Stage 3 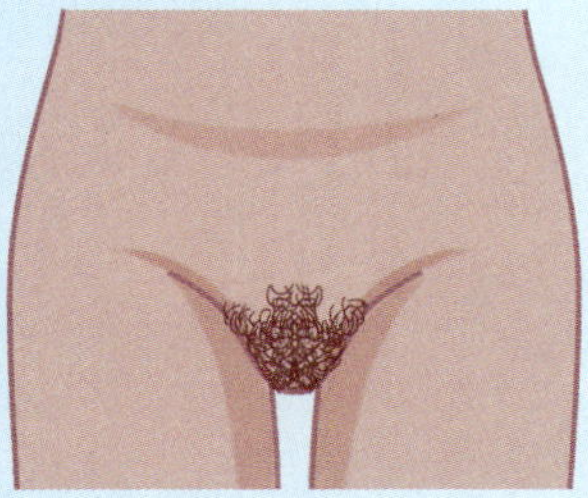	**Adolescent Stage** (ages 12 to 13) Pubic hair becomes darker, curlier, and spreads over the symphysis
Stage 4 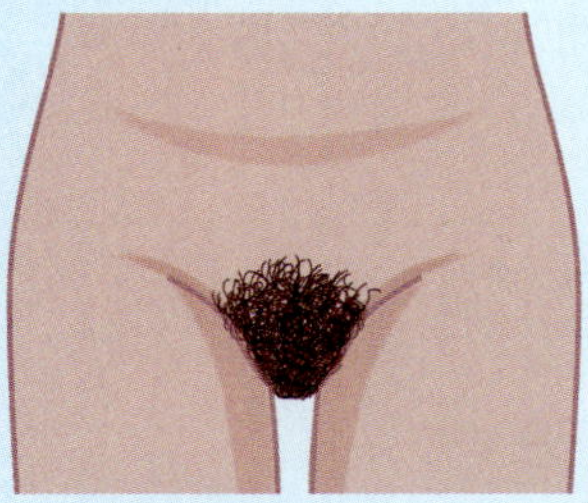	**Late Adolescent Stage** (ages 13 to 15) Texture and curl of pubic hair is similar to that of an adult but not spread to thighs
Stage 5 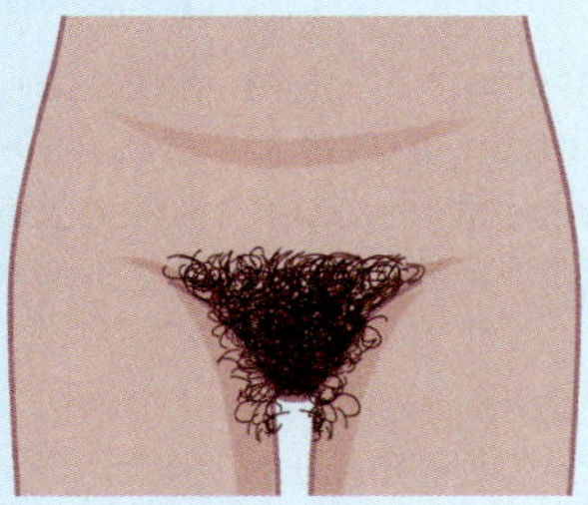	**Adult Stage** Adult appearance in quality and quantity of pubic hair; growth is spread to inner aspect of thighs and abdomen

NURSING TIP

Late Onset of Menarche

Late onset of menarche can result from a multiplicity of pathologies. If you encounter a client who has not experienced the onset of menstruation by 16 years of age or 14 years of age when secondary sex characteristics are present, this is called primary amenorrhea. Evaluate the client for the following:

1. Pregnancy
2. Inadequate nutrition or eating disorders
3. Chronic diseases such as Crohn disease, thyroid disease
4. Environmental stressors
5. Intensive athletic training (refer to Chapter 19 for a discussion of Relative Energy Deficiency in Sports (RED-S)
6. Use of opiates or steroids
7. Polycystic ovary syndrome
8. Autoimmune diseases
9. Anatomical obstruction to menstrual flow
10. Genetic or chromosomal syndromes
11. Hypothalamic-pituitary-ovarian axis disorders

HEALTH HISTORY

The female genitalia health history provides insight into the link between a client's life/lifestyle and female genitalia information and pathology.

CLIENT PROFILE

Diseases that are age-and race-specific for the female genitalia are listed.

Age Sexually transmitted infections (STIs) (increased incidence 15 to 24)
Uterine leiomyomas (30 to 50)
Cervical cancer (>35)
Endometrial cancer (50 to 60)
Ovarian cancer (postmenopause)
Vaginal cancer (>70)
Vulvar cancer (>70)
Uterine prolapse (postmenopause)
Cystocele (postmenopause)
Rectocele (postmenopause)
Atrophic vaginitis (postmenopause)

Race Leiomyomas (fibroids) are more common in Black females
Ethnicity (mutilation of the female genitalia, or cutting, is still practiced in some African nations)

CHIEF COMPLAINT

Common chief complaints for the female genitalia are defined, and information on the characteristics of each sign or symptom is provided.

1. Uterine Bleeding The presence of bleeding from the endometrium

Quality Odor, consistency, color, clotting

Quantity Amount (number and size of tampons or pads used in 24 hr), duration, and frequency of flow

Associated Manifestations Abdominal pain or cramping, passage of clots or tissue

Aggravating Factors Stress, anxiety, nonsteroidal anti-inflammatory drugs (NSAIDs) (e.g., aspirin, ibuprofen, naproxen), rapid weight loss or gain, obesity, sexual intercourse

Alleviating Factors Medications (e.g., NSAIDs, narcotics), dilation and curettage, surgery

Setting Traumatic abortion or dilation and curettage

Timing Relationship to menses (intermenstrual, oligomenorrhea, polymenorrhea, menometrorrhagia, metrorrhagia); use of intrauterine device (IUD); perimenopausal

2. **Vaginal Discharge** Discharge of fluid from the vagina
   Quality Color, consistency, odor
   Quantity Number and size of tampons or pads used in 24 hours
   Associated Manifestations Itching, presence of discharge in sexual partner, **dyspareunia** (painful sexual intercourse), dysuria, abdominal pain or cramping, spotting, rash on genitalia
   Aggravating Factors Tight pants, wet bathing suits, antibiotics, oral contraceptive pills (OCPs) (birth control pills), diet, pregnancy, deodorant tampons, bubble baths, chemical douches, lubricated condoms, contraceptive creams, pre-existing disease such as diabetes mellitus, increased number of sexual partners, semen, vaginal films, latex products
   Alleviating Factors Position, loose-fitting pants, cotton underpants, pantyhose with cotton crotch, medication
   Timing Postcoitus, while taking antibiotics
3. **Urinary Symptoms** Changes in the normal voiding pattern and characteristics of the urine
   Quality Color: straw, amber; microscopic or macroscopic hematuria
   Consistency: clear, cloudy; presence of particles; odor
   Quantity Polyuria, oliguria, or anuria
   Associated Manifestations Flank pain, abdominal pain or cramping, dysuria, abdominal distention, vaginal discharge, urgency and frequency in voiding, stress incontinence, pneumaturia, fever
   Aggravating Factors Douches, intravaginal devices, traumatic coitus, alcohol, caffeine, spices, delaying urination
   Alleviating Factors Medication, warm baths, hydration
   Setting Postcoitus, nocturia, use of unclean sex devices
   Timing At beginning, throughout, or end of stream
4. **Pelvic Pain** The subjective sense of discomfort in the pelvis
   Quality Stabbing, burning, cramping, aching, throbbing, drawing, pulling
   Associated Manifestations Abdominal distention, pelvic fullness, vaginal discharge or bleeding, gastrointestinal symptoms, menstruation, fever, ectopic pregnancy, urinary incontinence, pelvic inflammatory disease (PID)
   Aggravating Factors Exercise, sexual activity, cultural perception
   Alleviating Factors Rest, medication, surgery, heating pad, NSAIDs
   Setting During coitus, ovulation
   Timing Sudden or gradual onset, association with activity, duration, recurrence, relation to menstrual cycle

PAST HEALTH HISTORY

The various components of the past health history are linked to female genitalia pathology and female genitalia-related information.

Medical History

Female Genitalia Specific See Table 21-2

Nonfemale Genitalia Specific Diabetes mellitus, thyroid disease, incontinence, constipation, urinary tract infections (UTIs)

Surgical History Hysterectomy, myomectomy, salpingectomy, oophorectomy, dilation and curettage, laparoscopy, vulvectomy, tubal ligation, colpotomy, cesarean section, colposcopy, cryotherapy, uterine cryoablation, hysteroscopy

Allergies Numerous feminine hygiene products may cause allergic reactions or increase the incidence of *Candida* vaginosis. Be aware of any latex allergies; condoms and diaphragms are usually made of latex. The spermicide nonoxynol 9 may also cause allergic reactions.

Medications Antibiotics may increase incidence of *Candida* vaginosis and lessen the effectiveness of OCPs; hormonal contraception (oral, patch, vaginal ring, injection, IUD); emergency contraception; hormone replacement therapy (HRT) (oral, transdermal, topical gel, vaginal cream/ring/inserts)

Communicable Diseases STI: Gonorrhea, syphilis, herpes, HIV, hepatitis, *Chlamydia,* human papillomavirus, hepatitis B and C, Mpox, trichomoniasis, chancroid, molluscum contagiosum

Injuries and Accidents Abdominal trauma, rape, sexual abuse, vaginal trauma or injuries, pelvic fractures, lumbosacrococcygeal injuries

Differing Abilities Paraplegic and quadriplegic clients are at increased obstetric risk depending on level of injury, tone of uterus, and competency of cervix

Childhood Illnesses Fetal diethylstilbestrol (DES) exposure

Immunizations Human papillomavirus vaccine

FAMILY HEALTH HISTORY

Familial female genitalia diseases are listed.

Cervical, endometrial, and ovarian cancers, mother received DES while pregnant with client, transfer of STIs during delivery, placental transfer of hepatitis B virus and hepatitis C virus, HIV, multiple pregnancies, congenital anomalies

SOCIAL HISTORY

The components of the social history are linked to female genitalia factors and pathology.

Alcohol Use There is a significant positive correlation between alcohol use and date rape in the college-aged population

Tobacco Use There is an increased incidence of stroke and thrombotic events in females who concurrently smoke and use hormonal therapy. Smoking is a risk factor for cervical, vaginal, and vulvar cancers.

Recreational Drug Use Recreational drug use can impair cognitive function leading to increased sexual promiscuity, STIs, and HIV

Sexual Practice Sexual favors may be exchanged for narcotics, leading to increased rates of STIs. Prostitution increases the risk of STIs, HIV, hepatitis, Mpox, and cervical carcinoma (an increase in the number of partners increases the risk of human papillomavirus, which can lead to dysplasia and possible cervical cancer).

Home Environment Poor sanitation may lead to numerous forms of vaginitis and infections; overcrowding is an ideal condition for mite infestation

Hobbies and Leisure Activities Wearing wet bathing suits, sweaty workout clothes, or tight nylon underwear for extended periods may increase the likelihood of *Candida* vaginosis.

Strenuous equestrian sports and off-road cycling increase the likelihood of external genitalia trauma from saddle injuries. Female athletes may suffer from **amenorrhea** (absent menses).

Stress Stress can have significant effects on menstruation, causing amenorrhea and exacerbating genital herpes simplex

HEALTH MAINTENANCE ACTIVITIES

This information provides a bridge between health maintenance activities and female genitalia function.

Sleep Lack of sleep or extreme fatigue can lead to amenorrhea

Diet Increased levels of refined sugars, salt, and caffeine enhance PMS symptomatology. Extreme dieting can affect menstruation and lead to amenorrhea. Elevated sugar and lactose can lead to vaginal candidiasis. High-fat diet and obesity are risk factors for cervical, endometrial, and ovarian cancers.

Exercise Exercise may diminish **dysmenorrhea** (pain or cramping during menses) and **menorrhagia** (heavy menses)

Use of Safety Devices Condom use

Health Checkups Date of last Pap smear and results, HIV status, HPV status, hepatitis status, last STI screen, pessary check

Table 21-2 Female Reproductive Health History

Female Reproductive Health History	Information Collected
Menstrual History	• Age of menarche • Last menstrual period (LMP) • Length of cycle • Regularity of cycle • Duration of menses • Irregularities: amenorrhea, menorrhagia, dysmenorrhea, spotting, or missed menses • Presence of clots or vaginal pooling • Number and type of tampons or pads used
Medical History	• Vaginal infections/STIs • Yeast infections • Salpingitis • Endometritis/endometriosis • Pelvix inflammatory disease (PID) • Toxic shock syndrome • Pelvic pain • Cervicitis • Uterine fibroids/uterine prolapse • Ovarian cysts/polycystic ovary syndrome • Cancer of the reproductive organs • Infertility • Pap smear records
Obstetric History	See Chapter 24.
Premenstrual Syndrome (PMS)	• Duration of symptoms (occur 3–7 days before the onset of menses, with cessation of symptoms after second day of cycle) • Symptoms: breast tenderness; bloating; moodiness; cravings for salt, sugar, or chocolate; fatigue; weight gain; headaches; joint pain; nausea and vomiting
Menopause History	• Date of LMP • Beginning of menopause (1 year from LMP) • Postmenopausal spotting • Associated symptoms of menopause (such as hot flashes, palpitations, numbness, tingling, drenching sweats, mood swings, vaginal dryness, itching) • Treatment for symptoms (including estrogen replacement therapy) • Feelings about menopause
Vaginal Discharge	See Chief Complaint section and Table 21-3.
History of Uterine Bleeding	See Chief Complaint section.
Sexual Functioning	• Sexual preference for partner • Number of partners in lifetime • Number of current partners • Sexual desire • Satisfaction with sex life • Dyspareunia • Inorgasmia
Method of Birth Control	• Type of birth control currently using, if any • Types of birth control previously used and satisfaction • Frequency of use • Satisfaction with birth control • STI prevention methods • Problems with birth control or STI-prevention methods (reaction to the spermicides used with the vaginal sponges, diaphragms, and condoms)

NURSING CHECKLIST

General Approach to Female Genitalia Examination

Before the Examination

1. Observe Standard Precautions and don Personal Protective Equipment (PPE) such as gloves, gown, face shield, goggles, N-95 respirator mask or face mask if the client's status warrants these protective measures.
2. Ensure that the client will not be menstruating at the time of the examination, for optimal cytological specimen collection.
3. Instruct the client not to use vaginal sprays, to douche, or to have coitus 24 to 48 hours before the scheduled physical examination. The products of coitus and commercial sprays and douches may affect the Pap smear and other vaginal cultures.
4. Encourage the client to express any anxieties and concerns about the physical examination. Reassure the client by acknowledging anxieties and validating concerns. Remind the client that they are in control during the examination and that you will not proceed until they are comfortable. Virgins need reassurance that the pelvic examination should not affect the hymen.
5. Informed consent should be obtained.
6. Show the speculum and other equipment to the client and allow them to touch and explore any items that do not have to remain sterile. Answer any questions the client may have.
7. Inform the client that the examination should not be painful, but may be uncomfortable at times, and tell the client to inform you if they experience any pain.
8. Instruct the client to empty the bladder before the procedure.
9. The client should undress from the waist to the ankles and cover with a sheet/drape to maintain modesty. The client should remain draped until properly positioned.
10. Ensure that the room is warm enough to prevent chilling and provide additional draping material as necessary.
11. Place drapes or sheepskin over the foot stirrups to increase client comfort. If one is available, provide a pillow for the client's neck.
12. Have the client lie on their back on the examination table in the dorsal lithotomy position. Have the client place their feet in the foot supports and scoot down until the thighs are roughly perpendicular to the ground. The client's buttocks should be at the edge of the table.
13. Ensure that privacy will be maintained during the examination. Provide screens and a closed door.
14. Warm your hands with warm water before gloving.
15. Don clean gloves.
16. Warm the speculum with warm water or a warming device before insertion.

During the Examination

1. Inform the client of what you are going to do before you do it. Explain that the client may feel pressure when the speculum is opened and a pinching sensation when the Pap smear is done.
2. Adopt a nonjudgmental and supportive attitude.
3. Maintain eye contact with the client as much as possible to reinforce a caring relationship.
4. Provide the client with a mirror to see what you are doing and to educate the client about the body. Help the client with positioning the mirror during the examination so they will feel comfortable using this technique at home to inspect the genitalia.
5. Offer the client the opportunity to ask questions about the body and sexuality.
6. Encourage the client to use relaxation techniques such as deep breathing or guided imagery to prevent muscle tension during the examination.

After the Examination

1. Offer tissues with which to wipe away excess lubricant.
2. Assess whether the client needs assistance in dressing.
3. After the client is dressed, discuss the experience, invite questions and comments, listen carefully, and supply information regarding the examination.
4. Instruct the client on how the results of any laboratory tests that were performed will be communicated.
5. Explain that the client may experience a small amount of spotting following the Pap smear.

Assessment in Brief

Female Genitalia Examination

Inspection of the External Genitalia

- Pubic hair
- Skin color and condition
  - Mons pubis and vulva
- Clitoris
- Urethral meatus
- Vaginal introitus
- Perineum and anus

Palpation of the External Genitalia

- Labia
- Urethral meatus and Skene glands
- Vaginal introitus
- Perineum

Speculum Examination of the Internal Genitalia

- Cervix
  - Color
  - Position
  - Size
  - Surface characteristics
  - Discharge
  - Shape of the cervical os

Collecting Specimens for Cytological Smears and Cultures

- Pap smear
  - Endocervical smear
  - Cervical smear
- Chlamydia culture specimen
- Gonococcal culture specimen
- Saline mount or "wet prep"
- KOH prep
- Five percent acetic acid wash
- Anal culture

Inspection of the Vaginal Wall

- Color
- Texture

Bimanual Examination

- Vagina
- Cervix
- Fornices
- Uterus
- Adnexa

Rectovaginal Examination

- Rectal wall and rectovaginal septum texture
- Anal sphincter tone

NURSING TIP

Maintaining Gynecological Health

Encourage the client to adopt healthy gynecological practices:

1. Avoid douches and feminine hygiene sprays or films, or use sparingly because both products disrupt the natural vaginal flora and increase the vaginal pH.
2. Do not leave tampons in the vagina for longer than 8 hours at a time because of the increased risk of toxic shock syndrome.
3. Always wash and wipe the vaginal area from front to back to prevent contamination of the vagina and urethra with fecal material.
4. Thoroughly wash diaphragms, menstrual cups, pessaries (devices used to maintain the position of the uterus/bladder), and sexual aid devices before and after each use.
5. If using an intrauterine device (IUD) for birth control, perform monthly string checks.
6. Void immediately after coitus.

Equipment

Assemble items before placing the client on the examination table; materials should be arranged in order of use and within easy reach.

- Appropriate PPE
- Examination table with stirrups
- Stool, preferably mounted on wheels
- Large hand mirror
- Gooseneck lamp
- Clean gloves
- Linens for draping
- Vaginal specula (Fig. 21-6):
  - Graves' bivalve specula, sizes medium and large, useful for most adult sexually active females
  - Pederson bivalve specula, sizes small and medium, useful for non-sexually active females, children, menopausal females
- Cytological materials (Fig. 21-7):
  - Ayre spatulas
  - Cervical broom
  - Cytobrushes

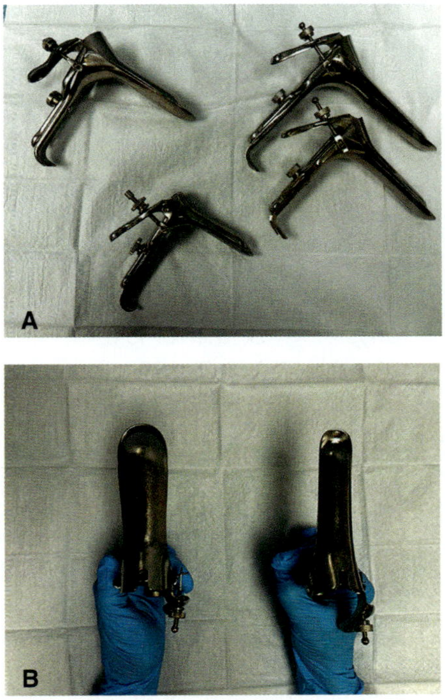

Figure 21-6 Vaginal specula. **A.** Lateral view. **B.** Superior view. Graves speculum (left), Pederson speculum (right).

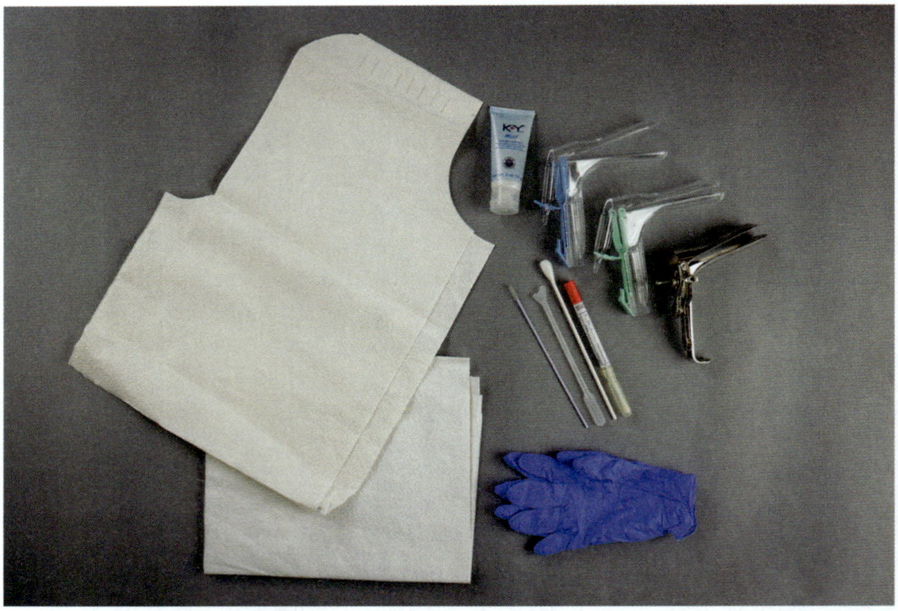

Figure 21-7 Materials needed for gynecological examination.

- Sterile cotton swabs/sterile culture tubes
- Liquid-based cytology vials
- Microscope slides, cover slips, culture probes labeled with the client's name, identification number, and date specimen was collected
- Cytology fixative spray, if not using liquid-based cytology
- Reagents: normal saline solution, potassium hydroxide (KOH), acetic acid (white vinegar)

- Warm water
- Water-soluble lubricant
- pH test tape
- Urine specimen cup for STI testing
- Microscope

NURSING TIP

Preparing for a Gynecological Examination

If you are a novice nurse or if you have not performed a gynecological examination:

- Ask another nurse to assist you with the first few examinations.
- Familiarize yourself with the equipment. Practice opening and closing the speculum. Plastic specula make significant audible clicking sounds when opening and closing, so you should prepare the client for this occurrence.
- Review the anatomy and physiology of the female genitalia; visualize the underlying structures of the anatomical landmarks.
- Review and practice any procedures to be done. Some nurses find it difficult to prepare slides and cultures without assistance if they are novices to these procedures.
- Know your institution's policies regarding the option of having a female nurse present if a male nurse is performing the gynecological examination.

Examination of the Female Genitalia

Examination of the female reproductive system consists of inspection and palpation only and includes an examination of the abdomen (see Chapter 18), an inspection of the external genitalia, palpation of the external genitalia, speculum examination of the internal genitalia, collection of specimens for laboratory analysis, an inspection of the vaginal walls, bimanual examination, and rectovaginal examination (see Chapter 23 for the complete rectal examination). The examination process requires somewhat uncomfortable positioning for the client; therefore, it should be completed as quickly and as efficiently as possible.

Inspection of the External Genitalia

1. Instruct the client to first sit on the examination table between the stirrups, facing away from the head of the table.
2. With the client seated, place a drape over the client's torso and thighs until positioning is completed.
3. Assist the client in assuming a dorsal recumbent or lithotomy position on the examination table. Assist the client in placing their heels in the stirrups, thus abducting their legs and flexing their hips.

4. Assist the client to move their buttocks down to the lower end of the examination table so that the buttocks are flush with the edge of the table. If the client desires, raise the head of the examination table slightly to elevate the head and shoulders. Provide a pillow for neck support. This position allows you to maintain eye contact with the client and prevents abdominal muscle tension (Fig. 21-8).
5. Readjust the drape to cover the abdomen, thighs, and knees; adjust the stirrups as necessary for client comfort. Push the drape down between the client's knees so you can see the client's face.
6. Sit on a stool at the foot of the examination table facing the client's external genitalia.
7. Adjust your lighting source and provide the client with a mirror. Before you touch the client's genitalia, explain how to hold the mirror to view the examination.
8. Remember to inform the client of each step of the examination process before it is performed, and be gentle.
9. Don clean gloves.

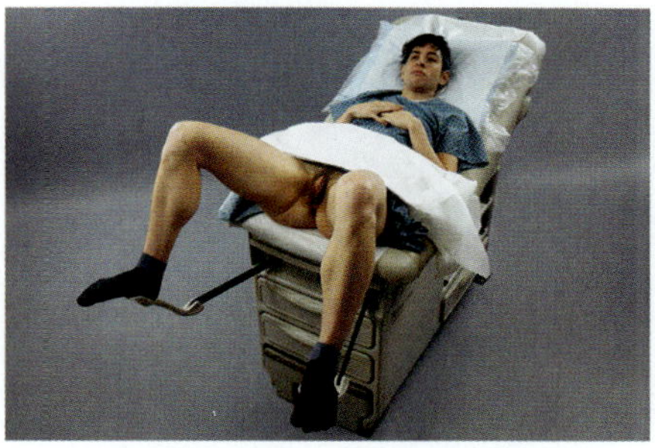

Figure 21-8 Client positioning and draping for gynecological examination.

NURSING TIP

Positional Variations for the Gynecological Examination

If a client has difficulty assuming the lithotomy position because of illness or disability, place the client in a left lateral or Sims position with the buttocks near the edge of the examination table and with the right knee flexed. Remember to limit questioning of the client in this position or the lithotomy position, because these positions often cause discomfort and embarrassment.

Pubic Hair

E 1. Observe the pattern of pubic hair distribution.
2. Note the presence of nits or lice.

N **The distribution of the female pubic hair should be shaped like an inverse triangle. There may be some growth on the abdomen and upper inner thighs. A diamond-shaped pattern from the umbilicus may be due to cultural or familial differences. There are no nits or lice.**

A A diamond-shaped pattern from the umbilicus, not associated with cultural or familial differences, is abnormal.

P A diamond-shaped pattern of pubic hair not associated with cultural or familial differences can occur with hirsutism, which is indicative of an endocrine disorder.

A Hair distribution is sparse or hair is absent at the genitalia area. This is called **alopecia,** and it is abnormal.

P Alopecia in the genital area may result from genetic factors, aging, or local or systemic disease. These include developmental defects and hereditary disorders, infection, neoplasms, physical or chemical agents, endocrine diseases, deficiency states (nutritional or metabolic), destruction, damage to the follicles, and obesity. *Note:* This variant may be expected if the client shaves or waxes this region.

A The presence of nits or lice is abnormal.

P Pubic lice (pediculosis pubis) is the infestation of the hairy regions of the body, usually the pubic area (Fig. 21-9), but it sometimes involves the hairy aspects of the abdomen, chest, and axillae.

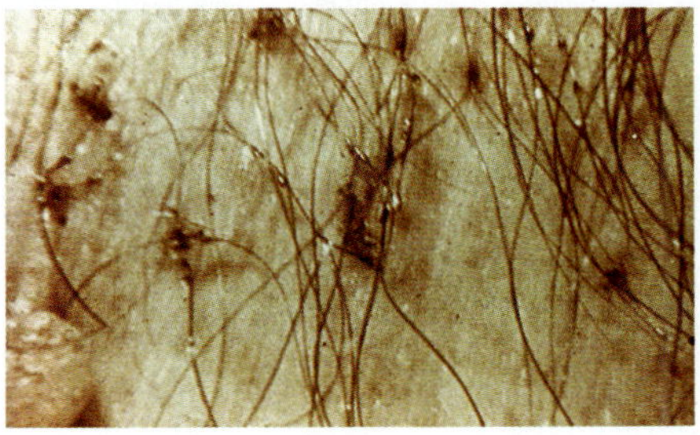

Figure 21-9 Pubic lice.

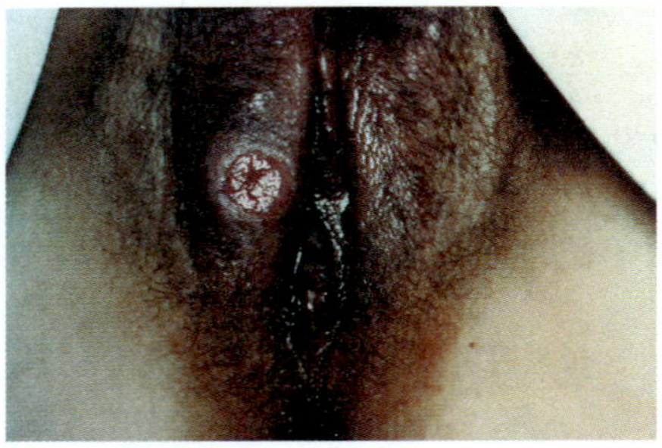

Figure 21-10 Syphilitic chancre.

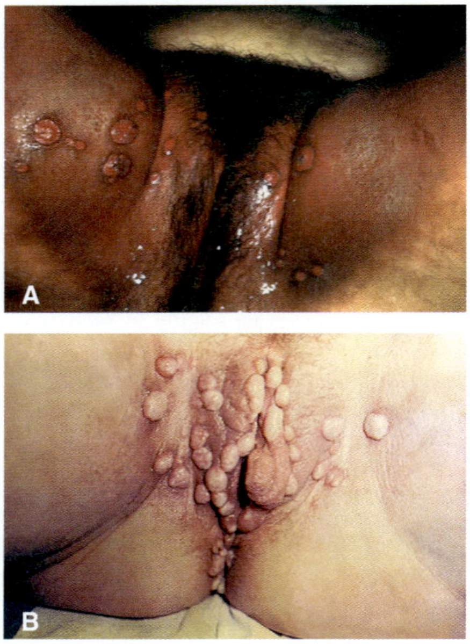

Figure 21-11 Condyloma latum in secondary syphilis. **A.** Note the raised, wart-like papules. **B.** Note the red-rimmed papules in the vulvar and anal regions.

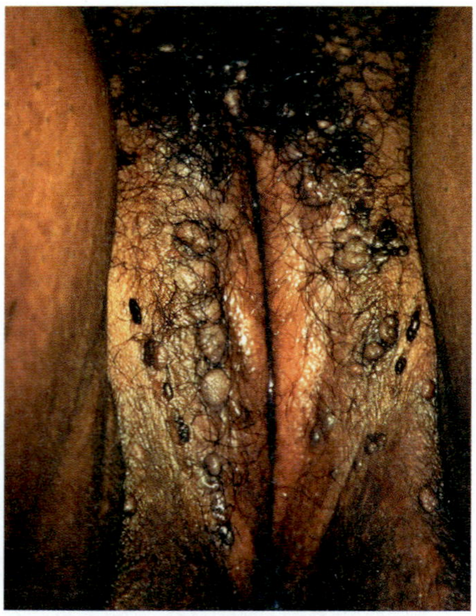

Figure 21-12 Genital warts (condyloma acuminatum).

Skin Color and Condition

Mons Pubis and Vulva

E
1. Observe the skin coloration and condition of the mons pubis and vulva.
2. Inform the client that you will touch the inside of their thigh before you touch the genitals.
3. With gloved hands, separate the labia majora using the thumb and index finger of the dominant hand.
4. Observe both the labia majora and the labia minora for coloration, lesions, or trauma.

N **The skin over the mons pubis should be clear except for nevi and normal hair distribution. The labia majora and minora should appear symmetrical with a smooth to somewhat wrinkled, unbroken, slightly pigmented skin surface. There should be no ecchymosis, excoriation, nodules, swelling, rash, or lesions. An occasional sebaceous cyst is within normal limits. These cysts are nontender, yellow nodules that are less than 1 cm in diameter.**

A Ecchymosis over the mons pubis or labia is abnormal.

P Ecchymosis over the mons pubis or labia may be due to blunt trauma from an accident or intentional abuse.

A Edema or swelling of the labia is an abnormal finding.

P Edema or swelling of the labia may be due to hematoma formation, Bartholin cyst, or obstruction of the lymphatic system.

A Broken areas on the skin surface are abnormal.

P Broken areas on the skin surface may be due to ulcerations or abrasions secondary to infection or trauma.

A Rash over the mons pubis and labia is abnormal.

P Rashes have multiple etiologies, including viral eruption, bacterial infection, contact dermatitis, and infestations.

A A nontender, reddish, round ulcer with a depressed center, and raised, indurated edges (**chancre**) is an abnormal finding (Fig. 21-10).

P A chancre appears during the primary stages of syphilis at the site where the *Treponema* enters the body. The chancre lasts for 4 weeks and then disappears.

A Flat or raised, round, wartlike papules that have moist surfaces covered by gray exudate (condyloma latum) are abnormal (Fig. 21-11).

P Condyloma latum lesions can occur during the secondary stage of syphilis.

A White, dry, cauliflower-like growths that have narrow bases are suggestive of condyloma acuminatum (Fig. 21-12) and are abnormal.

P Condyloma acuminatum warts are caused by the human papillomavirus and may be dysplastic.

A Small, swollen, red vesicles that fuse to form a large, burning ulcer that may be painful and itch (Fig. 21-13) are abnormal.

P Small, swollen, red vesicles that fuse to form large, burning ulcers are indicative of the herpes simplex virus (HSV). Primary HSV (or genital herpes) outbreaks can last up to 21 days. Recurrent HSV outbreaks are usually shorter in duration and last about 2 weeks. Serological

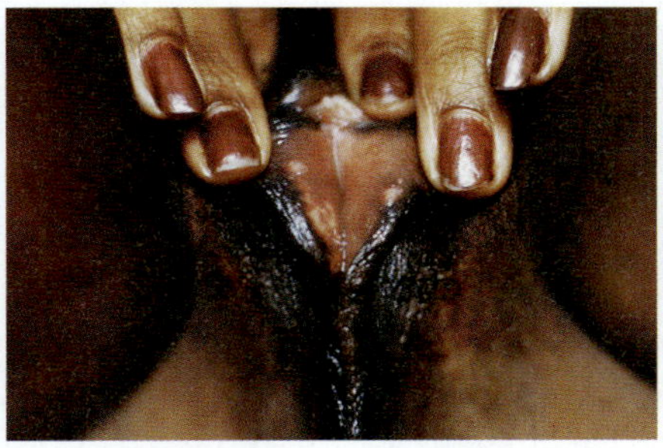

Figure 21-13 Genital herpes simplex virus. Gloves should always be worn when examining the genitalia.

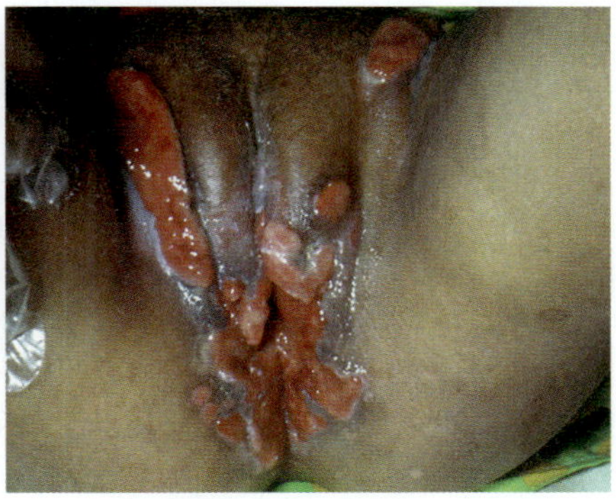

Figure 21-14 Granuloma inguinale.

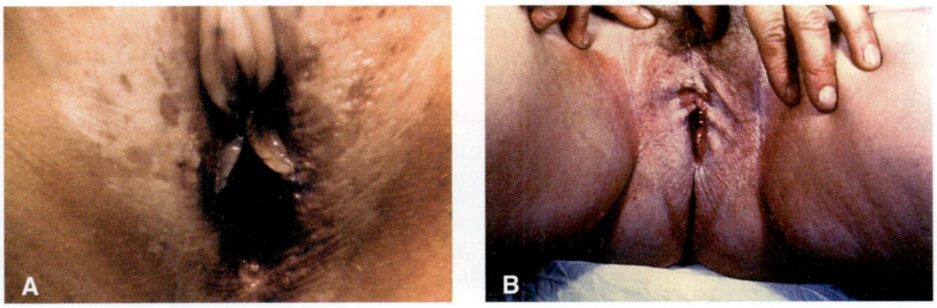

Figure 21-15 Lichen sclerosus. **A.** Early stage lichen sclerosus. **B.** Later stage lichen sclerosus. Gloves should always be worn when examining the genitalia.

testing can be performed to determine whether an eruption is HSV-1 or HSV-2.

A Firm, painless, papular, granular lesions that are beefy red are abnormal (Fig. 21-14).

P Granuloma inguinale is caused by the bacteria *Calymmatobacterium granulomatis*. It is also referred to as donovanosis and granuloma venereum. This STI tends to occur on the external genitalia, inguinal region, and anus.

A Small, white spots that are shiny and smooth may later grow into bigger patches, causing bright red or purple bruises are abnormal.

P Small, white, shiny, smooth spots that grow into bigger patches, causing bright red or purple bruises may be lichen sclerosus (Fig. 21-15). Lichen sclerosus is due to an overactive immune system. Hormonal issues may also play a role.

A Small white, pink, or flesh-colored bumps or growths with a dimple or pit in the center are abnormal (Fig. 21-16). The bumps are usually smooth and firm.

P Molluscum contagiosum is caused by a virus. Lesions resolve without treatment in 6 to 12 months. Molluscum contagiosum can also be transmitted via sexual contact and is then considered an STI.

A A painless mass that may be accompanied by pruritus or a mass that develops into a cauliflower-like growth is an abnormal finding.

P A painless mass that may be accompanied by pruritus or a mass that develops into a cauliflower-like growth is highly suggestive of a malignancy.

A Venous prominences of the labia may be abnormal.

P Varicose veins may develop due to a congenital predisposition, prolonged standing, pregnancy, or aging.

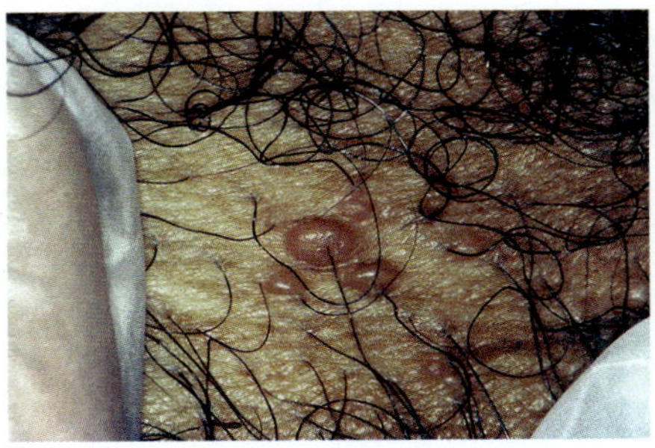

Figure 21-16 Molluscum contagiosum.

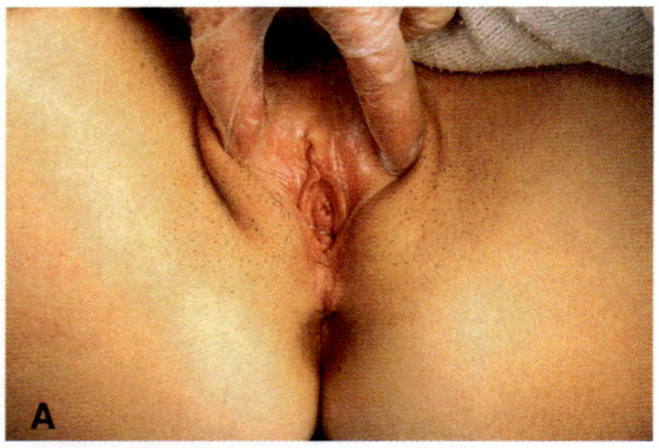

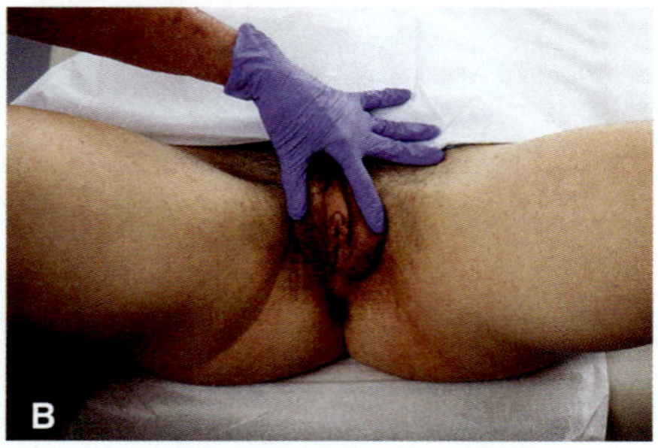

Figure 21-17 A. Inspection of the clitoris. **B.** Enlarged clitoris due to exogenous androgen use.

Clitoris

E
1. Using the dominant thumb and index finger, separate the labia minora laterally to expose the prepuce of the clitoris (Fig. 21-17A).
2. Observe the clitoris for size and condition.

N **The clitoris is approximately ¾ inch (2.0 cm) in length and ¼ inch (0.5 cm) in diameter and without lesions.**

A Hypertrophy of the clitoris is an abnormal finding.

P Hypertrophy of the clitoris may indicate female pseudohermaphroditism due to androgen excess (Fig. 21-17B).

A A reddish, round ulcer with a depressed center and raised, indurated edges (chancre) is an abnormal finding.

P Refer to the chancre discussion (Fig. 21-10).

A Excision of the clitoris is a postsurgical finding.

P Mutilation of the female genitalia (clitoridectomy), a practice in some cultures, can result in this finding.

Urethral Meatus

E
1. Using the dominant thumb and index finger, separate the labia minora laterally to expose the urethral meatus. Do not touch the urethral meatus; this may cause pain and urethral spasm.
2. Observe the shape, color, and size of the urethral meatus.

N **The urethral opening is slitlike in appearance and midline; it is free of discharge, swelling, or redness and is about the size of a pea.**

A Discharge of any color from the meatus is an abnormal finding.

P Discharge indicates possible urinary tract infection (UTI).

A Swelling or redness around the urethral meatus is an abnormal finding.

P Swelling indicates possible infection of the Skene glands, urethral caruncle (small, red growth that protrudes from the meatus, shown in Fig. 21-18), urethral carcinoma, or prolapse of the urethral mucosa (Fig. 21-19).

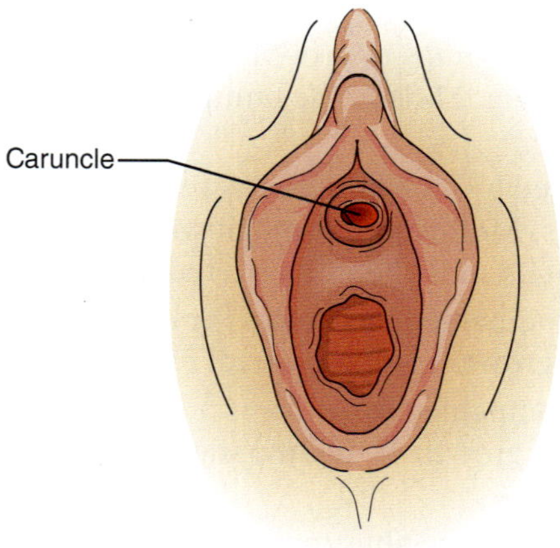

Figure 21-18 Urethral caruncle.

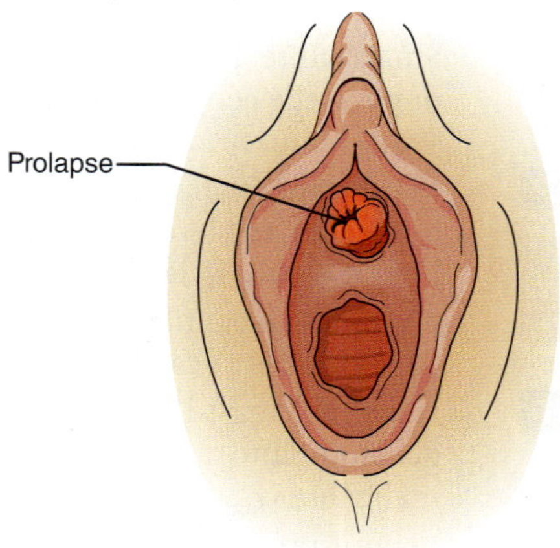

Figure 21-19 Prolapse of the urethral meatus.

Vaginal Introitus

E
1. Keep the labia minora retracted laterally to inspect the vaginal introitus.
2. Ask the client to bear down.
3. Observe for patency and bulging.
4. Apply pH test tape to any discharge and read the results based on the manufacturer's guidelines.

N **The introitus mucosa should be pink and moist. Normal vaginal discharge is clear to white and free of foul odor; some white clumps may be seen that are mass numbers of epithelial cells. The introitus should be patent and without bulging. Normal vaginal discharge is slightly acidic and has a pH of 4 to 4.5.**

A Pale color and mucosal dryness of the introitus occur in atrophic vaginitis.

P Postmenopausal females develop atrophic vaginitis as a result of decreased estrogen. Repeated use of topical steroids can also lead to this clinical finding.

A Foul-smelling discharge that is any color other than clear to slightly pale white is abnormal. Malodorous white, yellow, green, and gray discharge that may be purulent are some possible findings.

P Gonorrhea, *Chlamydia*, *Candida* vaginosis, *Trichomonas* vaginitis, bacterial vaginosis, atrophic vaginitis, or cervicitis are possible infectious processes or vectors (Table 21-3).

A The vaginal pH is greater than 4.5.

P Refer to Table 21-3. A higher pH promotes the growth of bacteria and fungal infections.

A An external tear or impatency of the vaginal introitus is abnormal.

Risk Factors

Vaginal Infections

The following may increase vaginal discharges and infections:

- Anatomy of the genital area
- Underlying skin diseases
- Increasing age
- Antibiotic use
- Immunodeficiency
- HIV
- OCP use
- Intravaginal contraceptive device
- Estrogen deficiency
- High sugar or milk intake
- Diabetes mellitus
- Steroid use
- Menses
- Douching
- Alkalinization from semen or chemical products
- Pregnancy
- Increased number of sexual partners
- Sexual abuse
- Hygiene

Table 21-3 Description of Vaginal Discharges

Discharge	Normal Physiological Discharge	Bacterial Vaginosis (BV)	Trichomonas	Candida	Gonococcal
Color	White	Gray	Grayish-yellow	White	Greenish-yellow
Odor	Absent	Fishy	Fishy	Absent	Absent
Consistency	Nonhomogenous	Homogenous	Purulent, often with bubbles	Cottage cheese-like	Mucopurulent
Location	Dependent	Adherent to walls	Often pooled in fornix	Adherent to walls	Adherent to walls
Vaginal pH	4–4.5	5–6	5–6	4–4.5	—
Anatomical Appearance					
Vulva	Normal	Normal	Edematous	Erythematous	Erythematous
Vaginal mucosa	Normal	Normal	Usually normal	Erythematous	Normal
Cervix	Normal	Normal	May show red spots	Patches of discharge	Pus in os

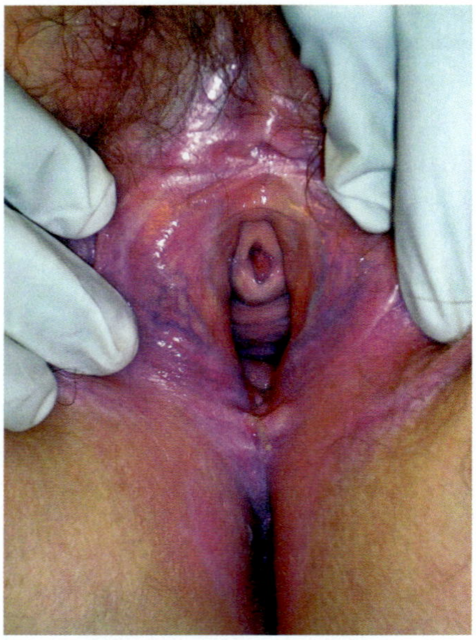

Figure 21-20 Cystocele. Also note the dry, pale appearance of the labia and the prominence of the urinary meatus.

P Possible causes of an external tear or impatency of the vaginal introitus include trauma and fissure of the introitus. An external tear may indicate trauma from sexual activity or abuse, and a fissure may indicate a congenital malformation or childbirth trauma.

A Bulging of the anterior vaginal wall indicates a **cystocele** (Fig. 21-20) and is abnormal.

P In a cystocele the upper two-thirds of the anterior vaginal wall, along with the bladder, push forward into the introitus due to weakened supporting tissues and ligaments. This can be caused by damage during vaginal childbirth.

A Closure of the vaginal introitus is abnormal.

P Trauma to the area and possible mutilation of the female genitalia are potential etiologies of closed vaginal introitus.

A Bulging of the anterior vaginal wall, bladder, and urethra into the vaginal introitus indicates a **cystourethrocele** (Fig. 21-21) and is abnormal.

P A cystourethrocele is usually caused by a weakening of the entire anterior vaginal wall. A fissure may define the urethrocele and cystocele.

A Bulging of the posterior vaginal wall with a portion of the rectum indicates a **rectocele** (Fig. 21-22) and is abnormal.

P A rectocele is caused by a weakening of the entire posterior vaginal wall.

Perineum and Anus

E
1. Observe for color and shape of the anus.
2. Observe texture and color of the perineum.

N **The perineum should be smooth and slightly darkened. A well-healed episiotomy scar is normal after vaginal delivery. The anus should be dark pink to brown and puckered. Skin tags are not uncommon around the anal area.**

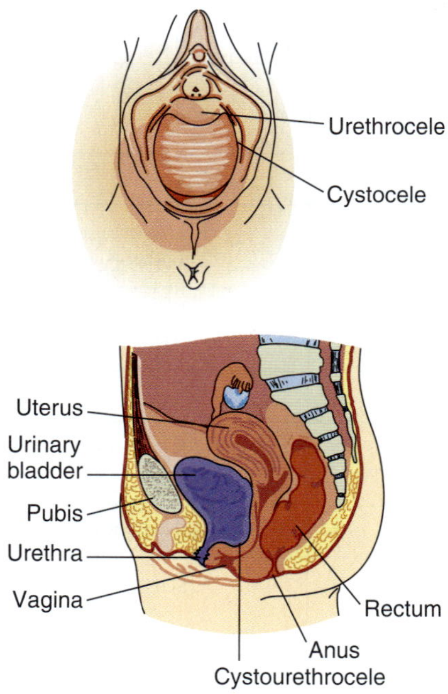

Figure 21-21 Cystourethrocele.

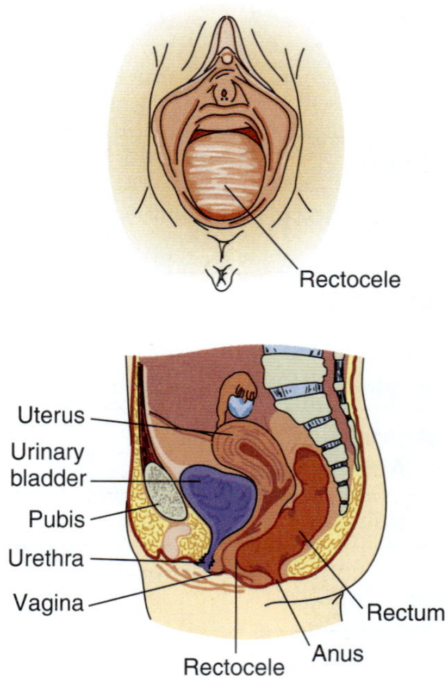

Figure 21-22 Rectocele.

A A fissure or tear of the perineum is an abnormal finding.

P Trauma, abscess, or unhealed episiotomy can lead to a fissure or tear of the perineum.

A Venous prominences of the anal area indicate external hemorrhoids and are abnormal.

P An external hemorrhoid is the varicose dilation of a vein of the inferior hemorrhoidal plexus and is covered with modified anal skin. A hemorrhoid can develop with excessive straining such as heavy lifting and constipation as well as consumption of a low fiber diet. Hemorrhoids frequently occur in weightlifters, pregnancy, and older adults.

A Painful, red ulcers that easily bleed on the labia, perineum, or thighs are abnormal (Fig. 21-23).

P Chancroids are caused by the bacteria *Haemophilus ducreyi*. This STI is not commonly found in the United States.

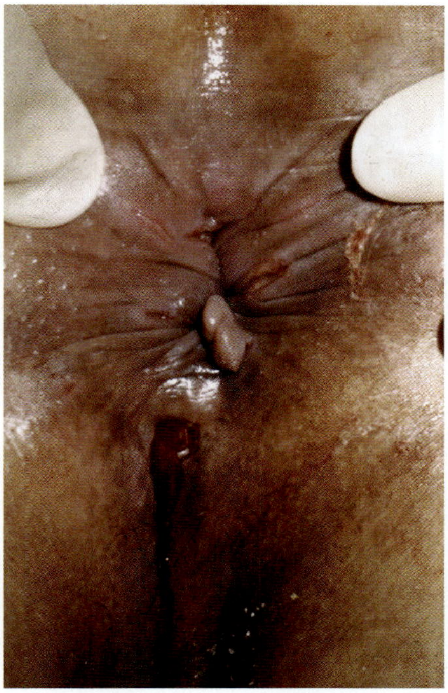

Figure 21-23 Perineal chancroid.

NURSING TIP

The Sexually Abused Client

No client, regardless of age, should be excluded from evaluation for sexual abuse. Physical signs of sexual abuse include bruising of the mons pubis, labia, or perineum, and vaginal or rectal tears. The presence of an STI in the very young or very old client suggests abuse. Emotional signs such as lack of eye contact during the examination, extreme anxiety or guarding during the examination, or refusing to assume certain positions may all indicate a history of abuse. Document all signs of suspected sexual abuse.

Know your institution's and state's policy regarding the reporting of sexual abuse. Most states have mandatory reporting policies for sexual abuse of children and teenagers. Some states require mandatory reporting of abuse of older adults.

Assure the client that they are safe with you and refer them to the appropriate social services or sexual assault services.

Palpation of the External Genitalia

Labia

E 1. Palpate each labium between the thumb and the index finger of your dominant hand.
2. Observe for swelling, induration, pain, or discharge from a Bartholin gland duct.

N **The labium should feel soft and uniform in structure with no swelling, pain, induration, or purulent discharge.**

A Swelling, redness, induration, or purulent discharge from the labial folds with hot, tender areas are abnormal findings (Fig. 21-24).

P Swelling, redness, induration, or purulent discharge from the labial folds with hot, tender areas indicate a probable Bartholin gland infection. Causative organisms include gonococci, *Chlamydia trachomatis*, and syphilis.

A A firm mass that is possibly painful in the labia majora is abnormal.

P A firm mass that is possibly painful in the labia majora can occur with an inguinal hernia. If this is suspected, repalpate the mass with the client in a standing position. See Chapter 22 for a more thorough explanation of hernias.

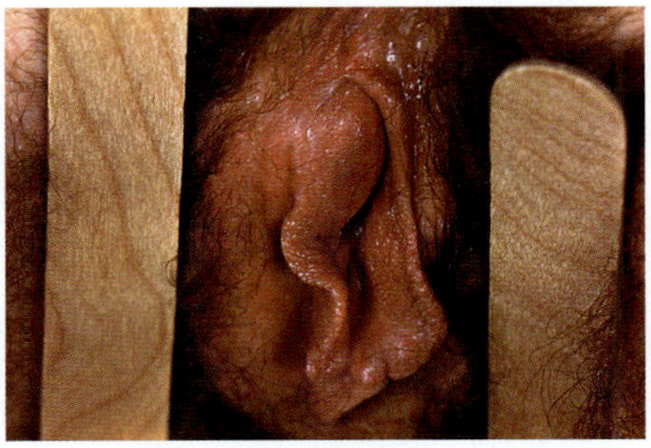

Figure 21-24 Bartholinitis of the right labia minora.

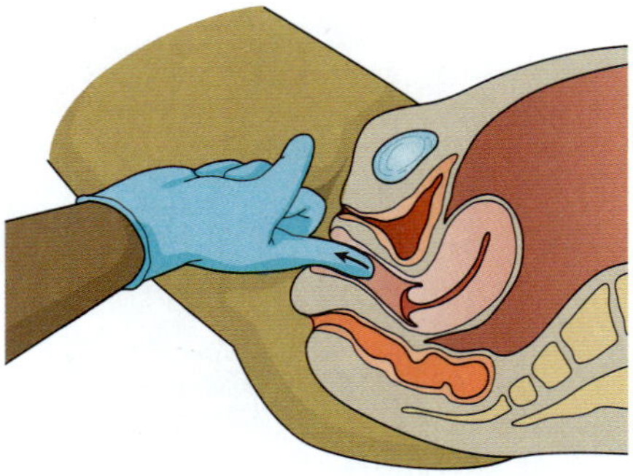

Figure 21-25 Milking the urethra.

Urethral Meatus and Skene Glands

E
1. Insert your dominant index finger into the vagina.
2. Apply pressure to the anterior aspect of the vaginal wall and milk the urethra (Fig. 21-25).
3. Observe for discharge. If discharge is noted from the urethra, use a cotton-tipped swab to obtain a sample and spread it on a microscope slide for further evaluation. A sterile culture tube can also be used to sample the discharge and sent for culture and sensitivity testing.

N **Milking the urethra should not cause pain or result in any urethral discharge.**

A Pain on contact and discharge from the urethra are abnormal findings.

P Pain on contact and discharge from the urethra indicate a Skene gland infection or urinary tract infection.

Vaginal Introitus

E
1. While your finger remains in the vagina, ask the client to squeeze the vaginal muscles around your finger.
2. Evaluate muscle strength and tone.

N **Vaginal muscle tone in a nulliparous woman should be tight and strong; in a parous woman, it will be diminished.**

A Significantly diminished or absent vaginal muscle tone and bulging of vaginal or pelvic contents are abnormal findings. Fig. 21-26 illustrates various degrees of uterine prolapse.

P Weakened muscle tone may result from injury, age, childbirth, or medication. Bulging results from cystocele, rectocele, or uterine prolapse.

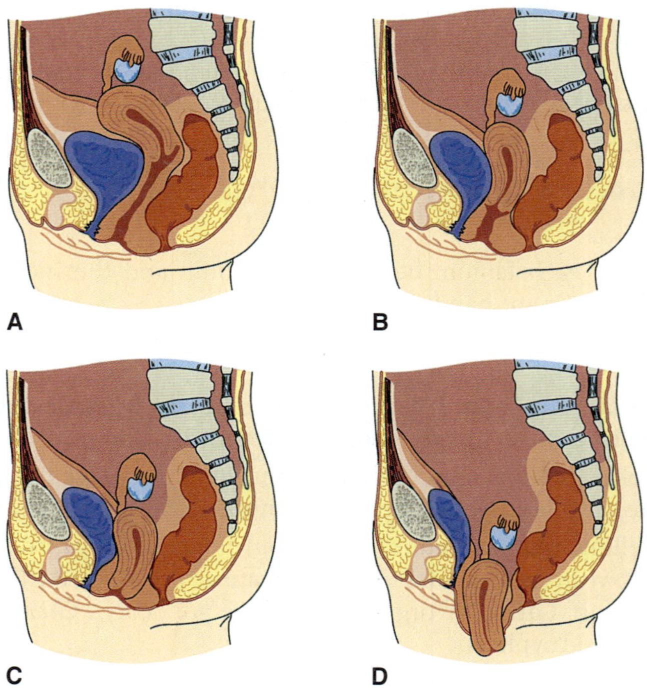

Figure 21-26 Uterine prolapse. **A.** Normal position of the uterus. **B.** In first-degree prolapse, the cervix is contained within the vagina with straining. **C.** In second-degree prolapse, the cervix is at the introitus with straining. **D.** In third-degree prolapse (complete prolapse), the cervix, uterus, and vagina are outside the introitus, even without straining.

Perineum

E 1. Withdraw your finger from the introitus until you can place only your dominant index finger posterior to the perineum and place the dominant thumb anterior to the perineum.
2. Assess the perineum between the dominant thumb and index finger for muscular tone and texture.

N **The perineum should be smooth, firm, and homogenous in the nulliparous female, and thinner in the parous female. A well-healed episiotomy scar is also within normal limits for a parous female.**

A A thin, tissue-like perineum, fissures, or tears are abnormal.

P A thin perineum is indicative of atrophy, and fissures and tears may indicate trauma or an unhealed episiotomy.

> **NURSING TIP**
> **Hernias in Females**
> Hernias can occur in females as well as males. Females typically develop femoral hernias. Be alert for this condition if the client complains of lower abdominal pain. Assess for a femoral hernia in the inguinal area by palpating the femoral area while the client bears down. A bulge or palpable mass may be present. Usually imaging such as an ultrasound is needed to confirm the presence of a femoral hernia in females. Inguinal hernias occur rarely in females.

Speculum Examination of the Internal Genitalia

Cervix

E 1. Select the appropriate-sized speculum. This selection should be based on the client's history, size of vaginal introitus, and vaginal muscle tone.
2. Lubricate and warm the speculum by rinsing it under warm water. Do not use other lubricants, because they may interfere with the accuracy of cytological samples and cultures.
3. Hold the speculum in your dominant hand with the closed blades between the index and middle fingers. The index finger should rest at the proximal end of the superior blade. Wrap the other fingers around the handle (Fig. 21-27), with the thumbscrew over the thumb.
4. Apply your nondominant index and middle fingers, ventral sides down, at 5 and 7 o'clock just inside the vagina, and apply pressure to the posterior vaginal wall. Be careful not to pull on pubic hair or pinch the labia.
5. Encourage the client to relax by taking deep breaths.
6. When you feel the muscles relax, insert the speculum at an oblique angle on a plane parallel to the examination table until the speculum reaches the end of the fingers that are in the vagina (Fig. 21-28A).
7. Remove the fingers of your nondominant hand.
8. Gently rotate the speculum blades to a horizontal angle and advance the speculum at a 45° downward angle against the posterior vaginal wall until it reaches the end of the vagina (Figs. 21-28B and C).
9. Using your dominant thumb, depress the lever to open the blades and visualize the cervix (Fig. 21-28D). Squamous epithelial cells should be visible.
10. If the cervix is not visualized, close the blades, withdraw the speculum ¾ to 1¼ inches (2 to 3 cm), and reinsert it at a slightly different angle to ensure that the speculum is inserted far enough into the vagina.

> **NURSING TIP**
> **Genital Self-Examination**
> Teach the client to inspect and palpate the external genitalia for lesions, irritations, and ulcerations, which may indicate disease. This self-examination should be done between menstrual periods. The use of a mirror and flashlight facilitates genital self-examination.

> **NURSING TIP**
> **Hormone Replacement Therapy in Menopause**
> Some clients may have concerns regarding the use of hormone replacement therapy (HRT) and the risks of a possible blood clot, heart attack, stroke, and breast cancer. Certain types of HRT have higher risks and each client's risk can vary. Recent findings suggest that although not entirely risk-free, HRT remains the most effective solution for relieving menopausal symptoms. Review with your client the benefits and risks of HRT keeping in mind the client's personal and family history.

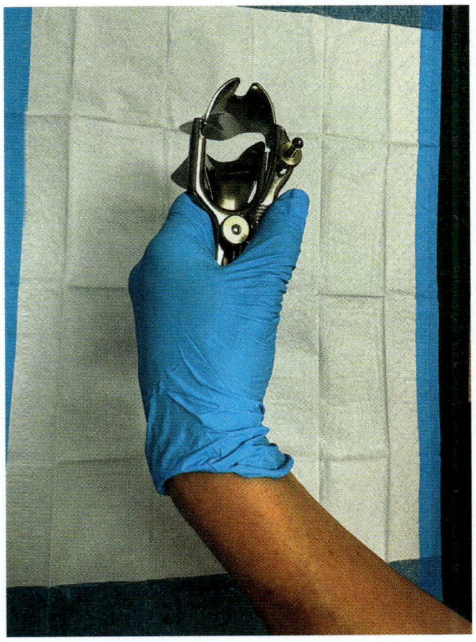

Figure 21-27 Holding the speculum.

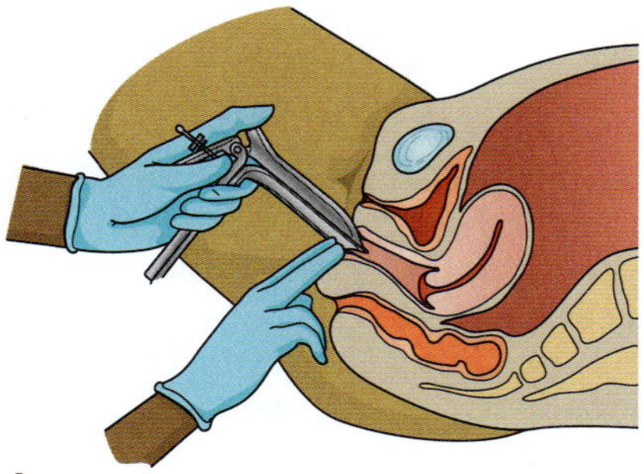

A Opening of the vaginal introitus

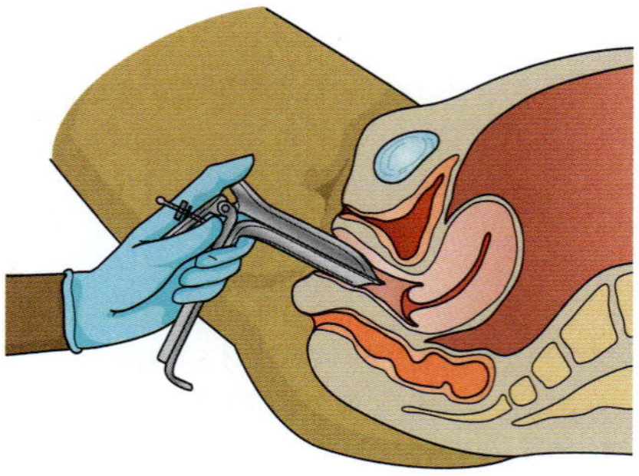

B Oblique insertion of the speculum

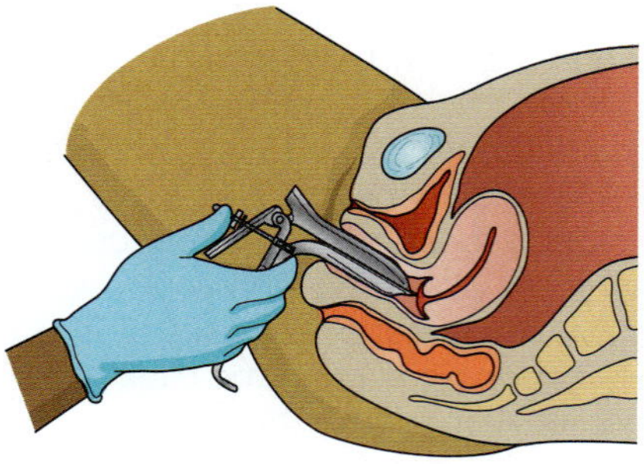

C Final advancement of the speculum

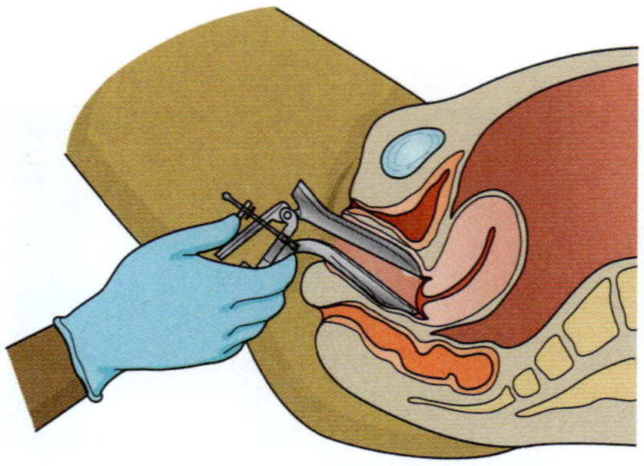

D Opening the speculum blades

Figure 21-28 Speculum examination.

11. Once the cervix is fully visualized, lock the speculum blades into place. The locking method varies based on the type of speculum being used.
12. Adjust your light source so that it shines through the speculum and the cervix is clearly visible.
13. If any discharge obstructs visualization of the cervix, clean it away with a cotton-tipped swab.
14. Inspect the cervix and the os for color, position, size, surface characteristics such as polyps or lesions, discharge, and shape.

Color

N **The normal cervix is a glistening pink (Fig. 21-29); it may be pale after menopause or blue (Chadwick sign) during pregnancy.**

A Cyanosis not associated with pregnancy is abnormal.

P Possible causes of a cyanotic cervix include venous congestion of the area or systemic hypoxia (as in congestive heart failure).

A Redness or a friable appearance is an abnormal finding (Fig. 21-30). This is frequently referred to as a "strawberry cervix."

P Possible causes of a red or friable appearing cervix include infection and inflammation, such as *Chlamydia*, gonorrhea, and trichomoniasis.

Position

N **The cervix is located midline in the vagina with an anterior or posterior position relative to the vaginal vault and projecting approximately 1 inch (2.5 cm) into the vagina.**

A Lateral positioning of the cervix may present as an abnormal finding.

P Tumors or adhesions can displace the cervix.

A Projection of the cervix into the vaginal vault further than normal limits is suspect.

P Uterine prolapse is caused by weakened vaginal wall muscles and pelvic ligaments and may push the cervix into the vaginal vault.

Size

N **Normal size is 1 inch (2.5 cm).**

A Cervical size greater than 1½ inches (4 cm) is indicative of hypertrophy and is abnormal.

P Inflammation or tumor can cause morbid enlargement of the cervix.

Surface Characteristics

N **The cervix is covered by the glistening pink squamous epithelium, which is similar to the vaginal epithelium. The deep pink**

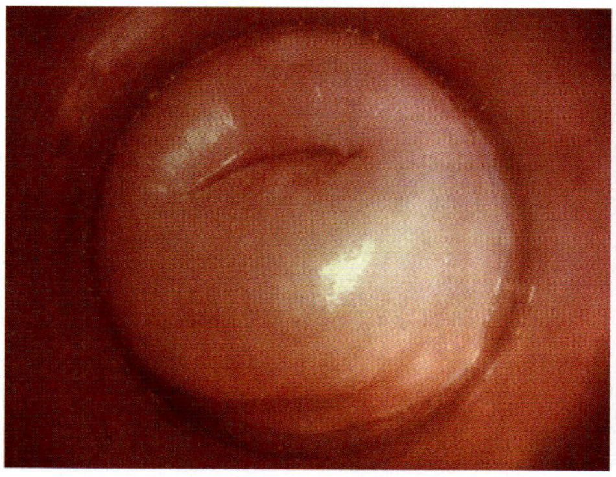

Figure 21-29 Normal appearing cervix.

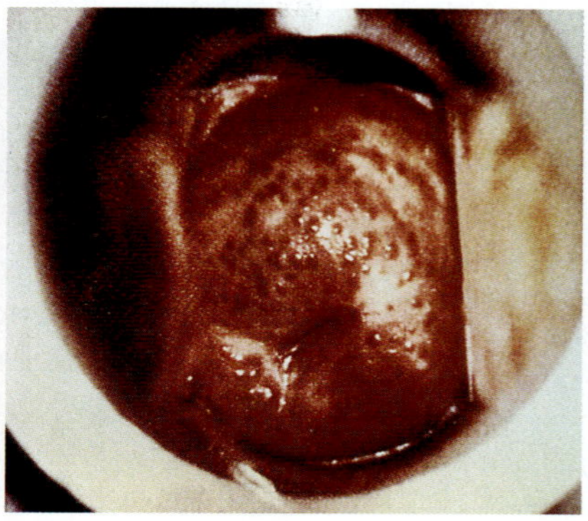

Figure 21-30 Strawberry cervix. Note the small vesicles on the cervix.

to red-columnar epithelium around the os is a continuation of the endocervical lining.

A A reddish circle around the os may be abnormal.

P A reddish circle around the os is known as **ectropion** or **eversion**. It occurs when the squamocolumnar junction appears on the ectocervix. It results from lacerations during childbirth or, possibly, from congenital variation.

A Small, cystic, yellow lesions on the cervical surface indicate **nabothian cysts** (Fig. 21-31), which are abnormal.

P Nabothian cysts are benign cysts that result from the obstruction of cervical glands.

A A bright red, soft protrusion through the cervical os indicates a cervical polyp (Fig. 21-32) and is abnormal.

P Polyps originate from the endocervical canal; they are usually benign but tend to bleed if abraded.

A Hemorrhages dispersed over the surface and known as strawberry spots are abnormal.

P Hemorrhages dispersed over the cervical surface may be seen in conjunction with trichomonal infections.

A Mucopurulent discharge, erythema, and friability of the cervix are abnormal (Fig. 21-33).

P Many females with *Chlamydia trachomatis* are asymptomatic; others have pelvic pain, fever, and dysuria. Chlamydia is the most common STI in the United States. Clients infected with this STI frequently also have gonorrhea.

A A whitish discharge or appearance in the cervical os is abnormal (Fig. 21-34).

P A whitish discharge or appearance in the cervical os occurs in cervical candidiasis.

A Irregularities of the cervical surface that may look cauliflower-like are an abnormal finding.

P Carcinoma of the cervix may manifest as a cauliflower-like overgrowth (Fig. 21-35).

A Columnar epithelium covering most of the cervix and extending to the vaginal wall (vaginal adenosis), and a collar-type ridge between the cervix and the vagina are abnormal (Fig. 21-36).

P Fetal exposure to DES results in columnar epithelium covering most of the cervix that extends to the vaginal wall with a collar-type ridge between the cervix and the vagina.

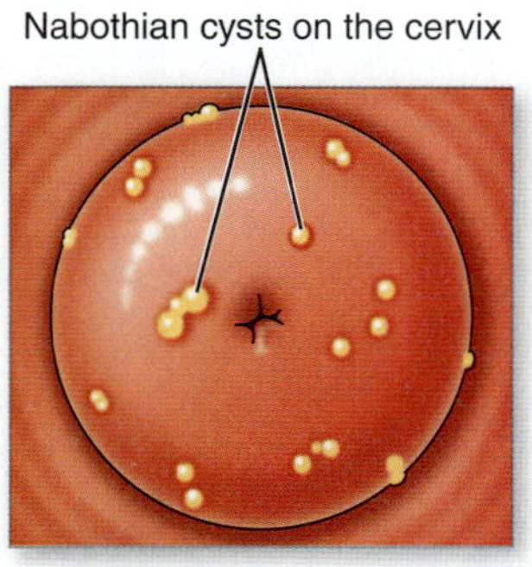

Figure 21-31 Nabothian cysts.

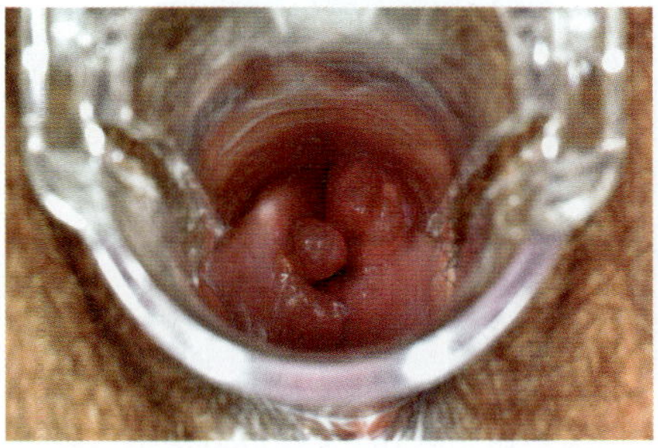

Figure 21-32 Cervical polyp.

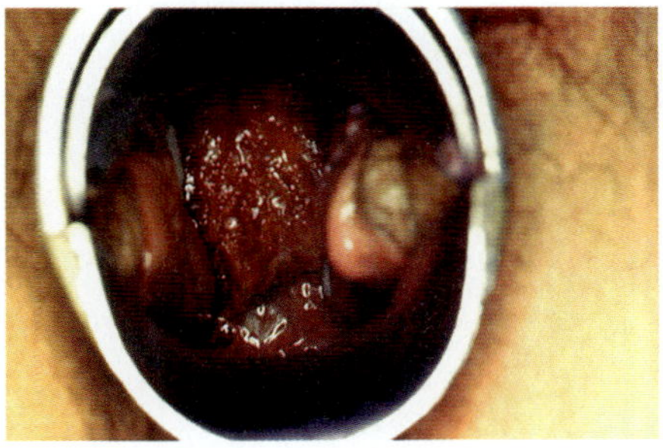

Figure 21-33 This woman's cervix is erythematous with erosions due to *Chlamydia*.

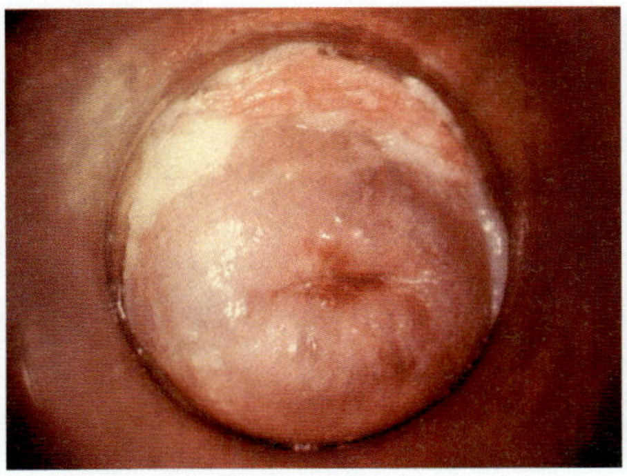

Figure 21-34 Cervical candidiasis.

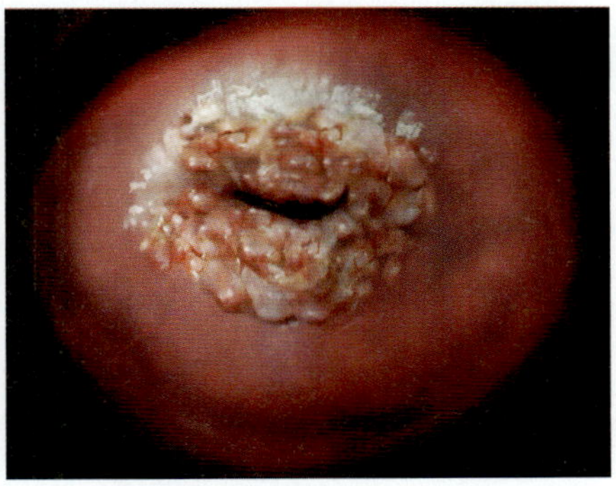

Figure 21-35 Cervical cancer.

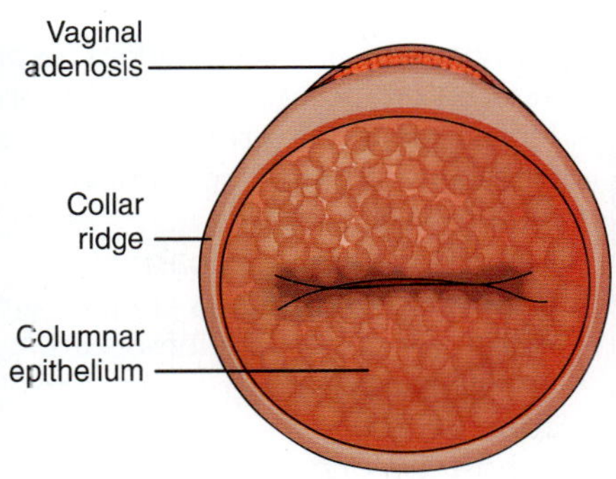

Figure 21-36 Fetal exposure to DES.

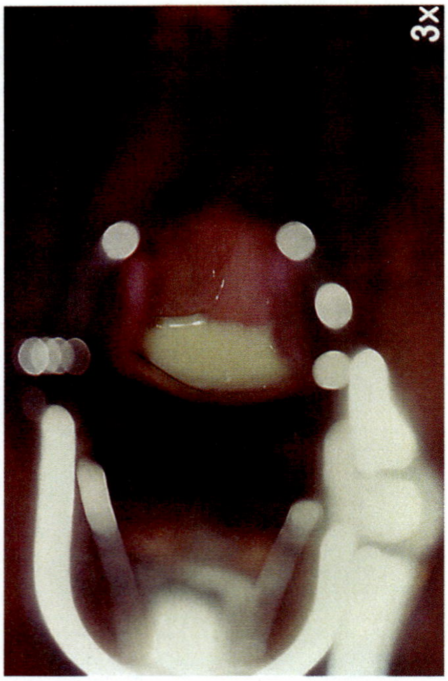

Figure 21-37 *Trichomonas vaginalis* is the cause of the purulent cervical discharge in this photo.

Discharge

E Note the characteristics of any discharge (Fig. 21-37).

N A P See Table 21-3.

Shape of the Cervical Os

N **In the nulliparous female, the os is small and either round or oval. In the parous female who has had a vaginal delivery, the os is a horizontal slit.**

A A unilateral transverse, bilateral transverse, stellate, or irregular cervical os is abnormal (Fig. 21-38).

P Possible causes of an irregularly shaped cervical os include cervical tears that occurred during rapid second-stage childbirth delivery, forceps delivery, and trauma.

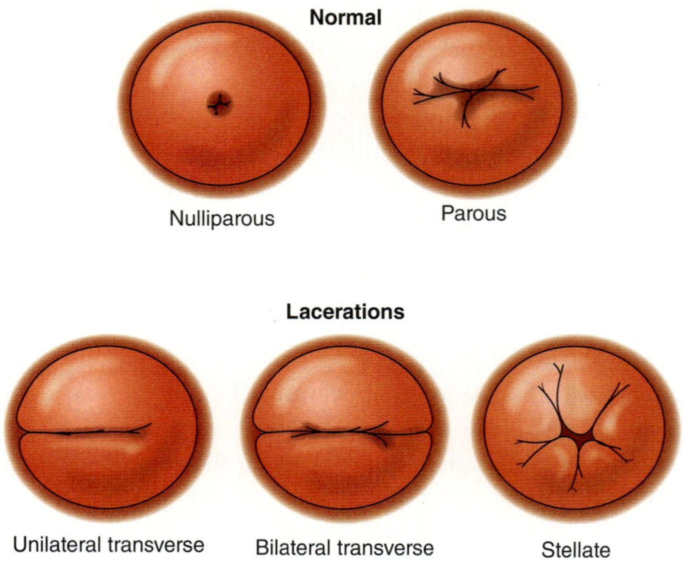

Figure 21-38 Shapes of the cervical os.

Risk Factors

Female Genitalia Cancer

Evaluate each client for risk factors, and counsel the client regarding diminishing risk factors that are behavior dependent. Suspected carcinoma of the female genitalia requires an immediate referral.

Cervical Cancer

- Age (>35 years)
- Early age at first intercourse (especially <18 years)
- Age 20 or younger at first full-term pregnancy
- More than 3 full-term pregnancies
- History of human papillomavirus (HPV)
- Multiple sex partners
- Having one high risk partner
- Prior history of herpes simplex virus
- History of chlamydia infections
- Family history of cervical cancer
- Tobacco use
- Long-term oral contraceptive use

- Daughters of females who took diethylstilbestrol (DES) during pregnancy (most clients with DES exposure were born before 1971)
- HIV
- Immunosuppression
- Females of lower socioeconomic status (due to lack of screening)

Endometrial Cancer

- Early or late menarche (before age 11 or after age 16)
- Age (50 to 60)
- Black females
- History of infertility/failure to ovulate
- Polycystic ovary syndrome
- Higher number of menstrual cycles
- Nulliparity
- History of endometrial hyperplasia
- Unopposed estrogen therapy
- Ovarian tumors (e.g., granulosa cell tumor)
- Use of tamoxifen
- Prior history of pelvic radiation therapy
- Obesity; high-fat diet
- Type 2 diabetes
- History of breast or ovarian cancer
- Family history of endometrial cancer
- Family history of hereditary nonpolyposis colon cancer (Lynch syndrome and Cowden syndrome)

Ovarian Cancer

- Advancing age (postmenopausal)
- Menses starting before age 12
- Menopause after age 52
- Nulliparity
- Endometriosis
- Inability to carry pregnancy to full term
- History of breast cancer
- Family history of ovarian, breast, or colorectal cancer
- Hereditary nonpolyposis colon cancer
- Family cancer syndromes (e.g., *BRCA1* and *BRCA2* mutations, Lynch syndrome)

Vaginal Cancer

- Advancing age (>70 years)
- Smoking
- HIV
- History of cervical cancer or precancer (cervical intraepithelial neoplasia or cervical dysplasia)
- Daughters of females who took DES during pregnancy
- Vaginal adenosis
- History of HPV
- Previous pelvic area radiation therapy

Vulvar Cancer

- Advancing age (>70 years)
- History of HPV
- HIV
- Smoking
- Vulvar squamous intraepithelial lesions
- Lichen sclerosus of the vulva
- History of cervical cancer

Adapted from *https://www.cancer.org/cancer/types/cervical-cancer/causes-risks-prevention/risk-factors.html*
https://www.cancer.org/cancer/types/endometrial-cancer/causes-risks-prevention/risk-factors.html
https://www.cancer.org/cancer/types/ovarian-cancer/causes-risks-prevention/risk-factors.html
https://www.cancer.org/cancer/types/vaginal-cancer/causes-risks-prevention/risk-factors.html
https://www.cancer.org/cancer/types/vulvar-cancer/causes-risks-prevention/risk-factors.html
Retrieved December 17, 2025.

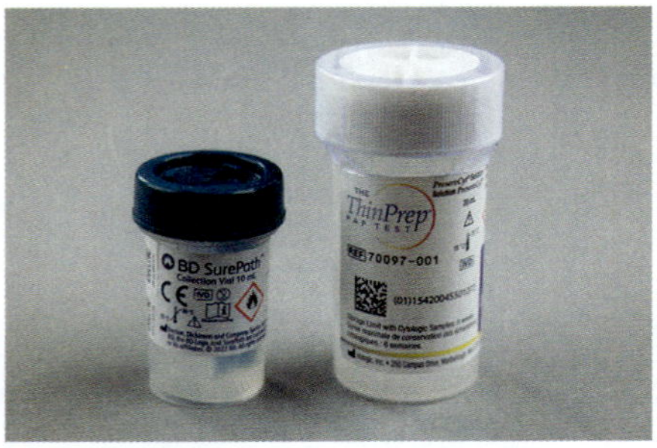

Figure 21-39 Liquid-based cervical cytology preparations.

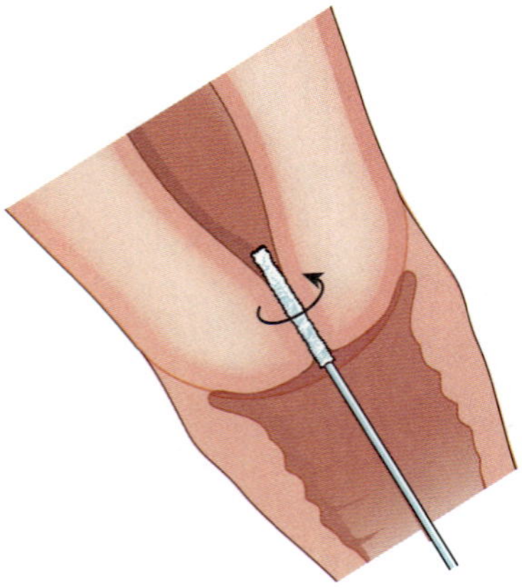

Figure 21-40 Endocervical smear.

Collecting Specimens for Cytological Smears and Cultures

After inspection of the cervix and the cervical os, obtain any laboratory specimens that are indicated.

Collect the Pap smear first, followed by the gonococcal and any other vaginal smears. There are many accepted variations among laboratories regarding the collection and fixing of vaginal specimens. It is prudent to identify the procedure recommended by the laboratory that will be testing the specimens.

Pap Smear

Cervical cancer screening has traditionally been conducted using the Papanicolaou Test (Pap test or Pap smear). Most institutions use liquid-based cytology, but conventional cytology with microscope slides and cytology fixative spray can be used. Both conventional cytology and liquid-based cytology have been shown to have similar sensitivity and specificity and are considered acceptable by the American College of Obstetrics and Gynecologists. The liquid-based cytology systems are the BD SurePath ™ (formerly known as Autocyte PREP System) and the ThinPrep system (Fig. 21-39). These systems clean the specimens for Pap smears by removing blood and mucus before the cells are mounted on the slide. The cell sample is placed in a preservative vial, and the specimen is centrifuged, filtered, or both at the laboratory. These liquid-based cytology tests also allow for testing for high-risk HPV genotypes. The Pap smear is collected from two sites: the endocervix and the cervix. If the client has had a hysterectomy, the specimen is obtained from the vaginal cuff. Refer to Table 21-4 for cervical cancer screening guidelines.

Endocervical Smear

E

1. Using your dominant hand, insert the Cytobrush or cervical broom through the speculum into the cervical os approximately 1 cm. Many clients find that this procedure causes a cramping sensation, so forewarn your client that they may feel discomfort during this element of the examination.
2. Rotate the Cytobrush between your index finger and thumb 360° clockwise, then counterclockwise. Keep the Cytobrush in contact with the cervical tissue (Fig. 21-40). *Note:* If you have to use a cotton-tipped swab instead of a Cytobrush, leave the applicator in the cervical os for 30 seconds to ensure saturation. If you use the cervical broom, rotate the broom 3–5 times clockwise. Place the broom or Cytobrush in the liquid-based cytology vial. Rotate the Cytobrush or broom ten times while pushing it against the wall and bottom of the vial. Swirl it vigorously and ensure that no material remains on the Cytobrush or broom.
3. Remove the Cytobrush and, using a rolling motion, spread the cells on the section of the slide marked E if a sectional slide is being used. Do not press down hard or wipe the Cytobrush back and forth, because doing so will destroy the cells.
4. Discard the brush/broom/swab.

N **Normal classifications for all cervicovaginal cytology should read "Specimen Adequacy—adequate for evaluation" and "General Categorization—negative for intraepithelial lesion or malignancy," using the Bethesda System 2001, which denotes a lack of pathogenesis. The Bethesda System was developed by a consensus conference in 2001 and is endorsed by the National Cancer Institute to report cervicovaginal cytological diagnoses.**

A A Pap report finding of benign cellular changes is abnormal.

P Benign cellular changes have a multiplicity of causes, including fungal, bacterial, protozoal, or viral infections.

Table 21-4 Cervical Cancer Screening Guidelines From ACS, ACOG, and USPSTF*

Age	ACS 2012	ACS 2025	ACOG	USPSTF
21–24	Pap test every 3 years	No Screening	Pap test alone every 3 years HPV testing is not recommended	Pap test every 3 years
25–29	Pap test every 3 years	HPV test every 5 years (preferred) HPV/Pap cotest every 5 years (acceptable) Pap test every 3 years (acceptable) HPV self-testing was endorsed in 2025 every 3 years if previous results were negative	Pap test alone every 3 years HPV testing alone can be considered but Pap tests are preferred	Pap test every 3 years
30–65	Pap test every 3 years (preferred) Pap test every 5 years (acceptable)	HPV test every 5 years (preferred) HPV/Pap cotest every 5 years (acceptable) Pap test every 3 years (acceptable) HPV self-testing was endorsed in 2025 every 3 years if previous results were negative	Pap test alone every 3 years or HPV test alone every 5 years or Pap test and an HPV test (cotesting) every 5 years	Pap test every 3 years HPV test every 5 years, or HPV/Pap cotest every 5 years
65+	No screening needed if a series of prior tests was normal	An average-risk client having a negative HPV test or negative co-test at ages 60 and 65 can cease cervical cancer screening or Cervical cancer screening can stop if client has had 3 consecutive negative cytology results with the last at age 65 when HPV testing is not available	No screening needed if a series of prior tests was normal and no history of moderate or severe abnormal cervical cells or cervical cancer	No screening needed if a series of prior tests was normal and not at high risk for cervical cancer

*Note: ACS: American Cancer Society; ACOG: American College of Obstetrics and Gynecologists; USPSTF: United States Preventive Services Task Force; HPV: Human Papillomavirus

The cervical cancer screening guidelines apply to clients with a cervix who do not have signs or symptoms of cervical cancer, regardless of sexual history or HPV vaccination status. These screening guidelines do not apply to clients who are immunocompromised, such as those with HIV infection, organ transplant, chemotherapy, chronic steroid use, prenatal exposure to diethylstilbestrol (DES), or history of high-grade cervical intraepithelial neoplasia (CIN). The ACS 2012 cervical cancer screening guidelines are shown to illustrate the differences with current guidelines.

American cancer Society (2025). American Cancer Society updates cervical cancer screening guideline: major changes include self-collection for HPV testing and guidance on exiting screening. Retrieved December 17, 2025, from https://www.newswise.com/articles/american-cancer-society-updates-cervical-cancer-screening-guideline-major-changes-include-self-collection-for-hpv-testing-and-guidance-on-exiting-screening/?sc=mwhr&xy=10069075

American College of Obstetrics and Gynecology. (2025). Cervical cancer screening. Retrieved December 17, 2025, from *https://www.acog.org/clinical/clinical-guidance/practice-advisory/articles/2021/04/updated-cervical-cancer-screening-guidelines*

National Cancer Institute. (2025). Cervical cancer screening. Retrieved December 17, 2025, from *https://www.cancer.gov/types/cervical/screening.*

United States Preventive Services Task Force A & B Recommendations (2025). Retrieved December 17, 2025, from *https://www.uspreventiveservicestaskforce.org/uspstf/recommendation-topics/uspstf-a-and-b-recommendations*

A A Pap report finding of "atypical squamous cells of undetermined significance" is abnormal.

P Causes of atypical squamous cells of undetermined significance (ASCUS) include inflammatory or infectious processes, a preliminary lesion, or an unknown phenomenon.

A A Pap result of epithelial cell abnormalities is aberrant.

P A Pap result of epithelial cell abnormalities is indicative of squamous intraepithelial lesion, which may or may not be transient; squamous cell carcinoma; or glandular cell abnormalities that are seen in postmenopausal females who are not on hormone replacement therapy.

NURSING TIP

HPV Vaccination

There are over 100 different strains of human papillomavirus (HPV), which have been divided into low- and high-risk subtypes. The low-risk types have been associated with genital warts and are identified as types 6, 11, 40, 42, 43, 44, 54, 61, 72, and 81. High-risk types are those associated with intraepithelial neoplasia, including types 16, 18, 31, 33, 35, 39, 45, 51, 52, 56, 58, 59, 68, and 69, and are considered cancer-causing. Types 16 and 18 have been found in 70% of cervical cancers.

Gardasil 9 is an HPV vaccine approved by the U.S. Food and Drug Administration and can be used for both girls and boys. It is the first vaccine shown to be effective in preventing infection of HPV genotypes 6, 11, 16, and 18. The vaccine offers protection against cervical cancer, cervical dysplasias, and vulvar or vaginal dysplasias caused by these four genotypes.

Children ages 11 to 12 years should receive two doses of the HPV vaccine, given 6 to 12 months apart. Younger adolescents ages 9 and 10 and teens ages 13 and 14 can also receive a vaccination on the two-dose schedule.

Children who start the HPV vaccine series on or after their 15th birthday need three doses, given over 6 months. The second dose should be given one to 2 months after the first dose with the third dose given 5 months after the first dose.

Teens and young adults who begin the vaccine series later, at ages 15 through 26, should receive three doses of the vaccine. The CDC recommends catch-up HPV vaccinations for all people through age 26 who aren't adequately vaccinated. In addition, some adults ages 27 to 45 may choose to get the HPV vaccine after consultation with their health-care provider (CDC, 2025).

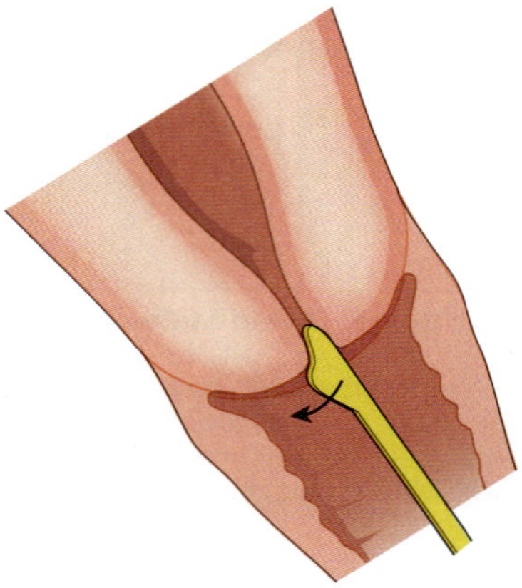

Figure 21-41 Cervical smear.

Cervical Smear

E

1. Insert the bifurcated end of the Ayre spatula through the speculum base. Place the longer projection of the bifurcation into the cervical os. The shorter projection should be snug against the ectocervix (Fig. 21-41).
2. Rotate the spatula 360° one time only. Make sure the transformation zone is well sampled.
3. Remove the spatula and gently spread the specimen on the section of the slide labeled C, if a sectional slide is being used. When using cytology-based liquid place the Ayre spatula into the vial and vigorously swirl it approximately 10 times. Discard the spatula.

N A P Refer to the Endocervical Smear description.

Chlamydia Culture Specimen

E

1. Have the client provide a urine specimen for chlamydia culture if laboratory testing is available.
2. If urine chlamydial testing is unavailable, then insert a sterile cotton-swab ⅜ inch (1 cm) into the cervical os.
3. Hold the swab in place for 20 seconds.
4. Remove the swab.
5. Place the swab in a viral, Chlamydia, or mycoplasma culture transport tube.
6. Submit the specimens to the appropriate laboratory per your institution's guidelines for culture specimens.

N **Cervicovaginal tissues are normally free of *Chlamydia trachomatis.***

A It is abnormal to find *Trachomatis,* serotypes D through K, or obligate, intracellular bacteria in cervicovaginal secretions.

P *Trachomatis* may invade the cervix or uterine tubes, and it is often asymptomatic in women.

Note: Nonculture laboratory test methods include direct fluorescent antibody (DFA), enzyme immunoassay (EIA), DNA probes, or polymerase chain reaction (PCR).

Gonococcal Culture Specimen

E 1. Have the client provide a urine specimen for gonococcal culture if laboratory testing is available.
2. If urine gonococcal testing is unavailable, then insert a sterile cotton-swab ⅜ inch (1 cm) into the cervical os.
3. Hold the applicator in place for 20 to 30 seconds.
4. Remove the swab.
5. Place the swab in a gonococcal or culture transport tube.
6. Submit the specimens to the appropriate laboratory per your institution's guidelines for culture specimens.

N **Cervicovaginal tissues are normally free of *Neisseria gonorrhoeae*.**

A It is abnormal to find a large number of gram-negative diplococci present in cervicovaginal secretions.

P *N. gonorrhoeae* are gram-negative diplococci organisms that prefer to invade columnar and stratified epithelium.

Saline Mount or "Wet Prep"

This test is performed for the rapid evaluation of white blood cells and protozoa.

E 1. Spread a sample of the cervical specimen onto a microscope slide, add one drop of normal saline solution, and apply a cover slip.
2. Examine under a microscope.

N **The sample should have fewer than 10 white blood cells (WBCs) per field.**

A A sample with more than 10 WBCs per field, protozoa (see Fig. 21-42), bacteria-filled epithelial cells (clue cells) (Fig. 21-43), or other organisms is abnormal.

P A large number of WBCs can be indicative of an inflammatory response, *Chlamydia trachomatis,* or a bacterial infection. Clue cells are seen in bacterial vaginosis. Protozoa are indicative of trichomoniasis.

KOH Prep

This test is performed for the rapid evaluation of *Candida.*

E 1. Spread a sample of the cervical specimen onto a microscope slide, add one drop of potassium hydroxide (KOH), and apply a cover slip. Examine under a microscope.
2. Note any odor.

N **Cervicovaginal tissues are normally free of *Candida albicans* except in a small percentage of females. There should be no odor.**

A The presence of yeast and hyphae forms (chains of budding yeast) is abnormal (Fig. 21-44).

P The presence of budding yeast is indicative of an overgrowth of *Candida.*

A An odor is abnormal.

P A fishy odor (the "whiff test") indicates bacterial vaginosis.

Five Percent Acetic Acid Wash

E After completing all other vaginal specimens, swab the cervix with a cotton-tipped applicator that has been soaked in 5% acetic acid.

N **The normal response is no change in the appearance of the cervix.**

A A rapid acetowhitening or blanching with jagged borders is an abnormal finding.

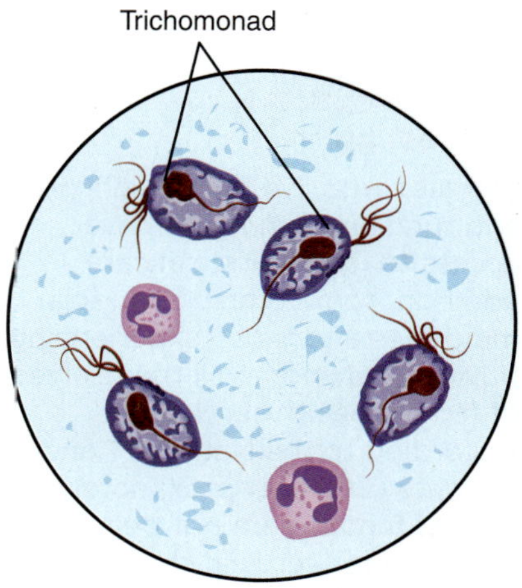

Figure 21-42 Microscopic view of *Trichomonas.*

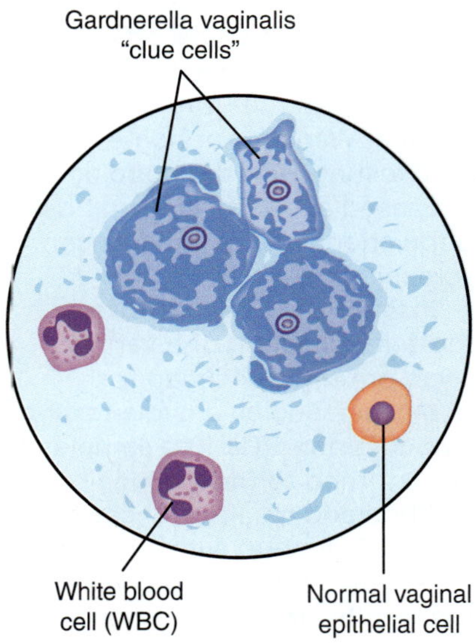

Figure 21-43 Microscopic view of clue cells.

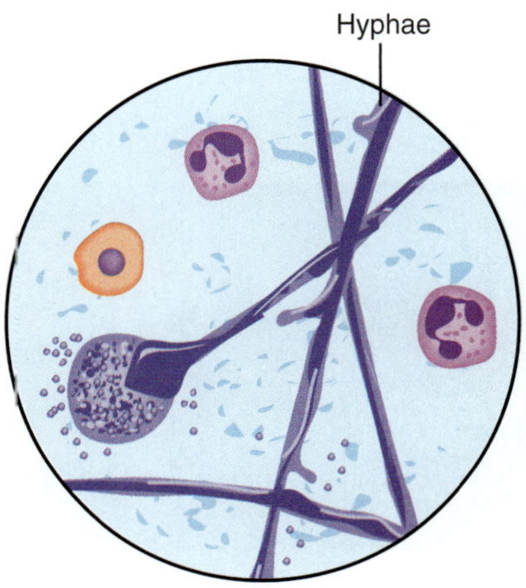

Figure 21-44 Microscopic view of hyphae.

> **NURSING TIP**
> **Self-Collection for HPV and STI Testing**
>
> Females who live in underserved and rural areas may not have access to gynecological care. In addition, some ethnic and racial minorities and those experiencing poverty may not avail themselves of female health services. According to the National Cancer Institute (2024) approximately 30% of females are not being screened for cervical cancer at designated intervals or they are not being tested at all. In May 2024 the FDA approved the self-collection of vaginal samples for HPV testing at health-care facilities (e.g., medical office, urgent care, pharmacies, etc.). In June 2025 the FDA approved the Teal Wand for at home HPV testing with the hope of increased accessibility for at risk populations for cervical cancer screening.
>
> In 2023 the FDA approved the self-collecting of a vaginal swab or urine specimen for gonorrhea and chlamydia testing, two common STIs. The samples are returned to the designated location and results are viewed online. Follow-up with a health-care provider is required when the results are inconclusive or positive.

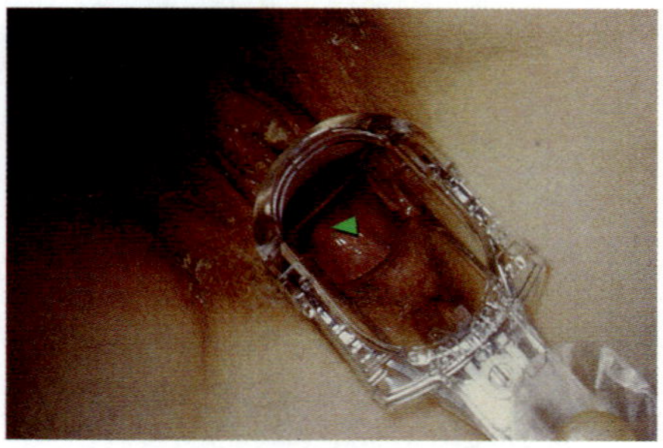

Figure 21-45 A chancroid on the posterior vaginal wall was seen as the speculum was withdrawn.

P Human papillomavirus, which is the causative agent of genital warts, may cause a rapid acetowhitening of the cervix. The borders of the cervix may have jagged borders.

Anal Culture

An anal culture can be performed in a client who engages in anal receptive type intercourse if there is concern about an anal STI such as gonorrhea or chlamydia.

E
1. Insert a sterile cotton swab ⅜ inch (1 cm) into the anal canal.
2. Hold the swab in place for 20 to 30 seconds and rotate the swab gently.
3. Remove the swab. If fecal material is collected, discard the cotton swab and start again.
4. Place the cotton swab in the specimen tube.
5. Submit the specimens to the appropriate laboratory per your institution's guidelines for culture specimens.

N **Anal tissues are normally free of *Neisseria gonorrhoeae.***

A The presence of a large number of gram-negative diplococci is abnormal.

P This is indicative of *N. gonorrhoeae.*

Inspection of the Vaginal Wall

E
1. Disengage the locking device of the speculum.
2. Slowly withdraw the speculum, but do not close the blades.
3. Rotate the speculum into an oblique position as you retract it to allow full inspection of the vaginal walls. Observe vaginal wall color and texture.

N **The vaginal walls should be shiny, pink, moist, deeply rugated, and without lesions or redness.**

A Decreased rugae in a mildly shortened and narrowed vagina is abnormal.

A Atrophic vaginitis caused by a decrease in estrogen in postmenopausal females leads to a mildly shortened and narrowed vaginal vault with thinning of the vaginal mucosal walls. The vaginal walls may not be shiny in appearance due to the dryness of the vaginal mucosal wall.

A Spots that appear as white paint on the walls are abnormal.

P A possible cause of white spots on the vaginal walls is leukoplakia from *Candida albicans.* Repeated occurrences even after treatment may indicate HIV infection.

A Pallor of the vaginal walls is abnormal.

P Pallor of the vaginal walls can be caused by anemia and atrophic vaginitis.

A Redness and abrasions of the vaginal walls are abnormal.

P Possible causes of vaginal erythema include inflammation, hyperemia, and trauma from tampon insertion or removal. Areas of vaginal abrasions that can bleed easily may be caused by decreased estrogen as occurs in atrophic vaginitis in many postmenopausal females. Mucoid discharge with scant specks of blood can sometimes be seen.

A Vaginal lesions or masses are abnormal findings (Fig. 21-45).

P Possible causes of vaginal lesions or masses include STIs, carcinoma, tumors, and DES exposure.

Bimanual Examination

E 1. Observe the client's face for signs of discomfort during the examination process.
2. Inform the client of the steps of the bimanual examination, and that the lubricant gel may be cold.
3. Squeeze water-soluble lubricant onto the fingertips of your dominant hand.
4. Stand between the legs of the client who is in the lithotomy position, and place your nondominant hand on the client's abdomen and below the umbilicus.
5. Insert your dominant index and middle fingers 1 cm into the vagina. The fingers should be extended with the palmar side up. Exert gentle posterior pressure.
6. Inform the client that pressure from palpation may be uncomfortable. Instruct the client to relax the abdominal muscles by taking deep breaths.
7. When you feel the client's muscles relax, insert your fingers to their full length into the vagina. Insert your fingers slowly so that you can simultaneously palpate the vaginal walls.
8. Remember to keep your thumb widely abducted and away from the urethral meatus and clitoris throughout the palpation to prevent pain or spasm.

Vagina

E Complete steps 1–8 of the bimanual examination. Rotate the wrist so that the fingers can palpate all surface aspects of the vagina.

N **The vaginal wall is nontender and has a smooth or rugated surface with no lesions, masses, or cysts.**

A The presence of lesions, masses, scarring, or cysts is abnormal.

P Vaginal lesions, masses, scarring, or cysts may be indicative of benign lesions such as inclusion cysts, myomas, or fibromas. The most common site for malignant lesions of the vagina is the upper one-third of the posterior vaginal wall.

Cervix

E 1. Position the dominant hand so that the palmar surface faces upward.
2. Place the nondominant hand on the abdomen approximately one-third of the way down between the umbilicus and the symphysis pubis.
3. Use the palmar surfaces of the dominant hand's finger pads, which are in the vagina, to assess the cervix for consistency, position, shape, and tenderness.
4. Grasp the cervix between the fingertips and move the cervix from side to side to assess mobility (Fig. 21-46).

N **The normal cervix is mobile without pain, smooth and firm, symmetrically rounded, and midline.**

A The presence of pain on palpation or the assessment of mobility is a positive **Chandelier sign** and is abnormal.

P Chandelier sign can be positive in pelvic inflammatory disease or ectopic pregnancy.

A Softening of the cervix (Goodell sign) is a significant finding.

P Goodell sign is seen in the fifth to sixth week of pregnancy.

A Irregular surface, immobility, or nodular surface structure of the cervix indicates abnormality.

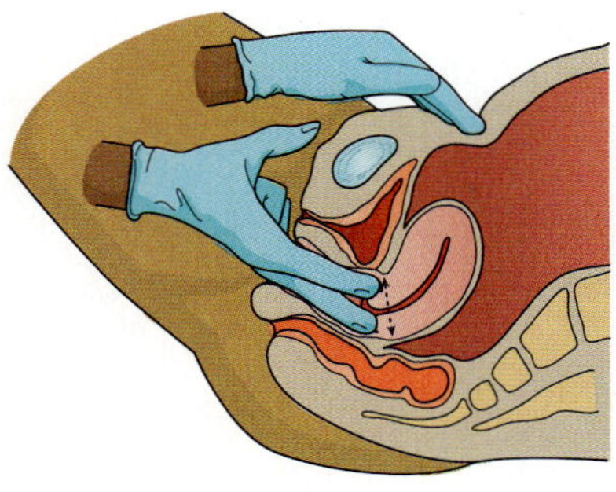

Figure 21-46 Assessment of cervical mobility.

NURSING TIP
Uterine Leiomyomas

Leiomyomas are smooth muscle tumors of the uterus, also known as fibroids. They are classified by their location in the uterus.

- Submucous—protrude into the uterine cavity and cause pain
- Intramural—within the myometrial wall
- Subserous—growing near the serous layer of the uterus
- Intraligamentous—located on the cervix or broad ligaments

Leiomyomas usually occur between puberty and menopause and are the leading cause of hysterectomy. Though usually benign, they may grow to be very large and painful. They are more common in Black females.

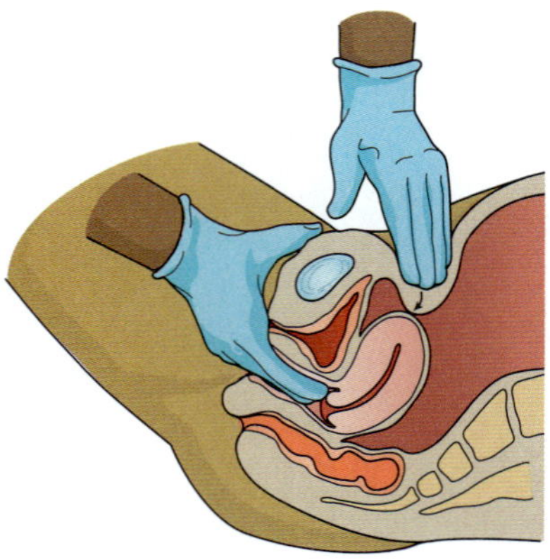

Figure 21-47 Uterine palpation.

P Possible causes include malignancy, fibroids, nabothian cysts, and polyps.

Fornices

E
1. With the fingertips and palmar surfaces of the fingers, palpate around the fornices.
2. Note nodules or irregularities.

N **The fornices' walls should be smooth and without nodules.**

A The presence of nodules or irregularities on the fornices' walls is abnormal.

P Possible causes of irregularities in the fornices' walls include malignancy, polyps, and herniations if the walls are impatent.

Uterus

E
1. With the dominant hand, which is in the vagina, push the pelvic organs out of the pelvic cavity and provide stabilization while the nondominant hand, which is on the abdomen, performs the palpation (Fig. 21-47).
2. Press the hand that is on the abdomen inward and downward toward the vagina, and try to grasp the uterus between your hands.
3. Evaluate the uterus for size, shape, consistency, mobility, tenderness, masses, and position.
4. Place the fingers of the intravaginal hand into the anterior fornix and palpate the uterine surface.

N **The size of the uterus varies based on parity; it should be pear-shaped in the nongravid client and more rounded in the parous client. The uterus should be smooth, firm, mobile, nontender, and without masses. For uterine positions, see Figure 21-3. A uterus may be nonpalpable if it is retroverted or retroflexed. The uterus in these positions can be assessed only via rectovaginal examination. A nonpalpable uterus in the older female may be a normal finding secondary to uterine atrophy.**

A Significant exterior enlargement and changes in the shape of the uterus are abnormal.

P Uterine enlargement indicates possible intrauterine pregnancy or tumor.

A Presence of nodules or irregularities indicates leiomyomas (see the Nursing Tip: Uterine Leiomyomas).

P Leiomyomas are tumors containing muscle tissue.

A An inability to assess the uterus can be a normal variant or an abnormality.

P A retroverted and retroflexed uterus is best assessed via the rectovaginal examination. A female who had a hysterectomy will not have a palpable uterus.

Adnexa

Uterine tubes are rarely palpable, and palpation of the ovaries depends on the client's age and size. Many times, the ovaries are not palpable, and this procedure can be painful to the client during the luteal phase of the menstrual cycle (postovulation) or due to normal visceral tenderness.

E
1. Move the intravaginal hand to the right lateral fornix, and the hand on the abdomen to the right lower quadrant just inside the anterior iliac spine. Press deeply inward and upward toward the abdominal hand.

2. Push inward and downward with the abdominal hand and try to catch the ovary between your fingertips.
3. Palpate for size, shape, consistency, and mobility of the adnexa.
4. Repeat these maneuvers on the left side (Fig. 21-48).

N **The ovaries are normally almond-shaped, firm, smooth, and mobile without tenderness.**

A Presence of enlarged ovaries that are irregular, nodular, painful, with decreased mobility, or pulsatile indicates pathology.

P Abnormal adnexal presentation may indicate ectopic pregnancy, ovarian cyst, pelvic inflammatory disease, or malignancy.

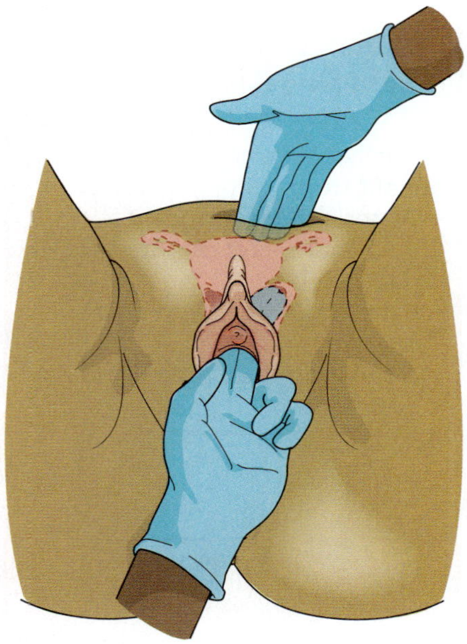

Figure 21-48 Palpation of the left adnexa.

NURSING TIP

Gynecological Examinations for Clients After Hysterectomies

If the client had a hysterectomy, follow the same examination sequence but omit the following items: cervical palpation, uterine palpation, endocervical smear, and cervical smear. The vaginal walls and adnexa are evaluated if they were not surgically removed during the hysterectomy. Some clients feel that it is unnecessary to have gynecological examinations after a hysterectomy. Many of these clients had surgery because of malignancy and therefore are at risk for recurrence. A client who had a hysterectomy must be encouraged to continue seeking gynecological examinations. Yearly monitoring helps to determine whether the malignancy has returned or if other pathologies have developed; for instance, a client whose ovaries were not removed in the hysterectomy is still at risk for ovarian cancer. A client who had a hysterectomy with the cervix removed and does not have a history of high-grade precancerous cervical lesions or cervical cancer does not need to continue to be screened for cervical cancer.

Rectovaginal Examination

E

1. Withdraw your dominant hand from the vagina and change gloves. Apply additional lubricant to the fingertips of your dominant hand.
2. Tell the client you will be inserting one finger into the vagina and one finger into the rectum. Remind the client that the lubricant jelly will feel cold and that the rectal examination will be uncomfortable.
3. Insert the dominant index finger back into the vagina.
4. Ask the client to strain down as when having a bowel movement, to relax the anal sphincter. Assess anal sphincter tone.
5. Insert the middle finger of the dominant hand into the client's rectum as they strain down (Fig. 21-49). If the rectum is full of stool, carefully remove the stool digitally from the rectum.
6. Advance the rectal finger forward while using the nondominant hand to depress the abdomen. Assess the rectovaginal septum for patency, the cervix and uterus for anomalies such as posterior lesions, and the rectouterine pouch for contour lesions.
7. On completion of the examination, withdraw the fingers from the vagina and rectum. If any stool is present on the glove, test for occult blood.
8. Provide the client with tissue to clean the genitalia and anal areas; when they have finished, assist the client back to a sitting position.

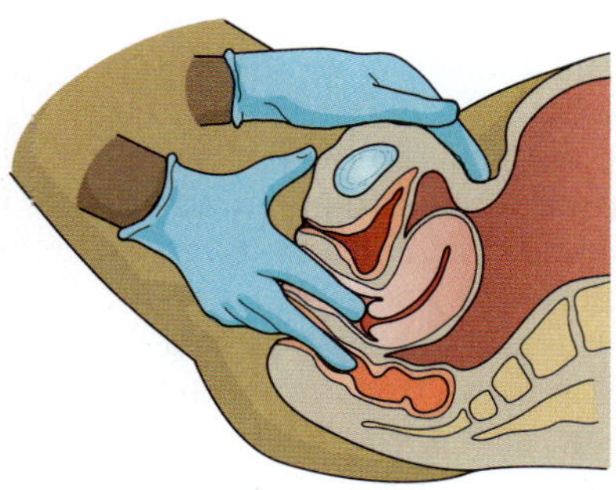

Figure 21-49 Rectovaginal examination.

N The rectal walls are normally smooth and free of lesions. The rectal pouch is rugated and free of masses. The anal sphincter tone is strong. The cervix and uterus, if palpable, are smooth. The rectovaginal septum is smooth and intact. Refer to Chapter 23 for further information on the complete rectal examination.

A The presence of masses or lesions indicates pathology.

P Possible causes of rectal masses or lesions include malignancy and internal hemorrhoids.

A Lax anal sphincter tone is an abnormal finding.

P Possible causes include perineal trauma from childbirth or anal intercourse and neurological disorders.

NURSING TIP

Maintaining Sexual Function in the Menopausal Female

Sexually active older females may benefit from:

- Water-soluble lubricant if vaginal secretions are decreased
- Extended foreplay to attain orgasm
- A reminder that there is no risk of pregnancy

NURSING TIP

Nursing Care of the Transgender Male Client

A general physical examination or gynecological/urological examination can be a source of extreme stress for some transgender male clients. Knowing the clinical status of the client is important to provide appropriate care. Some transgender clients dress in a manner consistent with their chosen gender identity. They may practice packing and the use of commercially available products that give the appearance of male genitals. Some clients use hormone replacement therapy as part of their transition. And some clients undergo surgery such as hysterectomy and salpingo-oopherectomy, colpectomy, metoidioplasty, phalloplasty (includes phallus, glansplasty, urethroplasty, and erectile prosthesis), and scrotoplasty with testicular implants. Surgery requires interdisciplinary care management involving multiple surgical disciplines. If the transgender client has not had the surgical removal of female reproductive organs, then a gynecological examination including a Pap smear needs to be done. Standards that guide these transitions can be found at the World Professional Association for Transgender Health (WPATH) *www.wpath.org.*

U.S. Preventive Services Task Force (USPSTF)

Grade A Recommendations:

- The USPSTF recommends screening for cervical cancer every 3 years with cervical cytology alone in women aged 21 to 29 years. For women aged 30 to 65 years, the USPSTF recommends screening every 3 years with cervical cytology alone, every 5 years with high-risk papillomavirus (hrHPV) testing alone, or every 5 years with hrHPV testing in combination with cytology (cotesting).
- The USPSTF recommends that clinicians screen for HIV infection in adolescents and adults aged 15 to 65 years. Younger adolescents and older adults who are at increased risk of infection should also be screened.
- The USPSTF recommends that clinicians prescribe pre-exposure prophylaxis using effective antiretroviral therapy to persons who are at increased risk of HIV acquisition to decrease the risk of acquiring HIV.
- The USPSTF recommends screening for syphilis infection in persons who are at increased risk for infection.

Grade B Recommendations:

- The USPSTF recommends that primary care clinicians assess women with a personal or family history of breast, ovarian, tubal, or peritoneal cancer or who have an ancestry associated with breast cancer susceptibility 1 and 2 (BRCA1/2) gene mutations with an appropriate brief familial risk assessment tool. Women with a positive result on the risk assessment tool should receive genetic counseling and, if indicated after counseling, genetic testing.
- The USPSTF recommends screening for chlamydia and gonorrhea in all sexually active women 24 years or younger and in women 25 years or older who are at increased risk for infection.
- The USPSTF recommends screening for hepatitis B virus (HBV) infection in adolescents and adults at increased risk for infection
- The USPSTF recommends screening for hepatitis C virus (HCV) infection in adults aged 18 to 79 years.
- The USPSTF recommends that clinicians screen for intimate partner violence (IPV) in women of reproductive age and provide or refer women who screen positive to ongoing support services.
- The USPSTF recommends behavioral counseling for all sexually active adolescents and for adults who are at increased risk for sexually transmitted infections (STIs).

Retrieved December 17, 2025 from *https://www.uspreventiveservicestaskforce.org/uspstf/recommendation-topics/uspstf-a-and-b-recommendations*

CASE STUDY

The Client With Atrophic Vaginitis

This case study illustrates the application and objective documentation of the female genitalia examination. Brenda Johnson is a 55-year-old postmenopausal female who has been a widow for over 5 years. She was married for 23 years and has two grown children who do not live near her. Since the death of her husband, Brenda had not been in a relationship nor was she sexually active until recently. She has been dating a male partner for the past 6 months whom she met at the gym. They have been sexually active for 1 month. Brenda presents with complaints of painful intercourse and urination after intercourse.

HEALTH HISTORY

CLIENT PROFILE

55-year-old widowed Black female

CHIEF COMPLAINT

"I feel like my vagina is on fire during and after intercourse."

HISTORY OF PRESENT ILLNESS

Ms. Johnson states she has recently resumed sexual intercourse after 5 years of celibacy after the death of her spouse. She has been postmenopausal for the last 3 years. In the past month, she has been sexually active once a week, however, each time it has not been pleasurable. She complains of vaginal dryness, itching, burning with penetration, and urination. There has been some spotting after sex. It's also hard for her to become lubricated. She has no hematuria, lower back pain, or fever. There has been no treatment for her symptoms.

PAST HEALTH HISTORY

Medical History Seasonal allergic rhinitis (SAR): Pollen and ragweed allergies: sneezing, runny nose, itchy eyes and ears

Female Reproductive Health History Menstrual history: Menarche at age 13, 28-day cycle with low/moderate flow for 4 days; last menstrual period (LMP) 3 years ago

Reproductive medical history: Denies any STIs, endometriosis, cancer of the reproductive organs, or abnormal Pap smears

Obstetric history: Gravida: 2; Para: Term: 2; Preterm:0; Abortion:0; Living children:2; Spontaneous vaginal delivery for both births,

Premenstrual syndrome: Denies

Menopause history: Last menses 3 years ago. Does not take HRT

Vaginal discharge: Clear

History of uterine bleeding: Complains of postcoital bleeding

Sexual functioning: Heterosexual, sexually active for 22 years, 4 lifetime partners; was with deceased husband for 23 years and current partner for 1 month, frequent dyspareunia at insertion and penetration

Method of birth control: Denies use

Surgical History Denies

Allergies NKDA; denies insect, bee sting, latex, and food allergies

Medications Levocetirizine 5 mg as needed spring, summer, and fall

Azelastine 137 mcg (0.1%) 2 sprays each nostril 1 to 2 times daily prn

Multivitamin daily

Communicable Diseases Denies

Injuries and Accidents Denies

Differing Abilities Denies

Blood Transfusions Denies

Childhood Illnesses Chickenpox as a child, unsure of age

Immunizations Annual flu shot; initial COVID vaccine June 2021, one booster in 2022; completed herpes zoster vaccines x 2 last year; Tdap last year

FAMILY HEALTH HISTORY

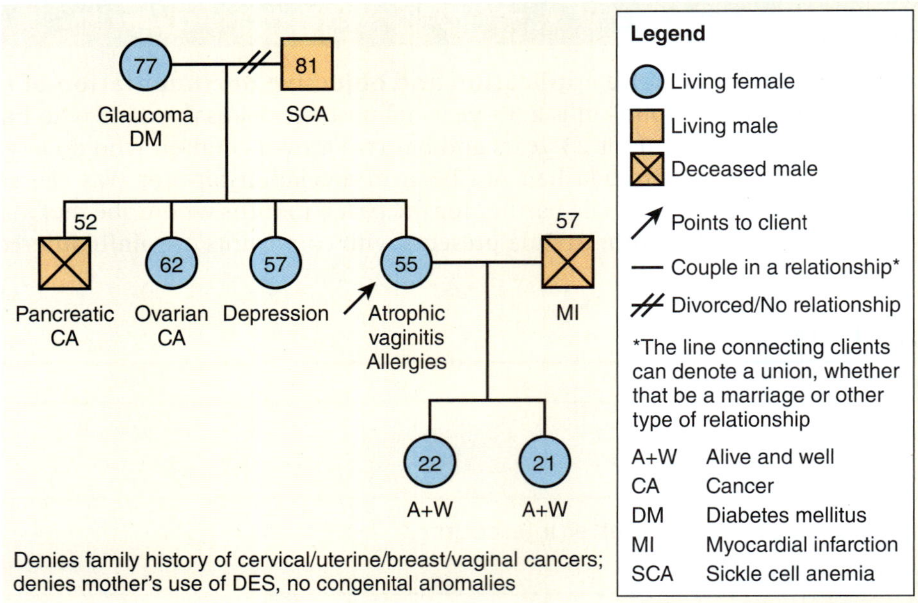

SOCIAL HISTORY

Alcohol Use Wine socially on weekends (2 glasses once a week)

Tobacco Use Denies

Recreational Drug Use Denies

Domestic and Intimate Partner Violence Denies

Sexual Practice Monogamous with all past partners

Travel History Family vacations to visit children out of state on holidays

Work Environment Works at local hospital as a social worker assisting clients with discharge planning and social services. Has been in the same job for 17 years. Enjoys her job and her colleagues

Home Environment Lives alone in single-family detached house; new construction with all modern conveniences. Checks smoke detector and carbon monoxide detector on her wedding anniversary

Hobbies and Leisure Activities Cycling and aerobic classes weekly at local gym; active member in her church, sings in the choir

Stress Concerned with painful intercourse. Does not want it to negatively impact her new relationship

Education Master's degree in social work

Economic Status Middle-upper income

Military Status Denies

Religion Presbyterian, active in church

Ethnic Background Black American

Roles and Relationships Mother, employee; states she is well equipped to juggle these roles, "I enjoy all aspects of my life."

Characteristic Patterns of Daily Living Wakes up at 6:00 AM to pray and have morning devotion. She prepares her breakfast and lunch before going to work. She drives to work at 7:30 AM to get to work by 8:00 AM. She has her regularly scheduled lunch at 12:00 PM, home by 4:30 PM, makes dinner by 6:00 PM. On certain evenings she has choir rehearsal, bible study, or goes to her gym to work out. Enjoys a "date night" every Saturday with new partner

HEALTH MAINTENANCE ACTIVITIES

Sleep 8 hr per night

Diet Well-balanced, low-fat diet

Exercise One-hour aerobic/cycling class on Saturday and occasional weeknights

Stress Management Prays and talks to friends

Use of Safety Devices Wears seat belts in the car; alarm system in home

Health Checkup Last gyn examination 3 years ago; Pap/HPV were negative
Last mammogram was 3 years ago: Negative
Performs monthly BSE
Vision and dental examinations annually

PHYSICAL EXAMINATION

Inspection of the External Genitalia

Pubic Hair Thin and faint, no nits or lice

Skin Color and Condition Mons pubis and vulva: clean, dry, intact; labia majora and labia minora are mildly erythematous with fissure-like lesions, brown skin color, free of discharge and odor

Clitoris No lesions

Urethral meatus Midline without swelling or discharge

Vaginal introitus Pink without lesions, scant mucoid discharge with specks of blood

Perineum and anus Pink-brown perineum, anus dark brown without hemorrhoids

Palpation of the External Genitalia

Labia Swollen, and mildly tender

Urethral Meatus and Skene Glands No pain or discharge

Vaginal Introitus Moderate muscle tone without protrusion of internal organs

Perineum Intact

Speculum Examination of the Internal Genitalia

Cervix
Color: Pink
Position: Midline
Size: 6 cm
Surface characteristics: Smooth, glistening pink
Discharge: None
Shape of the cervical os: Parous

Inspection of the Vaginal Wall Pale pink with decreased rugae and dry vaginal mucosa

Bimanual Examination

Vagina No masses, nontender

Cervix Nontender and mobile

Fornices No masses

Uterus Mobile, nontender, firm; anteflexed and parous

Adnexa Nontender

Rectovaginal Examination Deferred

CLINICAL JUDGMENT IN ACTION

1. What cues indicate that the client is having a disorder of the female genitalia?
2. What interventions have the highest priority?
3. What assessment findings indicate clinical improvement or decline in this client?

Review Questions

1. Which of the following substances is responsible for producing high levels of progesterone during the luteal phase of the female reproductive cycle?
   a. Luteinizing hormone
   b. Follicle-stimulating hormone
   c. Estrogen
   d. Corpus luteum

2. A 12-year-old client presents to the pediatrician for an annual physical examination. Which of the following physical findings would you expect to see if there have been no developmental delays?
   a. No pubic hair at this age
   b. Sparse growth of long, fine pubic hair
   c. Darker and curlier pubic hair that covers the symphysis pubis
   d. Hair growth that has spread to thighs and abdomen

3. A client presents to the clinic with complaints of dysuria, dyspareunia, and a vaginal discharge. The nurse assesses for which of the following conditions? Select all that apply.
   a. Gonorrhea
   b. Chlamydia
   c. Candida
   d. Cervical cancer
   e. Trichomoniasis

4. A 20-year-old college student presents to the student health center for an initial gynecological examination. The client has never been sexually active. The nurse should:
   a. Perform the genital examination only.
   b. Perform the genital examination and STI screening test since the client is a college student.
   c. Inform the client a genital examination is not necessary until the client is 21 years old.
   d. Decline to perform the examination until a parent is present.

5. A 35-year-old client presents for a well client visit with a complaint of vaginal discharge and spotting. In which order will the nurse perform the following tests?
   a. Bacterial vaginosis, Pap, gonorrhea/chlamydia, trichomoniasis
   b. Gonorrhea/chlamydia, bacterial vaginosis, trichomoniasis, Pap
   c. Pap, gonorrhea/chlamydia, trichomoniasis, bacterial vaginosis
   d. Trichomoniasis, bacterial vaginosis, gonorrhea/chlamydia, Pap

6. A sexually active client presents with a complaint of a foul-smelling vaginal discharge. The nurse detects a "fishy" odor upon examination. The nurse suspects that the client has which of the following conditions?
   a. Candidiasis
   b. Bacterial vaginosis
   c. Gonorrhea
   d. Normal physiological discharge

7. When performing a bimanual examination on a client, the nurse notices the client grimacing and wincing during the examination while palpating the cervix. The nurse's best course of action is:
   a. Continue with the examination because the response is normal.
   b. Document a positive Goodell sign because it is an expected response.
   c. Acknowledge the client's nonverbal behavior and ask what is being felt during the examination.
   d. Document a positive Chandelier sign as a normal response during the examination.

8. Mrs. Butrus brings an 8-year-old daughter, Zaina, in for an annual physical examination and immunizations. Mrs. Butrus inquires if Zaina should get the HPV vaccine today. The nurse's best response is:
   a. Yes. I can give it to Zaina today if you request it and sign the consent form.
   b. Yes. There may be an additional expense because Zaina was not scheduled for it.
   c. No, current guidelines recommend both boys and girls should initiate the HPV vaccination between the ages of 11 and 12 although a 9-year-old child may be eligible.
   d. No. Zaina needs to make a separate appointment for the vaccine because fasting is involved.

9. Which of the following are risk factors for cervical cancer? Select all that apply.
   a. History of chlamydia
   b. History of human papillomavirus
   c. Polycystic ovary syndrome
   d. Multiple sex partners
   e. Unopposed estrogen therapy
   f. Daughter of a woman who took DES during pregnancy

10. The nurse documents the presence of a cystocele. Which statement best describes this clinical finding?
    a. Bulging of the anterior vaginal wall by the bladder
    b. Bulging of the posterior vaginal wall with a portion of the rectum
    c. Bulging of the anterior vaginal wall, bladder, and urethra into the vaginal introitus
    d. Bulging of the cervix, uterus, and vagina outside the introitus

CHAPTER

22 Male Genitalia

Learning Outcomes

1. Identify the anatomy and physiology of the male genitalia.
2. Conduct a complete health history on a client with a male genitalia condition.
3. Perform a physical examination on a healthy adult and an adult with male genitalia pathology.
4. Differentiate between normal clinical findings from a client's physical examination of the male genitalia and the pathophysiology of abnormal clinical findings.
5. Identify risk factors for penile cancer.
6. Identify risk factors for testicular cancer.
7. Identify the United States Preventive Services Task Force recommendations for the male client.
8. Document a complete health history and physical examination of a client with male genitalia pathology.

The male reproductive system includes essential and accessory organs, ducts, and supporting structures (Fig. 22-1). The essential organs are the testes, or male gonads. The accessory organs include the seminal vesicles and bulbourethral glands. There are also several ducts, including the epididymis, ductus (vas) deferens, ejaculatory ducts, and urethra. The supporting structures include the scrotum, penis, and spermatic cords. The prostate is discussed in Chapter 23.

Anatomy and Physiology

Organs, ducts, supporting structures, and sexual development are discussed.

Essential Organs

The **testes**, or testicles, are two oval glands located in the scrotum. The average measurement is about 5 cm (2 inches) in length and 2.5 cm (1 inch) in width. The testes are partially covered by a serous membrane called the tunica vaginalis (Fig. 22-2). This membrane separates the testes from the scrotal wall. Interior to the tunica vaginalis is a dense, whitish membrane covering each testicle, called the tunica albuginea. This membrane enters the testes and divides each testis into sections called lobules, which contain tightly coiled tubules called the seminiferous tubules. These coiled structures are the main component of testicular mass, and they produce sperm by spermatogenesis.

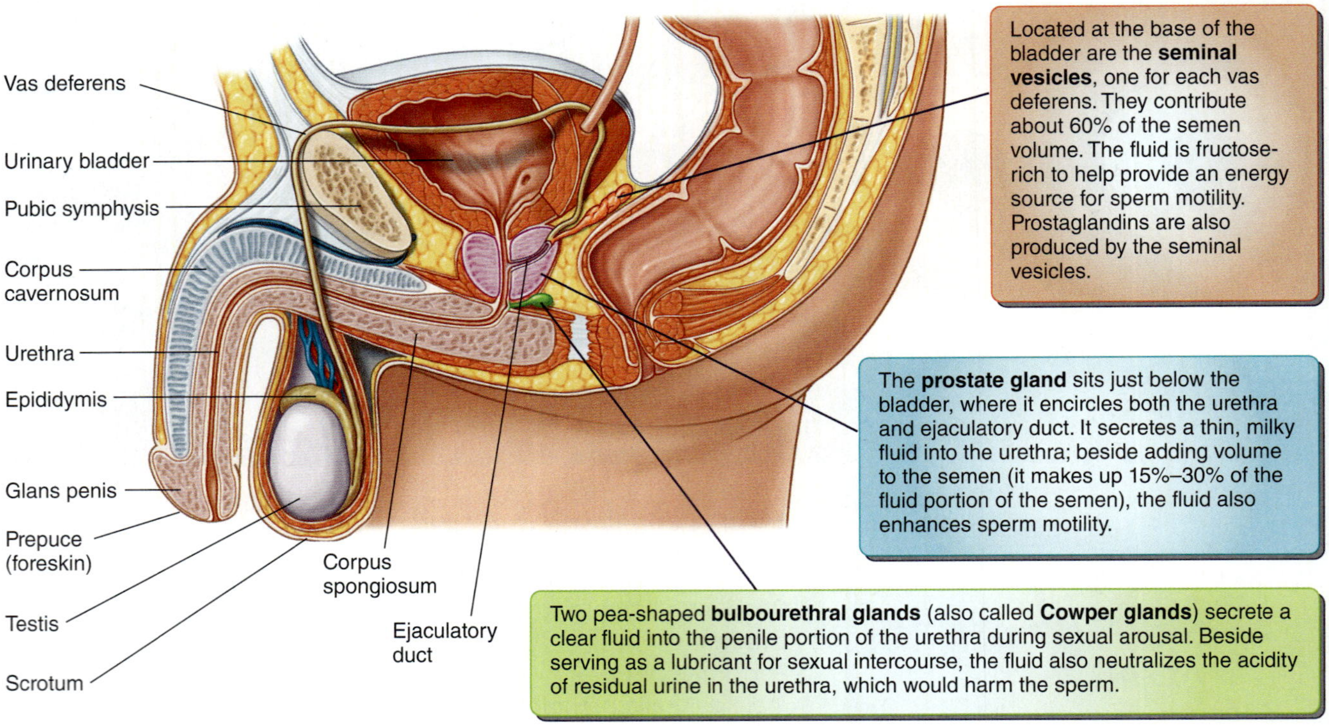

Figure 22-1 Male genitalia.

Accessory Organs

The **seminal vesicles** are two pouches located posterior to and at the base of the bladder and above the prostate. They contribute about 60% of the volume of semen. The fluid secreted by the seminal vesicles is rich in fructose and helps provide a source of energy for sperm metabolism. Prostaglandins, which contribute to sperm motility and viability, are also produced by the seminal vesicles.

The **bulbourethral glands**, or Cowper glands, are pea-sized glands located just below the prostate. Clear secretions are emptied from the bulbourethral glands at the time of ejaculation. The bulbourethral glands secrete an alkaline substance that protects sperm by neutralizing the acidity of the urine residue in the male urethra and the acidic environment of the vagina. These glands also provide lubrication at the end of the penis during sexual stimulation and intercourse.

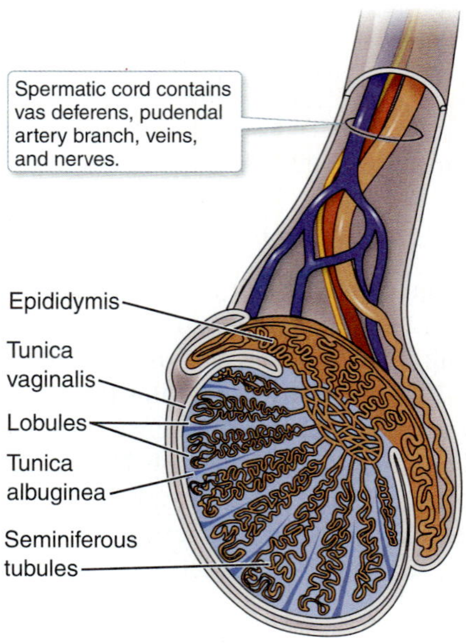

Figure 22-2 Testicle.

Ducts

The **epididymis** is a comma-shaped, tightly coiled tube that is located on top of and behind the testis and inside the scrotum. Each epididymis is composed of three parts: the head, which is connected to the testis; the body; and the tail, which is continuous with the vas deferens. Sperm mature and develop the power of motility as they pass through the epididymis.

The **ductus (vas) deferens** is an extension of the tail of the epididymis. Each duct ascends from the scrotum and permits sperm to exit from the scrotal sac upward into the abdominal cavity. The ductus deferens loops over the side and down the posterior surface of the bladder. This is where the duct enlarges into the ampulla of the vas deferens and joins the duct from the seminal vesicles to form the ejaculatory ducts.

The **ejaculatory ducts** are two short tubes posterior to the bladder. They descend through the prostate gland and terminate in the urethra. The ducts eject spermatozoa into the prostatic urethra just before ejaculation.

The **urethra** is the terminal duct of the seminal fluid passageway. It measures on average about 20 cm (8 inches) in length, passes through the prostate gland and penis, and terminates at the external urethral orifice (meatal opening).

Supporting Structures

The **scrotum** is a pouchlike supporting structure for the testes and consists of rugated, deeply pigmented, loose skin. Inside, the scrotum is divided by a single septum into two sacs, each containing a single testis. The production and survival of sperm require a temperature that is 34°F (1°C) cooler than normal body temperature 98.6°F (37°C). This is achieved by the scrotum's exposed location.

The **penis**, or male organ of copulation and urination, is hairless, slightly pigmented, and cylindrical in shape. It consists of three compartments of erectile tissue. The corpus spongiosum surrounds the urethra and is located ventromedially. The two corpora cavernosa are located on the dorsolateral sides of the corpus spongiosum. Distally, the corpus spongiosum expands to form the **glans penis**, or the bulbous end of the penis. In the uncircumcised male, a fold of loose skin, the **prepuce** (foreskin), covers the glans penis. The corona forms the border between the glans penis and the penile shaft. The penis contains the urethra, a slit-like opening on the tip of the glans. The urethra terminates at the urethral meatus and is the passageway for urine.

The **spermatic cord** is made up of testicular arteries, autonomic nerves, veins that drain the testicles, lymphatic vessels, and the cremaster muscle. The testicles are suspended by the spermatic cord and rarely present symmetrically as far as position in the scrotal sac. The cremaster muscle elevates the testes during sexual stimulation and exposure to cold. It also surrounds the testicles; its primary role is to keep the testes in a position that optimizes the temperature for sperm production.

The spermatic cord and ilioinguinal nerves pass through the inguinal canal into the abdomen. The inguinal canal is an oblique passageway in the anterior abdominal wall. The canal is about 4 to 5 cm (1.5 to 2 inches) long. It originates at the deep inguinal ring. The distal opening of the inguinal canal is called the external inguinal ring and is accessible to palpation. Superior to the inguinal canal lies the inguinal ligament, or Poupart ligament. The inguinal ligament extends from the anterior iliac spine to the pubic tubercle.

Sexual Development

Sexual development can be assessed according to the five stages described by Tanner (Table 22-1). Most of the changes in the male genitalia occur during puberty, starting between ages 9½ and 13½. The development of male genitalia to adult size and shape can take 2 to 5 years, with 3 years being the average.

Spermatogenesis

The primary function of the male reproductive system is to produce sperm to fertilize eggs. For this to be achieved, several essential features of male reproduction must take place. These are the production of sperm and the deposition of sperm into the female genital tract.

The testes produce sperm by a process called **spermatogenesis**. Specialized cells found between the seminiferous tubules, called the interstitial cells of Leydig, secrete the male hormone testosterone. Testosterone is an androgen and is responsible for the development of secondary sexual characteristics and the attainment of reproductive capacity. Testosterone is responsible for male sexual feelings, libido, and performance as well as muscle and skeletal development. The testes prepare for sperm production at approximately 13 years of age.

NURSING TIP
Males' Unique Health Issues

Nurses must understand the variability of masculine identity and behavior over the course of a male's life and consider how this behavior is formed by cultural and ethnic background, sexual identity, socioeconomic factors, and geographic location. Male socialization, social connectedness, and work-life balance also impact a male client's overall health. Males typically do not engage as frequently in routine health maintenance and have been conditioned to engage in health-care services much later when faced with illness, which often means presenting with later-stage illness.

Male's health is marginalized nationally; there is no national office for male's health that parallels the Office of Women's Health, which was established by the U.S. government in 1991. Males are more vulnerable to some conditions than females due to genetic and immunological differences (Channappanavar et al, 2017; Klein & Flanagan, 2016). The challenge for nurses is to remain engaged in the male's health arena, improve their own gender competency in the delivery of health and health-related services, and raise awareness that males have unique health issues that are not simply related to their reproductive organs.

Table 22-1 Sexual Maturity Rating (SMR) for Male Genitalia

Developmental Stage	Pubic Hair	Penis	Scrotum
1. 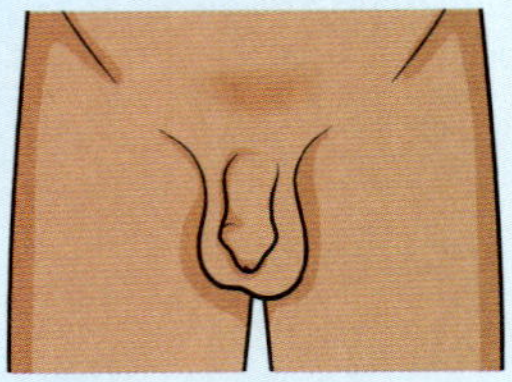	No pubic hair, only fine body hair (vellus hair)	Preadolescent; childhood size and proportion	Preadolescent; childhood size and proportion
2. 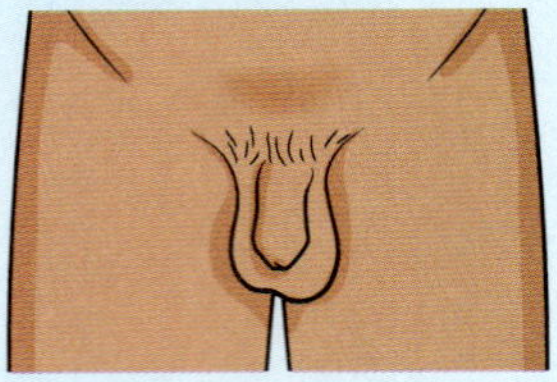	Sparse growth of long, slightly dark, straight hair	Slight or no growth	Growth in testes and scrotum; scrotum reddens and changes texture
3. 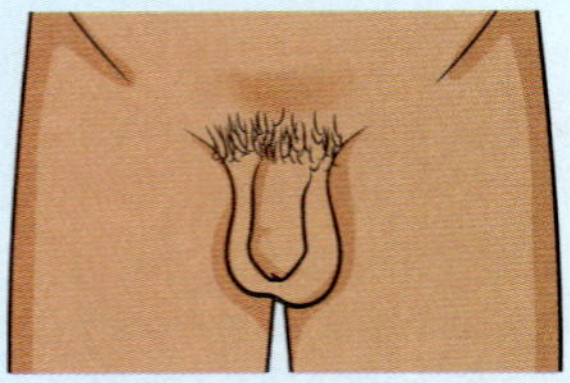	Becomes darker and coarser; slightly curled and spreads over symphysis	Growth, especially in length	Further growth
4. 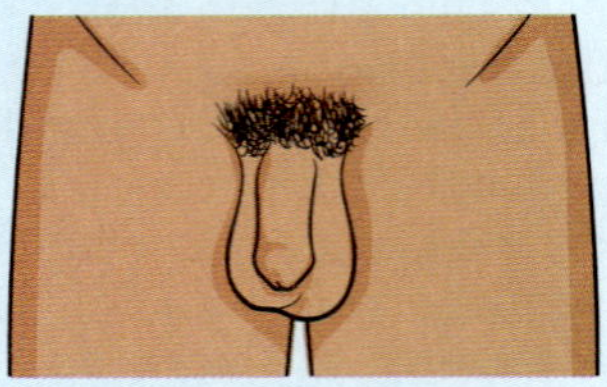	Texture and curl of pubic hair are similar to that of an adult but not spread to thighs	Further growth in length; diameter increases; development of glans	Further growth; scrotum darkens
5. 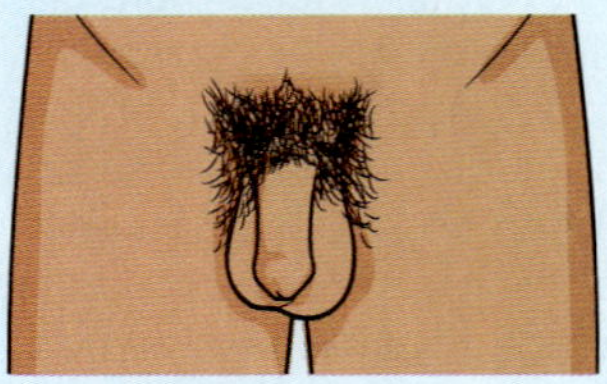	Adult appearance in quality and quantity of pubic hair; growth is spread to medial surface of thighs	Adult size and shape	Adult size and shape

Male Sexual Function

The male sexual act consists of four stages: erection, lubrication, emission, and ejaculation. Erection of the penis is the first stage and is achieved through either physical or psychogenic stimulation of sensory nerves in the genital area. Parasympathetic impulses from the sacral portion of the spinal cord cause a vascular effect. The arterioles dilate and blood fills the corpora cavernosa, causing the penis to expand and become rigid. The corpora cavernosa can hold from 20 to 50 mL of blood, or 40x the normal flow of a flaccid penis. The veins from the tissue are compressed to occlude venous outflow.

Parasympathetic impulses at the same time cause the bulbourethral glands to secrete mucus, which provides lubrication during intercourse. When the sexual stimulus reaches a critical intensity, the reflex centers of the spinal cord send sympathetic impulses to the genital organs, and an orgasm occurs. Emission begins with contraction of the epididymis and the vas deferens, causing expulsion of sperm into the internal urethra. Ejaculation follows with contractions of the penile urethra.

NURSING TIP
Erectile Function

Treatment for impotence varies greatly depending on the cause and may include any of the following:

- Patience and a relaxed atmosphere
- Oral medication: halotestin, yohimbine HCl, phosphodiesterase type 5 inhibitors
- Penile prosthesis
- Intracavernosal injections
- Vacuum erection device
- Transurethral suppositories

> **NURSING TIP**
> **Male Sexual History**
> Gender identity does not indicate sexual identity or suggest a specific sexual partner preference. The nurse should strive to provide inclusive interactions, accepting, and affirming an individual's identity, regardless of the clinical setting. When assessing sexual history and STI risk, begin questions by prefacing why the questions are needed and that they are of a sensitive and private nature.
> - "Do you have any general questions about safe sex practices?"
> - "Do you have any questions or concerns regarding your sexual health?"
> - "What are the genders of your partners (i.e., cisgender man, cisgender woman, trans man, trans woman, non-binary)?"
> - "What type of sex do you engage in—anal, oral, vaginal?"
> - "Do you have questions about your fertility potential or fertility preservation?"

HEALTH HISTORY

The male genitalia health history provides insight into the link between a client's life/lifestyle and male genitalia information and pathology.

CLIENT PROFILE

Diseases that are age- and race-specific for the male genitalia are listed.

Age

Testicular torsion (12 to 25)
Testicular cancer (20 to 45)
Penile cancer (>60)
Testicular lymphoma (>50)

Race

White, American Indian, Alaskan Native Higher risk for testicular cancer

CHIEF COMPLAINT

Common chief complaints for the male genitalia are defined, and information on the characteristics of each sign or symptom is provided.

1. Urethral Discharge Excretion or leakage from the urethra

Quality Color: clear, white, purulent, blood-tinged, green, yellow, pink
Consistency: thin, moderate, thick, mucoid; foul odor
Quantity Absent, scant, mild, moderate, copious
Associated Manifestations Dysuria, painful ejaculation, fever, urethral meatal discharge, change in frequency of urination, pruritus, conjunctivitis, arthritis, dermatological rash, sexually transmitted infection (STI)
Aggravating Factors Urethral trauma
Alleviating Factors Medications (antibiotics, analgesics)
Increased hydration; decreased constipation
Setting A new sexual partner in the last 6 months, multiple partners, a partner known to have other partners, unprotected intercourse, other high-risk sexual behaviors
Timing Varies with etiology

2. Palpable Mass A lump in the male genitalia

Quality Firm, smooth, stellate, soft, mobile, nonmobile, well-circumscribed, poorly circumscribed, "bag of worms," hard, heavy, transilluminating, nontransilluminating, fluctuant, separate from testes
Associated Manifestations Pain, scrotal enlargement, absence of pain, gynecomastia (if mass produces estrogen or human chorionic gonadotropin), nausea, vomiting, generalized edema, rash
Aggravating Factors Positioning, palpation or pressure, lifting, edema
Alleviating Factors Medications, surgical removal or repair, positioning
Setting Post-trauma, recurrent testicular pain
Timing Mumps orchitis present 7 to 10 days following parotitis

3. Scrotal Pain Discomfort in the scrotal sac

Quality Dull, sharp, heavy

Associated Manifestations Scrotal swelling, groin pain, lower abdominal pain, flank pain, dysuria, urinary frequency, fever, nausea, vomiting, pyuria, urethral discharge, scrotal edema, erythema, infertility, history of back issues

Aggravating Factors Sexual encounter, urinary tract infection (UTI), scrotal trauma, certain physical activities, posture

Alleviating Factors Medications (antibiotics, analgesics), bedrest, scrotal elevation, surgery

Setting New sexual partner months prior, unprotected intercourse, recent urinary instrumentation

Timing Epididymitis may present months following a new or unprotected sexual encounter; it may also present shortly after a UTI

4. Erectile Dysfunction The inability or decrease in ability to achieve and maintain a penile erection

Quality Inability to achieve erection (failed nocturnal tumescence test), ability to achieve with failure to maintain erection, inability to achieve complete erection

Associated Manifestations Anxiety, systemic disease (diabetes mellitus, hypertension, coronary artery disease), decreased libido, decreased or absent cremasteric reflex, decreased femoral pulses, trauma, prostatectomy, testicular atrophy, spinal cord injury, other neurological conditions, sickle cell disease

Aggravating Factors Medications (beta blockers, diuretics, reserpine, monoamine oxidase inhibitors, selective serotonin reuptake inhibitors, diazepam, alprazolam, chemotherapeutic agents, opioids), anxiety, unsupportive partner, work/home stress, alcohol, smoking, elevated blood sugar, hyperthyroidism, hypothyroidism, illicit drug use, gender dysphoria

Alleviating Factors Medications (e.g., hormone therapy, yohimbine, anxiolytics, phosphodiesterase type 5 [PDE 5] inhibitors, alprostadil), injections, implants, avoiding alcohol, smoking cessation, change in diet (avoiding foods high in saturated fat or cholesterol), maintaining ideal body weight, reducing tension and stress, vacuum erectile device, specialized sex therapy

Setting Uncomfortable physical environment, stress

Timing Nocturnal tumescence possible after COVID-19 infection (Kaynar et al, 2022)

5. Penile Lesion A growth on the penis

Quality Color: erythematous, hyperpigmented, hypopigmented, pink, brown, black

Presentation: flat, raised, indurated, papular, macular, multiple, isolated, ulcerated, warty, exudative (clear, purulent, bloody drainage)

Associated Manifestations Fever, malaise, inguinal lymphadenopathy, pain, prodromal numbness and tingling at lesion site, myalgias, headache, pruritus, immunosuppression, systemic illness, recurrent herpes simplex virus (HSV), human papillomavirus (HPV)

Aggravating Factors Stress, systemic illness, immunosuppression, postorgan transplant

Alleviating Factors Medications (antivirals, antibiotics), surgical removal, lifestyle changes

Setting Unprotected intercourse, multiple sexual partners

Timing Lymphogranuloma venereum: papule appears 1 to 3 weeks after inoculation

Primary HSV: lesions appear 2 to 7 days after inoculation, vesicles ulcerate in 3 to 4 days

Recurrent HSV: lesions appear a few hours to days after prodromal symptoms, lesions last approximately 10 days

PAST HEALTH HISTORY

The various components of the past health history are linked to male genitalia pathology and male genitalia-related information.

Medical History

Male Genitalia Specific Prior history of STI, prostatitis, UTI, nephrolithiasis, cryptorchidism, trauma, cancer of male genitalia/organ, benign prostatic hypertrophy (BPH), congenital or acquired deformity (epispadias, hypospadias), hydrocele, varicocele, spermatocele, epididymitis, orchitis, scrotal edema, testicular torsion, testicular tumor, phimosis, paraphimosis, priapism, premature ejaculation, erectile dysfunction, infertility vs paternity (inability to father children vs ability to father children)

Nonmale Genitalia Specific Mumps, rashes, joint pain, conjunctivitis, viral illness, renal disease, congestive heart failure, spinal cord injury, pelvic fracture, diabetes mellitus, hypertension, tuberculosis, multiple sclerosis, depression, anxiety, spinal cord injury

Surgical History Prostatectomy, transurethral prostatectomy, circumcision, orchiectomy, correction of malposition of testes, vasectomy, lesion or nodule removal, epispadias repair, hypospadias repair, hernia repair, retroperitoneal or pelvic surgery

Allergies Contact dermatitis from topical preparations, condoms, nonoxynol 9, or other spermicides

Medications Antibiotics, hormone replacements, 5-alpha-reductase inhibitors, antihypertensives, psychotropic agents, phosphodiesterase type 5 (PDE 5) inhibitors

Communicable Diseases HSV, HPV, HIV, Mpox, hepatitis, molluscum contagiosum, condyloma acuminata, syphilis, chlamydia, gonorrhea, ureaplasma

Injuries and Accidents Trauma, testicular torsion, spinal cord injury, pelvic injury

Differing Abilities Urinary incontinence, indwelling or intermittent urinary catheter, penile prosthesis, suprapubic urinary catheter

Childhood Illnesses Mumps: Orchitis, infertility

Immunizations HPV vaccine series

FAMILY HEALTH HISTORY

Familial male genitalia diseases are listed.

Varicocele, testicular cancer, hypospadias, infertility, mother's use of hormones (diethylstilbestrol [DES]) during pregnancy

SOCIAL HISTORY

The components of the social history are linked to male genitalia factors and pathology.

Alcohol Use Alcohol use impairs gonadotropin release and accelerates testosterone metabolism, causing impotence and loss of libido; large doses can acutely depress the sexual reflexes; chronic alcoholism causes high levels of circulating estrogens, which decrease libido; alcohol intoxication may impair judgment, decreasing incidence of safe-sex practices and increasing risk of exposure to STIs.

Tobacco Use Cigarette smoking increases risk of vascular disease, which may decrease penile blood flow; it is also associated with an increased risk of bladder and urothelial cancer.

Recreational Drug Use May impair judgment, increasing the risk of unsafe sex practices and STI exposure

Cocaine: priapism with chronic abuse, impotence, increased sexual excitability

Barbiturates: impotence

Amphetamines: increased libido and delayed orgasm in moderate users, impotence in chronic users

Sexual Practice Multiple partners, partner with multiple partners, new sexual partner, condom use (frequency and accuracy of use), sexual orientation, anal or oral intercourse

Work Environment Radiation exposure and exposure to environmental toxins have been linked to cancer of the male genitalia and male-factor fertility issues.

HEALTH MAINTENANCE ACTIVITIES

This information provides a bridge between health maintenance activities and male genitalia function.

Sleep Nocturia secondary to prostate enlargement

Diet Erectile dysfunction: Foods high in saturated fat or cholesterol, high in salt

Exercise Trauma or infection to the testicle or epididymis may cause a hydrocele

Use of Safety Devices Condoms used for vaginal and anal intercourse; supportive device worn while participating in sports

Health Checkups Testicular examination, prostate-specific antigen (PSA) level

NURSING CHECKLIST

General Approach to Male Genitalia Examination

1. Observe Standard Precautions and don Personal Protective Equipment (PPE) such as gloves, gown, face shield, goggles, N-95 respirator mask or face mask if the client's status warrants these protective measures.
2. Greet the client and explain the examination techniques that you will be using.
3. Ensure that the examination room is at a warm, comfortable temperature to prevent the client from chilling and shivering.
4. Use a quiet room that will be free from interruptions.
5. Ensure that the light in the room provides sufficient brightness to adequately observe the client.
6. Assess the client's apprehension level about the examination and reassure them that the examination is a normal process, if needed.
7. Instruct the client to remove pants and underpants and remain standing.
8. Stand to the client's right side or have the client stand in front of you while you are sitting.
9. Don clean gloves.
10. Expose the entire genital and groin area.

Assessment in Brief

Male Genitalia Examination

Inspection	Palpation	Auscultation	Advanced Techniques
• Sexual maturity rating • Hair distribution • Penis • Scrotum • Urethral meatus • Inguinal area	• Penis • Urethral meatus • Scrotum • Inguinal area	• Scrotum	• Prehn sign: Assessing for testicular torsion • Transillumination of the scrotum

Equipment

- Appropriate PPE
- Nonsterile gloves
- Penlight
- Stethoscope
- Urine collection cup

Examination of the Male Genitalia

Inspection

Sexual Maturity Rating (SMR)

E 1. Using the Tanner stages in Table 22-1, assess the developmental stage of the pubic hair, penis, and scrotum.
2. Determine the Sexual Maturity Rating.

N **Males usually begin puberty between the ages of 9½ and 13½. The average male proceeds through puberty in about 3 years, with a possible range of 2 to 5 years.**

A An SMR that is less than expected for a male's age is abnormal.

P Delayed puberty may be familial, caused by chronic illnesses, or may be influenced by treatment received as a child.

A A normally formed but diminutive penis is abnormal. There is a discrepancy between the penile size and the individual's age.

P A **microphallus** can result from a disorder in the hypothalamus or pituitary gland. It may be secondary to primary testicular failure due to partial androgen insensitivity. Maternal DES exposure has teratogenic effects caused by defects in nonandrogen-dependent regulatory agents. Microphallus can also be idiopathic in nature.

A It is abnormal when the penis appears larger than what is generally expected for the stated age. This condition is usually evident only before the age of normal puberty.

P Hormonal influence of tumors of the pineal gland or hypothalamus, tumors of the Leydig cells of the testes, tumors of the adrenal gland, or precocious genital maturity may cause penile hyperplasia.

A A testicle that is smaller and softer than normal (less than 5 cm × 2.5 cm [2 in. × 1 in.]) is abnormal in younger males.

P An atrophic testicle may be the result of Klinefelter syndrome (hypogonadism), previous injury, hypopituitarism, testosterone or antiandrogen therapy, a large varicocele, or a history of orchitis.

> **NURSING TIP**
>
> **Male Sexual Health Disparities**
>
> Male clients who identify as gay, bisexual, transgender, queer, questioning, or other sexual or gender minorities, face many health disparities, for both physical and mental health conditions, including reproductive health conditions. These disparities present as higher rates of illnesses, poorer health outcomes, and increased morbidity and mortality compared with their *cisgender* (sex assigned at birth is consistent with gender identity) and straight (heterosexual) peers. These disparities can be related to access to health care, comfort, insurance coverage, and the lack of inclusive health-care environments. A lack of training can contribute to this as well, and many members of the health-care workforce do not receive training relative to the health needs of LGBTQ clients as part of their prelicensure curricula (Makadon et al, 2015; Rossman et al, 2017; Wheldon et al, 2018).

Hair Distribution

E 1. Note hair distribution pattern.
2. Note the presence of nits or lice.

N **Pubic hair is distributed to the genitals and groin. It is sparsely distributed on the scrotum and inner thigh and is usually absent from much of the penile shaft. Genital hair is coarser than scalp hair. There are no nits or lice.**

A Hair distribution is sparse or hair is absent at the genitalia area **(alopecia)**.

P Alopecia in the genital area may result from genetic factors, aging, or local or systemic disease. These include developmental defects and hereditary disorders, infection, neoplasms, physical or chemical agents, endocrine diseases, deficiency states (nutritional or metabolic); destruction, damage to the follicles; advancing age.

A The presence of nits or lice is abnormal.

P See Chapter 10.

Penis

E 1. Inspect the glans, foreskin, and shaft for lesions, swelling, and inflammation. If the client is uncircumcised, ask the client to retract

NURSING TIP
Hygiene for the Uncircumcised Penis

During the penis examination, it is important to review proper hygiene. Instruct the client to retract the foreskin daily so that the underlying skin can be washed with soap and warm water. The skin should also be dried thoroughly and the foreskin returned to its original position.

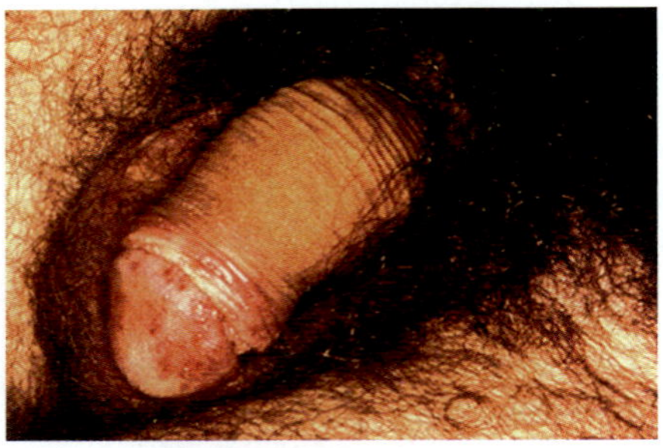

Figure 22-3 Balanitis of the glans penis.

the foreskin so that the underlying area can be inspected. After the examination, replace the foreskin.

2. Inspect the anterior surface of the penis first. Then lift the penis to check the posterior surface.
3. Note the shape of the penis.

N **Skin is free of lesions and inflammation. The shaft skin appears loose and wrinkled in the male without an erection. The glans is smooth and without lesions, swelling, or inflammation. The foreskin retracts easily and there is no discharge. A small amount of smegma, a white, cottage-cheese-like substance, may be present if uncircumcised, obese, or the penis is buried/retracted. The dorsal vein is sometimes visible. The penis is cylindrical in shape. The glans penis varies in size and shape and may appear rounded or broad.**

A Inflammation of the glans penis is abnormal.

P Inflammation of the glans penis is called balanitis (Fig. 22-3). The prepuce may also be affected. This is a bacterial infection that is associated with phimosis and is seen more commonly in diabetic men.

P Balanitis can occur with STIs, poor hygiene, obesity, and/or a buried penis.

A A small papular lesion that enlarges and undergoes superficial necrosis to produce a sharply marginated ulcer on a clean base is abnormal.

P The **chancre** is the lesion of primary syphilis (Fig. 22-4). It contains a multitude of *Treponema pallidum* spirochetes and is highly infectious. The tissue reacts to the organism with infiltration of lymphocytes, fibroblasts, and plasma cells that cause swelling and proliferation of the endothelial tissue, manifesting as a chancre. In secondary syphilis, the primary chancres are healing as the *Treponema pallidum* spreads throughout the body. Eruptions can present in many ways.

NURSING TIP
Male Genital Piercing

Awareness of the current types of genital piercings will help the nurse to educate and inform clients of possible complications of the procedure. The nurse can also educate clients about potential sexual partner reactions to the piercing.

The "Prince Albert" is one of the more popular types of genital piercings. The jewelry is inserted through the urethral meatus and exits through the base of the frenulum (the elastic band of tissue on the underside of the glans penis that connects the foreskin to the glans).

The frenum is another popular type of genital piercing. The piercing is through the frenulum membrane on the underside of the penis. Multiple piercings up the penile shaft are called a frenum ladder.

Other male genital piercings include the dydoe (lateral piercing of the glans penis; it is often done in pairs), ampallang (horizontal piercing of the glans penis above the urethra), apadravya (vertical piercing of the glans penis), guiche (piercing between the scrotum and anus), hafada (scrotal piercing), and foreskin (piercing passes through the foreskin only).

The most common complications of genital piercing are infection and bleeding. The Prince Albert piercing creates a fistula for urine to drain, and males may need to sit down to void due to the change in the urine stream and difficulty aiming. Site hypersensitivity is another commonly reported problem. Additional complications include urethral tears, paraphimosis, and postcoital bleeding. Sexual partners report painful sex, bleeding, and sensitivity reactions from the jewelry.

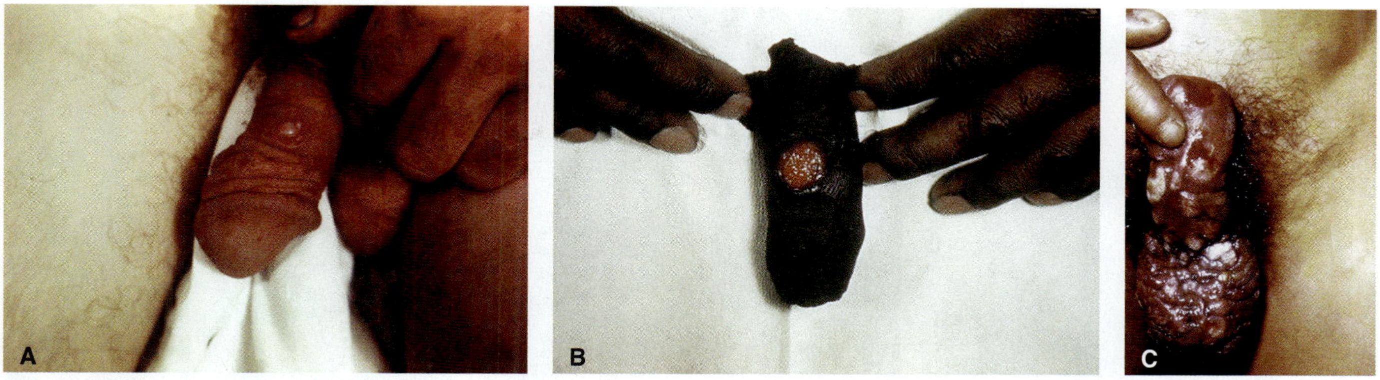

Figure 22-4 Syphilitic chancre in clients with different skin tones. Gloves should always be worn when examining the genitalia. **A.** Primary syphilitic chancre in a light-skinned penis. **B.** Primary syphilitic chancre in a dark-skinned penis. **C.** Secondary syphilis.

Risk Factors

Penile Cancer

- Age (>60 years)
- Intact foreskin, especially with phimosis
- Poor hygiene and smegma buildup
- History of HPV types 16, 18, and 31
- Tobacco use
- HIV
- Ultraviolet light treatment for psoriasis

Adapted from *https://www.cancer.org/cancer/penile-cancer.html* (retrieved November 26, 2025).

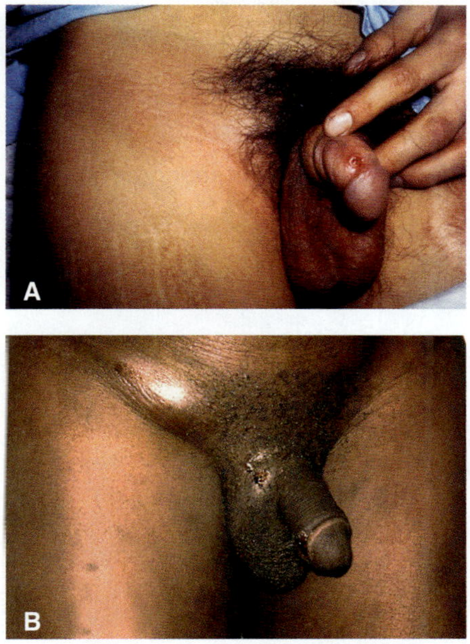

Figure 22-5 Chancroid of the penis in clients with different skin tones. Gloves should always be worn when examining the genitalia. **A.** Chancroid in a light-skinned penis. **B.** Chancroid in a dark-skinned penis.

A A tender, painful, ulcerated, exudative, papular lesion with an erythematous halo, surrounding edema, and a friable base is abnormal (Fig. 22-5).

P **Chancroid** is caused by inoculation of *Haemophilus ducreyi* through small breaks in epidermal tissue. Acute inflammatory response causes bubo formation. This is usually accompanied by inguinal adenopathy.

A Penile lesion that ranges from a relatively subtle induration to a small papule, pustule, warty growth, or exophytic lesion is abnormal. The distribution of lesions is most commonly on the glans and prepuce.

P Penile carcinoma (Fig. 22-6) usually begins with a small lesion that gradually extends to involve the entire glans, shaft, and corpora. Circumcision has been well established as a prophylactic measure that will decrease the risk of the occurrence of penile carcinoma.

A Pinhead papules to cauliflower-like groupings of filiform, skin-colored, pink, or red lesions are abnormal (Fig. 22-7).

P **Condyloma acuminatum** (genital warts) is caused by HPV infection of the epithelial cells. HPV may remain dormant for months to years after infection. There is a high incidence of recurrence of

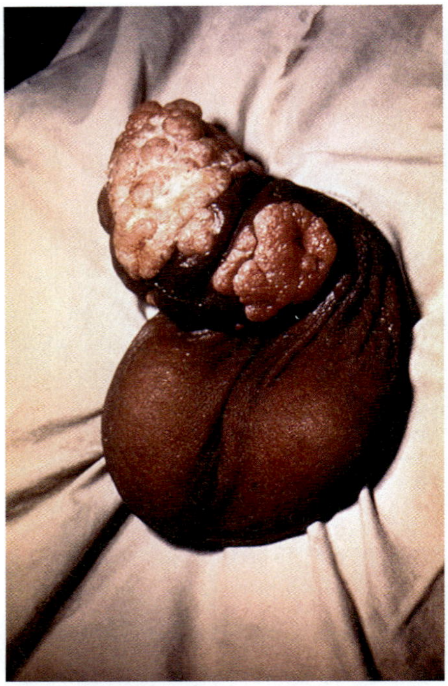

Figure 22-6 Penile carcinoma.

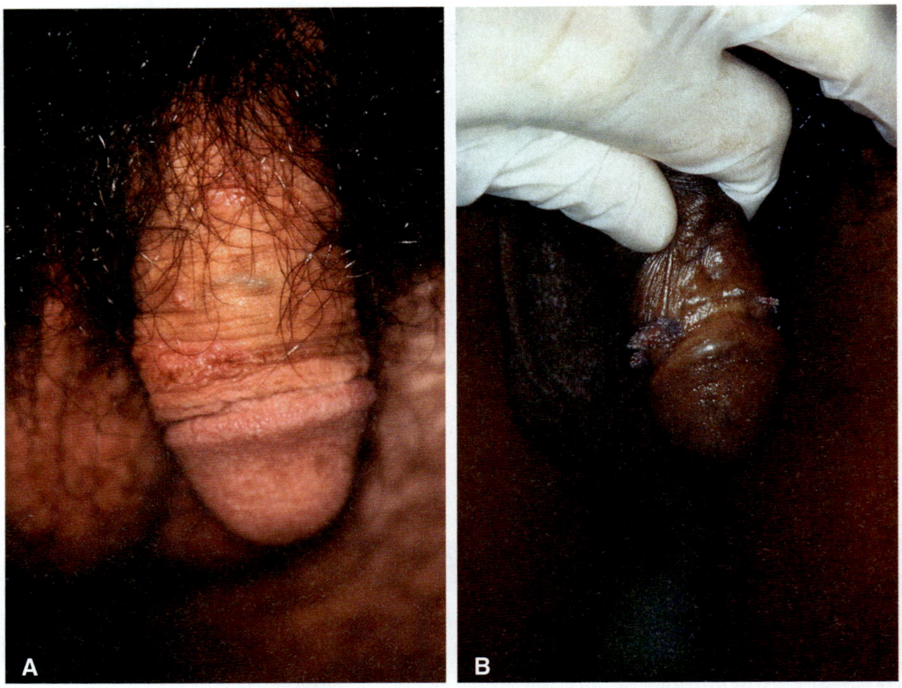

Figure 22-7 Genital warts in clients with different skin tones. **A.** Genital warts in a light-skinned penis. **B.** Genital warts in a dark-skinned penis.

Risk Factors

HIV

- Engaging in anal or oral sex with men who have sex with men, multiple partners, penetrative sex with any partner, or anonymous partners without using a condom
- Injecting drugs or steroids where needles/syringes are shared
- Having a STI such as syphilis, genital herpes, chlamydia, gonorrhea, bacterial vaginosis, or trichomoniasis
- Having been diagnosed with hepatitis, tuberculosis, or malaria
- Exchanging sex for drugs or money
- Exposure to the virus as a fetus or infant before or during birth or through breastfeeding from a mother infected with HIV
- Receiving a blood transfusion or clotting factor in the United States anytime from 1978 to 1985
- Engaging in unprotected sex with someone who has any of the preceding risk factors

NURSING TIP

HPV Vaccination

On October 16, 2009, the FDA licensed the HPV vaccine, HPV4, for use in males. Currently, the CDC advises males receive the 9-valent HPV vaccine at age 11 to 12 years through age 26. The vaccine can be started as early as age 9 years, especially if a sexual abuse/assault occurred or if the male has HIV. The HPV vaccine can also be given to males ages 27 to 45 based on shared clinical decision-making. The HPV vaccine is given for the prevention of genital warts caused by HPV types 6 and 11. Clients should be counseled that the HPV vaccination prevents new HPV infections but does not treat existing HPV infections or diseases. Clients should be encouraged to follow safe sex practices.

Retrieved November 26, 2025 from *https://www.cdc.gov/vaccines/schedules/index.html*

condyloma following appropriate treatment because of the persistence of latent HPV in normal-appearing skin

A Multifocal maculopapular lesions that are tan, brown, pink, violet, or white are abnormal.

P Multifocal maculopapular lesions that are tan, brown, pink, violet, or white describe intraepithelial neoplasia. HPV oncogenic types 16, 18, 31, and 33 infection causes epidermal proliferation and koilocytotic, dyskeratotic cells. Female partners may have a history of cervical intraepithelial neoplasm (CIN). The majority of lesions are distributed on the glans penis and prepuce. Changes of squamous cell carcinoma in situ are seen on histological examination.

A Erythematous, painful ulcers developing into vesicular lesions, which may become pustular, are abnormal (Fig. 22-8).

P HSV lesions are erythematous, painful ulcers that develop into vesicular lesions. Skin-to-skin contact infection of HSV 1 and HSV 2 causes epidermal degeneration, acanthosis, and intraepidermal vesicles. Moist or crusty lesions can become ulcerated and eroded. Epithelial changes resolve in 2 to 4 weeks and hyper- or hypopigmentation of these areas is common. Postinflammatory scarring is rare. Recurrent herpes lesions are smaller. Diagnosis may be confirmed by the Tzanck test for microscopic acanthocytes, viral culture, or serology for HSV antibodies.

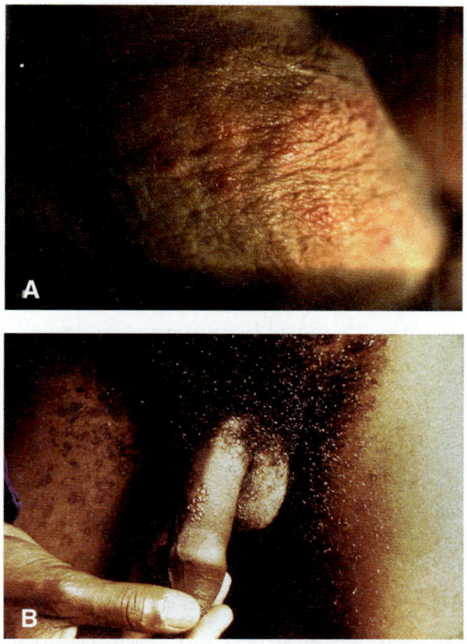

Figure 22-8 Penile HSV. **A** Light-skinned penis. **B** Dark-skinned penis.

NURSING TIP

Male Sexual Assault

Nurses need to be aware of the possibility that male clients have experienced male sexual assault (MSA). MSA is forced intercourse or sexual contact that occurs without consent by another person. MSA includes fondling, forced anal sex, forced oral sex, stimulation of an erection, stimulation of ejaculation, and oral-to-anal contact. Clients may present with genital injuries, lacerations to the anal sphincter, rectal tears, fissures, or hematomas. Nongenital injuries may include a black eye, fractured jaw, cerebral concussion, or facial contusions/lacerations. MSA victims may experience confusion about their sexual orientation, nightmares, suicidal ideation, and self-blame. You may need to offer the client referral to a therapist or counselor.

NURSING TIP

Guidelines for Screening of Men Having Sex with Men (MSM)

According to the CDC, routine laboratory screening is indicated for all sexually active MSM and transgender males and females. The CDC advises that sexual orientation, as well as the gender identity of individual persons and their sex partners, should be obtained during health-care visits. The following tests should be performed at least annually.

- HIV serology, if HIV negative or not tested within 1 year
- Syphilis serology
- A urine test for infection with *N. gonorrhoeae* and *C. trachomatis* in males who have had insertive intercourse during the last year (urine nucleic acid amplification test [NAAT] is preferred)*
- A test for rectal infections with *N. gonorrhoeae* and *C. trachomatis* in males who have had receptive anal intercourse in the past year (rectal NAAT is preferred)*
- A test for pharyngeal infections with *N. gonorrhoeae* in males who have had receptive oral intercourse during the past year (pharyngeal NAAT is preferred)*

In addition, the following tests can be considered in the MSM and transgender male and female populations:

- HSV 2
- Anal culture
- Frequent STI screening
- Hepatitis B infection
- Hepatitis C infection

The CDC recommends pre-exposure prophylaxis (PrEP) treatment for high-risk persons. When PrEP medications are taken as directed, they decrease the risk of sexually acquired HIV by 99% (CDC, 2025). Condom use is still advised to help protect against other STIs.

*regardless of condom use

Adapted from *https://www.cdc.gov/std/treatment-guidelines/msm.html* (retrieved November 26, 2025).

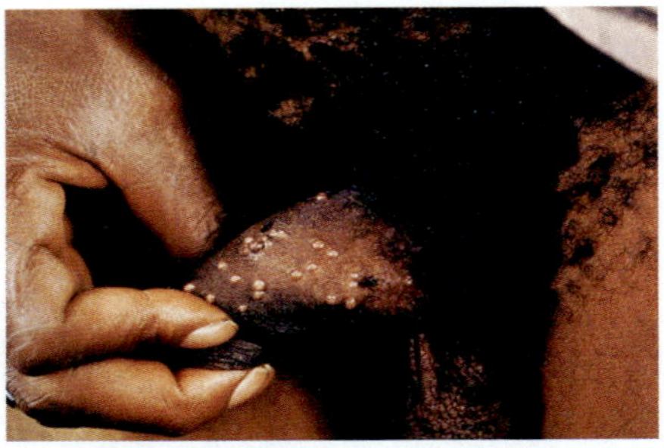

Figure 22-9 Molluscum contagiosum. Gloves should always be worn when examining the genitalia.

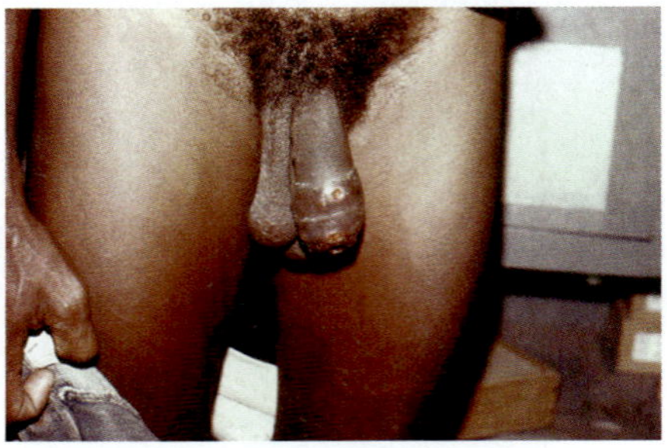

Figure 22-10 Granuloma inguinale.

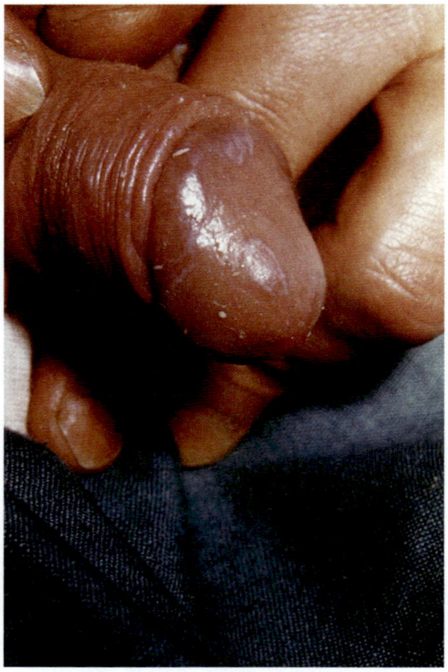

Figure 22-11 Lichen planus. Gloves should always be worn when examining the genitalia.

A Multiple, discrete, flat pustules with slight scaling and surrounding edema are abnormal.

P *Candida* is a superficial mycotic infection of moist cutaneous sites. Predisposing factors include moisture, diabetes mellitus, obesity, antibiotic therapy, and deficiencies in systemic immunity.

A Small white, pink, or flesh-colored raised bumps with a pit or dimple in the center (umbilicated) are abnormal (Fig. 22-9). The bumps are smooth and firm, are anywhere from 2 to 5 mm in diameter, and are usually painless. They may be found anywhere on the body and are not considered a STI, but if found in the genital area they usually are caused by sexual contact.

P Molluscum contagiosum is caused by a poxvirus and usually causes mild skin disease. The virus affects only the epithelial layer of the skin. The virus lives only in the skin, and once the growths are gone, the virus is gone and cannot be spread to others. Molluscum usually disappears in 6 to 12 months without treatment.

A Beefy, red, painless superficial ulcers on the penis are abnormal (Fig. 22-10).

P Donovanosis or granuloma inguinale is caused by the gram-negative rod-shaped bacterium *Calymmatobacterium granulomatis*. Lesions can bleed easily when touched. They occur in tropical climates.

A An annular purplish discoloration with thin white lines on the glans penis is abnormal (Fig. 22-11).

P Lichen planus of the penis may be itchy. Shiny, small papules that are flat-topped might also be present.

A Erythematous plaques with scaling; papular lesions with sharp margins, and occasionally clear centers; and pustules are abnormal.

P Tinea cruris is a fungal infection of the groin and genitals, usually caused by *Epidermophyton floccosum* or *Trichophyton rubrum*. Predisposing factors are a warm, humid environment, tight clothing, and obesity.

A An unusually long foreskin or one that cannot be retracted over the glans penis is abnormal.

P **Phimosis** occurs in uncircumcised males. Inability to retract the foreskin is normal in infancy (Fig. 22-12). In later years, an acquired constricting circumferential scar may follow the healing of a split foreskin.

A It is abnormal when the retracted foreskin develops a fixed constriction proximal to the glans (Fig. 22-13). The penis distal to the foreskin may become swollen and gangrenous.

P This is called **paraphimosis**, and it is a urological emergency. If the foreskin is retracted and not returned to its original position, paraphimosis can ensue (e.g., a client's penis is cleansed for indwelling catheter insertion, and the foreskin remains retracted). The foreskin acts as a circulatory constrictor, causing decreased blood flow, edema, and potential tissue necrosis.

A A continuous and pathological erection of the penis is abnormal.

P The cause of **priapism** is unclear in most clients; however, it does not occur as the result of sexual desire. Some of the cases are associated with leukemia, metastatic carcinoma, sickle cell anemia, intracavernous injection, alcohol abuse, genital trauma, illicit drugs, some prescription drugs (such as PDE5 inhibitors), and neurological disorders. Some drugs, such as antihypertensives, antipsychotics, and antidepressants, have also been associated with prolonged erections. The client may also present after having used medication for erectile dysfunction. Priapism is created by the positive imbalance between the arterial blood supply and its return, created by venous drainage.

A Penile curvature, or chordee, is either a ventral or a dorsal curvature of the penis and is abnormal.

P Curvature is usually congenitally caused by a fibrous band along the usual course of the corpus spongiosum. Ventral chordee is seen mostly with **epispadias** (Fig. 22-14) when the urethral meatus opens dorsally on the glans. In cases of congenital penile curvature without epispadias or **hypospadias** (when the urethral meatus opens ventrally on the glans), there is no additional tissue on or in any portion of the corpora cavernosa (Fig. 22-15). This is caused by congenital maldevelopment of the tunica albuginea of the corpora.

P Peyronie disease is a condition of penile curvature that occurs with erection (Fig. 22-16). The dorsal surface of the corpora cavernosa becomes hardened with palpable, nontender plaques. It may be the result of a distinct injury during sexual activity or mild injury that results in scarring over time.

Scrotum

E

1. Displace the penis to one side to inspect the scrotal skin.
2. Lift up the scrotum to inspect the posterior side.
3. Observe for lesions, inflammation, swelling, and nodules.
4. Note size and shape.
5. Have the client perform the Valsalva maneuver.
6. Observe for a mass of dilated testicular veins in the spermatic cord above and behind the testes.

N **Scrotal skin appears rugated and thin and more deeply pigmented than body color. The skin should hug the testicles firmly in the young male and become elongated and flaccid in the older adult male. The left scrotal sac is longer than the right in many males. All skin areas should be free of any lesions, nodules, swelling, or inflammation. Scrotal size and shape vary greatly from one individual to another. There should be no dilated testicular veins.**

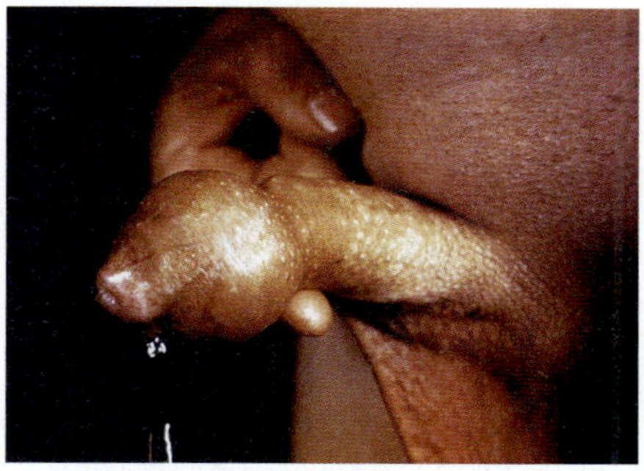

Figure 22-12 Phimosis. Gloves should always be worn when examining the genitalia.

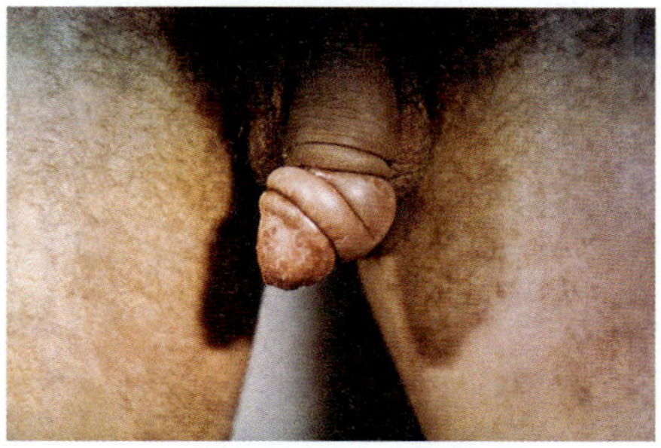

Figure 22-13 Paraphimosis.

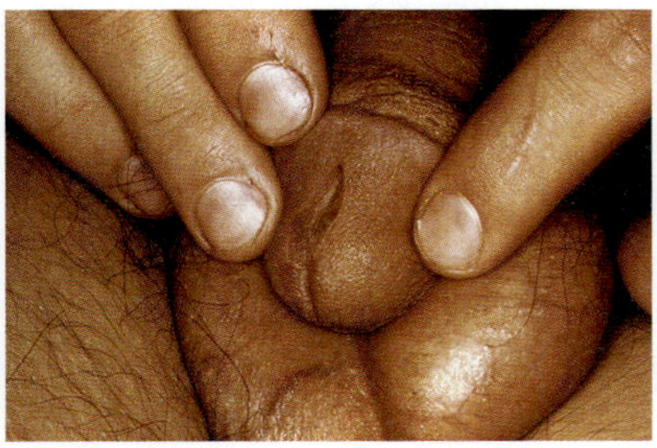

Figure 22-14 In epispadias the urethral meatus opens dorsally on the glans penis. Gloves should always be worn when examining the genitalia.

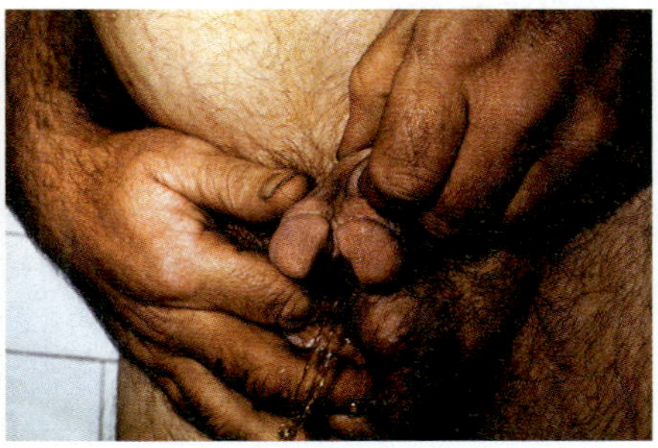

Figure 22-15 In hypospadias the urethral meatus opens ventrally on the glans penis; in addition, this man has a congenital bifid penis or diphallia. Gloves should always be worn when examining the genitalia.

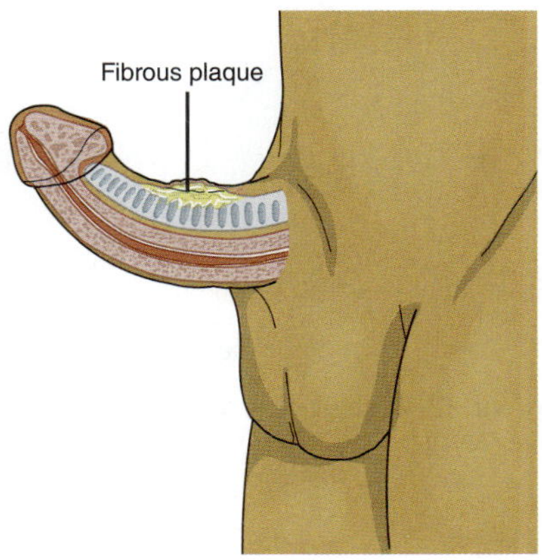

Figure 22-16 Dorsal curvature of the penis in Peyronie disease.

E Examination **N** Normal Findings **A** Abnormal Findings **P** Pathophysiology

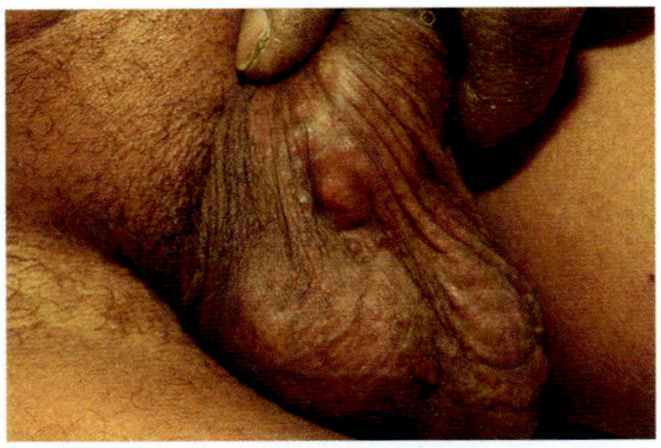

Figure 22-17 Scrotal condylomatous lesions. Gloves should always be worn when examining the genitalia.

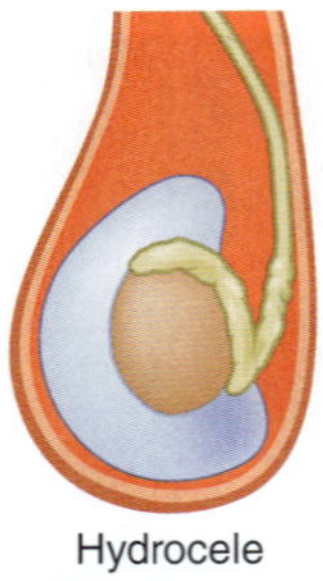

Figure 22-18 Representation of hydrocele.

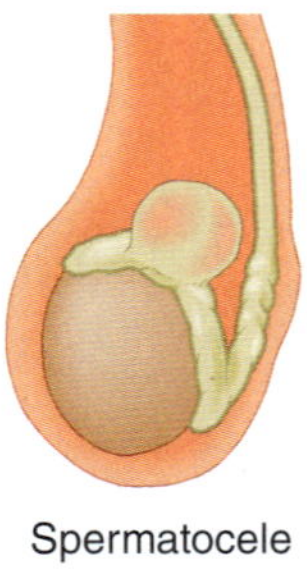

Figure 22-19 Representation of spermatocele.

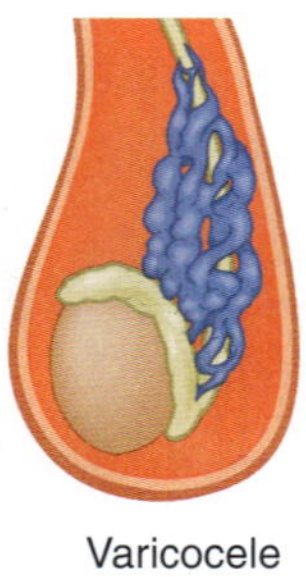

Figure 22-20 Representation of varicocele.

A P Condyloma acuminatum (Fig. 22-17), tinea cruris, and *Candida* are abnormal findings. See prior discussion.

A Enlargement of or masses within the scrotum is abnormal.

P Scrotal masses can arise from benign or malignant conditions. Scrotal swelling is seen with inguinal hernia, hydrocele, varicocele, spermatocele, tumor, and edema.

A A large, pear-sized mass in the scrotum is abnormal (Fig. 22-18). The scrotal skin is stretched, shiny, and erythematous, which may give the penis a shortened appearance.

P A **hydrocele** is created by the accumulation of fluid between the two layers of the tunica vaginalis. Hydroceles may be idiopathic or due to trauma, inguinal surgery, epididymitis, or testicular tumor.

A A well-defined cystic mass on the superior testis or in the epididymis is abnormal. It is usually <2 cm (¾ inch) in diameter (Fig. 22-19). Multiple masses may be present.

P A well-defined cystic mass on the superior testis or in the epididymis is called a **spermatocele**. Blockage of the efferent ductules of the rete testis causes the formation of sperm-filled cysts at the top of the testis or in the epididymis.

A In light-skinned individuals, a scrotal mass with a bluish discoloration is abnormal (Fig. 22-20).

P Dilated veins in the pampiniform plexus of the spermatic cord cause **varicocele** formation and can be accompanied by a decreased sperm count. Most appear in the left hemiscrotum; the remainder are bilateral. A right-sided varicocele may be indicative of an obstruction at the vena cava or right renal vein. Acute onset of a right-sided varicocele may be pathognomonic for a renal tumor extending into the renal vein or compression of the renal vein. It may increase in size with the Valsalva maneuver and decrease or disappear with supine positioning.

A Round, firm, cystic nodules confined within the scrotal skin are abnormal.

P A sebaceous cyst contains sebum, an oily, fatty matter secreted by the sebaceous glands. The cyst may result from an abrasion due to activity or tight clothing and closure of sebaceous glands or ducts.

Urethral Meatus

E

1. Note the location of the urethral meatus.
2. Observe for discharge.
3. Obtain a culture of any discharge (see Advanced Technique on urethral culture).
4. If the client complains of penile discharge but none is present, ask the client to milk the penis from the shaft to the glans. This maneuver may express a discharge that can then be cultured.

N **The urethral meatus is located centrally. It is pink and without discharge.**

A Erythema and swelling at the urethral meatus are abnormal (Fig. 22-21).

P Urethritis is a localized tissue inflammation resulting from bacterial, viral, or fungal infection as well as from urethral trauma.

A It is abnormal for the urethral meatus to be displaced dorsally (refer to Fig. 22-14).

P Epispadias is a congenital abnormality caused by a complete or partial dorsal fusion defect of the urethra.

A It is abnormal for the urethral meatus to open on the ventral aspect of the glans penis (refer to Fig. 22-15). The urethral meatus may also open at the perineum.

P Hypospadias is a congenital abnormality, usually associated with chordee. Complications of this defect include urethral meatal stenosis, inability to direct the urine stream, sexual dysfunction, and male factor fertility issues.

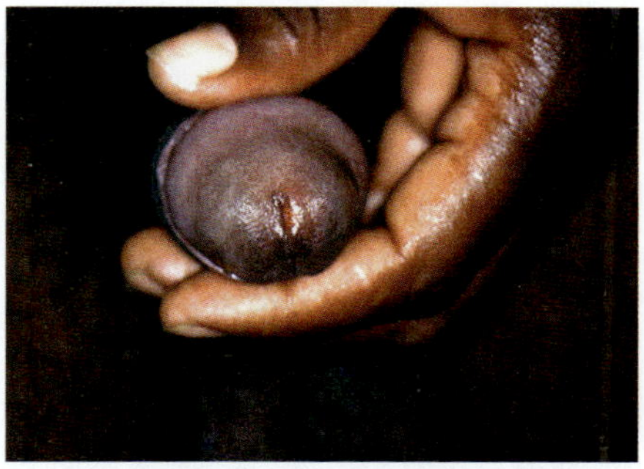

Figure 22-21 Urethritis. Gloves should always be worn when examining the genitalia.

Inguinal Area

E

1. If the client is supine, ask the client to stand.
2. Stand facing the client.
3. Observe for swelling or bulges.
4. Ask the client to bear down.
5. Observe for swelling or bulges.

N **The inguinal area is free of any swelling or bulges.**

A A bulge in the inguinal area is abnormal.

P Hernia pathology is discussed further in the section on palpation.

Palpation

Penis

E

1. Client should be standing. Stand in front of the client's genital area.
2. Don clean gloves.
3. Between the thumb and the first two fingers, palpate the entire length of the penis while gently stretching the phallus (Fig. 22-22).
4. Note any pulsations, tenderness, masses, or plaques.

N **Pulsations are present on the dorsal sides of the penis. The penis is nontender. No masses or firm plaques are palpated.**

A It is abnormal to palpate fibrotic plaques or ridges along the dorsal shaft.

P Plaques develop from perivascular inflammation between the tunica albuginea and the underlying spongy erectile tissue.

P Systemic disease, localized trauma, and localized disease may adversely affect normal blood flow in the penis.

A It is abnormal for the penis to be enlarged in a nonerect state. Generalized penile swelling may be present.

P Fluid accumulation in the loose tissue of the penile integument results from anasarcic states. Obstruction of the penile veins or inflammation of the penis results in local edema. Trauma to the penis may cause swelling secondary to penile contusion and extravasation of blood. Gentle finger pressure may cause pitting.

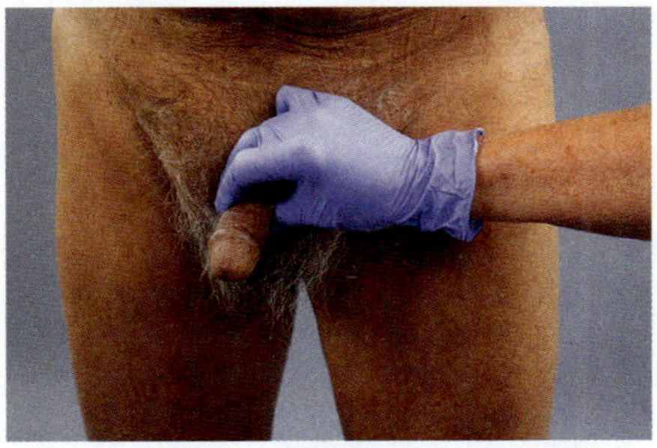

Figure 22-22 Palpation of the penis.

Urethral Meatus

E

1. Stand in front of the client's genital area.
2. Between the thumb and forefinger, grasp the glans and gently squeeze to expose the meatus (Fig. 22-23).

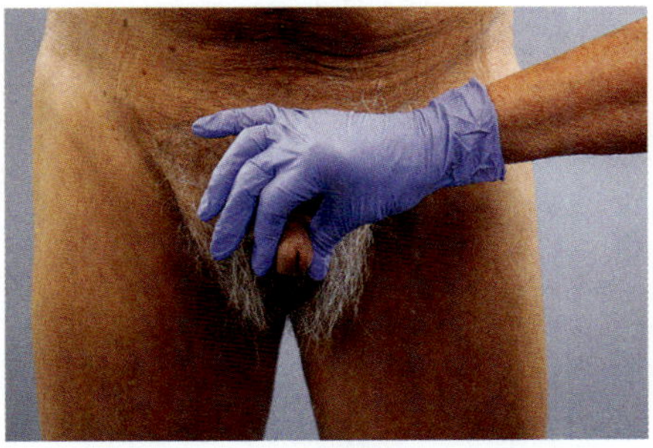

Figure 22-23 Palpation of the urethral meatus.

NURSING TIP

Warning Signs of STIs in the Male Client

- Urethral discharge, bloody or purulent
- Scrotal or testicular pain
- Burning or pain during urination
- Penile lesion

3. If discharge is seen, or if the client complains of a urethral discharge, a culture should be taken.

N **The urethral meatus is free of discharge and drainage.**

A A urethral discharge of pus and mucus shreds is abnormal (Fig. 22-24). The discharge may vary in color, consistency, and amount.

P Bacterial infection of the genitourinary tract causes inflammation and the formation of a liquid composed of albuminous substances, leukocytes, shedding tissue cells, and bacteria.

Scrotum

E
1. Between the thumb and the first two fingers, gently palpate the left testicle (Fig. 22-25).
2. Note the size, shape, consistency, and presence of masses.
3. Palpate the epididymis (Fig. 22-26).
4. Note the consistency and presence of tenderness or masses.
5. Between the thumb and the first two fingers, palpate the spermatic cord from the epididymis to the external ring.
6. Note the consistency and presence of tenderness or masses.
7. Repeat on the left side.

N **The scrotum contains on each side a testicle and an epididymis. The testicles should be firm but not hard, ovoid, smooth, and equal in size bilaterally. They should be sensitive to pressure but not tender. The epididymis is comma-shaped and should be distinguishable from the testicle. The epididymis should be insensitive to pressure. The spermatic cord should feel smooth and round.**

A A unilateral mass palpated within or about the testicle is abnormal (Fig. 22-27).

P Intratesticular masses should be considered malignant until proven otherwise. They are nodular and associated with painless swelling. The majority of intratesticular masses arise from germinal elements. Extratesticular tumors are uncommon and usually benign. They can arise from any of the surrounding structures, including the epididymis, the testicular tunica vaginalis, or the spermatic cord. Testicular cancer should be suspected if a hard, fixed nodule is palpated.

P Inguinal hernia is discussed in the "Inguinal Area" section.

P Refer to the section on scrotal inspection for a description of spermatocele.

A A large, pear-shaped mass that has a smooth wall is abnormal.

P Refer to the section on scrotal inspection for a description of hydrocele. The entire testicle must be palpated because underlying malignancies cause a small percentage of all hydroceles. Sonography must be performed if the entire testicle is not palpable.

A A soft testis is abnormal, but often seen with advancing age and when individuals are on testosterone replacement.

P This might indicate hypogonadism.

A A testicle that is smaller and softer than what is expected for the client's age is abnormal.

P An atrophic testicle may be found in Klinefelter syndrome, surgery for undescended testis at an older age, large varicocele, hypopituitarism, or orchitis, and in clients who are on estrogen therapy.

A Palpation of a scrotal mass superior to the testis that reveals a "bag of worms" is abnormal.

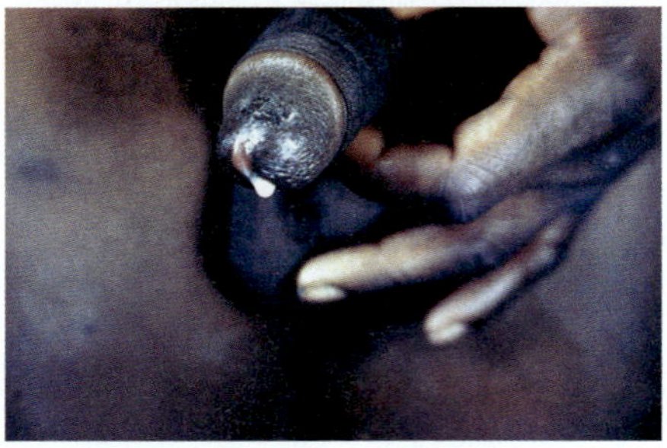

Figure 22-24 Purulent penile discharge from gonorrhea. Gloves should always be worn when examining the genitalia.

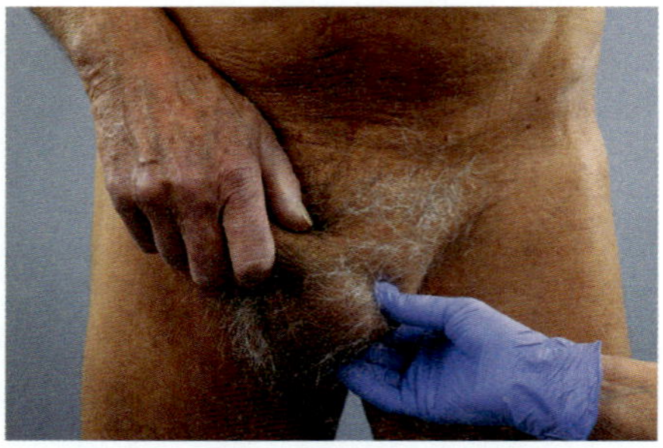

Figure 22-25 Palpation of the testicle.

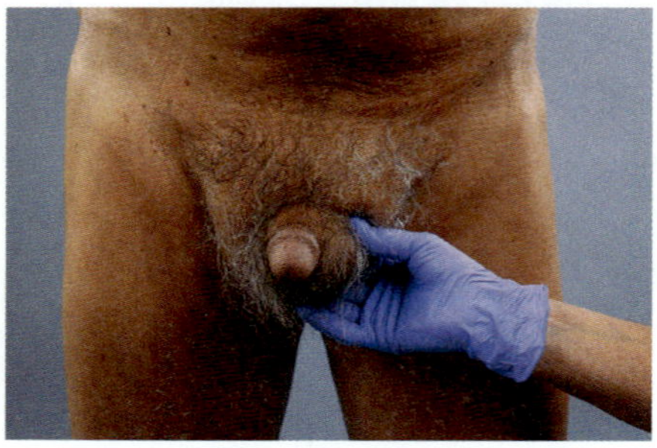

Figure 22-26 Palpation of the epididymis.

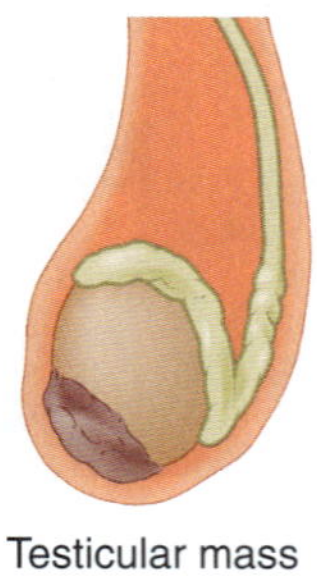

Figure 22-27 Representation of testicular tumor.

P Refer to the section on scrotal inspection for a description of varicocele.

A It is abnormal for the testicle to be enlarged, retracted, in a lateral position, and extremely sensitive (Fig. 22-28). Sometimes it is difficult to distinguish between testicular torsion and epididymitis. Refer to the Advanced Technique on Prehn Sign.

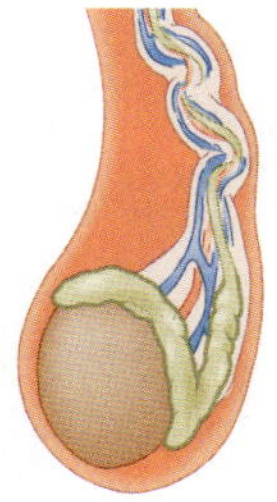

Figure 22-28 Representation of testicular torsion.

ADVANCED TECHNIQUE

Prehn Sign: Assessing for Testicular Torsion

E
1. Elevate the scrotum with towels until it is fully supported.
2. Observe the client's pain response, acknowledging that this test is not fully reliable.

N **The client with epididymitis will have decreased scrotal pain with scrotal elevation.**

A **P** The client with testicular torsion will not have any change in the scrotal pain with this maneuver.

P Testicular torsion is a surgical emergency. Twisting or torsion of the testis causes venous obstruction, secondary edema, and eventual arterial obstruction. Doppler ultrasonography reveals the absence of perfusion to the testicle.

A Palpation reveals an indurated, swollen, tender epididymis (Fig. 22-29).

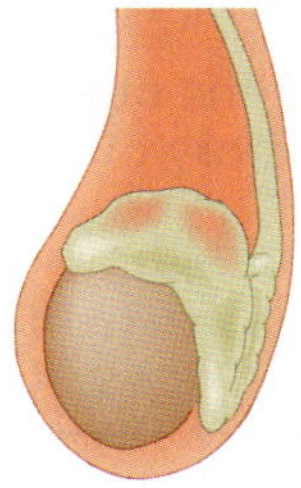

Figure 22-29 Representation of epididymitis.

P Epididymitis results from the retrograde spreading of pathogenic organisms from the urethra to the epididymis. The majority of infections are caused by bacterial pathogens such as *Chlamydia trachomatis* and *Neisseria gonorrhoeae*. An associated hydrocele may be present. The testis may also be enlarged and tender.

A It is abnormal for one or both testes to be undescended (Fig. 22-30).

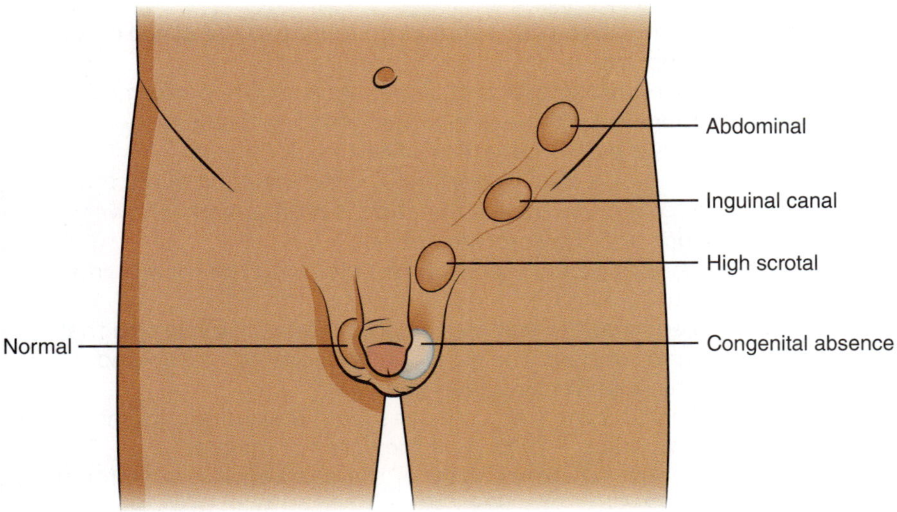

Figure 22-30 Representation of cryptorchidism.

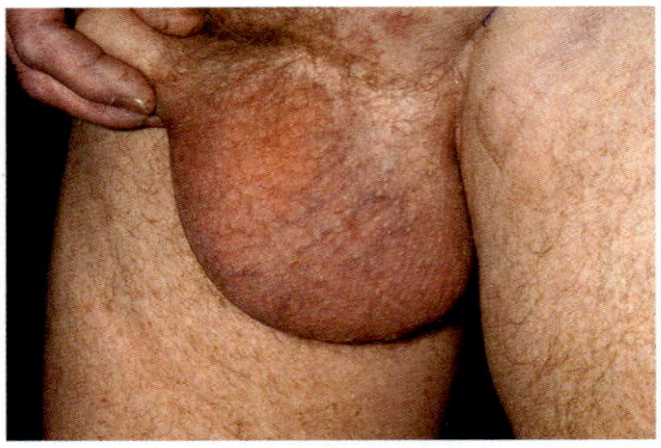

Figure 22-31 Scrotal edema. Gloves should always be worn when examining the genitalia.

Risk Factors

Testicular Cancer

- Race (White, American Indian, Alaskan Native)
- Age (most common between ages 20 and 45)
- History of cryptorchidism, even if an orchiopexy was performed
- Cancer of the other testicle
- Family history of testicular cancer
- HIV
- Carcinoma in situ of the testicle

Adapted from *https://www.cancer.org/cancer/testicular-cancer/causes-risks-prevention.html* (retrieved November 26, 2025).

P The causes of **cryptorchidism** are not established but may be multiple and related to testicular failure, deficient gonadotrophic stimulation, mechanical obstruction, or gubernacular defects. The undescended testis is usually smaller than its normally descended mate. Unilateral cryptorchidism is more common than bilateral. The undescended testicle is usually located in the inguinal canal or, less commonly, intra-abdominally. Spontaneous descent is unusual after 1 year of age.

A An acute, painful onset of swelling of the testicle along with warm scrotal skin is abnormal. The client may complain of heaviness in the scrotum.

P **Orchitis** can be caused by mumps, coxsackievirus B, infectious mononucleosis, and varicella. Involvement of the testes is via the hematogenous route. Orchitis is unilateral in the majority of cases, but onset in the second testicle may occur up to 1 week after that in the first.

A It is abnormal for the scrotum to be enlarged, taut with pitting edema. In light-skinned individuals, a reddened scrotum is abnormal (Fig. 22-31).

P Scrotal edema accompanies edema associated with the lower half of the body, such as in congestive heart failure (CHF), renal failure, and portal vein obstruction. Scrotal edema may also be the result of local inflammation. Scrotal contents are usually nonpalpable.

A Acute, painful, scrotal swelling may occur with a history of trauma.

P Trauma is a major cause of acute scrotal swelling. Scrotal or testicular hematoma formation as well as testicular rupture may be present. A small percentage of all diagnosed testicular tumors are diagnosed through medical attention for trauma; therefore, any intratesticular hematoma must be followed to rule out a neoplasm.

NURSING TIP

Teaching Testicular Self-Examination

Testicular self-examination (TSE) should be taught to the client during the scrotal examination.

- Ask the client if monthly testicular self-examination is performed.
- Explain the rationale for the examination. Monthly testicular examination allows earlier detection of testicular cancer.
- Tell the client to pick a date to perform the examination every month. The best time to perform the examination is after a warm shower when both hands and the scrotum are warm.
- Instruct the client to gently feel each testicle using the thumb and first two fingers (Fig. 22-32A).
- Remind the client that the testicles are ovoid and movable and that they feel firm and rubbery. The epididymis is located on top and behind the testis, is softer, and feels ropelike.
- Instruct the client to report any changes from these findings, including any lumps and nodules, especially if they are nonmobile.
- Instruct the client to squeeze the tip of the penis and observe for any discharge (Fig. 22-32B).

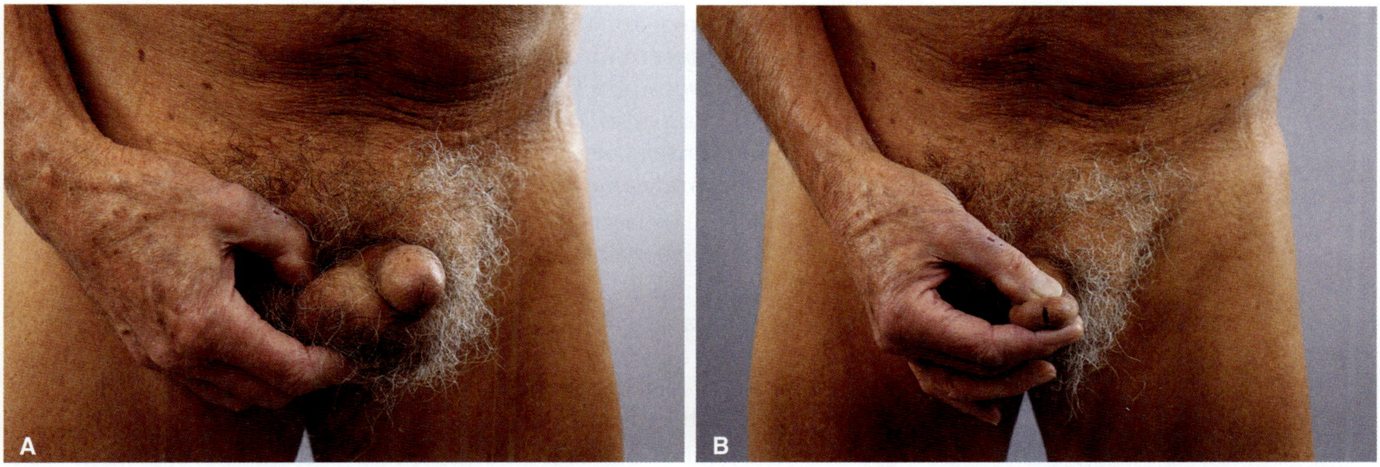

Figure 22-32 Testicular self-examination. **A.** Palpating the right testis. **B.** Assessing for penile discharge.

ADVANCED TECHNIQUE

Transillumination of the Scrotum: Assessing for a Scrotal Mass

If a scrotal mass or enlargement is detected, the scrotum should be transilluminated.

E
1. Tell the client what you are going to do and that it should not be painful.
2. Darken the room.
3. Using a penlight, apply the light source to the unaffected side behind the scrotum and direct it forward.
4. Apply the light source to the side of the scrotal enlargement or mass.
5. Note whether there is a transmission of a red glow (Fig. 22-33).

N **A normal testicle does not transilluminate (i.e., there is no red glow).**

A The transmission of a red glow indicates a serous fluid within the scrotal sac (Fig. 22-34). This can occur in hydrocele and spermatocele and is abnormal. Vascular structures such as a hernia and a tumor do not transilluminate.

P Refer to previous discussions of these conditions.

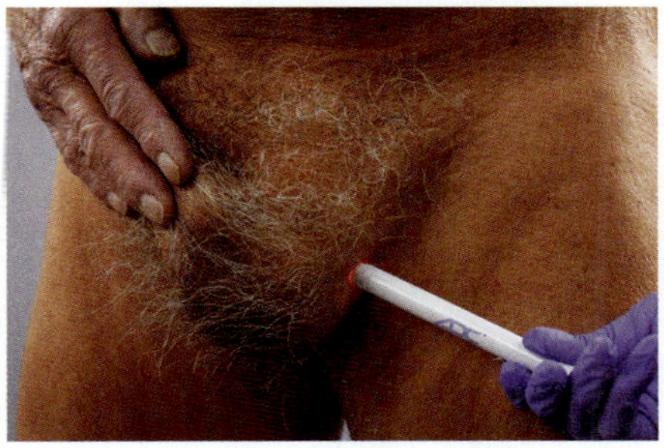

Figure 22-33 Technique for transillumination of the scrotum.

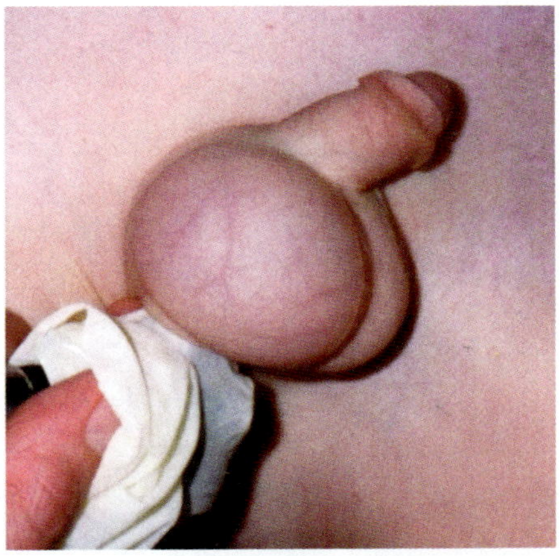

Figure 22-34 Transillumination of the scrotum. In this case, a transilluminator was not available. The nurse used a penlight with a rubber glove on top of it to illuminate the scrotal mass, which was a hydrocele.

Inguinal Area

E
1. With the index and middle fingers of the right hand, palpate the skin overlying the inguinal and femoral areas for lymph nodes.
2. Note size, consistency, tenderness, and mobility. Ask the client to bear down while you palpate the inguinal area.
3. Place the right index finger in the client's right scrotal sac above the right testicle and invaginate the scrotal skin. Follow the spermatic cord until you reach a triangular, slit-like opening (the external inguinal ring).
4. The finger is placed with the nail facing inward and the finger pad outward (Fig. 22-35).
5. If the inguinal ring is large enough, continue to advance the finger along the inguinal canal and ask the client to turn the head and cough.
6. Note any masses felt against the finger.
7. Repeat on the left side using the left hand to perform the palpation.
8. Palpate the femoral canal. Ask the client to bear down.

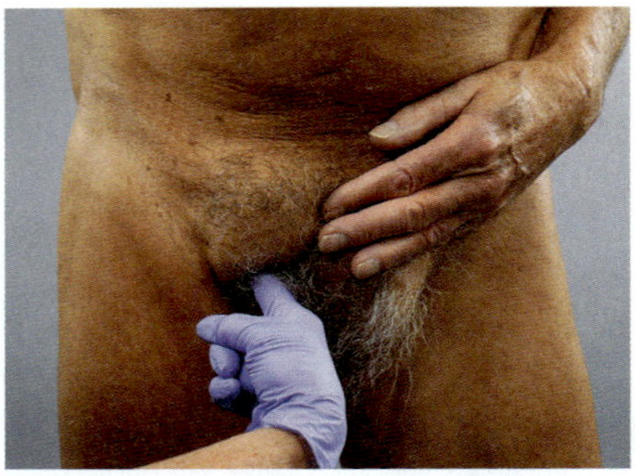

Figure 22-35 Palpating for an inguinal hernia.

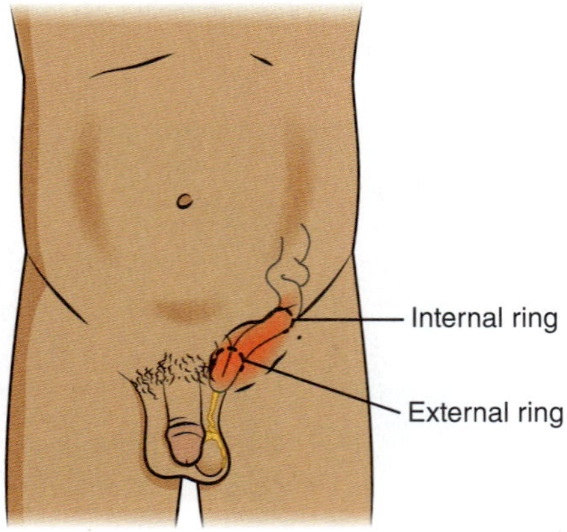

Figure 22-36 Schematic representation of indirect inguinal hernia.

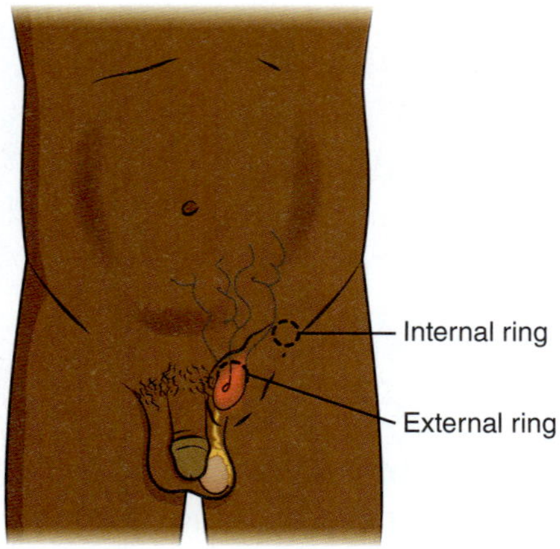

Figure 22-37 Direct inguinal hernia.

N **It is normal for there to be small (1 cm), freely mobile lymph nodes present in the inguinal area. There should not be any bulges present in the inguinal area. There should not be any palpable masses in the inguinal canal. No portions of the bowel should enter the scrotum. There should be no palpable mass at the femoral canal.**

A Unilateral enlargement of the lymph nodes along with erythematous overlying skin that may contain adhesions is abnormal.

P Three of the 15 strains of *Chlamydia trachomatis,* specifically L1, L2, and L3, cause lymphogranuloma venereum (LV). These serovars are more invasive and virulent and selectively infect lymphoid tissue rather than columnar epithelial cells. Firm inguinal masses result when buboes involute.

A Unilateral or bilateral enlargement of the inguinal lymph nodes is abnormal. The nodes may be tender or painless.

P Lymphadenopathy occurs when the immune system responds to bacterial infections, trauma, or carcinoma. Bacterial infections commonly associated with inguinal lymphadenopathy include syphilis, chancroid, and gonorrhea.

A An **indirect inguinal hernia** palpated at the inguinal ring is abnormal (Fig. 22-36). An impulse may be felt on the fingertip when the client is asked to cough. A larger indirect inguinal hernia may feel like a mass at the inguinal canal.

P Portions of the bowel or omentum enter the inguinal canal through the internal ring and exit at the external inguinal ring. All indirect hernias are congenitally related to a patent processus vaginalis. The severity of a combination of the congenital abnormality and a condition that increases abdominal pressure (e.g., obesity, chronic obstructive pulmonary disease [COPD], hard physical labor, coughing, ascites) determines the onset and degree of the hernia.

A Oval swelling found at the pubis on inspection represents a **direct inguinal hernia** and is abnormal (Fig. 22-37). Coughing causes enlargement on palpation of the mass.

P In direct hernias, portions of the bowel or omentum protrude directly through the external inguinal ring. Direct hernias are acquired masses that are influenced by increases in intra-abdominal pressure and weakening of the inguinal structures as part of the normal aging process. Other related factors include heavy lifting, obesity, and COPD.

A Palpation of a mass medial to the femoral vessels and inferior to the inguinal ligament is indicative of a **femoral hernia** and is abnormal (Fig. 22-38).

P A femoral hernia is caused by protrusion of the omentum or bowel through the femoral wall. The onset and size of the hernia may be affected by a congenitally large femoral ring, degradation of collagen and tissue attenuation associated with aging, increased intra-abdominal pressure, and the presence of preperitoneal fat.

Table 22-2 compares the different types of hernias.

Auscultation

Auscultation can be performed if a scrotal mass is found on inspection or palpation.

Scrotum

E 1. Place the client in a supine position.
2. Stand on the client's right side at the genitalia area.
3. Place your stethoscope over the scrotal mass.
4. Listen for the presence of bowel sounds.
5. Clean the headpiece of your stethoscope when finished.

N **No bowel sounds are present in the scrotum.**

A An indirect inguinal hernia is present if bowel sounds are present in the enlarged scrotum.

P Loops of bowel extending into the scrotum via an indirect hernia continue to produce bowel sounds unless the hernia is strangulated (lack of blood flow to bowel tissue) and bowel tissue becomes ischemic or necrotic.

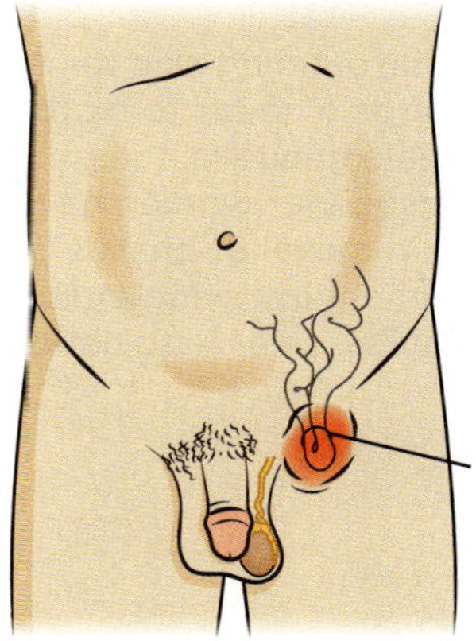

Figure 22-38 Schematic representation of femoral hernia.

Table 22-2 Comparison of Inguinal and Femoral Hernias

Feature	Indirect Inguinal Hernia	Direct Inguinal Hernia	Femoral Hernia
Occurrence	More common in infants <1 year and males 16–25 years of age	Middle-aged and older adult males	More frequent in females
Origin of Swelling	Above inguinal ligament Hernia sac enters canal at internal ring and exits at external ring. Can be found in the scrotum	Above inguinal ligament Directly behind and through external ring	Below inguinal ligament
Cause	Congenital or acquired	Acquired weakness brought on by heavy lifting, obesity, COPD	Acquired, due to increased abdominal pressure and muscle weakness
Signs and Symptoms	Lump or fullness in the groin that may be associated with a cough or crying	Lump or fullness in the groin area. It may cause an aching or dragging sensation.	Firm or rubbery lump in the groin. Pain may be severe.

NURSING TIP

Transgender Clients

Transgender individuals are those whose gender identity does not correspond with the sex they were assigned at birth. So as a nurse, you may have a client who was assigned male at birth (AMAB) who presents as female and is a transgender woman, or you may have a client who was assigned female at birth (AFAB) who presents as male and is a transgender man. Some transgender clients begin by dressing in a manner that is consistent with their chosen gender identity. Transgender clients may or may not have had gender-affirming treatment, which may include using hormones to replace the hormones of their genetic sex or surgery to affirm their gender. A general physical examination or urological examination can be a source of extreme stress for some clients, especially for those experiencing gender dysphoria. The nurse needs to be aware of the clinical status of a transgender client to provide appropriate care and be knowledgeable on practices that are followed. Before beginning the genitalia examination ask the client to share with you any concerns they have about their genitalia. For instance, some transgender women may practice tucking, which involves moving the scrotum and penis back and between the legs in the perineal region and moving testicles (if still present) into the inguinal canal. Clients may choose to secure their genitals by taping them in this position and then wearing tight-fitting underwear or specialized supportive underwear called gaffs. When examining the client who "tucks," visually inspect the surrounding skin for any irritation or infection. The client may experience testicular pain with tucking. The testicular pain needs to be further assessed for torsion, epididymitis, or orchitis. If the transgender female retains the male genitalia, the physical examination is unchanged from the cisgender male client.

Some transgender women have undergone feminizing genitoplasty surgery, which can include an orchiectomy, removal of phallus tissues, and creation of a neovagina and labia. Surgery requires interdisciplinary care management involving multiple surgical disciplines. Standards that guide these transitions can be found at the World Professional Association for Transgender Health (WPATH) *www.wpath.org.*

NURSING TIP

Phosphodiesterase Type 5 Inhibitors

Phosphodiesterase type 5 inhibitors (PDE 5) are available to treat erectile dysfunction, and they are available only by prescription. PDE 5 inhibitors improve vasodilation and smooth muscle relaxation in the penis. Libido is not affected by PDE 5 inhibitors. All PDE 5 inhibitors are contraindicated for men using organic nitrates.

Sildenafil (Viagra) was approved by the FDA in 1998. The medication is taken 30 to 60 minutes before initiating sexual activity, and it has a half-life of 4 to 5 hours. Sildenafil should be taken on an empty stomach or after a low-fat meal. Ingesting high-fat meat within 1 to 2 hours can reduce the onset of action by up to 70%. A blue discoloration of vision may be experienced.

Vardenafil (Levitra) received clearance from the FDA in 2003. Vardenafil is taken 1 hour before sexual activity, and its effects usually last 4 to 5 hours. All alpha blockers are contraindicated in clients taking vardenafil due to potential orthostatic hypotension. Vardenafil can be taken without regard to food.

Vardenafil HCl (Staxyn) was approved by the FDA in June 2010. Vardenafil HCl disintegrates on the tongue. It should be taken without liquid and may be taken with or without food. Vardenafil HCl should be taken about 1 hour before sexual activity. Caution should be used if the man also uses alpha blockers, as the combination may cause hypotension.

Tadalafil (Cialis) also became available in 2003. It is taken at least 2 hours before sexual activity. Tadalafil has a half-life of 17.5 hours, and clients will benefit from the medications for 36 hours or more. Men should not start new prescriptions for tadalafil and an alpha blocker at the same time. Tadalafil can be taken without regard to food. In January 2008, the FDA approved tadalafil for daily use, and it is an effective treatment for lower urinary tract symptoms for many men as well.

Side effects of all of the PDE 5 drugs may include headache, nasal congestion, and flushing, but these are less commonly reported with tadalafil. These side effects sometimes cause men to stop using the drug.

U.S. Preventive Services Task Force (USPSTF)

Grade A Recommendations:

- The USPSTF recommends that clinicians screen for HIV infection in adolescents and adults aged 15 to 65 years. Younger adolescents and older adults who are at increased risk of infection should also be screened. See the Clinical Considerations section for more information about assessment of risk, and screening intervals.
- The USPSTF recommends that clinicians prescribe preexposure prophylaxis using effective antiretroviral therapy to persons who are at increased risk of HIV acquisition to decrease the risk of acquiring HIV. See the Practice Considerations section for more information about identification of persons at increased risk and about effective antiretroviral therapy.
- The USPSTF recommends screening for syphilis infection in persons who are at increased risk for infection.

Grade B Recommendations:

- The USPSTF recommends screening for hepatitis B virus (HBV) infection in adolescents and adults at increased risk for infection. See the Practice Considerations section for a description of adolescents and adults at increased risk for infection.
- The USPSTF recommends screening for hepatitis C virus (HCV) infection in adults aged 18 to 79 years.
- See the Clinical Considerations section . . . for information on IPV in men.
- The USPSTF recommends behavioral counseling for all sexually active adolescents and for adults who are at increased risk for sexually transmitted infections (STIs). See the Practice Considerations section for more information on populations at increased risk for acquiring STIs.

Retrieved November 26, 2025, from *https://www.uspreventiveservicestaskforce.org/uspstf/recommendation-topics/uspstf-a-and-b-recommendations*

CASE STUDY
The Client With a Penile Lump and Peyronie Disease

This case study illustrates the application and objective documentation of the male genitalia examination. Liam is a 56-year-old landscape contractor who is concerned about his penis. His father had testicular cancer, and he is concerned that his penile lump could be malignant. He presents today for an evaluation.

HEALTH HISTORY

CLIENT PROFILE

56-year-old married White male

CHIEF COMPLAINT

"I have a lump in my penis."

HISTORY OF PRESENT ILLNESS

Client noticed a "pea-sized" penile lump, more than 6 months ago. The size has not changed. Noted pain in his penile shaft, but only during erections. Later a curvature to the left shaft developed that became more pronounced over about 2 months; client denies any pain except mild discomfort with sexual intercourse, which he attributes to the abnormal curvature of approximately 45° with an erection. The curvature causes his wife some occasional discomfort as well. He denies any traumatic injury or pain during intercourse before the onset of this condition. He reports a past episode of being hit in the genital area with a softball as a teenager. Monogamous with wife, denies STIs, discharge/odor, fever, malaise, swelling in groin. No change in scrotum, no history of UTIs or prostatitis; denies having been diagnosed with BPH. He also reports that his erection remains strong, despite the curvature to the left. Occasional nocturia, gets up 1x to 2x many nights.

PAST HEALTH HISTORY

Medical History Hyperlipidemia since age 42, on medication since that time
Hypertension since age 40, controlled on medication
Anaphylaxis age 30 from bee sting requiring emergency department visit; was given steroids and epinephrine, has carried epinephrine autoinjector since then. No recent use.

Surgical History Appendectomy, age 18, no complications. Vasectomy age 40, no complications

Allergies Bee sting: Hives and breathing difficulty
Sulfa: rash

Medications Rosuvastatin 10 mg daily, olmesartan 20 mg every morning, turmeric 500 mg daily, Co Q 10 300 mg daily, epinephrine autoinjector 0.3 mg/0.3 mL prn use—has never used it, expires in 3 months

Communicable Diseases Denies

Injuries and Accidents Fell 10 feet off a ladder last year with work, denies sequelae

Differing Abilities Hearing loss, needs to see audiologist

Blood Transfusions Denies

Childhood Illnesses Chickenpox (age 5), mumps (age 6)

Immunizations "Up to date," last tetanus 2018; gets annual flu shot, has received COVID-19 vaccine x 3, no booster, no shingles vaccine

FAMILY HEALTH HISTORY

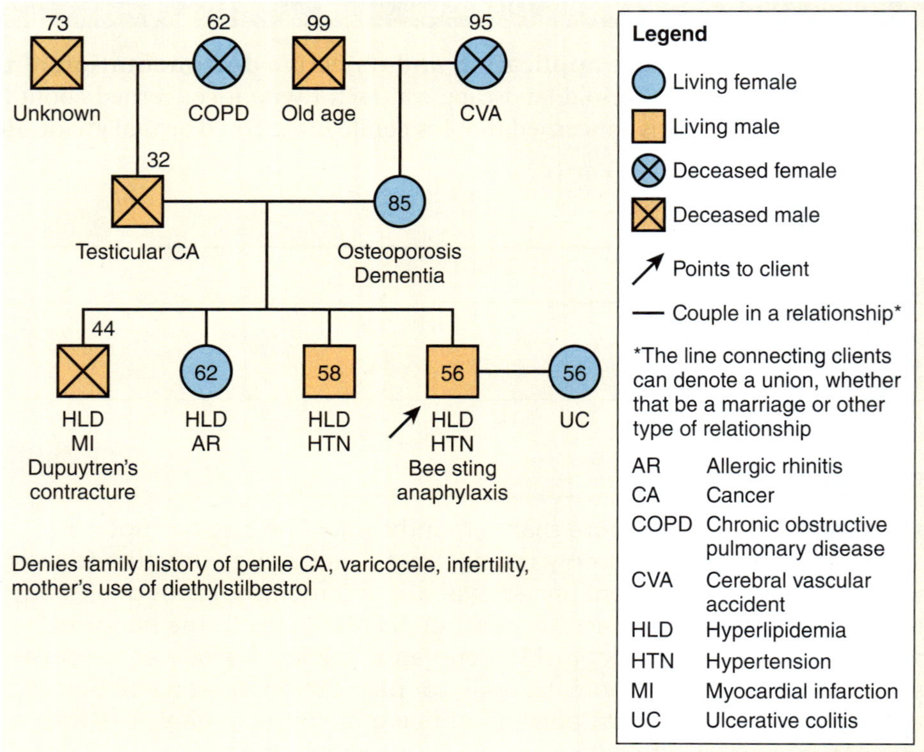

SOCIAL HISTORY

Alcohol Use 2 beers after work

Tobacco Use Cigars on the weekends

Recreational Drug Use Marijuana use in high school/college, denies recent use

Domestic and Intimate Partner Violence Denies

Sexual Practice Heterosexual; married for 26 years in monogamous relationship, 3 past sexual partners

Travel History Myrtle Beach every summer for 1 week

Work Environment Landscaper, designs and installs shrubs/trees; mows lawns and trims hedges, wears protective ear plugs and goggles

Home Environment Lives in a 20-year-old condo in the suburbs, has smoke and carbon monoxide detectors and checks them every New Year's Day

Hobbies and Leisure Activities Watching sports on TV

Stress Decreased clientele with current inflation

Education High school graduate, 1 year of community college

Economic Status "Things are tight right now"; denies food or shelter insecurity

Military Service None

Religion Nonpracticing Lutheran

Ethnic Background Welsh, no ethnic practices

Roles and Relationships Believes he is a good husband to his wife. Has little contact with siblings. Last saw his mother 18 mos ago. Mother has dementia and is being cared for by his sister in another state.

Characteristic Patterns of Daily Living Wakes up at 5:30 AM. Leaves for work at 6:30 AM. Has a 15-minute commute to the office and then he travels to different customers' residences/businesses to maintain the landscaping, has lunch in his truck. Arrives home by 5:00 PM. Goes to bed around 10:00 PM. Wakes twice a night to void

HEALTH MAINTENANCE ACTIVITIES

Sleep 7 hours/night

Diet Breakfast—cereal/toast; 2 days a week eats oatmeal for its cholesterol-lowering effects; lunch—packs a sandwich; dinner—wife prepares dinner most nights since she works from home. They try to eat healthy.

Exercise "My work is plenty of exercise!"

Stress Management Watching sports on television

Use of Safety Devices Wears seat belt while driving; does not use DEET when working outside but wears a long sleeve shirt and long pants with boots; showers when he gets home and looks for ticks (none found in past 3 mos)

Health Checkups Goes to his primary care provider twice a year for blood work and a checkup. Recently had first colonoscopy, which showed no polyps or tumors

PHYSICAL EXAMINATION

Inspection

Sexual Maturity Rating Tanner stage 5

Hair Distribution Distribution of pubic hair consistent with Tanner stage; no nits or lice

Penis Circumcised, no erythema at meatus, skin free of lesions, no inflammation, rounded glans penis with meatus slightly displaced ventrally and not centrally located, size equated with developmental stage, no penile plaque noted on inspection

Scrotum Scrotal skin rugated, no erythema, no edema, no lesions or masses; no dilated veins

Urethral Meatus Centrally located, no erythema or discharge

Inguinal Area No swelling or bulges

Palpation

Penis Pulsations present on dorsal aspect, nontender palpable plaques on the left shaft; 3 mm flesh colored, nontender firm mass on anterior penis 3 cm from glans

Urethral Meatus No discharge expressed from the urethral meatus

Scrotum No tenderness, testicles bilaterally firm, equal in size, no swelling/masses; epididymis nontender; spermatic cord smooth and round

Inguinal Area No inguinal nodes, no hernia masses

Auscultation Not performed

CLINICAL JUDGMENT IN ACTION

1. What cues indicate that the client is having a disorder of the male genitalia?
2. What interventions have the highest priority?
3. What assessment findings indicate clinical improvement or decline in this client?

Review Questions

1. What is the function of Cowper glands?
   a. To secrete viscous fluid that provides energy for sperm after ejaculation
   b. To function as a duct for transit of sperm
   c. To secrete alkaline fluid component of the ejaculate, to counteract vaginal acidity
   d. To support the position of the testes

2. The spermatic cords contain which of the following structures? Select all that apply.
   a. Testicular arteries
   b. Epididymis
   c. Lymphatic vessels
   d. Autonomic nerves
   e. Veins draining the testes

3. Which of the following are the functions of testosterone? Select all that apply.
   a. Influences male sexual behavior
   b. Promotes secondary sex characteristic development
   c. Produces sperm
   d. Promotes secretion of gonadotropins by the anterior pituitary gland
   e. Promotes musculoskeletal development

4. The nurse inspects a male client's genitalia. The nurse notes that there is sparse growth of long, slightly dark, straight pubic hair, no penile growth, and a slightly reddened scrotum. The nurse concludes that the client is in which stage of the Sexual Maturity Rating?
   a. Developmental Stage 1
   b. Developmental Stage 2
   c. Developmental Stage 3
   d. Developmental Stage 4

5. Which of the following are risk factors for penile cancer? Select all that apply.
   a. Age over 35
   b. Intact foreskin
   c. Smoking
   d. HPV types 16, 18, and 31
   e. Family history of penile cancer

6. The nurse performs a testicular examination on a 20-year-old male client. The nurse detects a varicocele on the right testicle. What does this clinical finding signify?
   a. The majority of varicoceles occur on the right testicle and do not require further investigation.
   b. A varicocele is considered a precancerous lesion of the testicle.
   c. A right-sided varicocele may indicate an obstruction at the vena cava.
   d. Varicoceles indicate poor testicular oxygenation.

7. Which of the following clients has the highest risk of developing testicular cancer?
   a. 15-year-old male
   b. Client with a history of hypospadias
   c. Asian male
   d. Client with a history of cryptorchidism

8. The nurse conducts an examination on a 55-year-old man. This client recently moved to a new condo and was lifting heavy boxes and furniture. A bulge is palpated above the inguinal ligament, directly behind and through the external ring. The nurse identifies this structure as which of the following?
   a. Direct inguinal hernia
   b. Indirect inguinal hernia
   c. Femoral hernia
   d. Umbilical hernia

9. A 30-year-old White male presents for a routine health examination and mentions that he has noticed that his left scrotum has become larger than his right scrotum, but it is painless, and he denies any recent trauma to his scrotum. The nurse suspects he is at risk for which condition?
   a. Left inguinal hernia
   b. Epididymitis
   c. Testicular tumor
   d. Testicular torsion

10. An 18-year-old male client presents for a routine screening physical before playing ice hockey. The client mentions that he has noticed that his left scrotum has a bluish tint and feels odd- like "a bunch of worms." The nurse knows that this may indicate which of the following conditions?
   a. An incarcerated hernia
   b. A large left varicocele
   c. A spermatocele
   d. Orchitis

CHAPTER

23 Anus, Rectum, and Prostate

Learning Outcomes

1. Identify the anatomy and physiology of the anus, rectum, and prostate.
2. Conduct a complete health history on a client with an anus, rectum, and prostate condition.
3. Perform a physical examination on a healthy adult and an adult with an anus, rectum, and prostate pathology.
4. Differentiate between normal clinical findings from a client's physical examination of the anus, rectum, and prostate and the pathophysiology of abnormal clinical findings.
5. Identify risk factors for anorectal cancer.
6. Identify risk factors for prostate cancer.
7. Identify the United States Preventive Services Task Force recommendations for the anus, rectum, and prostate.
8. Document a complete health history and physical examination of a client with anus, rectum, and prostate pathology.

The anorectal examination is an important part of the physical examination. In the male client, this includes examination of the anus, rectum, and prostate gland. In the female client, examination of the anus and rectum is performed. These examinations are usually performed last and should be performed regularly because they provide vital screening for anorectal and prostate cancers.

Anatomy and Physiology

Rectum

The large intestine is composed of the cecum, colon, rectum, and anal canal. The cecum and colon are discussed in Chapter 18. The sigmoid colon begins at the pelvic brim. Beyond the sigmoid colon, the large intestine passes downward in front of the sacrum. This portion is called the **rectum** (Fig. 23-1). The rectum contains three transverse folds, or valves of Houston. The function of these valves is to retain fecal material so it is not passed along with flatus.

Anus

The terminal 3 to 4 cm (1¼ to 1⅝ inches) of the large intestine is called the **anal canal**. The anal canal fuses with the rectum at the anorectal junction, or the dentate line, and together these structures form the **anorectum**. The anal orifice is located at the seam of the gluteal folds; it serves as the exit to the gastrointestinal tract and it is marked by corrugated

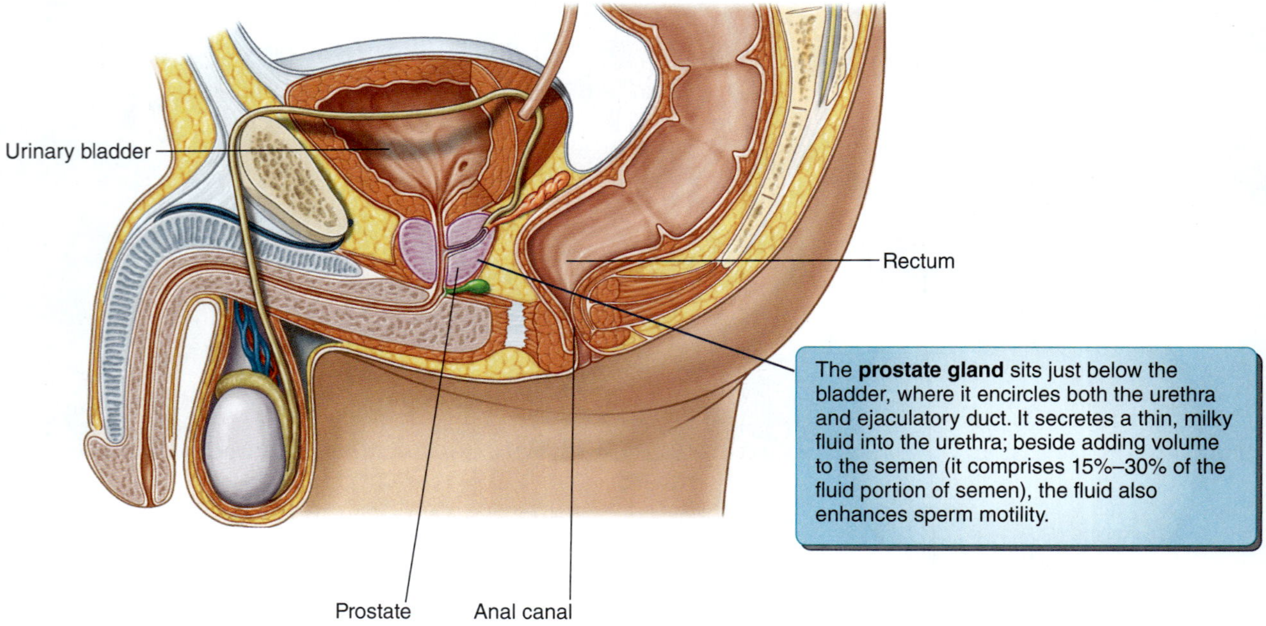

Figure 23-1 The anorectum and prostate.

skin. The anal orifice lies 2 cm (¾ inch) below the dentate line. The lower 2 cm of the anal canal is lined by **anoderm**, a thin, pale, stratified squamous epithelium that contains no hair follicles, sweat glands, or sebaceous glands.

In the superior half of the anal canal are **anal columns**, which are longitudinal folds of mucosa (also called columns of Morgagni). The **anal valves** are formed by inferior joining anal columns. Pockets located superior to the valves are called the **anal sinuses**. These sinuses secrete mucus when they are compressed by feces, providing lubrication that eases fecal passage during **defecation** (Fig. 23-2).

The anal canal opens to the exterior through the anus. Internal and external anal sphincter muscles surround the anus. Smooth muscle, which is under involuntary control, forms the internal sphincter. The skeletal muscle that forms the external sphincter is under voluntary control, allowing a person to control bowel movements.

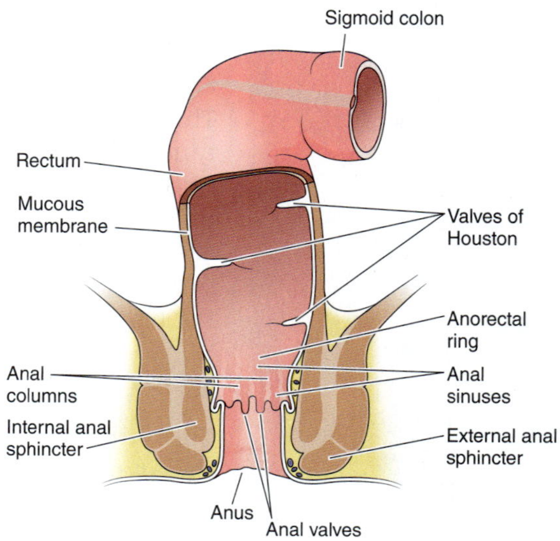

Figure 23-2 Anal canal.

The motility of the large intestine is controlled mainly by its nerves. There are two types of nerves: those that lie within the large intestine (the intrinsic nerves) and those that lie outside it (the extrinsic nerves). The rectum has more segmental contractions than the sigmoid colon. These contractions keep the rectum empty by the retrograde movement of contents into the sigmoid colon. As fecal material is forced into the rectum by mass peristaltic movements, the stretching of the rectal wall initiates the defecation reflex. A parasympathetic reflex signals the walls of the sigmoid colon and rectum to contract and the internal anal sphincter to relax. During defecation, the musculature of the rectum contracts to expel the feces.

Prostate

The prostate gland is contiguous with part of the anterior rectal wall in the male. The prostate is an accessory male sex organ the size and shape of a chestnut, approximately 3.5 cm (1⅜ inches) long by 3 cm (1¼ inches) wide. It consists of glandular tissue and muscle, and its small ducts drain into the urethra. The prostate lies just below the bladder and encircles the urethra like a doughnut (refer to Fig. 23-1).

The prostate has five lobes: anterior, posterior, median, and two lateral lobes. The median sulcus is the groove between the lateral lobes. The right and left lateral lobes are accessible to examination via the rectum.

Prostatic secretions are thin, milky, and alkaline. The secretions are made up of many different components. Citrate, a major component of prostatic fluid, provides a good transport medium for spermatozoa by maintaining the osmotic equilibrium of the seminal fluid. Prostatic fluid composes 15% to 30% of the ejaculate. Prostatic secretions have high prostatic acid phosphatase (PAP) levels and prostate-specific antigen (PSA).

The prostate is primarily involved in reproduction, but it also provides a certain measure of protection against urinary tract infections. Semen contains high levels of zinc, which is derived from the prostate. Zinc provides antibacterial properties to the prostate.

Within the prostatic cells, testosterone is converted to an androgen called dihydrotestosterone (DHT). DHT is the major androgen responsible for the benign enlargement of the prostate gland which occurs in males starting at age 40.

HEALTH HISTORY

The anus, rectum, and prostate health history provides insight into the link between a client's life/lifestyle and anal, rectal, and prostatic information and pathology.

CLIENT PROFILE

Diseases that are age-, sex-, and race-specific for the anus, rectum, and prostate are listed.

Age Pilonidal cyst or sinus (20 to 35)
Crohn disease of the anorectum (20 to 40)
Anal fissure (20 to 45)
Rectal condyloma acuminatum (20 to 50)
Ulcerative colitis (20 to 50)
Gonococcal proctitis (20 to 50)
Herpes proctitis (20 to 50)
Prostatitis (20 to 60)
Anal stenosis (>25)
Pruritus ani (>25)
Anal skin tags (<30)
Acute bacterial prostatitis (>30)
Anorectal abscess (30 to 40)
Anorectal fistula (30 to 40)

Hemorrhoids (>40)
Prostatic abscess (>40)
Fecal incontinence (>40)
Benign prostatic hypertrophy (>40)
Rectal cancer (>55)
Prostate cancer (>50)
Fecal impaction (>60)
Rectal prolapse (>65)

Sex

Female Rectal prolapse, fecal incontinence

Male Anorectal abscess, anorectal fistula, pruritus ani, rectal cancer, pilonidal cyst or sinus, hemorrhoids, gonococcal proctitis, herpes proctitis, benign prostatic hypertrophy (BPH), prostatitis, prostate abscess, prostate cancer

Race/Ethnicity

Black Prostate cancer (African American males and Caribbean males of African ancestry), anal cancer (Black males)

White Anal cancer (White females), Crohn disease of the anorectum, pilonidal cyst or sinus, BPH

CHIEF COMPLAINT

Common chief complaints for the anus, rectum, and prostate are defined, and information on the characteristics of each sign or symptom is provided.

1. Rectal Bleeding Discharge of blood from the rectum

Quality Occult, melena, hematochezia, massive hemorrhage

Quantity Scant, spotty, dripping, massive

Associated Manifestations Pain, absence of pain, malaise, fever, mass at anus

Aggravating Factors Defecation, constipation, diarrhea, minor trauma, pelvic irradiation, anal sex

Alleviating Factors Increased-fiber diet, bulk agents, exercise, increased fluid intake, hemorrhoidectomy

Setting Exposure to person with Mpox

Timing Constant, intermittent

2. Rectal Pain Subjective phenomenon of a sensation indicating real or potential tissue damage in the rectum

Quality Acute, sharp, tearing, burning, throbbing

Associated Manifestations Swelling, fever, blood, abdominal pain

Aggravating Factors Defecation, sitting, movement, foreign bodies, pregnancy, anal sex, constipation, hemorrhoids

Alleviating Factors High-fiber diet, bulk agents, exercise, increased fluid intake, warm sitz bath, topical emollients, surgery, removal of foreign body, lying down

Setting Exposure to person with Mpox

Timing More prominent with defecation; constant or episodic

3. Anal Incontinence Involuntary passage of stool

Associated Manifestations Diarrhea, constipation, urgency, rectal prolapse, prolapsed hemorrhoids, gaping anus

Aggravating Factors Diarrhea, impaction, cognitive impairment (e.g., dementia), anxiety, physical impairments (e.g., bedridden, impaired mobility), neurological disorders (e.g., stroke), trauma

Alleviating Factors Bulk fiber, constipating agents, laxatives, enemas, biofeedback, digital disimpaction, anal continence plugs

4. Constipation Infrequent, difficult passage of stool

Quantity Fewer than three bowel movements per week

Associated Manifestations Pain, blood, mucus, hard stool, straining with defecation, flatulence, abdominal bloating, decreased appetite

Aggravating Factors Low-fiber diet, lack of exercise, drugs (e.g., narcotics, calcium channel blockers), chronic use of laxatives, ignoring urge to defecate, weak abdominal muscles, inadequate fluid intake, rectocele, rectal prolapse, anal stenosis

Alleviating Factors High-fiber diet, bulking agents, increased fluid intake, defecation schedule, exercise, laxatives, digital removal, suppositories

5. **Diarrhea** Increased volume, fluidity, or frequency of bowel movements relative to the person's usual pattern

Associated Manifestations Abdominal pain, hematochezia, steatorrhea, weight changes, appetite changes

Aggravating Factors Viral infection, bacterial infection, antibiotics, laxatives, fecal impaction, Crohn disease, ulcerative colitis, lactose intolerance, specific foods (very individualized), irritable bowel syndrome, caffeine, alcohol

Alleviating Factors Constipating agents, anticholinergics, fluid replacement, certain foods (bananas, rice, apples, toast), antibiotics

Setting Stressful situations, recent ingestion of improperly stored or prepared food, recent travel abroad

6. **Pruritus** Itching of the anal and perianal skin

Associated Manifestations Erythema, edema, psoriasis, candidiasis, contact dermatitis, hemorrhoids, anal fissures, rectal carcinoma

Aggravating Factors Psoriasis, eczema, contact dermatitis, infections, parasites, oral antibiotics, diabetes mellitus, liver disease, obesity, poor hygiene, tight underclothes, wet clothing

Alleviating Factors Discontinuing current antibiotics and topical agents; eliminating coffee, tea, cola, milk, beer, and wine; discontinuing laxatives; rectal hygiene; loose clothing; nonmedicated talcum powder; topical fungicides

7. **Palpable Mass** Mass at the anus, in the anal canal, or on the prostate

Quality Firm, smooth, soft, mobile, nonmobile, nodular, fibrotic

Associated Manifestations Pain, absence of pain, blood, pus, mucus, fever, hemorrhoids, rectal prolapse

Alleviating Factors Warm sitz baths, high-fiber diet, bulk agents, surgery

PAST HEALTH HISTORY

The various components of the past health history are linked to anal, rectal, and prostatic pathology and anal-, rectal-, and prostatic-related information.

Medical History

Anorectal Specific Trauma, inflammatory bowel disease, prior history of sexually transmitted infections (STIs), polyps, rectal cancer, anal cancer, hemorrhoids, pruritus ani, constipation, diarrhea, fecal incontinence

Nonanorectal Specific Radiation, lymphogranuloma venereum, childbirth, arthritis, endocarditis, high serum PSA, endometrial cancer, ovarian cancer, breast cancer, cervical cancer, HIV infection, penile or vaginal STIs

Prostate Specific Prostate cancer, prostatitis, BPH

Surgical History

Anorectal Colectomy (partial or total), colonoscopy, rubber band ligation, injection sclerotherapy, hemorrhoidectomy, hemorrhoid banding, drainage of fistula or abscess

Prostate Prostatectomy, transurethral resection of the prostate (TURP), cystoscopy, prior urethral instrumentation

Allergies Contact dermatitis of perianal area

Medications Laxatives, constipating agents, alpha blockers, 5 alpha-reductase inhibitors, antifungals, astringent ointments, suppositories

Communicable Diseases HIV, *Neisseria gonorrhoeae, Treponema pallidum, Chlamydia trachomatis,* human papillomavirus (HPV), herpes simplex virus (HSV), Mpox

Injuries and Accidents Rectal trauma, foreign body in rectum

Childhood Illnesses Anal stenosis, Hirschsprung disease (with rectal pull-through)

FAMILY HEALTH HISTORY

Familial anal, rectal, and prostatic diseases are listed.

Rectal polyps, rectal cancer, pilonidal cyst, prostate cancer

SOCIAL HISTORY

The components of the social history are linked to anal, rectal, and prostatic factors and pathology.

Alcohol Use Excess intake of alcohol associated with pruritus ani; increased amount of alcohol associated with rectal and prostate cancers

Tobacco Use Cigarette smoking increases the risk of anal carcinoma and exacerbates Crohn disease.

Recreational Drug Use Illicit drug use may distort the user's perception, increasing the risk of unsafe sexual practices and STI exposure.

Sexual Practice Rectal penetration increases the risk of anal carcinoma and anorectal STIs.

Use of foreign objects in the rectum can lead to anal valve incompetence.

Work Environment Excessive sitting causes direct pressure and increases venous pooling, which can lead to hemorrhoids.

Hobbies and Leisure Activities Weightlifting (hemorrhoids, rectal prolapse), decreased mobility (constipation)

Stress Pruritus ani can be exacerbated by stress; diarrhea can be caused by stress; constipation can be caused by depression; irritable bowel and bladder symptoms can be exacerbated by stress.

HEALTH MAINTENANCE ACTIVITIES

This information provides a bridge between health maintenance activities and anal, rectal, and prostatic function.

Sleep Nocturia secondary to an enlarged prostate

Diet Diets high in vegetables, fruits, and whole grains, and low in red/processed meats may lower rectal cancer risk. Increased dairy consumption is associated with prostate cancer; Lycopene intake (raw tomatoes) may be preventive for prostate cancer.

Exercise Exercise promotes regular bowel evacuation.

Use of Safety Devices Condoms used with vaginal and anal intercourse

Health Checkups PSA level, digital rectal examination, guaiac fecal occult blood test (gFOBT), fecal immunochemical test (FIT), stool DNA test (sDNA-FIT), colonoscopy, CT colonography, flexible sigmoidoscopy

Assessment in Brief

Anus, Rectum, and Prostate Examination

Inspection

- Perineum and sacrococcygeal area
- Anal mucosa

Palpation

- Anus and rectum
- Prostate

Advanced Technique

- Anal Pap collection

Equipment

- Appropriate PPE
- Nonsterile gloves
- Water-soluble lubricant
- Hemoccult cards
- Gooseneck lamp

NURSING CHECKLIST
General Approach to Anus, Rectum, and Prostate Examination

1. Observe Standard Precautions and don personal protective equipment (PPE) such as gloves, gown, face shield, goggles, N-95 respirator or face mask if the client's status warrants these protective measures.
2. Greet the client and fully explain the examination techniques that you will be using.
3. Ensure that the examination room is at a warm, comfortable temperature to prevent the client from experiencing cold during the examination.
4. Use a quiet room that will be free from interruptions.
5. Ensure that the light in the room provides sufficient brightness to adequately observe the client. It may be helpful to have a gooseneck lamp available for additional lighting when lesions are observed.
6. Instruct the client to void before the examination.
7. Instruct the client to remove pants and underpants and to cover up with a drape or sheet.
8. Assess the client's apprehension level about the examination and reassure the client that apprehension is normal.
9. For inspection, place the client in the left lateral decubitus position and visualize the perianal skin (Fig. 23-3A). This position can also be used for palpation.
10. For palpation, leave the client in the left lateral decubitus position, or have the client stand at the side or end of the examination table, bending over the table, resting the elbows on the table, and spreading the legs slightly apart (Fig. 23-3B). As an alternative examination position for the client who cannot stand, have the client assume the knee-chest position (Fig. 23-3C). Have the woman who is undergoing a rectovaginal examination assume the lithotomy position. See Chapter 21.
11. Don nonsterile gloves.
12. Use a systematic approach every time the examination is performed. Proceed from the anus to the rectum in the female client. Proceed from the anus to the prostate in the male client.

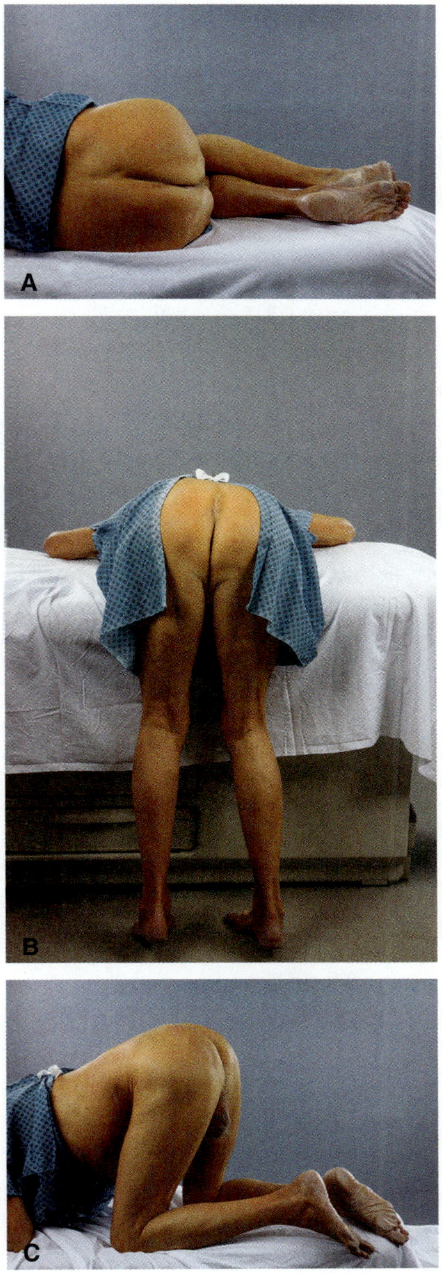

Figure 23-3 Client positions for the anus, rectum, and prostate examination. **A.** Left lateral decubitus. **B.** Standing. **C.** Knee-chest.

Examination of the Anus, Rectum, and Prostate

Inspection

As you examine the perineum and the sacrococcygeal area, perform a skin assessment. See Chapter 10 to review this examination.

Perineum and Sacrococcygeal Area

E Inspect the buttocks and sacral region for lesions, swelling, inflammation, and tenderness.

N **The buttocks and sacral region should be smooth and free of lesions, swelling, inflammation, and tenderness. There should be no evidence of feces or mucus on the perianal skin.**

A It is abnormal for one or several tiny openings to be seen in the midline over the sacral region, often with hair protruding from them.

P Pilonidal disease is an acquired condition of the midline coccygeal skin region induced by local stretching forces. There can be a cyst, an acute abscess (Fig. 23-4), or chronic draining sinuses in the sacrococcygeal area. Small skin pits representing enlarged hair follicles precede the development of the draining sinus or abscess. Lesions are often secondarily invaded by hair.

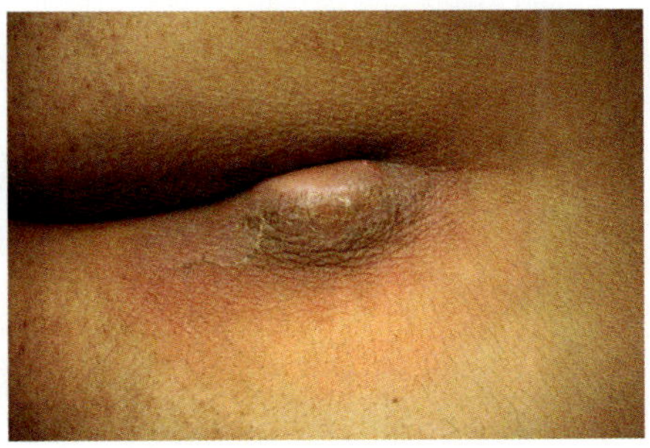

Figure 23-4 Pilonidal cyst.

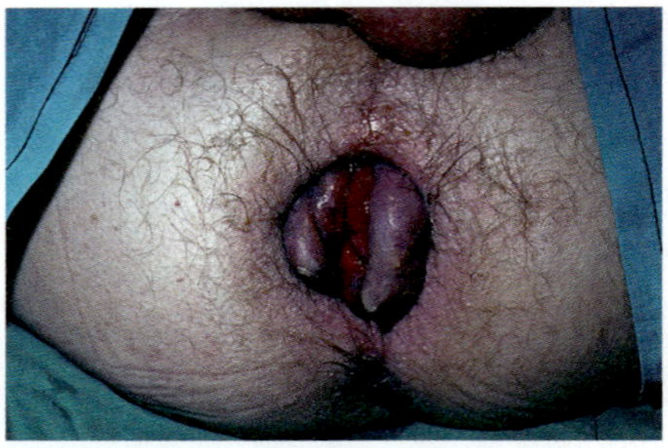

Figure 23-5 Hemorrhoid.

A Areas of hyperpigmentation, coupled with excoriation and thickened skin in the perianal area, are abnormal. The area may be intensely pruritic.

P Pruritus ani is caused by pinworms in children and by fungal infections in adults. The lesions are dull, grayish-pink.

A Well-demarcated, erythematous, sometimes itchy exudative patches of varying size and shape rimmed with small, red-based pustules are abnormal.

P **Candida albicans** occurs in sites where heat and maceration provide a fertile environment. Systemic antibacterial, corticosteroid, or antimetabolic therapy, pregnancy, obesity, diabetes mellitus, blood dyscrasias, and immunological defects increase susceptibility to candidiasis.

Anal Mucosa

E
1. Gently spread the client's buttocks apart with both hands, exposing the anus.
2. Instruct the client to bear down as though moving the bowels.
3. Examine the anus for color, appearance, lesions, inflammation, rash, and masses.

N **The anal mucosa is deeply pigmented, coarse, moist, and hairless. It should be free of lesions, inflammation, rash, masses, or additional openings. The anal opening should be closed. There should not be any leakage of feces or mucus from the anus with straining and there should not be any tissue protrusion.**

A A spherical, bluish lump that appears suddenly at the anus, and that ranges in size from a few millimeters to several centimeters in diameter (Fig. 23-5), is abnormal. The overlying anal skin may be tense and edematous. Pain and pruritus may be present in the perianal region.

P **Hemorrhoids** result from dilation of the superior and inferior hemorrhoidal veins. These hemorrhoidal veins form a hemorrhoidal plexus, or cushion, in the submucosal layer of the anorectum. An external hemorrhoid is located below the dentate line. Thrombosed external hemorrhoids (blood clots within subcutaneous hemorrhoidal veins) occur as a result of heavy lifting, childbirth, straining to defecate (which may be due to a low-fiber diet), or other vigorous activity. Bleeding may occur with defecation.

A Excess anal or perianal tissue of varying sizes that is soft, pliable, and covered by normal skin is abnormal.

P Anal skin tags are the result of residual resolved thrombosed external hemorrhoids, pregnancy, or anal operations. In some cases, there is no known cause.

A Fecal incontinence is abnormal.

P Fecal incontinence is usually a sign of an underlying acute medical problem. Some causes of fecal incontinence include fecal impaction, diarrhea, irritable bowel syndrome, neurogenic bowel dysfunction, stroke, dementia, multiple sclerosis, rectal prolapse, rectal trauma, and anorectal carcinoma.

A The perianal area may have erythema, excoriations, cracking, and bleeding. In chronic cases, the anal ring may have a shiny appearance.

P Pruritus ani is a condition in which itching around the rectum occurs. There are multiple causes of pruritus ani including poor anal hygiene, allergies, certain food, and drinks; however, excessive cleaning of the anal area is the most common cause. Moisture around the anus, associated with sweating or from the passage of abnormal feces, can also exacerbate or induce this problem. Other possible causes of pruritus ani include pinworms, psoriasis, eczema, dermatitis, hemorrhoids, anal fissures, and STIs.

A Linear tears in the epidermis of the anal canal, beginning below the dentate line and extending distally to the anal orifice, are abnormal (Fig. 23-6). Extreme pain, pruritus, and bleeding may accompany these findings.

P Anal fissures are the result of trauma, such as the forced passage of a large, hard stool, and anal intercourse, especially forced intercourse. Fissures occur most often in the area of the posterior coccygeal midline and less frequently in the anterior midline. This is because of weakness in the superficial external sphincter in these sectors. Predisposition to fissure is increased by perianal inflammation, which causes the anoderm to lose its normal elasticity. A sentinel skin tag may be visible inferior to the anal fissure and at the anal margin. Sphincter spasms may occur during the examination. The use of a local anesthetic may be necessary to thoroughly examine the area.

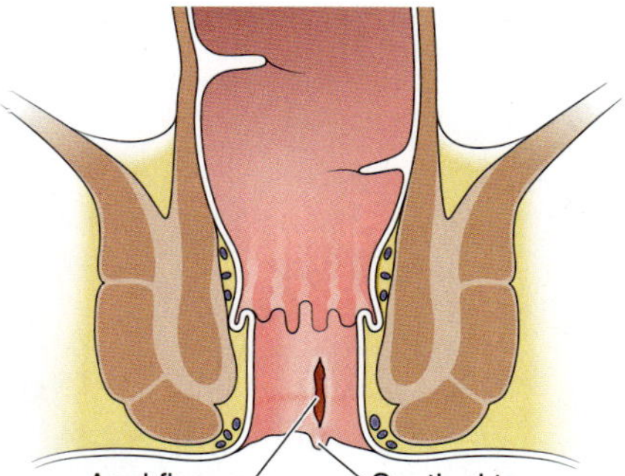

Figure 23-6 Anal fissure.

A Undrained collections of perianal pus in the tissue spaces in and adjacent to the anorectum are abnormal.

P The most common cause of an **anorectal abscess** is an infection of the anal glands, usually located posteriorly and situated between the internal and the external sphincters. These glands normally drain via the internal sphincter through small ducts and into anal crypts. When these ducts are occluded by impacted fecal material or trauma, ductal stasis and abscess formation result. An indurated mass with overlying erythema displaces the anus in cases of superficial abscess.

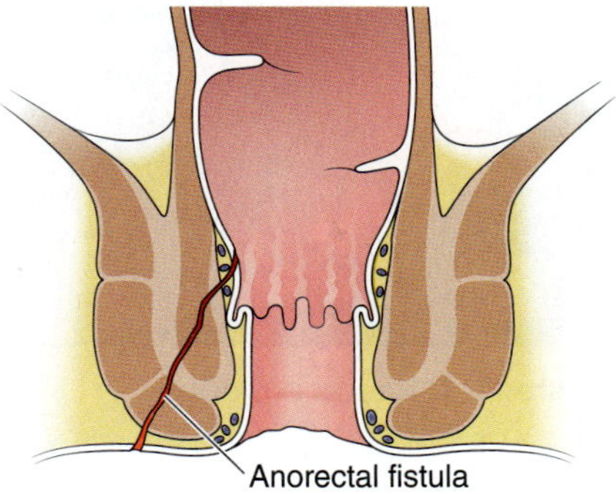

Figure 23-7 Anorectal fistula.

A An inflamed, red, raised area with purulent or serosanguineous discharge on the perianal skin is abnormal (Fig. 23-7).

P An **anorectal fistula** is a hollow, fibrous tract lined by granulation tissue and having an opening inside the anal canal or rectum and one or more orifices in the perianal skin. Fistulas are usually the result of incomplete healing of drained anorectal abscesses. However, they may occur in the absence of an abscess history. If this is the case, other causes of the fistula must be explored. Additional predisposing factors are inflammatory bowel disease, infectious disease, malignancy, Crohn disease, radiation therapy, chemotherapy, chlamydial infections, and trauma.

> **NURSING TIP**
> **Documenting Abnormalities of the Anus**
> When documenting any abnormalities found in the anus, describe them with regard to anatomical location: e.g., posterior toward the client's back; anterior toward the client's abdomen; right and left, respectively. Be sure to note client position and orientation.

A Soiling of the skin with stool and gaping of the anus are abnormal.

P **Anal incontinence** may be caused by neurological diseases, traumatic injuries, or surgical damage to the puborectalis or sphincter muscles. Perineal or intestinal disorders, diarrhea, fecal impaction, and constipating agents may also cause anal incontinence.

A The protrusion of the rectal mucosa (pinkish-red doughnut with radiating folds) through the anal orifice is abnormal (Fig. 23-8).

P **Rectal prolapse** is associated with poor tone of the pelvic musculature, chronic straining at stool, fecal incontinence, vaginal delivery, and, sometimes, neurological disease or traumatic damage to the pelvis. It is a condition more commonly associated with aging, occurring most frequently in those over age 65. A complete rectal prolapse involves the entire bowel wall. It is larger, red, and moist looking and has circular folds.

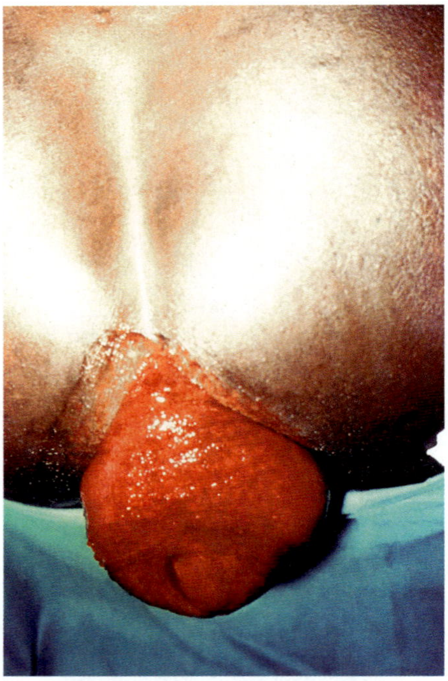

Figure 23-8 Rectal prolapse.

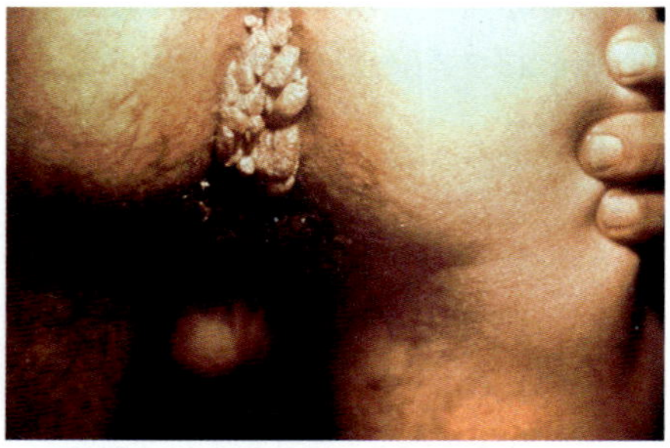

Figure 23-9 Human papillomavirus in the anal region.

A Erythematous plaques that develop into vesicular lesions that may become pustules and ulcerate are abnormal.

P These lesions are suggestive of HSV. Most anorectal herpes are due to HSV-2, and infections are related to anal intercourse.

A Warts or lesions that are beefy red, flesh-colored, irregular, and pedunculated are abnormal findings (Fig. 23-9). The lesions may involve the anoderm but may also extend deep into the anal canal and involve the rectal mucosa. There may be a few scattered lesions or extensive involvement of the entire anus.

P Condylomata acuminata are caused by HPV. Coital trauma allows entry into the anal epidermis in those in whom the wart virus is latent in the anorectum. Anal warts may also develop in females via an extension of genital warts along the perineum. Of the 50 strains of HPV, types 16, 18, and 31 have been associated with malignant lesions.

NURSING TIP

Assessing Risk Through Anal Pap

The anal Pap is a screening tool used to identify premalignant cytological changes in the anal epithelium in at-risk populations. Complete a comprehensive medical history with a focused anal cancer risk interview that facilitates the screening for risk factors. The interview should focus on:

- Sexual history, asking about anal intercourse and the number of sexual partners
- History of anal warts, genital warts, anal pain, anal discharge, anal dysplasia, or anal cancer
- Past history of an anal Pap; if yes, why, when, and the results

At-risk groups that may benefit from the anal Pap include:

- HIV-infected males with any history of receptive anal intercourse
- HIV-infected males with a history of injected drug use who might benefit from aggressive treatment
- Any recipient of allograft transplantation
- Males and females with a history of anogenital HPV infection, anal receptive intercourse, multiple sexual partners, and a history of STI or anal condyloma

ADVANCED TECHNIQUE

Anal Pap Collection

E

1. Inform the client to avoid enemas and receptive anal intercourse for 24 hours before specimen collection.
2. Colonic preparation is not required, but the rectum should be emptied before obtaining the sample.
3. Moisten a Dacron-tipped swab with tap water and gently insert the swab about 2 inches into the anal canal.
4. Perform 10 to 12 spiral rotation movements of the swab against the walls of the rectum and anus as the swab encircles the anal canal during slow withdrawal of the swab.
5. Remove the swab and swirl it for 15 seconds in a container of liquid cytology fluid.
6. Perform a digital rectal examination after the anal Pap to rule out any masses.

P Perineal chancroids (Fig. 23-10) are caused by *Haemophilus ducreyi*. Chancroids can be seen on the genitalia as well as the perineal and perianal regions.

A Mucoid or creamy exudate, possibly blood, from the rectum is abnormal.

P Gonococcal proctitis is most often seen in males who have sex with males as a result of direct inoculation, but it also occurs in females through contamination by vaginal discharge.

A Multiple perianal fissures and edematous skin tags of varying degrees are abnormal.

P Anorectal involvement occurs in the majority of clients with Crohn disease. Perianal disease may precede the onset of intestinal Crohn disease by several years. Perianal disease may proceed to anal stricture and incontinence. The development of perianal Crohn disease has no relation to other extraintestinal manifestations of the disease.

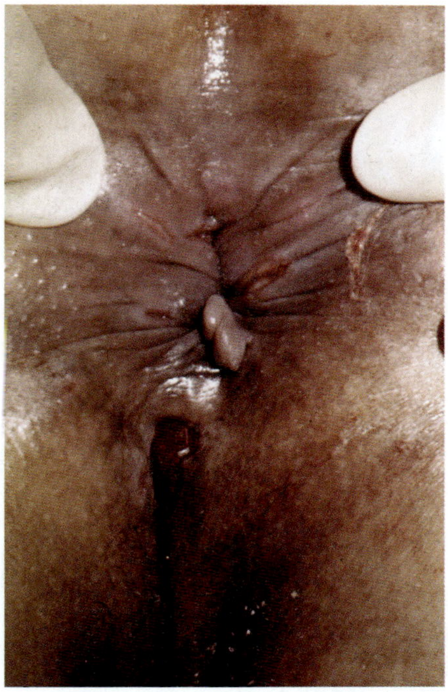

Figure 23-10 Perineal chancroid.

Palpation

The anorectal evaluation is usually reserved for the last portion of the examination after the nurse-client relationship has been established. A step-by-step explanation, description of expected sensations, reassurance, and a gentle technique will minimize client embarrassment and discomfort. It is also important for you to feel at ease about performing this examination.

Anus and Rectum

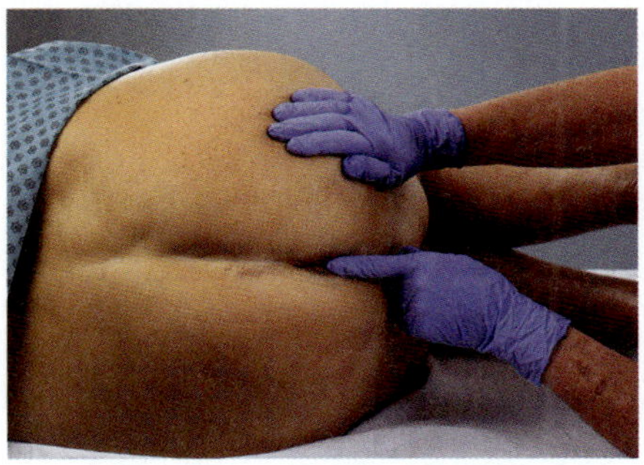

Figure 23-11 Position of the index finger for anorectal palpation.

E To perform anal and rectal wall palpation:

1. Have the client assume the most comfortable examination position (Fig. 23-3).
2. Reassure the client that sensations of urination and defecation are common during the rectal examination.
3. Lubricate a gloved index finger.
4. Place your finger by the anal orifice and instruct the client to bear down (Valsalva maneuver) as you gently insert the flexed tip of your gloved finger into the anal sphincter, with the tip of the finger toward the anterior rectal wall (pointed toward the umbilicus) (Fig. 23-11). The anus should never be approached at a right angle (with the index finger extended).

4 If the client tightens the sphincter, remove your finger, reassure the client, and try again, instructing the client to use a relaxation technique such as deep breathing.

5. Feel the sphincter relax. Insert your finger as far as it will go (Fig. 23-12). Note anal sphincter tone.
6. Palpate the lateral, posterior, and anterior walls of the rectum in a sequenced manner. The lateral walls are felt by rotating the finger along the sides of the rectum. Palpate for nodules, irregularity, masses, and tenderness. Ask the client to bear down again (which may help to palpate masses).
7. Slowly withdraw the finger; inspect any fecal matter on your glove and test it for occult blood. Refer to the Nursing Tip Common Causes of Rectal Bleeding. Table 23-1 lists common stool findings and etiologies.
8. Offer the client tissues to wipe off any remaining lubricant.

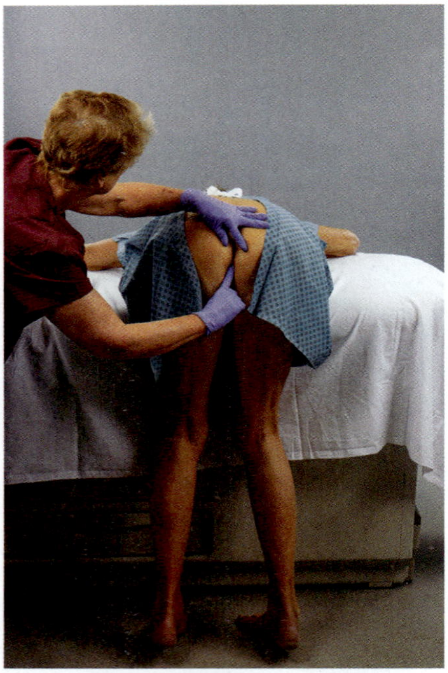

Figure 23-12 Position of the index finger in the anorectum.

NURSING TIP

Common Causes of Rectal Bleeding

Rectal bleeding is never a normal clinical finding; however, the etiology can be benign. Hemorrhoids, though painful for some clients, are not necessarily indicative of a more serious anorectal condition. Traumatic anal sexual practices as well as vigorous or forced anal intercourse can result in rectal bleeding from anal fissures. Inflammatory bowel disease, colorectal cancer, and benign colonic polyps can also result in rectal bleeding.

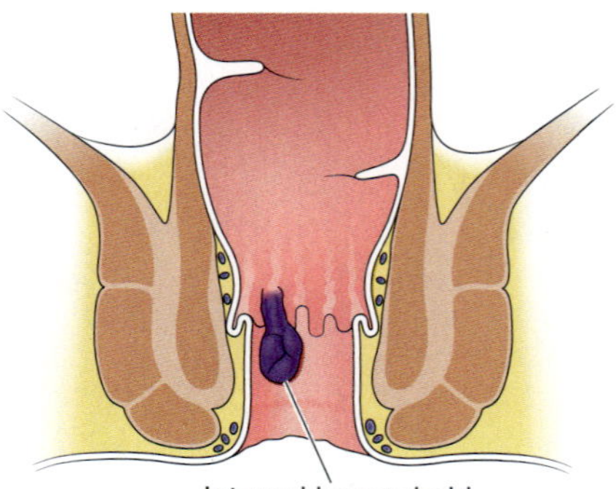

Figure 23-13 Internal rectal hemorrhoid.

Table 23-1 Common Stool Findings and Etiologies

Stool Finding	Etiology
Black, tarry (**melena**)	Upper gastrointestinal bleeding
Bright red	Rectal bleeding
Black	Iron or bismuth ingestion
Gray, tan	Obstructive jaundice
Pale yellow, greasy, fatty (**steatorrhea**)	Malabsorption syndromes (e.g., celiac disease), cystic fibrosis
Mucus with blood and pus	Ulcerative colitis, acute diverticulitis
Maroon or bright red stools	Diverticulosis/diverticulitis

NURSING TIP

Spotting Rectal Abuse

Suspect rectal abuse if you encounter any of the following in the examination: bruises around the buttocks and hip area; cuts, tears, or bleeding around the anal mucosa; or client refusal to undergo the rectal examination. Tell the client about your concern and consult your institution's policy regarding suspected abuse.

N **The rectum should accommodate the index finger. There should be good sphincter tone at rest and with bearing down. There should be no excessive pain, tenderness, induration, irregularities, or nodules in the rectum or rectal wall.**

A It is abnormal for the anal canal to be tight (making insertion of the index finger very difficult and painful or impossible).

P Anal stenosis can occur congenitally, but this condition usually is acquired. Anorectal operations, diarrheal disease, inflammatory conditions, and the habitual use of laxatives may cause anal stenosis. Chlamydial infections and malignancy must be excluded.

A Internal masses of vascular tissue in the anal canal are abnormal (Fig. 23-13).

P Internal hemorrhoids arise from the superior (internal) hemorrhoidal vascular plexuses above the dentate line; they are covered by mucosa. Internal hemorrhoids are usually painless unless they are thrombosed or prolapsed through the anal orifice.

A A soft nodule or nodules in the rectum are abnormal (Fig. 23-14).

P Rectal polyps occur frequently in the general population of the United States. Occasionally, they can be palpated, but more often they are diagnosed by proctoscopy/colonoscopy. They vary in size and may be accompanied by rectal bleeding. Rectal polyps are of two types: pedunculated (attached to a stalk) or sessile (adhering to the rectal mucosal wall). A biopsy of the tissue is required to determine whether the polyp is benign or malignant.

A A tender, indurated mass in the anorectum is abnormal.

P A tender, indurated mass in the anorectum may be an anorectal abscess. Refer to the preceding discussion on anorectal abscesses.

A An indurated cord palpated in the anorectum is abnormal.

P Anorectal fistula tracts may be palpated from the secondary orifice toward the anus. Digital rectal examination helps to determine the course of the tract. A drop of purulent drainage can be expressed from the opening if the opening is patent.

A A small, symmetrical projection 2 to 4 cm long from the rectum is abnormal.

P Rectal prolapse is best assessed with the client in a squatting position. The anal sphincter is lax, and palpation between the finger and thumb reveals only two layers of mucosa. Refer to the preceding description of rectal prolapse for additional information.

A Foreign bodies palpated in the rectum are abnormal.

P Thermometers, enema catheters, vibrators, bottles, and phallic objects may be introduced into the anus by accident, for erotic purposes, for concealment, for self-treatment, or by assault. Complications may include perforation of the rectum, obstruction, and pararectal infections.

A A hard mass in the anal canal is abnormal.

P A hard mass in the anal canal usually indicates anal carcinoma. There is a strong association between anal carcinoma (squamous cell) and HPV types 16 and 18.

A A firm, sometimes rocklike but often rubbery, puttylike mass is abnormal.

P In fecal impaction, the feces accumulate in the rectum because the colon does not respond to the usual stimuli promoting evacuation, or because accessory stimuli normally provided by eating and physical activity are lacking. Drugs, such as opiates, may compound the problem. Rectal sensitivity may be dulled by a habitual disregard for the urge to defecate. The prolonged use of laxatives or enemas may also decrease rectal sensitivity.

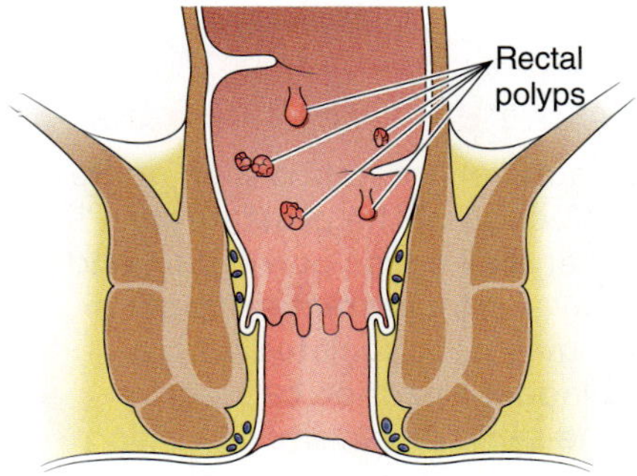

Figure 23-14 Rectal polyps.

Risk Factors

Anorectal Cancer

- HPV infection
- Anal warts
- HIV infection
- White females
- Females with cancer of the cervix, vagina, or vulva
- Black males
- Multiple sexual partners
- Smoking
- Decreased immune status from medications or disease process

Adapted from *https://www.cancer.org/cancer/anal-cancer/causes-risks-prevention/risk-factors.html* (retrieved December 18, 2025).

NURSING TIP

Risk of Prostate Cancer in Transgender Clients

The transgender client needs to be approached respectfully with sensitive history taking and appropriate physical examination. Whether the client has had gender-affirming surgery and hormonal therapy or not, their body status may not reflect their sense of gender and personal identity. Discuss with the client where they are in the transgender process to ascertain what anatomical parts are present so that appropriate care can be delivered. Transgender clients who identify as female but have not undergone gender affirmation surgery retain the prostate gland and are still at risk of prostate cancer. This needs to be well documented in the medical record, and the client is reminded that routine testing for prostate cancer should still be undertaken.

NURSING TIP

Prostate Examination Tip

A normal benign prostate gland feels different on palpation than a prostate gland with cancer. To become familiar with the difference, make a fist with your nondominant hand. Insert the index finger of your other hand into the space between your clenched thumb and index finger. Benign prostatic tissue feels soft and pliable like the tissue in this space. Next, feel along the top of your clenched thumb. Prostate cancer may feel firmer like this when palpated.

Prostate

E To perform prostatic palpation:

1. Position the client as tolerated (the standing position or left lateral decubitus positions are preferred).

NURSING TIP
Acute Bacterial Prostatitis

Bacterial prostatitis is an acute infection of the prostate gland that may cause pelvic pain and lower urinary tract symptoms. It may be associated with a bladder infection caused by the same organism. Obtaining a urine culture may identify the pathogen. Rectal examination should be avoided in known cases of acute bacterial prostatitis because of the possibility of bacteremia.

2. Reassure the client that sensations of urination and defecation are common during the prostatic examination.
3. Use a well-lubricated, gloved index finger.
4. Insert the gloved index finger and proceed as described in steps 4 and 5 of the "Palpation" section.
5. Perform a bidigital examination of the bulbourethral gland by pressing your gloved thumb into the perianal tissue while pressing your gloved index finger toward it (Fig. 23-15). Assess for tenderness, masses, or swelling.
6. Release pressure of the thumb and index finger. Remove your thumb from the perianal tissue and advance your index finger.
7. Palpate the posterior surface of the prostate gland (Fig. 23-16). Note the size, shape, consistency, sensitivity, and mobility of the prostate. Note whether the median sulcus is palpable.
8. Attempt to palpate the seminal vesicles by extending your index finger above the prostate gland. Assess for tenderness and masses.
9. Slowly withdraw the finger; inspect any fecal matter on your glove and test it for occult blood (if not previously performed).

N **The prostate gland should be small, smooth, mobile, and nontender. The median sulcus should be palpable.**

A A soft, nontender, enlarged prostate gland is abnormal (Fig. 23-17).

P The development of BPH is related to aging and the presence of testosterone, which converts to dihydrotestosterone and leads to prostatic cell growth. The size of the prostate gland on rectal examination is not always indicative of the degree of symptoms because the lobes may not be palpable or they may be causing an obstruction. In the client with BPH, the median sulcus may not be palpable.

A A firm, tender, or fluctuant mass on the prostate is abnormal.

P A high percentage of clients with prostatic abscess have diabetes mellitus. An abscess is suspected in the client with acute bacterial prostatitis or urinary tract infection who develops a spiked fever along with rectal pain. Prostatic abscesses are caused mainly by *Escherichia coli*.

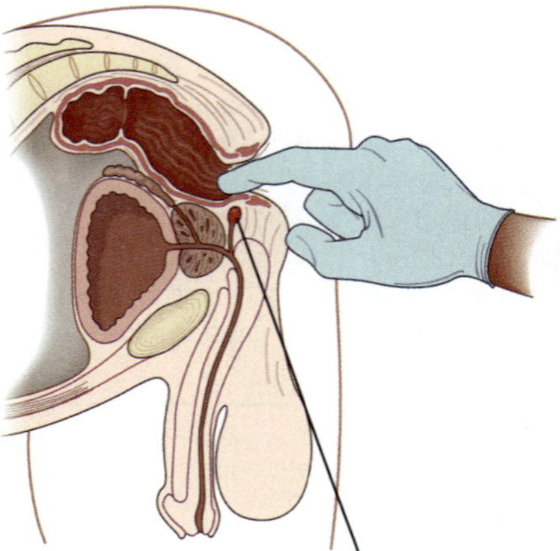

Figure 23-15 Bidigital palpation of the bulbourethral gland.

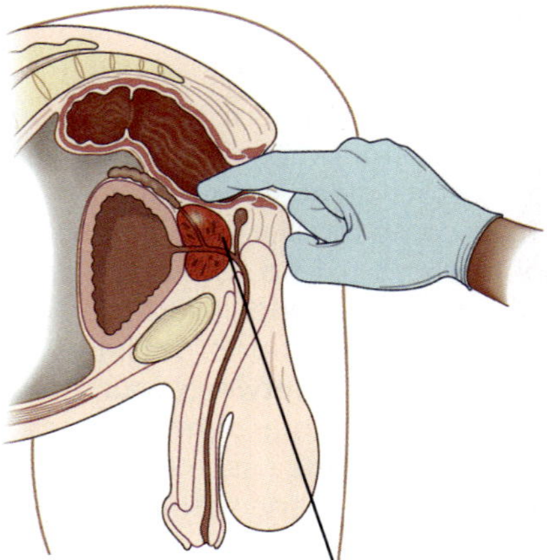

Figure 23-16 Prostatic palpation.

NURSING TIP
Prostate-Specific Antigen (PSA)

The normal value for a serum PSA is age-specific.

The recommended upper limits of normal serum PSA levels are: 2.5 ng/mL for 40 to 49 years, 3.5 ng/mL for 50 to 59 years, 4.5ng/mL for 60 to 69 years, and 6.5ng/mL for 70 to 79 years.

Serum PSA elevations occur as a result of disruption of the normal prostatic architecture, which allows PSA to diffuse into the prostatic tissue and gain access to the circulation. This can occur with prostate diseases such as prostate cancer, benign prostatic hypertrophy (BPH), and prostatitis. Prostate manipulation with prostate massage and prostate biopsy may also cause increases in the PSA level. However, a digital rectal examination causes no significant change in PSA.

Clients can have prostatic carcinoma with a normal PSA. Any time an abnormality (nodule, firmness, irregularity) is palpated during the prostate examination, a prostate biopsy must be performed to rule out carcinoma.

A Firm, hard, or indurated nodules on the prostate are abnormal (Fig. 23-18).

P The nodules of prostate cancer may be single or multiple. Early in the disease, the nodules may be small, but late in the disease, the entire prostate may seem irregular, hard, immobile, and quite large.

A An exquisitely tender and warm prostate is abnormal.

P Bacterial prostatitis is usually caused by *Escherichia coli.* When clients present with a sudden onset of high fever, chills, malaise, myalgias, and arthralgias, acute bacterial prostatitis is suspected.

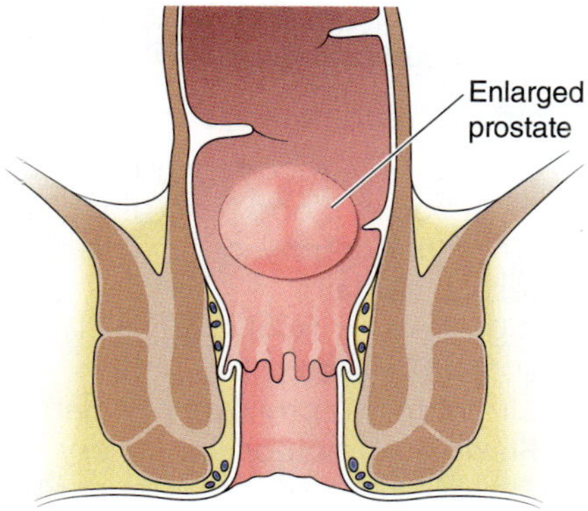

Figure 23-17 Benign prostatic hypertrophy.

Risk Factors

Prostate Cancer

- Age >50
- Family history of prostate cancer
- Race/ethnicity: African American males and Caribbean males of African ancestry
- Genetic risks: inherited mutations of *BRCA 1* and *BRCA 2* genes, Lynch syndrome
- Possibly with increased consumption of dairy products
- Possible risk for firefighters due to exposure to various chemicals

Adapted from *https://www.cancer.org/cancer/types/prostate-cancer/causes-risks-prevention/risk-factors.html* (retrieved November 23, 2025).

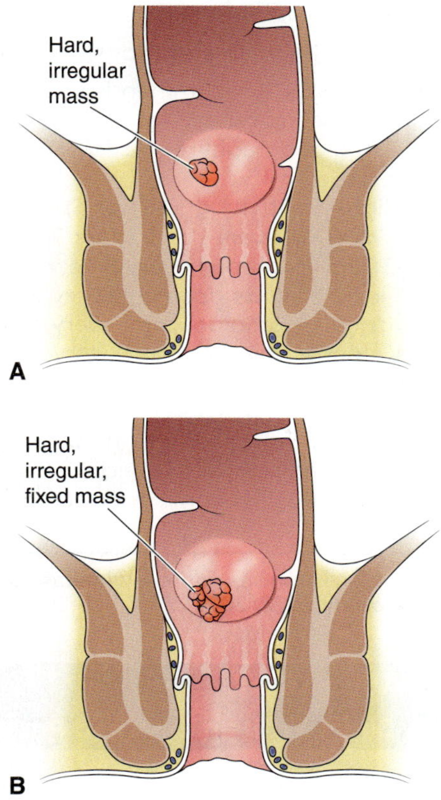

Figure 23-18 Cancer of the prostate. **A.** Single nodule. **B.** Multiple nodules.

NURSING TIP

Guidelines for Early Detection of Prostate Cancer

Screening for prostate cancer remains controversial with Guidelines for Prostate Cancer Screening being revised and differing between health-care groups.

The American Cancer Society (2023) recommends that males be allowed to make an informed decision with their health-care provider about whether to be screened for prostate cancer. This shared decision-making should be made after the client receives information about the uncertainties, risks, and potential benefits of prostate cancer screening. Prostate cancer screening includes the blood test prostate-specific antigen (PSA) and a digital rectal examination (though this may or may not be done depending on the client/and or clinician decision). Males should not be screened unless they have received this information. The discussion about screening should take place at:

- Age 50 for males who are at average risk of prostate cancer and are expected to live at least 10 more years.
- Age 45 for males at high risk of developing prostate cancer, including Blacks and males who have a first-degree relative (father or brother) diagnosed with prostate cancer at an early age (younger than age 65).
- Age 40 for males at even higher risk (those with more than one first-degree relative who had prostate cancer at an early age).

The frequency of PSA testing depends on the test result.

Adapted from *https://www.cancer.org/cancer/prostate-cancer/detection-diagnosis-staging/acs-recommendations.html* (retrieved November 23, 2025).

U.S. Preventive Services Task Force (USPSTF)

Grade A Recommendations

- The USPSTF recommends screening for colorectal cancer in all adults aged 50 to 75 years. with either a guaiac fecal occult blood test (gFOBT), fecal immunochemical test (FIT), stool DNA test (sDNA-FIT), colonoscopy, CT colonography, or flexible sigmoidoscopy in adults. Recommended intervals for colorectal cancer screening tests include:
  High-sensitivity gFOBT or FIT every year
  sDNA-FIT every 1 to 3 years
  CT colonography every 5 years
  Flexible sigmoidoscopy every 5 years
  Flexible sigmoidoscopy every 10 years + FIT every year
  Colonoscopy screening every 10 years
- The USPSTF recommends that clinicians screen for HIV infection in adolescents and adults aged 15 to 65 years. Younger adolescents and older adults who are at increased risk of infection should also be screened
- The USPSTF recommends that clinicians prescribe preexposure prophylaxis using effective antiretroviral therapy to persons who are at increased risk of HIV acquisition to decrease the risk of acquiring HIV.
- The USPSTF recommends screening for syphilis infection in persons who are at increased risk for infection.

Grade B Recommendations

- The USPSTF recommends screening for colorectal cancer in adults aged 45 to 49 years. with either a guaiac fecal occult blood test (gFOBT), fecal immunochemical test (FIT), stool DNA test (sDNA-FIT), colonoscopy, CT colonography, or flexible sigmoidoscopy. Recommended intervals for colorectal cancer screening tests include:
  High-sensitivity gFOBT or FIT every year
  sDNA-FIT every 1 to 3 years
  CT colonography every 5 years
  Flexible sigmoidoscopy every 5 years
  Flexible sigmoidoscopy every 10 years + FIT every year
  Colonoscopy screening every 10 years
- The USPSTF recommends behavioral counseling for all sexually active adolescents and for adults who are at increased risk for STIs.
- The USPSTF recommends screening for hepatitis B virus (HBV) infection in adolescents and adults at increased risk for infection
- The USPSTF recommends screening for hepatitis C virus (HCV) infection in adults aged 18 to 79 years.

https://www.uspreventiveservicestaskforce.org/uspstf/recommendation-topics/uspstf-a-and-b-recommendations (retrieved November 23, 2025).

CASE STUDY

A Client With an Enlarged Prostate and Hemorrhoid

This case study illustrates the application and objective documentation of the anus, rectum, and prostate examination. Hector Hatzis is a 55-year-old married American-born man with a history of ischemic heart disease, hypertension, hyperlipidemia, and psoriasis. Hector has no lower tract urinary symptoms. Hector comes to the office for a discussion and physical examination after being told that a recent blood test showed an elevated PSA. Hector is otherwise fit and well and is physically active.

HEALTH HISTORY

CLIENT PROFILE

55-year-old married White man.

CHIEF COMPLAINT

"I am here today because I was told my PSA blood test was too high and I need to get a prostate check."

HISTORY OF PRESENT ILLNESS

The nurse practitioner had a discussion with Hector at his last checkup about whether a PSA should be checked. Client agreed to have a PSA blood test last year and declined a prostate examination. Client's PSA was within normal limits at that time. Hector is feeling well and has no complaints. Hector reports no dysuria, frequency, or urgency. Client reports a good urinary flow and nocturia 1 to 2 times at night, which may be more frequent after having a few beers with his friends. Denies any sleep disturbance. In monogamous relationship with wife. Had 3 prior sexual partners. Denies any constipation, diarrhea, rectal pain, or rectal problems.

January 2022 PSA: 2.7 ng/mL
March 2024 PSA: 3.6 ng/mL
May 2026 PSA: 4.7 ng/mL

Client is not aware of any family history of prostate cancer. Hector's father had a "prostate problem" and had an operation, but recalls there was no cancer. Hector's sister was diagnosed with breast cancer in her 40s and had surgery and chemotherapy. Sister did not have any genetic testing for the BRCA gene mutation.

PAST HEALTH HISTORY

Medical History
Ischemic heart disease treated with coronary artery stent in 2019
Hyperlipidemia diagnosed 2019
Hypertension diagnosed 2019
Psoriasis since early adulthood

Surgical History Appendectomy (age 12)
Coronary artery stent insertion into left anterior descending coronary artery in April 2019

Allergies No known medication allergies
Denies any food or latex allergies

Medications Aspirin 81 mg enteric coated daily
Rosuvastatin 40 mg daily
Ramipril 5 mg daily
Triamcinolone 0.1% cream applied twice daily to affected areas as needed
Vitamin D 2,000 IU daily
Biotin 5,000 mcg daily
Mulitivitamin for eyes daily

Communicable Diseases Denies any STIs, has never undergone HIV testing
Had COVID-19 3 months ago, mild respiratory symptoms only, did not require hospitalization or treatment for this

Injuries and Accidents Denies

Differing Abilities Denies

Blood Transfusions Denies

Childhood Illnesses Remembers having chicken pox in first grade

Immunizations Reports usual childhood immunizations
Reports annual influenza vaccinations
Reports a total of 4 COVID-19 vaccines since 2021
Wants to get shingles vaccine

FAMILY HEALTH HISTORY

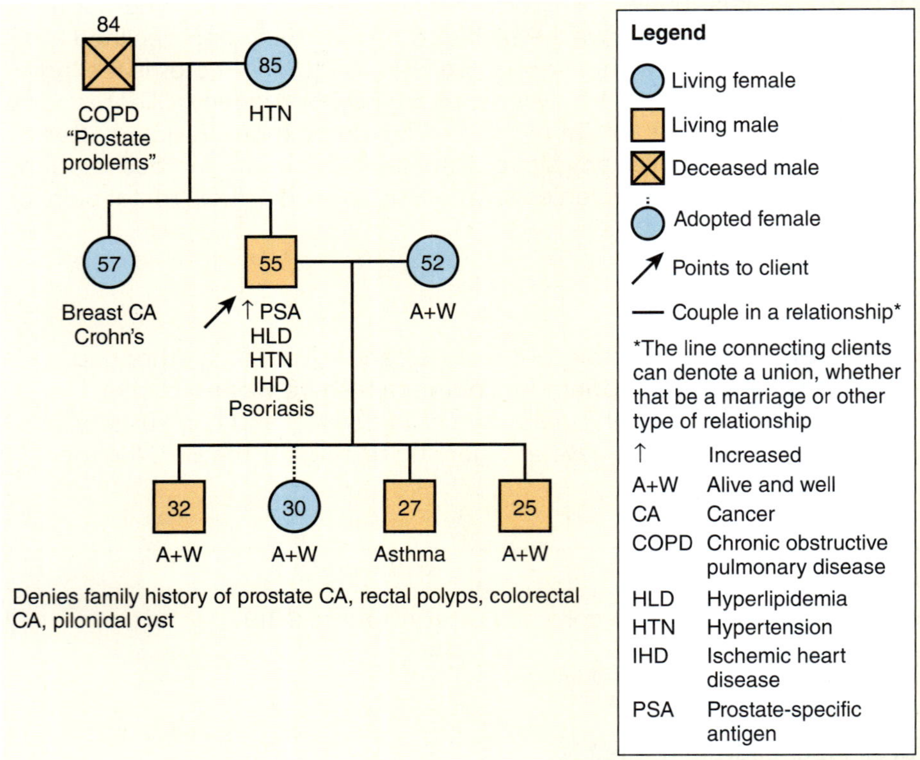

SOCIAL HISTORY

Alcohol Use Two 10 oz beers 2 to 3 nights/week, occasionally has four or five 10-oz beers on outings with his friends about once a month

Tobacco Use Smoked 10 to 20 cigarettes/day from age 18 to 25. None since. Denies vaping, use of e-cigarettes, and chewing tobacco

Recreational Drug Use Used to smoke an occasional (weekly) marijuana joint, but has not done this since age 30

Domestic and Intimate Partner Violence Denies

Sexual Practice Heterosexual. Had three sexual partners before meeting spouse. Married at age 24. They are still sexually active, and they have intercourse 1 to 2 times weekly. Reports erections are strong and sexual interaction is important to his identity as a male

Travel History Family beach holidays twice a year.

Work Environment Laborer with large building firm, reliable employment for now. Enjoys physical aspect of work, "Keeps me fit!"

Home Environment Client, wife, and 2 of their 4 children live in a townhouse. Client regularly checks the smoke detectors to make sure they are functioning; unsure if there is a carbon monoxide detector in the house. House is air-conditioned and has central heating

Hobbies and Leisure Activities Plays cards, enjoys building model planes, watching football and soccer on TV

Stress With the economy worries that layoffs may occur in the construction industry. Wife worries about the physical exertion of his job due to his "heart conditions"

Education Graduated from high school, then went straight into a building apprenticeship

Economic Status Can pay bills but does not have a lot left over

Military Service Denies

Religion Not particularly religious; was brought up Greek Orthodox religion

Ethnic Background Greek American; grandparents left Greece with the threat of war in 1939 and came to the United States. Hector's mother cooked traditional Greek meals for the family. Enjoyed large family gatherings as a child but now family lives on the other side of the country and has not seen them in many years

Roles and Relationships Married for 34 years, in a good relationship with wife. Four children: son aged 32 living close by, daughter aged 30 also living close by, two more sons aged 27 and 25 both still living at home. No grandchildren yet. Many good friends with whom client/wife socialize regularly. Has good friends at the workplace, but these tend to be short-term as coworkers frequently move from one building site to the next site

Characteristic Patterns of Daily Living Wakes early on workdays: 5:30 AM to be at the building site by 7:00; sleeps in until 8:00 AM on weekends

HEALTH MAINTENANCE ACTIVITIES

Sleep Midweek 6- to 7 hr, weekends 7 to 8 hr; sleeps well

Diet Client reports diet is much better since the diagnosis of hypertension, hyperlipidemia, and ischemic heart disease. Now most meals are plant-based with occasional chicken or meat. Tries to eat fish at least twice per week. Weight well maintained at 185 lb

Exercise Played in rec league soccer until age 26. Now goes for a run on the weekend, 2 to 3 miles. "I need to stay fit for my job."

Stress Management "Not sure. I rarely feel stressed. Suppose I talk to my wife if I do."

Use of Safety Devices Always uses seat belt

Health Checkups Regular health screening checks with internal medicine nurse practitioner and cardiologist

PHYSICAL EXAMINATION

Inspection

Perineum and Sacrococcygeal Area Skin smooth and even; intact without lesions, no inflammation or swelling

Anal Mucosa Lightly pigmented, coarse, moist, and hairless; one cm spherical mass at 9 o'clock position of anus, no odor or discharge, no inflammation, no rashes

Palpation

Anus and Rectum No pain or tenderness with rectal examination; positive sphincter tone, no nodules in the rectum or rectal wall

Prostate Enlarged; firm nodule on left, lobe; no tenderness, no pain with palpation

LABORATORY DATA (TODAY)

	Client's Values	Normal Range
PSA	5.0 ng/mL	0 to 3.5 ng/mL (for a 50- to 59-year-old male)
Hemoccult	Negative	Negative

CLINICAL JUDGMENT IN ACTION

1. What cues indicate that the client is having a disorder of the anus, rectum, and prostate?
2. What interventions have the highest priority?
3. What assessment findings indicate clinical improvement or decline in this client?

Review Questions

1. When performing inspection and palpation of the anus, rectum, and prostate on an adult, how should the client be positioned? Select all that apply.
   a. Standing, bending over the examination table
   b. Left lateral decubitus
   c. Prone
   d. Knee to chest
   e. Lithotomy
2. Which of the following factors may contribute to constipation? Select all that apply.
   a. Low-fiber diet
   b. Increased fluid intake
   c. Lack of exercise
   d. Medication such as a narcotic
   e. Caffeine ingestion
3. Which of the following structures form the anal sphincter? Select all that apply.
   a. Involuntary smooth muscle that forms the internal sphincter
   b. Voluntary smooth muscle of the anal sinuses
   c. Involuntary skeletal muscle of the anoderm
   d. Voluntary skeletal muscle that forms the external sphincter
   e. Involuntary folds of the valves of Houston
4. Which of the following are true statements about prostatic secretions? Select all that apply.
   a. Little is known about the function of prostatic secretions.
   b. Prostatic secretions compose 15 to 30% of fluid in the ejaculate.
   c. Prostatic secretions help maintain the osmotic equilibrium of seminal fluid.
   d. Prostatic secretions have spermicidal properties.
   e. Prostatic secretions have low levels of prostate-specific antigen.
5. Which of the following conditions may cause rectal bleeding? Select all that apply.
   a. Anal fissure
   b. Traumatic anal intercourse
   c. Benign prostatic hypertrophy
   d. Inflammatory bowel disease
   e. Benign colonic polyps
6. A 60-year-old woman reports some pain when having a bowel movement. There has been some blood on the toilet paper when wiping after passing the stool. On examination, anal skin tags are seen as well as a 5-mm bluish-colored lump visible at the anus. A thrombosed hemorrhoid is diagnosed. What factors may have contributed to this finding? Select all that apply.
   a. Heavy lifting
   b. Pruritus ani
   c. Constipation
   d. Childbirth
   e. Anal fissure
7. Fifty-three-year-old Manan asks whether testing for prostate cancer should be done at the annual physical examination. Which of the following are risk factors for prostate cancer? Select all that apply.
   a. Family history of prostate cancer
   b. Carrying the *BRCA 1* gene
   c. Family history of liver and pancreatic cancers
   d. Living for 10 years in South America
   e. Three previous episodes of gonorrhea
8. When performing an examination of a client's prostate, which of the following would be considered abnormal? Select all that apply.
   a. The prostate is firm and has a fluctuant mass.
   b. The prostate feels very firm and irregular.
   c. The prostate feels soft and is nontender.
   d. The prostate's median sulcus is not palpable.
   e. The prostate feels warm and is exquisitely tender.
9. A 95-year-old client is brought in by a family member because of anal incontinence. What may be some of the contributing factors for the anal incontinence? Select all that apply.
   a. The client has dementia.
   b. The client recently had a stroke.
   c. The client is very constipated.
   d. The client has a fecal impaction.
   e. The client has impaired mobility.
10. Pale, yellow, greasy, fatty stools may be seen in which of the following conditions?
    a. Upper gastrointestinal bleeding
    b. Iron ingestion
    c. Obstructive jaundice
    d. Celiac disease

UNIT

IV Special Populations

Chapter 24 The Pregnant Client, 784

Chapter 25 The Pediatric Client, 823

Chapter 26 The Older Adult Client, 889

The Pregnant Client

CHAPTER

24

Learning Outcomes

1. Identify the anatomical and physiological changes that occur in pregnancy.
2. Conduct a complete health history on a pregnant client.
3. Identify risk factors for pregnancy.
4. Perform a physical examination on a healthy pregnant client.
5. Differentiate normal clinical findings from a pregnant client's physical examination and the pathophysiology of abnormal clinical findings.
6. Identify the United States Preventive Services Task Force recommendations for the pregnant client.
7. Document a complete history and physical examination of a pregnant client.

Training is to teach nurses to know their business; that is, to observe exactly, to understand, to know, to do, to tell exactly, in such stupendous issues as life and death, health and disease.

Florence Nightingale

Pregnancy imposes many physiological, hormonal, and psychological changes on a person during the 280 days, or approximately 40 (normal range 37 to 42) weeks, of gestation. The pregnancy is subdivided into three trimesters of a little more than 13 weeks each, and various symptoms, problems, and client education can be specific to certain trimesters. You are encouraged to review Chapters 14 and 21 before beginning this chapter.

The focus when assessing a pregnant client is the wellness of the individual and the fetus. Much of prenatal care focuses on educating and reassuring the pregnant client and the family regarding physical changes that result from pregnancy. With the availability of accurate home pregnancy tests, an individual may know that they are pregnant within 2 weeks of conception. Ideally, nurses will provide preconception counseling, allowing early prenatal care, to ensure a healthy pregnancy. With active listening, a supportive attitude, and knowledge of evidence-based care, the nurse can play an important role in educating the family on what to expect during the prenatal and postpartum period, as well as educating the person and their families about warning signs of possible complications.

When complications arise or in the presence of certain risk factors, high-risk pregnancies may be managed in collaboration with a maternal-fetal medicine specialist.

Anatomy and Physiology

Physiological changes during pregnancy affect every system in the body. These changes occur to maintain maternal health and accommodate the growth of a healthy fetus. This chapter provides an overview of these changes and is not all-inclusive.

Skin and Hair

The skin is subjected to the influence of the hormones estrogen, progesterone, and melanocyte-stimulating hormone during pregnancy. There is an increased subdermal fat deposit, along with thickening of the skin. Acne may develop or improve during pregnancy. Other changes include an increase in sweat and sebaceous gland production, which, along with the increase in superficial capillaries and peripheral vasodilation, serves to dissipate heat by increasing perspiration. Existing pigmentation increases in the nipples, areolae, external genitalia, and anal region. The face may develop **melasma** (Fig. 24-1), known as the mask of pregnancy, which manifests as blotchy, irregular pigmentation. **Linea nigra**, or darkening of the linea alba, may present on the abdomen as a darkened vertical midline between the fundus and the symphysis pubis (Fig. 24-2). Linea nigra regresses, or fades, after delivery, but does not totally disappear. Nevi—circumscribed, pigmented areas of skin—may be stimulated to grow; and skin tags, molluscum fibrosum gravidarum, may develop from epithelial hyperplasia, especially on the upper body. With connective tissue changes of pregnancy, **striae gravidarum** (stretch marks) often develop on the abdomen, breasts, and upper thighs; after delivery, they regress or fade but do not totally disappear (Fig. 24-3).

Vascular changes reflected in the skin can include the development or enlargement of spider angiomas, hemangiomas, varicosities, and palmar erythema, which may become more pronounced as pregnancy progresses.

Facial hair may increase, but the scalp hair may shed and thin, especially in the postpartum period. The scalp hair may become oily.

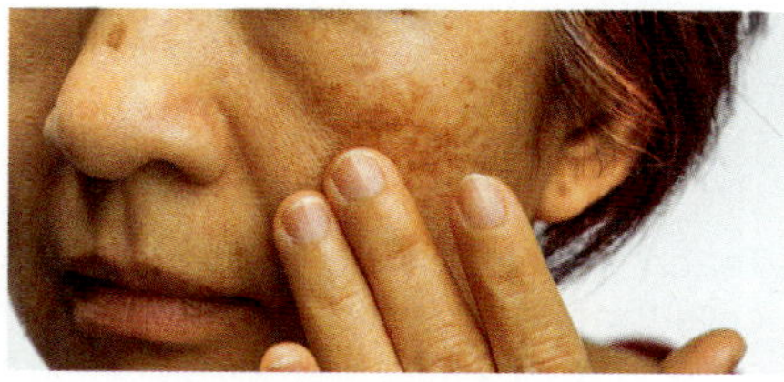

Figure 24-1 Melasma.

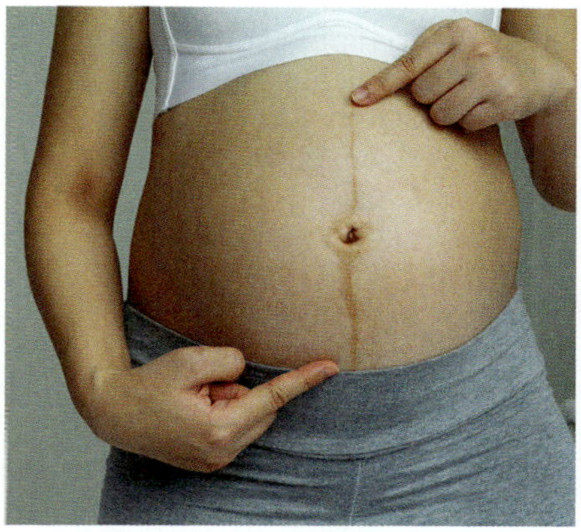

Figure 24-2 Linea nigra.

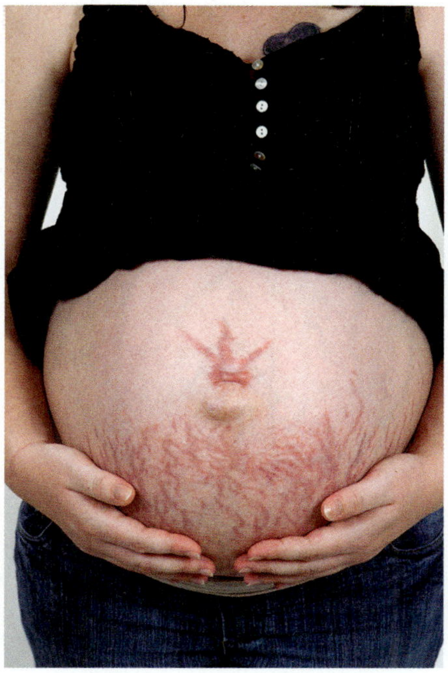

Figure 24-3 Striae gravidarum.

Head and Neck

The thyroid gland increases in size early in pregnancy and may be more prominent during physical examination. With the physiological changes to the thyroid, thyroid hormone production can be altered during pregnancy thus shifting thyroid test results.

> **NURSING TIP**
>
> **Pregnancy and Hair Treatments**
>
> Chemical hair treatments such as color and permanents are regarded by most experts as nontoxic during pregnancy. While a small amount of these chemicals can be absorbed through the scalp, there is limited research to demonstrate that these cause harm to the developing fetus. As a precaution, it can be recommended to avoid such chemicals during the first trimester, which is when the fetus is most susceptible to toxins. If hair treatments are performed while pregnant or breastfeeding, taking proper precautions such as appropriate use of products, proper hand hygiene, not eating/drinking while using products, and using in well-ventilated areas can reduce exposure to such chemicals.

Eyes, Ears, Nose, Mouth, and Throat

Corneal thickening and edema (especially in the third trimester) may occur, so the pregnant client may experience visual changes. Pregnant contact lens

> **NURSING TIP**
> **Breast Care During Pregnancy**
>
> Teach your clients to properly care for their breasts during pregnancy by:
>
> - Wearing a supportive bra that accommodates the breasts' changing size
> - Avoiding nipple stimulation, which may cause either leakage of colostrum, pain in already tender breasts, or premature contractions
> - Wearing nursing pads in the bra and air drying the breasts if colostrum leakage is significant

wearers may experience discomfort that they did not previously feel due to the changing curvature of the eye as well as shifts in the fluid levels of the eyes. These changes may be discussed with the client's ophthalmologist or optometrist, but pregnancy changes in vision are typically not treated because they are likely to resolve by 6 weeks postpartum.

Increased vascularity and increased mucus production often lead to nasal stuffiness, snoring, congestion and epistaxis, impaired hearing or fullness in the ears, and a decreased sense of smell. Nasal mucosa become more erythematous than oral mucosa and edematous. The pregnant client should be reassured that these are normal experiences that usually resolve after delivery.

Increased vascularity and hormonal changes often lead to soft, edematous, and bleeding gums, commonly noticed when brushing teeth. Epulis, or erythematous gingival nodules that bleed easily, may be present. **Ptyalism**, excessive secretion of saliva, may be an annoying symptom and, if noted, may require evaluation for other causes such as goiter. Vocal changes or cough may be noted due to hormonally induced changes in the larynx.

Breasts

Early breast changes may include enlargement, tingling, and tenderness secondary to hormonal changes. As the pregnancy progresses, the breasts continue to enlarge and may feel heavy as the mammary glands prepare for lactation after delivery (alveoli increase in both number and size, Montgomery tubercles enlarge, and lactiferous ducts proliferate). This may cause the breasts to feel more nodular on palpation than in the nonpregnant state. The areolae may darken. The nipples may become darker and more erect. **Colostrum**, a thick, often yellow discharge known as early breast milk, may be secreted as early as the second trimester. Veins in the breasts may become more apparent and blue as they become engorged from increased vascularization.

Thorax and Lungs

The demands of the physiological changes of pregnancy and the fetus lead to increased oxygen consumption and decreased carbon dioxide excretion. This helps to increase oxygen use by the fetus and facilitate the transfer of carbon dioxide from the fetus to the maternal circulation for elimination. With advancing pregnancy, the diaphragm elevates approximately 1⅝ inches (4 cm) and the movement of the diaphragm increases so that most respiratory effort is diaphragmatic. Stimulated by progesterone, the thoracic cage relaxes and expands by 2 to 3 inches (5 to 7 cm) in circumference to accommodate these increased respiratory demands, which may cause discomfort or pain as the intercostal muscles stretch. The tidal volume increases by 30% to 40% during pregnancy, probably due to the stimulatory effects of increased levels of progesterone. These physiological changes often lead to an increased respiratory rate, hyperventilation, or shortness of breath, especially on exertion such as climbing stairs.

Heart

In pregnancy, cardiac dilation occurs, reaching a maximum by 10 weeks gestation. The pregnant client's heart lies more horizontally and shifts upward and to the left along with the apical impulse. Heart rate increases by 10 to 20 beats per minute (bpm); a split first heart and S_3 sound may be heard, as well as a physiological systolic murmur of grade II/VI. In addition, especially near the end of the pregnancy, the increased breast vascularization may lead to a continuous murmur known as the "mammary souffle."

Peripheral Vasculature

Largely due to an increase in plasma, blood volume increases by 30% to 50% (more with multiple births), thus increasing cardiac output. This process begins at 12 weeks of gestation and peaks at 28 to 34 weeks. This increase protects the pregnant client from hemorrhage at delivery, increases oxygen transport, increases renal filtration, and dissipates fetal heat production.

The blood pressure varies according to position and trimester. Systolic pressure is not significantly different throughout pregnancy, whereas the diastolic pressure may lower by 5 mm Hg in the second trimester and then rise to first-trimester levels after midpregnancy. The lower blood pressure in the second trimester occurs as the body adjusts to the changes in the intravascular volume and to the hormonal effects on the vascular walls. Supine hypotension, resulting from the weight of the uterus on the inferior vena cava, is common. It is recommended that the pregnant client avoid a supine position starting at 20 weeks unless there is a uterine tilt to the side.

Monitoring of blood pressure during pregnancy is an important factor in determining complications such as preeclampsia. Many pregnant clients also experience dependent edema partially due to peripheral vasodilation and decreased vascular resistance. This swelling is most commonly seen in the feet, but may also occur in the hands and face. There is an increased stagnation of blood in the lower extremities, causing a tendency toward varicose vein formation in the legs, vulva, and rectum.

NURSING TIP

Avoiding Supine Hypotension and Lower Extremity Edema During Pregnancy

A side-lying position, with a pillow under the abdomen, behind the back, or between the legs, may provide the most comfort for the pregnant client (Fig. 24-4). Committed back sleepers may find comfort by placing a medium-sized pillow such as a body pillow underneath one side to displace uterine weight off the vena cava.

Edema may be especially noticeable after prolonged periods of sitting or standing in the pregnant client and may be minimized by increased rest on the left side to favor venous return, elevating the feet while sitting, and sitting for no longer than 1 hour at a time without walking.

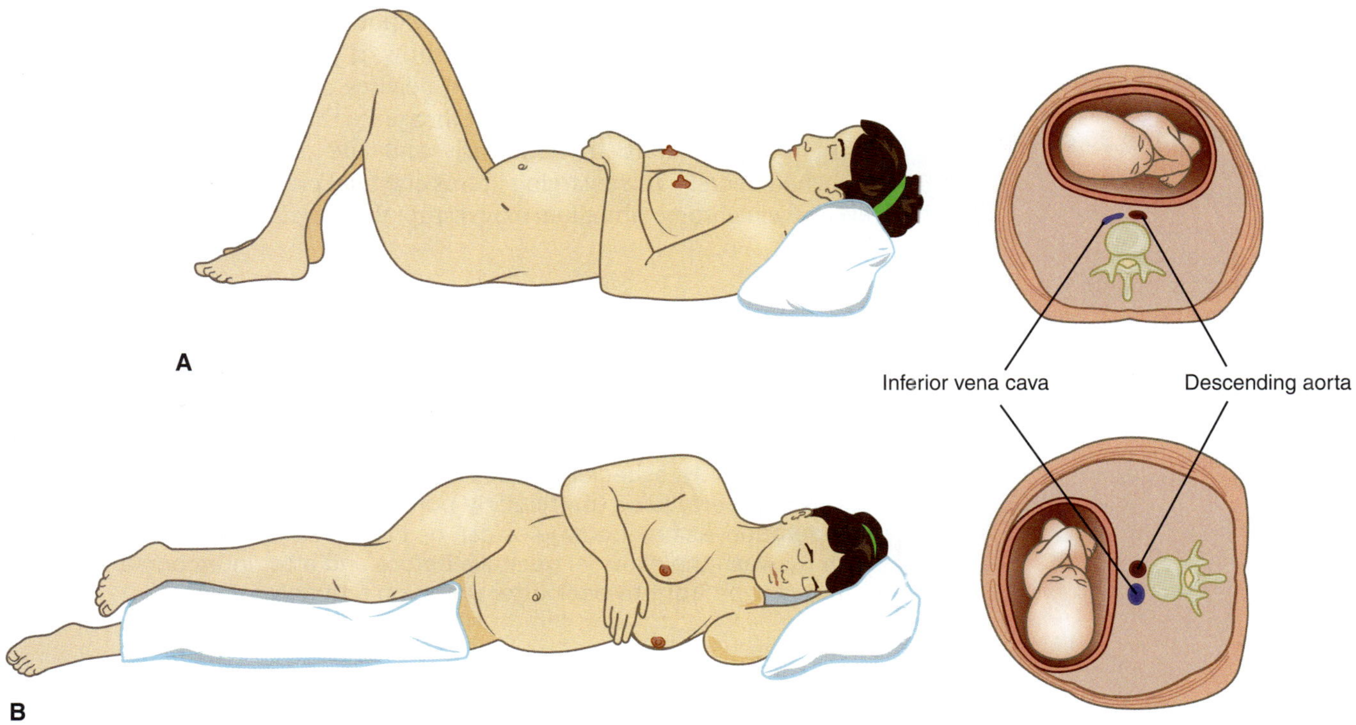

Figure 24-4 Effect of body position on the fetus in pregnancy. **A.** Supine hypotension can occur when the pregnant client is in the supine position. The weight of the gravid uterus may partially occlude the descending aorta and vena cava. **B.** Maintaining a lateral position alleviates compression on the descending aorta and vena cava.

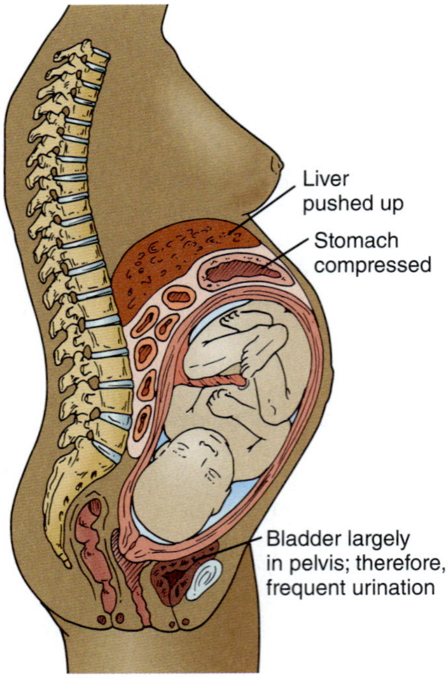

Figure 24-5 Crowding of abdominal contents by gravid uterus.

Abdomen

The growing uterus gradually displaces the abdominal contents, leading to decreased tone and motility, decreased bowel sounds, and an increased emptying time for the stomach and intestines (Fig. 24-5). These changes often bring about increased flatulence and constipation and can contribute to the development of hemorrhoids.

Indigestion and pyrosis (heartburn) are often experienced by the pregnant client due to the relaxation of the esophageal sphincter, subsequent reflux, and slowed gastric emptying. Bloating and constipation are also frequent complaints. Nausea and vomiting are common early in pregnancy and may even lead to weight loss in the first trimester. Peculiarities of taste and smell may aggravate abdominal discomfort.

Increased emptying time of the gallbladder and chemical changes in bile composition can put the pregnant client at increased risk for cholelithiasis, the presence or formation of bilestones or calculi in the gallbladder or duct. Hormonal levels of estrogen in pregnancy may augment any tendency to develop cholestasis (arrest of bile excretion), which is a complication of pregnancy that can lead to changes in prenatal care and delivery timing due to fetal risks.

Some pregnant clients will also experience a separation of the rectus muscle of the abdominal wall, known as **diastasis recti**, which may be asymptomatic and noticed only as a vertical protrusion midline. Diastasis recti requires no medical intervention during pregnancy. Postpartum, the pregnant client should be directed to be aware of proper core exercises, often with the assistance of a physical therapist, to ensure proper healing of the abdominal muscles.

NURSING TIP
Gastrointestinal Health During Pregnancy

Teach your pregnant clients to manage nausea, vomiting, constipation, and indigestion by:

- Eating several small, frequent meals
- Avoiding spicy and fatty foods and carbonated beverages
- Drinking 8 to 12 glasses of water a day (64 to 96 ounces)
- Increasing dietary fiber or supplemental fiber
- Exercising regularly
- Getting adequate rest
- Using antacids only in moderation and with health-care provider approval

Urinary System

Secondary to the increased intravascular volume, the glomerular filtration rate (GFR) increases by approximately 50%, and the reabsorption rate of various chemicals, especially sodium and water, changes. Urinary frequency usually increases in the first trimester.

Glycosuria, glucose in the urine, is common in pregnancy. There is also an increased loss of amino acids that may show as **proteinuria** on a urine dipstick. Dilation of the ureters and renal pelvises causing stasis, a decrease in bladder tone, and the short female urethra place the pregnant client at risk for urinary tract infections. In both early and late pregnancy, the bladder is encroached upon by the enlarging uterus and fetal presenting parts. **Nocturia**, or excessive nighttime urination, may disrupt the pregnant client's sleep pattern.

NURSING TIP
Maintaining Urinary Health During Pregnancy

Remind your pregnant clients to:

- Drink plenty of fluids, avoiding those with caffeine; 8 to 12 glasses of water (64 to 96 ounces) each day should be the minimum goal.
- Void frequently, especially after intercourse.
- Drink cranberry juice (particularly pure concentrated juice) but in moderation, as cranberry juice can be high in sugar content.
- Gently wash the external genitalia before and after intercourse.
- Always wipe front to back after urination and defecation.

Musculoskeletal System

The hormones relaxin and progesterone affect all joints in the pregnant client's body. This leads to a widening (and, occasionally, a separation) of the symphysis pubis at approximately 28 to 32 weeks, increased pelvic mobility to accommodate vaginal delivery, and an unsteady gait known as the "waddle of pregnancy." The pregnant client may experience pain over the symphysis pubis region as this widening occurs, which can create, at times, extreme discomfort upon movement and walking. These hormones also allow the thoracic cage to change shape, which can lead to concerns about upper back or rib pain.

Developing lordosis of the lumbar spine keeps the center of gravity over the legs and is often associated with lower back pain (Fig. 24-6). Sciatic nerve pain may also present as lower back pain, a shooting pain down the leg, or leg weakness. Late in pregnancy, aches in the neck, shoulders, and upper extremities occur because of shoulder slumping and anterior flexion of the neck accompanying lumbodorsal lordosis. For unknown reasons, muscle cramps, particularly in the calves, thighs, and buttocks, may develop, especially at night.

Shoe size may increase by as much as one full size as pregnancy progresses, due to edema and relaxation of foot joints. Fat deposits increase throughout the body and are most noticeable on the hips and buttocks.

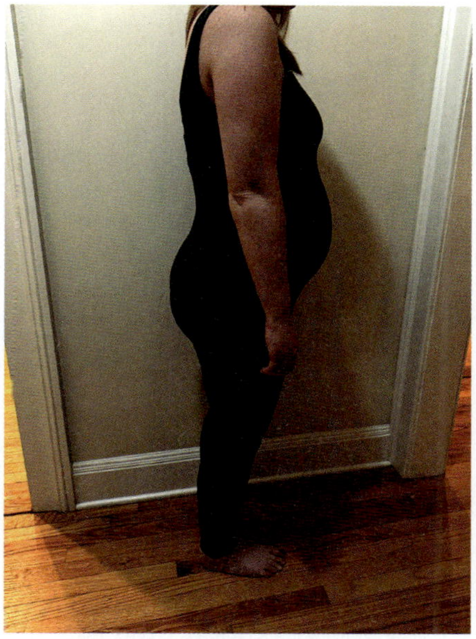

Figure 24-6 Lordosis in pregnancy.

NURSING TIP

Avoiding Muscle Cramps During Pregnancy

Encourage pregnant clients to:

- Practice proper muscle-stretching exercises.
- Wear low-heeled shoes.
- Consume adequate dietary calcium.
- Ensure proper hydration with water throughout the day (8 to 12 glasses or 64 to 96 ounces as a daily minimum).
- Avoid excessive milk intake (higher phosphorus content may cause muscle cramps).
- Take a calcium carbonate supplement if necessary and if approved by the health-care provider.

NURSING TIP

Center of Balance During Pregnancy

Warn the pregnant client regarding the vulnerability to falls and accidents because of the change in the center of balance. Pregnant clients should exercise caution when changing position, moving over uneven surfaces, ascending and descending stairs, and participating in activities such as riding a bicycle.

Neurological System

The most commonly experienced neurological changes of pregnancy include headaches, numbness, and tingling. The more bothersome neuropathies include carpal tunnel syndrome, footdrop, facial palsy, fatigue, and difficulty remaining asleep at night. After ruling out any underlying disorder, reassure the client that these are temporary symptoms. Headaches may be relieved by small, frequent meals; adequate rest; and posture and work environment adjustments. If headaches are persistent despite these comfort measures, clients should discuss this with their health-care provider. Seizure activity with no prior history may indicate the development of **eclampsia**, or new onset seizures associated with hypertensive disorders of pregnancy. Dizziness and lightheadedness may be due to the pressure of the fetus on the vena cava. Memory lapses are common, including decreased attention and concentration, but the etiology is poorly understood.

Female Genitalia

The pelvic organs experience vascular, hormonal, and structural changes during pregnancy. Uterine vessels dilate and at term can hold one-sixth of the maternal circulation, with a blood flow of 500 mL/min. With the increased blood flow, the pregnant client may note a feeling of pelvic congestion as well as vulvar edema. Amenorrhea, secondary to the hormonal changes of pregnancy, is generally the first noticeable sign.

The pregnant client's enlarging uterus begins as a pelvic organ; becoming palpably enlarged at 6 to 7 weeks (Fig. 24-7), as determined by bimanual examination, and progresses to become an abdominal organ at approximately 12 weeks of gestation. At 16 weeks the fundus of the uterus is midway

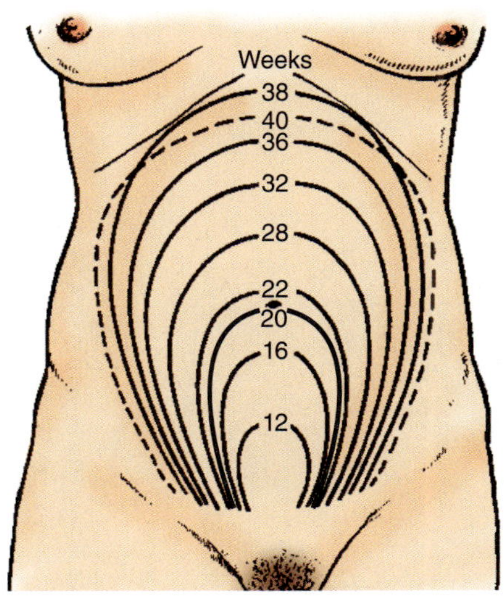

Figure 24-7 Uterine and abdominal enlargement of pregnancy.

> **NURSING TIP**
>
> **Avoiding Vaginal Yeast Infections During Pregnancy**
>
> Teach your clients good perineal care during pregnancy:
>
> - Avoid clothing that fits tightly in the pelvic region such as spandex and leggings.
> - Choose underwear made from cotton rather than other materials such as nylon, spandex, and silk.
> - Remove a wet bathing suit promptly.
> - Monitor sugar and simple carbohydrates in the diet, if prone to yeast infection.
> - Report recurrent yeast infections, which could suggest the possibility of glucose intolerance.

between the symphysis pubis and the umbilicus, and at 20 weeks the fundus is typically at the umbilicus or just above.

Between weeks 18 and 32 of gestation, the height of the uterine fundus above the symphysis pubis is measured in centimeters and is used to confirm the gestational age in weeks. After 32 weeks, although still used, this measurement is less accurate. This measurement can be affected by a full bladder, a person's habitus, the fetal position, and the amniotic fluid index. As such, this measurement should be used as just one part of the clinical assessment of a pregnant client's gestational age and growth.

The round and broad ligaments elongate to accommodate the growing fetus and may cause the client lower quadrant abdominal pain. **Lightening**, also called dropping, is a decrease in fundal height due to the descent of the presenting fetal part into the pelvis. This typically occurs approximately 3 weeks before the onset of labor in a nulliparous client and is often indicated by increased pressure in the pelvis and increased frequency of urination. In a multiparous client, lightening may not occur until after active labor begins. **Braxton Hicks contractions**, which are irregular and sometimes painless, may begin as early as the first trimester. Although Braxton Hicks contractions are often referred to as "practice contractions," these can be an uncomfortable experience for the pregnant client. Proper education as it relates to labor warning signs is important to help the client distinguish between Braxton Hicks contractions and true labor.

The cervix experiences increased vascularity and increased **friability**, or susceptibility to bleeding, especially following a pelvic examination or intercourse. Table 24-1 lists additional changes in the cervix and uterus in pregnancy. The endocervical glands increase in number and size. This causes a softening of the cervix. Mucus production occurs to form an endocervical protective plug, and the vaginal mucosa thickens secondary to hormonal changes. Throughout pregnancy, the vaginal discharge increases and is typically of a white, milky consistency. From 36 weeks on, vaginal discharge may become noticeably thicker and clumps may be present when the mucus plug is expelled. The hormonally induced changes in the vaginal environment lead to an increased risk of yeast infection.

Anus and Rectum

Decreased gastrointestinal tract tone and motility produce a sense of fullness, indigestion, constipation, bloating, and flatulence. The development of hemorrhoids is common and can become very problematic. As pregnancy progresses and the uterus enlarges, mechanical pressure may aggravate constipation and hemorrhoids. Vitamin and iron supplementation may increase these symptoms and commonly darken the stool.

Table 24-1 Changes in Pelvic Organs in Pregnancy

Name	Gestational Age	Description
Ladin sign	5–6 weeks	Softening of cervical-uterine junction
Goodell sign	6 weeks	Cervical softening
McDonald sign	7–8 weeks	Easy flexion of fundus on cervix
Chadwick sign	8 weeks	Cervical bluish hue
Hegar sign	8 weeks	Softening of uterine isthmus

Hematological System

Common hematological changes include increased white blood cell (WBC) count, increased total red blood cell (RBC) volume, increased plasma volume, decreased number and increased size of platelets, and increased fibrinogen and clotting factors VII through X. The relatively larger increase in plasma volume compared with RBC volume leads to physiological anemia during pregnancy. The coagulation changes protect against hemorrhage at birth but may also put the pregnant client at increased risk for thromboembolic conditions such as deep vein thrombosis (DVT).

Endocrine System

The basal metabolic rate (BMR) increases by 15% to 25% due to increased oxygen consumption and fetal metabolic demands. This can often lead to feelings of warmth and heat intolerance.

As pregnancy progresses, increased resistance to insulin develops and peaks in the late second to third trimester as the placenta grows. This is caused by human placental lactogen (hPL) and other diabetogenic hormones. This process occurs to ensure adequate amounts of glucose for fetal and placental demands. As a result of this phenomenon, gestational diabetes screening tests are used to rule out or diagnose gestational diabetes in all pregnancies. If a client experiences gestational diabetes during pregnancy, it dramatically increases the risk of developing type 2 diabetes later in life. Glycosuria may be noted because the distant renal tubules cannot respond to the increased amounts and duration of glucose in the circulatory system. The maternal immunological system is also less resistant to infection, due to a decreased cellular immune response.

NURSING TIP

Identifying Abuse in Pregnant Clients

Abusive relationships are much more common in our society, across all socioeconomic groups, than is generally believed, and abusive situations often intensify when a person announces a pregnancy. Suspect abuse if the pregnant client:

- Has a pattern of frequent visits, especially with vague complaints
- Presents with complaints inconsistent with a known injury (any unusual pattern of bruises on the head, neck, breasts, chest, abdomen, and genitalia)
- Frequently misses appointments
- Fails to plan appropriately for the baby's arrival
- Is always accompanied by an overly solicitous partner

HEALTH HISTORY

The pregnant client's health history provides insight into the link between a client's life/lifestyle and pregnancy-related information and pathology.

The health history of the pregnant client is generally taken in a way that is specific to pregnancy. This history intake may contain information on the client from a preconception visit through delivery, as well as on the newborn. The history covers the standard health history questions, any prior gynecological and obstetric history, genetic predispositions, current signs and symptoms (including those of pregnancy), any change in normal routine, initial prenatal visit physical examination, subsequent visits, and laboratory data. This comprehensive approach is essential for directing risk factor assessment and developing a plan of management. Table 24-2 illustrates a typical reproductive health history.

CLIENT PROFILE

Diseases that are age- and race-specific for pregnancy are listed.

Age Pregnant clients who are younger than age 16 or older than age 35 are at risk for various pregnancy complications such as hypertensive disorders, gestational diabetes, genetic disorders, multiple gestation, miscarriage, operative delivery, and preterm labor and/or delivery.

Race/Ethnicity

Black: sickle cell trait or disease, increased risk for hypertension, low birth weight, and preterm delivery

People of Asian, Asian Indian, or Mediterranean origin (Greece, Italy, Cyprus, Middle East): Thalassemias

Ashkenazi Jews: Tay-Sachs and Gaucher diseases

French Canadians (and possibly Cajuns): Tay-Sachs disease

Black, Hispanic, clients from Caribbean islands, Central/South America, Arabs, Egyptians, Asian Indians: Sickle cell disease/trait

White (Northern Europeans, Celtic populations), Ashkenazi Jewish clients: Cystic fibrosis

CHIEF COMPLAINT

The pregnant client may have a myriad of complaints as discussed throughout the chapter. The most common chief complaints have been discussed in previous chapters.

PAST HEALTH HISTORY

The various components of the past health history are linked to pregnancy pathology and pregnancy-related information. The health-care team must obtain a comprehensive health history of all pregnant clients. Below are some components that are additionally important when caring for the pregnant client.

Medical History Obtain a comprehensive medical history including past or present history of: asthma, diabetes mellitus, hepatitis, hospitalizations, cardiac disease, renal disease, seizure disorder, autoimmune disorders, bleeding disorders, hypertension, thyroid disorders, previous postpartum depression, psychiatric disorders

Surgical History Obtain a comprehensive surgical history including uterine surgery, cone or excisional biopsy of the cervix, abdominal surgery leading to internal or external scarring or adhesions (e.g., appendectomy)

Allergies Symptoms may change with pregnancy; it is best to review all current allergy medications to ensure compatibility with pregnancy. Ask about latex allergies or sensitivities.

Medications Certain medications for chronic conditions may be continued during pregnancy, such as methyldopa and hydralazine for hypertension. Other medications may be changed due to the teratogenic effect on the fetus; for example, warfarin (Coumadin) would be changed to heparin, and an oral diabetic agent may be changed to insulin. Medications for seizure disorders or psychiatric conditions should be discussed with the health-care provider in terms of risk-benefit ratio for both the client and the fetus, as well as any possible alternate medications for use preconceptually and during pregnancy. Some OTC medications such as acetaminophen are considered safe during pregnancy, but any pregnant (or possibly pregnant) client should consult a health-care provider before taking any medications, herbs, supplements, or homeopathic therapies. Obtain information regarding all medications, supplements, herbs, and homeopathic therapies being used by the pregnant client including during the preconception period.

Communicable Diseases

TORCH diseases (toxoplasmosis, rubella, cytomegalovirus, herpes), measles, varicella, mumps, human parvovirus B19, HIV, hepatitis B, hepatitis C.

A rubella titer, RPR or VDRL, and hepatitis B surface antigen are routinely drawn on pregnant clients. HIV testing is recommended using an "opt-out" on all pregnant clients. Many states are now requiring HIV testing on all pregnant clients; see your specific state guidelines.

Rubella (German measles), especially in the first trimester, and syphilis during pregnancy can cause anomalies and complications. Other infectious diseases may affect the pregnancy, depending on their severity and the gestational age at which the disease is contracted—e.g., varicella may present a problem to the fetus if active at the time of delivery. Other infectious diseases to review include tuberculosis and any history of sexually transmitted infections (STIs).

Injuries and Accidents Any trauma that leads to abdominal scarring, injury to the pelvic organs themselves, or injury to the musculoskeletal systems in the pelvic region (hips, pelvis, sacrum) may affect the pregnancy; injuries to the head and back may also be of concern.

Differing Abilities Disabilities and handicaps do not generally interfere with pregnancy; however, these are important in caring for the whole person. Some neuromuscular disorders such as myasthenia gravis may affect muscle response as pregnancy progresses and during labor. Paralysis does not interfere with pregnancy other than with regard to the client's decreased ability to note significant changes in physical status, e.g., change in vaginal discharge or increase in uterine contractions.

Access to language services and resources for the hearing impaired (such as American Sign Language [ASL] interpreters) is required by statute.

Childhood Illnesses Rheumatic heart disease, if mitral valve prolapse (MVP) develops, may put the client at risk for endocarditis with an extremely long or complicated labor or delivery and could require prophylactic antibiotics with delivery. Knowledge of childhood diseases leading to immunity may decrease anxiety if exposure to those illnesses occurs during pregnancy.

Immunization Vaccines that contain live-attenuated viruses are not recommended during pregnancy. Other types of vaccines that have inactive antigens or toxoids are considered safe in pregnancy and can be administered. Examples of vaccines that are considered safe and are recommended in pregnancy include the influenza, Tdap, and COVID-19 vaccines. Any unavoidable travel to an area with known infectious disease risk requires a discussion of the risk-benefit ratio of immunization. Immune status testing should be encouraged at any preconceptual visit. If the immune status is unknown or immune status testing reveals a lack of adequate titers, rubella and varicella immunizations should be given in the preconceptual period, along with instructions to avoid pregnancy for 3 months. If the client is already pregnant, rubella and varicella vaccinations should be deferred until postpartum.

FAMILY HEALTH HISTORY

Familial pregnancy-related conditions and diseases are listed.

Preterm labor or delivery; hypertensive disorders of pregnancy; diethylstilbestrol (DES) exposure; multiple births in female relatives of the client's mother; chromosome abnormalities such as Down syndrome; genetic disorders such as Tay-Sachs, Gaucher diseases, or sickle cell disease; inheritable diseases such as Huntington chorea; congenital anomalies such as cleft lip or palate; neural tube defects; cardiac deformities; blood disorders; diabetes (gestational, type 1 diabetes, type 2 diabetes); neuromuscular diseases; psychiatric disorders; any history of abuse, neglect, or substance abuse; preeclampsia or eclampsia; cause of death for deceased parents or siblings

Family history of the biological partner: genetic, hereditary, or chromosomal disorders, abuse or neglect, substance abuse

SOCIAL HISTORY

The components of the social history are linked to pregnancy factors and pathology.

Alcohol Use Alcohol use can lead to fetal alcohol syndrome (FAS). The absolute safe level of alcohol consumption is unknown. Problems have been documented with more than 2 oz of alcohol per day and with binge drinking.

Tobacco Use Smoking can lead to low-birth-weight infants, preterm labor, spontaneous abortions, and lower Apgar scores (refer to Chapter 25). The effects are dose-related, and tobacco use during pregnancy should be discontinued. Referral to a smoking cessation program may be beneficial. With a history of smoking or secondary smoke exposure, status should be checked frequently throughout pregnancy. These same precautions apply to any tobacco product, e-cigarettes, and vaping.

Recreational Drug Use Drug effects on the fetus vary according to the drug(s) used and the gestational age at time of use. The most common complications are spontaneous abortion, preterm delivery, congenital anomalies, and stillbirth. Some illicit drug use can lead to neonatal abstinence syndrome (NAS), a spectrum of withdrawal symptoms, requiring treatment of the newborn by the pediatric team upon birth. Cocaine use is associated with a higher incidence of placental and cord accidents and preterm delivery. Marijuana is often reported and asked about among clientele as this is medically legal and recreational in many areas. As data are limited on the safety of marijuana use in pregnancy, it is advised to discontinue its use, even medicinally, during pregnancy and lactation.

Sexual Practice Sexual expression or practice throughout pregnancy is not contraindicated unless there are high-risk restrictions. Sexual intercourse should be avoided after the membranes have ruptured. The pregnant client should be encouraged to maintain safe sex practices for the prevention of STIs.

Travel History Ask about travel outside the United States or to regions at risk for infectious diseases. Travel more than 1½ hours from home during the last month of pregnancy should be avoided. Air travel should be taken only in pressurized cabins. Pregnant clients should move about every hour, drink plenty of liquids, and travel with enough food for small, frequent meals or snacks.

Work Environment Prolonged sitting or standing; heavy lifting; an extremely loud, cold, or wet environment; work with chemicals (e.g., lead or mercury); or a one-way commute greater than 1 hour may put the pregnant client at risk for preterm labor or congenital anomalies in the newborn.

Home Environment Stairs may make domestic chores even more difficult for the pregnant client. The pregnant client should avoid toxic chemicals; exposure to toxoplasmosis should be avoided by not cleaning cat litter boxes and by wearing gloves and washing hands after gardening. Household chores should be avoided if they either lead to excessive contractions or aggravate pregnancy discomforts.

Hobbies and Leisure Activities May be continued during the pregnancy unless they present a physical risk (such as certain high-risk sports, including skiing and horseback riding).

Stress The client's perception of more stress in life than can be comfortably coped with should be addressed by practicing relaxation techniques, seeking counseling if needed, and using family and social support systems. Excessive stress may be a risk factor for preterm labor and low-birth-weight infants.

HEALTH MAINTENANCE ACTIVITIES

This information provides a bridge between health maintenance activities and pregnancy.

Sleep Increased demand, complicated frequently by nocturia, active fetus, or difficulty in finding and maintaining a comfortable position

Diet All meats should be well cooked, and all dairy products should be pasteurized to prevent infections such as toxoplasmosis and listeria. Identify type of vegetarianism if practiced. Avoid fish with high mercury levels. Avoid raw eggs to prevent possible salmonella contamination.

Exercise Normal activities may be continued and exercise may help with some of the common complaints such as constipation. Exercise done in moderation is beneficial, but any exercise should be discontinued or modified if pain occurs; intensity and duration may have to be decreased from prepregnancy exercise levels (e.g., heart rate should not exceed 150 bpm or moderate levels of perceived exertion). Low birth weight is associated with prolonged, strenuous activities in pregnancy. Care should be taken to avoid overheating, especially in humid weather, and water intake should be increased as needed. Physically dangerous exercises, such as waterskiing, downhill skiing, horseback riding, and scuba diving, should be discontinued. Activities requiring balance and coordination, such as surfing and mountain climbing, may have to be discontinued.

Use of Safety Devices Seat belts are recommended, with the lap portion worn below the pregnant abdomen and across the upper thighs. The shoulder belt should be positioned snugly between the breasts. The steering wheel should be positioned 10 inches from the sternum to prevent airbag trauma to the growing uterus.

Health Checkups Gynecological evaluations; avoid X-rays

NURSING TIP

Drug Safety Categories in Pregnancy

Previously, the Food and Drug Administration (FDA) classified drugs into safety categories using a lettering system (A, B, C, D, and X), which indicated their level of safety for the fetus. However, this system did not elaborate on what is known about the safety of these drugs on the human fetus. In 2015, the FDA replaced the categorical labeling system with the Pregnancy/Lactation Labeling Rule (PLLR). This required three components of drug safety: (1) pregnancy, (2) lactation, and (3) females and males of reproductive potential. Each category is required to have subsections according to the area they are referring to (pregnancy: fetal risk summary, clinical considerations, background data; lactation: risk summary, clinical considerations, background data; female/males of reproductive potential: risks, clinical considerations). This new labeling system allows for a more comprehensive review of drug safety based on the available evidence.

NURSING TIP

Obstetric Abbreviations

Pregnant clients can be classified according to their obstetric outcomes by using the TPAL acronym. In the past, the terms *Gravida* and *Para* referred to a client's pregnancies rather than to the fetus, thus failing to identify one pregnancy resulting in a twin delivery or fetal loss. At the first prenatal visit, many facilities use a more comprehensive detailed approach to document obstetric history, the TPAL. Gravida (**G**) keeps the same meaning (any pregnancy, regardless of duration, including present pregnancy) and Para (**P**) is described using the acronym **TPAL**.

T Number of TERM infants born: number of infants born at 37 weeks gestation or greater.
P Number of PRETERM infants born: number of infants born at 20 weeks 0 days to 36 weeks 6 days gestation; whether viable or nonviable, living, or stillborn.
A Number of pregnancies ending in either spontaneous or induced ABORTION.
L Number of current LIVING children to whom the client has given birth.

Examples

Francesca Akol Sanchez is pregnant for the fourth time. Francesca has a child who was born at term. A second pregnancy ended at 12 weeks gestation. Francesca then gave birth to twins at 34 weeks. One of the twins died soon after birth. Using the TPAL approach, the obstetric history would be recorded as: Gravida 4 Para 1212.

Maria Domestici is a Gravida 2 Para 2002. Maria delivered two full-term infants, both of whom are currently alive, and had no preterm births or abortions.

Sunny Oh is a Gravida 6 who delivered one full-term live birth, one full-term stillbirth, one premature live birth, and premature triplets of whom two lived and one died. Sunny has had two abortions. This would be recorded as Gravida 6 Para 2424.

Table 24-2 Reproductive History

Reproductive History	Obstetric History

• Menstrual history: menarche, cycle frequency, cycle duration; first day of last menstrual period (LMP),
• Sexual history (sexarche, number of partners, sex with male/female/both, history of rape and sexual abuse, history of STIs)
• Health history since LMP (e.g., fever, rashes, disease exposure, abnormal bleeding, nausea and vomiting, medication use, toxic exposure)
• Signs and symptoms of pregnancy
• Use of fertility drugs
• Contraception (current and past use)
• Genetic predispositions
• Gynecology history including information about past Pap smears
• Estimated date of delivery (EDD) or estimated date of confinement (EDC)*
	• Gravidity/gravida (number of pregnancies). Often represented as "G"
	  • Parity/para (TPAL system). Often represented as "P"
	  • Detailed information about each pregnancy including date, outcome, duration of weeks in pregnancy, type of delivery, length of labor (if applicable), medications and anesthesia used, complications during pregnancy/labor/delivery/postpartum, infant weight/sex/Apgar scores (if applicable), type of feeding (specifics for breastfeeding include length of time or difficulties/complications)
	  • High-risk factors for pregnancy (see Table 24-3)

*Use Naegele rule to determine EDD: subtract 3 months from the first day of the LMP, then add 7 days. Naegele rule is based on a 28-day cycle and may have to be adjusted for shorter or longer cycles. For example, if the LMP is September 1: 09/01 - 3 months = 06/01 + 7 days = 06/08; the EDD for this client is June 8.

A pregnancy wheel may also be used (Fig. 24-8). While Naegele rule and pregnancy wheels have long been used in estimating clinical dates during pregnancy, electronic calculators (via apps, integrated into electronic health records, etc.) are now favored to remove the possibility of human error.

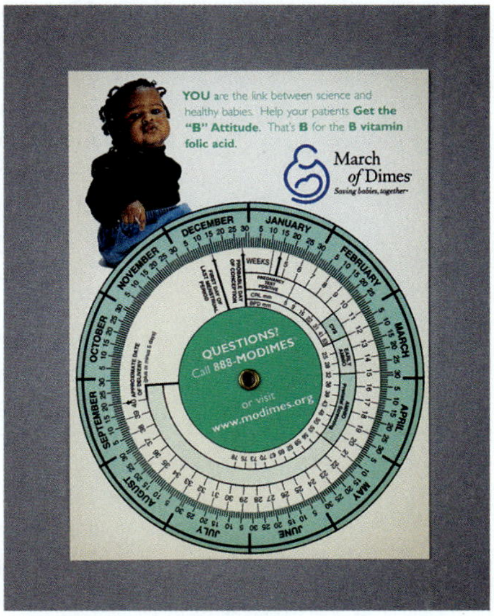

Figure 24-8 Gestation calculation wheel used to determine EDD. "First day of LMP" arrow is placed on that date. The other arrow, labeled "expected delivery date," shows the expected date of delivery.

Table 24-3 High-Risk Factors for Pregnancy

Many risk factor tools and scoring systems are available, and they have varying degrees of sensitivity and specificity. Some prenatal risk screenings are obtained during the health history intake.

Risk Factors	Considerations
Maternal factors	• Age less than 16 or older than 35 • Unplanned pregnancy or conflict about pregnancy (or both) • Without a partner (single) • Living at high altitude • Less than 1 year since previous birth • Abusive relationship and other violence or family stressors • Below the federal poverty level • Low educational level • Long working hours/commute/trips • Stress or unusual anxiety (or both) • Height less than 5 ft • Body mass index (BMI) less than 18.5 kg/m^2 or greater than 30 kg/m^2 • Inadequate diet • Smoking, excessive caffeine intake (more than 6 cups of caffeinated beverage per day), alcohol consumption, drug addiction
Medical conditions	• Hypertension • Renal disease, pyelonephritis, asymptomatic bacteriuria • Diabetes mellitus • Heart disease • Pulmonary disease • Sickle cell disease • Anemia • Neurological disorder • Autoimmune disorder • Hematological disorder • Gastrointestinal disorder • Endocrine disorder • Cancer
Reproductive history	• More than one prior abortion (some risk tools differentiate first and second trimester) • Uterine anomaly • Molar pregnancy/hydatidiform mole • Myomas (leiomyomas) • Sexually transmitted infections • Perinatal death • Preterm labor or delivery or both • Delivery of infant less than 2,500 g • Delivery of infant greater than 4,000 g • Delivery of infant with congenital or perinatal disease • Delivery of infant with isoimmunization or ABO incompatibility • Gestational diabetes • Operative delivery • Diethylstilbestrol (DES) exposure • Cervical incompetence • Prior cerclage
Present pregnancy	• Late/inadequate/no prenatal care • Low/excessive weight gain • Abdominal surgery • Bleeding • Previous cesarean section • Placenta previa • Premature rupture of membranes • Anemia • Hypertension • Preeclampsia/eclampsia

Table 24-3 High-Risk Factors for Pregnancy—cont'd

Risk Factors	Considerations
	• Hydramnios • Multiple gestations • Abnormal glucose screen • Rh-negative sensitization • Teratogenic exposure • Viral infections (especially fever-rash with first trimester) • Sexually transmitted infections • Bacterial infections • Protozoal infections • Abnormal fetal presentations at approximately 36 weeks • Postdates

NURSING TIP

Gestational Age at Birth

When determining the parity with TPAL on a pregnant client, the terminology for preterm and term is broad. However, there are definitions specific to weeks' gestation of pregnancy. These definitions have been correlated to neonatal outcomes and are relevant to the historical information of the pregnant client.

Gestational Age	Definition
<32 weeks	Very preterm
32 weeks 0 days – 33 weeks 6 days	Moderately preterm
34 weeks 0 days – 36 weeks 6 days	Late preterm
37 weeks 0 days – 38 weeks 6 days	Early term
39 weeks 0 days – 40 weeks 6 days	Full term
41 weeks 0 days – 41 weeks 6 days	Late term
>42 weeks	Post term

NURSING CHECKLIST

General Approach to Examination of the Pregnant Client

1. Observe standard precautions and don personal protective equipment (PPE) such as gloves, gown, face shield, goggles, N-95 respirator mask or face mask if the client's status warrants these protective measures.
2. Greet the client and explain how the examination will proceed.
3. Ensure that the examination room is ready, and supplies are at hand. Ensure that the examination room is at a warm, comfortable temperature to prevent the client from chilling and shivering.
4. Use a quiet room that will be free from interruptions.
5. Ensure that there is adequate lighting, including a light that is appropriate for the pelvic examination.
6. Before the physical examination, complete the health history and the nutritional and psychosocial assessments. (This is usually done in an office before proceeding to the examination room.)
7. Ask the client to void before the examination, both for client comfort and to facilitate uterine and adnexal evaluation (which can be impeded by a full bladder). The urine should be saved and evaluated based on institutional guidelines.
8. For the physical examination, instruct the client to remove all street clothes, don an examination gown, and cover the lap with a drape or sheet.
9. Perform the initial examination in a head-to-toe manner. Try to minimize the client's time in the supine position—ask questions later. Assist the client in assuming the lithotomy position via verbal guidance and by assisting in placing the feet in the foot or leg pedals (stirrups) if the client desires to use them. Always inform the client before touching them of what you will be doing and what to expect ("you will feel my hand on your thigh," "you may feel some pressure," and so on). Special sensitivity should be considered for the first pelvic examination, if a history of sexual assault exists, and with the LGBTQIA+ populations. The client may be dizzy upon sitting up or upon standing. It may be beneficial to assist the client to a sitting position. The client should be cautioned not to stand or sit up abruptly.

Assessment in Brief

Examination of the Pregnant Client*

*Only pregnancy-specific examinations are listed. All other examination skills are performed as described in Chapters 9–23.

Fundal Height

- Measure in centimeters using a tape measure

Fetal Heart Tone

- Fetal Doppler
- Fetoscope
- Ultrasound

Leopold Maneuvers

- First maneuver
- Second maneuver
- Third maneuver
- Fourth maneuver

Equipment

- Appropriate PPE
- Stethoscope
- Doppler or **fetoscope**
- Centimeter tape measure
- Watch or smartphone with a second hand
- Nonsterile gloves
- Speculum
- Genital culture supplies
- Pap smear supplies (see Chapter 21)
- Sphygmomanometer
- Urine cup
- Urine dipsticks

Examination of the Pregnant Client

Assessment of the pregnant client includes a complete initial examination as well as subsequent specific follow-up prenatal visits. The initial examination is done when the pregnant client first seeks care. Encourage clients to seek prenatal care in the first trimester or as soon as pregnancy is suspected. Optimally, this should be preceded by a visit with the health-care provider to assess health status before conception. This is especially important for clients with preexisting medical conditions such as diabetes mellitus, cardiac disease, or seizure disorders. The American College of Obstetricians and Gynecologists (ACOG) recommends the following schedule for prenatal visits: every 4 weeks for weeks 6 to 28 of gestation, every 2 weeks for weeks 28 to 36 of gestation, and weekly from 36 weeks until delivery. Clients going beyond the 40th week of gestation require additional evaluations. The following examination guidelines discuss how each system examination is different for the pregnant client than for the nonpregnant client. See the previous chapters for the specific examination of each system. The goal of the examination is not only to confirm pregnancy and gestational age but also to evaluate general health so any needed intervention can be provided and to educate the client to maintain and promote their own health as well as that of the fetus. See Table 24-4 for signs and symptoms of pregnancy. In addition, prenatal care provides guidance for the labor and delivery process and can be viewed as the foundation for a healthy family.

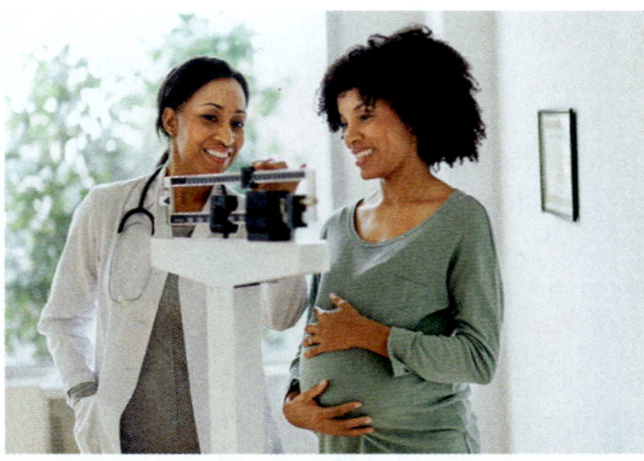

Figure 24-9 The client's weight is determined at each prenatal visit.

General Assessment, Vital Signs, Height, and Weight

E

1. Conduct a general assessment, including obtaining vital signs.
2. Obtain the client's height and weight (Fig. 24-9).
3. Calculate the client's BMI.

Table 24-4 Signs and Symptoms of Pregnancy

Presumptive*	Probable†	Positive‡
Amenorrhea	Abdominal enlargement	Fetal heartbeats
Breast tenderness and enlargement	Uterine changes	Fetal movement
Fatigue	Cervical changes	Fetal outline
Changes in skin pigmentation	Braxton Hicks contractions	Ultrasound
Nausea, vomiting, or both	Ballottement	
Urinary frequency	Chloasma	
Quickening	Hegar sign Chadwick sign Goodell sign Positive pregnancy test–HCG in blood or urine	

***Presumptive:** Maternal physiological changes that are associated with pregnancy but are not conclusive.
†**Probable:** Signs or symptoms that are more indicative of pregnancy, including maternal physiological symptoms and anatomical examination changes.
‡**Positive:** Signs or symptoms that are directly attributable to a fetus and confirm a definite pregnancy by the examiner.

N **See Chapter 9 for normal general assessment and the Anatomy and Physiology section of this chapter for blood pressure changes that occur in pregnancy. See Chapter 7 for the recommended weight gain in pregnancy. See Table 24-5 for common complaints of pregnancy.**

A Hypertension at any time in pregnancy is considered abnormal. In pregnancy, hypertension is defined as a systolic pressure greater than 140 and a diastolic pressure greater than 90. This is assessed by taking the blood pressure twice, at least 4 hours apart. If a prepregnancy blood pressure is unknown, the greater than 140/90 criterion is used. Hypertension noted before 20 weeks is most likely chronic hypertension. After 20 weeks, blood pressure elevation is related to hypertensive disorders of pregnancy. See Table 24-6 for additional information on hypertensive disorders during pregnancy.

P The pathophysiology of hypertensive disorders of pregnancy is still being researched. It is widely thought that vasospasms occurring throughout the vasculature contribute.

A A weight gain that is more than the recommended amount is abnormal.

P Excessive weight gain may be due to increased caloric intake, gestational diabetes, multiple pregnancies, polyhydramnios, and edema secondary to hypertension.

A A weight gain that is less than or more than the Institute of Medicine's recommendations (2009) is abnormal.

P Weight loss or insufficient weight gain in pregnancy can be due to hyperemesis gravidarum, decreased caloric intake, and malabsorption syndromes.

NURSING TIP

Differentiating Hypertensive Disorders of Pregnancy From Chronic Hypertension

Retinal examination may help in differentiating chronic hypertension from hypertensive disorders of pregnancy. With chronic hypertension, hemorrhage, exudates, angiosclerosis, and vascular tortuosity may be noted, whereas with hypertensive disorders of pregnancy, arterial constriction may be the only finding.

Table 24-5 Common Complaints in Pregnancy

Complaint	Relief Measures
Backache, sciatic pain, femoral nerve pain	For posture, stand with abdomen pulled in and buttocks tucked in. Do cat-arch exercises and stretching exercises for legs, gluteal muscles, and back. Avoid bending at waist—bend at knees to pick up objects from floor. If available, attend pregnancy exercise class or program. Many pregnancy exercises and stretches can be found on the Internet if classes are not available. Wear flat, comfortable shoes. A maternity or pregnancy support belt can be helpful, as can local heat and massage.
Bleeding gums	Maintain good dental hygiene. Use a soft toothbrush.
Breast soreness, tenderness, or tingling	A well-fitting, supportive brassiere, worn as much as 24 hr a day.
Constipation	High-fiber diet and 8 to 12 glasses (64 to 96 ounces) of water a day plus exercise.
Difficulty sleeping	Pillows for support, between legs, under abdomen, and under shoulders. Exercise, a warm bath before bed. Avoid caffeine. Go to bed at the same time every night.
Dizziness	Avoid sudden position changes or prolonged standing, especially in heat or a closed room. Eat small meals or snacks frequently. Ensure adequate hydration throughout the day.
Edema	Left lateral position for rest. Plenty of fluids.
Fatigue	Increased rest and relaxation, which may necessitate a different division of duties at home or work and prioritization of projects and chores.
Headache	Frequent meals and increased rest. If severe, further evaluation is required.
Heartburn	Small, frequent meals; avoid foods that aggravate heartburn, for example, spicy or fatty foods, carbonated drinks. If severe, further evaluation is required.
Hemorrhoids	Avoid constipation. Local treatment with a witch hazel-type product may reduce burning and itching, at least temporarily. Rest in left lateral position.
Increased vaginal discharge	It is acceptable to wash more often with plain tepid water, or mild, nonirritating, unscented soap and water. Always avoid douching. Panty liners may be necessary but can also cause vaginal irritation or itching. Vaginal odor, itching, or unusual discharge needs to be investigated. Report any episode of bleeding.
Leg cramps	Make sure dietary calcium is sufficient (dairy products, dark, leafy vegetables); there can even be an excess of milk intake (calcium in the form of phosphate); calcium carbonate supplement may be indicated (as well as for cases of lactose intolerance). Stretching exercises, flexing calf muscle; avoid hyperextending calf muscle.
Lapses or changes in memory	Lists! A sense of humor. Explain to family, friends, and coworkers that short-term memory is frequently affected by pregnancy. Store items like keys in the same place. Develop the habit of mentally checking for needed items (cell phone, wallet, and grocery list) before leaving the house.
Loss of balance	Flat shoes. Avoid activities where loss of balance could present a serious problem (e.g., bicycle riding). Use caution when changing position.
Pelvic or abdominal discomfort or pressure	After ruling out a complication, increased rest, leg elevation, and maternity support devices may be beneficial.
Nausea or vomiting, or both	Small, frequent meals. Avoid foods that trigger nausea. A protein snack at bedtime or crackers before getting up in the morning can help. If severe nausea and vomiting is associated with weight loss, or if they persist past the first trimester, additional measures may need to be initiated. Avoid smoking and alcohol.

Table 24-5 Common Complaints in Pregnancy—cont'd

Complaint	Relief Measures
Shortness of breath	Extra pillows under head, shoulders, or upper back may help relieve pressure on the diaphragm, especially late in pregnancy.
Sweating/acne/melasma/ptyalism	Dress in layers. Fans may help at home or desk. Maintain hygiene, but avoid overcleaning, especially face so as not to irritate skin. Avoid prolonged sun exposure. Wear sunscreen when outside.
Urinary changes (increased frequency, urinary incontinence)	Maintain fluid intake. Arrange work and errands to allow for restroom breaks or stops. Dysuria or abnormal discharge warrants further evaluation.
Stuffy nose	Avoid allergens (e.g., cats, sleeping with window open) when possible. Saline nasal products may be helpful.
Varicose veins	Left lateral position for rest. Frequent movement of legs if work requires prolonged standing or sitting. Support hose or even antiembolism-type hose may be necessary.

Table 24-6 Hypertensive Disorders of Pregnancy

Hypertensive Disorder	Onset of Hypertension	Diagnostic Criteria
Gestational hypertension	≥ 20 weeks gestation of pregnancy or within the first 24 hr postpartum	Systolic blood pressure ≥ 140 mm Hg and/or diastolic blood pressure ≥ 90 mm Hg on 2 separate occasions 4 or more hours apart in the absence of proteinuria or other signs of preeclampsia (Jones, et al 2025).
Preeclampsia	≥ 20 weeks gestation of pregnancy	Systolic blood pressure ≥140 mm Hg and/or a diastolic blood pressure ≥ 90 mm Hg on 2 separate occasions 4 hours apart in a woman ≥ 20 weeks gestation with previously normal blood pressure. OR Systolic blood pressure ≥160 mm Hg or diastolic blood pressure ≥ 110 mm Hg confirmed in 15 minutes *AND one of the following:* • Proteinuria: ≥ 300 mg of protein on a 24-hr urine collection • Protein/creatinine ratio of ≥ 0.3 • Urine dipstick reading ≥ 2+ protein *OR any of the following** • Platelet count < 100,000 µL • Renal insufficiency characterized by a serum creatinine level > 1.1 mg/dL or 2X baseline serum creatinine level

Continued

Table 24-6 Hypertensive Disorders of Pregnancy—cont'd

Hypertensive Disorder	Onset of Hypertension	Diagnostic Criteria
		• Impaired liver functions characterized by elevated liver transaminases (ALT, AST) to twice the normal level • Pulmonary edema • New onset headache unresponsive to medications not related to an alternative diagnosis OR visual symptoms (Jones, et al 2025).
Hemolysis, Elevated Liver Enzymes, Low Platelets (HELLP) Syndrome	≥ 20 weeks gestation of pregnancy	A severe form of preeclampsia diagnosed by: LDH elevated to 600 IU/L or more AST and ALT elevated more than twice the upper limits of normal Platelet count less than 100,000 μL Most common complaints include right upper quadrant pain, generalized malaise, and nausea and vomiting
Eclampsia	After or with the onset of preeclampsia	Preeclampsia plus the new onset of seizures in the absence of other diagnoses or conditions
Chronic hypertension	Prior to pregnancy or < 20 weeks gestation of pregnancy	In absence of pre-pregnancy blood pressure values, the parameters of systolic blood pressure of 140 mm Hg or greater or a diastolic blood pressure of 90 mm Hg or greater are used
Chronic hypertension with superimposed preeclampsia (with or without severe features)	Prior to pregnancy or < 20 weeks gestation of pregnancy	A diagnosis of chronic hypertension with the manifestations of preeclampsia as listed above

*Proteinuria is not required for the diagnosis of preeclampsia (with or without severe features) if the client exhibits blood pressure criteria and one (or more) additional severe feature as listed above.

Adapted from Jones, D.W., Ferdinand, K.C., Taler, S.J., Johnson, H.M.et al. (2025**).** 2025 AHA/ACC/AANP/AAPA/ABC/ACCP/ACPM/AGS/AMA/ASPC/NMA/PCNA/SGIM Guideline for the Prevention, Detection, Evaluation and Management of High Blood Pressure in Adults: A Report of the American College of Cardiology/American Heart Association Joint Committee on Clinical Practice Guidelines. *Hypertension.* August 14, 2025. doi:10.1161/HYP.0000000000000249.

Skin and Hair

E N **See Chapter 10 and the Anatomy and Physiology section of this chapter.**

A Atopic eruptions of pregnancy are dermatoses generally characterized by intense pruritis (itching) which can include eczema, prurigo, and pruritic folliculitis. These lesions are generally papular involving the face, neck, bends of elbows and knees, trunk, abdomen, and hands and feet. These lesions most commonly appear in the first or second trimester but can occur at any point and generally resolve in the postpartum period.

P Etiology is poorly understood but is likely related to hormonal changes that impact the integumentary system during pregnancy. Atopic eruptions of pregnancy have no known adverse effects on maternal or fetal outcomes. These can be safely treated with topical corticosteroids, moisturizers, and lukewarm showers with mild soap.

A Polymorphic eruptions in pregnancy (PEP), also known as pruritic urticarial papules and plaques of pregnancy (PUPP), is a common skin condition seen in the third trimester and generally resolves spontaneously. The rash is characterized by red, painfully pruritic urticarial papules most commonly seen on the trunk, abdomen, and extremities.

P The pathophysiology of PEP/PUPP is likely related to the excessive stretching of skin leading to tissue damage in combination with high levels of estrogen and progesterone during pregnancy. While PEP or PUPPs can be very uncomfortable for the pregnant client, there are no known adverse effects on maternal or fetal outcomes. These conditions can be treated with topical steroids and antihistamines. In rarely severe cases, systemic corticosteroids can be considered.

A Erythematous plaques that develop into vesicular lesions that may become pustular are abnormal.

P Primary herpes (see Chapter 10) contracted in the first trimester places the fetus at risk for abnormalities, as it is more virulent and likely to cross the placental barrier during that time. Recurrent genital herpes lesions contain fewer viral particles and carry less severe outcomes throughout the pregnancy. At the time of delivery, if lesions are present in the genital area, vaginal delivery is contraindicated due to the potential for severe complications for the newborn should they develop a viral infection associated with the maternal outbreak. Therefore, cesarean delivery is recommended in the presence of a maternal outbreak at the time of delivery.

A Rashes are generally abnormal and should be further investigated.

P Rashes should be evaluated for infectious, collagen, or other disease etiologies as described in Chapter 10.

A Pallor and bronze/yellow skin color, as well as petechiae, ecchymoses, and bruising, are abnormal, and their etiology in the pregnant client should be established.

P Refer to Chapter 10.

A Edema is often observed, especially in the mid to late third trimester.

P Edema in pregnancy is often related to impaired venous circulation and increased venous pressure as a result of the enlarging uterus in addition to hormonal effects on maternal circulation. Previously, edema was a factor indicative of preeclampsia. While edema is no longer a part of the diagnostic criteria, it should be assessed and clinically correlated appropriately.

Head and Neck

E N **See Chapter 11 and the Anatomy and Physiology section of this chapter.**

A A new diagnosis of hyperthyroidism and hypothyroidism is abnormal in pregnancy.

P Neoplastic disorders such as choriocarcinoma, ovarian teratoma, and hydatidiform mole, as well as a single active thyroid nodule or multinodular goiter, should be considered when a pregnant client is diagnosed with hyperthyroidism.

Eyes, Ears, Nose, Mouth, and Throat

E N **See Chapters 12 and 13 and the Anatomy and Physiology section of this chapter.**

A Arterial constriction of retinal vessels is abnormal. This may lead to blurred vision, scotomata, and, rarely, retinal detachment.

P Arterial constriction of retinal vessels can occur in hypertensive disorders of pregnancy.

A Any growth in the mouth is abnormal.

P Some pregnant clients develop pregnancy tumors in their mouths. These growths are usually benign. Vascular proliferation occurs secondary to hormonal changes. They may not resolve at the end of pregnancy.

> **NURSING TIP**
> **Nipple Assessment**
> Assess nipples at the initial visit and again in the third trimester for any changes. The assessment may change as the breasts enlarge with advancing pregnancy. Inverted nipples may be helped using a nursing cup (breast shield) that is held in place by the brassiere; the nipple is pushed forward through the hole in the base of the cup.

Breasts

E

1. Wash hands before beginning the examination.
2. Examine the breasts as described in Chapter 14.
3. Assess the shape of each nipple; erect, flat, or inverted (Fig. 24-10) while also assessing for spontaneous discharge, cracking, or bleeding. Do not squeeze the nipple to attempt to elicit discharge.
4. Instruct the client on how to become breast self-aware (refer to Chapter 14). This will familiarize the client with their breasts and help them prepare for breastfeeding.

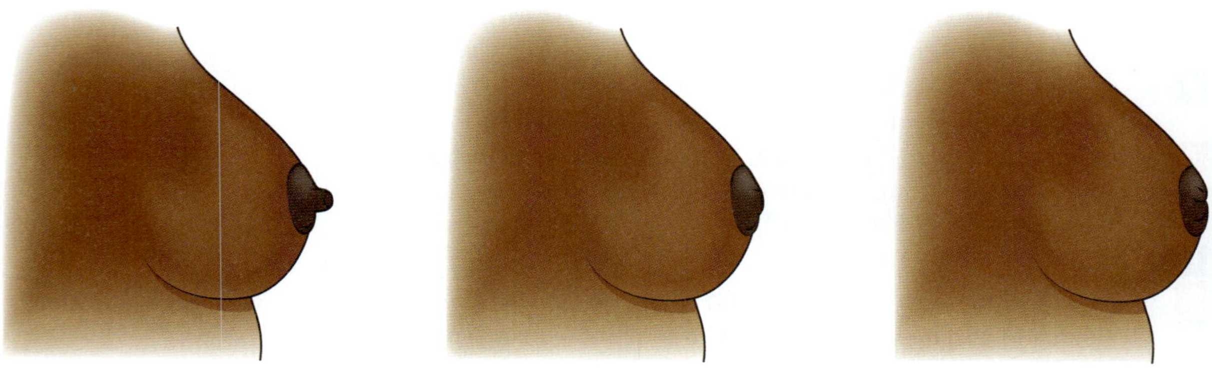

Figure 24-10 Assessing for protractivity of the nipple.

N **Refer to Chapter 14 and the Anatomy and Physiology section of this chapter. Nipples normally protract when stimulated.**

A Accessory breast tissue (supernumerary nipple), if present, is unusual but does not present a problem. Refer if there is evidence of inflammation.

P Accessory breast tissue is a result of abnormal embryological development but does not present a problem in pregnancy. These areas may develop during pregnancy along with the normal breast tissue which may lead to reported discomfort as the accessory mammary tissue attempts to develop.

A Orange-peel appearance (Peau d'orange), redness, heat, or cracked/fissured nipples are abnormal.

P All of these conditions are abnormal and should be evaluated further, as they may affect breast health and breastfeeding. Refer to Chapter 14.

Thorax and Lungs

E N **Refer to Chapter 15 and the Anatomy and Physiology section of this chapter.**

A P Pathology noted in Chapter 15 would also be considered abnormal for the pregnant client.

Heart

E N **Refer to Chapter 16 and the Anatomy and Physiology section of this chapter.**

A A client with a thrill, an irregular heart rhythm, a gallop rhythm, or extra sounds should be referred to a specialist.

P Refer to Chapter 16.

Peripheral Vasculature

E N **Refer to Chapter 17 and the Anatomy and Physiology section of this chapter.**

A Generalized edema, in contrast to the dependent edema of pregnancy, is abnormal.

P The most common causes for edema are standing or sitting too long. Edema can also be indicative of hypertensive disorders of pregnancy. This disease decreases the colloid osmotic pressure within the vasculature, thus allowing fluid to leak into the tissues. Other potential causes to be considered are kidney disease and cardiovascular diseases such as cardiomyopathy.

Abdomen

E N **Refer to Chapter 18 and the Anatomy and Physiology section of this chapter.**

A Severe nausea and vomiting (**hyperemesis gravidarum**) leading to a significant weight loss in pregnancy is abnormal.

P Hyperemesis gravidarum is a disease of unknown etiology. It usually presents in the first trimester and may continue throughout the pregnancy. This is more severe than morning sickness and may persist throughout the day, leading to nutritional deficiencies.

Diagnostic criteria for hyperemesis gravidarum include persistent vomiting, dehydration or ketonuria, weight loss greater than 5% of initial weight, and electrolyte imbalance. There may be an associated hyperthyroid state, which generally resolves spontaneously. There are several risk factors thought to be associated with hyperemesis gravidarum including history in a previous pregnancy, hyperthyroid disorders, gastrointestinal diseases, and multifetal gestations.

A Epigastric pain is abnormal.

P Epigastric pain is usually a result of liver inflammation or necrosis which can be a result of hypertensive disorders of pregnancy. It must be differentiated from cholecystitis or other liver disorders. It may be confused with commonly experienced pregnancy heartburn, but pain resulting from liver pathology is often over the right upper quadrant of the abdomen, whereas heartburn is felt more midline in the epigastric region.

Urinary System

E
1. Obtain a complete urinalysis and culture with sensitivities at the initial prenatal visit.
2. It is common (but not proven to affect the outcome of pregnancy) to assess urine for protein, glucose, and ketones at each subsequent prenatal visit. The presence of leukocytes and nitrites can also be assessed.

N **The urine may turn a brighter yellow as a result of prenatal vitamins. Trace amounts of protein may be noted. Glycosuria may be noted without pathology, but the possibility of diabetes mellitus cannot be ignored. Ketones, leukocytes, and nitrites are normally absent. The urine culture should have no notable pathogens.**

A Nitrites or large amounts of leukocytes are abnormal.

P Nitrites, a breakdown product of bacteria, and large amounts of white blood cells (leukocytes) may indicate a urinary tract infection.

A Ketonuria is abnormal.

P Ketonuria can occur in diabetes mellitus or a compromised nutritional state such as hyperemesis gravidarum.

A Dysuria that presents as any of the following is abnormal: difficulty in initiating urinary flow, increased urinary frequency, and a feeling of being unable to empty the bladder.

P Dysuria results most commonly from a bacterial infection, inflammation of the bladder (cystitis), or urinary tract infection.

A Pain in the flank area (costovertebral angle tenderness) is abnormal.

P The pregnant client is more prone than the nonpregnant client to develop pyelonephritis from a lower urinary tract infection secondary to the dilation of the ureters and renal pelvises, along with decreased tone and peristalsis, which lead to stasis. This results from the physiological changes that occur during pregnancy.

A Asymptomatic bacteriuria is abnormal.

P A clean-voided urine specimen containing more than 100,000 organisms of the same species per milliliter of urine is consistent with infection. Asymptomatic bacteriuria sometimes progresses to acute symptomatic infection unless treated. Through poorly understood mechanisms, bacteriuria is associated with an increased rate of preterm labor and birth.

A Proteinuria greater than trace as shown on a urine dipstick is abnormal.

P The most common cause of proteinuria is hypertensive disorders of pregnancy. The vasospasms that occur also affect the kidneys and their ability to filter substances. Other possible causes are collagen disorders or kidney diseases.

Musculoskeletal System

E N **Refer to Chapter 19 and the Anatomy and Physiology section of this chapter.**

A P Abnormalities and pathology described in Chapter 19 are also considered abnormal for the pregnant client.

Neurological System

E N **Refer to Chapter 20 and the Anatomy and Physiology section of this chapter.**

A Seizures are abnormal.

P Eclampsia is the most common cause of seizures in the pregnant client. Other less common causes are stroke, tumors, or epilepsy. The coagulation and vascular changes associated with pregnancy may exacerbate preexisting conditions.

A Hyperreflexia and clonus are abnormal.

P Hypertensive disorders of pregnancy can cause hyperreflexia and clonus.

Female Genitalia

E
1. For the initial prenatal visit, perform the examination as described in Chapter 21.
2. Perform cultures as indicated in Table 24-7.
3. Postdate pregnancies and pregnancies complicated by preterm labor symptoms or preterm labor risk factors may require a cervical examination at each visit.

N **See Chapter 21 for normal findings of the female genitalia examination. The multiparous vulva and vagina may appear more relaxed in tone, with a shorter perineum. There is often a visible, white, milky discharge during pregnancy (called leukorrhea), and the cervix may show more ectropion (also called eversion and friability). Ectropion is the condition in which the columnar epithelium extends from the os past the squamocolumnar junction, often producing a red, possibly inflamed appearance. See Table 24-1 for additional changes in pelvic organs.**

Manual examination should show uterine size appropriate for gestational age, and the uterus may be slightly more tender than in a nonpregnant client. The retroverted and retroflexed uterus may be more difficult to examine. Palpation of the adnexa may demonstrate a slight tenderness and enlargement of the ovulatory ovary secondary to the corpus luteum of pregnancy.

A Persistent abdominal pain or tenderness is abnormal and should be evaluated.

P Persistent abdominal pain or tenderness may indicate many underlying disorders related or unrelated to pregnancy. Hypertensive

> **NURSING TIP**
> **Ectopic Pregnancy**
>
> A positive home urine pregnancy test, late menstruation followed by vaginal bleeding, an abnormal last period, and abdominal or pelvic soreness or pain that is typically one-sided should alert you to the possibility of an ectopic pregnancy. The pain is often perceived as a cramping sensation or intense localized pain.
>
> On physical examination, there may be cervical motion tenderness (CMT) and enlargement and tenderness in the affected area, although this is truer for a tubal pregnancy than for an abdominal pregnancy. There may or may not be blood on the cervix or in the vagina. If a tubal pregnancy has ruptured (a true emergency), the client may be in shock.
>
> The client should receive a pelvic ultrasound and be put on immediate "ectopic precautions"; that is, the client should be told to call immediately should any increased pain or bleeding occur and be advised not to travel any significant distance away from the local hospital. While serial quantitative serum HCGs or ultrasound, or both, are pending, the client should be informed that a ruptured ectopic pregnancy is often a surgical emergency. Some tubal pregnancies resolve on their own or with medical intervention but all require close supervision. Any tissue passed from the vagina should be saved.

Table 24-7 Laboratory Tests and Values in Pregnancy

Test	Timing
Prenatal Panel includes	
Blood type	Initial visit
Rh factor	Initial visit
Antibody screen	Initial visit; as needed at 28 weeks
RPR (rapid plasma reagent) or VDRL (venereal disease research laboratory)	Initial visit; repeated in the third trimester
Rubella	Initial visit
Hepatitis B surface antigen	Initial visit; repeated in the third trimester
HIV (many states are mandating this test; it should be offered)	Initial visit; repeat based on history or exposure as well as in the third trimester
Varicella	Initial visit if uncertain history
Human parvovirus B19 (fifth disease)	May be done on initial visit or as indicated by exposure
Hepatitis C antibody	Initial visit and as indicated by exposure
CBC, to include: HGB HCT MCV Platelets	Initial visit; repeat at 26–28 weeks and 36 weeks
Hemoglobin electrophoresis	As indicated by race, ethnic background, or demonstrated anemia
Maternal serum alpha fetal protein (MSAFP) or Quad marker screen*	15–20 weeks; 16–18 weeks is optimal
Cystic fibrosis screening	Ideally, before pregnancy; if not, at initial prenatal visit
Thyroid stimulating hormone	Initial visit if risk factors or thyroid disease is present; may repeat each trimester if indicated
Illicit drug screen	Offer at initial visit; may repeat as needed
Toxoplasma IgG	As indicated by any history of exposures and symptoms
Glucose screen	26–30 weeks for all pregnant clients and an early test, preferably with initial prenatal panel, for a client with a family history of diabetes, a prior macrosomic baby, or a client who is 34 years or older or has a BMI of 30 kg/m^2 or more
3-hr glucose tolerance test	If indicated by elevated screening glucose or with history of failure in screening in prior pregnancies
Chlamydia by DNA probe or culture	Initial visit; repeated in the third trimester
Gonorrhea by DNA probe or culture	Initial visit; repeated in the third trimester
Culture for Group ß Streptococcus (GBS)	Vaginal/rectal culture between 35–37 weeks
Urinalysis	Initial visit; as needed per symptoms and history
Urine culture	Initial visit; as needed per symptoms and history

*Both are maternal blood screening tests. MSAFP screens for neural tube defects and ventral wall defects, an elevation being a positive screen. As a screening test, there are false negatives (misses 20% of actual defects) and false positives, which may result from inaccurate dates, multiple-fetus pregnancy, or bleeding with pregnancy. The MSAFP incidentally picks up 20% of Down-affected infants, as the alpha fetal protein will be diminished. Poorly understood is the association of an increased MSAFP with a normal fetus but increased pregnancy complications such as preterm labor or delivery or hypertensive disorders of pregnancy. The Quad screen adds estradiol, HCG, and inhibin A to the test and thus increases the detection of Down to approximately 80%. Adding a nuchal translucency ultrasound at 11 weeks gestation may increase detection of Down syndrome to 90%.

disorders of placental abruption are the most common causes of pain related to pregnancy. Pain is secondary to the hepatic involvement and is often localized in the right upper quadrant of the abdomen. When placental abruption occurs, pain is from the retroplacental bleeding of the placental separation. The pregnant client may experience unrelenting abdominal pain with a rigid abdomen. Disorders unrelated to pregnancy include ulcers, cholecystitis, appendicitis, and pancreatitis.

A Painful adnexal masses are abnormal.

P In early pregnancy, painful adnexal masses may indicate an **ectopic pregnancy** (pregnancy other than intrauterine, such as in the abdomen or fallopian tube), infection, or cancerous growth. Pain associated with an adnexal mass may be elicited via cervical motion during a bimanual examination.

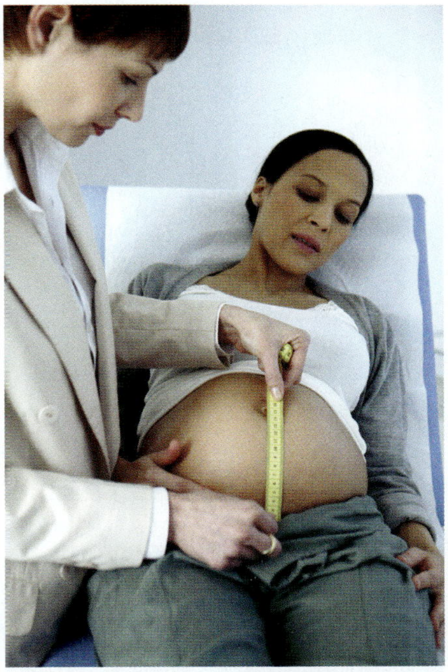

Figure 24-11 Measuring fundal height.

Uterine Size

Uterine size is determined by an internal pelvic examination on the initial prenatal visit, by palpation if less than 18 weeks, and by fundal height in centimeters for subsequent visits. If the initial visit is late in pregnancy, it will include the internal pelvic examination and fundal height.

Fundal Height by Centimeters

E
1. Place the client in a supine position.
2. Place the 0-cm mark of the tape measure at the symphysis pubis in the midline of the abdomen.
3. Palpate the top of the fundus and pull the tape measure to the top (Fig. 24-11).
4. Note the centimeter mark.

N **A 16-week uterus is between the symphysis pubis and umbilicus, a 20-week uterus is at or just above the umbilicus (20 cm), and from 18 to 32 weeks the size is equal to the centimeter height of the uterine fundus. After 32 weeks, although still used, this measurement is less accurate. Fundal height measurement is generally equal to the weeks' gestation though +/– 2 cm is normal. If the measurement is outside this allotted range, further evaluation should be considered.**

A Uterine size larger than expected for the established LMP is abnormal.

P A uterine size larger than expected may indicate hydatidiform mole or molar pregnancy (especially in the absence of fetal heart tones); multiple gestations; inaccurate dating; uterine pathology (fibroid); polyhydramnios; or, later in pregnancy, **macrosomia** (newborn weighing greater than 4,000 g).

A Uterine size smaller than expected for the established LMP is abnormal.

P A uterine size smaller than expected may indicate a nonviable pregnancy; inaccurate dating; or, later in pregnancy, fetal growth restriction (FGR) or transverse lie of the fetus.

Fetal Heart Tone

E
1. Place the client in the supine position.
2. Before placing the Doppler or fetoscope (Fig. 24-12), the provider should evaluate the pregnant abdomen with Leopold maneuver (see

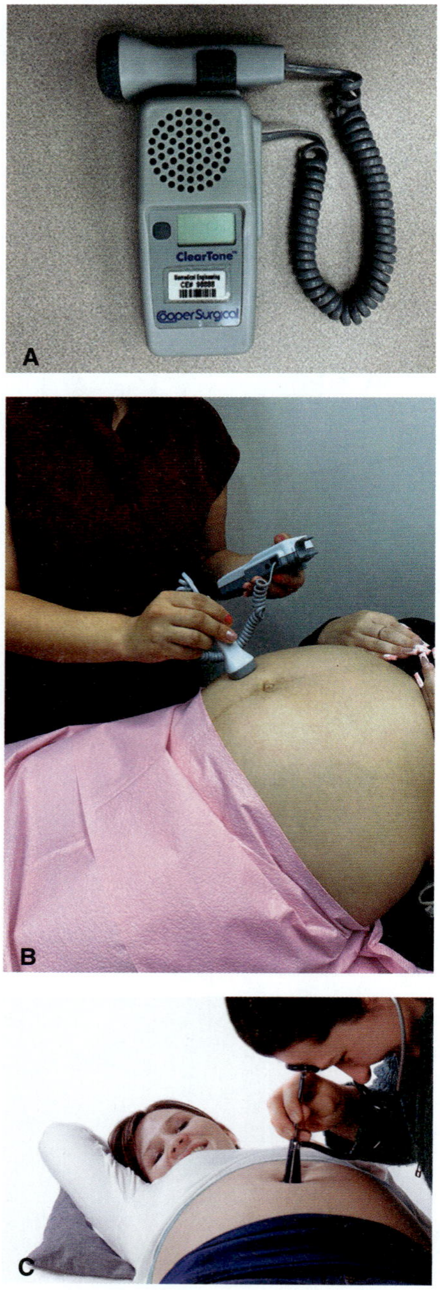

Figure 24-12 Equipment used for fetal heart tone determination. **A.** Doppler. **B.** Auscultating fetal heart tones with a Doppler. **C.** Auscultating fetal heart tones with a fetoscope.

next section) to evaluate fetal position if far enough along in gestational age. Refer to Figure 24-13 to see the best location for auscultation based on fetal position. Place the Doppler or fetoscope on the abdomen and slowly angle the device until fetal heart tones are heard.

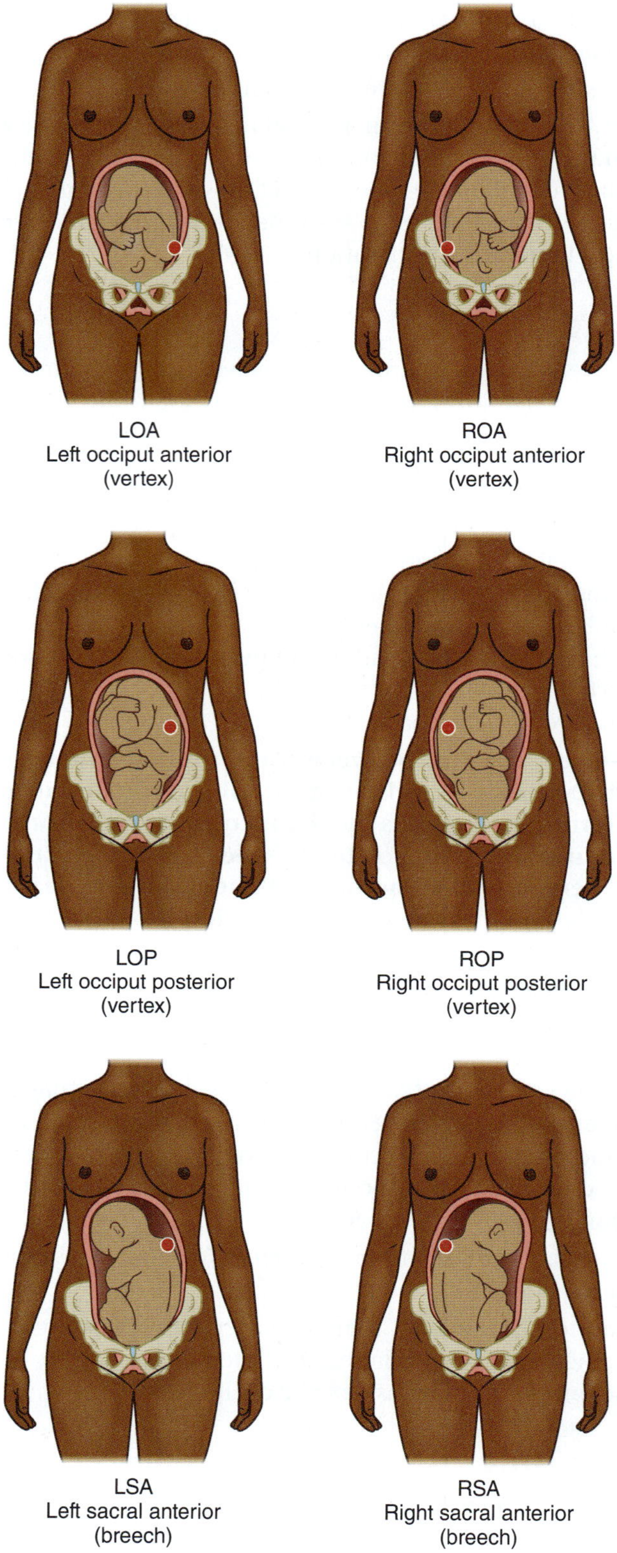

Figure 24-13 Locations for auscultating fetal heart tones.

3. Count the fetal heart tone for sufficient time to determine the rate and absence of an irregularity (optimally 1 minute).

N **During early gestation, the fetal heart is generally heard in the midline area between the symphysis pubis and the umbilicus. It can be heard via Doppler by approximately 10 to 12 weeks (and maybe as early as 9 weeks). Use Doppler to auscultate fetal heart tones before 20 weeks; a fetoscope can be used after 20 weeks. Doppler is commonly used throughout pregnancy, as it is more convenient and also allows the client to hear fetal heart tones. The normal rate is 110 to 160 bpm. If the fetal heart tone seems low, check the client's pulse rate to verify that you are listening to the fetal heart tone and not the client's heart rate. Near-term fetal heart tones are generally heard at maximum intensity in the left or right lower quadrant. If fetal heart tones are best heard above the umbilicus, one should suspect a breech presentation. The fetal heart tone is best heard through the fetal back, which can be located by performing Leopold maneuver (see next section).**

A Fetal heart tone below 110 bpm indicates bradycardia, which is abnormal.

P Bradycardia may be a sign of fetal distress or maternal drug use. A fetal heart tone of 60 bpm or below may be indicative of a heart block. These conditions may be benign and convert to normal after delivery, but a consultation with a perinatologist is advised for consideration of intervention with the newborn.

A Absence of fetal heart activity is abnormal.

P Absence of fetal heart tones after 12 weeks gestation may indicate a missed abortion, fetal demise, or a molar pregnancy.

A Fetal heart tone above 160 bpm indicates tachycardia, which is abnormal.

> **NURSING TIP**
> **FHT AKA FHR**
> The term *fetal heart tone* (FHT), described in beats per minute, is commonly used in antepartum assessment, whereas in much of the literature, especially intrapartum discussions, the term *fetal heart rate* (FHR) is used.

> **NURSING TIP**
> **Documentation of FHTs**
> Document the location of the FHTs by identifying the abdominal quadrants (RUQ, RLQ, LUQ, LLQ), what instrument was used, and indicate the fetal heart tone heard either as an exact number or a range. For example: FHT: RLQ, 140s by Doppler or FHT: LUQ, 145 bpm by fetoscope.

P Tachycardia may indicate cardiac dysrhythmia, maternal fever, or maternal drug use. Before approximately 28 weeks of gestation, tachycardia is a natural consequence of the immaturity of the fetal nervous system. In early gestation, the parasympathetic system exerts a greater influence. As the fetus matures, the sympathetic and parasympathetic systems mature and the fetal heart tone should remain within the normal range of 110 to 160 bpm.

Leopold Maneuver

Beginning at approximately 30 weeks, determine fetal presentation using Leopold maneuver (Fig. 24-14).

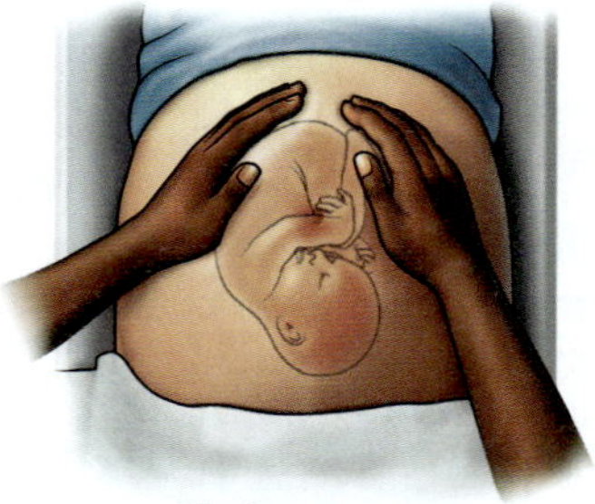

First maneuver

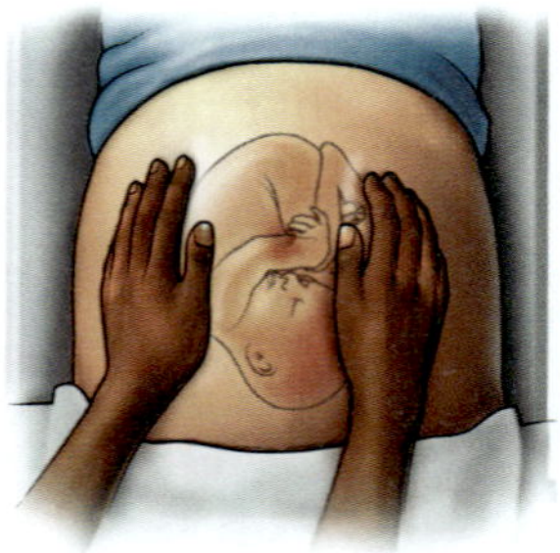

Second maneuver

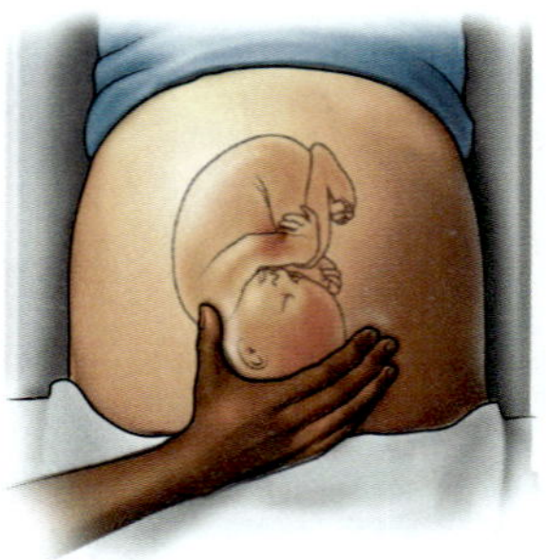

Third maneuver

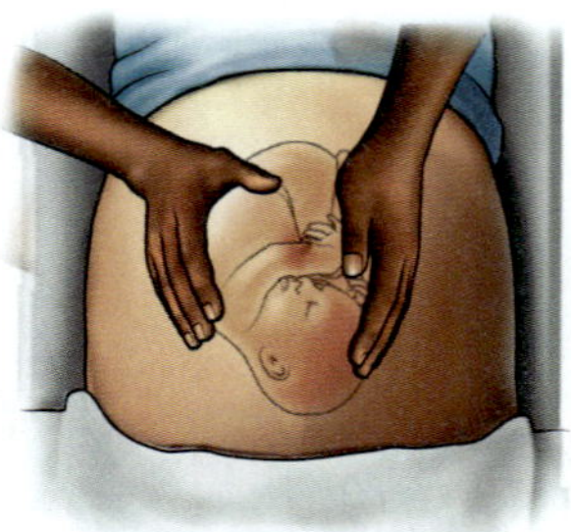

Fourth maneuver

Figure 24-14 Leopold maneuver.

First Maneuver

E
1. Place the client in a supine position with the knees slightly bent.
2. Stand to the client's side facing their head.
3. Keeping the fingers of your hand together, palpate the uterine fundus.
4. Determine which fetal part presents at the fundus.

Second Maneuver

E
1. Move both hands to the sides of the uterus.
2. Keep your one hand steady and palpate the client's abdomen with your other hand.
3. Determine the positions of the back and small parts of the fetus.
4. Repeat the process with your opposite hand on the opposite side of the abdomen.

Third Maneuver

E
1. Place one hand above the symphysis pubis with your thumb on one side of the fetus's presenting part and your fingers on the other side.
2. Gently palpate the presenting part.
3. Determine whether the buttocks or the head is the presenting part in the pelvis. (This should confirm the findings of the first maneuver.) This maneuver is called Pawlik grip and can sometimes be uncomfortable for the pregnant client.

Fourth Maneuver

E
1. Change your position so you are facing the client's feet.
2. Place your hands on each side of the uterus above the symphysis pubis and attempt to palpate the cephalic prominence (forehead or back of the head). This will assist you in determining the fetal lie (the long axis of the fetus in relation to the long axis of the mother) and attitude (head flexed or extended).

N **The fetus's head is usually the presenting part. It feels firm, round, and smooth. The head can move freely when palpated. If the fetus is in a breech position, the buttocks feel soft and irregular. With palpation, the fetus's whole body seems to move, but not with as much facility as the head. The fetus's back is firm, smooth, and continuous. The limbs are bumpy and irregular. The long axis is vertical, and the fetal head is flexed. A fetus not in a vertex presentation can affect the type of delivery; for example, a fetus in a persistent transverse or oblique lie will have to be delivered by cesarean. A breech fetus may be delivered vaginally or by cesarean, depending on the health-care provider's comfort with and experience in doing a vaginal breech delivery. Breech presentation, if uncorrected (i.e., by external version [the manual turning of the fetus by the health-care provider]), is associated with an increased rate of perinatal morbidity and mortality, prolapsed umbilical cord, placenta previa, fetal anomalies and abnormalities (which may not manifest immediately after birth), and uterine anomalies.**

A Inability to determine fetal outline is abnormal.

P Polyhydramnios and maternal habitus can lead to an inability to outline the fetus.

Refer to a textbook on obstetrics for more specific information.

Anus, Perineum, and Rectum

Inspection and Palpation

E

1. Observe for color and shape of the anus.
2. Observe texture and color of the perineum.
3. Palpate the rectum as described in Chapter 23. A digital rectal examination may be part of the bimanual examination in pregnancy.

N **The anus should be dark pink to brown and puckered. Skin tags are a normal variant and hemorrhoids may be seen with pregnancy, especially as the fetus enlarges. The perineum should be smooth and slightly darkened. A prior episiotomy scar may be visible. The perineum may vary significantly in length. The rectum should be free of masses and blood; however, constipation is common in early pregnancy. Discomfort is common with this examination.**

A Warty growths or abnormal lesions, fissures, or tears are not normally found.

P Possible causes of fissures and tears are trauma, abscess, or unhealed episiotomy. Warty growths can represent HPV. Abnormal lesions can represent a malignancy.

Hematological System

E **N** **See Table 24-7.**

Endocrine System

E **N** **See Table 24-7 for information on the glucose screen.**

A Glucose screen greater than 130 to 140 mg/dL after glucola is abnormal. Exact cut-off values vary by institution.

P Normal physiological changes that occur during pregnancy affect glucose metabolism. In some pregnant clients, these changes accentuate and lead to gestational diabetes. These changes affect the client with diabetes by altering the need for insulin throughout the pregnancy. The client with diabetes is at an increased risk for hypertensive disorders, infection, macrosomia or fetal growth restriction (FGR), fetal demise, polyhydramnios, and postpartum hemorrhage.

Nutritional Assessment

E **N** **A** **P** See Chapter 7.

Special Antepartum Tests and Evaluations

Table 24-8 lists special antepartum tests and evaluations that can be performed on pregnant clients.

Psychosocial Assessment and Learning Needs

The diagnosis of pregnancy can normally lead to very mixed feelings. These feelings can range from ambivalence to anger, fear, or excitement. Crying for no apparent reason and mood swings are common in pregnant clients. Feelings of dependency may also present. Early physical changes such as nausea and fatigue may accentuate these feelings. Among the changes confronting the pregnant client and significant others are role expectations (e.g., lifestyle and career); relationship expectations, definitions, and requirements (e.g., parent versus lover); and physiological changes.

> **NURSING TIP**
>
> **Perinatal Depression**
>
> Clinical depression can negatively impact pregnancy and newborn care and development. It is important at prenatal visits to screen, and postpartum to monitor, for symptoms of depression. Screening questions may include a personal or family history of depression or anxiety, prior or current use of antidepressants, difficulty dealing with life stress, lack of support, relationship problems, equivocal feelings about pregnancy, and/or significant premenstrual moodiness.

E Examination **N** Normal Findings **A** Abnormal Findings **P** Pathophysiology

Table 24-8 Special Antepartum Tests and Evaluations

Test	Description
Ultrasound	At any time for pregnancy dating, although more accurate for dates early in pregnancy. Confirm or rule out placenta previa, multiple pregnancies; confirm presenting fetal part. Evaluate fetal anatomy. Evaluate amniotic fluid volume or fetal growth (especially to rule out fetal growth restriction (FGR) or discordant growth with a multiple pregnancy). Evaluate for ectopic pregnancy or fetal demise.
Genetic testing: chorionic villi sampling (CVS), early amniocentesis, amniocentesis, chromosome studies	CVS for chromosome studies is best done at approximately 9-week gestational age, while early amniocentesis is done at approximately 13–16 weeks and traditional amniocentesis between 16–20 weeks, timing being the only difference between the two techniques. Early amniocentesis may carry a higher incidence of abortion. There may be an approximately 1% increased risk of limb deformities associated with CVS, as well as a 1% increased risk of spontaneous abortion. Blood or tissue chromosome studies can be done at any time but are best done with a known family history or advanced maternal age.
Nonstress test (NST) or contraction stress test (CST) for fetal well-being, e.g., with decreased fetal movement, known decreased fluid volume, history of certain maternal diseases (insulin-dependent diabetes, collagen vascular disease), or obstetric complications such as FGR, postdates, preeclampsia, discordant twin, or multiples	For a nonstress test, an electrical fetal monitor is applied to the abdomen, with a tocodynamometer to monitor and record uterine activity and a Doppler to monitor and record FHR, looking at fetal heart response to fetal movement (and any spontaneous uterine contractions). Timing is typically 1 or 2 times per week, and may start as early as 28–32 weeks depending on the risk factor. With a contraction stress test, uterine activity is induced by timed breast nipple stimulation (which induces uterine contractions) and, failing adequate uterine stimulation from nipple stimulation, pitocin intravenously via a pump is used to induce uterine activity. (Relative contraindications for a contraction stress test include any risk for uterine rupture, e.g., previous vertical cesarean section; premature delivery risk; any bleeding risk such as known placenta previa; or any unexplained vaginal bleeding.) Timing is typically once per week after 36 weeks.
Amniotic fluid index (AFI) is most commonly ordered with postdate pregnancies or in the presence of risk factors.	Ultrasound measurement of AFI using an index to determine normal, increased, or decreased fluid levels.
Biophysical profile	A composite test that includes amniotic fluid index, nonstress test, fetal breathing movements, fetal limb movements, and fetal tone; each rated on 0–2 score. This study is done most commonly for the same reasons as an NST or CST.
Fetal movement count	Can be done by all pregnant clients, requires no equipment, and incurs no direct cost. There are many methods of doing fetal movement or kick counts, e.g., number of movements during the day or at certain times of the day, or noting the amount of time to discern 10 separate fetal movements after dinner.

Feelings may fluctuate throughout the pregnancy depending on the trimester and can be predicated on a change in medical status such as the development of a high-risk condition. Early in pregnancy, the client often focuses on self-care and on how these changes are affecting their physical state and lifestyle. As pregnancy progresses, the client usually shifts the focus from self to the fetus as an individual and to the fetus's well-being. The client's age, prior history, family history, and prior pregnancy experience, whether the pregnancy was planned or accidental, and any known risk factors all affect their state of mind. Social support systems, socioeconomic status, environmental hazards, and culture are also influencing factors.

The learning needs of the pregnant client also change throughout pregnancy, and your assessments and teaching must change accordingly. Many communities offer pregnancy-related classes that start with early pregnancy and progress through the childbirth process, breastfeeding, infant care, and sibling involvement. The first-trimester classes typically focus on the physiological changes occurring during pregnancy and what the client must do to develop a healthy infant (for example, nutrition, rest, exercise, and behaviors to avoid). During the second trimester, the emphasis shifts to information on danger signs and symptoms (Table 24-9). At 24 to 26 weeks, the

Table 24-9 Danger Signs of Pregnancy

Sign or Symptom	Action
Vaginal bleeding*	Call health-care provider immediately. Small amounts of bleeding may require only rest and observation at home. More significant bleeding or significant cramping, pain, or fever may require intervention at a hospital. Concerns would be for miscarriage, preterm labor, and placenta previa.
Leaking or gush of watery fluid*	Call health-care provider immediately. Nothing should be put in the vagina unless the provider inserts a sterile speculum to evaluate for rupture of membranes. A sample of the fluid can be evaluated with the nitrazine test to evaluate if it is amniotic fluid.
Abdominal or pelvic pain or cramping*	Call health-care provider immediately after consideration of the normal discomforts of pregnancy (e.g., round or broad ligament pain). It is important for the client to describe the quality of the pain, duration, and location. Concerns would be for premature labor, ectopic pregnancy, placenta abruptio, or urinary tract infection.
Severe headache or blurring of vision	Call health-care provider immediately because of the concern for hypertensive disorders of pregnancy. Evaluation would include blood pressure and labs (blood chemistries, liver function tests, and platelet count).
Persistent chills or fever greater than 102°F (38.9°C)	Call health-care provider. Associated symptoms may be helpful in determining underlying cause and its significance (e.g., infection, dehydration). Acetaminophen may be used to decrease the fever.
Persistent vomiting	Call health-care provider immediately. Need to determine underlying cause (e.g., gastritis, food poisoning) and treat symptoms before dehydration.
Decreased fetal movement or lack of fetal movement	Call health-care provider immediately. At 20–24 weeks, lack of fetal movement could require an ultrasound to confirm dates and fetal viability. Decreased fetal movement or lack of movement later in pregnancy would require evaluation for fetal well-being.
Change in vaginal discharge or pelvic pressure before 36–37 weeks*	Call health-care provider to evaluate for preterm labor.
Frequent (more than four per hour) uterine contractions or painless tightenings between 20 and 37 weeks*	Call health-care provider. Rest, fluids, or snack may be recommended if uterine activity is not excessive or for prolonged period of time. If either is true, evaluation for preterm labor is required.

*Associated with preterm labor.

client should be provided verbal and written information on the signs and symptoms of preterm labor and other danger signs of pregnancy.

Third-trimester classes focus on the preparation for childbirth and the care of a newborn infant. The topic of breastfeeding should be introduced in the first trimester and discussed throughout the pregnancy. The client should be informed of available childbirth education classes.

Adolescents may need additional support and educational reinforcement. Many school districts offer special programs for pregnant teens in addition to their normal school courses. Such programs typically encompass childbirth preparation and infant care assistance while the teen finishes school.

Learning needs must be assessed on an ongoing basis so that interventions can occur at the appropriate times. A social services consultation may be indicated for certain clients, such as those with a history of physical, emotional, or sexual abuse; those experiencing current drug and/or alcohol abuse; and those requiring help with basic housing and food needs. Learning may require reinforcement and educational needs should be reviewed and documented throughout the pregnancy. Appropriate written or visual information should be used to reinforce verbal discussions.

Any client or family who suffers a fetal loss, whether intrauterine, stillborn, or newborn demise, should be offered supportive follow-up. Many communities have support groups, or the client may seek help from a counselor or religious leader. People who experience early miscarriages often find that society does not allow them to grieve their losses; supportive follow-up should thus be offered in these situations.

Sexual relations during pregnancy are often viewed as a taboo subject. Intercourse, unless specifically proscribed, is considered safe during pregnancy, although it may not always be easy or comfortable. During the first trimester, there may be no changes in libido. During the second trimester, the pregnant client may even experience increased libido, whereas the physical and psychological changes of the third trimester may decrease the client's interest in sexual relations. As the pregnancy advances, the client may find that sexual intercourse is most comfortable in a side-lying position, perhaps with a pillow under the abdomen, facing away from the partner. This position may decrease the depth of penetration. Partners may express concern about injuring the fetus or the pregnant client's perceived discomfort.

> **NURSING TIP**
> **Fetal Movement**
>
> At approximately 18 to 22 weeks in a primigravida pregnancy and as early as 16 to 18 weeks in a subsequent pregnancy, the pregnant client notices the first fetal movements in utero, known as **quickening**. These are felt as fluttering or kicking, and initially may be difficult to differentiate from other pregnancy symptoms such as gas and ligament stretching. Failure on the part of the pregnant client to notice fetal movement by approximately 22 weeks should alert the nurse to the possibility of either inaccurate dating or, in the absence of FHTs, nonviable pregnancy. Beginning at approximately 28 weeks, fetal kick or movement self-monitoring should be introduced. The most common method of movement monitoring is for the pregnant client to assess 10 fetal movements in a 2-hr period. If this does not occur, the pregnant client should be advised to contact their health-care provider. The pregnant client's sensation of fetal movement may change in the third trimester, going from "somersaults," to rolling from side to side, to kicks or subtle shifts; however, the actual number of fetal movements should not decrease dramatically. Any decrease in fetal movement requires rapid evaluation.

Subsequent or Return Prenatal Visits

Return prenatal visits include vital signs, FHR, fundal height, documentation of fetal movement appropriate for gestational age, weight, urine dipstick, assessment of any edema, assessment of uterine activity, assessment of any vaginal discharge or pelvic pain or pressure, and cervical examination, if done. Other issues discussed at return visits include concerns of weight gain, diet, childbirth preparation, breastfeeding, family planning, preparedness of the home, any family issues, and blood and other tests as appropriate to the gestational age.

> **NURSING TIP**
> **Pregnancy, Childbirth, Breastfeeding, and Sibling Education**
>
> Early in the pregnancy, encourage relevant preparation classes. These are offered by most health-care systems and hospitals. The fees, if charged, vary widely. Give the pregnant client a packet of information at the first visit and include information on the classes available and contact numbers to register for them. Some facilities offer a special class on pain relief and anesthesia. This initial packet may also include information on optimal nutrition, importance of normal weight gain, avoidance of excessive weight gain, safe activities during pregnancy, and warning signs of complications and preterm labor. Clients often enjoy pamphlets or books that show fetal development and pregnancy symptoms at various stages of the pregnancy.

Each laboratory, ultrasound, and/or genetic test may require a specific explanation or education. At approximately 20 weeks, in addition to advising the pregnant client to avoid sleeping on their back, you can again stress the importance of registering for preparation classes.

Some facilities also offer a class for siblings. These classes provide an opportunity for siblings to explore their feelings about changes in their parent's behavior and the possibility of a new person intruding into their world. The classes often offer tips to help the siblings adjust. Expectant parents may not have explored this issue and how to best parent the newborn and siblings.

Some clients may need encouragement to take breastfeeding classes because they perceive that it is a natural process and therefore should require no teaching. If a pregnant client is planning to breastfeed, classes should be highly encouraged because they can be very beneficial to help understand the physical and hormonal changes being experienced, not to mention the benefits of breastfeeding to the newborn.

At about 24 to 28 weeks is the best time to review the signs and symptoms of preterm labor and appropriate action, in addition to expected laboratory studies. Handouts are generally available. You can also teach the pregnant client the fetal movement (kick) counting technique.

U.S. Preventive Services Task Force (USPSTF)

Grade A Recommendations:

- The USPSTF recommends that all persons planning to or who could become pregnant take a daily supplement containing 0.4 to 0.8 mg (400 to 800 mcg) of folic acid.
- The USPSTF recommends screening for hepatitis B virus (HBV) infection in pregnant women at their first prenatal visit.
- The USPSTF recommends that clinicians screen for HIV infection in all pregnant persons, including those who present in labor or at delivery whose HIV status is unknown.
- The USPSTF strongly recommends Rh(D) blood typing and antibody testing for all pregnant women during their first visit for pregnancy-related care.
- The USPSTF recommends early screening for syphilis infection in all pregnant women.
- The USPSTF recommends that clinicians ask all pregnant persons about tobacco use, advise them to stop using tobacco, and provide behavioral interventions for cessation to pregnant persons who use tobacco.

Grade B Recommendations:

- The USPSTF recommends screening for anxiety disorders in adults, including pregnant and postpartum persons.
- The USPSTF recommends the use of low-dose aspirin (81 mg/day) as preventive medication after 12 weeks of gestation in persons who are at high risk for preeclampsia.
- The USPSTF recommends screening for asymptomatic bacteriuria using urine culture in pregnant persons.
- The USPSTF recommends providing interventions or referrals, during pregnancy and after birth, to support breastfeeding.
- The USPSTF recommends screening for chlamydia and gonorrhea in all sexually active women 24 years or younger and in women 25 years or older who are at increased risk for infection.
- The USPSTF recommends screening for depression in the adult population, including pregnant and postpartum persons, as well as older adults.
- The USPSTF recommends screening for gestational diabetes in asymptomatic pregnant persons at 24 weeks of gestation or after.
- The USPSTF recommends that clinicians offer pregnant persons effective behavioral counseling interventions aimed at promoting healthy weight gain and preventing excess gestational weight gain in pregnancy.
- The USPSTF recommends screening for hypertensive disorders in pregnant persons with blood pressure measurements throughout pregnancy.
- The USPSTF recommends that clinicians screen for intimate partner violence (IPV) in women of reproductive age and provide or refer women who screen positive to ongoing support services.
- The USPSTF recommends that clinicians provide or refer pregnant and postpartum persons who are at increased risk of perinatal depression to counseling interventions.
- The USPSTF recommends repeated Rh(D) antibody testing for all unsensitized Rh(D)-negative women at 24 to 28 weeks' gestation, unless the biological father is known to be Rh(D)-negative.
- The USPSTF recommends screening for unhealthy alcohol use in primary care settings in adults 18 years or older, including pregnant women, and providing persons engaged in risky or hazardous drinking with brief behavioral counseling interventions to reduce unhealthy alcohol use. The USPSTF recommends screening by asking questions about unhealthy drug use in adults aged 18 years or older. Screening should be implemented when services for accurate diagnosis, effective treatment, and appropriate care can be offered or referred.

Retrieved December 18, 2025, from *https://www.uspreventiveservicestaskforce.org/uspstf/recommendation-topics/uspstf-a-and-b-recommendations*

CASE STUDY
The Pregnant Client

This case study illustrates the application and objective documentation of the pregnant client examination. Rose is a 37-year-old Haitian-born Black female with a positive home pregnancy test 10 days ago. Rose is a walk-in client who came to the clinic for a pregnancy blood test confirmation. Rose recently immigrated to the United States from Mexico after traveling from Chile. Rose is unsure of how long she has been pregnant. Today's date is March 1, 2026.

HEALTH HISTORY

CLIENT PROFILE

37-year-old married Black cisgender female

REASON FOR SEEKING HEALTH CARE

Positive home pregnancy test

PRESENT HEALTH

Currently without any active disease, feels "good"

Unplanned pregnancy. Recently immigrated to the United States from Mexico

REPRODUCTIVE HISTORY

Menstrual History

Menarche age 14; menstrual cycles: every 28 to 60 days, lasting 5 to 7 days

LMP: 12/9/2025 (client is sure of date)

Sexual History Became sexually active at age 24. Monogamous relationship with same male partner x 10 years. Two previous male partners; denies rape or sexual abuse; denies recent STI

Health History Since LMP No bleeding or cramping since LMP; denies fevers, rashes, exposure to communicable diseases; denies exposure to dangerous chemicals, heavy metals, or radiation

Signs/Symptoms of Pregnancy Amenorrhea, breast tenderness, nausea

Use of Fertility Drugs Denies; previously used Depo-Provera injections

Contraceptive History Has not been on contraception in 4 years

Genetic Predisposition Denies any known familial genetic conditions

Gynecological History

Denies history of gynecological problems. Unsure of date of last Pap smear and denies history of abnormal results

Denies history of STI

Estimated Date of Delivery Current working EDD 09/16/2026

Obstetrical History Gravida 3 Para 1011

- G1: 09/18/2021: 39 weeks spontaneous vaginal delivery. Labored for 12 hours. Delivered in Haiti. Unmedicated labor and delivery. Infant weight unknown, does not recall the baby being weighed. Denies complications with pregnancy, delivery, or postpartum. Child is healthy and doing well
- G2:2023: 10-week spontaneous abortion; required surgical treatment which was done in Mexico, no complications
- G3: Current pregnancy. 11 weeks and 5 days by date of LMP; current working EDD 09/16/2026

  Denies history of hypertensive disorders of pregnancy, glucose intolerance, bleeding or postpartum hemorrhage, isoimmunization, or postpartum depression. No history of hyperemesis gravidarum

PAST HEALTH HISTORY

Medical History Denies any medical problems

Surgical History 2023 dilation and curettage for spontaneous abortion

Allergies No known drug allergies.

Medications Not taking any medications, prenatal vitamins, or folic acid

Communicable Diseases Denies history of TB, measles, mumps, or exposure to ill children or viral illnesses. Denies history of hepatitis, cytomegalovirus, and toxoplasmosis. Denies risk factors for HIV

Injuries and Accidents Burned left arm with hot iron at dry cleaning job last month, now healed

Differing Abilities Haitian Creole is primary language; speaks some Spanish, little to no English

Blood Transfusion Denies

Childhood Illnesses Positive for varicella and fifth disease at age 7

Immunizations States had "everything" for immigration to U.S. Not sure of last tetanus booster. Received COVID-19 vaccines x 2 doses in Chile in late 2021

FAMILY HEALTH HISTORY

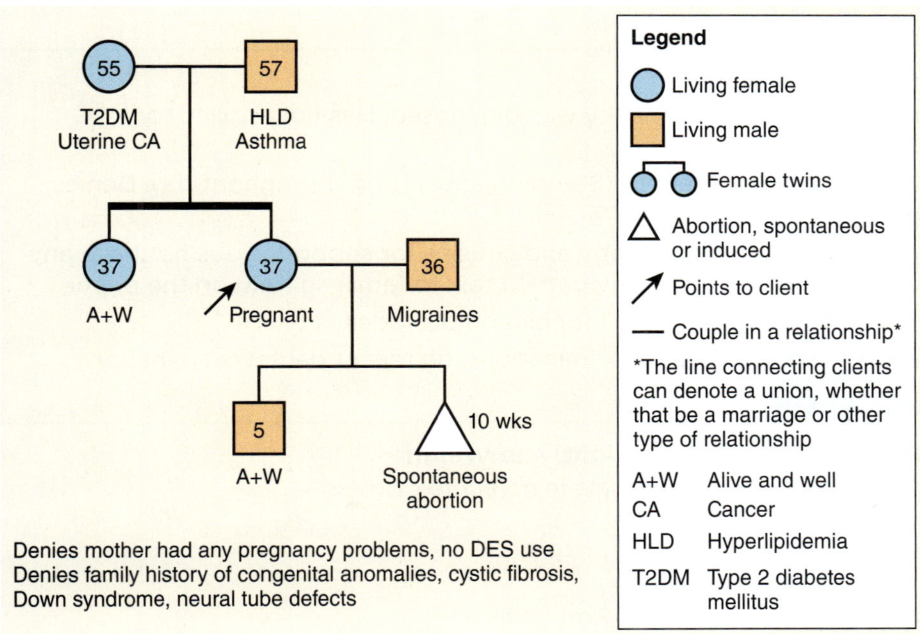

SOCIAL HISTORY

Alcohol Use Occasional beer with friends; none since pregnancy discovered; no binge or heavy drinking

Tobacco Use Denies ever using. Father of baby does not smoke. Denies secondary smoke exposure

Recreational Drug Use Client and father of baby deny use

Domestic and Intimate Partner Violence Denies history of verbal, physical, emotional, or sexual abuse or neglect with husband. One previous male partner verbally abused her and hit her a few times—this abuse led to client leaving this partner 15 years ago. No contact with ex-partner since then

Sexual Practice Heterosexual

Travel History Born in Haiti. Started immigration process to United States 4 years ago. Traveled to Chile where she lived for 2 years, then moved to Mexico for 2 years. Entered the United States legally 3 months ago

Work Environment Long hours mostly standing at dry cleaners pressing clothes

Home Environment Secure and safe, comfortable. Lives with husband and their one child in a rental house with 4 other people who are described as cousins. They do not have any animals living in the home.

Hobbies and Leisure Activities Being involved in her church; enjoys homemaking

Stress Working long hours at a dry-cleaning business. Father of baby is a day worker, sometimes unemployed. Misses family back in Haiti, especially twin sister

Education Completed fourth grade

Economic Status "Not too good. I need help."

Military Service Denies

Religion Christian, Pentecostal

Ethnic Background She is Black, non-Hispanic, of Haitian descent. Father of baby is also Black, non-Hispanic of Haitian descent

Roles and Relationships Client and father of baby share parenting and working roles; relying on her cousins who babysit on occasion

Characteristic Patterns of Daily Living Rises at 5:30 AM, showers, has eggs and plantains for breakfast and a glass of milk; takes the bus to work, arrives 7:30 AM. Takes a lunch break at noon; usually eats rice, pork, beans, or a sandwich. Finishes work 5:00 PM; takes bus home. Client and father of baby take turns cooking dinner and cleaning up; may watch TV, do some chores; goes to bed about 11:30 PM

HEALTH MAINTENANCE ACTIVITIES

Sleep 6 to 8 hours every night

Diet No change in diet since pregnancy was diagnosed. Has not applied for WIC supplements

Exercise Walks to and from bus stop. Standing and sitting throughout day. Denies heavy lifting

Stress Management Has father of baby and cousins for support. Does not have any other family in the area. Occasionally gets to talk to family in Haiti on the phone

Use of Safety Devices Uses car seat for child on bus rides

Health Checkups No recent health examinations, no recent dental examination

PHYSICAL EXAMINATION

General Assessment, Vital Signs, Height, and Weight

Well-developed, well-nourished female in no acute distress
Temperature: 98.3°F (36.8°C)
Pulse: 88 bpm
Respirations: 18 breaths per minute
Blood Pressure: 102/75 mm Hg left arm sitting
Weight: 223 lb (101.2 kg)
Height: 70 inches (178 cm)
Body mass index: 32 kg/m^2

Skin and Hair Intact without lesions, rashes, bruises

Head and Neck Thyroid without enlargement, no lymphadenopathy

Eyes, Ears, Nose, Mouth, and Throat Within normal limits

Breasts Tender with everted nipples

Thorax and Lungs Breath sounds clear, no wheezing or crackles

Heart Regular rhythm, no murmur/gallop/rub

Peripheral Vasculature No peripheral edema

Abdomen Positive bowel sounds, no bruits; no masses, nontender; no hepatosplenomegaly

Urinary System Clean-catch urinalysis and urine culture sent to laboratory; negative glycosuria/proteinuria/ketonuria in dipstick; negative for leukocytes and nitrites

Musculoskeletal System No limitations in range of motion

Neurological System Cranial Nerves II–XII grossly intact, funduscopic deferred; mental status intact; upper and lower extremities strength equal and 5/5; cerebellar intact; deep tendon reflexes 2+/4+ bilaterally

Female Genitalia External genitalia: Without lesions, abnormalities, or tenderness

Internal genitalia: Vagina and cervix without lesions or abnormalities, with softening of the cervix and cervical/uterine junction, the uterus is 8 weeks post LMP size. Pap smear collected with cotesting as well as gonorrhea and chlamydia testing.

Anus, Perineum, and Rectum Within normal limits

Hematological System Prenatal panel requisition given

Endocrine Early glucose tolerance test ordered with prenatal laboratory panel due to pregravid body mass index greater than 30 kg/m^2

Nutrition Reports now eating several small meals; fairly balanced diet; without physical signs/symptoms of malnutrition; body mass index 32 kg/m^2

PSYCHOSOCIAL ASSESSMENT AND LEARNING NEEDS

Unplanned pregnancy at 11 weeks and 5 days by date of LMP of 12/09/2025; current working EDD 09/16/2026. Referral for social services offered. Encouraged to access free childbirth, infant care, and breastfeeding classes at Health Department. Has concerns about steady income to support family

CLINICAL JUDGMENT IN ACTION

1. What cues indicate the client's unique health-care needs?
2. What risk factors contribute to the client having a high-risk pregnancy?
3. What are the client's learning needs?

Review Questions

1. A client presents to the clinic reporting that they found out they are pregnant via a home pregnancy test. The client remembers that the first day of their last menstrual period was September 8, 2025. Using Naegele Rule, what would the client's estimated due date be?
   a. June 1, 2026
   b. December 1, 2026
   c. June 15, 2026
   d. December 15, 2026
2. A primigravida pregnant client presents to the clinic for a routine prenatal visit at 37 weeks gestation. The client is concerned about a thick, yellow-colored substance leaking from their nipples. What is the nurse's best response to this client?
   a. "You are already producing your milk, don't worry."
   b. "This is called colostrum. This can be secreted starting as early as the second trimester."
   c. "If it's okay with you, we should do an examination to make sure this is normal."
   d. "This could indicate an infection."
3. A pregnant client who is 40 weeks and 6 days gestation is in labor. The client's gestational age is referred to as:
   a. Full term
   b. Post dates
   c. Post term
   d. Late term
4. During pregnancy, a client reports to the nurse that a blotchy, irregular discoloration of the face has developed. The nurse knows that this is called:
   a. Rosacea
   b. Linea nigra
   c. PUPPS
   d. Melasma
5. A pregnant client presents to the clinic for a new pregnancy visit. While obtaining the obstetrical history, the nurse learns that the client had two babies born on their due dates, who are alive and well. The client also reports that a miscarriage occurred a couple of years ago. The nurse would document the client gravida (G) and para (P) using the TPAL system as:
   a. G4 P2012
   b. G3 P2012
   c. G3 P3002
   d. G4 P2002

6. During a physical examination of a pregnant client at 10 weeks gestation, the nurse notes that the cervix has a blueish hue in appearance. The nurse knows that this is called:
   a. Hegar sign
   b. Chadwick sign
   c. Goodell sign
   d. Friability
7. The nurse is going to perform a brief assessment on a pregnant client. What are the components of a brief assessment of a pregnant client? Select all that apply.
   a. Fundal height
   b. Fetal heart tones
   c. Heart auscultation
   d. Leopold maneuvers
   e. Liver palpation
8. A healthy pregnant client with no medical history presents to the clinic at 35 weeks gestation. The client reports "not feeling well" the last couple of days at home and has been tracking their blood pressure. The client shows the nurse the blood pressure logs with readings of 135/90, 152/99, 140/85, and 133/88. What complications of pregnancy is the nurse concerned about? Select all that apply.
   a. Gestational hypertension
   b. Chronic hypertension
   c. Preeclampsia
   d. HELLP Syndrome
9. A primigravida pregnant client is 17 weeks gestation and reports concerns related to fetal movement. The client has not felt fetal movement and is concerned that something may be wrong with the baby. Which statement is true related to fetal movement?
   a. Pregnant clients begin feeling fetal movement around 18 to 22 weeks gestation.
   b. The client will need an ultrasound to verify if a missed abortion has occurred.
   c. Pregnant clients begin feeling fetal movement around 15 to 18 weeks gestation.
   d. It is not important if a pregnant client can feel fetal movement or not.
10. A client presents to the clinic reporting there has been no menses for the last 2 months. The client admits to regular, monthly periods before this. The client reports nausea, vomiting, breast tenderness, and fatigue for the last 3 weeks. The nurse knows that these symptoms are called:
   a. Probable signs and symptoms of pregnancy
   b. Positive signs and symptoms of pregnancy
   c. These signs and symptoms are not associated with pregnancy
   d. Presumptive signs and symptoms of pregnancy

CHAPTER

25 The Pediatric Client

Learning Outcomes

1. Describe the physical growth of a child through the pediatric years.
2. Identify the anatomy and physiology of the pediatric client.
3. Elicit a complete health history from a client or caregiver using standard components of a pediatric health history.
4. Identify personal-social, language, and fine and gross motor findings when using the Revised Denver Developmental Screen II.
5. Perform a physical examination on a healthy pediatric client and a pediatric client with pathology.
6. Differentiate between normal clinical findings from a pediatric client's physical examination and the pathophysiology of abnormal clinical findings.
7. Identify risk factors for adolescent suicide.
8. Identify the effects of COVID-19 on the pediatric client.
9. Identify the United States Preventive Services Task Force recommendations for the pediatric client.
10. Document a complete health history and physical examination of a pediatric client.

Children are unique individuals who undergo rapid changes from birth through adolescence. Physical growth, motor skills, and cognitive and social development are evidence of the numerous changes family members, friends, and health-care professionals observe throughout a child's maturing years. In your examination of the pediatric client, you must be aware of these changes as you continually reassess what is considered to be within normal limits for the child.

Physical Growth

One important set of parameters required for pediatric health examination is physical growth. The parameters of weight, length or height, and head circumference (dependent on age) are essential in serial physical growth measurements. (Chest circumference is of less importance). For example, by plotting a child's growth on a chart (Fig. 25-1), you can determine normal or abnormal growth curves according to the child's age. Special growth charts are available for genetic syndromes such as Down or Turner syndrome, achondroplasia, and Prader-Willi syndrome. It is also important to adjust for prematurity when assessing physical and developmental growth (see Nursing Tip, Adjusting Chronological Age).

The Centers for Disease Control and Prevention (CDC) currently recommend the use of the World Health Organization (WHO) growth standards and growth charts to monitor growth for infants and children ages 0 to 2 years of age in the United States. The rationale for using the WHO growth standards is that they establish the growth for breastfed infants as the norm for growth and they identify how children should grow when provided optimal nutrition and other environmental conditions. In addition, the research-based WHO standards better reflect infants' physiological growth and not children's typical growth patterns during a specific period. The CDC growth charts are recommended to record the growth of children ages 2 to 20 years of age.

Growth charts were revised in 2000 by the National Center for Health Statistics (NCHS), the National Center for Chronic Disease Prevention and Health Promotion (NCCDPHP), and various other experts. WHO growth charts were revised in 2006. One addition, the Body Mass Index (BMI) for Age Percentiles chart, is used to decide whether a child's weight is appropriate for their height. The BMI growth chart is available for use with children aged 2 years and older. The charts are used to compare a child's growth to the growth of children in the United States. For example, you are plotting the growth of a 5-year-old female whose BMI is 17.3 kg/m^2 (Fig. 25-1G). This would indicate that her BMI is higher than that of approximately 90% of 5-year-old girls in the United States. In December 2022, the Centers for Disease Control and Prevention, National Center for Health Statistics, introduced an updated BMI-for-age growth chart that extended to a BMI of 60 kg/m^2 for children ages 2–20 (Fig. 25-1 I, Fig. 25-1 J). The BMI-for-age growth chart previously ended at the 97th percentile. The new chart extends to the 99.99th percentile. Sadly, the need for this alteration arose from an obesity epidemic in the country's children. In the years 2017–2018, the CDC (2022) estimated that over 4.5 million children ages 2 to 20 had severe obesity, necessitating this change.

For infants, the average birth weight is 7.5 pounds (3.4 kg), length is 19 to 21 inches (48 to 53 cm), and head circumference is 13.7 inches (35 cm). Infants should double their birth weight by 6 months and triple their birth weight by 1 year of age, although it is not uncommon for infants to be at double their birth weight at 4 months. An infant's height increases about 1 inch (2.5 cm) per month for the first 6 months and then slows to ½ inch (1.3 cm) per month until 12 months. Head circumference increases by around 0.4 inches (1 cm) per month during the first year. The most rapid growth occurs during the first 6 months of life, and most head growth is completed by 4 years of age.

Growth in the toddler period (12–24 months) begins to slow. The birth weight usually quadruples by 2.5 years of age, with an average weight gain during the toddler period of 4 to 6 pounds (1.8 to 2.7 kg) per year. The toddler usually grows 3 inches (7.6 cm). One-half of adult height is usually reached by 24 to 30 months.

Preschoolers (2–6 years) gain an average of 5 pounds (2.3 kg) per year. Height increases between 2.5 and 3 inches (6.4 to 7.6 cm) per year. The preschooler's birth length usually is doubled by 4 years of age. In contrast, the school-age child (6–12 years) grows 1 to 2 inches (2.5 to 5 cm) per year and gains 3 to 6 pounds (1.4 to 2.7 kg) annually.

School-age (6-12) children steadily grow at least 2 inches (5 cm) per year and gain around 6.5 pounds (3 kg) pounds per year. There is typically a slowed height velocity in late school age for males, which can predispose them to obesity, while females are hitting their "growth spurts" and often surpass males in weight and height during late school age.

Infancy and adolescence (13–18 years) are two periods of rapid growth in the pediatric client. Rapid growth in the adolescent is called the growth spurt. Females commonly experience this between ages 10 and 14, whereas in males it occurs somewhat later, between 12 and 16 years of age.

NURSING TIP

Adjusting Chronological Age

For the infant born prematurely, you will need to adjust the chronological age on the growth chart. For instance, the corrected age for a 6-month-old infant who was born 2 months prematurely would be 4 months. Plot the obtained weight and length on the growth chart under the child's corrected age, and mark "corrected" above the weight. There is no current consensus regarding how long to continue age correction, varying from 18 to 40 months depending on prematurity.

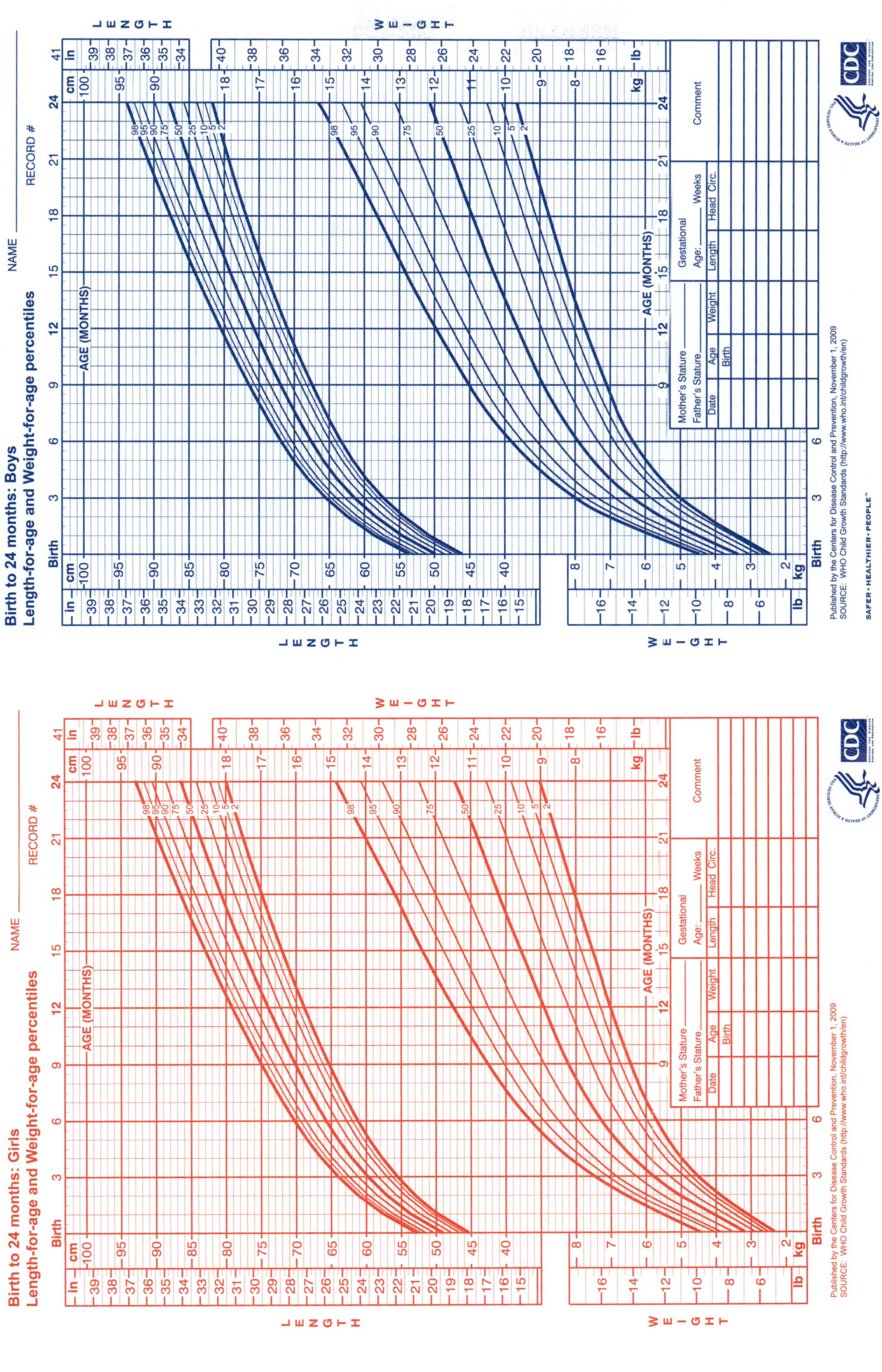

Figure 25-1 Physical growth charts. **A.** Girls: Birth to 24 months (length and weight) (WHO). **B.** Boys: Birth to 24 months (length and weight) (WHO).

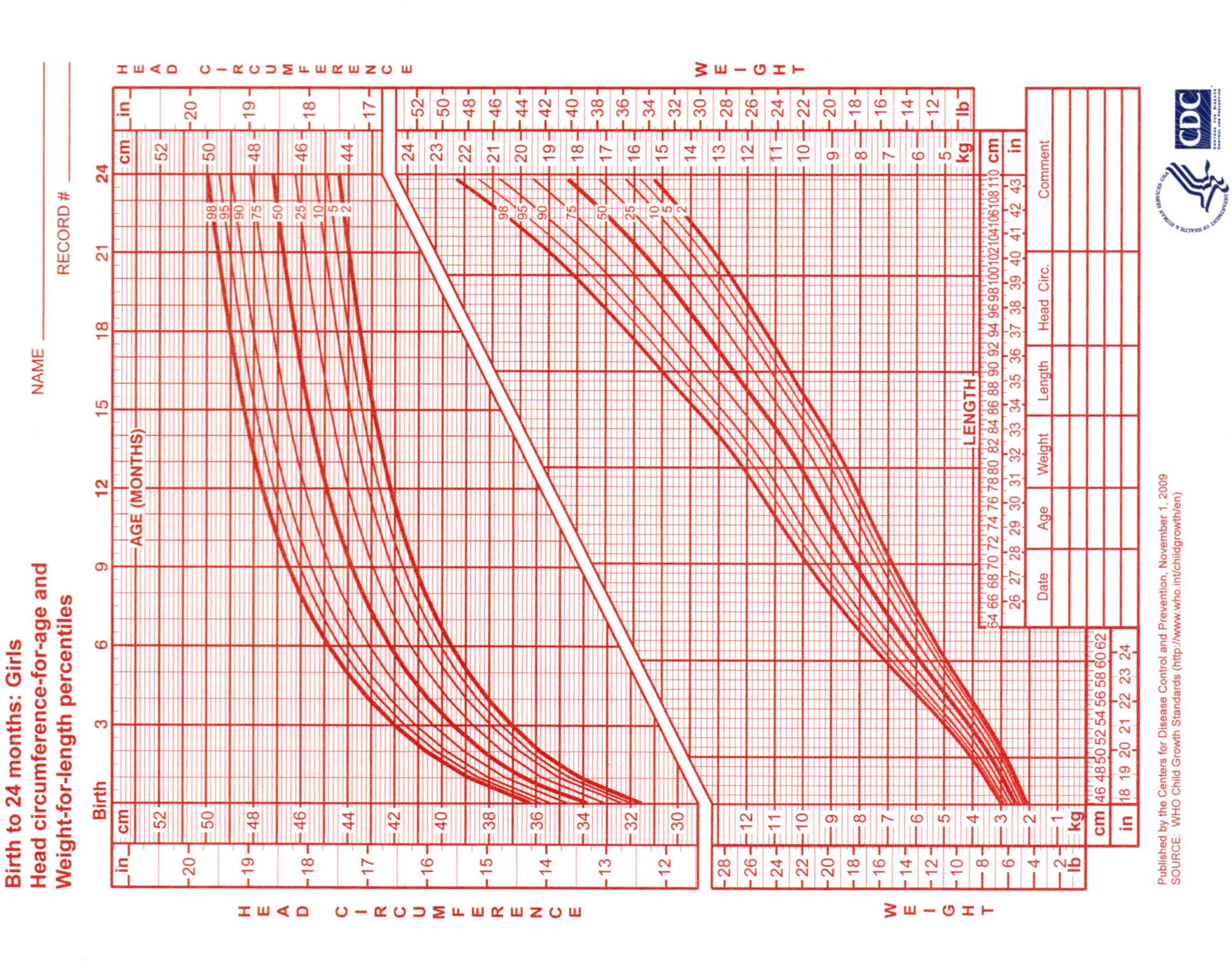

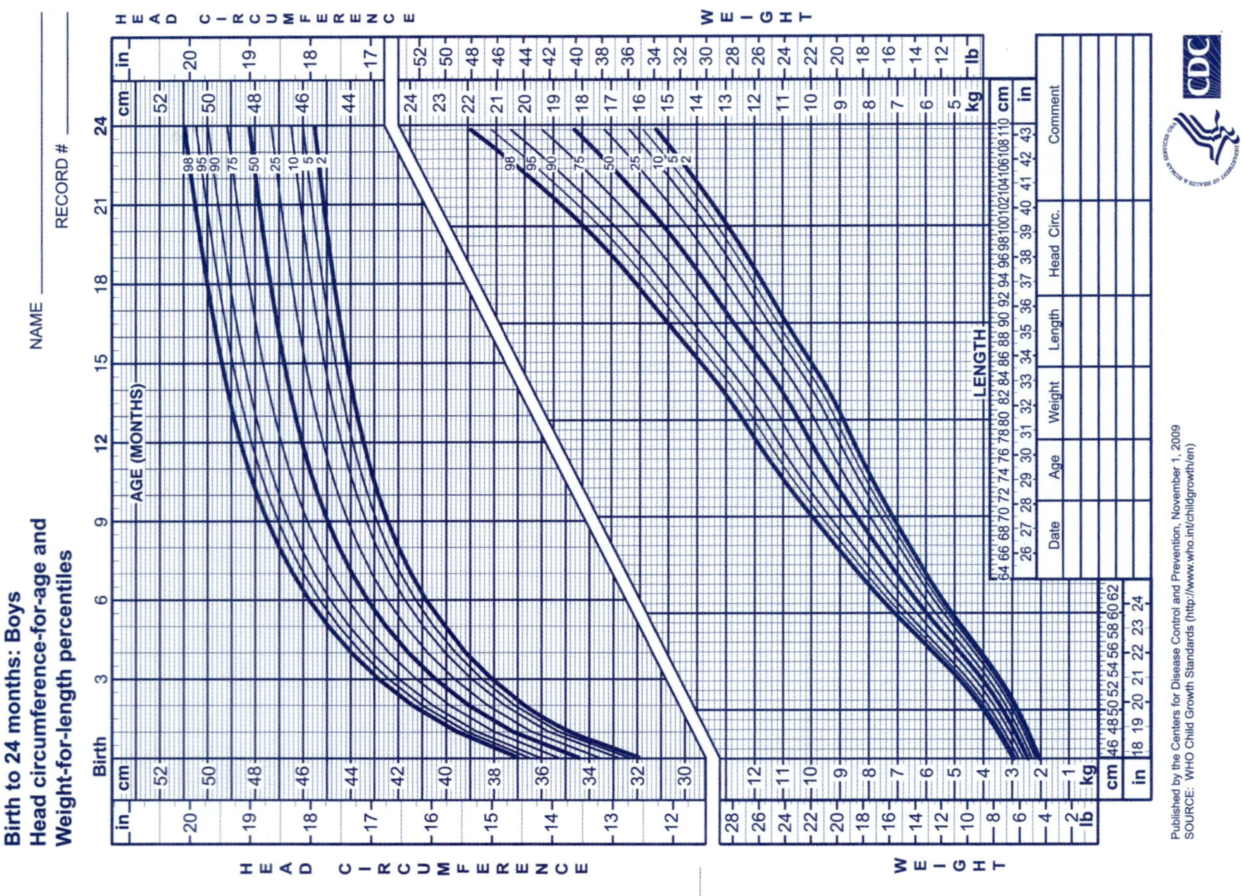

Figure 25-1—cont'd C. Girls: Birth to 24 months (head circumference) (WHO). **D.** Boys: Birth to 24 months (head circumference) (WHO).

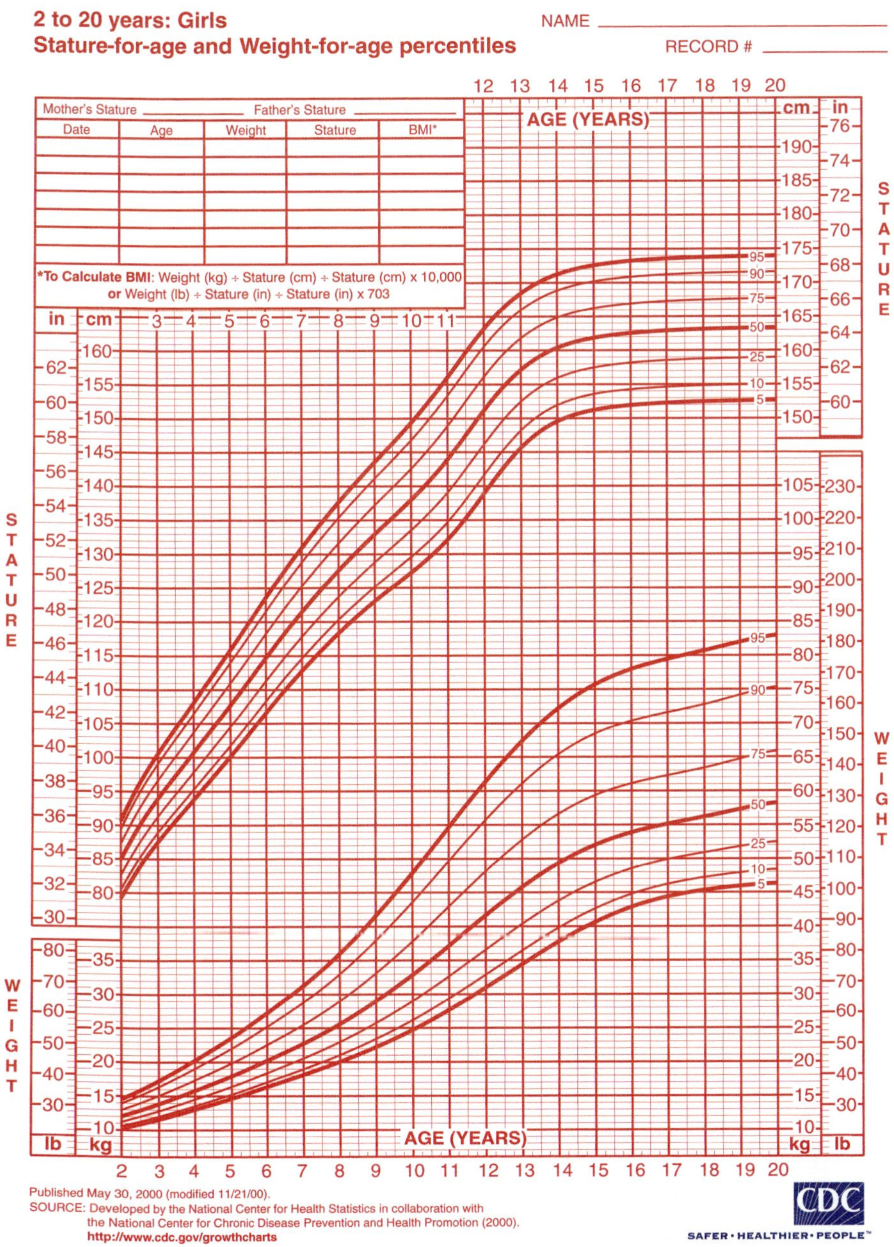

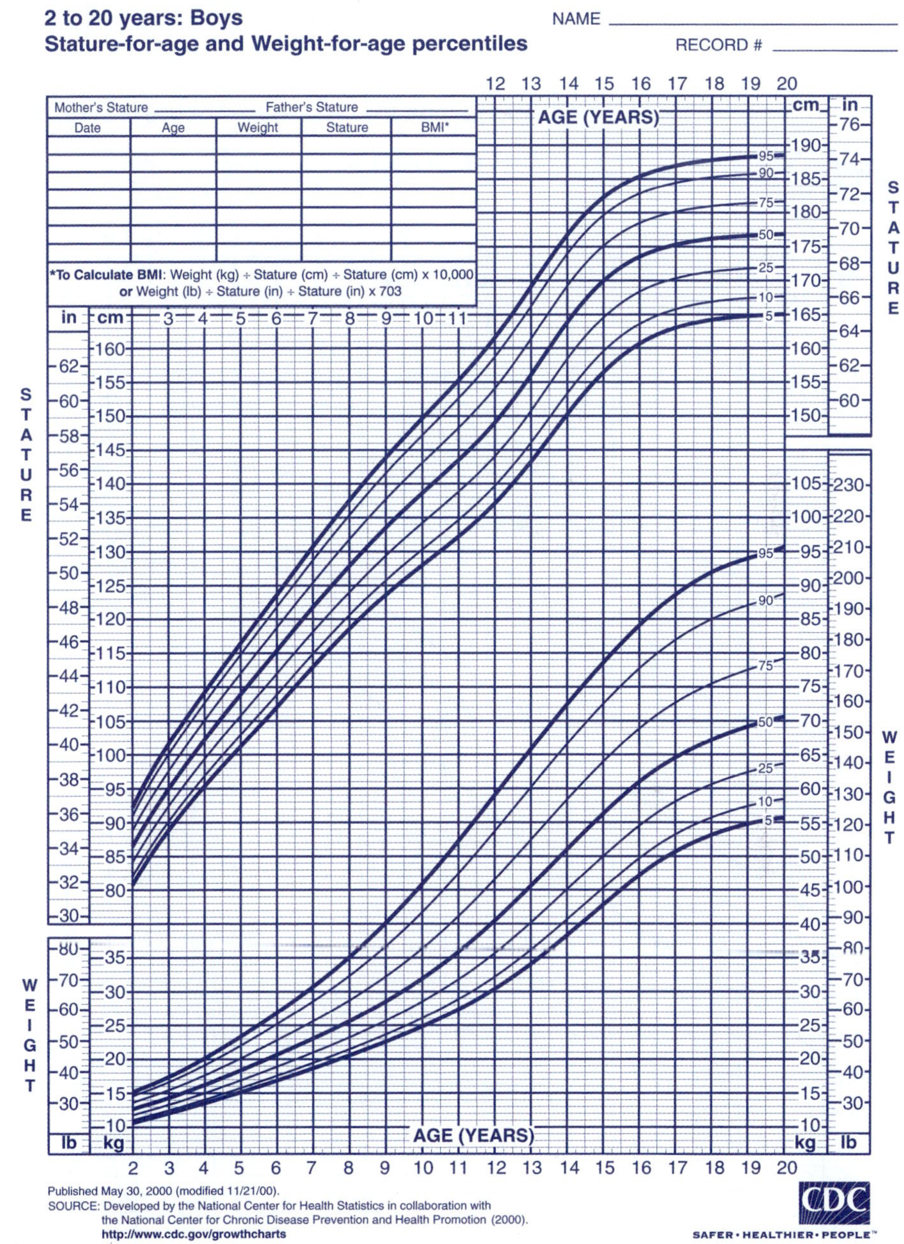

Figure 25-1—cont'd E. Girls: 2 to 20 years (stature and weight) (CDC). **F.** Boys: 2 to 20 years (stature and weight) (CDC).

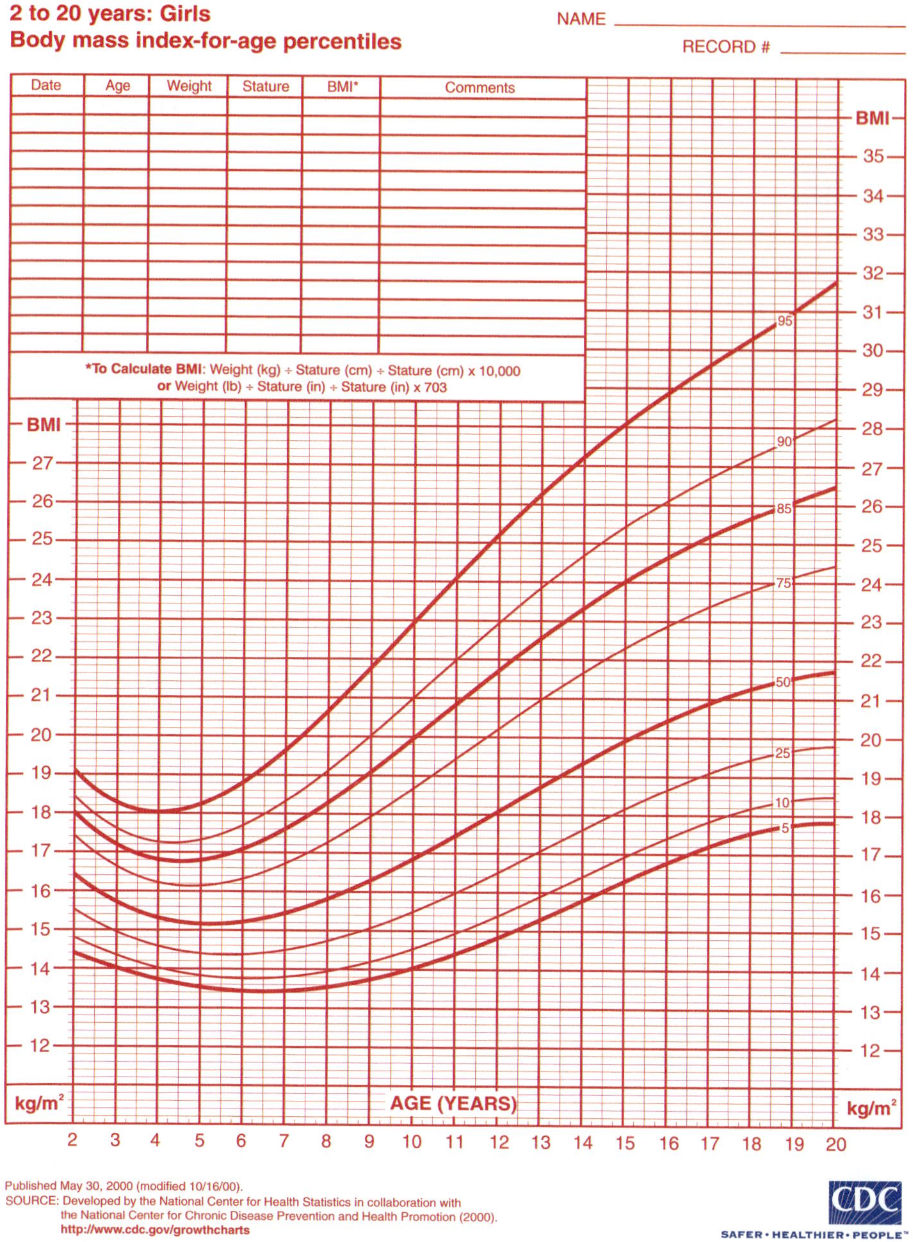

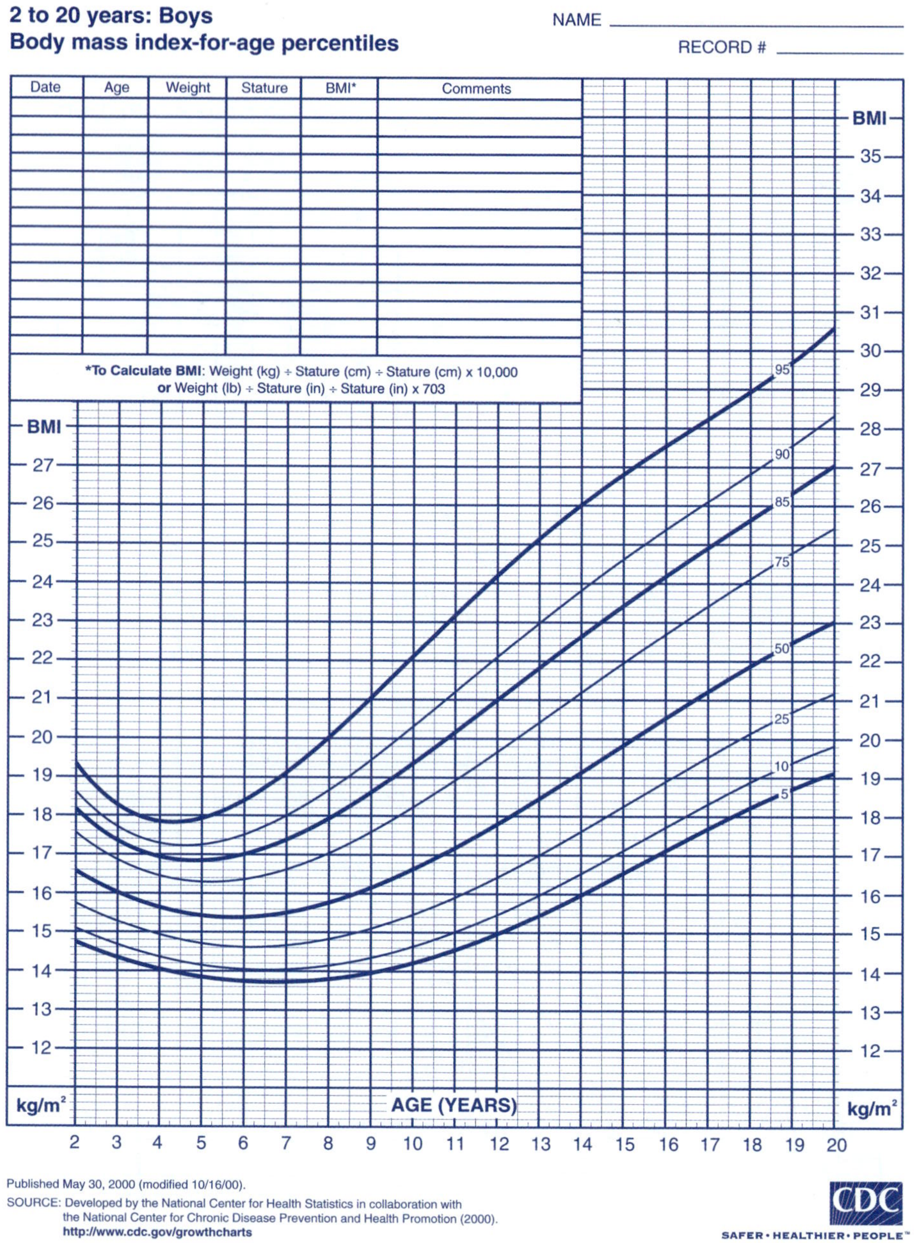

Figure 25-1—cont'd G. Girls: 2 to 20 years (body mass index for age) (CDC). **H.** Boys: 2 to 20 years (body mass index for age) (CDC).

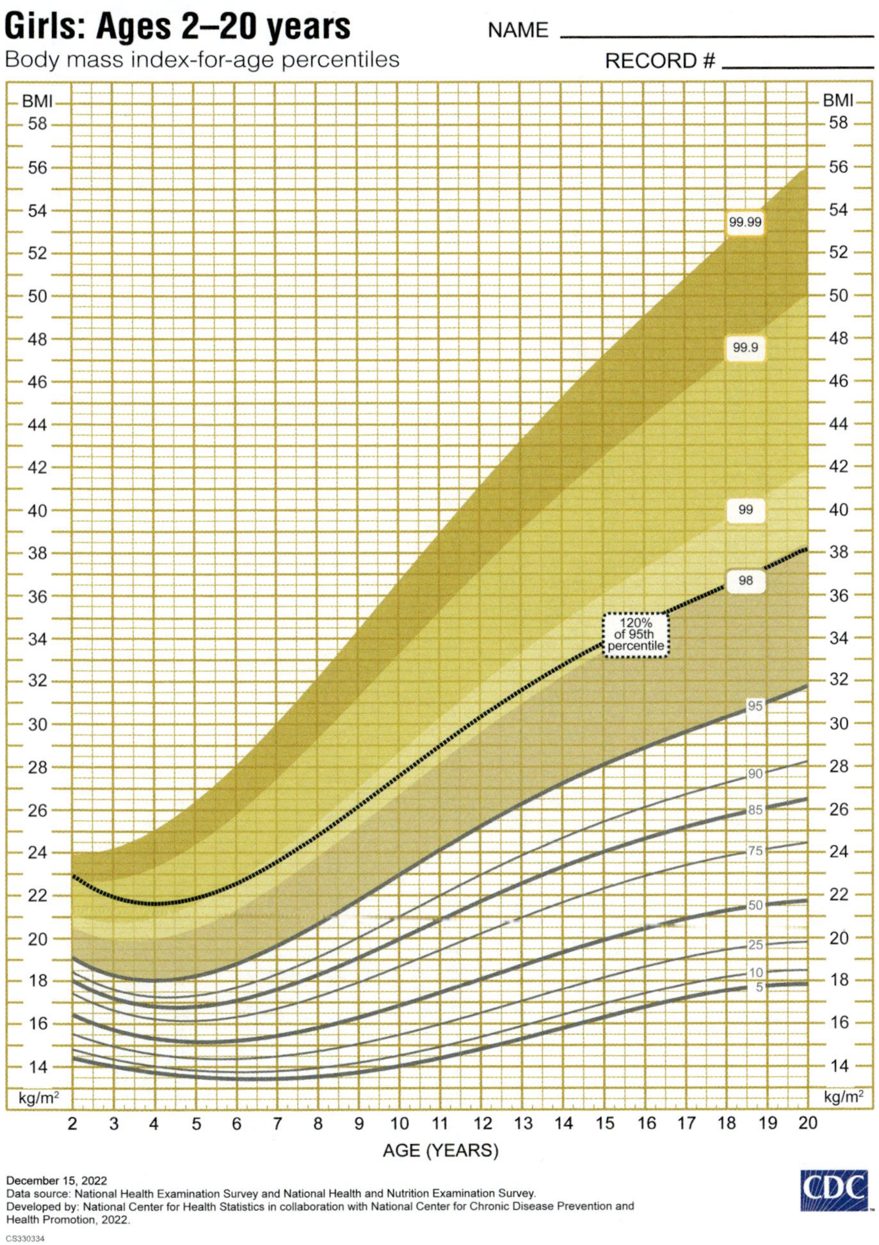

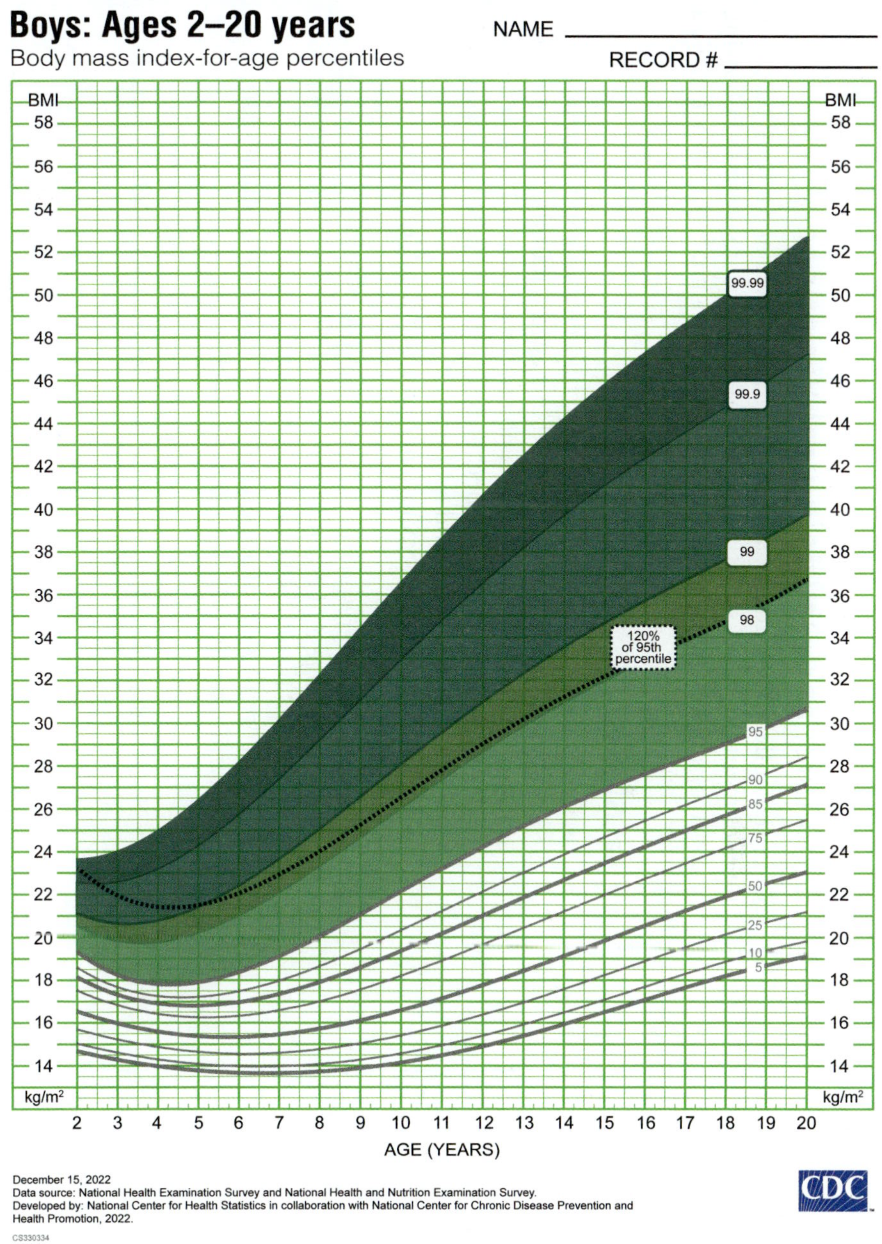

Figure 25-1—cont'd I. Girls: 2 to 20 years (body mass index for age percentile) (CDC). **J.** Boys: 2 to 20 years (body mass index for age percentile) (CDC).

Anatomy and Physiology

Structural and Physiological Variations

Children differ from adults and among themselves at various stages of development in their structural and physiological makeups. Following is a list of important variations that occur from birth through a child's maturation.

Vital Signs

- One notable difference in the way children and adults regulate temperature is the inability of infants aged 6 months and younger to shiver in the face of lower ambient temperature. The absence of this important protective mechanism puts infants at risk for hypothermia, bradycardia, and acidosis.
- By age 4, temperature parameters are comparable to those seen in adults.
- Both pulse and respiratory rates in children tend to decline with advancing age and reach levels comparable to those found in adulthood by adolescence.
- In children 1 year of age and older, an easy rule of thumb for determining normal systolic blood pressure is:

  $$\text{normal systolic BP (mm Hg)} = 80 + (2 \times \text{age in years}).$$

- Normal diastolic blood pressure is generally two-thirds of systolic blood pressure.
- Blood pressure charts for children ages 1 to 17 years provide systolic and diastolic readings using the sex, age, and height percentile (refer to Table 9-5; *https://www.nhlbi.nih.gov/files/docs/guidelines/child_tbl.pdf*).

NURSING TIP

Allaying Childhood Fears

Throughout childhood, children exhibit various fears and behaviors in response to past and present health-care encounters. The following nursing tips will help you calm fears and behaviors children may exhibit during an examination.

Infant

The fear of parents leaving the room begins at around 6 months of age but increases significantly after the acquisition of object permanence. Older infants experience a fear of strangers called stranger anxiety.

Tip: Allow parents to be present and to hold their child during the examination; speak in a calm, reassuring voice, and allow the child to use security objects such as a pacifier, blanket, or stuffed animal during the examination. Try to listen to the lungs and heart when the child is calm and not crying.

Toddler

Fear of strangers and parents leaving the room continues in the toddler age-group. Clinginess is prevalent in toddlers. They may also become upset if their parent is feeling stressed. Additionally, fear of pain and discomfort usually begins in the toddler years.

Tip: Allow parents to be present and to hold their child during the examination; speak in a calm, reassuring voice; allow the use of security objects such as a pacifier, blanket, or stuffed animal during the examination; explain what is happening in simple words, and allow time for the toddler to play, explore, and express their feelings. Allowing choices gives the toddler a feeling of control. Try to listen to the lungs and heart when the child is calm and not crying. Save intrusive examinations until the end.

Preschooler

This age-group fears being left alone and experiencing pain. Behaviors exhibited include clinginess, temper tantrums, asking for help with things that were once done without help, baby talk, or thumb sucking (regression-type behaviors).

Tip: Allow parents to be present and to hold their child during the examination; speak in a calm, reassuring voice; let the child know what is going to be examined, allow manipulation of examination equipment; be honest about what is going to happen next and how it may feel. Save intrusive examinations until the end.

School-Age

Behaviors once thought to be outgrown may often come back as mechanisms for coping with stress. Fears include separation from parents, pain, and losing control. Some behaviors seen in school-age children include asking for help with things that were once done without help, acting out by yelling or screaming, and attention seeking. Anxiety and fears may present with somatic complaints, such as "tummy aches," during this stage.

Tip: Allow parents to be present, allow time for play or manipulation of examination equipment. Let the child ask questions, acknowledge feelings, allow choices, and set limits for losing control. Most school-age children are now able to have a traditional head-to-toe examination.

Adolescent

Adolescents may be skeptical concerning truth-telling and think health-care professionals avoid telling the truth. The fear of pain and losing control may persist during adolescence. Privacy is a big factor during adolescent examinations.

Tip: Involve the adolescent in planning and decision making. Allow the choice of the parent leaving during the examination, and encourage expressions of feelings. Be upfront regarding confidentiality parameters from the beginning of the visit.

Skin and Hair

- **Lanugo**, a fine, downy hair, may be present on the skin of a newborn. The lanugo is most prominent over the temples of the forehead and on the upper arms, shoulders, back, and pinna of the ears. Dark-skinned newborns have an increased amount of lanugo, which is readily evident as very dark black hair.
- **Vernix caseosa**, a thick, cheese-like, protective integumentary deposit that consists of sebum and sheds epithelial cells, is present on the newborn's skin.
- Relative to an adult, a child has a higher ratio of body surface area to body surface mass. This impacts temperature regulation and predisposes the infant and young child to hypo- and hyperthermia.

Head

- Suture ridges are palpable until approximately 6 months of age, at which time unionization occurs.
- The posterior fontanel, which is triangular in shape and is formed by the junction of the sagittal and lambdoidal sutures, is typically no longer palpated after 2 months of age (Fig. 25-2).
- The junction of the sagittal, coronal, and frontal sutures forms the anterior fontanel. It is diamond-shaped. This fontanel should close by 10 to 24 months of age.

Eyes, Ears, Nose, Mouth, and Throat

- At birth, the newborn's peripheral vision is intact. Visual acuity is approximately 20/200. The child's visual acuity is usually 20/20 at 6 years of age.
- Newborns do not produce tears until their lacrimal ducts open, at around 2 to 3 months of age.
- The external auditory canal of a child is shorter than that of an adult, and it is positioned upward, necessitating the need to pull down and back for the otoscopic examination.
- The eustachian tube is wider, shorter, and more horizontal than that of an adult. These factors increase the likelihood of middle ear infections caused by the migration of pathogens from the nasopharynx.
- Only the ethmoid and maxillary sinuses are present at birth, although their volume increases steadily throughout childhood and adolescence. At approximately 7 years of age, the frontal

NURSING TIP

Sleep Position Recommendations

Instruct caregivers to decrease the risk of sudden infant death syndrome (SIDS) by placing infants on the back when sleeping in an infant sleep product that meets federally approved safety standards. In 2025, the American Academy of Pediatrics (AAP) revised its recommendations on sleep positioning. Its goal is to guide caregivers in creating a safe sleep environment for infants, thus reducing the risk of all sleep-related infant deaths, including SIDS. The AAP's current recommendations include the use of a firm, noninclined, sleep surface, breastfeeding, room-sharing without bed-sharing, routine immunizations, and offering of a pacifier at nap time and bedtime. In addition, soft bedding, overheating, infant head covering, and exposure to tobacco smoke, marijuana, alcohol, and illicit drugs are to be avoided. Furthermore, supervised, awake tummy time is encouraged to assist in infant development and minimize the risk of positional plagiocephaly (Moon, Carlin, & Hand, 2022). **Plagiocephaly** is a unilateral flattened head or back of the head.

sinuses develop. The sphenoid sinuses do not develop until after puberty (Fig. 25-3).

- Eruption of the first lower central incisors occurs between 5 and 7 months of age. By 2.5 years of age, toddlers have 20 primary or deciduous, teeth. By puberty, permanent teeth and four molars have replaced the primary teeth. Wisdom teeth normally appear between 18 and 21 years of age (Fig. 25-4).
- Salivation starts at about 3 months, and the infant drools until the swallowing reflex is more coordinated.

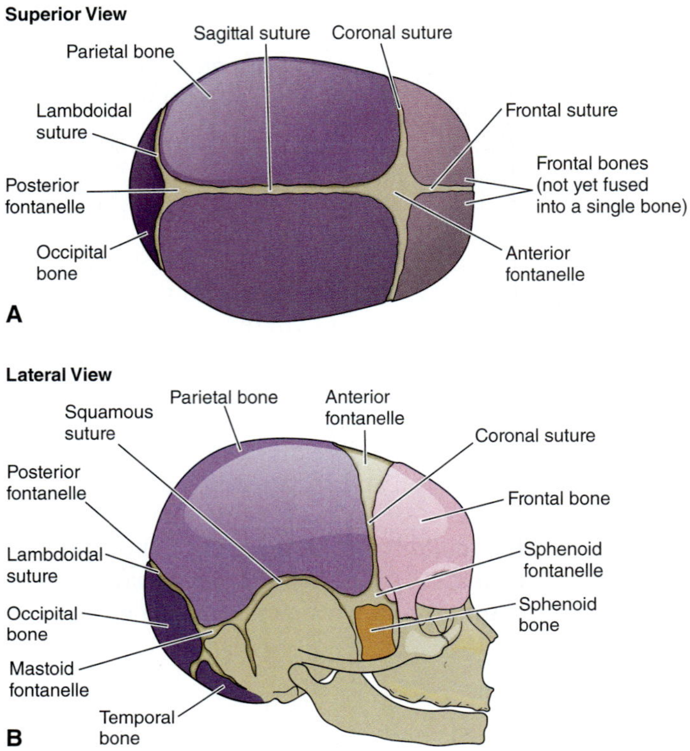

Figure 25-2 Infant head structures. **A.** Superior view. **B.** Lateral view.

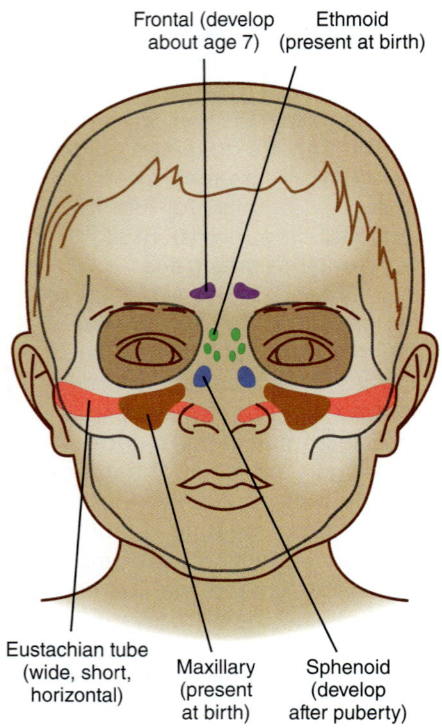

Figure 25-3 Position of sinuses and eustachian tubes in children.

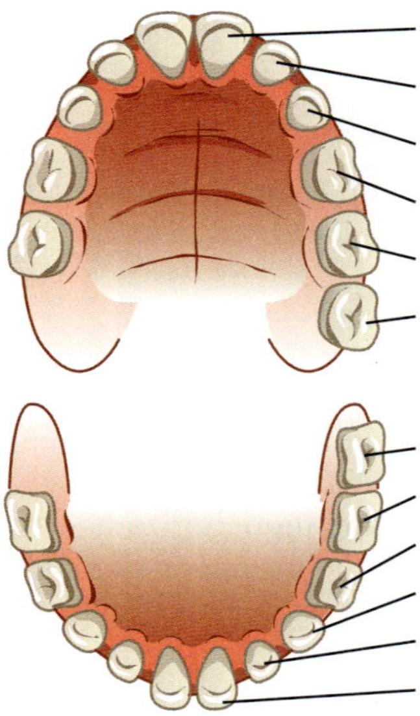

Upper teeth	Erupt	Shed
Central incisor	6–8 mos.	6–7 yrs.
Lateral incisor	8–12 mos.	7–8 yrs.
Canine (cuspid)	16–20 mos.	10–12 yrs.
First molar	10–16 mos.	9–11 yrs.
Second molar	20–30 mos.	10–12 yrs.
Third molar	18–21 yrs.	

Lower teeth	Erupt	Shed
Third molar	18–21 yrs.	
Second molar	20–30 mos.	10–12 yrs.
First molar	14–18 mos.	9–11 yrs.
Canine (cuspid)	14–18 mos.	9–12 yrs.
Lateral incisor	7–12 mos.	7–8 yrs.
Central incisor	5–7 mos.	6–7 yrs.

Figure 25-4 Ages for deciduous teeth eruption and shedding.

Breasts

- Breast tissue in the female starts to develop between 8 and 10 years of age. Mature adult breast tissue is achieved between 14 and 17 years of age. Refer to Table 14-1 for Tanner's Sexual Maturity Rating.
- In early puberty development, boys can experience unilateral or bilateral breast nodules that are tender-to-touch and firm. These nodules usually follow the pattern of physiological gynecomastia in puberty and often decrease in size over a couple of years.

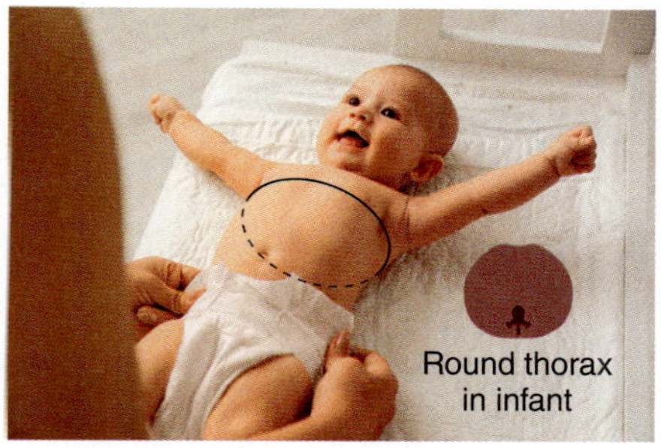

Figure 25-5 Infant chest configuration.

Thorax and Lungs

- A newborn's chest is circular because the anteroposterior and transverse diameters are approximately equal (Fig. 25-5). The transverse diameter increases with age. A continued barrel-shaped chest after the age of 12 to 24 months should elicit an examination for underlying pathology, such as cystic fibrosis.
- Decreased muscularity is responsible for the thin chest wall in infants.
- Ribs are displaced horizontally in infants.
- The trachea is short in the newborn. By 18 months of age, it has grown from the newborn length of 2 inches (5 cm) to 3 inches (7.6 cm). Toward the latter part of adolescence, the trachea will have grown to adult size, normally 4 to 5 inches (10.2 to 12.7 cm).
- Until 3 to 4 months of age, infants are totally dependent on breathing through their noses.
- During infancy and the toddler period, abdominal breathing is always prevalent over thoracic breathing.
- Rapid breathing with occasional pauses is common in sleeping infants.
- Assessment of respiratory rate in infants should occur over a full minute due to the periodic breathing common during this age.

Heart

- The heart in an infant, toddler, and preschooler lies more horizontally than an adult's heart; thus, the apex is higher, at about the left fourth intercostal space.

Peripheral Vasculature

- The fetal circulation changes to pulmonary circulation when the umbilical cord is separated from the maternal (or gestational parent) circulation. In utero, the ductus venosus allows blood to flow from the placenta into the right heart. Blood flows from the right side of the heart to the left through an opening called a foramen ovale. This opening is a flap valve located on the atrial septum between the septum secundum and septum primum. The ductus arteriosus, located between the left pulmonary artery and the descending aorta, allows blood to flow from the pulmonary artery to the aorta. Normally, the three fetal shunts (ductus venosus, foramen ovale, and ductus arteriosus) close at birth or shortly thereafter.
- The cardiac output of an infant is normally 1 liter/minute. Toward the end of the toddler period, it increases to 1.5 liters/minute. At the age of 4 years, it is 2.2 liters/minute. By 15 years of age, cardiac output has reached the adult level of 5.5 liters/minute.
- Infants have a higher circulating blood volume (normally around 85 mL/kg) compared with that of an adult (65 mL/kg).

NURSING TIP

Reducing Salmonellosis

Reptiles, including pet turtles, shed salmonella in their feces. Thus, direct contact with a reptile or its cage poses a serious health risk to children of all ages, especially immunocompromised children. This information should be shared with parents and school officials because the incidence of reptile pets is increasing. If a child is in contact with a reptile, thorough hand washing is needed. In addition, the reptile should be confined to a particular space, and food preparation areas should be off-limits. Salmonellosis can occur from fomite contact alone.

Abdomen

- At birth, the neonate's umbilical cord contains two arteries and one vein.
- The infant's liver is proportionately larger in relation to the abdominal cavity than the liver of an adult.
- Infants' and toddlers' abdomens are more protuberant, but this does not necessarily indicate pathology.

Musculoskeletal System

- Bone growth ends for females around 2.5 years after menarche. For males, bone growth ends around age 20, when the epiphyses close.

Neurological System

- The neurological system of the infant is incompletely developed. The autonomic nervous system helps maintain homeostasis as the cerebral cortex develops.
- In the first 2 years, the neurons become myelinated, and primitive motor reflexes are replaced by purposeful movement. The myelinization occurs in a cephalocaudal and proximodistal manner (head and neck, trunk, and extremities).
- Myelinization in the bowel and bladder allows the child to control these functions and facilitates toilet training.

Urinary System

- In infancy, the urinary bladder is between the symphysis pubis and umbilicus.
- Infants and young children are unable to concentrate urine, predisposing them to dehydration and electrolyte abnormalities.

Female Genitalia

- Development of pubic hair in the female begins at puberty, between 8 and 12 years of age. Within about 1 year, the pubic hair becomes dark, coarse, and curly, although it is not considered fully developed. Axillary hair follows 6 months later. After about age 13 to 15, pubic hair distribution approaches adult quantity and consistency. See Sexual Maturity Rating in Table 21-1.

Male Genitalia

- The testes usually descend by the age of 1 year, but should always be "descendible."
- Puberty usually starts between the ages of 9½ and 13½ and can last 2 to 5 years. Testicular enlargement is usually the first area of sexual development to occur. Within about 1 year, the pubic hair becomes dark, coarse, and curly, although it is not fully developed. Axillary hair follows 6 months later. Facial hair follows approximately 6 months after the emergence of axillary hair. See Sexual Maturity Rating in Table 22-1 for additional information.

HEALTH HISTORY

The same principles that apply in obtaining an adult health history, such as questioning, listening, observing, and integrating, apply to obtaining a pediatric history. Because the historian in a pediatric history is less often the child and more likely the caregiver, it is very important to document the historian's relationship to the child. The following serves only to expand on the adult health history by providing information not previously discussed but relevant to the child.

BIOGRAPHICAL DATA

Client Name In addition to the client's name, obtain the full name of the legal guardian. Occasionally, the caregiver is not the legal guardian (e.g., when the child is a ward of the court or state).

Address and Phone Number Obtain the address, phone number, and e-mail of the caregiver if different from those of the client.

Source of Information Other than the client or caregiver, information can be obtained from medical and school records, diaries, clinic notes, children's agencies, public health departments, and home health agencies. Written consent is needed to release records to a third party.

CHIEF COMPLAINT

The caregiver is often the individual who seeks health care for the child and provides a description of the perceived problems, especially for infants, toddlers, and young preschoolers whose age and mental status prevent them from offering genuine descriptions of their problems. You must frequently rely on the caregiver's intuition in such cases. The caregiver is usually acutely aware of cues to the child's illness. For instance, changes in sleeping patterns (difficulty falling asleep, reversion to night waking), regression to outgrown behaviors (bedwetting, finicky eating, thumb sucking), and unusual physical complaints in an otherwise healthy child (headaches, stomachaches) are important signs that the child may be experiencing stress or illness and warrant further investigation. The older preschooler, school-age child, and adolescent can provide verbal descriptions of their complaints. Refer to Chapter 9 for pain rating scales that are used for children.

PAST HEALTH HISTORY

Much of the information outlined in the past health history for an adult applies to a child. Additional pertinent information should be elicited regarding the birth history, including prenatal, labor and delivery, and postnatal history.

Birth History Obtaining the birth history may be one of the more sensitive topics of the past health history. You must feel comfortable and show sensitivity when inquiring whether the pregnancy was planned, the date prenatal care was first sought, and the birth order of pregnancy, taking into account miscarriages and abortions. It is important to determine whether the child was adopted or born via surrogacy and, if so, what is known about the past medical history of the birth mother (or gestational parent).

Prenatal

1. Did you plan your pregnancy for ______ (insert name)?
2. How many weeks after thinking that you were pregnant did you go to a health-care provider for a checkup?
3. How many children have you carried to full term?
4. Were there any pregnancies that you were not able to carry to full term? What happened?
5. Did you take any prescribed or over-the-counter medications during pregnancy, including ibuprofen products?
6. Did you drink alcohol or caffeine or smoke cigarettes or vape during pregnancy?
7. Did you take any drugs during pregnancy, such as marijuana, crack cocaine, amphetamines, or hallucinogens such as LSD and mescaline? If so, what were the amounts and frequency of use?
8. Were there any problems or illnesses that either you or your health-care provider worried about during pregnancy (hypertensive disorders of pregnancy, HELLP syndrome, preeclampsia/eclampsia, preterm labor, gestational diabetes, group ß streptococcus [GBS], TORCH infection [toxoplasmosis, rubella, cytomegalovirus, and herpes], or an abnormal finding on a prenatal ultrasound)?
9. Was the pregnancy conceived naturally?

Labor and Delivery

1. How many weeks did you carry the baby before delivering?
2. Was the labor spontaneous or induced?
3. How many hours was the labor?
4. Was the baby delivered vaginally or by cesarean? If by cesarean, why?
5. Was any analgesia or anesthetic used?
6. Did you hold your baby immediately after delivery? (This question will provide information about the neonate's condition at delivery).
7. Immediately following delivery, what was the baby's color?
8. What were the baby's Apgar scores at 1 and 5 minutes? (See section on Apgar scoring later in this chapter).
9. What were the birth weight and length of the baby?
10. Was a partner, family member, or friend with you at the baby's birth?
11. Where was the baby born (home, hospital, automobile, or other location)?

Postnatal

1. Did you and your baby go home together? (If answered no, inquire as to the reason for separate discharges).
2. If hospital delivery, how long was the hospitalization for you and the baby?
3. Did the baby have any breathing or feeding problems during the first week?
4. To your knowledge, did your baby receive any medications during the first week?
5. How would you describe the baby's color at 1 week? (For light-skinned babies, ask if the skin was pale, pale pink, blue, or yellow. For the dark-skinned baby, inquire about the color of the sclera, oral mucosa, and nailbeds).
6. Did the baby receive any intervention for jaundice?
7. Was the baby circumcised?
8. Did you start breast- or bottle feeding your baby?
9. Were there any problems with your choice of feeding?
10. Did you or the baby have a fever after delivery?
11. Did the baby lose more than 10% of their birth weight?
12. Did the baby regain their birth weight by 10 to 14 days?
13. How did you feel 1 to 2 weeks after delivery?
14. Did you have anyone to help you take care of the baby in the first few weeks after delivery?
15. Did you or anyone else involved in caring for the baby have any signs or symptoms of postpartum depression or "baby blues"? Was treatment or counseling sought?

Medical History Inquire about the circumstances and outcomes of any hospitalizations or emergency department visits. Keep in mind that some children's caregivers may use the emergency department for episodic health care and may not have a primary care provider.

Surgical History Inquire if the child has ever had any surgery or surgical procedures

Communicable Diseases Measles was officially eliminated from the U.S. in 2000 (CDC, 2024). In 2024 the CDC (2024a) alerted communities of the increase in the number of measles cases and measles outbreaks in the U.S. 67% of these cases were in children with no immunization or had an unknown measles immunization status. Unvaccinated persons, travel to an endemic area, and the influx of unvaccinated people to the U.S. accounts for this situation (CDC, 2024b). In December 2025 the CDC reported an increase of infected people. There were 1,912 confirmed measles cases in 43 states. A small number of these cases were international visitors to the U.S. (CDC, 2025).

Injuries and Accidents Determine whether the child has a pattern of frequent injuries or accidents. Repeat trauma may indicate abuse.

Childhood Illnesses Document past and current exposure to measles, mumps, rubella, pertussis, chickenpox, COVID-19, and respiratory syncytial virus (RSV).

Immunizations Immunizations protect against many contagious diseases of childhood. The mother's (or gestational parent's) antibodies pass through the placenta and breast milk, offering the baby limited protection from disease. Table 25-1 lists a schedule of immunizations recommended by the Advisory Committee on Immunization Practice for children aged birth to 18 years (CDC, 2025). Many health-care providers follow the immunization schedule as a guide for well-child checkups. A record of immunizations is often important for school admission and to avoid repeat vaccinations. Many children fall behind on their immunization schedule, particularly during and after the COVID-19 pandemic, while immigrants to the United States may not have received some of the recommended immunizations. Dengue and Mpox vaccinations are administered to children under the age of 18 when specific criteria are met. The RSV monoclonal antibody, nirsevimab, is administered to infants if the pregnant person did not receive the RSV vaccine at gestational age 32 to 36 weeks in the months of September through January.

FAMILY HEALTH HISTORY

See Family Health History in Chapter 3. In addition, be sure also to ask about a family history of sudden infant death syndrome (SIDS), congenital disorders or defects, and cognitive, physical, or mental health conditions.

SOCIAL HISTORY

Work Environment Day-care facilities and schools are the child's equivalent of a work environment. Inquire about the number of hours the child attends a day-care facility or school per week, whether the day-care facility is licensed, private, or commercial and the number of children in the facility. Inquire about the child's academic performance. In addition, ask if the child is home alone before or after school.

Home Environment Ask about potential exposure to lead in chipping paint, because lead is harmful to the developing brain and nervous system of fetuses and young children. This group is four to five times more likely to absorb lead by ingestion than older children.

The next series of questions pertain to gun safety.

"Is there a gun in the home?"

"Where is the gun stored?"

"Is it locked?"

"Is the ammunition kept separate?"

Families are encouraged to ASK if there is an unlocked gun in any home the child may enter (Schaechter, 2023).

Child's Personal Habits

1. Determine what activities the child enjoys.
2. Ask how the child copes with stress and if a security object (blanket, stuffed toy) helps calm the child.
3. Determine whether the child is prone to temper tantrums and what type of discipline is used.

Domestic and Intimate Partner Violence Adolescents are not immune to intimate partner violence (IPV). Specific questions about IPV can be asked during the Home Environment section. Refer to Chapter 3 for detailed information.

1. Do you have a significant other?
2. What happens when one disagrees with the other?
3. Have you ever been hurt by someone you know?

HEALTH MAINTENANCE ACTIVITIES

Preventive health maintenance is essential for optimal health in the pediatric population. For a complete guide to pediatric preventive care, see the American Academy of Pediatrics' *Recommendations for Preventive Pediatric Health Care* at: *https://publications.aap.org/pediatrics/article/150/1/e2022058044/188302/2022-Recommendations-for-Preventive-Pediatric?_ga = 2.205738579.171541094.1663175585-61461165.1651090390*

Sleep

1. Determine the number of hours the child sleeps per day, including naps.
2. Ask if the child shares a bed and if so, with whom. Likewise, ask if the child shares a bedroom and if so, with whom.
3. Ask whether the child experiences night terrors or nightmares.
4. Ask whether the child sleepwalks.
5. Ask if the child remains dry during the night and if this is an issue for the child or the family. Primary nocturnal enuresis can be common in school-age children.

Diet Questions concerning diet must be tailored to the child's developmental level. See Chapter 7 for additional information.

Safety Childproofing the environment, especially for young children, is an essential practice. Incorporate these questions into your interview:

1. Tell me how you have childproofed your home.
2. Do you have gates on the top and bottom of the stairs?
3. Are the slats on the crib less than 2⅜ inches (6 cm) apart?
4. Have you removed the crib mobile for an infant who is trying to reach for objects (usually around 3 months)?
5. Is all sleepwear flame retardant?
6. Is the hot water thermostat turned down to 120° F (49°C)?
7. Have you installed potty locks to keep the toilet lid down?
8. Do you keep curtain and blind strings out of reach?
9. Have you placed all sharp items, such as razors and knives, out of reach of the child?
10. Do you sit within arm's reach of your child's bath? Do you always drain the water in the tub after getting the child out?
11. Do you have lead paint in your living quarters (homes built before 1978) or use items from other countries for feeding or playing?
12. Have you placed cushioned covering on the tub's water faucet and drain lever?
13. Do you use a nonskid bath mat in the tub?
14. Are there outlet covers on every outlet in the house?
15. When you are cooking, do you keep the pot or pan handles turned in?
16. Have you removed tablecloths from all tables?
17. Do you keep electrical cords out of reach?
18. Is the slack taken up on all electrical appliances and lamp cords?
19. If you have a raised hearth, have you covered it with bumpers, pads, or towels?
20. Are all of your plants out of reach?
21. Are your deck slats covered with a mesh net?
22. Are slip protectors under all rugs?
23. If you have a pool in the yard, is it fenced in, or is a protective cover on the top? Is there a functional alarm system for the pool? Do you assign a sober adult to watch the pool when children are swimming?
24. Do you empty pails that contain liquid after using them?
25. Are medications, cosmetics, pesticides, gasoline, cleaning solutions, paint thinner, detergents, batteries, and all other poisonous/dangerous materials out of the child's reach?
26. Do you have your local poison control center's telephone number next to each landline phone and entered into your mobile phone?
27. Do you have syrup of ipecac in the house? AAP recommended against using syrup of ipecac in the home setting starting in 2003.
28. Do you have smoke detectors close to or in the child's bedroom and on each floor of the house?
29. Do you have a fire extinguisher on each floor?
30. Have you devised and practiced an escape route plan in case of fire?
31. Are you and other caregivers of the child trained in cardiopulmonary resuscitation (CPR)?

32. What would you do in case of an emergency?
33. Where do you place your child's car seat—in the front or back seat, facing front or rear? What type of car seat is utilized (infant, 5-point harness, booster, etc.)? Do you place your child in the car where an airbag is supplied? Do you need or use a locking clip?
34. Does your child use protective gear such as a helmet or knee or elbow pads if participating in an activity in which injuries may occur?
35. Do you keep plastic dry cleaner overwraps, latex balloons (unattended by a caregiver), plastic trash bags, and grocery bags out of the child's reach?
36. Do you have a carbon monoxide detector in the house?
37. Do you give your child nutritional supplements or herbal remedies? If so, name the type and amount given.
38. Do you have a dog? Is the dog child friendly? Do you keep the dog on a leash when other children are visiting your home?
39. Are there other pets in the house? Which?

Table 25-1 Recommended Child and Adolescent Immunization Schedule for Ages 18 Years or Younger, United States, 2025

These recommendations must be read with the notes that follow. For those who fall behind or start late, provide catch-up vaccination at the earliest opportunity as indicated by the green bars.
To determine minimum intervals between doses, see the catch-up schedule (Table 2).

Vaccine and other immunizing agents	Birth	1 mo	2 mos	4 mos	6 mos	9 mos	12 mos	15 mos	18 mos	19–23 mos	2–3 yrs	4–6 yrs	7–10 yrs	11–12 yrs	13–15 yrs	16 yrs	17–18 yrs
Respiratory syncytial virus (RSV-mAb [Nirsevimab])	1 dose depending on maternal RSV vaccination status (See Notes)					1 dose (8 through 19 months), See Notes											
Hepatitis B (HepB)	1st dose	←2nd dose→			←3rd dose→												
Rotavirus (RV): RV1 (2-dose series), RV5 (3-dose series)			1st dose	2nd dose	See Notes												
Diphtheria, tetanus, acellular pertussis (DTaP <7 yrs)			1st dose	2nd dose	3rd dose			←4th dose→				5th dose					
Haemophilus influenzae type b (Hib)			1st dose	2nd dose	See Notes		←3rd or 4th dose (See Notes)→										
Pneumococcal conjugate (PCV15, PCV20)			1st dose	2nd dose	3rd dose		←4th dose→										
Inactivated poliovirus (IPV)			1st dose	2nd dose	←3rd dose→							4th dose					See Notes
COVID-19 (1vCOV-mRNA, 1vCOV-aPS)					1 or more doses of 2024–2025 vaccine (See Notes)												
Influenza (IIV3, ccIIV3)					1 or 2 doses annually								1 dose annually				
or																	
Influenza (LAIV3)											1 or 2 doses annually		1 dose annually				
Measles, mumps, rubella (MMR)					See Notes		←1st dose→					2nd dose					
Varicella (VAR)							←1st dose→					2nd dose					
Hepatitis A (HepA)					See Notes		2-dose series (See Notes)										
Tetanus, diphtheria, acellular pertussis (Tdap ≥7 yrs)														1 dose			
Human papillomavirus (HPV)														See Notes			
Meningococcal (MenACWY-CRM ≥2 mos, MenACWY-TT ≥2years)			See Notes											1st dose		2nd dose	
Meningococcal B (MenB-4C, MenB-FHbp)													See Notes				
Respiratory syncytial virus vaccine (RSV [Abrysvo])														Seasonal administration during pregnancy (See Notes)			
Dengue (DEN4CYD: 9–16 yrs)													Seropositive in endemic dengue areas (See Notes)				
Mpox																	

Range of recommended ages for all children; Range of recommended ages for catch-up vaccination; Range of recommended ages for certain high-risk groups or populations; Recommended vaccination can begin in this age group; Recommended vaccination based on shared clinical decision-making; No Guidance/Not Applicable

Page 2

Centers for Disease Control and Prevention. (2025). Child and adolescent immunization schedule by age. Retrieved December 18, 2025, from *https://www.cdc.gov/vaccines/schedules/hcp/imz/child-adolescent.html*

Growth and Development

Refer to Chapter 4 for a summary of motor, language, and sensory tasks that normal children from infancy through adolescence can accomplish.

Developmental Assessment

A commonly used tool for assessing the development of the child from birth through 6 years of age is the Revised- Denver II (Fig. 25-6) (Frankenburg, 1990). The test is composed of four sections: personal-social, fine motor-adaptive, language, and gross motor. There are a total of 125 items described on the test. Some items can be accomplished easily by observing the child without commands from the observer. For instance, the child may be smiling spontaneously, saying words other than "mama" or "dada," or sitting with the head held steady. Certain items can be given an automatic pass mark if the caregiver indicates that the child can accomplish the corresponding item, such as drinking from a cup, washing and drying hands, or dressing without help. Other commonly used assessments include the CDC's Developmental Milestones (2024) and Ages and Stages Questionnaire for parents. (See Chapter 4 for more detail.)

Before administering the test, determine the child's chronological age and draw a straight line through the four sections intersecting the age intervals on the top and bottom of the sheet. This line indicates which items are to be tested for the child's chronological age. Begin testing by assessing the item that is three items to the left of the age line. Documentation is reflected by using a "P" for pass, "F" for fail, "R" for refuses, and "NO" for no opportunity. Give up to three trials before documenting the score for that particular item on the Revised-Denver II. At the end, complete the five test behavior questions. A normal test consists of no delays and a maximum of one caution. A caution is failure of a client to perform an item that has been achieved by 75% to 90% of children the same age. A delay is a failure of any item to the left of the age line. A suspect test has one or more delays or two or more cautions; in these instances, retest the child in 1 to 2 weeks.

Keep in mind that current illness, lack of sleep, fear and anxiety, language barriers, deafness, or blindness can affect a child's performance. If these or other logical rationales can explain a child's failure to complete a series of Revised-Denver II items during a session, readminister the test in 1 month if the preexisting condition has been resolved (as appropriate). If the child does have a developmental disability, early detection can lead to appropriate intervention and assistance.

Pediatric Pain Assessment

Research has shown that pain in children is often poorly assessed and not thoroughly addressed. Pain increases a child's sense of fear and vulnerability, an emotion that is already felt whenever a child is sick or injured. Thus, for children who cannot easily verbalize or communicate their experiences, pain potentially compounds the child's fear and feelings of vulnerability. Nurses' lack of adequate knowledge about assessment techniques and age-appropriate pain assessment tools has been identified as a reason for inadequate pain management in children. Although several pain assessment tools have been developed and are available, none have been identified as the best in all situations. The individual child's age and developmental level should be taken into consideration when choosing a pain assessment tool. Two tools that have been successful in assessing children's pain are the Wong-Baker FACES Rating Scale (FACES) (Fig. 9-19) and the Oucher Scale (Fig. 9-20). Assessment tools should be used to assist in establishing and documenting a child's pain. However, they should be used in conjunction with nurses' observational and assessment skills. Nurses should also be aware of behavioral and physiological signs that may indicate a child is in pain; these include grimacing, posture, and positioning of affected areas of the body (Fig. 25-7). Parents and caregivers can also help determine whether their child's behavior indicates discomfort or pain.

NURSING TIP
HEEADSSS 3.0 Assessment

A valuable tool that is easily remembered during the adolescent's health history is the HEEADSSS 3.0 assessment. This tool highlights vital areas of an adolescent's daily life that can affect physical and mental well-being. The letters in this acronym represent the first letter in the subject area that is to be asked about. The HEEADSSS acronym stands for:

- **H** Home environment
- **E** Education/Employment
- **E** Eating and Exercise
- **A** Activities
- **D** Drugs, Substances, and Alcohol
- **S** Sexuality
- **S** Suicide/Depression
- **S** Safety

NURSING TIP
Prevalence of Birth Defects

One in every 33 babies in the United States is born with a birth defect. The most common of these defects involves the heart (congenital heart defects), spine (spina bifida), lip/palate (cleft lip and/or palate), and urinary meatus (hypospadias). Taking a thorough family history of major birth defects enables the health-care provider to better assess potential risk factors and give advice on preventive measures for future pregnancies. For example, a mother (or gestational parent) whose baby was born with spina bifida can be counseled to take folic acid supplementation before conception to reduce the risk of having another child born with a neural tube defect.

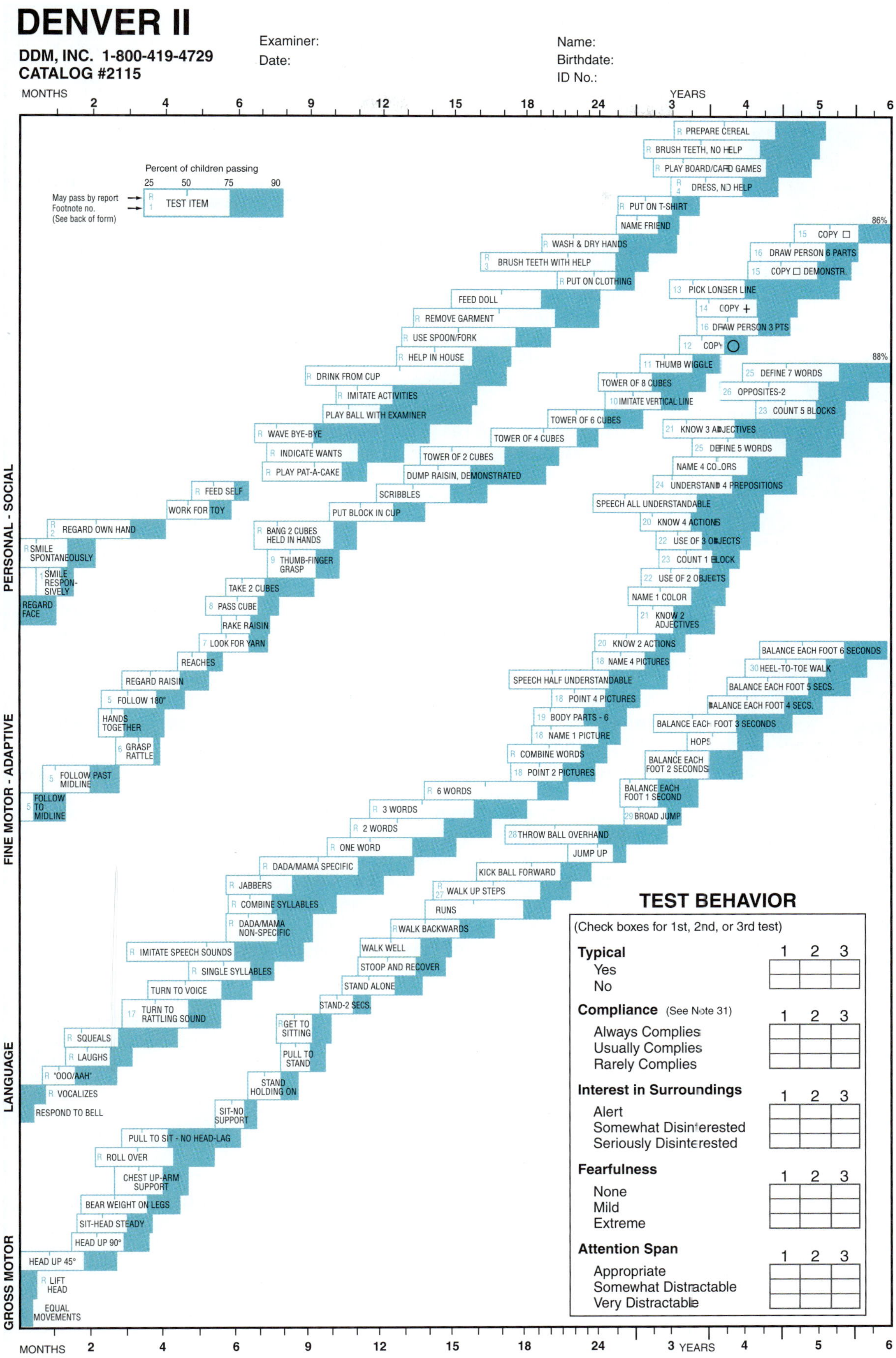

©1969, 1989, 1990 W. K. Frankenburg and J. B. Dodds ©1978 W. K. Frankenburg ©2009 Wilhelmine R. Frankenburg

Figure 25-6 Revised-Denver II.

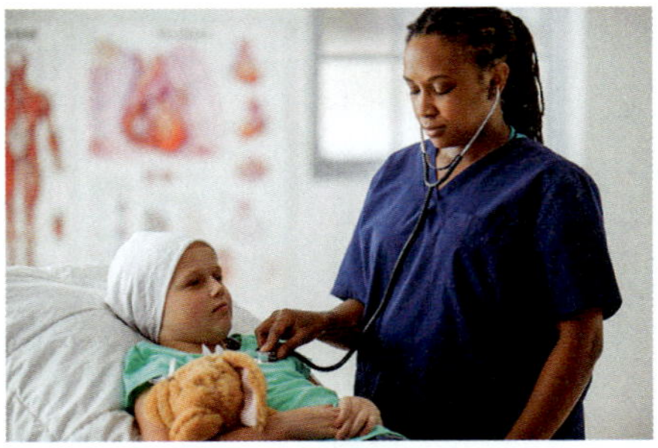

Figure 25-7 The nurse can assess the child's pain level while providing care.

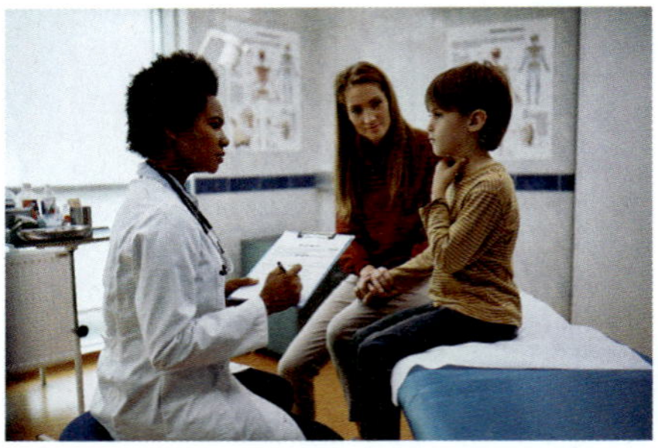

Figure 25-8 Having a parent or caregiver present during the examination can decrease the child's anxiety.

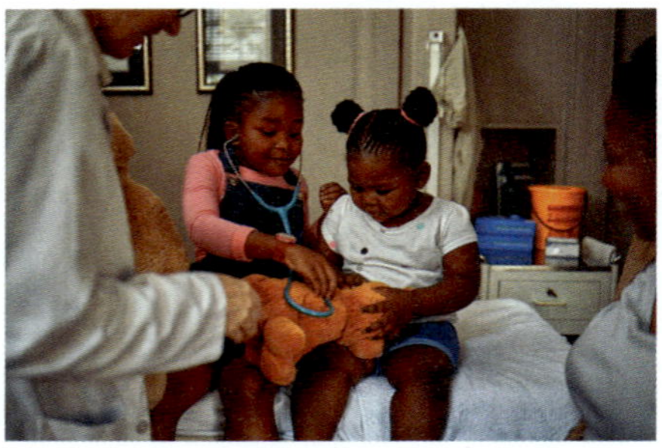

Figure 25-9 Allowing the young child to touch equipment and use pretend play goes a long way in alleviating anxiety during the examination.

NURSING CHECKLIST

General Approach to Pediatric Physical Examination

1. Observe Standard Precautions and don personal protective equipment (PPE) such as gloves, gown, face shield, goggles, N-95 respirator mask or face mask if the child's status warrants these protective measures.
2. Examine the client in a warm, quiet room. To prevent hypothermia, always keep infants under the age of 6 months warm during the examination.
3. Use natural lighting, if available, during the examination. Fluorescent lighting makes assessing varying degrees of cyanosis and jaundice difficult.
4. To help reduce anxiety and uncooperativeness (especially when examining young children), have a familiar caregiver present during the examination (Fig. 25-8).
5. Talk to the child in a soothing voice; even an infant who cannot understand your words will take comfort in a calm and supportive approach.
6. Explain all procedures in developmentally appropriate terms and allow older infants, toddlers, preschoolers, and younger school-age clients to touch or manipulate medical equipment (Fig. 25-9).
7. To promote the child's feeling of security, allow the infant who cannot sit up and the younger child to sit on the caregiver's lap for as much of the examination as possible.
8. Until the infant or toddler is comfortable, maintain eye contact with the caregiver while the examination is taking place. Maintaining eye contact with a child who experiences anxiety in the presence of strangers can interfere with the completion of the examination. Maintain eye contact with the caregiver if other means of alleviating the client's fears are not successful.
9. Interview the older school-age child or adolescent separately, without the caregiver. Talking to the individual without the caregiver present may yield important information not gained during a group interview (e.g., that the client is using drugs).
10. Adolescents are often reluctant to discuss issues such as substance use or sexuality with unfamiliar adults. Therefore, when discussing private and/or sensitive matters with adolescent clients, use an honest, nonjudgmental approach. Be sure to clarify confidentiality parameters at the beginning of any visit.
11. Respect the client's modesty.
12. Warm your equipment (e.g., stethoscope, hands).
13. Avoid making abrupt movements, because these may startle a child.
14. If the child is sleeping, take advantage of the situation by performing simple procedures (length, head circumference) and system examinations that require a quiet room (such as the cardiac and respiratory examinations) first.
15. Perform all invasive or uncomfortable procedures (ear inspection, hip palpation) last because they may cause discomfort, crying, fear, and increased heart rate.
16. Always provide comfort measures during and following pain. It is especially helpful to allow the caregiver the opportunity to provide supportive measures. This shows the child that you are genuinely concerned about their feelings.
17. To prevent falls, always keep one hand on any infant or toddler who is placed on the examination table.
18. Before completing the examination, ask the caregiver and client what questions they have.

Assessment in Brief

Pediatric Examination*

**Only pediatric-specific examinations are listed. All other examination skills are performed as described in Chapters 9–23.*

Developmental Assessment

- Denver II

Physical Growth

- Weight
- Length or height
- Head circumference
- Chest circumference

Apgar Scoring

- Heart rate
- Respiratory rate
- Tone
- Reflex irritability
- Color

Physical Examination

- Head
  - Inspection
    - Head control
  - Palpation
    - Anterior fontanel
    - Posterior fontanel
    - Suture lines
    - Surface characteristics
- Eyes
  - Vision screening
  - Red reflex
  - Tumbling E chart
  - Strabismus screening
  - Color vision screening
- Breasts
  - Sexual maturity rating
- Musculoskeletal system
  - Inspection
    - Tibiofemoral bones
  - Palpation
    - Feet (metatarsus varus)
    - Hip and femur (Barlow/Ortolani maneuver)

Physical Examination (cont.)

- Neurological system
  - Rooting reflex
  - Sucking reflex
  - Palmar grasp reflex
  - Tonic neck reflex
  - Stepping reflex
  - Plantar grasp reflex
  - Babinski reflex
  - Moro (startle) reflex
  - Galant reflex
  - Placing reflex
  - Landau reflex
- Genitalia
  - Sexual maturity rating
- Anus
  - Anal reflex

Advanced Techniques

- Assessing for hydrocephalus and anencephaly: Transillumination of the skull
- Assessing for coarctation of the aorta

Equipment

- Appropriate PPE
- Equipment listed in Chapters 9–23
- Scale (infant and stand-up)
- Appropriate-sized blood pressure cuff
- Snellen E and Tumbling E charts
- Color vision charts
- Ophthalmoscope
- Otoscope, speculum (2.5 to 4 mm), pneumatic attachment
- Pediatric stethoscope
- Growth charts
- Small bell
- Brightly colored object
- Revised-Denver II materials
- Clean gloves
- Disposable centimeter tape measure

> **NURSING TIP**
> **Facilitating the Pediatric Examination**
> - Use game playing and distraction to increase client cooperativeness. It is important to have available different items of distraction that can be used when a client is uncooperative or focusing on what will be done next. Distractions include small toys that easily hook onto a stethoscope, wind-up musical toys, and humming, whistling, or whispering.
> - Demonstrate procedures on a doll, stuffed toy, or even the caregiver before performing them on the child.
> - If available, consult with and/or utilize Child Life professionals when dealing with difficult, anxiety-producing, or uncomfortable experiences.

> **NURSING TIP**
> **Obtaining Blood Pressure in Children**
> Never use the phrases "take your blood pressure" or "hug your arm" with a younger pediatric client, because they may mislead a child. Say instead, "This cuff is going to squeeze your arm" or, to the older child, "I am going to measure your pressure."

Physical Examination

Many examination techniques for the child are similar to those for the adult. Refer to the specific system chapters for detailed explanations of examination techniques covered in those chapters.

Techniques for approaching the pediatric client vary from one age-group to the next. A basic principle during any physical examination is building a trusting relationship; this can be done in a variety of ways. First, always explain what will be done before each portion of the examination and answer questions honestly. Second, praise the client for positive behaviors (for example, cooperating during examination of the middle ear). Displaying a caring attitude will greatly influence both the client's and the caregiver's sense of trust. Show respect for the client as an individual and allow expression of feelings (whimpering, crying).

Vital Signs

General Approach

1. The act of measuring vital signs is often disturbing to a young child. Past experiences influence the degree of cooperation you will encounter.
2. Vital signs may be obtained at the beginning of the examination or during the examination of a certain system. Blood pressure and rectal temperature measurements are more threatening and should be performed toward the end of the examination, preferably before using the otoscope.
3. If the child is particularly anxious, it is best to integrate the assessment of vital signs into the overall examination.

Temperature

You need to be proficient in measuring axillary, rectal, oral, temporal artery, noncontact infrared, and tympanic temperatures. A rectal temperature is not appropriate in all instances; for example, it is contraindicated in a child who presents with a history of diarrhea or in a child who is immunocompromised. Accurate oral temperature is difficult to obtain in most toddlers and preschoolers. Axillary temperature, though quick and painless, is often less reliable than rectal or oral temperatures. Temporal artery, tympanic, and noncontact infrared temperatures are quick, painless, and accurate if performed correctly. In addition, the temporal artery and noncontact infrared temperatures can be obtained in a noninvasive manner. Refer to Chapter 9.

Axillary

E
1. When taking axillary temperature, have the child sit or lie on the caregiver's lap to free your hands for other observations or to prepare for the next area of examination.
2. Explain to the child that this type of temperature measurement does not hurt. To pass time, ask the caregiver to read the child a story.

N **A** **P** See Chapter 9.

Rectal

E
1. Children dislike having rectal temperature taken, so your approach to explanation should be matter-of-fact: "I need to measure your temperature in your bottom. You need to hold very still while I do this. Your caregiver will be right here with you."

2. Place the child in either a side-lying or a prone position on the caregiver's lap or place the child on the back of the examination table and firmly grasp the feet with your nondominant hand.
3. After lubricating the stub-tipped thermometer, insert it gently into the child's rectum: ½ inch (1.3 cm) for newborns, ¾ inch (1.9 cm) for infants, and 1 inch (2.5 cm) for preschoolers and older children. Hold the thermometer firmly between your fingers to avoid accidentally inserting it too far. Firmly hold the buttocks together during measurement to prevent expelling the thermometer prematurely. Be sure to have a protective chux under the child as this often stimulates a bowel movement.

N A P See Chapter 9.

Respiratory Rate

E
1. Try to obtain the respiratory rate early in the examination, when the child is most cooperative and not crying.
2. If the child is crying, the measurement will not be accurate and should be retaken.
3. Remember to observe the expansion of the abdomen in infants and toddlers.
4. For infants, count for a full minute due to physiological periodic breathing.

N A P See Chapter 9.

Physical Growth

Weight

Use the same scale at each visit, if possible, to prevent variations in serial weight checks.

E
1. If using an infant scale, cover it with a paper protector.
2. Balance or zero the scale (if the child is wearing a clean diaper, make sure to zero the scale with another clean diaper of the same size; change any dirty diapers before weighing).
3. Place infants supine and young toddlers seated on the scale (Fig. 25-10). Always keep one hand on the child to prevent falls and lift your hand slightly when obtaining the actual weight reading.
4. Preschoolers and young school-age children can wear street clothes to be weighed (Fig. 25-11). Have the older child undress, don a paper or cloth gown, and step on the standard platform scale, if the scale is in the room. If the scale is outside the room, have the child remain in lightweight clothing and remove shoes.
5. Note and record weight.

N **Refer to the growth charts in Figs. 25-1A and B and Figs. 25-1E and F. Usually, neonates lose approximately 10% of birth weight by the third or fourth day after birth, then regain it by 10 to 14 days of age. This expected change in weight is called physiological weight loss, and it is due to a loss of extracellular fluid and meconium, a dark-green, sticky, stool-like substance excreted from the rectum within the first 24 hours after birth.**

A A newborn weight less than the 10th gestational age percentile is considered abnormal.

P A newborn whose growth has been inhibited in utero is referred to as small for gestational age (SGA). Potential causes include alcohol, drug, or tobacco abuse by the mother (or gestational parent), or certain genetic syndromes.

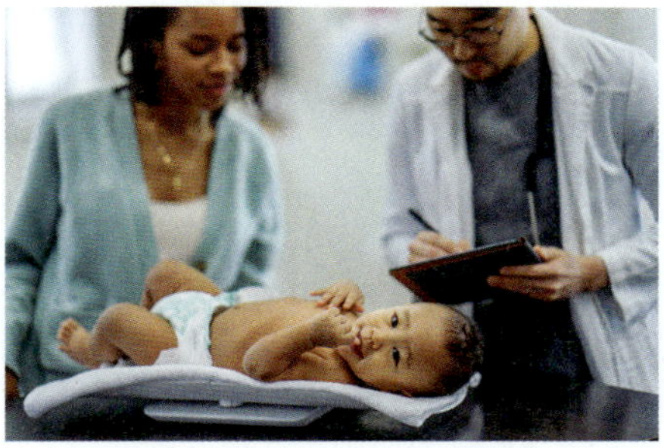

Figure 25-10 Measuring weight in the infant.

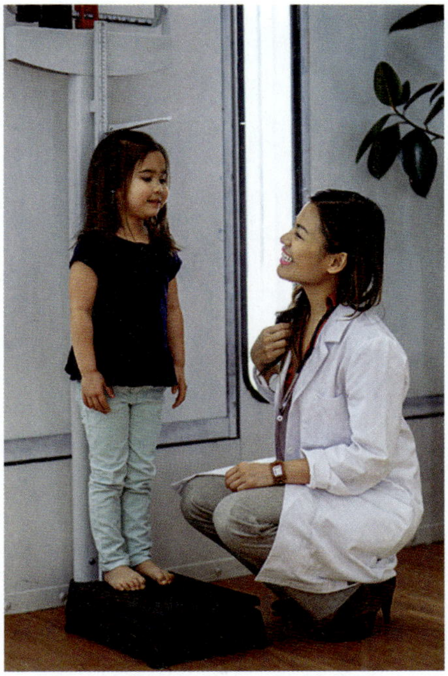

Figure 25-11 Measuring weight in the preschooler.

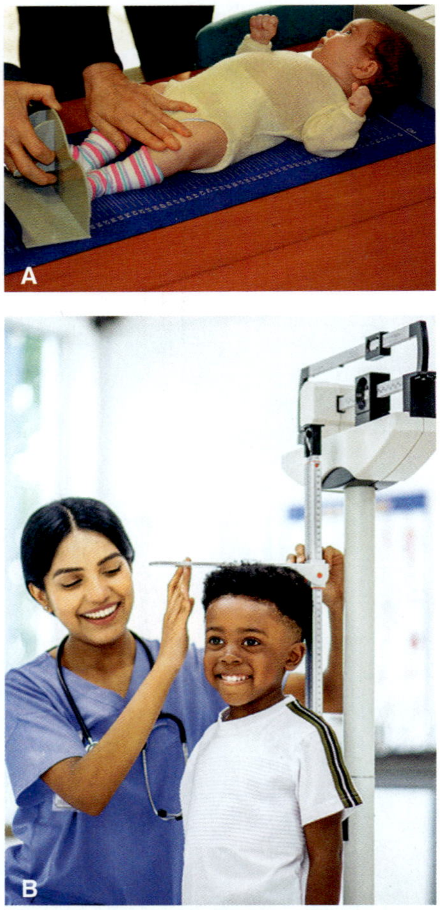

Figure 25-12 Measuring length and height in children. **A.** Recumbent length in an infant. **B.** Height in preschooler.

A A newborn weight greater than the 90th gestational age percentile is abnormal.

P A mother (or gestational parent) with diabetes or a genetic predisposition may give birth to a large for gestational age (LGA) newborn.

A A weight below the 5th or above the 95th percentiles warrants investigation, as does the child who falls 2 standard deviations below their own established curve. Any such finding is abnormal.

P Possible causes of weight below the 5th percentile include organic or nonorganic failure to thrive, congenital or cyanotic heart disease, cystic fibrosis (CF), fetal alcohol syndrome, and malabsorption diseases. Weight above the 95th percentile is caused by overeating and decreased physical activity in the majority of children, though genetic/hormonal causes must be considered.

Length or Height

Recumbent length is measured for children less than 2 years old.

E
1. Position the measuring board flat on the examination table.
2. Place the child's head at the top of the board and the child's heels at the foot of the board, making sure the legs are fully extended (Fig. 25-12A).
3. Measure and record the length.
4. If a board is not available, place the child in a supine position and mark lines on the paper at the tip of the head and the heel, making sure the legs are fully extended.
5. Measure between the lines and record.

Height for all other age-groups can be measured in the same fashion as for an adult.

Fig. 25-12B shows a preschooler's height being measured.

N **See the growth charts in Figs. 25-1A and B and Figs. 25-1E and F.**

A A height below the 5th or above the 95th percentile warrants investigation, as does the child who falls 2 standard deviations below their own established curve. Any such finding is abnormal.

P Possible causes of height below the 5th percentile include organic or nonorganic failure to thrive, congenital or cyanotic heart disease, CF, fetal alcohol syndrome, and malabsorption diseases. Height above the 95th percentile may be familial though genetic/hormonal causes must be considered.

Head Circumference

Head circumference is measured in all children less than 2 years of age or serially in children with known or suspected hydrocephalus. Measuring head circumference is an invaluable tool in the infant with suspected cessation of brain growth.

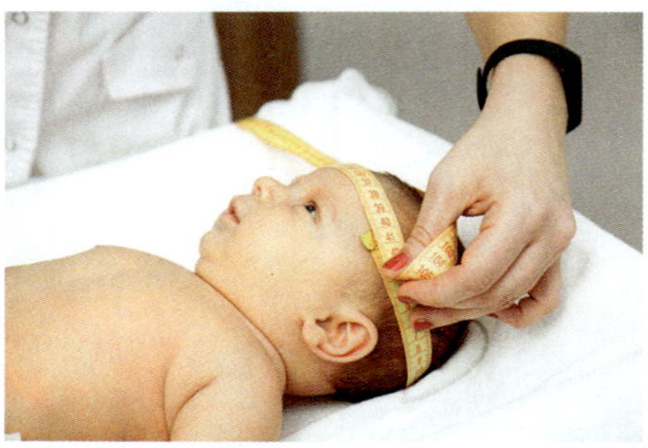

Figure 25-13 Measuring head circumference.

E
1. Place the child in a sitting or supine position.
2. Using a tape measure, measure anteriorly from above the eyebrows and around posteriorly to the occipital protuberance (Fig. 25-13).

N **Refer to Figs. 25-1C and D. Normal average head growth is $3/8$ to $5/8$ inches (1 to 1.5 cm) per month during the first year. Premature infants often have small head circumferences.**

A **Microcephaly**, a condition characterized by a small brain with a resultant small head, is an abnormal finding.

E Examination N Normal Findings A Abnormal Findings P Pathophysiology

P Microcephaly is a congenital finding associated with a mental deficit. Microcephaly can be caused by a variety of disorders, including intrauterine infections (such as the Zika virus), drug or alcohol ingestion (fetal alcohol syndrome) during pregnancy, and genetic defects.

A **Hydrocephalus** (enlarged head) is indicated when an infant's or young child's head circumference is above the 95th percentile and crosses over the child's established percentile lines from one serial measurement to the next. Hydrocephalus is abnormal. Note if the eyes are looking downward ("setting sun" sign) and the sclera is visible above the iris.

P Hydrocephalus is characterized by an imbalance in cerebrospinal fluid (CSF) production and reabsorption. Hydrocephalus may result from embryological malformations of the nervous system. Congenital hydrocephalus can also be caused by syphilis, rubella, toxoplasmosis, or cytomegalovirus. Bacterial meningitis or tumors are acquired causes of hydrocephalus. The setting sun sign results from progressive enlargement of the lateral and third ventricles related to excessive accumulation of CSF.

Chest Circumference

If necessary and requested by a provider, chest circumference can be measured. This measurement by itself provides little information but is compared with the head circumference to evaluate the child's overall growth.

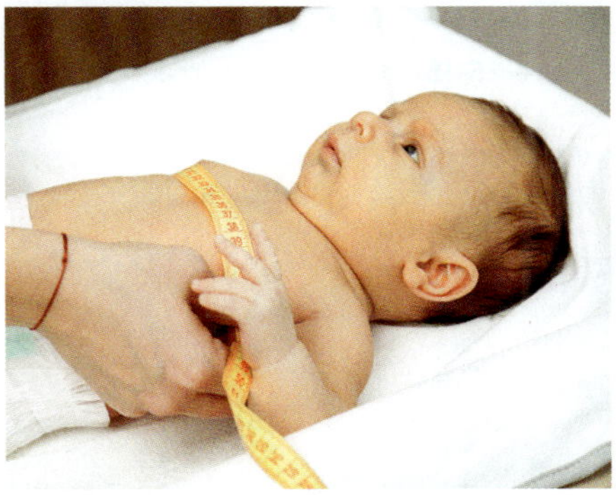
Figure 25-14 Measuring chest circumference.

E
1. Stand in front of the supine child.
2. Measure the chest circumference by placing the tape measure around the chest at the nipple line (Fig. 25-14).
3. Measure during exhalation.

N **From birth to about 1 year, the head circumference is greater than the chest circumference. After age 1, the chest circumference is greater than the head circumference.**

A A measured chest circumference below normal limits is abnormal.

P A below-normal chest circumference for age can be attributed to prematurity.

Apgar Scoring

The **Apgar score** system provides a quick method to assess the need for newborn resuscitation in the delivery room. An Apgar score is given to a newborn at 1 and 5 minutes after birth. Perform steps 1 through 5 at 1 minute following birth; add the score in each category for the total. Repeat at 5 minutes following birth.

E
1. Auscultate the heart rate for 1 full minute.
2. Measure the degree of respiratory effort.
3. Evaluate muscle tone by attempting to straighten each extremity individually.
4. Evaluate the newborn's reflex irritability. Use a flicking motion of two fingers against the newborn's sole to rate reflex irritability.
5. Inspect the newborn's color.

N **A score of 8 to 10 demonstrates that the newborn is in good condition. Table 25-2 outlines the scoring system for each of the five areas assessed.**

Table 25-2 Apgar Scoring

Heart Rate	Respiratory Rate	Tone	Reflex Irritability	Color
Absent = 0	Apnea = 0	Flaccid = 0	No response = 0	Cyanosis = 0
< 100 = 1	Slow, irregular rate = 1	Some degree of flexion = 1	Grimace = 1	Body pink, extremities acrocyanotic = 1
> 100 = 2	Crying vigorously = 2	Full flexion = 2	Crying = 2	Completely pink = 2

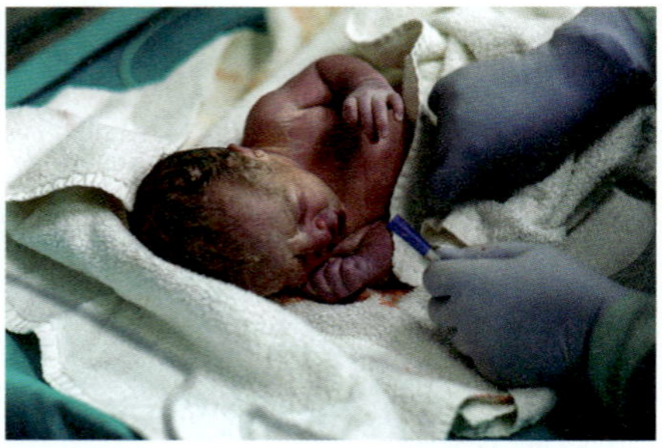

Figure 25-15 Acrocyanosis in a newborn.

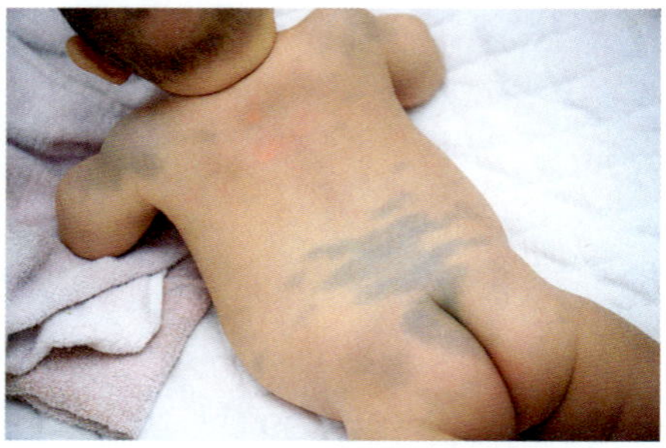

Figure 25-16 Congenital dermal melanocytosis (formerly known as Mongolian spots).

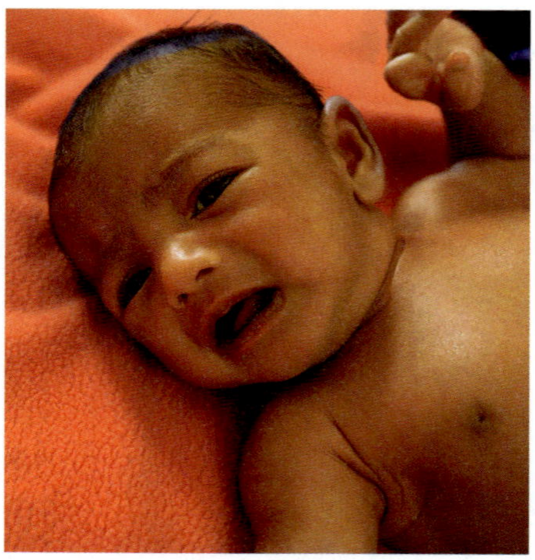

Figure 25-17 Physiological jaundice of a newborn.

A A moderately depressed newborn earns a score of 4 to 7. A score of 0 to 3 indicates that the newborn is severely depressed and needs immediate resuscitation. Either finding is abnormal.

P A low score can be the result of one or numerous problems. Prematurity, central nervous system depression, blood or meconium in the trachea, maternal or (gestational parent) history of drug abuse, certain drugs that are given to the mother (or gestational parent) in preparation for delivery and that cross over and cause fetal depression, congenital complete heart block, and congenital heart disease are some of the potential etiologies for a low Apgar score.

Skin

Inspection

Color

E Observe the color of the body, especially at the tip of the nose, the external ear, the lips, the hands, and the feet. In darker-skinned individuals, assess the conjunctiva, palms, soles, and tongue. These areas are prominent locations for detecting cyanosis or jaundice.

N **In light-skinned newborns the integument is reddish in color for the first 24 hours and then changes to varying shades of pale pink to pink to brown or black, depending on the child's race. It is normal for dark-skinned newborns to have a ruddy appearance and for light-skinned newborns to exhibit a bluish-purple color of the hands and feet while the rest of the body remains pink. This is called acrocyanosis (Fig. 25-15). It may disappear with warming. Congenital dermal melanocytosis (formerly known as Mongolian spots) is a deep blue pigmentation over the lumbar and sacral areas of the spine, over the buttocks, and sometimes over the upper back or shoulders in newborns of African, Hispanic, or Asian descent (Fig. 25-16), are extremely common and not to be confused with ecchymosis or signs of child abuse.**

A A blue hue is abnormal in light-skinned newborns. In darker-skinned infants, cyanosis may present as whitish-gray, especially around the mouth.

P Cyanosis in the newborn is often associated with a congenital heart defect secondary to the abnormal mixing of arterial and venous blood. In the older child with unrepaired heart disease, cyanosis may be a sign of decreasing levels of oxygen saturation.

A A yellowing of the skin or sclera is abnormal. In darker-skinned individuals, jaundice may appear as greenish-yellow of the skin (Fig. 25-17).

P Physiological jaundice of the newborn occurs on the second or third day of life. This type of jaundice results from increased levels of serum bilirubin. The newborn's body is unable to remove the bilirubin, thus producing a yellow cast or hue to the skin of light-skinned infants and the sclera of both light- and dark-skinned infants.

P Pathological jaundice of the newborn occurs within the first 24 hours of life. Possible causes of pathological jaundice include Rh/ABO incompatibility and infections (rubella, herpes, syphilis, or toxoplasmosis) in the mother (or gestational parent). The pathophysiological response occurs because there is a deficiency or inactivity of bilirubin glucuronyl transferase in the newborn.

P Breast milk jaundice occurs within the first 2 weeks of life, with the onset being 4 to 5 days after birth. The etiology is not clear, but breast milk may contain an inhibitor of bilirubin conjugation.

A It is abnormal when the light-skinned newborn lies on one side and the dependent half becomes red or ruddy and the upper half turns pale. In dark-skinned children, the dependent half may become a ruddy color and the upper half seems normal.

P **Harlequin color change** is a benign condition thought to be a result of poor vasomotor control. It occurs between 48 and 96 hours after birth.

A Erythema of the palms or soles, edema of the hands or feet, or periungual desquamation is found in children presenting with Kawasaki disease (mucocutaneous lymph node syndrome). For a practitioner to diagnose Kawasaki disease, the child must present with a fever for 5 days and with four of the five diagnostic criteria. Signs other than those previously mentioned include bilateral, nonexudative conjunctival injection; at least one of several possible mucous membrane changes, including injected or fissured lips, injected pharynx, or strawberry tongue; polymorphous exanthema; and acute nonsuppurative cervical lymphadenopathy.

P The cause of Kawasaki disease is unknown. Coronary artery vasculitis is a major concern as the disease progresses.

Lesions

E N See Chapter 10.

A Lesions that are usually symmetrical, scaly, erythematous patches or plaques with possible exudation and crusting are abnormal.

P Eczema or atopic dermatitis (AD) is a common abnormal skin disorder involving inflammation of the epidermis and superficial dermis (Fig. 25-18). Inhaled allergens, such as pollens, molds, or dust mites, or food allergens are thought to induce mast cell responses that cause AD.

A Small, maculopapular lesions on an erythematous base, wheals, and vesicles that erupt on the newborn are abnormal.

P Erythema toxicum is a benign rash. The cause is unknown.

A Flat, deep, irregular, localized, pink areas in light-skinned children and deeper red areas in dark-skinned children are abnormal.

P Pink nevus simplex, commonly known as stork bites, angel kiss, or salmon patch, appear on the forehead, back of the neck, lower occiput, upper eyelids, and nasolabial (Fig. 25-19). They do not require treatment and often fade within this first year of life. The cause is capillary dilation.

A Diffuse redness, papules, vesicles, edema, scaling, and ulcerations on the area covered by a baby's diaper are abnormal.

> **NURSING TIP**
> **Integumentary Signs of Child Abuse**
> - When examining the skin, observe for injuries in a location the child cannot reach, such as the back.
> - Examine for "item" marks, such as marks produced by irons, belts, electrical cords, cigarettes, or teeth.
> - Check for excessive bruising and numerous bruises in various stages of healing.
> - Look for hot water scalding marks, which present as even lines across the skin (usually on the legs or buttocks), often termed stocking or glove patterns on feet and hands.
> - Check extremities for a limited range of motion and tenderness, which can be related to fractures.

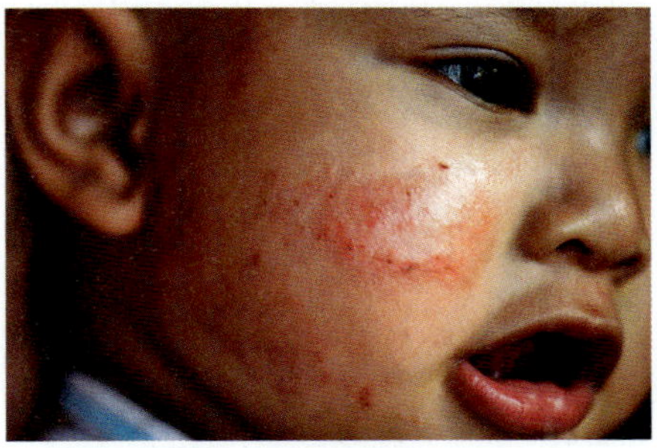

Figure 25-18 Atopic dermatitis in an infant.

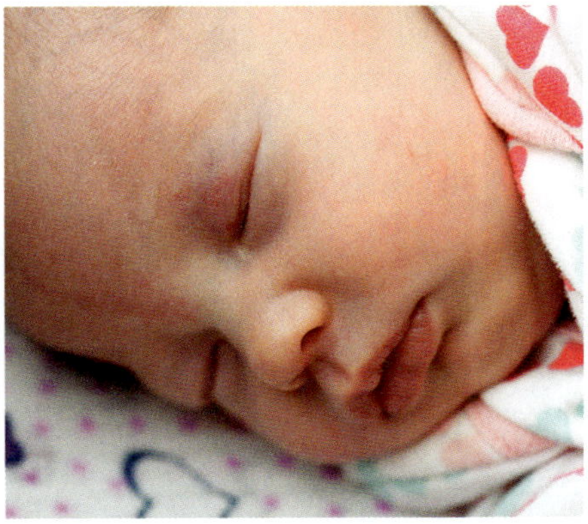

Figure 25-19 Pink nevus simplex.

NURSING TIP

Adoption and Foster Care

Many families choose to adopt or foster children from within the United States; others choose to adopt children from other countries. Foster care and adoptions often result in multiracial or multicultural families. Millions of children have joined their families via adoption in the United States. In addition to providing the child with a sense of safety and security, families have the responsibility of providing children with knowledge about their ethnic origins, culture, and values. The American Academy of Pediatrics recommends the following ways to instill a sense of pride and allow children to experience their heritage: visit cultural programs and ethnic restaurants as a family; include multiethnic food, art, and objects as a part of the family's home; and read multicultural books and literature to all children in the family (American Academy of Pediatrics, 2019, 2020).

To assure a successful and healthy adoption, families planning international adoption should carefully consider all aspects of the adoption process, including cultural, legal, and medical aspects. All available information regarding the child's family and medical histories should be obtained to aid health-care providers in meeting the child's health-care needs and to better understand any health issues for which the child may be at risk.

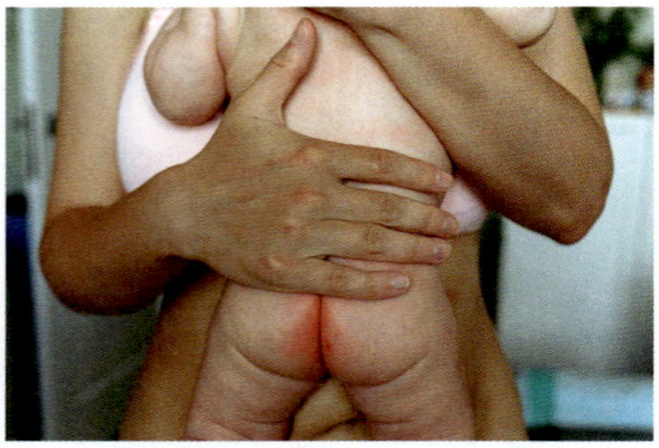

Figure 25-20 Diaper dermatitis.

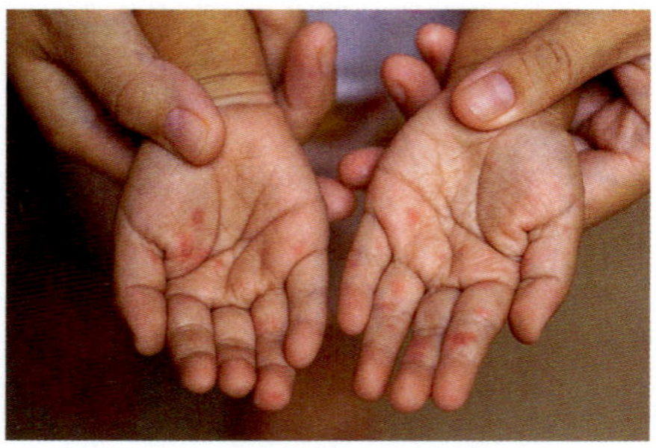

Figure 25-21 Hand vesicles on a child with hand-foot-mouth disease.

P Possible causes of diaper dermatitis (Fig. 25-20) include fecal enzymes, irritated skin, stool consistency and frequency, *Candida,* cleansing agents, sensitive skin, and poor nutrition.

A Vesicles located on the palms of hands (Fig. 25-21), soles of feet, and in the mouth are abnormal. A papular erythematous rash may also be on the buttocks.

P Hand-foot-mouth disease is caused by coxsackievirus A16.

A A dark black tuft of hair or a dimple over the lumbosacral area is abnormal.

P The neural tube fails to fuse at about the fourth week of gestation and causes a vertebral defect known as spina bifida occulta.

A A myelomeningocele is an open spina bifida lesion in which there is either no skin covering or neural tissue covered only by a thin membrane (Fig. 25-22A and B).

P Myelomeningocele has been associated with maternal (or gestational parent) diabetes mellitus, obesity, fever, hyperthermia, and the use of valproic acid and carbamazepine. The increased incidence of neural tube defects seen in some lower socioeconomic groups suggests that nutritional deficiencies, particularly lack of folic acid, may play a significant role in etiology. Neural tube defects are presumably caused by failure of the neural tube to close between the third and fourth week of gestation, resulting in abnormalities of the brain and spinal cord.

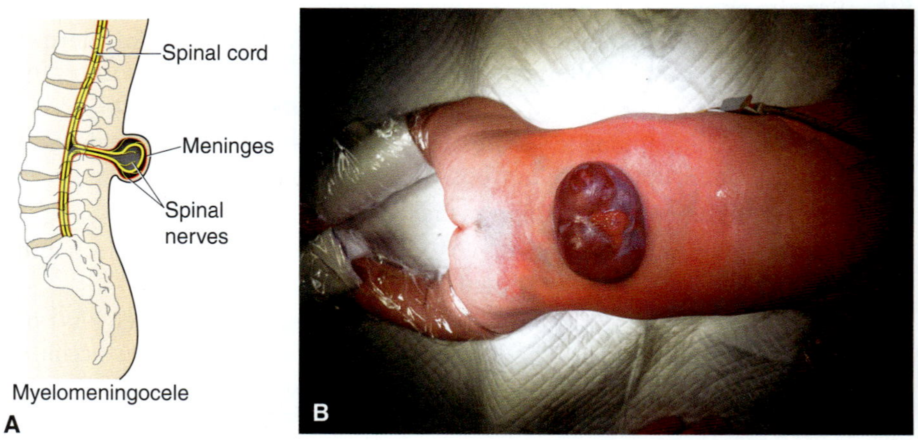

Figure 25-22 Myelomeningocele. **A.** Schematic anatomic representation. **B.** Myelomeningocele in an infant.

Palpation

Texture

E
1. Use the finger pads to palpate the skin.
2. The technique of palpating the skin of a younger child can be accomplished by playing games. For example, use the finger pads to "walk" up the abdomen and touch the nose.

N **The skin of the pediatric client normally is smooth and soft. Milia, plugged sebaceous glands, present as small, white papules in the newborn (Fig. 25-23). Milia occurs mainly on the head, especially the cheeks and nose. Preterm infants have vernix caseosa (Fig. 25-24).**

A An oily texture and appearance to the skin, particularly the face, chest, and back, can start as early as 8 to 9 years of age as puberty is beginning.

P Oily skin during puberty is caused by a surge of sex hormones called androgens. Genetics also plays a role in the amount of oil that oil glands produce.

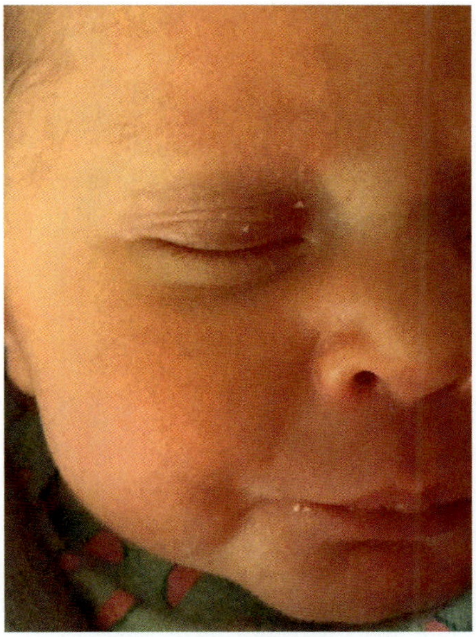

Figure 25-23 Milia in a newborn.

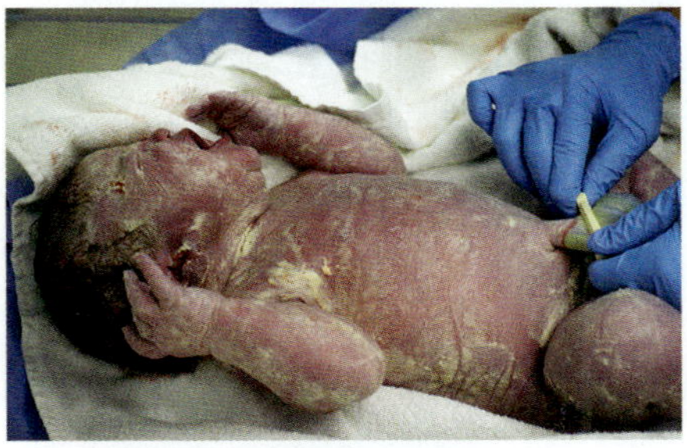

Figure 25-24 Vernix caseosa in a preterm infant.

Hair

Inspection

Lesions

E **N** See Chapter 10.

A Yellow, greasy-appearing scales on the scalp of a light-skinned infant are abnormal. In dark-skinned infants, the scaling is light gray.

P Seborrheic dermatitis (**cradle cap**) is possibly related to increased epidermal tissue growth (Fig. 25-25A and B). It can also extend to the forehead, eyebrows, and ears.

Head

Inspection

Shape and Symmetry

E With the child sitting upright either in the caregiver's arms or on the examination table, observe the symmetry of the frontal, parietal, and occipital prominences.

N **The shape of a child's head is symmetrical without depressions or protrusions. The anterior fontanel normally may pulsate with every heartbeat.**

A A flattened occipital bone with resultant hair loss over the same area is abnormal.

P A prolonged supine position places pressure on the parietal or occipital bone and can cause positional plagiocephaly.

Head Control

E
1. Assess head control while the infant is in the position used for assessing shape and symmetry.
2. With the head unsupported, observe the infant's ability to hold the head erect.

N **At 3 months of age, the infant can hold the head steady without lag.**

A Lack of head control is evidenced by the infant who is unable to hold the head steady while in a sitting position and is abnormal. Head lag beyond 4 to 6 months of age should be further investigated.

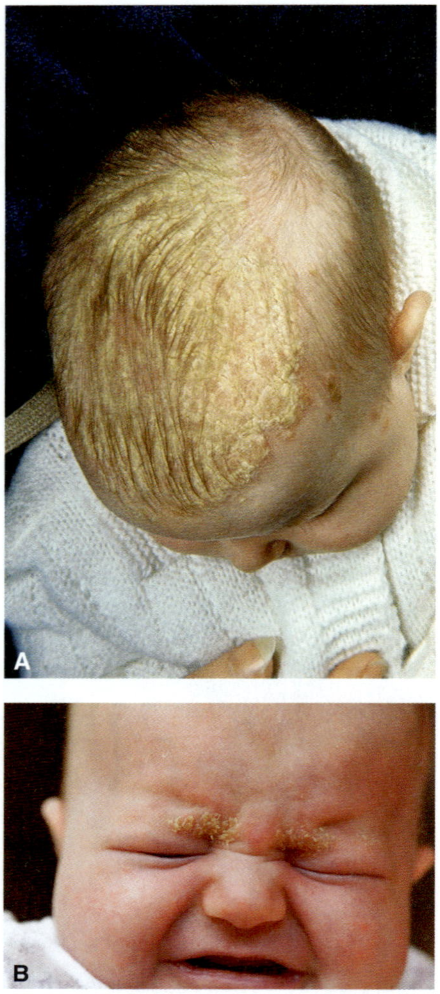

Figure 25-25 Seborrheic dermatitis. A. Cradle cap on the scalp. B. Seborrheic dermatitis on the eyebrows of an infant.

P Documented prematurity, hydrocephalus, and illnesses causing developmental delays are possible causes of head lag.

Palpation

Fontanel

E
1. Place the child in an upright position.
2. Using the second or third finger pad, palpate the anterior fontanel at the junction of the sagittal, coronal, and frontal sutures.
3. Palpate the posterior fontanel at the junction of the sagittal and lambdoidal sutures.
4. Assess for bulging, depression, pulsations, and size. To obtain accurate measurements, the infant should not be crying. Crying will produce a distorted, full, bulging appearance.

N **The anterior fontanel is soft and flat. Size ranges from 1½ to 2½ inches (4 to 6 cm) at birth. The fontanel gradually closes between 10 and 24 months of age. The posterior fontanel is also soft and flat. The size ranges from ¼ to ⅝ inches (0.5 to 1.5 cm) at birth. The posterior fontanel gradually closes after birth and typically cannot be felt after 2 months of age. It is normal to feel pulsations related to the peripheral pulse. Premature infants' fontanelles often have a later closure time.**

A Palpation reveals a bulging, tense fontanel, which is abnormal.

P A bulging, tense fontanel can be a sign of increased intracranial pressure associated with meningitis and an elevated amount of cerebrospinal fluid (CSF).

A A sunken, depressed fontanel is abnormal.

P A sunken, depressed fontanel is a sign of dehydration.

A A wide anterior fontanel in a child older than 2½ years is an abnormal finding.

P An anterior fontanel that remains open after 2½ years of age may indicate disease, such as rickets, or it can be a normal variant. In rickets, there is a low level of vitamin D relative to decreased phosphate levels. Other causes of enlarged fontanel include congenital hypothyroidism, Down syndrome, increased intracranial pressure, primary megalocephaly, and hydrocephalus.

Suture Lines

E
1. With the finger pads, palpate the sagittal suture line. This runs from the anterior to the posterior portion of the skull in a midline position.
2. Palpate the coronal suture line. This runs along both sides of the head, starting at the anterior fontanel.
3. Palpate the lambdoidal suture. The lambdoidal suture runs along both sides of the head, starting at the posterior fontanel.
4. Ascertain if these suture lines are open, united, or overlapping.

N **Grooves or ridges between sections of the skull are normally palpated up to 6 months of age.**

A Suture lines that overlap or override one another, giving the head an unusual shape, warrant further investigation.

P **Craniosynostosis** is premature ossification of suture lines, whereby there is early formation and fusion of skull bones. Craniosynostosis may be caused by metabolic disorders or may be a secondary consequence of microcephaly.

Surface Characteristics

E 1. With the finger pads, palpate the skull in the same manner as the fontanels and suture lines.
2. Note surface edema and contour of the cranium.

N **The skin covering the cranium is flush against the skull and without edema.**

A A softening of the outer layer of the cranial bones behind and above the ears combined with a ping-pong-ball sensation as the area is pressed in gently with the fingers is indicative of **craniotabes**, an abnormal finding.

P Craniotabes is associated with prematurity, rickets, syphilis, hydrocephaly, or hypervitaminosis A.

A A resonant or "cracked pot" sound is produced upon percussion of the skull in an older infant.

P This is Macewen's sign. It is a normal finding in young infants when the cranial sutures are open. After early infancy, hydrocephalus and other pathologies that cause increased intracranial pressure cause cranial suture separation. This is when Macewen's sign may be elicited.

A A localized, subcutaneous swelling over one of the cranial bones of a newborn is referred to as a **cephalohematoma** and is abnormal (Figs. 25-26A and B). This abnormality differs from other surface characteristics in that edema does not cross suture lines with this condition. Varying degrees of swelling can persist for up to 3 months.

P Cephalohematomas acquired during forceps deliveries are due to subperiosteal bleeding and usually resolve within a couple of weeks, but may persist longer.

A Swelling over the occipitoparietal region of the skull is abnormal.

P **Caput succedaneum** results from pressure over the occipitoparietal (crosses suture lines) region during a prolonged delivery (Fig. 25-27). It usually resolves within 1 to 2 weeks after birth.

A **Molding** can occur in conjunction with caput succedaneum (Fig. 25-28).

P The parietal bone overrides the frontal bone as a result of induced pressure during delivery. It should resolve within 1 week of delivery.

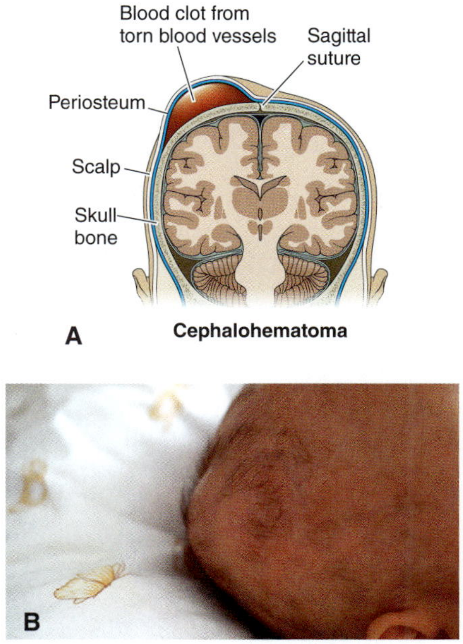

Figure 25-26 Cephalohematoma. **A.** Schematic representation of cephalohematoma. **B.** Cephalohematoma in an infant.

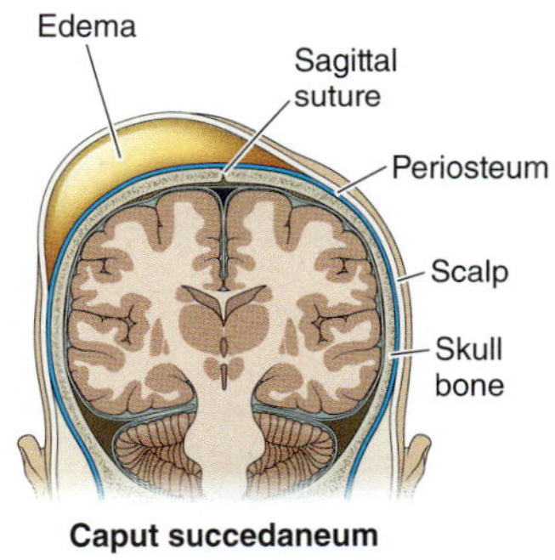

Figure 25-27 Caput succedaneum.

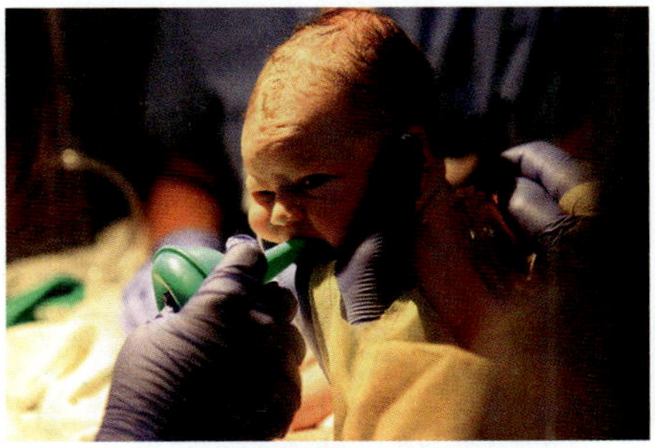

Figure 25-28 Molding

Eyes

General Approach

1. From infancy through about 8 to 10 years of age, you should assess the eyes toward the end of the examination, except for testing vision, which should be done first. Remember that the child's attention span is short, and attentiveness decreases the longer you evaluate. Children generally are not cooperative for eyes, ears, and throat examinations.
2. Place the young infant, preschool, school-age, or adolescent client on the examination table. The older infant or the toddler can be held by the caregiver.
3. Become proficient at performing funduscopic examinations on adults before examining the pediatric client.

> ## ADVANCED TECHNIQUE
> ### Assessing for Hydrocephalus and Anencephaly: Transillumination of the Skull
>
> Transillumination of the infant's head to rule out hydrocephalus or anencephaly can be performed as a temporary alternative to diagnostic imaging if the head circumference is not within normal limits.
>
> **E**
> 1. Support the child in an elevated or sitting position.
> 2. Darken the room.
> 3. Place a flashlight with cranial transillumination or a soft, flexible, rubber end directly against the frontal, parietal, and occipital areas of the skull.
> 4. Note the size of the light over the various areas.
> 5. Result should be confirmed with an ultrasound of the head or other diagnostic imaging.
>
> **N** **A normal finding over the frontal and parietal bones is a circle of light no larger than ¾ inches (2 cm) around the flashlight. Over the occipital area, a circle of light no larger than ⅜ inches (1 cm) is considered within normal limits. Normal findings are the same for light- and dark-skinned children.**
>
> **A** It is abnormal for the illuminated area to be more than ⅜ inches (1 cm) in the occipital area and ¾ inches (2 cm) elsewhere.
>
> **P** **Anencephaly** is an abnormal finding whereby the cortex or cranium does not develop. The fetal nervous system thus fails to develop normally. Between the 18th and 24th day of gestation, the neural tube fails to close, resulting in anencephaly. These clients usually do not live more than 24 hours.
>
> **P** Excess fluid in the cranial vault, as in hydrocephalus, may lead to positive transillumination.

Vision Screening

General Approach

1. The adult Snellen chart can be used on children as young as kindergarten or first grade, provided they can read the alphabet. The Tumbling E chart is used for a child over 3 years of age or any child who cannot read the alphabet (Fig. 25-29).
2. Test every 1 to 2 years through adolescence.
3. Each eye should be assessed separately while covering the opposite eye with a hand or eye patch, as well as both eyes concurrently.
4. If the child resists wearing a cover patch over the eye, make a game out of wearing the patch. For example, the young child could pretend to be a pirate exploring new territory. Use your imagination to think of a fantasy situation.

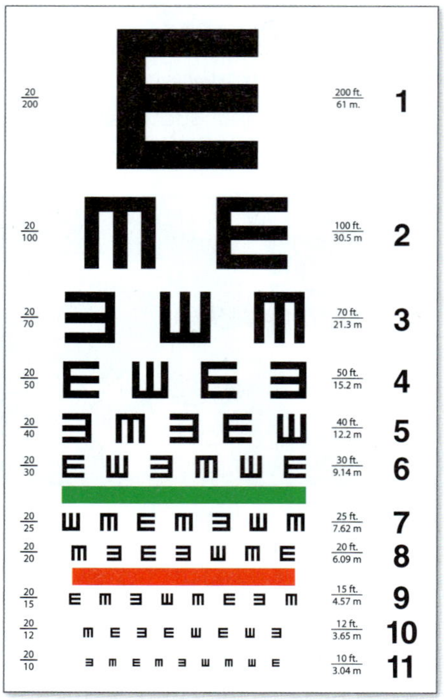

Figure 25-29 Tumbling E chart.

Tumbling E Chart

E
1. Ask the child to point an arm in the direction the E is pointing.
2. Observe for squinting.

N **Vision is 20/40 from 2 to approximately 6 years of age when it approaches the normal 20/20 acuity. Refer the child to an ophthalmologist if results are 20/50 or worse in a child 3 years of age, 20/40 or worse in a child 4 years of age, or 20/30 or greater in a child 6 years or older, or if results vary by two or more lines between eyes even if in the passing range.**

A **P** See Chapter 12.

Strabismus Screening

The Hirschberg (corneal light reflex) test and the cover/uncover test assess eye alignment. The latter is the more definitive test.

Hirschberg Test

E N See Chapter 12.

A It is abnormal for the light reflection to be displaced to the outer margin of the cornea as the eye deviates inward (Fig. 25-30).

P Esotropia is thought to be congenital. Some theories suggest that neurological factors contribute to its development.

A It is abnormal for the light reflection to be displaced to the inner margin of the cornea as the eye deviates outward.

P Exotropia can result from eye muscle fatigue or can be congenital.

A It is abnormal for the light reflection to be inferiorly displaced.

P Hypertropia can result from cranial nerve IV palsy, Brown syndrome, or Duane syndrome.

Cover/Uncover Test

E Conduct the examination in the same manner as for an adult.

N **Neither eye moves when the occluder is being removed. Infants less than 6 months of age display intermittent strabismus due to poor neuromuscular control of eye muscles.**

A It is abnormal for one or both eyes to move to focus on the penlight during the examination. Assume that strabismus is present.

P Constant strabismus or intermittent strabismus after 4 months of age is abnormal and requires referral to an ophthalmologist. It may indicate eye muscle weakness, cataracts, cranial nerve abnormalities, chorioretinitis, or retinoblastoma.

Color Vision

Preschoolers aged 3 to 6 years should have their ability to distinguish colors assessed during the annual well-child examination. The two most commonly used color vision assessment tools are the Ishihara color test

> **NURSING TIP**
> **Pseudostrabismus**
> Some infants have an epicanthal fold that gives the false appearance of strabismus. The Hirschberg (corneal light reflex) test reveals a tropia in true strabismus. A tropia is absent in pseudostrabismus.

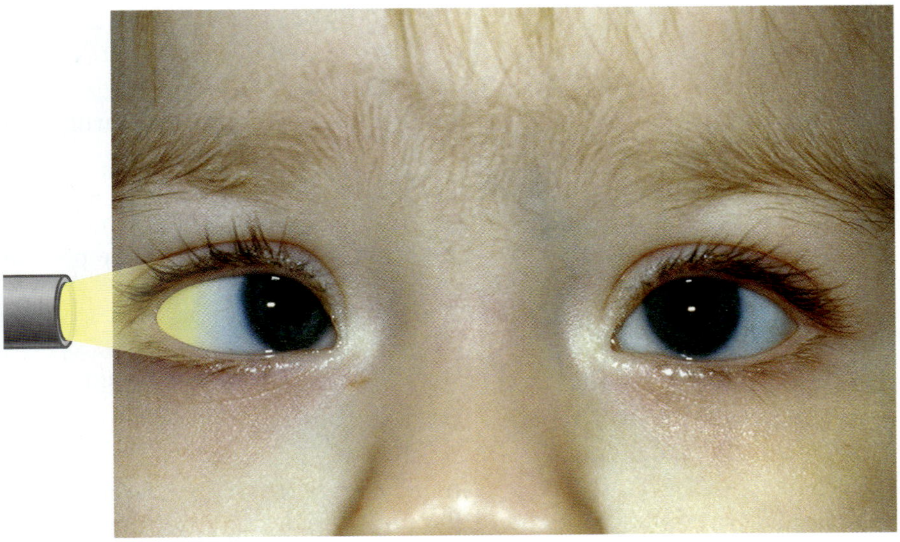

Figure 25-30 Infantile esotropia.

E Examination **N** Normal Findings **A** Abnormal Findings **P** Pathophysiology

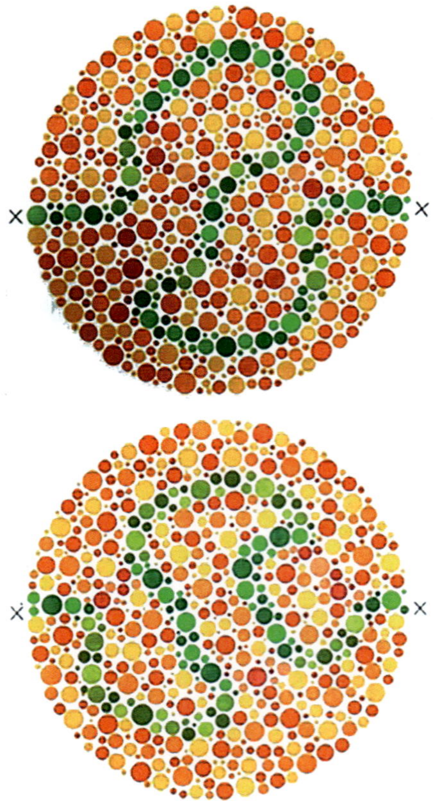

Figure 25-31 Pseudoisochromatic-colored background for color vision testing.

and the Color Vision Testing Made Easy test. The Ishihara test places numbers on a pseudoisochromatic-colored background. The Color Vision Testing Made Easy tool also uses a pseudoisochromatic-colored background but uses objects that are readily recognizable by a preschooler, such as a car, boat, house, and dog. Fig. 25-31 illustrates a simplistic curvy line on a pseudoisochromatic-colored background that can be used.

E
1. Show the child the color vision test plate.
2. Have the child identify the number or object within 3 seconds.

N **The child should be able to correctly identify the number or object within 3 seconds.**

A If the child is unable to correctly identify the number or object within 3 seconds, a color vision deficiency, or color blindness, should be suspected.

P A color vision abnormality is a congenital finding in a small percentage of children and is more prevalent in males. A small number of individuals with color blindness acquire the condition through eye, nerve, or brain conditions.

Inspection

Eyelids

E
1. Sit at the client's eye level.
2. Observe for symmetrical palpebral fissures and the position of eyelids in relation to the iris.
3. Lid eversion is not performed in children unless assessing for an infection or foreign body. If performed, the technique is the same as for an adult.

N **The palpebral fissures of both eyes are positioned symmetrically. The upper eyelid normally covers a small portion of the iris, and the lower lid meets the iris. Epicanthal folds can be normal in many people, particularly in infants and those of various ethnicities. When not physiologically occurring, they may be related to various syndromes (including but not limited to fetal alcohol syndrome, Down syndrome, and Turner syndrome).**

A It is abnormal for a portion of the sclera to be seen above the iris.

P The sclera is exposed above the iris in hydrocephalus. As the forehead becomes prominent, the eyebrows and eyelids are drawn up, creating a setting sun appearance of the child's eyes.

A A fold of skin covering the inner canthus and lacrimal caruncle is abnormal.

P During embryonic development, the fold of skin slants in a downward direction toward the nose. This is seen in a child with Down syndrome. Epicanthal folds and short palpebral fissures are present in a child with fetal alcohol syndrome.

Lacrimal Apparatus

E N Conduct the examination in the same manner as for an adult.

A The child's caregiver reports that the child is unable to produce tears, an abnormal finding.

P The lacrimal ducts should be patent by 3 months of age. Dacryocystitis results when the distal end of the membranous lacrimal duct fails to open or a blockage occurs elsewhere.

Anterior Segment Structures

Sclera

E Conduct the examination in the same manner as for an adult.

N **The newborn exhibits a bluish-tinged sclera related to the thinness of the fibrous tissue. The sclera is white in light-skinned children and a slightly darker color in some dark-skinned children.**

A **P** See Chapter 12.

Iris

E Conduct the examination in the same manner as for an adult.

N **Up to about 6 months of age, the color of the iris is blue or slate gray in light-skinned infants and brownish in dark-skinned infants. Between 6 and 12 months of age, a complete transition of iris color has occurred.**

A Small white flecks, called **Brushfield spots**, noted around the perimeter of the iris are abnormal.

P Brushfield spots are found on the iris of the client with Down syndrome. The spots develop during embryonic maturation.

Pupils

E Conduct the examination in the same manner as for an adult.

N **When the pupils' reaction to light is assessed, a newborn will normally blink and flex the head closer to the body. This is called the optical blink reflex.**

A **P** See Chapter 12.

Lens

E Conduct the examination in the same manner as for an adult.

N **The lens is transparent.**

A A white or pearly gray appearance is abnormal.

P A white or pearly gray lens can be caused by a congenital or acquired cataract.

Posterior Segment Structures

General Approach

1. The examination is easier to accomplish if the infant or toddler is lying supine on an examination table. The assistance of another individual, such as the caregiver, to hold the child in position is essential. The older child may be allowed to sit, if cooperative.
2. Observe the red reflex, retina, and optic disc. The red reflex may appear red, orangish-red, or perhaps grayer than red (in darkly pigmented individuals). Any abnormality of the red reflex necessitates referral to an ophthalmologist.

Inspection

Red Reflex

E **N** See Chapter 12.

A An absent red reflex is abnormal.

P Chromosomal disorders, intrauterine infections, and ocular trauma are possible causes of cataracts in newborns.

A A yellowish or white light reflex (cat's eye reflex) is abnormal.

P Retinoblastoma is a malignant glioma located in the posterior chamber of the eye.

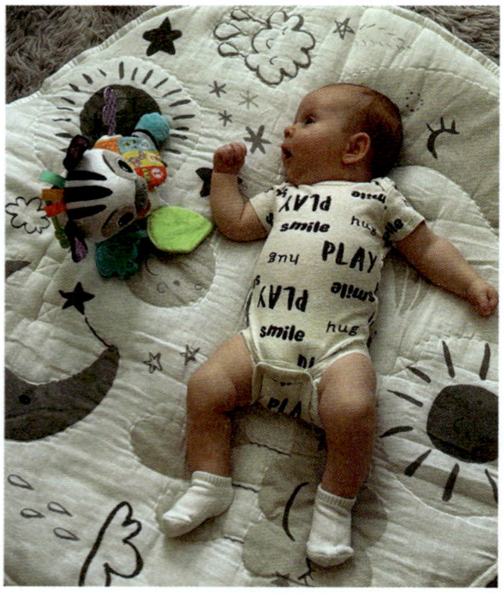

Figure 25-32 This 3-month-old infant turns to the toy playing music.

Retina/Optic Disc

E N See Chapter 12.

A A red to dark-red color is abnormal. Some areas may be rounded or flame-shaped.

P Retinal hemorrhage is seen in trauma. Bleeding into the optic nerve sheath is found in children who have been physically shaken. This is called shaken baby syndrome.

Ears

Auditory Testing

General Approach

1. Universal hearing screening of all newborns is recommended in the United States. Before 3 years of age, the following are a few parameters for evaluating hearing.
   a. Does the child react to a loud noise? (Fig. 25-32)
   b. Does the child react to the caregiver's voice by cooing, smiling, or turning eyes and head toward the voice?
   c. Does the child try to imitate sounds?
   d. Can the child imitate words and sounds?
   e. Can the child follow directions?
   f. Does the child respond to sounds not directed at them?
2. Perform auditory testing at about age 3 to 4 years of age or when the child can follow directions. A whisper test or more formal diagnostic testing can be conducted when there is a concern for a hearing deficit.

External Ear

Inspection of Pinna Position

E N See Chapter 13.

A The top of the ear is below the imaginary line drawn from the outer canthus to the top of the ear.

P Kidneys and ears are formed at the same time in embryonic development. If a child's ears are low set, renal anomalies must be ruled out. Low-set ears can also occur in Down syndrome.

Internal Ear

Inspection

E

1. A cooperative child may be allowed to sit for the examination. A young child may be held as shown in Fig. 25-33.
2. Restrain the uncooperative young child by placing the child supine on a firm surface or the caregiver's lap. While in the caregiver's lap, the child's legs should be braced between the caregiver's legs, with the head turned to the side, and firmly braced against the shoulder or chest. Instruct the caregiver or assistant to hold the child's arms up near the head, embracing the elbow joints on both sides of either arm. Restrain the infant by having the caregiver hold the infant's hands down.
3. With your thumb and forefinger grasping the otoscope, use the ulnar side of the hand to brace against the forehead or face to prevent the head from jerking. Your other hand can also be used to stabilize the child's head.
4. Pull the lower auricle down and out to straighten the canal. This technique is used in children up to about 3 years of age. Use the adult technique after age 3.

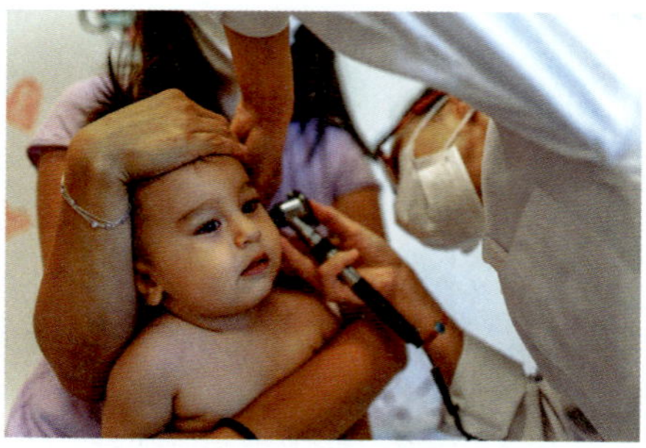

Figure 25-33 Securing the child for the otoscopic examination.

5. Insert the speculum about ¼ to ½ inch (0.6 to 1.3 cm), depending on the child's age.
6. Suspected otitis media must be evaluated with a pneumatic bulb attached to the side of the otoscope's light source.
7. Select a larger speculum to make a tight seal and prevent air from escaping from the canal.
8. If a light reflex is present, focus on it.
9. Gently squeeze the bulb attachment to introduce air into the canal.
10. Observe the tympanic membrane for movement.

N A P See Chapter 13.

> **NURSING TIP**
> **False Impression of Otitis Media**
> If the client is screaming and crying, a flush or erythema on the tympanic membrane will be present. After allowing the caregiver to comfort the child, attempt to reexamine. The flush or erythema can give false impressions of otitis media. Assessing the movement of the tympanic membrane (TM) via pneumatic otoscopy can elicit valuable data. The normal TM will move slightly inward and outward with positive and negative pressure. Middle ear effusions can result in no or exaggerated movement. A perforated TM can result from trauma, increased middle ear pressure, foreign body, or surgical placement of pressure-equalizing tubes.

Nose

Inspection

General Approach

Conduct the inspection of the nose utilizing the same positioning used for the adult ear examination. Observe the mucosa, nasal septum, and presence of drainage.

E 1. Gently push the child's nose upward with one finger. Insert the speculum gently into the naris. Avoid touching the nasal septum with the speculum.
2. Note the color of the mucosa, color and consistency of drainage, presence of septal deviation, or foreign body.

N **The nasal mucosa is pink or dull red. There is no evidence of polyps, foreign bodies, nasal drainage, or septal deviation.**

A Nasal mucosa that is pale pink, gray, or blue is abnormal.

P The child with pale pink, gray, or blue nasal mucosa is frequently seen in allergic rhinitis. Allergic rhinitis is triggered by breathing in an allergen such as pollen or dust.

A A pearly gray-colored, grape-like growth noted within the nasal mucosa is abnormal.

P The cause of polyps is unknown but may be attributed to several factors including allergies and rhinosinusitis. Some individuals, including those with asthma, chronic rhinosinusitis, or cystic fibrosis, are at greater risk for developing polyps.

A Persistent odor and unilateral nasal drainage in a child with a suspected foreign body warrant further evaluation by a trained clinician.

P A foreign body lodged in a nasal cavity may need to be removed while the child is placed under light sedation.

A A nasal septum that is not straight is abnormal. The septum may appear bowed into the nasal passage.

P Septal deviation may be congenital or caused by an injury. Septal deviation can cause snoring, difficult nasal breathing, excessive nasal drainage, nosebleeds, rhinosinusitis, and headaches.

Mouth and Throat

Inspection

Lips

E 1. Follow the same technique described in Chapter 13.
2. Observe if the lip edges meet.

N **The lip edges should meet. A newborn may have a blister (Fig. 25-34) on the upper lip caused by vigorous sucking during**

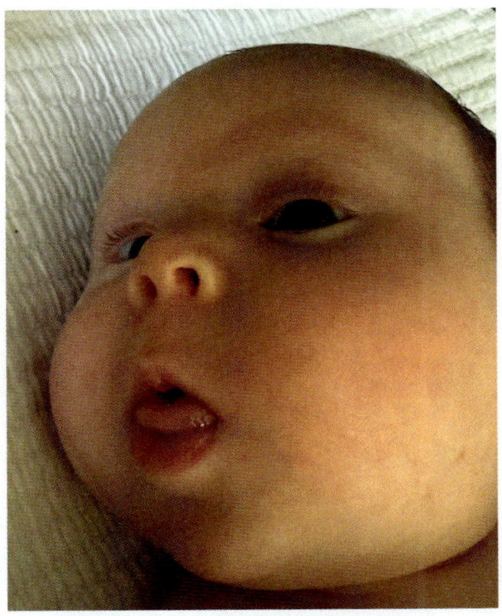

Figure 25-34 Newborn lip blister

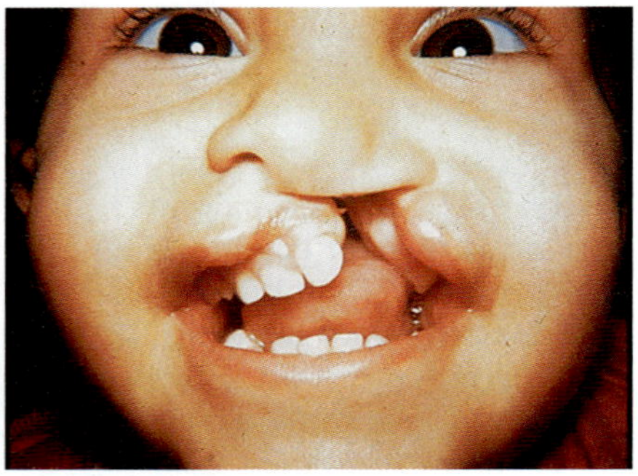

Figure 25-35 Cleft lip.

breastfeeding. It is usually harmless and goes away on its own. Occasionally a blister may appear on the lower lip.

A It is abnormal if the lip edges do not meet.

P A cleft lip is seen as a separated area of lip tissue (Fig. 25-35). It involves the upper lip and sometimes extends into the nostril. A cleft lip is an obvious finding during the examination of a newborn. It occurs mainly on the left side and is more frequently found in males. A cleft lip develops during the fifth to sixth week after fertilization. Genetics plays a small role in etiology.

A A thin upper lip is abnormal.

P A child with fetal alcohol syndrome exhibits a thin upper lip, as well as a flat and elongated philtrum.

Buccal Mucosa

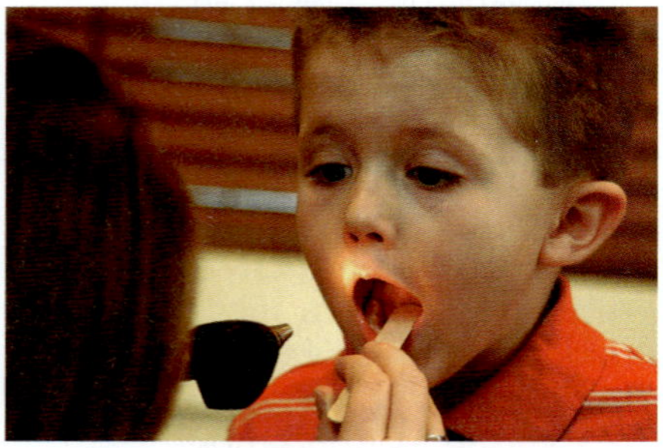

Figure 25-36 The nurse uses a light source and tongue depressor to examine the child's mouth and throat.

E Use the same technique as for an adult (Fig. 25-36). If the child is unable to open the mouth on command, use the edge of a tongue blade to lift the upper lip and move the lower lip down.

N **See Chapter 13.**

A A thick, curd-like coating on the buccal mucosa or tongue is abnormal (Fig. 25-37).

P Thrush can be acquired when a newborn passes through the vagina during delivery. Thrush after the neonatal period can be caused by breastfeeding from a yeast-infected breast, antibiotic use, or immune system pathology.

Teeth

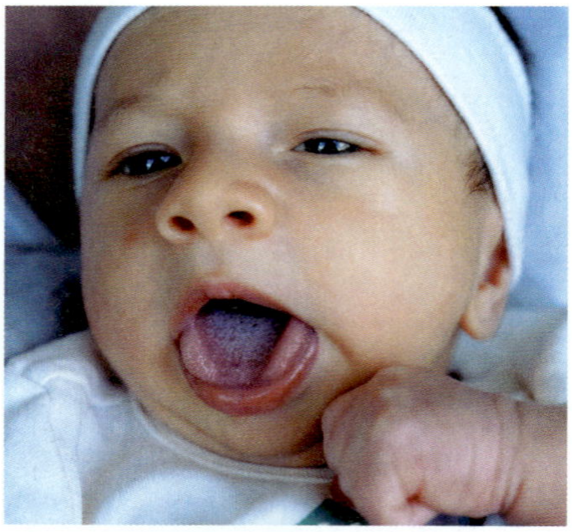

Figure 25-37 Thrush in an infant.

E N See Chapter 13.

A A lack of visible teeth coupled with roentgenographic findings revealing the absence of tooth buds is abnormal.

P The absence of deciduous teeth beyond 16 months of age signifies an abnormality most commonly related to genetic causes.

A It is abnormal for the teeth to turn brownish black, possibly with indentations along the surfaces of the teeth.

P Carbohydrate-rich fluid (from milk or juice) causes severe caries when a child falls asleep with a bottle in the mouth.

Hard and Soft Palate

E
1. Observe the palate for continuity and shape.
2. For infants, you will need to use a tongue depressor to push the tongue down and examine it with a light source. Infants usually cry in response to this action, which allows visualization of the palates.

N **The roof of the mouth is continuous and has a slight arch.**

A It is abnormal if the roof of the mouth is not continuous. This anomaly is called cleft palate (Fig. 25-38).

P Cleft palates vary greatly in size and extent of malformation. The degree of malformation is classified into two groups. A midline malformation may involve the uvula or extend through the soft or hard palates or both. If associated with a cleft lip, the malformation may extend through the palates and into the nasal cavity. Cleft palates form between the sixth and tenth week of embryonic development, during the fusion of the maxillary and premaxillary processes. Genetics plays a small role in etiology.

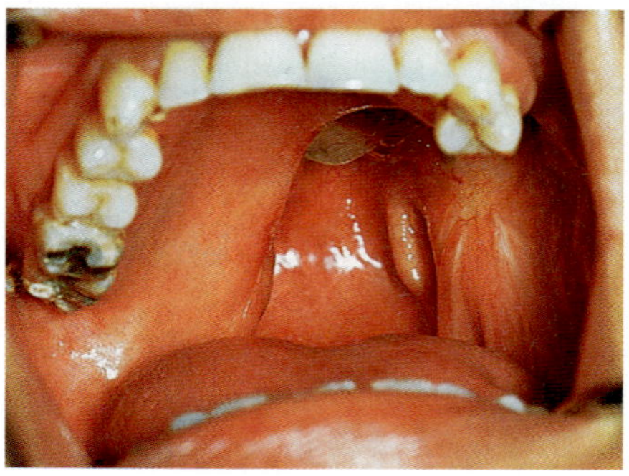

Figure 25-38 Cleft palate.

A The roof of the mouth is abnormally arched. On inspection, the shape resembles an upside-down letter "V."

P High palates are usually associated with a particular syndrome such as trisomy 21, trisomy 18, and Noonan syndrome.

A Intraoral epithelial occlusion cysts are quite common in newborns, occurring in up to 90% of infants. **Epstein's pearls** are small white cysts that appear on the hard palate. They may feel hard when palpated. Small, white cysts called **Bohn nodules** may appear on the gums of a newborn.

P These keratin-filled cysts typically resolve within a few months.

Oropharynx

E Conduct the examination in the same manner as for an adult.

N **Up to the age of 12 years, a tonsil grade of 2+ is considered normal. Around puberty, tonsillar tissue regresses. Tonsils should not interfere with the act of breathing.**

A Excessive salivation is an early sign of a tracheoesophageal fistula (TEF). Drooling is accompanied by choking and coughing during the child's feeding.

P In a tracheoesophageal fistula the esophagus failed to develop as a continuous passage during embryonic formation.

A Exudative pharyngitis is present in infectious mononucleosis. Other symptoms include fever, sore throat, splenomegaly, petechiae on the palate, and cervical adenitis.

P Mononucleosis is caused by the Epstein-Barr virus.

A Hypertrophy of lymphoid tissue occurs in the posterior pharyngeal wall, causing a condition known as enlarged or hypertrophied adenoids.

P Excessive lymphoid tissue interferes with the passage of air through the nose, resulting in snoring and apnea. Obstruction of the eustachian tubes by enlarged lymphoid tissue can lead to otitis media. Sinusitis can occur when lymphoid tissue blocks the clearance of nasal mucus.

Neck

Inspection

General Appearance

E
1. Observe the neck in a midline position while the child is sitting upright.
2. Note shortening or thickness of the neck on both the right and left sides.
3. Note any swelling.

N **There is a reasonable amount of skin tissue on the sides of the neck. There is no swelling.**

A Additional weblike tissue found bilaterally from the ear to the shoulder is abnormal.

P Webbed necks are associated with congenital syndromes. One example is Turner syndrome, noted in female children.

A Unilateral or bilateral swelling of the neck below the angle of the jaw is abnormal (Fig. 25-39).

P Enlargement of the parotid gland occurs in parotitis, or mumps, an inflammation of the parotid gland. There is pain and tenderness in the affected area.

A Torticollis is observed.

P Torticollis can be congenital and acquired. An infant who is always placed on the same side when supine can develop a lateral deviation at the neck with decreased range of motion.

> **NURSING TIP**
> **Preventing Choking in Children**
> The infant's or toddler's airway is small, approximately the size of their "pinky" finger. Fresh grapes, uncut hot dogs with the skin on, popcorn, and peanuts are common foods that can cause choking. These foods should not be given to young children. Caregivers should be encouraged to only allow children to eat or drink while seated.

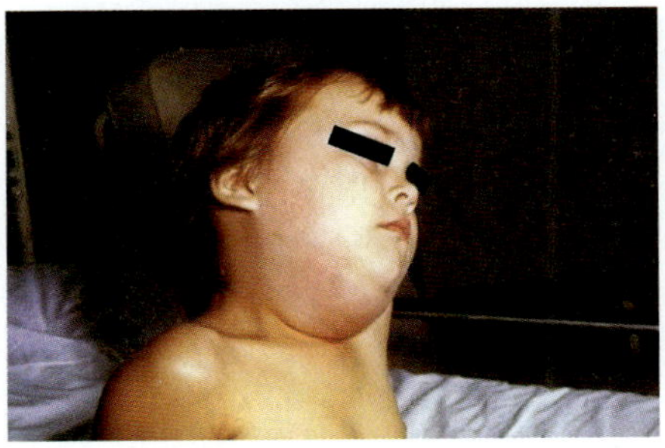

Figure 25-39 Parotitis (mumps).

Palpation

Thyroid

E 1. Use the same technique as for an adult except use the first two finger pads on both hands.
2. Have the younger child who is unable to swallow on command take a sip from a bottle or cup.

N A P The normal findings, abnormal findings, and pathophysiology are the same as for an adult.

Lymph Nodes

E 1. Because of the infant's short neck, you must extend the chin upward with your hand before proceeding with palpation.
2. With the finger pads, palpate the submental, submandibular, tonsillar, anterior cervical chain, posterior cervical chain, supraclavicular, preauricular, posterior auricular, and occipital lymph nodes.
3. Use a circular motion. Note the location, size, shape, tenderness, mobility, and associated skin inflammation of any swollen nodes palpated.

N **Lymph nodes are generally not palpable. Children often have small, movable, cool, nontender nodes referred to as "shotty" nodes. These benign nodes are related to environmental antigen exposure or residual effects of a prior illness and have no clinical significance.**

A Enlargement of the anterior cervical chain is abnormal.

P Enlargement of the anterior cervical chain occurs in bacterial infections of the pharynx (such as Group A β-hemolytic streptococcus- strep throat) or viral infections (mononucleosis).

A Enlargement of the occipital nodes or posterior cervical chain nodes is abnormal.

P Enlargement of the occipital nodes or posterior cervical chain nodes occurs in infectious mononucleosis, tinea capitis, and acute otitis externa.

Breasts

Inspection of the breasts is performed throughout childhood. Palpation is not usually performed on the client until puberty unless otherwise indicated.

Sexual Maturity Rating (SMR)

E Using the Tanner stages in Table 14-1, assess the developmental stage of a female's breasts.

N **Breast development usually starts between the ages of 8 and 10 and is finished after 14 to 17 years of age.**

A An SMR that is less than expected for a female's age is abnormal.

P Pituitary pathology should be considered if the SMR is less than expected for a female's age. Familial predisposition must also be considered.

Thorax and Lungs

General Approach

Remove the child's clothes or gown. Keep the infant warm during the examination by placing a blanket over the chest until ready for this portion of the examination.

Inspection

Shape of Thorax

E Conduct the examination in the same manner as for an adult.

N **The infant has a barrel chest; by age 6, the chest attains the adult configuration.**

A If a school-age child has an abnormal chest configuration, suspect pathology.

P In addition to the conditions discussed in Chapter 15, cystic fibrosis (CF) can lead to an altered anteroposterior-transverse diameter.

Retractions

E
1. In children, it is important to evaluate intercostal muscles for signs of increased work of breathing.
2. If at all possible, perform this examination when the child is quiet because forceful crying will mimic retractions.

N **Retractions are not present.**

A In respiratory distress, retractions are seen as an inward collapse of the chest wall. Retractions can be seen in the suprasternal, supraclavicular, subcostal, and intercostal regions of the chest wall. Other signs of respiratory distress include (but are not limited to) nasal flaring, stridor, expiratory grunting, head bobbing, and wheezing.

P Respiratory distress is a result of abnormal function or disruption of the respiratory pathway or within organs that control or influence respiration. Infants with RSV frequently present with retractions.

> **NURSING TIP**
>
> **Stridor in Children**
>
> Stridor is indicative of upper airway obstruction, particularly edema in children. They can present with a barking, seal-like cough. Inspiration accentuates these stridorous sounds. Children who present with stridor should be promptly evaluated to rule out epiglottitis (a medical emergency). Other causes of stridor in children are croup-like illnesses (e.g., laryngotracheobronchitis, RSV, COVID-19), anatomical defect, mass, external compression to the neck, or foreign body.

Palpation

Tactile Fremitus

If present, fremitus can be easily felt when a child cries. If the infant or young child is not crying, it is advisable to defer this procedure until later in the examination, perhaps after the throat and ear examinations, which usually produce crying.

Percussion

E Conduct the examination in the same manner as for an adult.

N **Normal diaphragmatic excursion in infants and young toddlers is one to two intercostal spaces.**

A P See Chapter 15.

Auscultation

Breath Sounds

E Use the same examination techniques as for an adult (Fig. 25-40A and B). Sometimes, it is difficult to differentiate the various adventitious sounds because a child's respiratory rate is rapid; for example, differentiating expiratory wheezing from inspiratory wheezing can be difficult. Mastering the technique takes time and practice.

N **Of the three types of breath sounds—bronchial, bronchovesicular, and vesicular—the bronchovesicular are normally heard throughout the peripheral lung fields up to 5 to 6 years of age because the chest wall is thin with decreased musculature. Lung fields are clear and equal bilaterally.**

A Crackles are abnormal.

P Conditions such as bronchiolitis, CF, pneumonia, and bronchopulmonary dysplasia produce crackles.

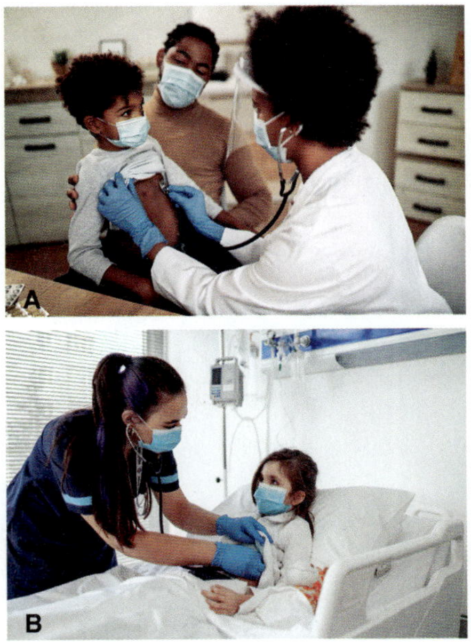

Figure 25-40 Lung auscultation. **A.** The nurse auscultates the child's thorax. **B.** Auscultation should always be skin-to-skin. Maintaining modesty in tweens and teens is essential.

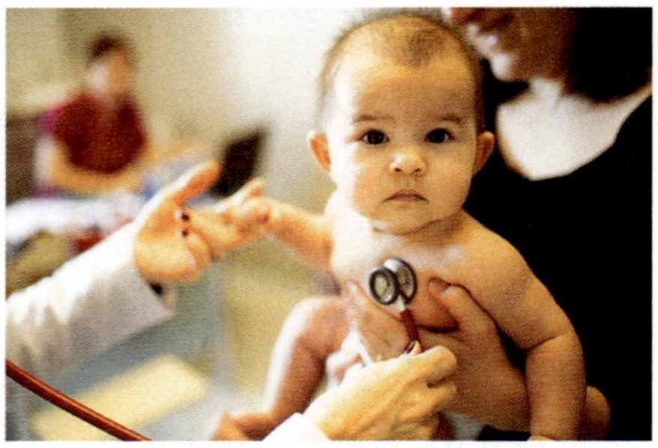

Figure 25-41 Heart auscultation of an infant.

A Wheezing is abnormal.

P Clients with CF and bronchiolitis may present with wheezing. Infants with RSV usually present with wheezing. Other causes of wheezing in children can be malacia, gastroesophageal reflux disease, foreign body aspiration, and asthma.

Heart

General Approach

1. Examine the child's general appearance first. Signs of concern related to the cardiovascular system include cyanosis, increased respiratory rate, increased respiratory effort, diaphoresis during feedings, and precordial bulge. Clubbing may be present in infants older than 12 months and indicates chronic hypoxia. As with adults, jugular venous distention, peripheral edema, and enlarged liver may indicate right ventricular dysfunction. Failure to gain weight, shortness of breath at rest and with activity, and developmental delays are also frequent clues to an undiagnosed cardiac condition.
2. It is best to perform the cardiac examination near the beginning of the examination, when the infant or young child is relatively calm (Fig. 25-41).
3. Do not get discouraged during the examination. The novice nurse is not expected to identify a murmur and its location within the cardiac cycle. Be patient because skill will come only with practice.
4. During the examination, note physical signs of a syndrome such as a distinct facies in a child with trisomy 21 or Down syndrome. Many children with Down syndrome have associated atrioventricular (A-V) canal malformations. These defects each involve an atrial septal defect (ASD), ventricular septal defect (VSD), and a common A-V valve.
5. Cardiac landmarks change when a child has dextrocardia. In this condition, the apex of the heart points toward the right thoracic cavity; thus, heart sounds are auscultated primarily on the right side of the chest.

Inspection

Apical Impulse

E Conduct the examination in the same manner as for an adult.

N **In newborns, the apical pulse is best noted at the lower left sternal border and may be palpated with the heel of the hand. In both older infants and toddlers, the apical impulse is located at the fourth intercostal space at the left midclavicular line. The apical impulse of a child 7 years or older is at the fourth or fifth intercostal space, left midclavicular line. The impulse may not be visible in all children, especially in those who have increased adipose tissue or muscle.**

A **P** See Chapter 16.

Precordium

E Observe the chest wall for any movements other than the apical impulse.

N **There should be no movements other than the apical impulse.**

A Lifting of the cardiac area is abnormal.

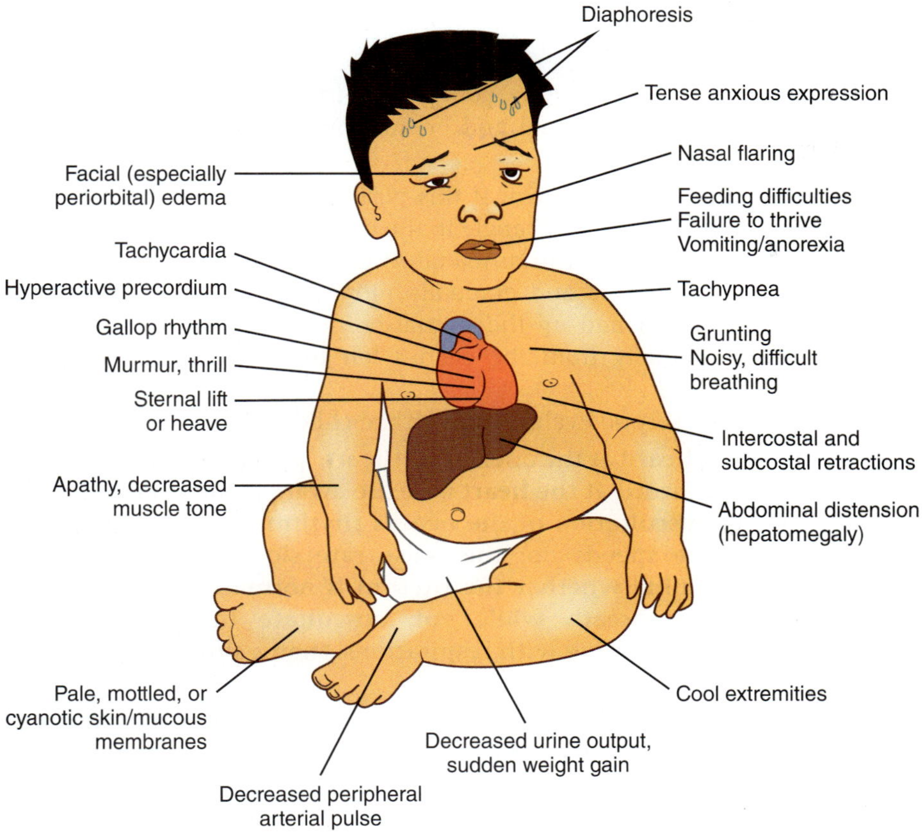

Figure 25-42 Infant with congestive heart failure.

P Heaves are associated with volume overload. A child with congenital heart disease is at risk for developing congestive heart failure (CHF) with associated volume overload. Fig. 25-42 depicts the manifestations of CHF in children. Large left-to-right shunt defects, such as a VSD, cause right ventricular volume overload.

Palpation

Thrill

E

1. Palpate as for an adult or use the proximal one-third of each finger and the areas over the metacarpophalangeal joints. Many nurses find that the latter method yields greater sensitivity to the presence of thrills.
2. Place the hand vertically along the heart's apex and move the hand toward the sternum.
3. Place the hand horizontally along the sternum, moving up the sternal border about ½ to 1 inch (1.3 to 2.5 cm) each time.
4. When at the clavicular level, place the hand vertically and assess for a thrill at the heart's base.
5. Use the finger pads to palpate a thrill at the suprasternal notch and along the carotid arteries.

N **A heave, tap, or thrill noted on the chest wall is not found in the healthy child.**

A P Thrills may indicate valve dysfunction, abnormal ventricular dysfunction, or compromised hemodynamic status. Thrills occur with grade IV-VI murmurs and are always abnormal.

See Chapter 16 for additional information.

Auscultation

Heart Sounds

Auscultating the infant's or the young pediatric client's heart is difficult because the heart rate is rapid and breath sounds are easily transmitted through the chest wall.

E

1. Have the child lie down. If this position is not possible, the child should be held at a 45° angle in the caregiver's arms.
2. Use the "Z" pattern to auscultate the heart. Place the stethoscope in the apical area and gradually move it toward the right lower sternal border and up the sternal border in a right diagonal line. Move gradually from the client's left to the right upper sternal borders.
3. Perform a second evaluation with the child in a sitting position.

N **S_1 is best heard at the apex of the heart, left lower sternal border. S_2 is best heard at the heart base. Be aware of sinus arrhythmias during auscultation of the heart's rhythm. On inspiration, the pulse rate speeds up; the pulse rate slows with expiration. To determine whether the rhythm is normal, ask the child to hold their breath while you auscultate the heart. If the pulse stops varying with respirations, then a sinus arrhythmia is present.**

Approximately half of all children develop an innocent murmur at some time in their lives. Less than 1% of all pediatric heart murmurs are related to congenital cardiac disease, leaving most murmurs "innocent" in nature. See Table 25-3. Innocent murmurs are accentuated in high cardiac output states such as fever, stress, or pregnancy. When the client is sitting, murmurs are heard early in systole at the second or third intercostal space along the left sternal border and are softly musical in quality. They disappear when the client lies down.

A A fixed or increasing split S_2 sound is abnormal

P If the S_2 split is fixed with the act of respiration, you can suspect an atrial septal defect. In children, S_2 physiologically splits with inspiration and becomes single with expiration. This phenomenon is due to a greater negative pressure in the thoracic cavity.

A In children, S_3 often sounds like the three syllables of the word "Kentucky," especially when accompanied by tachycardia.

P A loud third heart sound may be present in children with CHF or a VSD. S_3 is produced by rapid filling of the ventricle.

A With tachycardia, S_4 sounds like a gallop resembling the word "Tennessee."

P S_4 is not normally heard in children. If detected, aortic stenosis may be present. The left ventricle's ability to pump blood through the stenotic valve produces a dilation within the left ventricular muscle resulting in decreased ventricular compliance.

A A systolic ejection murmur is heard between the first and second heart sounds over the aortic or pulmonic areas.

P Ejection murmurs occur in aortic and pulmonic valvular stenosis. The murmur is the result of blood passing through stenotic valves.

A Holosystolic murmurs are heard maximally at the left lower sternal border. They begin with S_1 and continue until the second heart sound, S_2, is heard.

Table 25-3 Innocent Heart Murmurs

Type	Age	Intensity/Location	Quality	Other Characteristics
Stills	>2 yr	< III/VI midsystolic located at LLSB or between LLSB and apex	Twanging, squeaking, buzzing, musical, harp-like or vibratory sound	Low frequency heard with the bell with child in supine position, softer when the child is standing or sitting
Pulmonary flow murmur	3 yr–adolescence	< III/VI, low-pitched ejection systolic murmur located at LUSB, radiating to back/axillae	Soft-blowing, low-pitched murmur"	Ejection-type murmur; prominent in high output states; intensity increases with inspiration and while supine; decreases when standing and with Valsalva maneuver
Peripheral pulmonary arterial stenosis	1st year of life, especially in premature babies	I-II/VI midsystolic, RUSB/LUSB radiating to axillae	Short, soft	Intensity of murmur and split of S_2 generally increases with the severity of the obstruction. However, neonates with severe pulmonic stenosis may present with a very soft murmur due to the decreased flow through the pulmonary valve.
Venous hum	2–8 yr	< III/VI continuous murmur, audible in right or left infraclavicular and supraclavicular areas	Humming	Originates from turbulence in jugular venous system, low-pitched, heard in upright position, disappears in supine position, obliterated by rotating the head or gently occluding neck veins

LLSB = left lower sternal border, LUSB = left upper sternal border, RUSB = right upper sternal border.

ADVANCED TECHNIQUE

Assessing for Coarctation of the Aorta

If coarctation of the aorta is suspected (as when a brachial-femoral pulse lag is present, with upper extremity hypertension, or absent/decreased pedal pulses), obtain blood pressures and compare the right upper and left lower extremity readings. Pulse oximetry measurement may also be helpful. It is important to remember that signs and symptoms of coarctation of the aorta may not present until 2 to 3 weeks of life with the onset of respiratory distress, as this is the common time when the patent ductus arteriosus closes completely.

E
1. Take the upper extremity blood pressure in the right arm.
2. Because weak or absent leg pulses accompany coarctation, measurements are difficult to obtain. Use a Doppler transducer to intensify the sound of the pulse. Until you feel proficient, the Doppler technique requires two people for accurate measurement. Have the caregiver hold the child's leg still while you assess the pulse.
3. Locate the right posterior tibial pulse with the Doppler transducer and make an "X" with a pen where the pulse is felt or heard.
4. Obtain the blood pressure measurement in the left leg with the cuff ½ to 1 inch (1.3 to 2.5 cm) above the pulse location. Only the systolic number is obtained with this technique.
5. Repeat the steps on the left side of the body.

N **Upper and lower extremity blood pressures are equal.**

A If the systolic blood pressure in the leg is lower than that in the arm and femoral, popliteal, posterior tibial, or dorsalis pedis pulses are weak or absent, you can suspect that coarctation of the aorta is present. If undiagnosed, as the child becomes older, the upper extremity pulses will be bounding.

P During the fifth or sixth week of embryonic development, the aorta may form abnormally.

P Holosystolic or pansystolic murmurs are heard in children with a VSD, where blood flows from a chamber of higher pressure to one of lower pressure during systole.

A Diastolic murmurs are heard between S_2 and S_1.

P Diastolic murmurs are classified into early diastolic, middiastolic, and presystolic. Early diastolic murmurs are high-pitched and blowing. They occur in aortic regurgitation and subaortic stenosis. A middiastolic murmur is a low-pitched rumble. These occur in mitral stenosis or VSDs with large left-to-right shunts. A presystolic murmur is heard in children with mitral stenosis or tricuspid stenosis.

A Continuous murmurs heard throughout the cardiac cycle are abnormal.

P Collateral blood flow murmurs are heard radiating throughout the back, such as in pulmonary atresia.

A Continuous murmurs are present in coronary artery fistulas.

P Palliative shunt murmurs are normal and should be heard. If they are not heard, there is a possibility of a clotted shunt. These murmurs are heard over the right or left upper chest in the respective area where surgically placed. A palliative shunt is created temporarily until the client is ready for corrective surgery. A palliative shunt may be needed in a small infant with a combination of tetralogy of Fallot and pulmonary atresia or a hypoplastic pulmonary artery.

Peripheral Vasculature

Palpation

Peripheral Pulses

E
1. Use the same finger to examine each peripheral pulse. The sensation of one finger pad versus another can be different.
2. Use the finger pads to palpate each pair of peripheral pulses simultaneously (Fig. 25-43), except for the carotid pulse.
3. Palpate the brachial and femoral pulses simultaneously.

N **Pulse qualities are the same in the adult and the child.**

A A brachial-femoral lag, when femoral pulses are weaker than brachial pulses when palpated simultaneously, is abnormal.

P Coarctation of the aorta is due to a narrowing of the aorta before, at, or just beyond the entrance of the ductus arteriosus. Thus, blood flow to the lower body is reduced.

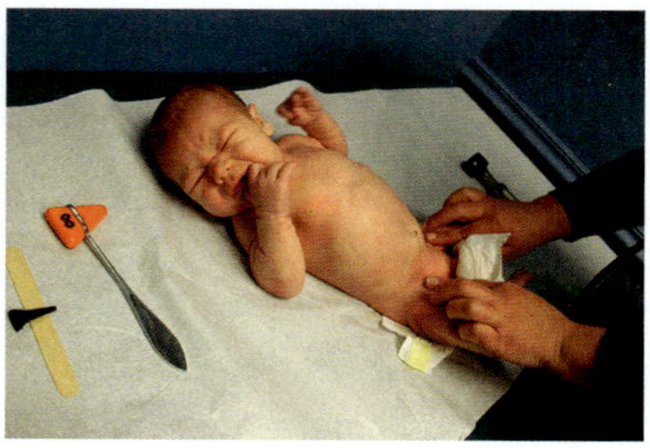

Figure 25-43 The nurse is assessing bilateral femoral pulses.

Abdomen

General Approach

E
1. If possible, ask the caregiver to refrain from feeding the infant before the examination, because palpation of a full stomach may induce vomiting.
2. Physically able children should be encouraged to empty their bladder before the examination.
3. The young infant, school-age child, or adolescent should lie on the examination table. For the toddler or preschooler, have the caregiver hold the child supine on the lap, with the lower extremities bent at the knees and dangling.
4. If the child is crying, encourage the caregiver to help calm the child before proceeding with the examination.

5. Observe nonverbal communication in children who are not able to verbally express feelings. During palpation, listen for a high-pitched cry and look for a change in facial expression (Fig. 25-44) or for sudden protective movements that may indicate a painful or tender area.
6. If the child is upset and crying, assess the umbilicus for an outward projection, which is indicative of an umbilical hernia (Fig. 25-45). If an umbilical hernia is present, palpate the area to determine whether the hernia reduces easily. Approximate the size of the inner ring (the diameter of the hernia) (see Chapter 18).

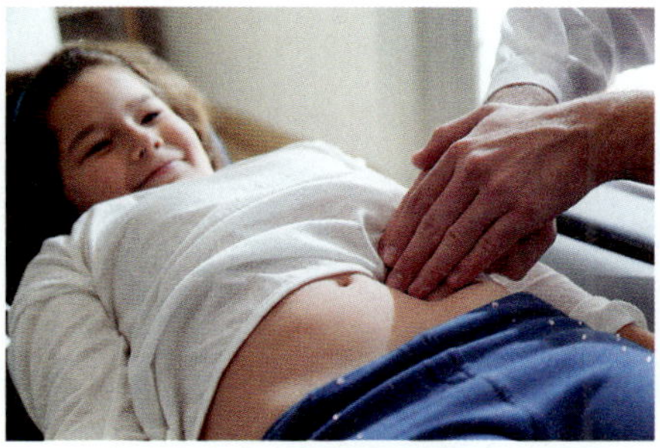

Figure 25-44 During palpation of the child's abdomen the nurse observes for facial grimacing or other signs of discomfort.

Inspection

Contour

E Conduct the examination in the same manner as for an adult.

N **The young child may have a "potbelly."**

A **P** Refer to Chapter 18.

Peristaltic Wave

E **N** See Chapter 18.

A Visible peristaltic waves seen moving across the epigastrium from left to right are abnormal.

P Obstruction at the pyloric sphincter causes a condition called pyloric stenosis. The pyloric muscle hypertrophies, obstructing embryonic development. Signs and symptoms during infancy include projectile, nonbilious vomiting, with the child being hungry afterward. This can predispose the child to dehydration and electrolyte abnormalities.

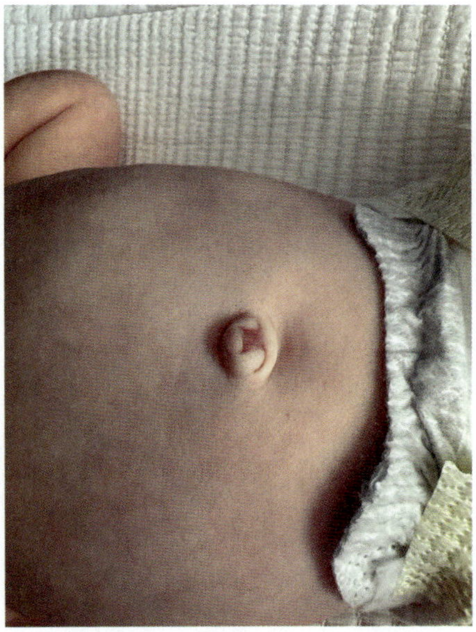

Figure 25-45 Umbilical hernia.

Auscultation

After performing auscultation of the lungs, it is helpful to proceed to auscultating the abdomen because doing so allows you to complete a good portion of auscultation all at once. If the child is not cooperating, a simple distracting phrase such as "I can hear your breakfast in there" is helpful during auscultation. Remember, just as with adults, auscultation should always precede palpation or percussion so as not to create artificial bowel sounds.

Palpation

General Palpation

E **N** See Chapter 18.

A On palpation, an olive-shaped mass felt in the epigastric area and to the upper right of the umbilicus is abnormal.

P An olive-shaped mass felt in the epigastric area and to the upper right of the umbilicus is indicative of pyloric stenosis.

A Abdominal distention coupled with palpable stool over the abdomen and the absence of stool in the rectum is abnormal.

P An aganglionic segment of the colon is responsible for Hirschsprung disease.

A Bowel sounds heard in the thoracic cavity, a scaphoid abdomen, an upwardly displaced apical impulse, and signs of respiratory distress are abnormal findings in the newborn.

P Approximately in the eighth week of embryonic development, the diaphragm fails to fuse, creating a **diaphragmatic hernia**. This condition results in protrusion of the intestines into the thoracic cavity.

> **NURSING TIP**
>
> **Measuring the Abdomen in Children**
>
> If abdominal distention is seen during inspection, evaluate its circumference. Place the tape measure around the abdomen at the level of the umbilicus. Use a marking pen to indicate the location where the tape measure was placed if serial abdominal circumference measurements are to be taken.

Liver Palpation

E For infants and toddlers, use the outer edge of your right thumb to press down and scoop up at the right upper quadrant. For the remaining age-groups, use the same technique as for an adult.

N **The liver is not normally palpated, although the liver edge can be found ⅜ inches (1 cm) below the right costal margin in a normal, healthy child. The liver edge is soft and regular.**

A It is abnormal for the liver edge to be palpated more than ⅜ inches (1 cm) below the right costal margin and be full with a firm, sharp border.

P Hepatomegaly occurs in several disease states, such as viral or bacterial illnesses, tumors, congestive heart failure, and fat and glycogen storage diseases. Viral and bacterial illnesses and tumors cause liver cells to multiply in number, creating an enlarged liver. In heart failure, the hepatic veins and sinusoids enlarge from congestion, resulting in hemorrhage and fibrosis of the liver. In fat and glycogen storage diseases, fat and glycogen accumulate within the liver, and fibrosis ensues.

Musculoskeletal System

General Approach

1. The extent or degree of the examination depends greatly on the child's or caregiver's complaints of musculoskeletal problems. Be aware that during periods of rapid growth, children complain of normal muscle aches.
2. Try to incorporate musculoskeletal examination techniques into other system examinations. For instance, while inspecting the integument, inspect the muscles and joints.
3. Inspecting the musculoskeletal system in the ambulatory child is accomplished by allowing the child to move freely about and play in the examination room while you inquire about the health history. Your observations of the child enable you to assess posture, muscle symmetry, and range of motion of muscles and joints.
4. Do not rush through the examination. Throughout the examination, incorporate game playing that facilitates evaluation of the musculoskeletal system.
5. Observe the range of motion and joint flexibility as the child undresses.

> **NURSING TIP**
>
> **Palpating Muscle Strength in Children**
>
> Playing games will assist you if the child is resistant to formal examination. For example, you can test plantar flexion by asking the child to pretend that the feet are pushing the brake on a car while you bear the force with your hands.

Inspection

Muscles

E

1. Have the child disrobe down to a diaper or underwear.
2. To evaluate the small infant's shoulder muscles, place your hands under the axillae and pull the infant into a standing position. The infant should not slip through your hands. Be prepared to catch the infant if needed.
3. Evaluate the infant's leg strength in a semistanding position. Lower the infant to the examination table so the infant's legs touch the table.
4. Place the infant older than 4 months in a prone position. Observe the infant's ability to lift the upper body off the examination table using the upper extremities.

N **The degree of joint flexibility and range of motion are the same for the child as for the adult.**

A Increased muscle tone (spasticity) is abnormal.

P Cerebral palsy (CP) results from a nonprogressive abnormality in the pyramidal motor tract. One of the more common contributing factors, perinatal asphyxia, causes abnormal posture and gross motor development and varying degrees of abnormal muscle tone.

A The inability to rise from a sitting to a standing position is abnormal. In attempting to rise from a supine position, the child first turns over onto the abdomen and raises the trunk to a crawling position. Then, with the aid of the arms, the child places the feet firmly on the floor and gradually elevates the upper part of the body by climbing up the legs with the arms.

P The inability to rise from a sitting to a standing position is called Gower's sign. Gower's sign occurs in Duchenne muscular dystrophy (MD) early in childhood. An abnormal gene in the short arm of the X chromosome is responsible for this condition.

Joints

E Conduct the examination in the same manner as for an adult.

N **The infant's spine is C-shaped. Head control and standing create the normal S-shaped spine of the adult. Lordosis is normal as the child begins to walk. A toddler's protruding abdomen is counterbalanced by an inward deviation of the lumbar spine.**

A Extra fingers or toes are abnormal (refer to Fig. 19-69B).

P Supernumerary digits, or polydactyly, may be found in certain congenital syndromes such as Carpenter, fetal hydantoin, orofaciodigital syndrome, Smith-Lemli-Opitz, trisomy 13, and VACTERL.

A A fusion between two or more digits is abnormal (refer to Fig. 19-69C).

P Syndactylism is also associated with certain congenital syndromes, such as Aarskog, Apert, Carpenter, Russell-Silver, and orofaciodigital syndrome. Look for other physical signs of a syndrome if either syndactyly or polydactyly is present.

A It is abnormal for a young male (usually 2 to 12 years old) to present with a painless limp from the affected hip. The limp is accompanied by limited abduction and internal rotation, muscle spasm, and proximal thigh atrophy.

P Legg-Calvé-Perthes disease, also called coxa plana, is caused by an interruption in the blood supply to the capital femoral epiphysis. Avascular necrosis of the femoral head results.

A The affected hip has a loss of flexion. The client is unable to rotate the hip inward. The affected leg turns outward and may appear shorter compared with the other leg while in a standing position. The adolescent often presents with a limp.

P In slipped capital femoral epiphysis the ball at the upper end of the femur slips from its normal position in a backward direction. This is due to the weakness of the growth plate. It commonly develops during periods of accelerated growth, shortly after the onset of puberty. Slipped capital femoral epiphysis occurs with greater frequency in males and children who are overweight.

A An exaggerated lumbar curvature of the spine is abnormal after 6 years of age.

P Lordosis can be attributed to bilateral developmental dislocation of the hip or postural factors such as the progression of congenital kyphosis or can occur secondary to contractures of hip flexors.

Tibiofemoral Bones

E
1. Instruct the child to stand on the examination table with the medial condyles together.
2. Stand at eye level of the client's knees.
3. Measure the distance between the two medial malleoli.
4. Measure the distance between the two medial condyles.

N **The distance between the medial malleoli is less than 2 inches (5 cm). The distance between the medial condyles is less than 1 inch (2.5 cm). Knock-knee, or genu valgum, is common between 2 and 4 years of age. Bowleg, or genu varum, is normally present in many infants up to 12 months of age.**

A Genu valgum persisting after 6 years of age is abnormal (refer to Fig. 19-55). The distance between the medial condyles is less than 1 inch (2.5 cm), and the distance between the medial malleoli is more than 2 inches (5 cm).

P The cause of genu valgum is usually physiological.

A The measured distance between the two medial condyles is greater than 1 to 2 inches (2.5 to 5 cm).

P Genu varum persisting after 2 years of age is abnormal and may be caused by rickets (refer to Fig. 19-56).

Palpation

Joints

E **N** See Chapter 19.

A Knee pain aggravated by any motion or activity that puts undue pressure on the joint is abnormal. Palpation of a slight elevation of the tibial tuberosity is abnormal.

P The deformed tubercle in Osgood-Schlatter disease is caused by repetitive stress on the area. A fibrocartilage microfracture may cause joint pain.

A Swollen, inflamed, painful joints are abnormal.

P Juvenile idiopathic arthritis causes synovial inflammation and degeneration of the joint. Its cause is unknown.

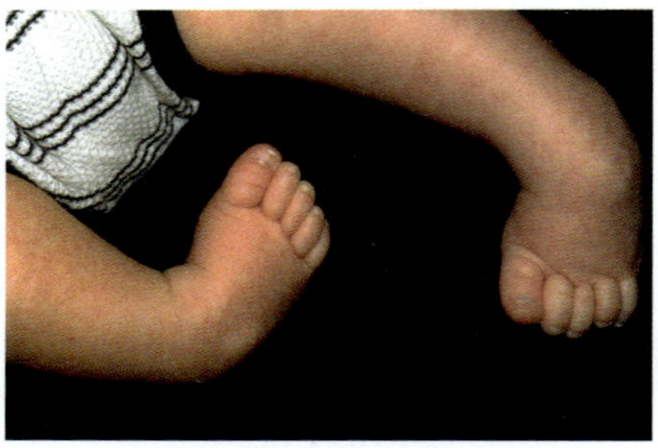

Figure 25-46 Talipes equinovarus (clubfoot).

Feet

E
1. Place the child on the examination table or the caregiver's lap.
2. Stand in front of the child.
3. Hold the right heel immobile with one hand while pushing the forefoot (medial base of great toe) toward a midline position with the other hand.
4. Observe for toe and forefoot adduction and inversion.
5. Repeat on the left foot.

N **The toes and forefoot are not deviated.**

A Toes or forefeet that are deviated are abnormal.

P **Metatarsus varus** is a medial forefoot malalignment. In **talipes equinovarus** (clubfoot), there is heel inversion, forefoot adduction, and plantar flexion of the foot (Fig. 25-46). Heredity plays a role in the etiology, as does the abnormal intrauterine position of the fetal foot.

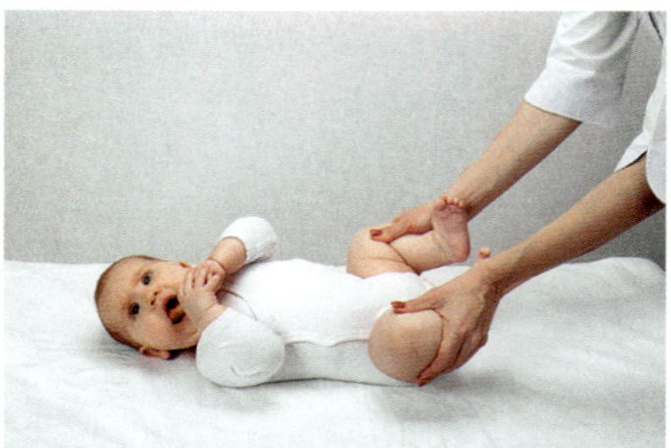

Figure 25-47 Assessing for DDH (developmental dislocation of the hip) with Ortolani maneuver.

Hip and Femur

Barlow and Ortolani maneuvers should be performed near the end of the examination because they may produce crying (Fig. 25-47). These assessments are performed on one hip at a time. Evaluate the hips up until 18 months of age or until the child is an established walker.

E

1. Place the infant supine on an examination table with the feet facing you.
2. Stand directly in front of the infant.
3. With the thumb, hold the inner thigh of the femur and with the index and middle fingers, hold the greater trochanter. These two fingers should rest over the hip joint.
4. For the Barlow maneuver, begin by adducting the hip to the midline, while applying posterior pressure. A positive finding results in a palpable clunk if the femoral head subluxes. This finding demonstrates a femoral head resting in the acetabulum but with pathological instability.
5. For the Ortolani maneuver, slowly press outward and abduct until the lateral aspects of the knees nearly touch the table. The tips of the fingers should palpate each femoral head as it rotates outward.
6. Listen for an audible clunk (positive Ortolani sign) as the femoral head relocates.
7. With the fingers in the same locations, adduct the hips to elicit a palpable clunk (positive Ortolani sign). As each hip is adducted, it is lifted anteriorly into the acetabulum.
8. Compare leg lengths in full extension.
9. Place both of the infant's feet flat on the examination table with the knees together.
10. Observe the height of the knees. Unequal knee height is termed Galeazzi's sign.
11. Turn the infant to a prone position and observe the levels of the gluteal folds.

N **A clunk is not audible or palpated with these maneuvers. Legs should be of equal lengths, and the knees should be at the same height as the feet on the examination table. The gluteal folds are at approximately the same level.**

A Abnormal findings include a positive Ortolani's sign; a sudden, painful cry during the test; asymmetrical thigh skin folds; uneven leg length or knee level; and limited hip abduction.

P Epidemiology of **developmental dislocation of the hip** (DDH) is related to familial factors, maternal (or gestational parent) hormones associated with pelvic laxity, firstborn children, oligohydramnios, and breech presentations.

A Knees that are not at the same level are abnormal.

P Knees that are not at the same level can potentially detect DDH.

A Unequal gluteal folds are abnormal.

P Unequal gluteal folds can be present in DDH.

A The affected hip has a loss of flexion and the child is unable to rotate the hip inward. The affected leg turns outward and may appear shorter compared with the other leg while in a standing position. The gait may be antalgic.

P These findings can occur in the slipped capital femoral epiphysis. Trauma, genetics, endocrine disorders, and rapid growth all play a part in the development of slipped capital femoral epiphysis.

Neurological System

General Approach

1. Some aspects of the neurological examination are different for the infant and the young child compared with the adult. An infant

> **NURSING TIP**
>
> **Neonatal Abstinence Syndrome**
>
> Neonatal Abstinence Syndrome (NAS) is a syndrome of withdrawal seen in neonates exposed to opioids and other substances in utero. There are both short- and long-term consequences depending on the substance, duration, and timing of exposure. Polysubstance use is of particular concern during pregnancy. Clinical signs and symptoms in the neonate with NAS can include high-pitched cry, sleep/wake cycle disturbances, tone or movement abnormalities, feeding difficulties, weight loss, irritability, gastrointestinal symptoms such as reflux, vomiting, and diarrhea, respiratory abnormalities, and failure to thrive. Maternal (or gestational parent) screening can be helpful in diagnosis and management plan, but infant screening often yields inconclusive results. A multidisciplinary, multimodality approach to management is key to improving outcomes (Jansson, 2025).

functions mainly at the subcortical level. Memory and motor coordination are about three-fourths developed by 2 years of age when cortical functioning is acquiring dominance.

2. Incorporate findings for fine and gross motor skills previously tested during the musculoskeletal examination. In addition, use the Revised-Denver II to assess personal-social and language skills. Refer to normal developmental milestones (see Chapter 4) and extrapolate warning signs of neurological development lag.
3. Because the infant cannot verbally express level of consciousness, instead assess the newborn's ability to cry, level of activity, positioning, and general appearance.
4. Only reflex mechanisms and cranial nerve testing are described in this section. Refer to the adult neurological examination for all other testing.

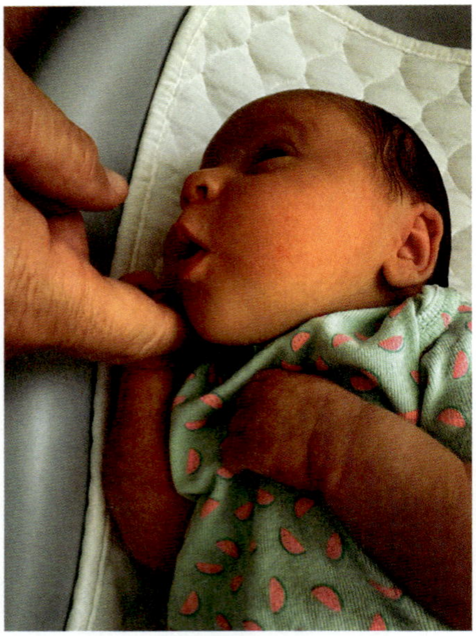

Figure 25-48 Rooting reflex.

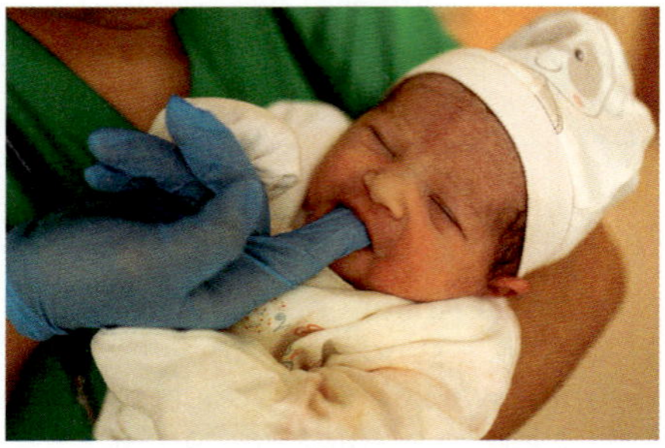

Figure 25-49 Sucking reflex.

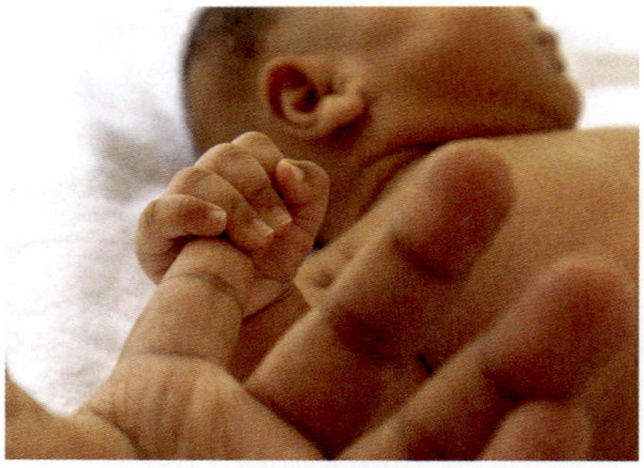

Figure 25-50 Palmar grasp reflex.

Reflex Mechanisms of the Infant

Neonatal reflexes must be lost before motor development can proceed.

Rooting Reflex

E
1. Place the infant supine with the head in a midline position.
2. With your forefinger, stroke the skin located at one corner of the mouth (Fig. 25-48).
3. Observe the movement of the head.

N **Up until 3 or 4 months of age, the infant will turn the head toward the side that was stroked. In the sleeping infant, the rooting reflex can be present normally until 6 months of age.**

A An absent rooting reflex from birth through 3 to 4 months is abnormal.

P Central nervous system disease such as frontal lobe lesions accounts for an absent rooting reflex.

Sucking Reflex

E
1. Place the infant in a supine position.
2. With your forefinger, touch the infant's lips to stimulate a response (Fig. 25-49).
3. Observe for a sucking motion.

N **The sucking reflex occurs up to approximately 10 months.**

A Absence of the sucking reflex is abnormal.

P A premature infant or a breastfed infant of a mother (or gestational parent) who ingests barbiturates does not exhibit the reflex secondary to CNS depression.

Palmar Grasp Reflex

E
1. Place the infant supine with the head in a midline position.
2. Place the ulnar sides of both index fingers into the infant's hands while the infant's arms are in a semiflexed position (Fig. 25-50).
3. Press your fingers into the infant's palmar surfaces.

N **Normally, the infant grasps your fingers in flexion.**

A Presence of the palmar grasp reflex after 4 months of age is abnormal.

P Presence of the palmar grasp reflex after 4 months of age is attributed to frontal lobe lesions.

Tonic Neck Reflex

E 1. Place the infant in a supine position on the examination table.
2. Rotate the head to one side and hold the jaw area parallel to the shoulder.
3. Observe for movement of the extremities.

N **The upper and lower extremities are on the side to which the jaw is turned extend, and the opposite arm and leg flex (Fig. 25-51). Sometimes this reflex does not show up until 6 to 8 weeks of age.**

A After 6 months of age, the tonic neck reflex is abnormal.

P Cerebral damage is suspected if the tonic neck reflex is seen after 6 months of age.

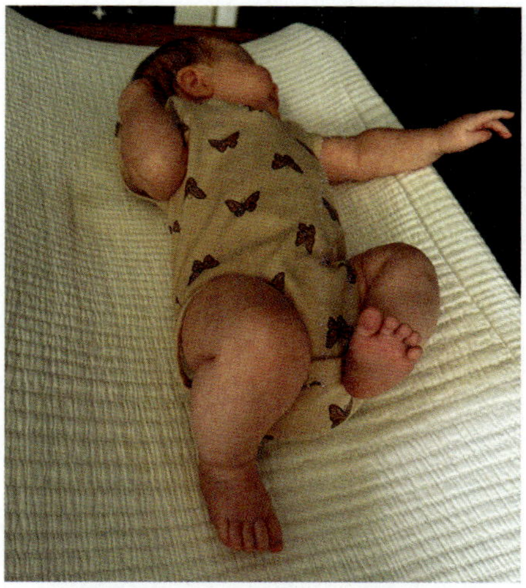

Figure 25-51 Tonic neck reflex.

Stepping Reflex

E 1. Stand behind the infant, grasp the infant under the axillae, and bring the body to a standing position on a flat surface. Use the thumbs to support the back of the head if needed.
2. Push the infant's feet toward a flat surface and simultaneously lean the infant's body forward (Fig. 25-52).
3. Observe the legs and feet for stepping movements.

N **Stepping movements are made by flexing one leg and moving the other leg forward. This reflex disappears at about 3 months of age.**

A Presence of the stepping reflex beyond 3 months of age is abnormal.

P Children with CP demonstrate a stepping reflex beyond 3 months of age.

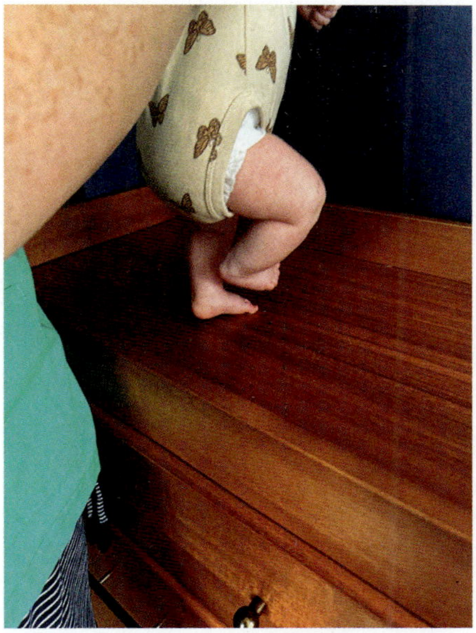

Figure 25-52 Stepping reflex.

Plantar Grasp Reflex

E 1. Position the infant supine on the examination table.
2. Elevate the foot to be examined.
3. Touch the infant's foot on the plantar surface beneath the toes (Fig. 25-53).
4. Repeat on the other side.

N **The toes curl down until 8 months of age.**

A It is abnormal for the plantar grasp reflex to be absent on one or both feet.

P An obstructive brain lesion such as an abscess or tumor can cause the plantar grasp reflex to be absent on the affected side. Bilateral absence can occur in CP.

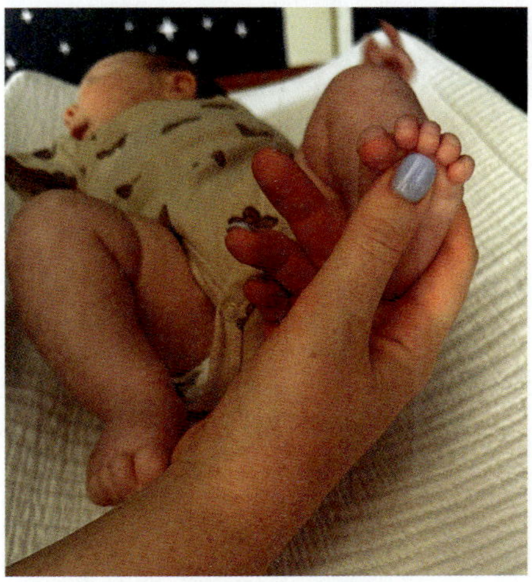

Figure 25-53 Plantar grasp reflex.

Babinski Reflex

E 1. Position the infant supine on the examination table.
2. Elevate the foot to be examined.
3. Stroke the plantar surface of the foot from the lateral heel upward with the tip of the thumbnail.

N **A child less than 15 to 18 months of age normally fans the toes outward and dorsiflexes the great toe (Fig. 25-54).**

A After the child masters walking, presence of the Babinski reflex is abnormal.

P Presence of the Babinski reflex after 18 months of age can be indicative of a perinatal insult such as cerebral palsy.

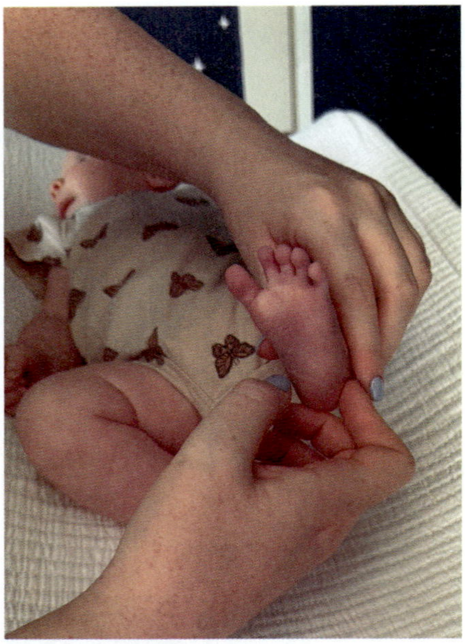

Figure 25-54 Babinski reflex.

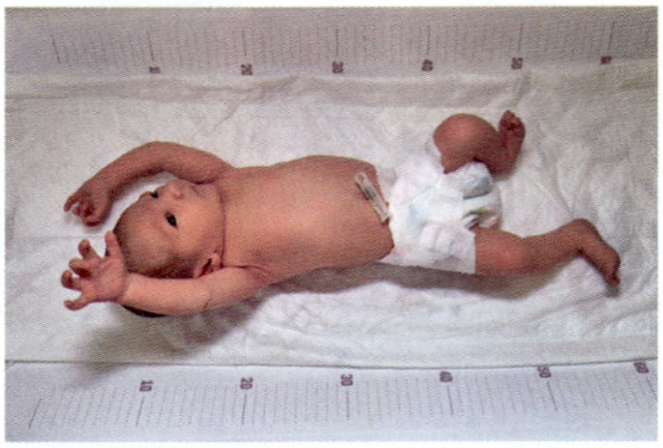

Figure 25-55 Moro reflex.

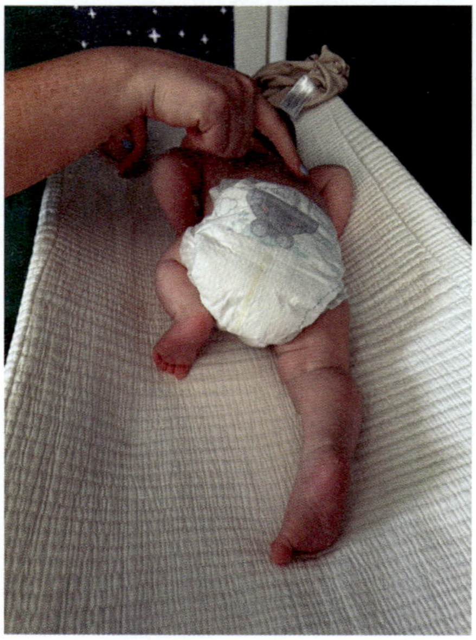

Figure 25-56 Galant reflex.

Moro (Startle) Reflex

E
1. Place the infant supine on the examination table.
2. Make a sudden, loud noise, such as hitting your hand on the examination table.
3. Another technique is to brace the infant's neck and back on the undersurface of your arm while holding the undersurface of the buttocks with the other hand and then mimicking a falling motion by quickly lowering the infant.

N **The infant under 4 months of age quickly extends then flexes the arms and fingers while the maneuver is performed. The thumb and index fingers form a C shape (Fig. 25-55).**

A Presence of the startle reflex after 4 to 6 months of age is abnormal.

P Neurological diseases such as CP can cause a positive response after the normal age of disappearance.

Galant Reflex

E
1. Place the infant prone, with the infant's hands under the abdomen.
2. Use your index finger to stroke the skin along the side of the spine (Fig. 25-56).
3. Observe the stimulated side for any movement.

N **An infant less than 1 to 2 months of age will turn the pelvis and shoulders toward the stimulated side.**

A Lack of response from an infant less than 2 months of age is abnormal.

P A spinal cord lesion is suspected if there is no response from an infant less than 2 months of age.

Placing Reflex

Do not test the placing and stepping reflexes at the same time, because they are two different reflexes.

E
1. Grasp the infant under the axillae from behind and bring the body to a standing position. Use the thumbs to support the back of the head if needed.
2. Touch the dorsum of one foot to the edge of the examination table (see Fig. 25-57).
3. Observe the tested leg for movement.

N **The infant's tested leg will flex and lift onto the examination table. This reflex typically is gone by 1 year of age.**

A Lack of response is abnormal.

P It is difficult to elicit this reflex in breech-born babies and in those with paralysis or cerebral cortex abnormalities

Landau Reflex

E
1. Carefully suspend the infant in a prone position, supporting the chest with your hand.
2. Observe for extension of the head, trunk, and hips.

N **The arms and legs extend during the reflex. The reflex appears at about 3 to 4 months of age.**

A Presence of the Landau reflex beyond 3 years of age is abnormal. Also, it is abnormal for the infant to assume a limp position.

P A retained Landau reflex can indicate a motor development condition.

Cranial Nerve Function

A thorough examination of cranial nerve function is difficult to perform on an infant who is less than 1 year old. Difficulty is also encountered with toddlers and preschoolers because they often cannot follow directions or are not willing to cooperate. Testing for the school-age child or the adolescent is carried out in the same manner as for an adult.

Infant (Birth to 12 Months)

E
1. To test cranial nerves (CN) III, IV, and VI, move a brightly colored toy or black toy along the infant's line of vision. An infant older than 1 month responds by following the object. Also, evaluate the pupillary response to a bright light in each eye.
2. CN V is tested by assessing the rooting or sucking reflexes.
3. CN VII is tested up until 2 months by assessing the sucking reflex and by observing symmetrical sucking movements. After 2 months of age, an infant will smile, allowing assessment of the symmetry of facial expressions.
4. A positive Moro reflex in an infant less than 6 months old is evidence of normal functioning of CN VIII.
5. CNs IX and X are examined by using a tongue blade to produce a gag reflex. Do not test if a positive response was already elicited by using a tongue blade to view the posterior pharynx.
6. To test CN XI, evaluate the infant's ability to lift the head while in a prone position.
7. CN XII is assessed by allowing the infant to suck on a pacifier or a bottle, abruptly removing the pacifier or bottle from the infant's mouth, and observing for lingering sucking movements.

N A P See Chapter 20.

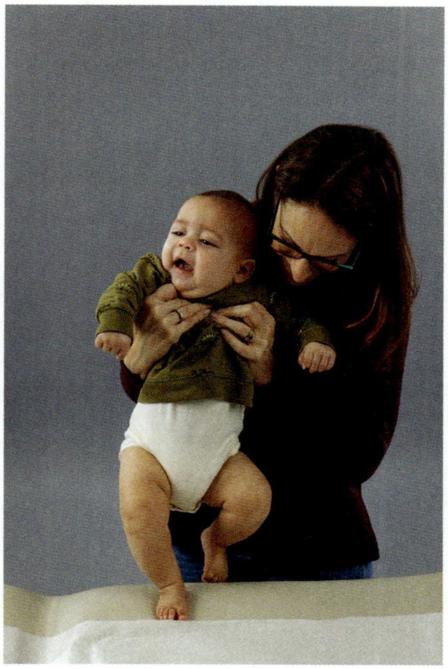

Figure 25-57 Placing reflex.

Toddler and Preschooler (1 to 5 Years)

1. The older preschooler can identify familiar odors. Most children readily identify the smells of orange and chocolate. (Assess for food allergies before using food in a test.) Test CN I one side at a time by asking the child to close their eyes and to identify a familiar smell. Test each nostril with different substances while occluding the other nostril with your finger can also test for nasal patency and CN I at the same time.
2. Test vision (CN II) by having the child identify and match common objects on cards.
3. CNs III, IV, and VI are tested in the same fashion as for the infant.
4. CN V is tested by giving the child something to eat and evaluating chewing movements. Sensory responses to light and sharp touch are still not easily interpreted in these age-groups.
5. Observe facial weakness or paralysis (CN VII) by making the child smile or laugh. An older preschooler may cooperate by raising the eyebrows, frowning, puffing the cheeks out, and closing the eyes tightly on command.
6. To evaluate CN VIII, ring a small bell out of the child's vision and observe the response to unseen sounds.
7. Test CNs IX and X in the same manner as for the infant.
8. CN XII can be assessed by asking the child to stick out their tongue and push against their cheek.

N A P See Chapter 20.

> **NURSING TIP**
> **Fat Intake in Young Children**
> The caregiver should not restrict or limit fat intake until after 2 years of age because fat is needed for myelin development. After 2 years of age, the caregiver should switch the child to 2% milk; after 6 years of age, a switch to skim milk can be made. Six years of age coincides with the time the brain has achieved its greatest growth potential.

Female Genitalia

General Approach

1. Place the up-to-preschool-age child on the caregiver's lap or examination table. Ask the caregiver to assist by holding the child's legs in a froglike position. Place the child older than 4 years on the examination table in a semilithotomy position, without the feet in

NURSING TIP

Accidental Marijuana Poisoning in Children

With the increased decriminalization of state marijuana laws and increase in the mechanism of delivery, in particular with edible products, an increase in accidental marijuana ingestion in the pediatric population is being observed and anticipated to increase in prevalence. Marijuana-related emergency room visits are increasing (CDC, 2023). Marijuana can be consumed in many forms: via inhalation, topical absorption, and orally in the form of edibles, oils, tinctures, and capsules. Of particular concern for the pediatric population is the route of edibles, such as brownies or gummies, as these appeal to younger children in their presentation and are easily consumed. In a 2023 study, Tweet, Nemanich, and Wahl reported a 1375% increase in edible cannabis product ingestion in children under the age of six. Furthermore, tetrahydrocannabinol (THC), the active ingredient in the marijuana plant that produces psychoactive properties, also contributes to CNS toxicities. THC is often more highly concentrated in edibles. Children under the age of 6 typically present with neurological signs and symptoms, including, but not limited to, tremor, ataxia, and a decreased level of consciousness (lethargy, stupor, and/or coma). In contrast, older children usually present with tachycardia, tachypnea, hypertension, nystagmus, ataxia, slurred speech, dry mouth, conjunctival injection, and increased appetite. Other signs and symptoms seen include pallor, hypotonia, bradycardia, irritability, nausea, and vomiting. Almost all of the cases present with some sort of delayed effect of altered mental status after ingestion. Nurses must be familiar with the common products seen in their practice area, as well as be vigilant to assess for possible ingestion in children presenting with any of the aforementioned signs and symptoms. Of note, synthetic marijuana is difficult to detect and quantify via standard methodologies, making detection even more challenging. Education and advocacy for this vulnerable population will become even more important as the legalization and decriminalization of marijuana increase across the U.S. in future years.

stirrups. Reserve the lithotomy position with the feet in stirrups for the older adolescent.

2. Explain the procedure before the examination. Never ask the caregiver of the infant or young school-age child to leave the room during this portion of the examination because the caregiver is a source of comfort to the child.
3. The child should be told before the genitalia examination that it is all right for the provider to touch the genitals with the parent present but not for anyone else to do so for any reason.
4. Drape the older-than-preschool-age child.
5. A vaginal and pelvic examination is not routinely performed on young females. A vaginal examination is warranted, however, when signs of possible sexual abuse are present. See the Nursing Tip on Signs of Sexual Abuse in Children in this chapter. The examination is undertaken by a health-care provider who is trained to perform pediatric vaginal examinations and can evaluate the clinical findings.
6. Any female who has reached menarche needs to be evaluated for a pregnant uterus when dictated by the health history.

NURSING TIP

Alternative Alcohol Consumption

Be alert for new ways in which children and adolescents abuse substances such as alcohol. Some individuals may choose to get drunk via an alcohol enema. Others may use "backpacking." In "backpacking" a tampon is soaked in some type of alcohol, frequently vodka, and inserted into the rectum. Females may also insert the alcohol-infused tampon into their vaginas. Due to the blood supply in the rectum and vagina, rapid absorption of the alcohol occurs and the individual may exhibit signs/symptoms of intoxication. This method of getting "a buzz" avoids an alcohol odor to the breath and is therefore attractive to underage individuals. Acute alcohol poisoning has resulted from alcohol enemas and "backpacking" because the amount of alcohol absorbed is not readily quantified by the user.

Inspection

Sexual Maturity Rating

E
1. Using the Tanner stages in Table 21-1, assess the developmental stage of the pubic hair.
2. Determine the SMR.

N **Female adolescents usually start developing pubic hair by 8 to 12 years of age. Females' pubic hair usually reaches the adult stage by age 15.**

A An SMR that is less than expected for a female's age is abnormal.

P Delayed puberty may be familial, genetic, or caused by chronic illnesses.

> **NURSING TIP**
>
> **Sexually Transmitted Infection Education for Adolescents**
>
> The following preventive guidelines are essential to discuss during your interview. To fit appropriately into the context of the interview, inquiry is preferable after questioning about sexual relationships and the use of contraceptives.
>
> - If the adolescent is sexually active, discuss their feelings on the subject.
> - Talk about the various sexually transmitted infections (STIs) (e.g., human immunodeficiency virus (HIV), chlamydia, herpes simplex virus (HSV), human papillomavirus (HPV), gonorrhea), including their symptoms and sequelae.
> - Mention that abstinence is the only certain method of preventing STIs and pregnancy.
> - If the individual cannot comply with abstinence, then discuss proper condom or other barrier application and use.
> - Encourage the client to avoid having sex with anyone who claims to be infected.
> - Discuss facilities that offer confidential testing if the individual believes they or a partner has contracted an STI.
> - Discuss the dangers of oral or anal sex without condom/barrier product use.

Perineal Area

E Conduct an examination in the same manner as for an adult.

N **The female infant's labia minora are sometimes larger than the labia majora. The hymen is sometimes intact up until the point of sexual activity.**

A It is abnormal for the female infant to display a rudimentary penis in the clitoral area.

P Genital ambiguity occurs during embryonic development as a consequence of genetic causes, androgens, or androgen inhibitors that reverse genital characteristics.

A A bloody discharge noted at the vaginal opening or on the diaper is abnormal.

P It is not uncommon to note pseudomenstruation in an infant under 2 weeks of age. Maternal (or gestational parent) hormones such as estrogen are the cause.

Male Genitalia

General Approach

1. Female nurses may encounter difficulty examining a reluctant male adolescent. Be firm when explaining that this portion is a required part of his examination. Infants and toddlers do not object to the examination. Be sure to explain to the preschool-age child and older that it is only permissible for a medical professional to look at or touch private areas with the caregiver in the room.
2. Have a diaper or disposable cloth available to catch the stream of urine in case the infant or toddler urinates during the examination.
3. The older school-age child and the adolescent should be draped to maintain modesty.

Inspection

Sexual Maturity Rating

E
1. Using the Tanner stages in Table 22-1, assess the developmental stage of the pubic hair, penis, and scrotum.
2. Determine the SMR.

> **Risk Factors**
>
> **Adolescent Suicide**
>
> - Verbalizing ways to commit suicide
> - Giving personal items away to friends and family
> - Withdrawing from friends and family
> - Demonstrating difficulty with accepting individual failures or disappointments
> - Exhibiting an attitude of disgust or discouragement with day-to-day living
> - Feelings of burdensomeness
> - Recent hospitalization for nonfatal self-harm
> - Sleep disturbances
> - History of mental health issues
> - Psychosocial stresses
> - Sexual orientation and gender identity dysphoria
> - Family instability
> - Diagnosis of a chronic medical condition

NURSING TIP
Male Circumcision

In August 2012, the American Academy of Pediatrics (AAP) published its recommendation that the benefits of newborn male circumcision outweigh the risks of the procedure. Evidence-based studies show that a circumcised male has a decreased risk of contracting HIV, STIs (e.g., HSV, HPV, and syphilis), and penile cancer. There is also a decreased occurrence of urinary tract infections (UTIs) in the circumcised male. The AAP states that the decision of whether to circumcise a male infant ultimately rests with the family of the newborn.

N **Males usually begin puberty between the ages of 9½ and 13½. The average male proceeds through puberty in about 3 years, with a possible range of 2 to 5 years.**

A An SMR that is less than expected for a male's age is abnormal.

P Delayed puberty may be familial or caused by genetics and chronic illnesses.

A A normally formed but diminutive penis is abnormal. There is a discrepancy between the penile size and the age of the individual.

P A **microphallus** penis can result from a disorder in the hypothalamus or pituitary gland. It may be secondary to primary testicular failure due to partial androgen insensitivity. In-utero exposure to diethylstilbestrol (DES) has teratogenic effects on the fetus. Microphallus may also be idiopathic in nature.

A It is abnormal when the penis appears larger than what is generally expected for the stated age. This condition is usually evident only before the age of normal puberty.

P Hormonal influence of tumors of the pineal gland or hypothalamus, tumors of the Leydig cells of the testes, tumors of the adrenal gland, or precocious genital maturity may cause penile hyperplasia.

A A testicle that is smaller and softer than normal (less in the fully developed male) is abnormal.

P An atrophic testicle may be the result of Klinefelter syndrome (hypogonadism), hypopituitarism, estrogen therapy, or orchitis.

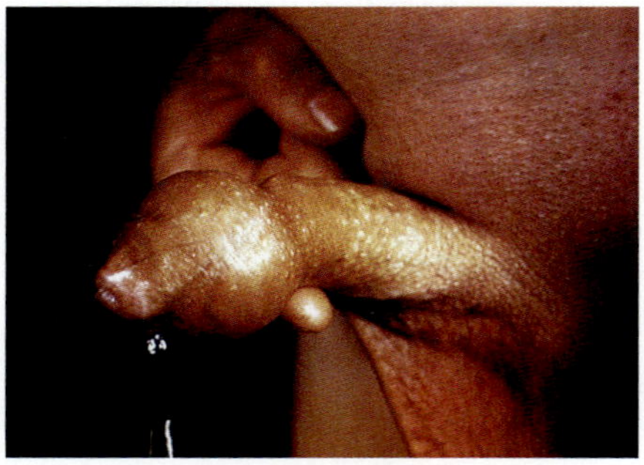

Figure 25-58 Phimosis.

Penis

E
1. Note the appearance of the penis. If you are not able to determine circumcision status, ask the caregiver if the child was circumcised.
2. Note the position of the urethral meatus.

N **The meatus is normally found on the tip of the penis. A disappearing penis phenomenon occurs normally in infants with increased adipose tissue in the area surrounding the penis. Reassure the caregiver that this is normal and will resolve after adipose tissue is lost.**

A An unusually long foreskin or one that cannot be retracted over the glans penis is abnormal.

P **Phimosis** (Fig. 25-58) occurs in uncircumcised males. The inability to retract the foreskin is normal in infancy. In later years, an acquired constricting circumferential scar may follow the healing of a split foreskin.

A It is abnormal for the meatal opening to be on the dorsal surface of the penis.

P During the third month of fetal development, the urethral meatus fails to move toward the glans penis, causing an epispadias deformity (Fig. 22-14).

A It is abnormal for the urethral meatus to be located behind or along the ventral side of the penis.

P During the third month of fetal development, the urethral meatus fails to move toward the glans penis, creating a condition known as hypospadias (Fig. 22-15). Children at greater risk for hypospadias are those whose mothers (or gestational parents) were on hydantoin for epilepsy during pregnancy.

Scrotum

E 1. Evaluate scrotal size and color.
2. Note if the testes are seen in the scrotal sac.

N **The scrotum appears proportionately large compared with the penis. The sac color is brown or black in dark-skinned children and pink in light-skinned children. Two testes should be present, but, in infants, they may retract into the inguinal canal or abdomen due to various stimuli, including cold and palpation.**

A P See Chapter 22.

Palpation

Scrotum

E 1. Place the infant in a supine position on the examination table. Instruct the young child to sit cross-legged to inhibit the cremasteric reflex from occurring. The older child may be allowed to stand for this portion of the examination.
2. Locate each testis within the scrotal sac by using the fingers of one hand in a milking motion to cause the testes to descend.
3. Palpate and note the size, shape, and mobility of each testis.

N **See Chapter 22.**

A It is abnormal to be unable to palpate the testes.

P **Cryptorchidism** is a failure of a testis to descend into the scrotal sac. One or both testes failing to descend within the inguinal canal occurs during embryonic development.

A An enlargement of the scrotum is abnormal.

P A congenital hydrocele (Fig. 22-34) results from failure of the male reproductive tract to develop properly while the fetus is in utero. This mass will transilluminate and the fluid will often clear during the first year of life.

Inguinal Hernia

E 1. Place the infant supine on the examination table if unable to stand. All other children should stand during the examination.
2. Use the little finger for the infant's and the index finger for the younger child's examination.
3. Follow the inguinal canal as is done on an adult male.
4. If possible, perform the examination on a crying infant.
5. Have preschoolers and early school-age children attempt to blow out a pretend candle while you palpate the inguinal areas.
6. Palpate the inguinal areas while the older school-age child or adolescent coughs.

N A P See Chapter 22.

> **NURSING TIP**
>
> **Signs of Sexual Abuse in Children**
>
> The following are signs of possible sexual abuse in children:
> - A strong fear of the examination
> - Presence of STIs
> - Abnormal genital discharge or odor
> - Anorectal tears
> - Absent or delayed anal reflex
> - Anorectal ecchymosis, pruritus, scarring, HPV, or bleeding
> - In the female child, a broken hymen can be a sign of sexual abuse. Keep in mind that a broken hymen can also occur from foreign objects being placed into the vagina by the child, forceful use of diaper wipes during a diaper change, tampon use, and strenuous exercise such as gymnastics and horseback riding
> - Vaginal tears or other signs of trauma

Anus

As a rule, rectal examinations are not performed on children unless an abnormal clinical finding is detected or there is suspicion of sexual abuse. In these cases, refer children for further evaluation if you are not trained specifically for this procedure and follow your institution's guidelines.

Inspection

E 1. Ask the child to lie on the abdomen.
2. Gently separate the buttocks to allow direct visualization of the anal opening.

3. Observe for bleeding, fissures, prolapse, skin tags, hemorrhoids, lesions, and pinworms.
4. During separation of the buttocks, observe any movement of the anus.
5. Stroke the perianal area with your finger and note any movement. This is called the anal reflex or anal wink.

N **No bleeding, fissures, prolapse, skin tags, hemorrhoids, lesions, or pinworms should be present. An anal reflex is observed.**

A An absent anal reflex is abnormal.

P Conditions such as a spinal cord lesion, trauma, and tumors that interrupt nervous innervation to the anal sphincter cause this finding.

P Anal trauma, such as that which occurs in sexual assault, manifests as poor anal sphincter control. Consider sexual abuse if a child exhibits an absent or slow anal reflex.

COVID-19 Effects on the Pediatric Client

While the entire world has been affected by the COVID-19 pandemic, children have unique considerations due to their developmental levels that predispose them to significant consequences from the virus. More than 1.5 million children worldwide have experienced primary or secondary orphanhood from their parents'/caretakers' COVID-19 illness or death (Hillis et al, 2022). In the U.S. more than 140,000 children under the age of 18 lost their caretaker to COVID-19 (NIH, 2021). The pandemic also affected access to health care, schooling, socialization, and well-child and immunization recommended schedules. Many children were less active during the pandemic due to forced isolation being indoors. Furthermore, the pandemic's stress on caregivers and children has led to increased depression, anxiety, behavioral concerns, and significant impacts on social determinants of health (food insecurity, housing insecurity, caregiver job loss, loss of health insurance, etc.). Due to these effects, children are at increased risk for developmental delays, communicable diseases, obesity, diabetes, hypertension, poor academic outcomes, and mental health disorders. Not to be overlooked is the increase in neglect, abuse, risk-taking behaviors (Lundahl et al, 2021), and suicide ideation. Nurses must recognize the deleterious effects the pandemic had on child, now even years later (Crawford et. al, 2022).

U.S. Preventive Services Task Force (USPSTF)

Grade A Recommendations:

- The USPSTF recommends screening for cervical cancer every 3 years with cervical cytology alone in women aged 21 to 29 years.
- The USPSTF recommends that all persons planning to or who could become pregnant take a daily supplement containing 0.4 to 0.8 mg (400 to 800 mcg) of folic acid.
- The USPSTF recommends that clinicians screen for HIV infection in adolescents and adults aged 15 to 65 years. Younger adolescents . . . who are at increased risk of infection should also be screened.
- The USPSTF recommends screening for hypertension in adults 18 years or older with office blood pressure measurement (OBPM). The USPSTF recommends obtaining blood pressure measurements outside of the clinical setting for diagnostic confirmation before starting treatment.
- The USPSTF recommends prophylactic ocular topical medication for all newborns to prevent gonococcal ophthalmia neonatorum.
- The USPSTF recommends screening for syphilis infection in persons who are at increased risk for infection.

Grade B Recommendations:

- The USPSTF recommends screening for anxiety in children and adolescents aged 8 to 18 years.
- The USPSTF recommends screening for chlamydia and gonorrhea in all sexually active women 24 years or younger . . . who are at increased risk for infection.
- The USPSTF recommends screening for major depressive disorder (MDD) in adolescents aged 12 to 18 years.
- The USPSTF recommends screening for hepatitis B virus (HBV) infection in adolescents and adults at increased risk for infection.
- The USPSTF recommends screening for hepatitis C virus (HCV) infection in adults aged 18 to 79 years.
- The USPSTF recommends that clinicians provide or refer children and adolescents 6 years or older with a high body mass index (BMI) (≥95th percentile for age and sex) to comprehensive, intensive behavioral interventions.
- The USPSTF recommends that clinicians screen for HIV infection in adolescents and adults aged 15 to 65 years. Younger adolescents and older adults who are at increased risk of infection should also be screened.
- The USPSTF recommends that clinicians screen for intimate partner violence (IPV) in women of reproductive age and provide or refer women who screen positive to ongoing support services. [See the USPSTF website for information on IPV in men]
- The USPSTF recommends that clinicians screen for obesity in children and adolescents 6 years and older and offer or refer them to comprehensive, intensive behavioral interventions to promote improvements in weight status.
- The USPSTF recommends that primary care clinicians apply fluoride varnish to the primary teeth of all infants and children starting at the age of primary tooth eruption.
- The USPSTF recommends that primary care clinicians prescribe oral fluoride supplementation starting at age 6 months for children whose water supply is deficient in fluoride.
- The USPSTF recommends behavioral counseling for all sexually active adolescents and for adults who are at increased risk for sexually transmitted infections (STIs).
- The USPSTF recommends counseling young adults, adolescents, children, and parents of young children about minimizing exposure to ultraviolet (UV) radiation for persons aged 6 months to 24 years with fair skin types to reduce their risk of skin cancer.
- The USPSTF recommends that primary care clinicians provide interventions, including education or brief counseling, to prevent initiation of tobacco use among school-aged children and adolescents.
- The USPSTF recommends screening for unhealthy alcohol use in primary care settings in adults 18 years or older, including pregnant women, and providing persons engaged in risky or hazardous drinking with brief behavioral counseling interventions to reduce unhealthy alcohol use.
- The USPSTF recommends screening by asking questions about unhealthy drug use in adults age 18 years or older. Screening should be implemented when services for accurate diagnosis, effective treatment, and appropriate care can be offered or referred. (Screening refers to asking questions about unhealthy drug use, not testing biological specimens.)
- The USPSTF recommends vision screening at least once in all children aged 3 to 5 years to detect amblyopia or its risk factors.

Note: USPSTF Recommendations relating to pregnancy can be found in Chapter 24, The Pregnant Client. Retrieved December 18, 2025 from *https://uspreventiveservicestaskforce.org/uspstf/recommendation-topics/uspstf-a-and-b-recommendations*

CASE STUDY

The Client With Ear Pain and a Hydrocele

This case study illustrates the application and objective documentation of the pediatric examination. The Gonzalez family emigrated from Venezuela to the U.S. 7 years ago due to limited job opportunities back home. Daniela and Luis Gonzalez have 3 children. Daniela and Luis speak little English. Spanish is their primary language. Daniela brings the youngest child, Mauricio, to the health clinic for an illness.

HEALTH HISTORY

LEGAL GUARDIAN

Daniela Gonzalez

SOURCE OF INFORMATION

Ms. Daniela Gonzalez (Mother); Ms. Maria Hernandez (Interpreter)

CLIENT PROFILE

Mauricio Gonzalez, 10-month-old male

CHIEF COMPLAINT

"I'm worried my son has an ear problem."

HISTORY OF PRESENT ILLNESS

Mauricio was in good health until 2 days ago. Mother reported the baby has been cranky, congested, and pulling at the left ear for 2 days. Last night he had a fever of 38.9°C (102°F). Mother denies the child has had any cough, difficulty breathing, color changes, vomiting, or diarrhea. Mauricio has been breastfeeding more often but for shorter periods and often pulls off the breast crying.

PAST HEALTH HISTORY

Birth History Mauricio is the third of 3 children. Mother denies alcohol, drug, ibuprofen, caffeine, or tobacco use during her pregnancies. Mauricio was carried to full term at 40 weeks without any complications during labor, home delivery, or postpartum. There were no health problems or developmental problems during the neonatal period.

Medical History No known medical conditions

Surgical History Denies

Allergies No known allergies

Medications No routine medications per mother's report; mother gave infant liquid acetaminophen — a small spoonful (exact quantity unknown) last night and this morning to manage fever

Communicable Diseases None that the mother knows about

Injuries and Accidents None

Differing Abilities None identified

Blood Transfusions None

Childhood Illnesses At 2 mos of age the mother reports child had a breathing virus for a few days but recovered quickly

Immunizations Daniela believes Mauricio is current, "he gets what is given to at the health department"

FAMILY HEALTH HISTORY

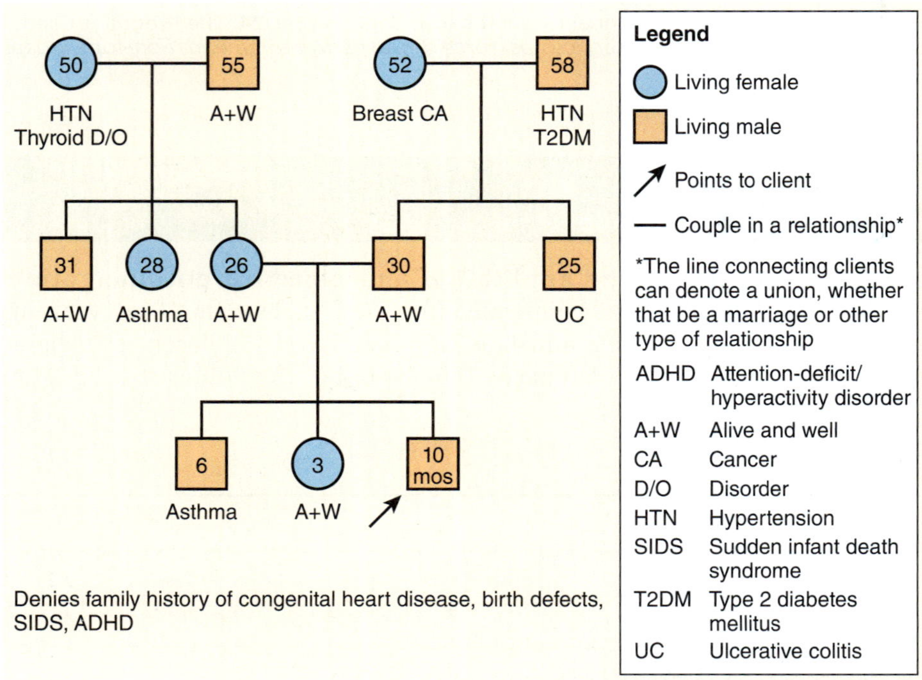

Denies family history of congenital heart disease, birth defects, SIDS, ADHD

SOCIAL HISTORY

Alcohol, Tobacco, and Recreational Drug Use Denies

Domestic and Intimate Partner Violence Denies

Sexual Practice Denies

Travel History Daniela and Luis are originally from Venezuela. They came to the U.S. 7 yrs ago and have not left the country since then. The children have never been outside the U.S. Mother refused to provide additional details.

Home Environment The Gonzalez family lives in a 3-bedroom, 2-bathroom apartment with another Venezuelan family of 3 people. Apartment has modern appliances but no air conditioning. The kitchen is shared. The Gonzalez family has no guns in home; mother denies use of alcohol and recreational drugs; no pets

Economic Status Daniela is at home caring for the 3 children. Luis is a day laborer with unsteady work. They frequently acquire food from the Catholic Charities food pantry. The family has no savings and no health insurance; they rely on public transportation.

Religion The family practices Roman Catholicism and attend weekly Mass. They pray the rosary every night together as a family.

Ethnic Background Family observes Venezuelan cultural events/celebrations.

Roles and Relationships Daniela and Luis want to provide a safe life for their children in the U.S. and have them get a good education. Daniela and Luis support each other. They miss their family and friends back home.

HEALTH MAINTENANCE ACTIVITIES

Sleep Baby shares a bed with parents. Sleeps through the night, although has been awakening the past two nights crying and wanting to nurse. Other 2 children share a bed.

Diet Breastfeeds ad lib, 2 meals of vegetables, fruits, and grains each day- a mix of baby and table food. Drinks tap water from a bottle.

Use of Safety Devices Transportation to appointments via public transportation. Baby does not have car seat.

Safety The family feels safe in their apartment. The apartment has a smoke detector, but it is not known if the battery is active. Not sure if there is a carbon monoxide detector. There is a fire extinguisher in the hallway by the elevator.

Health Checkups Health care is usually obtained at the health department, but it was closed today for an unknown reason.

DEVELOPMENT

All gross motor, fine motor, social language skills are well developed and appropriate for age: pulls to stand, crawls, sits unsupported; utilizes 2-finger grasp to retrieve cheerios, bangs objects together, claps hands, waves 'bye-bye'; babbles, nonspecific; plays peek-a-boo

PHYSICAL EXAMINATION

General Survey and Vital Signs

General survey: Male infant in no apparent distress
Temperature: 101.8°F (38.8°C) temporal artery
Heart rate: apical pulse: 120
Respirations: 32
Blood pressure: not measured
SpO_2: 98%

Physical Growth

Weight: 18 lb, 8 oz (8.4 kg) (25th percentile)
Height: 28 inches (71 cm) (25th percentile)
Head circumference: 17.75 inches (45 cm) (50th percentile)
Weight-for-length: 50th percentile

Skin

Inspection Skin appropriate for ethnicity; no cyanosis or jaundice noted; no erythema, papules, vesicles, or edema

Palpation Soft, warm, and moist. Extremities warm with 2-second capillary refill in all 4 extremities

Hair and Nails

Inspection and Palpation Black, soft hair. Nails clean, nailbeds intact

Head

Inspection Normocephalic, symmetrical, round. No plagiocephaly. Face symmetrical, no involuntary movements

Palpation Nontender, no masses or lesions. No overriding sutures. Anterior fontanel soft and flat. Posterior fontanel nonpalpable

Eyes

Inspection No ptosis or lid lag

Sclera white, conjunctiva without injection, no discharge, cornea smooth and transparent, iris brown, extraocular movements (EOM) intact

Pupils equally reactive to light and accommodation (PERRLA), positive red reflex, optic disc creamy without hemorrhages

Ears

Auditory Testing Responds to conversational tones

Inspection (External Ear) Top of pinna positioned at level of outer canthus bilaterally, pinna without lesions or masses

Palpation (External Ear) No pain with movement

Inspection (Internal Ear) External canals with no cerumen, lesions, erythema. Right tympanic membrane (TM) pearly gray without retraction, bulging, perforation, fluid, or air bubbles, TM moves with insufflation, landmarks intact, positive light reflex. Left TM erythematous, bulging, opaque, no landmarks, scattered light reflex, no movement on insufflation.

Nose

Inspection Nares patent. Mucosa pink, septum midline, no edema of turbinates. Mucoid-yellowish discharge bilaterally

Mouth and Throat

Inspection Lips pink, moist, no lesions, edges meet; buccal mucosa pink, moist, no lesions; 4 teeth present in good condition, no visible caries. Tongue pink, midline. Normal positioned palate, hard and soft palates intact, no lesions. Tonsils 1+/4+. Pharynx pink, no lesions. Uvula midline. Uvula and soft palate rise symmetrically on phonation.

Neck

Inspection Symmetrical, full active range of motion (AROM), no edema; no torticollis

Palpation Thyroid nonpalpable, trachea midline, <1 cm left posterior auricular lymph node mobile, nontender node; no other lymph nodes palpable

Breasts and Regional Lymph Nodes

Inspection Within normal limits (WNL)

Palpation Axillary nodes nonpalpable

Thorax and Lungs

Inspection Thorax without lesions, retractions; no barrel chest

Palpation Nontender

Percussion Resonant bilaterally

Auscultation Clear breath sounds equal bilaterally; bronchial sounds over trachea, vesicular sounds throughout peripheral lung fields. No adventitious sounds

Heart

Inspection Apical impulse at left 4th intercostal space (ICS) at midclavicular line (MCL), no heaves/precordial lifts

Palpation Apical impulse at left 4th ICS MCL, regular rhythm

Auscultation Apical heart rate even and regular, normal S_1 and S_2, no S_3 or S_4 audible, no murmur noted

Peripheral Vasculature

Inspection No digital clubbing, negative jugular venous distention

Palpation Pulses 2+/3+ bilaterally. No brachial-femoral lag

Abdomen

Inspection Rounded and symmetrical, abdominal musculature continuous. No masses, no lesions, no hernias noted

Auscultation Positive bowel sounds in all 4 quadrants, no venous hums, no bruits at femoral, iliac, renal, or aortic areas

Percussion Tympanic in all 4 quadrants

Palpation Soft, nontender, no masses, no hepatosplenomegaly, kidneys nonpalpable

Musculoskeletal

Inspection AROM in all 4 extremities

Palpation Joints without tenderness, crepitus, warmth, edema. Hips: negative Barlow/Ortolani; equal leg lengths, knee heights, and thigh folds

Neurological

Inspection Appropriate bulk and tone; CN II–XII grossly intact. Fine motor and gross motor skills intact. Deep tendon reflexes (DTRs) 2+/3+ all 4 extremities. Babinski present

Male Genitalia

Inspection Tanner I, uncircumcised. Testicles descended. The right scrotum is enlarged.

Palpation No scrotal or testicular tenderness, no hernias; both testicles are firm and palpable

Rectum and Anus Deferred

Advanced Technique Positive transillumination of the right scrotal sac

CLINICAL JUDGMENT IN ACTION

1. What cues indicate the child is having some health issues?
2. What interventions have the highest priority?
3. What assessment findings indicate clinical improvement in this client?

Review Questions

1. You are seeing a 12-month-old for a well-child visit with no prior health records. The child weighs 24 lb, 8 oz. The parent asks if this is normal for a child who was 8 lb at birth. An appropriate response would be:
   a. "We expect children to double their birth weight by 12 months."
   b. "We expect children to triple their birth weight by 12 months."
   c. "Without seeing the past medical records, there is no way to answer this question."
   d. "As long as your child is not losing weight, there is no concern."
2. The parents of a 2-month-old want to create an alternative immunization schedule for their child. The best response by the nurse would be:
   a. "This is totally your decision. As long as the child gets all the immunizations before school, you are fine."
   b. "I don't blame you, giving all these vaccines at once overloads the immune system."
   c. "The vaccine schedule has been well studied and choosing an alternate schedule carries increased risks. Please tell me what makes you hesitant to follow the schedule?"
   d. "A lot of these diseases don't even exist in the U.S. currently, so an alternative schedule is no big deal."

3. A 3-year-old child is brought to the emergency room in the middle of the night with a history of a recent cold and parental concern about difficulty breathing. Upon entering the room, you find the child sitting comfortably in the parent's lap, coughing a barky, seal-like cough. Which of the following signs would lead the nurse to suspect laryngotracheobronchitis?
   a. Crackles in the lower left lobe of the lung
   b. History of the child choking on a cracker
   c. Audible stridor on inspiration
   d. Erythematous, 3+/4+ tonsils, petechiae on the soft palate, with cervical lymphadenopathy

4. A 12-month-old is seen for a well-child visit. Which of the following clinical findings warrant concern and additional follow-up? Select all that apply.
   a. Bilateral red reflex present
   b. Positive Babinski reflex
   c. Unequal thigh folds
   d. Right undescended testicle
   e. III/VI diastolic murmur

5. A 4-year-old child is seen in the office with upper respiratory symptoms of mucoid rhinorrhea and productive cough for 2 days. Which assessment would the nurse not include?
   a. Examining bilateral tympanic membranes
   b. Assessing mucous membranes and skin turgor
   c. Palpating the thyroid for tenderness
   d. Auscultating anterior, posterior, and lateral lung fields

6. The parents of a 2-month-old child present to the urgent care clinic after they noticed that their child was lethargic and difficult to arouse. The nurse should be most concerned about which of the following clinical findings? Select all that apply.
   a. Yellow, greasy-appearing scales on the scalp
   b. A strawberry hemangioma on the right knee
   c. A papular rash on bilateral cheeks
   d. Bruises on the head
   e. Multiple ecchymoses on the legs
   f. The left humerus is not anatomically aligned

7. Mara is a 1-year-old who is in the office for a 12-month well-child physical examination. Which approach to the physical examination would be most appropriate for the nurse to use?
   a. Place Mara on the examination table wearing only a diaper
   b. Take Mara to a treatment room for her examination
   c. Allow Mara to remain in the parent's lap for the examination
   d. Have Mara's parent step out of the room during the examination

8. The nurse assesses the newborn baby 5 minutes after delivery. The following is observed: heart rate of 120, crying vigorously, tone has some degree of flexion, and has pink body color. What Apgar score does the nurse assign this newborn?
   a. 10
   b. 9
   c. 8
   d. 7

9. The nurse assesses a 1-month-old child's fontanels. Which of the following does the nurse recognize as an abnormal clinical finding that warrants additional follow-up?
   a. The anterior fontanel is 5 cm in size.
   b. The posterior fontanel is soft and flat.
   c. The anterior fontanel is sunken and depressed.
   d. The posterior fontanel is 1 cm in size.

10. The nurse places the infant supine on the examination table and makes a sudden noise by hitting the examination table. In a normally developing infant, what is the expected response to this stimulus?
    a. The infant extends the arms and the leg
    b. The infant's leg flexes on the examination table
    c. The infant turns the pelvis and shoulders toward the stimulus
    d. The infant quickly extends, then flexes the arms and fingers when the examination table is hit while the thumb and index fingers form a C shape

CHAPTER

26 The Older Adult Client

Learning Outcomes

1. Identify the structural and physiological aging variations of the older adult.
2. Conduct a complete health history on an older adult client.
3. Perform a physical examination on a healthy older adult client and an older adult client with pathology.
4. Differentiate between normal clinical findings from an older adult client's physical examination and the pathophysiology of abnormal clinical findings.
5. Identify the United States Preventive Services Task Force recommendations for the older adult.
6. Document a complete health history and physical examination of an older adult client with pathology.

The examination of the older adult is presented in this chapter. Many of the skills used to assess the older adult client are the same examination techniques used with the younger adult. Specialized examinations will be presented in addition to their appropriate use in the care of the older adult. The nurse must understand the variations within this special population and its differences compared with the younger adult. The nurse will often need to modify the approach and individualize the examination of the older adult.

Epidemiology

According to the U.S. Census Bureau (2020), the number of older adults is increasing exponentially. The first Baby Boomers reached 65 years in 2011, and their numbers have continued to rapidly increase. Older adults are usually grouped as young-old, those aged 65 to 75 years; old, those aged 75 to 85 years; and old-old, those aged 85 and older, which is the group whose numbers are increasing most rapidly (U.S. Census Bureau, 2020). Older individuals will be seen at all levels of the health-care system, and nurses must address their unique health-care needs, keeping in mind that people living to an older age may have one or more chronic conditions that affect their ability to function. Although disability increases with the increased number of chronic conditions, much of the aging population remains highly functional.

Older adults are a unique population who experience specific changes in their bodies related to age (Fig. 26-1). Consequently, they will have different and unique presentations in their normal healthy status and in their disease states. The older an individual is, the more differences

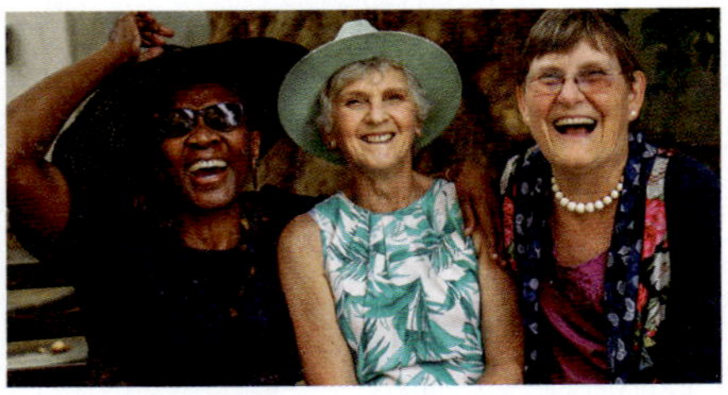

Figure 26-1 Older adults are the population group increasing at the fastest rate. Adults age in their own way and at their own pace.

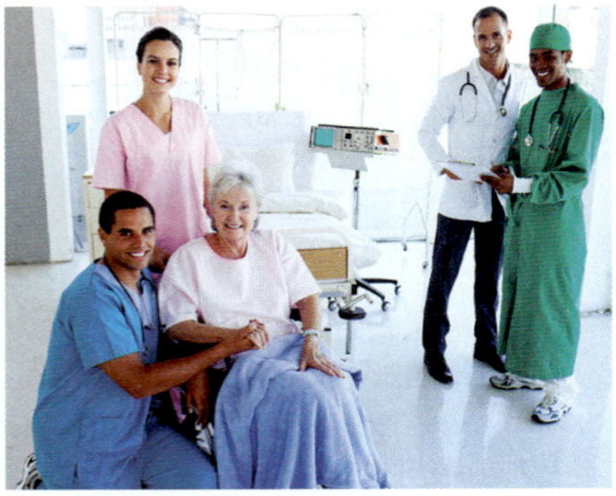

Figure 26-2 Quality care of the older adult is best provided in an interdisciplinary setting.

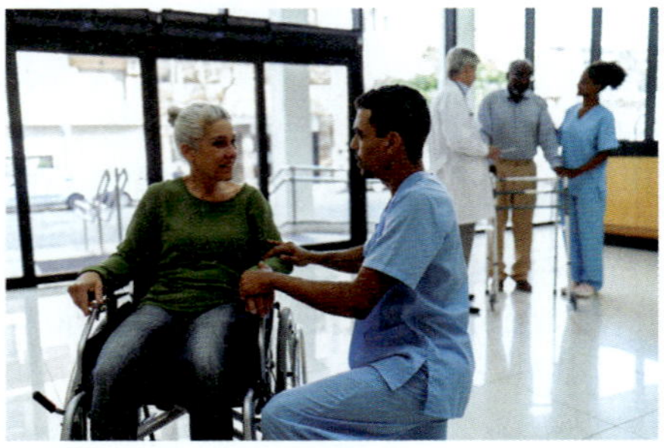

Figure 26-3 This older adult is receiving care in an acute rehabilitation facility.

among individuals will be seen, as well as differences in rates of decline related to both physiology and disease. To correctly care for a given individual, the nurse must be able to differentiate between the normal changes of aging and pathological processes. It is essential to identify how the changes of aging have affected the older adult so that care can be modified appropriately. It is vital that the nurse be acutely aware of these changes and incorporate them into the examination and care planning of each older adult client. Optimal care for this population is most effectively delivered in an interdisciplinary setting (Fig. 26-2), after a carefully organized, methodical examination.

Deterioration of the human organism begins around the fourth decade. This deterioration, though significant, is usually not detectable clinically; one may notice graying hair and decreasing visual acuity, but overall function is not affected. All presentations and complaints should be addressed and assessed and not automatically attributed to age. A healthcare provider's failure to recognize a treatable condition may result in long-term pain, suffering, loss of function, and a decreased quality of life for the client.

Variations in Presentation

The older population resides in a variety of venues. Most older adults live in their own homes independently. They may be in their own homes with a caregiver (informal: spouse, adult child, or other family member or neighbors; or formal: paid help). The small minority lives in an organized setting (2%). These range from senior congregate living (also independent) with no assistance offered, to senior living where there are varying levels of services (U.S. Census Bureau, 2020). These services range from assisted living with varying levels of assistance and foci, to long-term nursing home residence (3% to 5%) (Johnson et al, 2021). Older adults may spend short periods of time in acute rehabilitation or skilled nursing home rehabilitation to receive physical therapy, occupational therapy, speech therapy, or nursing care during a postillness recovery or after hospitalization (Fig. 26-3). Many older adults have more than one comorbid chronic condition, and a large number have more than two conditions. These may or may not affect the older adult's functioning. An older adult with a single diagnosis, such as advanced dementia, may require complete care, whereas an older adult who has multiple health issues, such as arthritis, congestive heart failure, and prostate enlargement, may live and function independently with few or no limitations.

Disease and disability are not automatic consequences of the aging process. The number of chronic or comorbid diseases and conditions one has generally increases with age. However, most older adults' functional abilities remain intact. Vulnerability to functional decline and poorer outcomes in the presence of major health events increase. Increasing age results in an extreme variability of that decline when it occurs. The incidence of vague complaints or symptoms—and neglect by clients, family, and healthcare providers—also places the older adult at increased risk of functional decline and frailty. Decreased organ function and declining homeostatic mechanisms further increase the older adult's susceptibility to disease and disability.

Frequently, the presentation of disease in the older adult is not obviously attributable to a specific pathology. Older adults have a high rate of absent or atypical presentations of illness and disease. One such example is myocardial infarction: One-third of older adults have a typical symptom presentation; one-third have atypical symptoms, such as shortness of breath, gastrointestinal upset, or new confusion; and one-third have no symptoms at all (Boyd & McNabney, 2022). Poor management of chronic conditions, as well as nonspecific presentations, predispose the older person to an even higher risk of disability. The older population, having lived through several hardships and life experiences, may also erroneously attribute specific symptoms to normal aging and delay seeking treatment. Older adults do not always present with the same signs and symptoms as younger persons. The most common complaints tend to be somewhat nonspecific and vague, frequently general lethargy or weakness, loss of appetite, or generalized fatigue.

Issues compromising the recognition of disease are, in some cases, the gradual onset and vague symptomatology with which diseases present. Many caregivers see symptoms of disease as a normal change in aging. The stoicism of the older adult and misperception of normal aging are impediments to reporting developing symptoms, as are the worry about testing and the fear of bad news. Fears of possible expense, physical discomfort, and loss of independence are all concerns commonly expressed by older adults. Reporting may also be hampered by cognitive impairment, inability to verbalize symptoms, and concerns of not being taken seriously by the healthcare provider.

Anatomy and Physiology

Structural and Physiological Variations

Every cell, tissue, organ, and organism is affected by the process of aging. Most systems have specific changes, while a few systems have vague, deregulatory changes. These changes are due to a combination of factors, among them genetics, environment, nutrition, and activity. Changes in aging are not harmful in isolation, but physiological resilience is compromised primarily due to loss of reserves. Homeostasis becomes more difficult to maintain in times of stress such as injury, illness, or surgery. These changes are more commonly seen in the very old or frail older adult. Although most changes seen in the older adult are part of the normal aging process, many can also indicate underlying systemic or localized disease. Therefore, it is prudent not to generalize changes as routine.

Vital Signs

Respirations

The normal respiratory rate is between 12 and 24 breaths per minute. An elevated respiratory rate frequently precedes the usual symptoms of upper respiratory infection or a developing illness.

Pulse

The resting heart rate remains constant in the older adult, but the maximum heart rate declines. Reflex tachycardia is delayed due to a blunted baroreceptor reflex.

Temperature

The older adult may have an abnormally low body temperature and greater variations in temperature. Diurnal variations are not affected by age. Frail older adults may present with an infective process with the absence of fever.

Blood Pressure

Both diastolic and systolic blood pressure rise due to the loss of elasticity in the vasculature of the older adult. The emergence of new diastolic hypertension in an older person usually has a secondary etiology, which should be explored. In addition, approximately 20% of older individuals exhibit postural hypotension. Postprandial hypotension is more commonly seen in older adults than in younger adults. A widening of the pulse pressure also occurs.

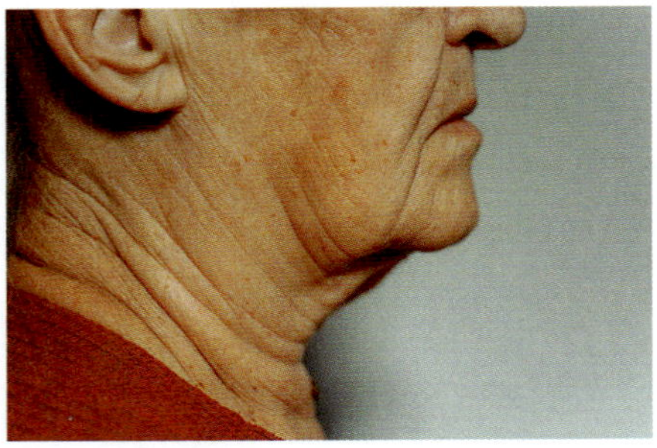

Figure 26-4 Skin changes in the older adult may lead to wrinkles.

Skin, Hair, and Nails

The most visible signs of aging are manifested in the skin and hair. These signs include wrinkles, sagging skin folds, graying hair, and hair loss. Light-skinned individuals appear to manifest the changes of aging more rapidly than do dark-skinned individuals, and these changes are accelerated by sun exposure. Skin disorders are also more likely to occur as a person ages.

With aging, the epidermis thins and elastic fibers that provide support to the dermis degenerate and lead to sagging skin folds (Fig. 26-4). The vascularity of the skin declines, which can lead to senile purpura. Because the number of sweat and sebaceous glands diminishes, a disruption in the body's thermoregulation occurs. There is also an increased incidence of hypothermia due to vasodilation and vasoconstriction of the dermal arterioles and loss of subcutaneous fat. The loss of subcutaneous tissue over bony prominences increases the risk of skin breakdown in the older adult.

A diminished inflammatory response and a diminished perception of pain increase the risk of adverse effects from noxious stimuli in the older adult. Thus, the older adult is at a greater risk for frostbite and burns because of their diminished pain perception, and their injuries are more serious because of the thinning of the epidermis and prolonged wound healing.

Wrinkling is the change most associated with aging. Wrinkles are most prominent on the face and neck because these areas have the greatest sun exposure. Other factors leading to wrinkling are loss of subcutaneous fat and diminished elasticity of the skin.

Senile pruritus is the most common skin affliction in older adults. Pruritus is due to a decrease in the skin's water content, a decrease in the number of sebaceous glands, and atrophy of the eccrine glands. The latter contributes to the risk of hyperthermia in the older adult. Dryness and itching are exacerbated during winter because the humidity is low, indoor temperatures are high, and drying winds are present. The condition is aggravated by frequent bathing in hot water, which robs the skin of moisture. Generalized itching is also associated with systemic diseases such as diabetes mellitus, atherosclerosis, liver disease, renal disease, thyroid dysfunction, lymphoma, and multiple myeloma. The number and thickness of terminal hairs generally diminish, and there is a conversion of vellus hair to terminal hair in areas such as the rims of the ears and nose in males, and on the upper lip and chin in females. Decreased melanin production decreases the melanocytes at the hair follicles and leads to hair pigment loss manifested as graying hair.

The nails in the older adult may thicken, split, and become more yellow and dull. There may be an overcurvature of the toenails if tight shoes were worn for a large portion of the adult's life

Head, Neck, and Regional Lymph Nodes

Loss of subcutaneous fat and musculoskeletal changes due to the aging process affect the appearance and function of the head and neck. Wrinkles are more prominent. Facial symmetry may be altered because of the presence of dentures or loss of teeth. Due to the reabsorption of mandibular bone, a change in facial appearance is to be expected. Neck veins may be more prominent due to the loss of fat.

The head, neck, and lower jaw may be thrust forward, especially with a kyphotic posture. A "buffalo hump" may appear as an accumulation of fat over the posterior cervical vertebrae. This is seen in clients with osteoporosis or a kyphotic posture. The range of motion of the head may be limited, painful, or possible only with a jerking or "cogwheel" motion. Dizziness accompanying the movement of the head may create safety problems. All of these changes may affect the older adult's ability to maintain normal activities of daily living.

Eyes

Visual impairments are among the most prevalent chronic conditions in the older adult. Sight provides information to enable people to function in the environment. Thus, prevention of sensory impairment and resulting handicaps are challenges for the individual and health-care providers.

During the aging process, the eye undergoes significant changes. First, by the age of 42, the lens cortex becomes denser, compromising its ability to change shape and focus. This condition, **presbyopia**, is responsible for farsightedness and the need for bifocals. A decrease in aqueous humor secretion and increased vitreous gel debris lead to decreased cleansing of the lens and cornea as well. Next, there is a tendency for the lens to yellow and become cloudy. This change impairs a person's ability to discern colors, especially blues and greens. In addition, pupils become smaller, causing the amount of light reaching the retina to be reduced. Consequently, older adults need more light to see and their eyes take longer to accommodate to darkness and glare. Peripheral vision is decreased, and an upward gaze may be limited, which can create safety issues for driving and other activities.

Externally, the older adult has a loss of pigment in the iris, decreased orbital fat, and thinning of the eyelid tissue. Decreased corneal sensitivity and a decreased corneal reflex, in conjunction with the presence of entropion, ectropion, or ptosis, can result in corneal abrasion or infection. The globe appears to be deeper in the eye socket, and the lacrimal gland may be visible because of the loss of subcutaneous fat around the eye.

Ears

Hearing loss, or **presbycusis**, is a common condition among older adults. Conductive hearing loss occurs in the outer or middle ear and usually makes things sound softer. High-pitched tones are lost first. However, the more common age-related hearing loss is sensorineural, which involves the inner ear. Ossicular joint deterioration occurs; there is a degeneration of hair cells in the inner ear; and vestibular structures, the cochlea, and the organ of Corti all atrophy. These bilateral ear changes can also result in an increased risk of balance and equilibrium deficits.

Externally, the pinna increases in length and width in the older adult and cerumen production decreases. This can lead to ear dryness and cerumen impaction. An otoscopic examination may reveal more pronounced landmarks if atrophic or sclerotic changes have occurred.

Nose

Nasal hairs are coarser, and less efficient filtration occurs as a person ages. This can lead to sinus and respiratory conditions. In addition, the sense of smell declines rapidly after age 50. The smaller number of smell receptors is less efficient, and smells must be more intense to be perceived. This diminished sense of smell may result in decreased appetite and weight loss.

Mouth and Throat

Common alterations in the mouth of an older adult are precancerous and cancerous lesions; untreated caries (due to decreased saliva production, lack of funds to obtain dental care, and neglect of oral hygiene); periodontal disease (e.g., receding gum lines, gingivitis); tooth loss, which can affect the closure of the mouth; worn tooth surfaces; and orofacial pain. Dysphagia or swallowing problems increase in part due to decreased saliva production. In addition, side effects from medications (e.g., xerostomia from anticholinergic medications and antihistamines, possible oral candidiasis from inhaled steroids) can alter the normal anatomy of the mouth.

Taste may not diminish with age, but it may become less reliable due to a decreased number of taste buds and a decline in their function. Specifically,

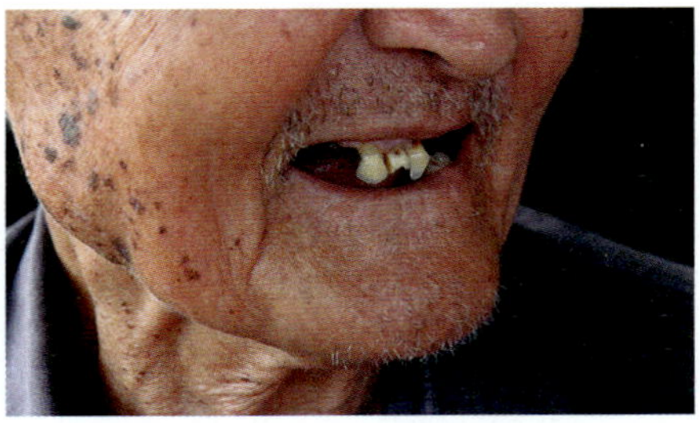

Figure 26-5 Older adults may develop severe dental disease, especially in clients with cognitive conditions.

the older adult has a more difficult time discriminating the tastes of sweet, sour, salt, and bitter.

There is a higher incidence of loss of teeth and periodontal disease in the older adult population than in the younger age-groups (Fig. 26-5). Those wearing dentures may not realize that their dentures might require adjustment every year or two due to changing mandibular bone structure. Oral hygiene practices should be assessed on each comprehensive visit. Frequently heard symptoms with which the older adult client may present are foul breath and sensitivity to extremes of temperature. Periodontal disease may be the cause and should always be evaluated, as this is a major cause of tooth loss. The same symptoms, however, can be presentations of sinusitis or a pulmonary infection.

Breasts and Regional Lymph Nodes

The adipose tissue of the breast atrophies with age and is replaced with connective tissue. The glandular tissue gradually decreases, causing the breasts to feel granular instead of lobular. Breast tissue mass decreases with age and becomes pendulous and wrinkled. The nipples become smaller and flatter. Ductal tissue becomes more palpable, especially around the nipples, and may become firm and stringy. In addition, the musculature around the breasts tends to atrophy, which contributes to the overall droopiness of the breasts.

There is an increased incidence of breast cancer after the age of 50. In women, breast cancer is the second major cause of cancer death, exceeded only by lung cancer (Centers for Disease Control and Prevention, 2025a, 2025b).

Thorax and Lungs

The older adult undergoes changes that involve the external and internal anatomy of the thorax and lungs. As a result, the physiology of the respiratory system becomes altered. The resulting state of the client depends on the extent of the changes and the presence of comorbid conditions. Variations of the respiratory system include four broad areas: anatomical changes, alveolar gas exchange, regulation of ventilation, and lung defense mechanisms.

Older adults experience degeneration of the intervertebral discs, stiffening of ligaments and joints, and calcification of the costochondral cartilage. These changes limit chest wall expansion during the respiratory cycle. Muscles atrophy and become weaker and the diaphragm flattens out, leading to decreased respiratory endurance for the older adult. Strenuous exercise is taxing secondary to the decrease in oxygen uptake and decreased elastic recoil of the lung parenchyma. Most older adults will have some degree of a barrel chest and some kyphosis. Forced vital capacity decreases, residual volume and functional residual capacity increase, and the total lung capacity remains unchanged.

The second major change in the older adult occurs in alveolar gas exchange. The lung's decreased elastic recoil causes the closure of airways for a portion of the respiratory cycle. This occurs particularly in the lower lobes of the lungs. As a result, the apices and the bases of the lungs have a ventilation-perfusion mismatch. Other factors contributing to this loss of alveolar gas exchange are the loss of lung tissue and alveolar capillaries and pulmonary wall thickening. In essence, this creates a situation in which there is less surface area for diffusion, and the surface area that is present is thicker. In addition, hemoglobin's affinity for oxygen decreases, which leads to a decrease in the partial pressure of oxygen.

The aging adult experiences changes in the regulation of ventilation. The medulla is less sensitive to changes in carbon dioxide and oxygen levels, which normally trigger the respiratory drive. There is a compromised acid-base balance. Neural output to respiratory muscles is decreased. Both peripheral and central chemoreceptors are affected.

The last area of change in the older adult is in lung defense mechanisms. There is less ciliary and macrophage activity, which increases susceptibility to infection. The cough reflex decreases, and the risk of aspiration increases.

Heart

As adults age, their cardiovascular system undergoes physiological changes that in many instances are complicated by disease processes (Fig. 26-6). In the older adult, the size of the cardiac muscle decreases with age. As fibrotic and sclerotic changes take place in the atria and the ventricles, cardiac output can fall by as much as 35% at rest after the age of 70. Skeletal changes such as osteoporosis, kyphosis, or collapsed vertebrae can alter the position of the heart within the thoracic cavity, giving rise to changes in the electrocardiogram (ECG). Obesity leads to increased abdominal girth and diaphragm elevation, which can also displace the heart within the chest.

With the aging process, cardiac valves may develop calcifications or fibrosis, which results in systolic or diastolic murmurs. A systolic ejection murmur commonly found at the left lower sternal border is of no diagnostic significance. If the left ventricle has thickened or enlarged, thus losing its compliance, an S_4 heart sound can be auscultated. Changes in the conduction system resulting from electrolyte imbalance, pharmacotherapy, debilitating states, or thickened myocardial fibers can cause cardiac irritability, leading to a variety of dysrhythmias. The older adult also has a reduced β-adrenergic response.

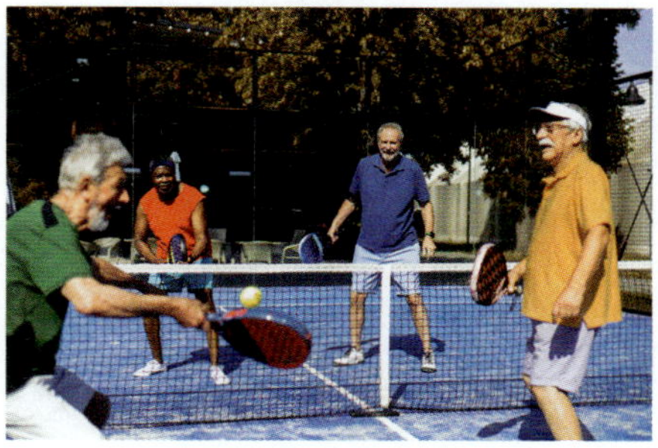

Figure 26-6 It is essential that older adults keep active to maximize cardiovascular health. Pickleball has become very popular!

Peripheral Vasculature

Vascular integrity is also affected in the aging process. The arterial system becomes increasingly rigid as the blood vessels become fibrotic. If a pathological process such as atherosclerosis is present, the insult to the vasculature becomes even greater. Elasticity is lost, the vessel lumen is narrowed, and peripheral vascular resistance is increased, thus impeding blood flow. Conditions such as smoking, which cause vascular spasm, contribute to a further decrease in vascular flow. In the venous system, there is intimal thickening with dilation and loss of valve competency. Venous return to the heart is affected, and edema or varicosities may develop. The baroreceptors located in the aortic arch and the carotid sinuses are also affected by vascular integrity. Impaired compliance alters the ability of these structures to respond to blood pressure changes. A dilated aorta and cool extremities are commonly found with decreased peripheral pulses.

Abdomen

In the process of aging, the abdominal musculature diminishes in mass and loses much of its tone. At the same time, the fat content of the body increases, leading to increased fat deposition in the abdominal area. The mucosal lining of the gastrointestinal tract becomes less elastic, and changes in gastric motility result in alterations in digestion and absorption.

Decreased esophageal motility and lower esophageal sphincter pressure can lead to complaints of gastroesophageal reflux disorder (GERD) symptoms. Pancreatic, enzymatic, and hormonal secretions decrease, and there is an atrophy of antral cells, causing a decreased secretion of hydrochloric acid and intrinsic factor. These can cause malabsorption, altered digestion, and a cobalamin deficiency. A decrease in intestinal motility can lead to constipation, one of the most frequent complaints of the older adult.

As the intestinal wall weakens, diverticuli increase. These can progress to inflammation and obstruction resulting in diverticulitis and possible bowel perforation.

There is little evidence that liver function changes significantly with age. However, hepatic weight, blood flow, and regenerative capacity decrease progressively with age. The decrease in liver mass and blood flow alters the pharmacokinetics of medications.

Musculoskeletal System

Bone density decreases in the older adult due to an increased rate of reabsorption, which exceeds the rate of bone replenishment. Both cortical and trabecular bone mass decrease. These changes lead to a weaker bone that is more susceptible to fracture. Bone density loss is accentuated in the postmenopausal female due to an estrogen deficiency. Other manifestations of bone density loss are thoracic kyphosis and a reduction in height. Thoracic kyphosis will cause a change in the older adult's center of gravity, making the individual more prone to loss of balance and falls. Refer to Chapter 19 for a list of osteoporosis risk factors.

With age, muscle fibers deteriorate and are replaced by fibrous connective tissue. Muscle atrophy is accompanied by a reduction in muscle mass, a loss of muscle strength against resistance, and a reduction in overall body mass. The fat content of the body increases, with particular distribution around the waistline. For this reason, even a very thin older adult may have a larger-than-expected waist circumference.

There is a decrease in the water content of cartilage, which leads to a narrowing of joint spaces; thinning of intervertebral discs; and possibly pain, crepitus, and decreased movement of the affected area. The ability of cartilage to repair itself following trauma or surgery is also reduced. Articulating cartilage will deteriorate due to a lifetime of wear and tear.

Mental Status and Neurological System

Neuronal changes occur with aging. The myelin sheath surrounding each nerve begins to degenerate, decreasing impulse transmissions and nerve conduction rates. This can lead to a decreased reaction time manifested in slowed deep tendon reflexes (DTR) and decreased vibratory sense. The axons of the neuron become smaller. Biochemically, the amount of neurotransmitter produced in the neuron is diminished, and the activity of the enzymes that degrade the neurotransmitter increases. Changes in neurotransmitters are known to affect sleep, temperature control, and mood. Depression, for example, is associated with decreased levels of norepinephrine.

Total brain weight, the number of synapses, and the number of neurons diminish with aging, beginning at age 50. Most of the loss occurs in the cerebral cortex and the cerebellum, with less loss in the brainstem. The brain atrophies, causing a widening of the sulci and gyri, especially in the frontal lobes. The tendency of the brain to atrophy increases the size of the subdural space, leaving the cortical bridging veins vulnerable to trauma, bleeding, and the formation of a chronic subdural hematoma. The ventricles increase in size and the amount of cerebrospinal fluid increases to fill the space.

Cognitive changes characteristic of aging include a decline in mental flexibility, abstract thinking, recall, and visual-spatial ability. However, recognition, attention, and language skills remain unchanged. The older adult typically has an extended learning and word retrieval time. Short-term memory may decrease slightly, but this must be evaluated because it may not be due to a decline in neurological function. In addition, changes in affect, mood, and orientation must be investigated, as they may be signs of dementia, delirium, or acute mental confusion, especially in the older adult suffering from infection, dehydration, or central nervous system (CNS) damage. Cognitive screening should be a part of each interaction with the older adult client, and any abnormal findings should be investigated.

Urinary System

Renal

In the older adult, the kidney shrinks. Renal function can be altered due to glomerular degeneration, thickening of glomerular and tubular basement membranes, decreased length of proximal and distal tubes, and decreased renal blood flow. As a result, the glomerular filtration rate decreases by 60% to 70% by age 75. The kidney does not respond as efficiently to vasopressin, and the ability to dilute, concentrate, and acidify urine is compromised. Impaired sodium regulation can also occur.

Bladder

The bladder becomes less elastic because of reduced muscle tone from the aging process. Because the older adult has a bladder with a smaller capacity and delayed perception of voiding signals, urinary incontinence is a frequent occurrence. In addition, the bladder has increased detrusor muscle instability, a weakened urinary sphincter, and involuntary contractions. Increased nocturnal production of urine leads to nocturia in both men and women.

Female Genitalia

The older female adult undergoes definite physical changes in the internal and external genitalia and reproductive organs. These changes begin with menopause, which usually occurs between the ages of 45 and 55. Menopause is characterized by low estrogen levels, which cause the cessation of menses. As aging progresses, a generalized atrophy of the external and internal female reproductive organs evolves.

Atrophy of the internal reproductive organs causes the ovaries and uterine tubes to diminish in size so that they are rarely palpable. The uterus atrophies so that it may be difficult to palpate. Also, a delayed and reduced production of vaginal secretions may cause alterations in sexual response. These changes in the vagina may cause the female to complain of dyspareunia. An increase in the pH of the vaginal secretions and a decrease in the normal vaginal flora lead to an increase in vaginal infections in older adult females. However, the older female adult experiences no change in sexual desire or pleasure or in the ability to experience orgasm.

The pelvic muscles also atrophy, causing a decrease in the support of the pelvic organs. These muscles are often already weakened by trauma from childbirth; thus, prolapse of the uterus and vaginal walls is common. Incontinence is not a normal change of advancing age; however, due to the changes of aging accompanied by childbirth, there is a higher incidence of urinary incontinence in the older female. The condition should be assessed to identify effective interventions. These interventions range from scheduled toileting, to exercises to strengthen the pelvic floor, to surgical interventions.

Male Genitalia

Testicular degeneration seems to occur in a patchy distribution, which allows normal spermatogenesis to be present in the majority of males until 70 years of age when sperm count and motility decline. Sperm output may be slightly decreased.

Typically, the older male adult has no change in sexual desire or satisfaction, but the ability to obtain or maintain an erection is affected. Also, erection is often not as complete. Testosterone levels decline slightly with age but are related to impotence in only a small minority of males who have low hormone levels. An absence or marked reduction of ejaculatory fluid emission is often seen in the older adult male. The refractory period before rearousal, after a cycle of erection and ejaculation, lengthens with age. This physiological change in what used to be an almost automatic erection is often perceived by males as the onset of impotence. Anxiety levels rise, thus further triggering erectile dysfunction. Physiological impotence can be caused by vascular disease, diabetes mellitus, and hypogonadism. The older male may also suffer from urinary incontinence, usually at a slightly lower rate than the older female. Incontinence at any age should be evaluated for etiology and effective treatment.

Anus, Rectum, and Prostate

Anorectal function changes in the older adult are due to the loss of muscle elasticity in the rectum. Older adults have reduced maximum tolerated volumes in the rectum, with higher rectal pressures in response to distention. Rectal prolapse is most commonly seen in older adult females. Constipation commonly occurs due to a decline in large bowel transit time and decreased fecal water excretion.

Fecal incontinence may develop due to denervation associated with an increase in the motor unit fiber density and degeneration of the rectal wall's afferent neuron. This interferes with the ability to detect changes in pressure and creates a decrease in internal sphincter tone. Fecal incontinence in the older adult is usually the result of impairment of more than one of the factors that ordinarily maintain continence. Fecal incontinence can be caused by fecal impaction, diarrhea, irritable bowel syndrome (IBS), rectal prolapse, anorectal carcinoma, anorectal trauma, stroke, diabetes, dementia, and multiple sclerosis.

The prostate begins to enlarge after the age of 40 and often leads to the development of benign prostatic hypertrophy. The prostate capsule may contract and prostatic urethral tone may increase, resulting in urinary obstruction. There are lower levels of zinc in the prostatic fluid of older males, which appear to reduce the amount of prostatic antibacterial factor, therefore making the older male more susceptible to urinary tract infections.

Interview of the Older Adult

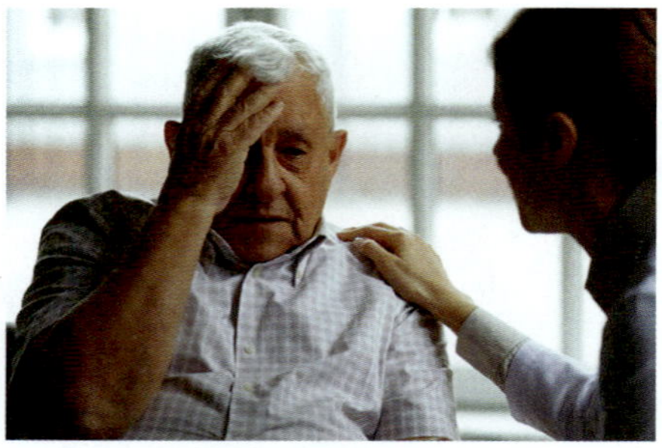

Figure 26-7 The health history interview of the older adult may pose a unique challenge to nurses.

The older adult population spans a lengthy time, from age 65 years to 100+. Chronological age should not be the major factor considered in the approach to the older adult client. The ability to function and interact will be as diverse as individuals themselves, regardless of age. Those young-old adults, ages 65 to 75, in most cases, will be highly functional, independent individuals, and the nurse's approach will require only minimal modification. However, old-old adults, those 85 and older, may have limitations that will call for modification of both the interview and the examination itself (Fig. 26-7). The presence of frailty may mandate multiple appointments for the completion of a comprehensive examination. Additional time should be incorporated into the interview to allow for an accurate interpretation of the information requested and the responses.

Assurance of accurate communication is essential in providing care to any client in any setting. Older clients face additional challenges in terms of normal changes of aging that affect their ability to accept and interpret visual, auditory, and sensory stimuli. Health-care facilities should have readily available equipment that effectively enhances communication with older adults who have vision loss or a hearing impairment. Nurses should be aware of what assistive devices are available and take the time to access and use them. Hearing deficits may be ameliorated by using a stethoscope—in the client's ears.

A communication phenomenon called "elderspeak" is often seen from those working with older adults. This type of communication features simplistic vocabulary and grammar, shortened sentences, slowed speech, elevated pitch and volume, and inappropriately intimate terms of endearment (Shaw & Gordon, 2021). This infantilizing communication used with older adults precipitates communication breakdowns with cognitively intact clients and has significant negative outcomes. Older adults exposed to negative stereotypes, such as those inherent in elderspeak, perform worse on memory and balance assessments. Self-perception and esteem declined in the presence of continued demoralizing interactions. Elderspeak compromises interactions with the older client. Minimizing the use of elderspeak reduces stereotyped messages that older adults are weak, dependent, and incapacitated.

Improved communication enhances the cognitive and functional abilities of older adults.

The health history of the older adult encompasses the same major areas as the health history of a younger client; however, there are some basic differences. Reasons for seeking care may be a chronic condition or a new issue or problem. Issues of depression, weakness, or self-care deficits may be more difficult to identify but will emerge from a thorough, skilled examination. New pains or discomfort should never be attributed to "getting old," and client teaching should emphasize this point. Past health history for the older client is similar to that for the younger adult. The length of time covered is extended, however, and therefore the interview may take more time to complete. Medication should always be carefully evaluated; if possible, the client should bring all prescription medications, over-the-counter (OTC) medications, and vitamins/supplements to the appointment (Fig. 26-8). Multiple providers (and lack of communication among them) can result in multiple medications being prescribed to treat similar conditions, which can increase the risk of drug interactions and adverse drug effects. Family history may be less helpful in the older adult. Its utility is especially questionable in the very old client because the main purpose of collecting it is to identify conditions that might cause premature illness and death—concerns that are no longer applicable in such a client. Table 26-1 identifies strategies to enhance the health history interview and examination of the older adult.

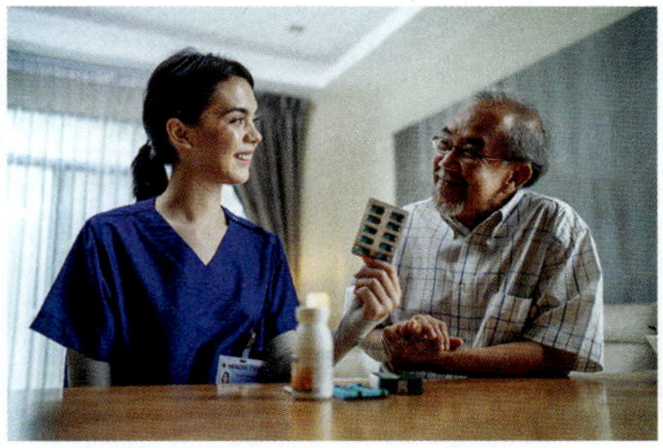

Figure 26-8 Older adults should be encouraged to bring all their prescription and nonprescription medications with them to each health-care appointment.

The psychosocial aspect of the interview is similar to that of the younger adult, with some areas receiving increased focus. Current living situation and the older adult's satisfaction with the living arrangements should be elicited. Engagement with friends and family should be explored, as should spousal issues that may present.

Older adults experience many life changes, and these changes may accelerate with age. Their ability to cope with the stressors associated with aging, such as retirement, moving, illness, or deaths of significant others, should be assessed. The nurse should also assess for depression, personality changes, or other signs of cognitive issues (Fig. 26-9). Cognitive issues may result from medical issues and thus be amenable to treatment. The normal examination findings should be emphasized, and client teaching should occur regarding commonly experienced issues of aging.

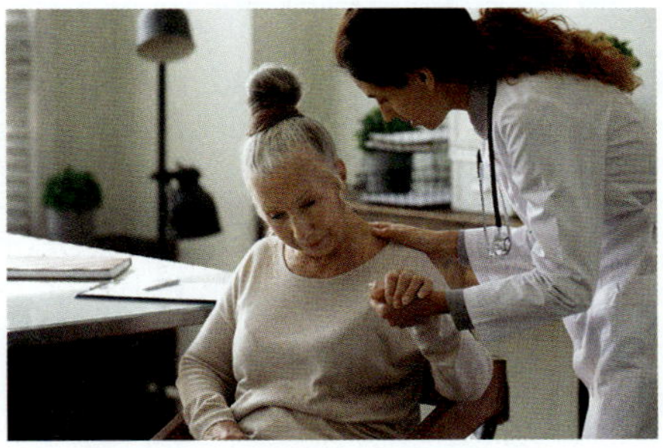

Figure 26-9 Assessment for cognitive changes and depression in the older adult should occur at each nursing visit.

Table 26-1 Guide to Enhanced Interview and Examination

Potential Deficit	Goal	Intervention
Vision	Maximize visual component of communication	Sit facing client to ensure clear view of your face. Avoid light behind you. Provide bright, indirect light without glare. Ensure that client has clean glasses (clean as needed). Provide written material in 14-point font on matte paper with clear contrast between text and background.
Hearing	Maximize auditory component of communication and enhance information gathering	Provide quiet environment with no background noise. Ask if there is a hearing deficit and which ear is better. Speak directly to the good ear. Address the client by the correct title and last name at the initiation of new or returning conversation. Assist with the use of working hearing aids. If needed, use alternate mechanisms for communication such as writing, signing, or using a stethoscope as an assistive device. Validate that information is understood.

Continued

Table 26-1 Guide to Enhanced Interview and Examination—cont'd

Potential Deficit	Goal	Intervention
Mobility	Promote independence and autonomy	Explain what parts of the examination will be done. Plan to reinforce the explanation during the examination. Allow extra time for the client to prepare for the examination. Ask if the client would like assistance in preparation. Ask who the client would like present during the examination, if anyone. If a designated individual is present during the interview, observe the interaction between this person and the older adult.
Fatigue	Enhance quality of information and accuracy and efficacy of examination	Allow flexibility in scheduling so client can select the best time of day. May need to break comprehensive examination into sections and allow for rest periods as needed or schedule on separate days. Ensure that positioning is not adding to fatigue. Client may have less fatigue if examination is done in semirecumbent position.
Eliciting minimal information	Enhance quality of information and accuracy and efficacy of examination	Ensure that preceding issues are addressed adequately. Ask open-ended questions that cannot be answered yes/no.
Difficulty with focus	Enhance quality of information and accuracy and efficacy of examination	Limit questions with essential subjective information to closed-ended questions. Organize reminiscences to enhance data gathering.
Pain	Promote comfort and enhance quality of information	Allow client to assume position of most comfort. Provide client with available interventions to enhance comfort.

Special Assessments

Developmental Assessment

Many older adults fear the aging process. It is often seen as a time of uselessness and decline. However, older adults are not useless, and they have their own developmental tasks to accomplish. Older adults demonstrate tremendous flexibility in their thinking, learning, and adaptive ability. They have to be resilient to incorporate the aging process into their self-image (Fig. 26-10). Growing old is a time of enormous individual growth. Coping with the losses

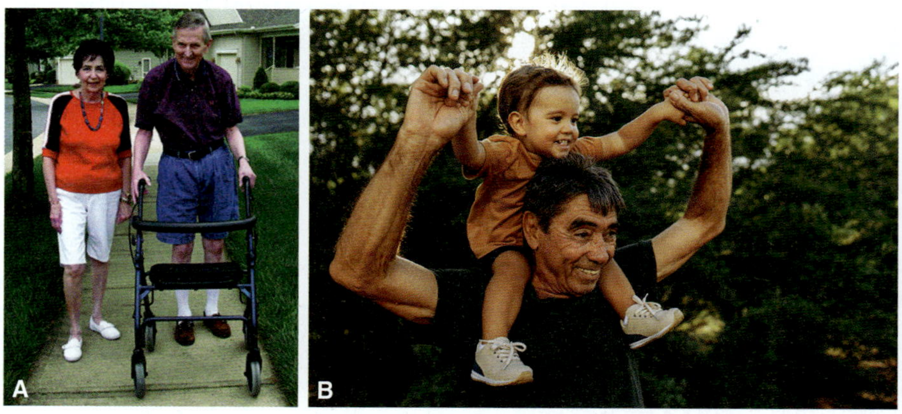

Figure 26-10 Developmental tasks of the older adult. **A.** All older adults should continue to be active, despite any changes in their mobility. **B.** The oldest and youngest members of the family are enjoying their time together.

of spouse, family, and friends through death, illness, or relocation; adjusting to altered living arrangements; retiring; and adjusting to changing sexual and physical function are just a few examples of the developmental work that older adults accomplish. Refer to Chapter 4 for a summary of the developmental tasks of the older adult.

Assessment of the older adult's functioning may allow the nurse to assist the client in adapting to these changes or in compensating and planning for the future (Fig. 26-11). Assessing functionality, nutrition, sleep, and caregiver strain will improve the quality of life and adaptation of the older client. Reliable and valid tools for use with the older population may be found on the Hartford Institute for Geriatric Nursing website: *https://hign.org*. These tools include the Mini-Cog, the CAM (Confusion Assessment Method), the Katz Index of Independence in Activities of Daily Living (ADL), the Lawton Instrumental Activities of Daily Living Scale (IADL), the Mini-Nutritional Assessment (MNA), the Pittsburgh Sleep Quality Index (PSQI), and the Modified Caregiver Strain Index (CSI).

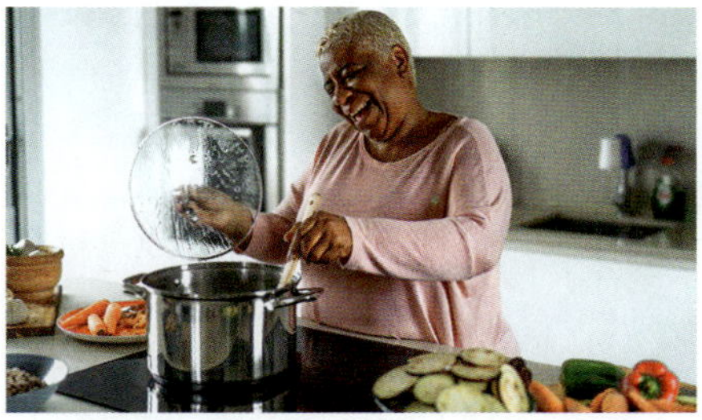

Figure 26-11 Preparing meals is one of the functional abilities that is assessed in older adults.

Cultural Assessment

The number of minority older adults is increasing at a rate similar to the increase in the population as a whole. Some ethnic groups experience a higher rate of specific disorders. For example, Black and Hispanic older adults have a higher rate of dementia than Whites (Rajan et al, 2021). Just as older clients present with great variation, there is a large amount of variety among ethnic groups. Older individuals with non-U.S. cultural origins may have different health practices and beliefs (Fig. 26-12).

Assessment may be complicated further by the lack of a common language between the nurse and the non-English-speaking older adult. As a sign of respect, all older adults should be addressed by title and last name. Validation of understanding of answers to questions in addition to instructions is essential. Many cultures nod "yes" without understanding. When addressing topics that are private in other cultures, the nurse should explain that it is necessary to discuss these topics to deliver appropriate care.

Attempts should be made to assess and honor individual beliefs and attitudes regarding health and illness. This will facilitate the development of respect and rapport with the older client. Cognitive examination instruments can be affected by ethnicity, education, language, and socioeconomic status (Luth & Prigerson, 2022).

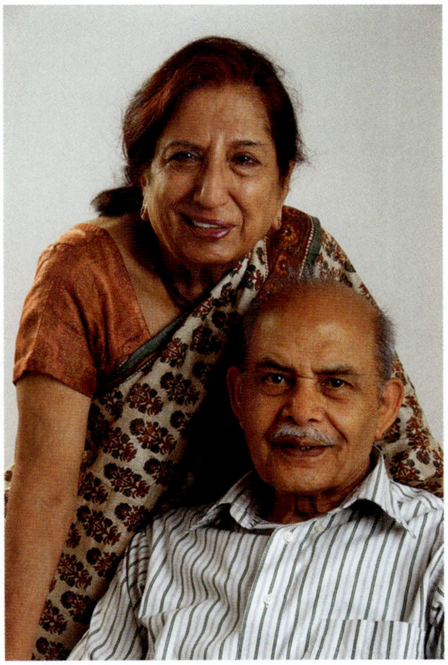

Figure 26-12 An older adult's culture must be assessed to deliver holistic nursing care.

Spiritual Assessment

A strong link between faith and health has been documented by researchers (refer to Chapter 6). When older adults are questioned, many believe in the healing power of prayer, that faith can facilitate recovery, and that their faith and religious practices are important means of coping with illness and disability. Just as faith is an individual perception and practice at a younger age, so it is with the older adult. Older adults do not become more religious as they age. Rather, they maintain the same support and belief system that has supported them throughout their lives (Fig. 26-13).

The spiritual history and assessment is the same as for the younger adult and should include the key concepts of the older adult's idea of a higher power, the meaning of illness, the mechanisms used to maintain hope, and support system. Refer to Chapter 6 which discusses the FICA spiritual assessment tool.

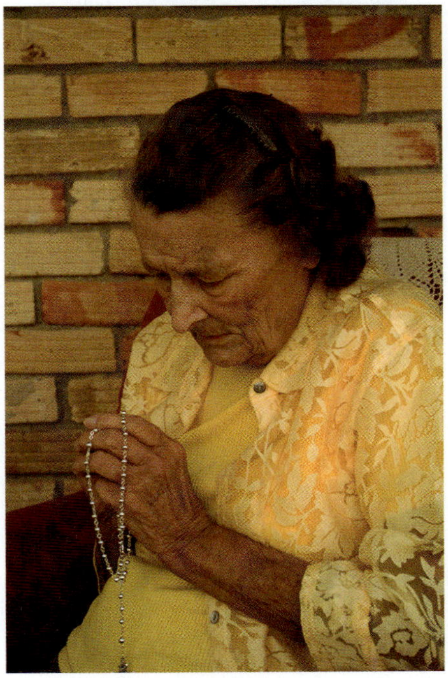

Figure 26-13 Many older adults maintain their belief system as they age.

Geriatric Syndromes

Normal aging changes increase the older adult's risk of developing geriatric syndromes. Prevalent problems that may be experienced at a higher rate by

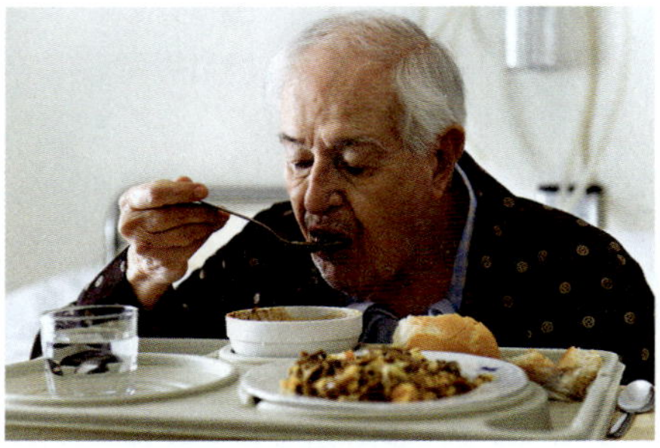

Figure 26-14 The older adult faces unique challenges in attempting to maintain good nutritional intake.

older adults include nutritional disorders, sleep disorders, falls, and pain. Familiarity with these commonly occurring disorders helps the nurse prevent unnecessary iatrogenesis and promote the optimal function of the aging client. Flagging conditions for further assessment allows the nurse to implement preventive and therapeutic interventions.

Nutritional Assessment

A nutritional assessment should be performed on the older adult. Specific, identified nutritional deficits, risk factors placing the individual at risk for nutritional deficiencies, and weight loss are the main stimuli. The older adult faces unique challenges in attempting to maintain good nutritional intake (Fig. 26-14). For instance, caloric requirements decline with age, and older adults may have decreased or blunted taste perception in addition to less efficient intestinal absorption. Chewing and swallowing issues are most prevalent in this age-group. Food preparation may pose challenges. Financial constraints in shopping and food-buying habits are frequently seen in older adults living on a fixed income, and the loss of partners, friends, and spouses decreases the many social aspects of eating.

The nutritional assessment should be performed as for the younger adult, with the elicitation of additional information on medications, social interactions, living arrangements, and functional ability. Food and drug interactions are more common in this age-group. Single living, loneliness, and loss of a spouse or significant other are major risk factors for inadequate nutrition. A nutritional assessment of the older adult may be conducted using a standardized evidence-based tool such as the Mini-Nutritional Assessment (MNA), which may be found at *https://www.mna-elderly.com/sites/default/files/2021-10/mna-mini-english.pdf*. Refer to Chapter 7 for the comprehensive nutritional assessment.

Sleep Assessment

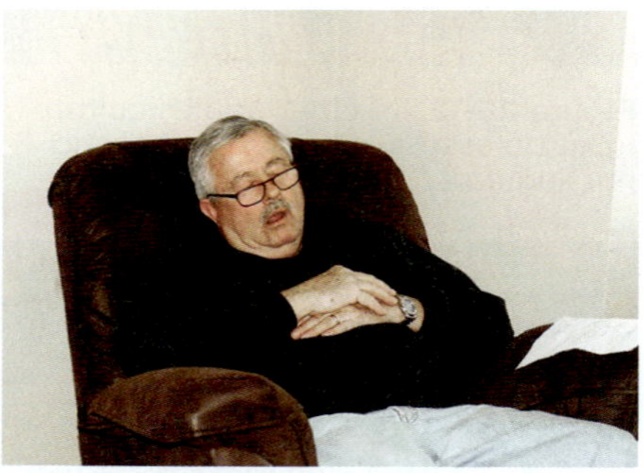

Figure 26-15 Many older adults have difficulty sleeping all night because of daytime napping.

Sleep is part of the rhythm of life and necessary for function, but older adults are at higher risk of having sleep disturbances. Normal aging changes may interfere with the quality of sleep, while health and medication use can negatively affect sleep patterns. Without adequate, good-quality sleep, the body loses the ability to revitalize. The mind is less effective when tired and mood may become depressed. Sleep disorders may present as excessive sleepiness: somnolence, hypersomnia, excessive daytime sleepiness, or subjective sleepiness. Sleepiness may be experienced as a symptom in several medical, psychiatric, and primary sleep disorders, but also as a normal physiological state over any given 24-hour period. The older adult may report feeling tired all the time or having no energy (Fig. 26-15). This can be due to difficulty falling asleep, intermittent or early awakening, or sleep fragmentation. The most common conditions disturbing sleep in older adults are nocturia, pain due to degenerative joint disease, obstructive sleep apnea, insomnia, and restless legs syndrome. Many disorders share excessive sleepiness as a symptom. Sleep difficulties should be assessed using valid and reliable tools for the older adult such as the Epworth Sleepiness Scale (Johns, 1991). The scale can be found at *https://epworthsleepinessscale.com/*.

Falls Assessment

Falls occur at a higher rate in the older adult population but are not a normal consequence of aging. Falls are viewed as a geriatric syndrome that has multiple complex causes. Nearly one-third of community-dwelling older adults fall each year in their homes. The highest fall incidence occurs in the institutional setting. Falls are a leading cause of accidental injury and are the leading cause of traumatic death in older adults. Fall risk factors are diverse. Intrinsic factors include cognitive, vision, gait, or balance impairment, and high-risk/contraindicated medications. Extrinsic factors are predominantly environmental and include nonsturdy furniture or equipment, poor lighting, and uneven or slippery surfaces. Falls and falls risk assessments have been extensively studied and several resources exist on this subject. The Centers for Disease Control and Prevention (CDC) (2021) initiated the Stopping Elderly Accidents, Deaths & Injuries (STEADI) program. The CDC website contains a falls risk screening tool as well as resources for health-care providers working in various clinical settings. Another fall risk assessment tool is the Hendrich Fall Risk Assessment (*https://hign.org/consultgeri/try-this-series/fall-risk-assessment-older-adults-hendrich-ii-fall-risk-model*). The National Patient Safety Center (*https://www.patientsafety.va.gov/professionals/onthejob/falls.asp*) has abundant free resources for client assessment and interventions.

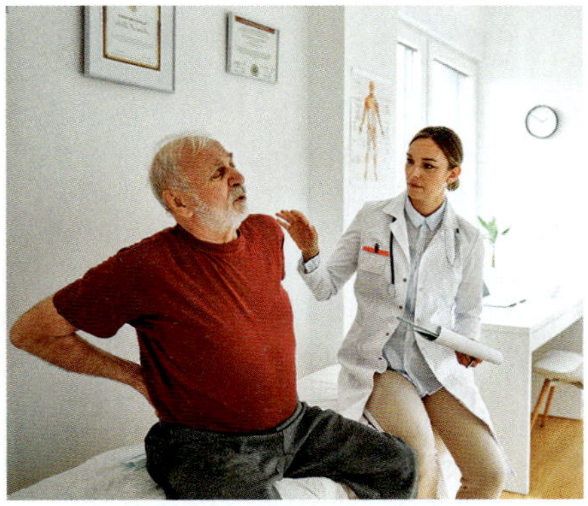

Figure 26-16 The older adult's pain level must be assessed at regular intervals, just as in a younger client.

Pain Assessment

Always ask the older client about pain (Fig. 26-16). Many older clients assume that pain is an inevitable part of aging. Older adults may use other words, such as *discomfort, soreness,* or *achiness,* when describing their pain to you.

Assessment of pain should include asking:

- How long has the pain been a problem?
- Is this new pain, or have you had it before?
- Where is the pain? Does it radiate? Where is it the worst?
- How severe is the pain? (Ask the person to rate the pain using the Numeric Rating Scale, refer to Chapter 9).
- Is the pain sharp, stabbing, dull, or aching?
- Is there any numbness or tingling associated with the pain?
- Has the pain interfered with any activities?
- What makes the pain worse or better?
- What have you tried to relieve the pain? Did it work?

Use of a valid and reliable pain assessment instrument will improve the rating of the pain and evaluation of the effectiveness of treatment. Examples of tools that can be used may be found at *https://hign.org/*.

Clients with severe cognitive impairments may not be able to communicate or describe their pain. Specific pain assessment instruments are available for use with this population. Two pain assessment tools for clients with cognitive impairments are the Checklist of Non-Verbal Pain Indicators (CNPI) (Feldt, 2000) and PAINAD (Warden, et al, 2003). The PAINAD tool can be found at *https://hign.org/sites/default/files/2020-06/Try_This_Dementia_2.pdf*.

Pain should be reassessed at regular intervals to evaluate the effectiveness of interventions.

> **NURSING TIP**
> **Emergency Response System**
> Many older adults wear an electronic device (e.g., watch, bracelet, necklace) that is used to activate emergency care when warranted. Frequently this device is worn on a chain around the client's neck and is activated by pushing a button. Depending on the company, some type of response is initiated when the client activates the device. Note the presence of such a device and verify that the client knows how to use it. There should also be a plan to check the device's functionality.

Self-Determination Assessment

Self-determination is the ability and right to decide what would happen if a client cannot communicate their health care wishes at any time. Older adults have the right to make decisions about their bodies and their health care and are presumed to have decision-making capacity until proven otherwise. Although all people have the risk of not being able to verbally communicate their care wishes, the older adult is at higher risk. All clients who can participate in a conversation, either verbally or through an alternate means of communication, should be approached to discuss and record their treatment preferences and wishes. Health-care professionals can improve end-of-life care for older clients by encouraging the use of advance medical directives. Discussion regarding their availability allows older adults to provide directions about the kind of medical care they do or do not want if they become unable to make decisions or communicate their wishes (Fig. 26-17). These documents provide guidance to health-care professionals, families, and health-care surrogates about the person's wishes. The documents may also provide immunity from civil and criminal liability when health-care professionals follow the advance medical directive in good faith.

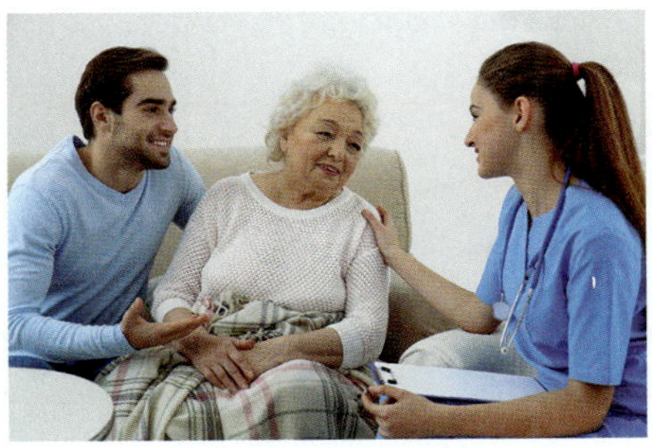

Figure 26-17 Discussing an advance medical directive with family members and health-care professionals allows older adults to express their wishes if they are not able to do this.

NURSING TIP

Older Adults and Driving

Independence is highly valued by older adults and driving is a key component of this independence. Older adults' health conditions and effects/side effects of medications may impact driving skills. Physiological changes may include limitations in movement, speed of response, slowed maneuvering and braking, less acute vision, and loss of hearing. These changes can be evaluated and possibly ameliorated at an older adults driver's assessment clinic, where driving skills can be evaluated by a driving specialist, an occupational therapist or other trained professional. The American Automobile Association (AAA) offers a "Road Wise Driver Course," designed to assist older adults adjust to age-related physical changes and prolong their safe driving abilities. Many older adults are self-aware of their driving challenges and self-limit the hours, time of day, and distance they drive.

If an individual experiences increasing near misses, fender benders, or accidents, and increasing insurance premiums and does not self-limit their driving, a difficult discussion may be necessary, regarding the need to stop or limit one's driving. Learn about local community resources to help those no longer able to drive safely. The National Highway Traffic Safety Administration (NHTSA) has a helpful guide to assist concerned individuals and their families begin a discussion *(https://www.nhtsa.gov/road-safety/older-drivers)*.

There are two types of advance medical directives: (1) a durable power of attorney for health care and (2) a living will. The use of a durable power of attorney allows the older adult to designate an individual, called a health-care proxy, an agent, or a surrogate, to make health-care decisions in the event the client loses the ability to make decisions or communicate their wishes. A living will provides specific instructions about particular kinds of health-care treatment an individual would or would not want. Living wills are often used to declare a wish to refuse, limit, or withhold life-sustaining treatment. Although these documents are usually in writing, oral directives are allowed in some states.

An advance medical directive or living will may contain instructions for no resuscitation or "Do Not Resuscitate" (DNR). This allows health-care personnel to respect an individual's wishes to not have attempts made to restart the heart or breathing should cardiopulmonary arrest occur. A DNR does not mandate or imply nontreatment of any other medical conditions. There is a trend in the community to change the DNR term to "Allow Natural Death" (AND). Older adults requiring advanced life support have a low survival rate both outside and inside the hospital setting. Further information is available at *https://hign.org/consultgeri/try-this-series/working-families-hospitalized-older-adults-dementia*.

Palliative Care

Palliative care is a type of care that can coexist with a client's usual care. It is given predominantly for a chronic condition that causes the client discomfort in some way. With palliative care, medical illness continues to be treated, but symptoms of pain, nausea, shortness of breath, or other discomfort may be treated aggressively. This care may progress to hospice care, although this is not a requirement. Hospice care is used when the burdens of the treatment outweigh their benefits or the treatments or interventions are futile. The older adult sets priorities for life, and those priorities are honored as much as possible.

NURSING CHECKLIST

General Approach to Examination of the Older Adult

1. Observe Standard Precautions and don personal protective equipment (PPE) such as gloves, gown, face shield, goggles, N-95 respirator mask or face mask if your client's status warrants these protective measures.
2. Examine the older adult in an environment that is warm, comfortable, and welcoming.
3. Always address questions to the older adult even in the presence of the caregiver. If the caregiver is not allowing the client to speak, assure the client their concerns will be addressed.
4. Use bright, indirect light to enhance the client's ability to function. Ensure a quiet environment with minimal background noise.
5. Minimize interruptions in the interview and examination.
6. Allow adequate time for the examination. A comprehensive examination of the frail older client may require an extended visit with rest periods, or multiple visits.
7. Allow the older adult to maintain independence in all activities related to the examination even if it increases the time needed.
8. Before assisting the older client, ask the client whether they would like assistance preparing for the examination.
9. Instruct the older adult to remove all items of clothing for a full examination and provide a gown with instructions for its use. Always respect client modesty.
10. Provide a warmer temperature. Offer a blanket if the room temperature cannot be adjusted.

11. Ascertain that the older adult has clean glasses (clean as needed) and working hearing aids. If a hearing aid would enhance the examination, offer a temporary amplification device if available. If no amplification is wanted or available, ask the client which ear has better hearing. Speak with a low-pitched, normal-volume voice to the client's better ear. Validate that all information presented to the client has been heard correctly.
12. Ask the frail older adult if the caregiver should remain during the examination.
13. Allow the older adult to select a position of comfort. Frail older adults may be less fatigued and more comfortable if examined in a semirecumbent position.
14. Maximize the visual cues the older adult can use by ensuring a clear view of your face without bright background glare.
15. Ask open-ended questions and avoid "yes/no" questions to ensure completeness of the interview and examination.
16. After the examination, elicit essential subjective information related to answers to the closed-ended questions to validate the findings.
17. Use evidence-based tools specific to the older adult to ensure accuracy of information.
18. Always conclude the examination by asking if there are other concerns that have not been addressed or if the client has questions about anything discussed.

Assessment in Brief

Older Adult Examination

Special Assessments

- Developmental assessment
- Cultural assessment
- Spiritual assessment
- Geriatric syndromes
  - Nutritional assessment
  - Sleep assessment
  - Falls assessment
  - Pain assessment
- Self-determination assessment

Physical Examination*

- Quick screen
- Functional assessment
- Cognitive assessment

**All other examination skills are performed as described in Chapters 9–23.*

Equipment

- Appropriate PPE
- Equipment listed in Chapters 9–23
- Equipment/forms needed to conduct cognition and functional assessments

Physical Examination

The older adult population is an extremely heterogeneous group. Life experiences, coupled with genetics, exposures, lifestyles, and diverse culture, diet, recreation, education, environmental influences, and work types, all affect an individual's health and wellness status. Key to the assessment of older clients is their functional ability within their environment and community.

> **NURSING TIP**
> **Alzheimer Client Safety**
> The Alzheimer's Association sponsors the Safe Return Program for Alzheimer clients. The client wears an identification bracelet that contains the client's name, states that the wearer is memory impaired, and includes the phone number of the National Missing Persons Bureau. In the event that the client wanders from their surroundings, the Missing Persons Bureau is alerted, and it is through this agency that the person responsible for the client is contacted.

There is no specific age at which the aging process routinely warrants screening. The older adult may have unique concerns and requirements secondary to disability, comorbid conditions, normal changes of aging, and personal coping strategies.

An essential facet of care of the older adult is incorporating the caregiver into the examination. Care should be taken to defer to the wishes of the older adult regarding the need to involve another individual in assessment and care. Communication should always be directed toward the client while still attending to the caregiver or family input.

Functional testing and cognitive testing should be conducted at each visit with the older adult. Table 26-2 offers a quick screening tool to assess the health of the older adult. Many of the components of the Older Adult Quick Screen are also incorporated into the Medicare Annual Wellness visit for people who are 65 years and older.

Functional Assessment

Functional assessment may be accomplished using any of several valid and reliable tools. Refer to *https://hign.org/consultgeri-resources/try-this-series*. The tool selected should be specific to the older population and the older adult's situation. If the older adult is living independently, the Lawton IADL scale should be used, as it covers all activities needed to maintain oneself at home and maintain independence safely. If the older adult resides in an institution offering assistance or resides with and receives assistance from caregivers, the narrower focus of the Katz ADL index may be more appropriate. These tests may be accessed at *https://hign.org/*. If the individual resides in a facility with a high level of care and the major concern is safety, the "Get Up and Go" test allows evaluation of the older adult's ability to be mobile safely. This test can be accessed at *http://www.gericareonline.net/tools/eng/falls/attachments/Falls_Tool_2_Get_Up_and_Go_Test.pdf*.

Table 26-2 Older Adult Quick Screen

Assessment	Screen
Function	Positive response to one or more questions, when asked, "Do you need help with ..." Shopping? Doing light housework? Walking across a room? Washing in shower or bath? Doing finances?
Mobility	Perform "Timed Get Up and Go Test" (should be completed in <20 seconds)
Nutrition	Weight loss of more than 10 pounds (4.5 kg) in the past 6 months without trying (or) Body mass index <20 kg/m^2
Vision	Check ability to read newspaper headline and one sentence with correction. If unable, check each eye with Snellen chart.
Hearing	Unable to hear fingertip friction at 6 inches (15 cm) in both ears (or) If audioscope available, check for 40 dB at 1,000–2,000 Hz in one or both ears or either in one ear.
Cognition	Mini-Cog test: three-item recall, clock drawing, and recheck recall without reminder. Clients recalling none of the three words are classified as demented (score = 0). Clients recalling all three words are classified as nondemented (score = 3). Clients with intermediate word recall of 1–2 words are classified based on the Clock Drawing Test (CDT) (Abnormal = demented; Normal = nondemented).
Depression	Positive answer to "Do you often feel sad or depressed?" requires further assessment and followup.

Cognitive Assessment

Early identification of cognitive impairment has a significant influence on the quality of life in the older adult (Fig. 26-18). Because safety is affected by cognitive function, the ability to function independently is, too. Some erroneous stereotypes of aging are almost completely based on cognitive function and decline. This is more complex than perceived by some health-care providers. Cognitive function consists of the processes by which the older adult perceives, recognizes, registers, stores, retrieves, and uses information. These processes are made up of perception, memory, and thinking. Older adults more commonly suffer from cognitive alteration, and it is essential that the nurse differentiate the entity being seen. Stereotyping cognitive impairment as the aging norm is common—and harmful.

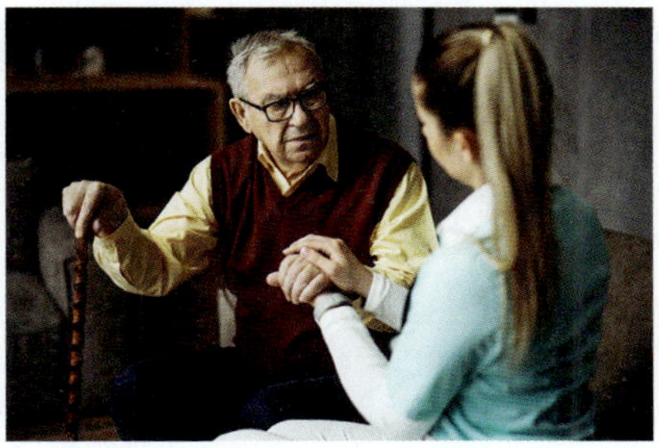

Figure 26-18 The nurse needs to assess the older adult's cognitive status at each encounter.

The major cognitive entities fall into three diagnoses: dementia, delirium, and depression. Each of these cognitive entities has different clinical features (Table 26-3). Delirium is considered a medical emergency and early diagnosis leads to improved outcomes. Depression also benefits from early diagnosis and treatment. No treatment currently exists for dementia. It is imperative also to remember that older adults may have other etiologies that account for their behavior, such as thyroid disease, altered glucose metabolism, electrolyte imbalance, and **polypharmacy** (the simultaneous use of numerous medications to treat medical conditions). In the presence of cognitive impairment, a full organic work-up is warranted.

Cognition may be assessed using several reliable and valid tools specific to the older adult. The Folstein Mini-Mental State Examination (Folstein et al, 1975) is the gold standard of cognitive tests for all ages even though it is susceptible to educational and cultural bias (Ng et al, 2018).

The Mini-Cog is a valid, reliable screening tool for assessing cognitive status that takes 3 to 5 minutes to complete and shows no bias toward educational level or cultural background. Cognitive impairment of dementia and delirium may also be assessed using the Mini-Cog, which is available at *https://hign.org/consultgeri/try-this-series/mental-status-assessment-older-adults-mini-cog*.

Delirium can be objectively assessed using the Confusion Assessment Method (CAM). Delirious older adults will have a labile level of consciousness, drifting in and out during the examination. They may be able to perform cognitive testing well during lucid periods but still demonstrate impairment on testing. The etiology may be infection, metabolic abnormalities, CNS damage, cranial lesions, or the addition of new medications. Withdrawal from medicines, both prescribed and OTC, must also be considered. Older adults exhibiting signs of delirium should be questioned about alcohol use. A complete work-up is indicated to determine the etiology. Secondary treatment includes assessment and maintenance of client safety and symptomatic treatment. The CAM can be found at: *https://hign.org/consultgeri/try-this-series/confusion-assessment-method-cam*.

Depression may be easily screened for using the Geriatric Depression Scale. Refer to Table 26-4. This tool is available at *https://hign.org/consultgeri/try-this-series/geriatric-depression-scale-gds*. Adults who score 5 or higher should receive further evaluation and treatment. The presence of depression should always prompt the nurse to ask about suicidal ideation before the older adult departs the examination. Geriatric depression responds as well to treatment as depression in a younger population does. The client's safety is paramount and must be ensured.

Vital Signs

Vital signs should be assessed in the same manner as in the younger adult client. Usually performed at the initiation of the encounter, vital sign assessment is an introduction to the examination almost universally accepted and expected by the older adult. This allows the nurse to introduce personal touch and establish rapport.

Table 26-3 Differentiating Delirium, Dementia, and Depression in the Older Adult

	Delirium	Dementia	Depression
Onset of Symptoms	Sudden	Gradual	Gradual but may present more quickly than dementia
Progression	Rapid unless cause treated	Slow and progressive, vascular dementia (VD) may present with more abrupt declines	May be rapid or gradual
Duration	Hours to months	Months to years	Months to years depending on treatment given and response
Attention	Impaired and distracted	Decreases as disease worsens	Easily distracted; difficulty concentrating
Level of Consciousness	Waxing and waning	Stable state of consciousness	Normal, may be hypervigilant
Orientation	May be disoriented with altered perceptions	Disorientation to place and time common	Normal
Memory	May or may not be impaired	Short-term memory usually impaired first. Long-term memory declines from recent to distant	Detailed complaints of memory problems, but relatively normal performance on clinical tests if motivation is adequate
Thought Processes	Frequently disorganized	Impaired judgment; difficulty with abstractions	Intact but may express feelings of hopelessness, helplessness. May have suicidal ideation
Perception	Delusions, auditory and visual hallucinations common; difficulty differentiating between reality and perceptions	Delusions and hallucinations possible depending on etiology	Delusions and hallucinations may be present but less common
Mood	Variable; fluctuating	May be depressed, especially in early stages; may have inappropriate affect	Depressed, self-absorbed
Speech	Disorganized, may be rambling or incoherent	Will decline over course of disease from trouble with word finding to aphasia and muteness	Generally normal, may be slowed
Behavior During Assessment	Distracted and difficult to assess; answers based on perceptions	Tries very hard to give correct answers, may deny problems, wants to get it right	Often displays little effort on clinical tests; often responds "I don't know," but can give the correct answer upon further probing

Table 26-4 Geriatric Depression Scale

Directions: Have the patient reflect over the last week and choose the best answer for how they have felt. Score 1 point for each shaded answer.

1.	Are you basically satisfied with your life?	YES	**NO**
2.	Have you dropped many of your activities and interests?	**YES**	NO
3.	Do you feel that your life is empty?	**YES**	NO
4.	Do you often get bored?	**YES**	NO
5.	Are you in good spirits most of the time?	YES	**NO**
6.	Are you afraid that something bad is going to happen to you?	**YES**	NO
7.	Do you feel happy most of the time?	YES	**NO**
8.	Do you often feel helpless?	**YES**	NO
9.	Do you prefer to stay at home rather than going out and doing new things?	**YES**	NO
10.	Do you feel you have more problems with memory than most?	**YES**	NO
11.	Do you think it is wonderful to be alive now?	YES	**NO**
12.	Do you feel pretty worthless the way you are now?	**YES**	NO
13.	Do you feel full of energy?	YES	**NO**
14.	Do you feel that your situation is hopeless?	**YES**	NO
15.	Do you think that most people are better off than you are?	**YES**	NO

A score of 5 points or greater indicates depression and further evaluation is indicated.
Adapted from Development of a Comprehensive Assessment Toolbox for Stroke, by P. W. Duncan, 1999, *Clinics in Geriatric Medicine, 15*(4), pp. 885–894.

Pulse

As in the younger client, the radial artery is used for heart rate assessment. If the client has an irregular heart rate, the apical pulse is assessed. An older adult's heart rate is the same as that of a younger adult. Refer to Chapter 9.

Temperature

An older adult with severe cognitive impairment may be unable to comprehend the instruction to hold the thermometer under the tongue. An axillary, tympanic, or noncontact infrared temperature may be easier to obtain (Fig. 26-19).

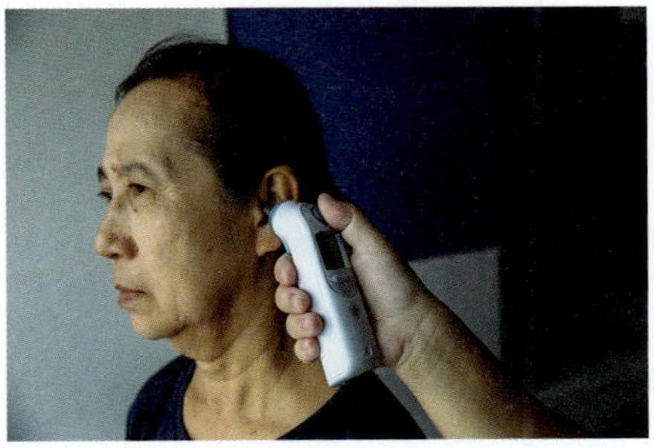

Figure 26-19 The tympanic thermometer can be used with ease in the older adult.

E Refer to Chapter 9.

N **The older adult may normally have a lower body temperature, down to 96°F (35.6°C).**

A **P** Refer to Chapter 9.

Blood Pressure

Blood pressure should be measured in the supine and standing postures, especially if the client is taking antihypertensive medication.

E Refer to Chapter 9.

N **Increased systolic and diastolic pressures may be seen. Widening of pulse pressure is common.**

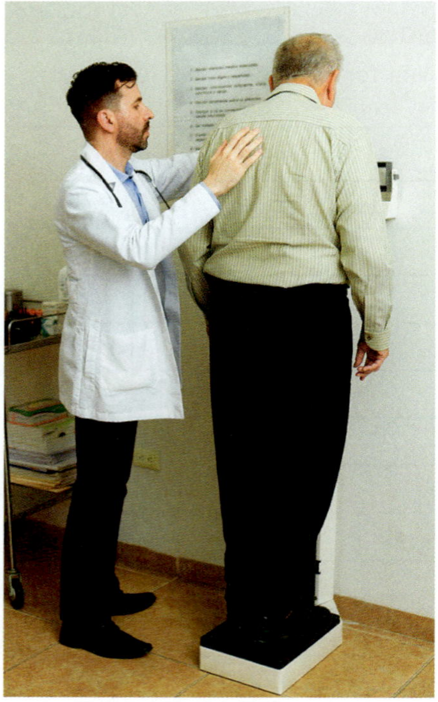

Figure 26-20 The older adult may need assistance stepping on a scale.

A fall in diastolic blood pressure is seen more frequently in older adults with risk factors for hypotension. Decreases may range from 20 to 40 mm Hg.

A Bilateral differences in blood pressure from each arm may be present.

A Isolated systolic hypertension is a blood pressure of greater than 160 mm Hg (systolic) over less than 90 mm Hg (diastolic).

P These blood pressure changes can occur because of atherosclerosis and arteriosclerosis.

Height and Weight

The frail or weak older adult may require assistance with getting weighed (Fig. 26-20). A modified standing or sitting scale may be necessary. Older adults may note that their height is decreasing as they age; this is due to osteoporosis. Older adults may also lose weight. Weight should be assessed at each client interaction and carefully documented and monitored. Unexplained weight loss should be investigated.

E N A P Refer to Chapter 7.

Skin

Skin should be monitored for hydration status, lesions, bruising, and changes in temperature, turgor, color, and pigmentation as described in Chapter 10. Intertriginous areas should be examined for fungal infections. Monitor feet for the need for podiatry interventions. Older clients should be examined regularly for skin breakdown and assessed for the risk of skin breakdown. Appropriate interventions should be implemented. Clients and families may be following the usual norms of daily hot showers, which are not indicated for aging skin.

E Refer to Chapter 10.

N **The following changes can be observed in the older adult:**

- **Skin may be drier and may or may not be accompanied by less perspiration.**
- **A thin, parchment-like appearance of the skin with wrinkles and sagging skin folds may be present.**
- **Liver spots, also called senile lentigo or solar lentigo, are irregular, flat, deeply pigmented macules that appear in sun-exposed areas (Fig. 26-21). They result from the inability of melanocytes to produce an even pigmentation of the skin. Larger areas, called lentigines, are generally seen on the backs of the hands and wrists of light-skinned people and are related to the degree of sun exposure.**
- **Sebaceous hyperplasia presents as flattened papules with a central depression and is usually yellowish.**
- **Seborrheic keratoses are characterized by overgrowth of the horny layer. Lesions are raised but flattened growths with a wart-like appearance (Fig. 26-22). They commonly appear somewhat greasy and as though they could easily be scraped from the skin's surface. They may be scaly and dry in presentation and range from pale white to brownish in color. They are usually not premalignant.**
- **Senile purpura is a bluish-purple spot that develops on the older adult's skin, especially in areas of trauma, even slight trauma.**

> **NURSING TIP**
> **Skin Changes in the Older Adult**
> Hypothermia and hyperthermia occur more frequently in the older adult client. The older adult has a decreased ability to compensate for changes in temperature because of impaired vasoconstriction or vasodilation and the normal loss of subcutaneous fat. Decreased dermatome activity, inflammatory response, and pain perception increase the risk of frostbite and burns.

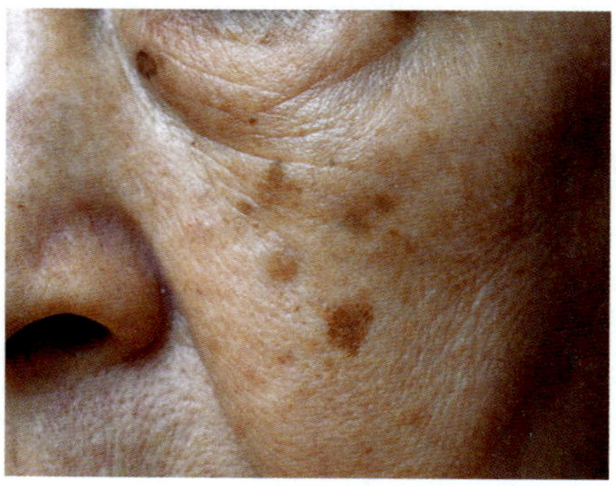

Figure 26-21 Senile lentigo.

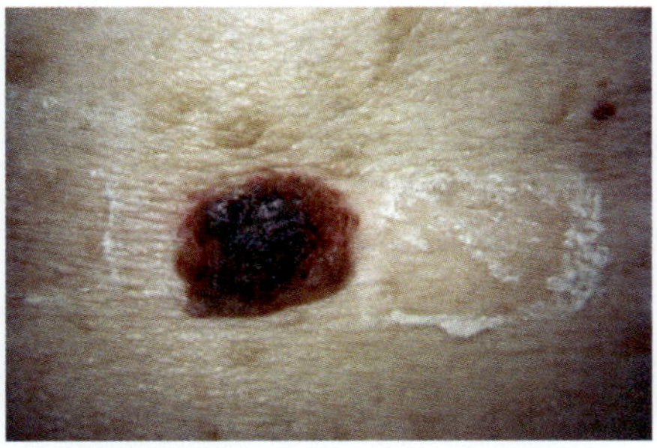

Figure 26-22 Seborrheic keratosis.

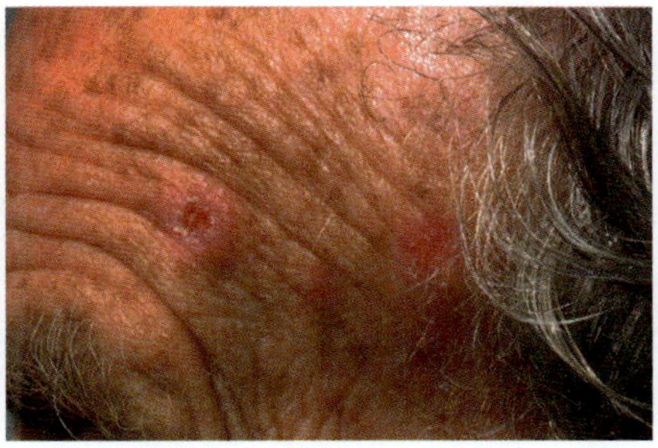

Figure 26-23 Actinic keratosis.

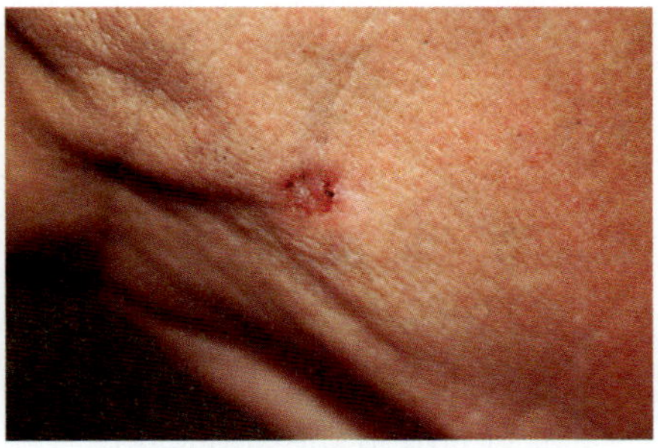

Figure 26-24 Basal cell carcinoma.

A Actinic keratosis, or solar keratosis, is seen in areas of the greatest sun exposure and is premalignant to squamous cell carcinoma (SCC). These lesions are superficial, flattened papules covered by dry scales, which may be irregular in shape and pink or tan in color (Fig. 26-23).

A Basal cell carcinoma (BCC) is more common among the older adult population (Fig. 26-24). The majority of BCC occur on the head and neck. White males are at highest risk, especially those with prolonged exposure to the sun and tanning salons, and previous therapy with ionizing radiation. The lesions can be pigmented or pearly white or pink, and they frequently bleed or scab.

A Squamous cell carcinoma (SCC) tends to occur on the backs of the hands, scalp, and top of the pinna (Fig. 26-25). The SCC lesion often appears red and has an inflamed base. The lesion is mobile with well-defined borders.

P Actinic keratosis, BCC, and SCC are associated with sun exposure. UVB radiation is a risk factor for SCC, as is damage from thermal burns or chronic inflammation.

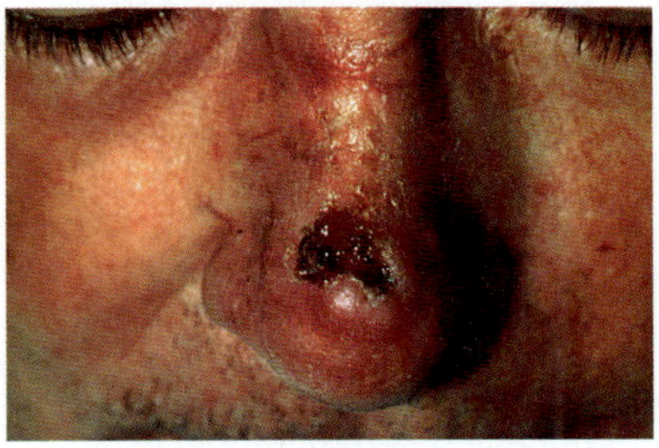

Figure 26-25 Squamous cell carcinoma.

Hair

E Refer to Chapter 10.

N **The hair becomes thinner and coarser, possibly with some degree of alopecia, in the older adult (Figure 26-26). Facial hair may be seen on females.**

A P Refer to Chapter 10.

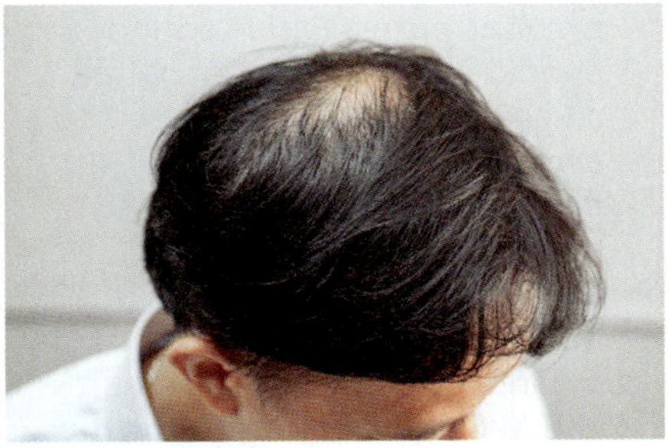

Figure 26-26 Thinning hair and patches of alopecia are common in older adults.

Nails

E Refer to Chapter 10.

N **Nails commonly become thicker, harder, and yellowish in the older adult. Nails may develop ridges and split into layers.**

A P Refer to Chapter 10.

Head and Neck

In the older adult, range of motion of the neck should be assessed using a single motion at a time to diminish the possibility of dizziness. Monitor for pain, crepitus, and dizziness in addition to range of motion.

E Refer to Chapter 11.

N **There should be a full range of motion. In addition, there may be an altered appearance of the face due to tooth loss and the absence or presence of dentures.**

> **NURSING TIP**
>
> **Safety Tips to Help the Older Adult Client Avoid Integumentary Damage**
>
> - Assist older adult clients in identifying hazards in the home that could cause trauma (e.g., loose rugs, sharp table edges, glass items in the bathroom, stoves, electric appliances, etc.).
> - Remind older adult clients that sensation to temperature diminishes with age and that they may therefore wish to check their bath water with a thermometer (should not be warmer than 105°F [40.6°C]).
> - Advise older adult clients to wear multiple layers of clothing in cooler temperatures and gloves and socks to protect the distal extremities from hypothermia and frostbite.
> - Remind older adults to keep electric blankets and heating pads on a medium setting to prevent burns. Older adults should exercise caution when sleeping with a heating pad to avoid skin damage/burns.
> - Advise older adult clients to apply emollient lotions to decrease xerosis and pruritus but to avoid lotions with a high alcohol content, as these can cause further drying of the skin.
> - Warn older adult clients that their skin will tear more easily and be prone to shearing because their epidermal layers are thinner, and that because the integumentary system is slower to recover from trauma, healing from such injuries will take longer.

A Range of motion may be limited. A stiff neck may indicate the presence of cervical arthritis.

P Cartilage and ligaments become less elastic and may be prone to calcification as a person ages. Tendons and muscles lose elasticity and tone. Cervical intervertebral discs lose water and disc space narrows.

Eyes

Inspection

E Refer to Chapter 12.

N **The following changes can occur in the older adult's eyes as part of the normal aging process and may be noted on inspection:**

- **Graying of eyebrows and eyelashes**
- **Diminished tearing**
- **Loss of pigment in the iris**
- **Diminished or absent corneal reflex**
- **Decreased peripheral vision**
- **Altered color perception; difficulty discriminating blue, green, and violet colors**
- **Arcus senilis, a grayish or whitish arc or circle around the limbus not associated with an underlying condition**

A The lower eyelid can drop away from the eye (ectropion) in the older adult.

P Genetic predisposition, lid muscle dysgenesis, trauma, infection, and autoimmune causes can lead to ectropion.

A The lower lid can turn inward (entropion) in the older adult.

P Laxity of medial and lateral muscles, cranial nerve (CN) III or CN VII paralysis, Bell palsy, herpes zoster, or CN lesions—in addition to trauma, infection, and autoimmune disorders—are etiologies of entropion.

A Decreased central vision can occur in the older adult. This can occur in conjunction with the older adult looking forward when addressing someone who is standing to the side.

P Macular degeneration is often age-related and is a common vision problem affecting the older adult. The older adult will require significant magnification to compensate for the central loss. An altered head position maximizes available vision.

Anterior Chamber and Lens

E **N** Refer to Chapter 12.

A The pupil may have a pearly gray appearance.

P A lens that is pearly gray in appearance may indicate cataract formation.

P Acute-angle glaucoma occurs in older adults at a higher rate than in younger adults. It may be caused by an inhibition of the flow of fluid from the posterior to the anterior chamber or by "plateau iris syndrome" with iris laxity, which comes into close proximity to the angle. Other causes are anterior uveal displacement, posterior segment inflammation, or tumors.

Pupil

E Refer to Chapter 12.

N **The older adult may have a decreased pupil size with slow accommodation.**

A An irregularly shaped pupil, either bilaterally or unilaterally, is abnormal.

P Cataract repair will alter the shape of the surgical pupil.

Posterior Segment Structures

E Refer to Chapter 12.

N **The older adult's posterior segment structures may have the following changes:**

- **Dullness of retinal structures**
- **Pale blood vessels**
- **Narrower light reflex of arterioles**
- **Straighter and narrower retinal vessels**

A **P** Refer to Chapter 12.

Ears

During the examination, the older client's ears should be assessed for wax buildup and impaction, which can be removed by irrigation and curette. Ensure that any hearing aids are functional, with working batteries and correct placement. If impairment is noted and the client has not had an audiological examination, encourage the client to get that examination. Face the older adult client when speaking to them. Ensure there is no background glare obscuring the older client's view. Speak slowly, in a low-pitched voice, and avoid raising your voice or yelling. Eliminate as much background noise as possible.

Auditory Testing

Ask the older adult about hearing problems. Consider using standardized tools to assess the individual's perception of hearing, such as the Brief Hearing Loss Screener (which may be found at *https://hign.org/consultgeri/try-this-series/hearing-screening-older-adults*).

E **N** Refer to Chapter 13.

A Some hearing loss or presbycusis is common in the older adult.

P Conductive hearing loss can occur in the outer ear because of foreign body obstruction (including cerumen) or due to the loss of elastic tissue in the tympanic membrane. Conductive hearing loss can occur in the middle ear because of rigidity of movable bones in the inner ear, which mutes sound.

P Sensorineural loss is common in the older adult and involves inner ear dysfunction.

External Ear

E Refer to Chapter 13.

N **Pendulous earlobes that are wrinkled can develop normally in the older adult. Wiry hair protruding from the auditory canal is normal (Fig. 26-27). Cerumen is dry, which leads to an increased incidence of impaction.**

A Skin lesions on the external ear may be premalignant or malignant (SCC or BCC) and should be evaluated by a dermatologist or other qualified professional.

P The external ear receives a significant amount of sun exposure, especially in males, which predisposes the external ear to dermatological changes (Fig. 26-28).

NURSING TIP
Visual Limitations

Visual limitations have the potential to limit driving, ambulation, and safety. In the social setting, visual changes affect social interactions and safety in the home. A home safety inspection can facilitate remediation with lighting and hazard elimination. The older individual should be educated on the importance of regular eye examinations to preserve vision. The older adult should also be provided information about positive lighting changes that can enhance function, newly developing driving hazards, and fall-prevention techniques.

Visual acuity should be assessed using an increased level of indirect lighting, and color discrimination should be assessed more frequently than in the younger population. Additional questions should be asked of the older adult during the health history regarding visual difficulties while driving or on stairs, loss of peripheral vision, loss of night vision, and difficulty distinguishing colors. Ask if the client is having any eye dryness/burning, and increased/decreased tearing.

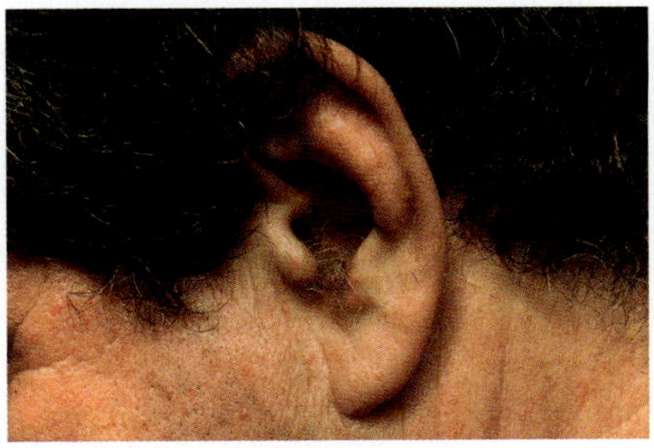

Figure 26-27 Wiry ear hair.

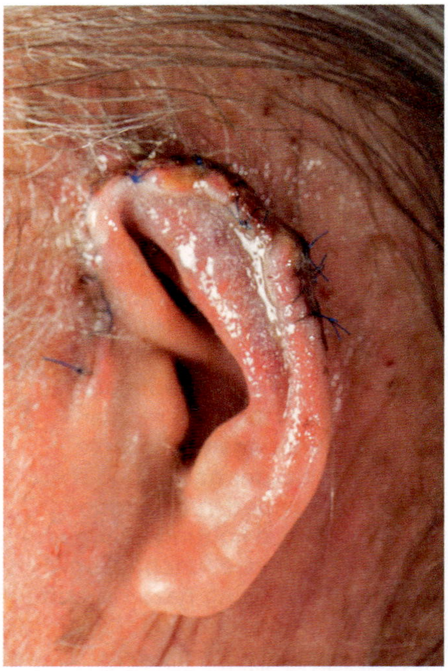

Figure 26-28 This client has sutures in the ear helix after having a melanoma excised.

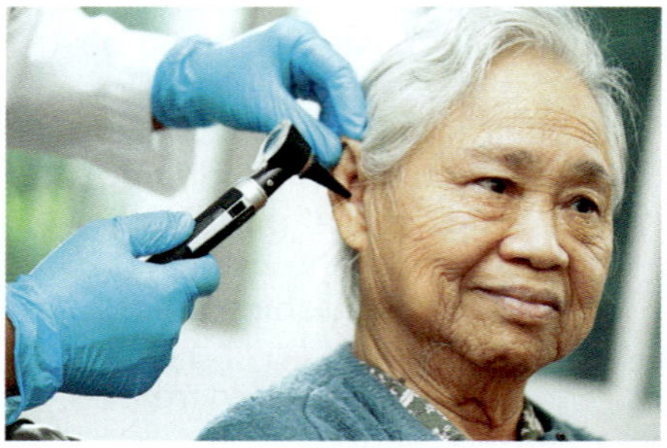

Figure 26-29 The nurse may find a slightly altered appearance to the tympanic membrane in the older adult.

Internal Ear

E Refer to Chapter 13.

N **The older adult's normal ear may have pronounced landmarks if atrophic or sclerotic changes have occurred (Fig. 26-29). The tympanic membrane may appear white, opaque, and thickened. It may be less mobile.**

A P Refer to Chapter 13.

Nose

E Refer to Chapter 13.

N **The following are changes in the nose of an older adult:**
- **The nose increases in size due to increased cartilage formation.**
- **Nasal hairs are coarser.**
- **There is a decrease in the sense of smell because the number of sensory cells in the nasal lining decreases.**

A P Refer to Chapter 13.

Mouth and Throat

If the older adult has dentures, the mouth and oral cavity should be examined both with dentures and without.

E Refer to Chapter 13.

N **The following changes occur in the older adult:**
- **Lip surface develops deep wrinkling, with an increase in the granular lining on the lips and cheeks.**
- **The buccal mucosa thins, with a decrease in its vascularity.**
- **Gums are paler in color with recession.**
- **Saliva production decreases (may be partly due to medications).**
- **Fissuring of the tongue increases with atrophy of the papilla.**
- **Taste sensation diminishes due to atrophy and loss of taste buds.**
- **Gingival tissue has less elasticity.**
- **Dental roots may become exposed.**

A Fissures may develop at the corners of the mouth.

P Fissures at the corners of the mouth may be due to a vitamin deficiency or yeast infection (due to impaired immunity).

A Lesions on the lips, especially for clients who are or were smokers, are abnormal and should always be investigated.

P Lips are exposed to the environment and sun damage. Tobacco use increases the risk of oral cancer.

Breasts

Breast examinations should continue throughout the lifespan.

E Refer to Chapter 14.

N **The following are breast changes in the older adult female:**
- **Breasts may appear flattened and elongated due to relaxation of suspensory ligaments.**
- **The nipples may be smaller and flatter.**
- **Cystic breasts may feel smoother as the female ages and glandular tissue decreases.**
- **The inframammary ridge thickness increases in prominence.**

A Masses or lesions should be evaluated. Refer to Chapter 14.

P Increased incidence of breast cancer occurs with advancing age.

Thorax and Lungs

The thorax and lung examination may necessitate frequent breaks for the older adult, to avoid fatigue and hyperventilation (Fig. 26-30).

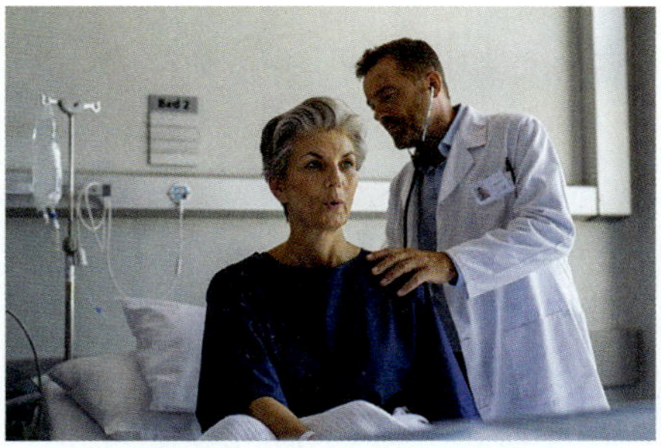

Figure 26-30 The nurse may need to give the older adult frequent rest periods when examining the lungs.

E Refer to Chapter 15.

N **Expansion of the chest wall decreases with increased inspiratory effort in the older adult.**

A P Refer to Chapter 15.

Heart

The older adult's heart functions without compromise under normal stress. However, it has reduced reserve and may not be able to compensate for stress, blood loss, extreme exertion, or high fever.

E Refer to Chapter 16.

N **The apical impulse may be displaced due to a decrease in the size of the heart in the older adult. A systolic ejection murmur may be auscultated at the left lower sternal border due to stiffening of the ventricles and valvular leaflets.**

A An S_4 heart sound is a common finding.

P Left ventricular thickening and/or enlargement resulting in loss of compliance result in the S_4.

Peripheral Vasculature

E N Refer to Chapter 17.

A Decreased pulse volume may be present. Limbs may be cool.

P Decreased pulse volume and cool limbs can be due to arteriosclerosis and atherosclerosis.

Abdomen

E Refer to Chapter 18.

N **Abdominal musculature diminishes in mass and tone in the older adult. The fat content of the body increases with age, leading to increased deposits in the abdomen. The liver decreases in size.**

A Increased incidence of urinary and fecal incontinence commonly occurs but is not a normal change of aging and should be evaluated.

P Incontinence is secondary to changes of aging such as thinning of perineal tissues secondary to loss of estrogen, damage from childbirth, surgery, prostate problems, neurological disorders, and functional disability. Refer to Table 18-4 for information on types of urinary incontinence.

Musculoskeletal System

Health of the musculoskeletal system can dramatically affect the quality of life of the older adult. Assessment should include mobility, fine and gross motor skills, and activities of daily living (ADL). The examination should be carefully performed to ensure joint stabilization. Slow, gentle, passive movements should be used to assess range of motion (ROM). Regular exercise should be encouraged, and information regarding the components of a program should be discussed with the client. Maximal benefit will occur when the client includes aerobic exercise in addition to muscle strengthening and balance. The older client garners significant benefits from physical or occupational therapy consultation and information on environmental modifications to maximize function.

> **NURSING TIP**
> **Elder Abuse and Neglect**
> The Centers for Disease Control and Prevention (CDC) (2024) defines elder abuse as "an intentional act or failure to act that causes or creates a risk of harm to an older adult. An older adult is someone age 60 or older. The abuse occurs at the hands of a caregiver or a person the elder trusts." Abuse can be physical, sexual, psychological, emotional, financial, or neglect. There is an increased incidence of abuse and neglect among older adults. Approximately 10% of adults aged 60 and older who live at home are victims of abuse (CDC, 2024). Etiological factors include stress related to financial difficulties, multiple family members residing in limited space, the lack of nearby family members, and dealing with an older relative who has dementia or incontinence. Possible indications of physical abuse include unexplained bruises, swelling, hematomas, burns, fractures, poor hygiene, and poor nutritional status. Health-care providers are obligated to investigate these symptoms further when they are unexplained or when the explanation is inappropriate for the location and severity of the trauma. Be familiar with your institution's policy on elder abuse (Daly & Butcher, 2018).

Inspection

E Refer to Chapter 19.

N **The following changes occur in the musculoskeletal system with the aging process:**

- **Posture changes to a more flexed position, which changes the center of gravity.**
- **Steps tend to be smaller, with a wider base in males; females maintain a narrow standing base. The step height is reduced.**
- **The gait has a higher risk for unsteadiness due to changes in the center of gravity and changes in the ear cochlea that result in a decreased ability to compensate.**
- **Transfers in and out of a sitting position will be more difficult for the older adult because of vertebral inflexibility and reduced muscle strength.**

A A reduction in height occurs in the older adult. Kyphosis may be present.

P Intervertebral discs lose water, causing narrowing of the disc space and a resultant loss of 1½ to 3 inches (3.8 to 7.6 cm) in height.

A The lordotic curve of the back flattens, and both flexion and extension of the back decrease.

P Bone mass loss and bone density loss due to increased rate of bone reabsorption, and slowed bone cell replacement lead to these musculoskeletal changes.

Muscles

E Refer to Chapter 19.

N **Reduced muscle mass and loss of strength, especially against resistance, occur in the muscles of the older adult.**

A **P** Refer to Chapter 19.

Joints

E **N** Refer to Chapter 19.

A Decreased range of motion of individual joints and pain at rest and with range of motion can occur with the aging process. Crepitus may be present with joint movement.

P There is a decrease in the water content of cartilage and a narrowing of joint space with age. A lifetime of wear and tear results in deterioration.

Mental Status and Neurological System

Changes of aging gradually affect the nervous system. The changes are both structural and functional.

Mental Status

E Refer to Chapter 20.

N **A slight decline in short-term memory is normal in the aging adult. There is minimal cognitive decline in normal aging.**

A There is an increased incidence of depression in the older adult (Fig. 26-31).

P Decreases in the neurotransmitters norepinephrine and serotonin, caused by changes in dendrite distribution and decreased enzymatic activity, can lead to depression.

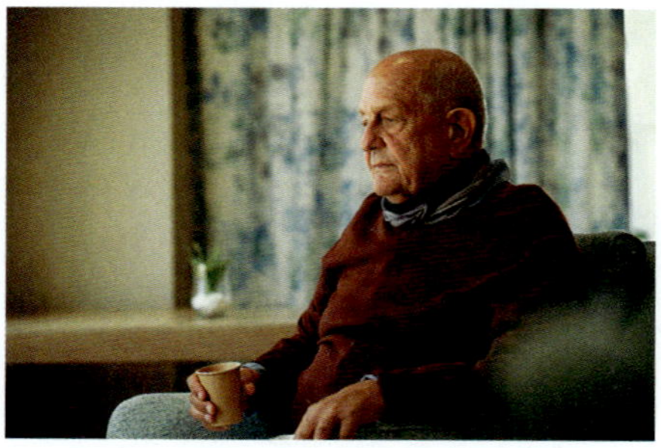

Figure 26-31 A change in neurotransmitters and neurophysiology in the brain can lead to depression in the older adult.

Sensory Assessment

E Refer to Chapter 20.

N **The following changes are seen in the sensory assessment of the older adult:**
- **Reduced sensation of vibrations**
- **Reduced sensation of cold/heat**
- **Reduced sensation of touch discrimination, especially fine touch; some older adults develop an increased sensitivity to light touch due to thinner skin**
- **Decline in proprioception**

A **P** Refer to Chapter 20.

Cerebellar Function

E Refer to Chapter 20.

N **The older adult commonly has some balance impairment and may have an altered gait. There may be a decline in coordination.**

A Abnormal gait accompanied by new incontinence or confusion is abnormal.

P Normal-pressure hydrocephalus is more frequently seen in the older adult.

Deep Tendon Reflexes

E Refer to Chapter 20.

N **In the older adult, there may be a decline in deep tendon reflexes, and the Achilles reflex may be extinguished.**

A **P** Refer to Chapter 20.

Female Genitalia

Examination of the pelvis should not be avoided in the older adult. The focus of the examination changes to evaluation for incontinence, pelvic relaxation, irritation, dryness, or rectal conditions. Always screen for cancer if intact reproductive organs remain, if consistent with the goals of care and national guidelines. A smaller speculum may be needed for the internal examination.

Inspection

E Refer to Chapter 19.

N **These changes may be found during inspection of the older adult female's genitalia:**
- **The clitoris and labia become smaller.**
- **The labia become flatter and lose pigmentation.**
- **The labial skin becomes thin, shiny, avascular, and dry.**
- **Pubic subcutaneous fat is lost.**
- **Pubic hair becomes sparse and turns gray or white.**

A **P** Refer to Chapter 21

Palpation

E Refer to Chapter 21.

N **These changes may be found during palpation of the older adult female's genitalia:**
- **The ovaries and uterine tubes may not be palpable due to shrinkage.**
- **The uterus atrophies and may be difficult to palpate.**

> **NURSING TIP**
>
> **STIs in the Older Adult Population**
>
> The incidence of sexually transmitted infections (STIs) such as gonorrhea, chlamydia, and syphilis has greatly increased in adults over age 55 in the past decade (CDC, 2024, Epps et al, 2023). Many older adults underestimate the risk of acquiring a STI and believe STIs are only a concern for young adults. Condom use is not consistently or ever used. With advancing age, the older adult regards sexual activity differently. An older female does not need to worry about pregnancy in later adulthood. Older adult males may have erectile dysfunction but can take phosphodiesterase type 5 inhibitor medications to rectify this. Older adults are living longer have may have more sexual partners. Lifestyles have changed. Retirement communities offer readily available partners. Many dating apps cater to the older adult population. Clinicians need to remember that sexual activity is an important quality of life for many older adults and sexual history needs to be addressed. The nurse has an opportunity to provide age-appropriate sexual health education.

- **The cervix becomes smaller, paler, and less mobile.**
- **The cervical os becomes smaller but remains palpable.**
- **The vagina shortens, narrows, and thins.**
- **The introitus constricts due to atrophy.**
- **The vaginal wall loses rugae and elasticity.**
- **Vaginal secretions are delayed, and production is reduced.**

A The risk of a prolapsed uterus and vagina increases with age.

P Prolapsed uterus and vagina are caused by the atrophy of pelvic muscles, which leads to a decrease in pelvic organ support. Ligaments and connective tissue of the pelvis also lose muscle tone. This is not an uncommon finding in females who experienced pregnancy.

A Uterine enlargement, nodularity, irregularity, or induration are abnormal.

P Advancing age is a risk factor for malignancies such as ovarian, cervical, and endometrial cancers.

Male Genitalia

Inspection

E Refer to Chapter 22.

N **The following changes may be found during inspection of the older adult male's genitalia:**

- **The pubic hair thins and turns white or gray.**
- **The penis atrophies.**
- **The scrotal sac loses elasticity and elongates.**
- **The testicles may be smaller.**

A P Refer to Chapter 22.

Palpation

E Refer to Chapter 22.

N **The testicles are smaller and atrophic.**

A P Refer to Chapter 22.

Anus, Rectum, and Prostate

Palpation

E Refer to Chapter 23.

N **The older male adult typically has a smooth and rubbery prostate that is enlarged.**

A P Refer to Chapter 23.

U.S. Preventive Services Task Force (USPSTF)

Grade A Recommendations

- The USPSTF recommends screening for colorectal cancer in adults aged 50 to 75 years.
- The USPSTF recommends screening for hypertension in adults 18 years or older with office blood pressure measurement (OBPM). The USPSTF recommends obtaining blood pressure measurements outside of the clinical setting for diagnostic confirmation before starting treatment.
- The USPSTF recommends that clinicians prescribe preexposure prophylaxis using effective antiretroviral therapy to persons who are at increased risk of HIV acquisition to decrease the risk of acquiring HIV.
- The USPSTF recommends screening for syphilis infection in persons who are at increased risk for infection.
- The USPSTF recommends that clinicians ask all adults about tobacco use, advise them to stop using tobacco, and provide behavioral interventions and US Food and Drug Administration (FDA)–approved pharmacotherapy for cessation to nonpregnant adults who use tobacco.

Grade B Recommendations

- The USPSTF recommends 1-time screening for abdominal aortic aneurysm by ultrasonography in men aged 65 to 75 years who have ever smoked.
- The USPSTF recommends screening for anxiety disorders in adults.
- The USPSTF recommends that primary care clinicians assess women with a personal or family history of breast, ovarian, tubal, or peritoneal cancer or who have an ancestry associated with breast cancer susceptibility 1 and 2 (BRCA1/2) gene mutations with an appropriate brief familial risk assessment tool. Women with a positive result on the risk assessment tool should receive genetic counseling and, if indicated after counseling, genetic testing.
- The USPSTF recommends that clinicians offer to prescribe risk-reducing medications, such as tamoxifen, raloxifene, or aromatase inhibitors, to women who are at increased risk for breast cancer and low risk for adverse medication effects.
- The USPSTF recommends biennial screening mammography for women aged 50 to 74 years.
- The USPSTF recommends screening for chlamydia and gonorrhea in all sexually active women ... 25 years or older who are at increased risk for infection.
- The USPSTF recommends screening for colorectal cancer in adults aged 50 to 75 years.
- The USPSTF recommends screening for depression in the adult population ... as well as older adults.
- The USPSTF recommends exercise interventions to prevent falls in community-dwelling adults 65 years or older who are at increased risk for falls.
- The USPSTF recommends offering or referring adults with cardiovascular disease risk factors to behavioral counseling interventions to promote a healthy diet and physical activity.
- The USPSTF recommends screening for hepatitis B virus (HBV) infection in ... adults at increased risk for infection.
- The USPSTF recommends screening for hepatitis C virus (HCV) infection in adults aged 18 to 79 years.
- The USPSTF recommends that clinicians screen for HIV infection in ... older adults who are at increased risk of infection.
- The USPSTF recommends that clinicians screen for intimate partner violence (IPV) in women and provide or refer women who screen positive to ongoing support services. [See the USPSTF website for information on IPV in men].
- The USPSTF recommends behavioral counseling for all sexually active adults who are at increased risk for sexually transmitted infections (STIs).
- The USPSTF recommends that clinicians prescribe a statin for the primary prevention of CVD for adults aged 40 to 75 years who have 1 or more CVD risk factor (i.e., dyslipidemia, diabetes, hypertension, or smoking) and an estimated 10-year risk of a cardiovascular event of 10% or greater.
- The USPSTF recommends annual screening for lung cancer with low-dose computed tomography (LDCT) in adults aged 50 to 80 years who have a 20 pack-year smoking history and currently smoke or have quit within the past 15 years. Screening should be discontinued once a person has not smoked for 15 years or develops a health problem that substantially limits life expectancy or the ability or willingness to have curative lung surgery.
- The USPSTF recommends screening for osteoporosis to prevent osteoporotic fractures in women 65 years or older.
- The USPSTF recommends screening for prediabetes and type 2 diabetes in adults aged 35 to 70 years who have overweight or obesity. Clinicians should offer or refer patients with prediabetes to effective preventive interventions.
- The USPSTF recommends screening for unhealthy alcohol use in primary care settings in adults 18 years or older and providing persons engaged in risky or hazardous drinking with brief behavioral counseling interventions to reduce unhealthy alcohol use.
- The USPSTF recommends screening by asking questions about unhealthy drug use in adults age 18 years or older. Screening should be implemented when services for accurate diagnosis, effective treatment, and appropriate care can be offered or referred. (Screening refers to asking questions about unhealthy drug use, not testing biological specimens.)
- The USPSTF recommends that clinicians offer or refer adults with a body mass index (BMI) of 30 or higher (calculated as weight in kilograms divided by height in meters squared) to intensive, multicomponent behavioral interventions.

Retrieved December 30, 2025, from *https://www.uspreventiveservicestaskforce.org/uspstf/recommendation-topics/uspstf-a-and-b-recommendations*

CASE STUDY
The Older Adult With Pneumonia and Altered Mental Status

This case study illustrates the application and objective documentation of the older adult client examination. Mr. Joseph Anderson, a 98-year-old male, is brought to the urgent care clinic by his daughter and wife due to worsening respiratory symptoms and altered mental status.

HEALTH HISTORY

CLIENT PROFILE

98-year-old married Black male

CHIEF COMPLAINT

Client's daughter: "Please help my Dad. He does not know who he is or what year it is!"

HISTORY OF PRESENT ILLNESS

History provided by client's daughter and wife; electronic health record consulted for additional information. Client has had episodes of weakness and shortness of breath for 5 to 7 days with a productive cough developing 4 days ago. Sputum has been a thick green. Fever to 101°F (38.3°C). Client had shaking chills last night for the first time. Initially self-treated by increasing fluids, taking vitamin C and acetaminophen 1,000 mg every 6 hours with minor improvement in the fever to 99.5°F (37.5°C). In the past 24 hours, client has had little oral fluids and no food. Client has rested in bed and taken naps, which is not the norm. Client's wife called their daughter today when client became confused as to where he was and did not recognize her. Client's daughter drove over to the parents' house and found the client in bed and talking incomprehensibly. Usually, client is oriented and very "sharp" as he knows exactly what day it is and all the current events of the day from the newspaper.

PAST HEALTH HISTORY

Medical History

- Diverticulitis in May 2012—treated outpatient with ciprofloxacin and clear liquid diet, symptoms resolved within a week
- Degenerative joint disease for past 20 years, managed with OTC medication
- Hypertension (HTN) for past 30 years, controlled on medications

Surgical History Appendectomy aged 21 without complications

Allergies Erythromycin caused diarrhea in the past, but no angioedema or anaphylaxis

Medications

Prescription: Irbesartan-hydrochlorothiazide 300/25 mg orally every morning

OTC: Acetaminophen 500 mg orally every 8 to 12 hours as needed; psyllium 2 tablespoons in water at lunchtime; multivitamin daily

Communicable Diseases No documented HSV, STI, HIV, hepatitis or other communicable diseases

Injuries and Accidents None

Differing Abilities Hard of hearing, has bilateral hearing aids

Blood Transfusions None

Childhood Illnesses Usual childhood diseases

Immunizations Pneumococcal vaccine polyvalent 23 in 2001; diphtheria/tetanus in 2019; recombinant herpes zoster- completed 2 shot series in 2018; high-dose flu shot annually; COVID-19 had initial 2 shot series, RSV vaccine last year, gets additional vaccines when advised to do so

FAMILY HEALTH HISTORY

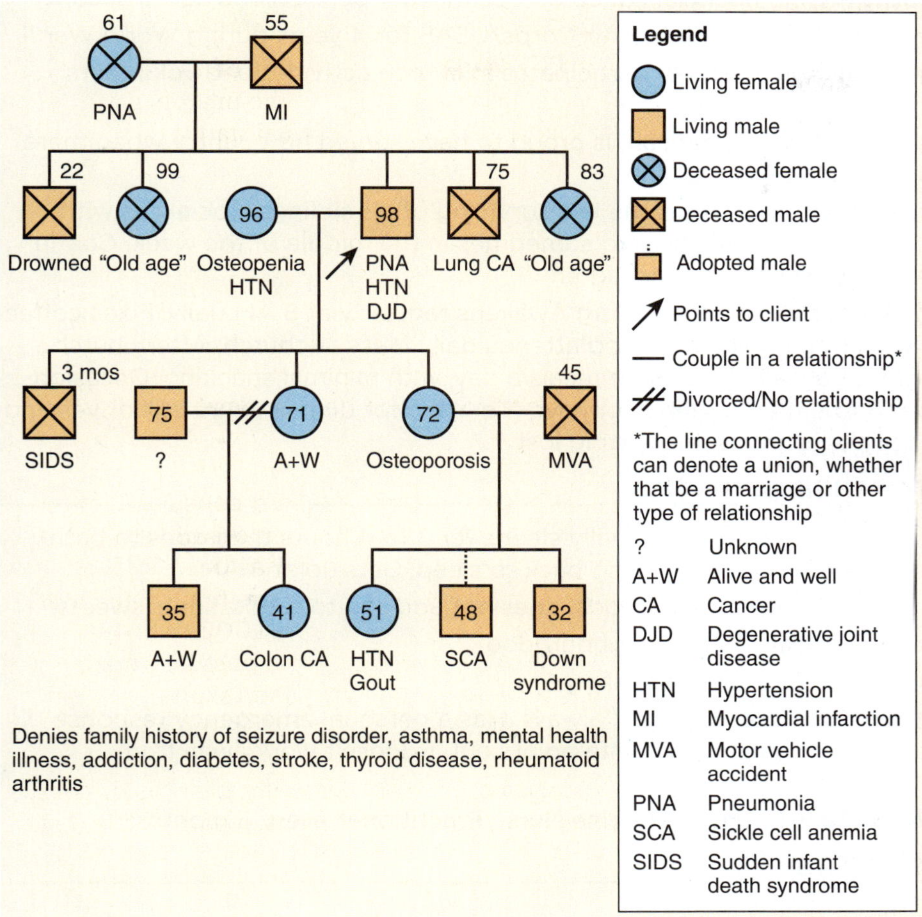

SOCIAL HISTORY

Alcohol Use 6 ounces of red wine daily

Tobacco Use 4-year-pack history; quit in 1946 (picked up smoking habit while serving in the military)

Recreational Drug Use No history of illicit drug use

Domestic and Intimate Partner Violence Married to his wife of 76 years; denied intimate partner violence at recent wellness check

Sexual Practice Monogamous heterosexual male

Travel History Traveled to granddaughter's wedding 3 weeks ago out of state, 4 hours away. Was stationed at many overseas locations when in the military

Work Environment Retired U.S. Army Air Corps/USAF. After the military worked for a government contractor doing defense contract work. Retired at age 67. Now client works in his workshop doing furniture repair and refinishing

Home Environment Lives with his wife in 3-bedroom ranch house with all essential services on the first floor. Does own repair work/maintenance on their house, including mowing lawn and landscaping. Has cleaning service every 2 weeks

Hobbies and Leisure Activities

Enjoys working on the furniture. Also enjoys spending time with his 2 daughters and grandchildren

Walking in the neighborhood and local parks. Attends his church and is active in many volunteer roles

Stress Denies

Education Master's degree in engineering

Economic Status Has no financial concerns, has military pension and social security

Military Service Served in the Army Air Corps/USAF for 4 years during World War II

Religion Roman Catholic; actively participates in church activities and volunteers regularly

Ethnic Background Black American. Is proud to have served his country when there were few Blacks in the service

Roles and Relationships Client is the last surviving of his siblings. Socializes with friends at church every weekend and sometimes in the middle of the week. Continues to drive. Enjoys seeing grandchildren

Characteristic Patterns of Daily Living Awakens regularly at 8 AM daily. Fixes coffee for self and wife. Reads the paper and attends daily Mass at church. After church goes with wife for a walk. Eats three meals a day, with minimal snacking. Occasionally they go out to eat with friends or have friends in for dinner. Client still drives and has had no accidents and is not getting lost

HEALTH MAINTENANCE ACTIVITIES

Sleep Goes to bed around 10 PM. Usually sleeps for 3 to 4 hours then goes to bathroom. Sometimes has difficulty falling back to sleep. Gets up at 8 AM

Diet Regular diet with low-sodium foods, does not add salt to foods, limits sweets

Exercise Walks 1 mile daily in the neighborhood

Stress Management No stress per wife

Use of Safety Devices Uses seat belt always. Has a personal emergency response system that he wears reliably, but wife points out it doesn't work away from home

Health Checkups Sees Internal Medicine Nurse Practitioner every 6 months

SPECIAL ASSESSMENTS

Deferred

PHYSICAL EXAMINATION

Functional Assessment (from records at wellness visit 2 months ago)

Independent in all activities and functions at an extremely high level; uses no assistive devices
KATZ ADL 6/6, no deficits
Lawton IADL 8/8, no deficits
"Get Up and Go" test: Unable to assess due to client's altered mental status
Mini-Mental State Examination (MMSE) from most recent PCP visit: 30/30, clock drawing normal
Geriatric Depression Score from most recent PCP visit: 0/15 (not depressed)

General Survey and Vital Signs

Black male who looks younger than stated age who is disoriented and irritable
Height: 74 inches (188 cm)
Weight: 170 lb (77.3 kg)
Temperature: 102°F (38.9°C) noncontact infrared
Pulse: 122
Respiratory Rate: 28
Blood Pressure: 99/58 mm Hg (Left arm sitting)
101/62 mm Hg (Left arm supine)
105/64 mm Hg (Right arm sitting)

Skin, Hair, and Nails Thinning hair on legs, skin very warm to touch without diaphoresis; smooth texture, decreased turgor on chest, hair gray; nails clean and clipped, no clubbing

Head Normocephalic, without lesions, masses, depressions, or tenderness; face symmetrical, without involuntary movement or swelling; scalp shiny with some keratoses and age spots; TMJ articulates smoothly, no crepitus or clicking

Eyes Acuity-deferred

Eyebrows bushy and gray, full and coarse, eyelashes evenly distributed and without inflammation; no ptosis or lid lag; lacrimal apparatus without inflammation; corneal light reflex symmetrical without strabismus; cover/uncover test deferred-client unable to follow directions, EOMI, no nystagmus, conjunctiva pink, no foreign bodies, no tearing, sclera white without exudate, arcus senilis present bilaterally, PERRLA at 3 mm

Ears Gross hearing intact with bilateral hearing aids; pinna without masses, lesions, nodules, inflammation, or tenderness; EAC with dry wax, without inflammation; TMs shiny, positive light reflex, Weber/Rinne deferred

Nose and Sinuses No deformities, bleeding, lesions, masses, or swelling; nares patent, nontender, septum midline without perforation, mucosa pale; maxillary and frontal sinuses without tenderness and resonant

Mouth and Throat Lips pink, without swelling; gums without erythema; mucosa pink and dry; teeth in good repair; tongue midline, well papillated, and without fasciculation, lesions, swelling, or bleeding; hard and soft palates intact without lesions or masses; pharynx pink and nonedematous; uvula midline and rises with phonation; gag reflex intact

Neck Supple without masses or spasms and with FROM, neck symmetrical without masses or tenderness, no lymphadenopathy, trachea midline, thyroid nontender without enlargement or masses, no bruits, no JVD at 90°, 45°, and supine

Thorax and Lungs Anteroposterior: transverse diameter = 1:1; chest wall symmetrical, costal angle > 90°, angle of ribs with sternum > 45°.

No bulging of ICS, retractions present; some use of sternocleidomastoid, trapezius, and abdominal muscles; respirations regular and mildly labored, positive tactile fremitus at posterior bases, bilateral crackles at bases anteriorly and posteriorly

Heart Precordium without pulsations/heaves/thrills, apical pulse 116, apical impulse ⅜ inches (1 cm) at 5th ICS at left MCL, S_1 and S_2 present, SEM II/V at LLSB, no S_3 or S_4, no radiation

Peripheral Vasculature No edema or ulcerations, Homan sign negative, no pulsus paradoxus, no bruits

	Carotid	Brachial	Radial	Femoral	Popliteal	Dorsalis Pedis	Posterior Tibial
Right	3+	3+	3+	3+	3+	3+	3+
Left	3+	3+	3+	3+	3+	3+	3+

Scale = 0–4+

Abdomen Round; no dilated veins, scars, incisions; bowel sounds in 4 quadrants, no bruits, venous hum, or friction rub; tympanic throughout except dullness superior to symphysis pubis for 1¼ inches (3 cm); abdomen soft, no masses, positive tenderness left lower quadrant to deep palpation; liver span—unable to obtain, negative bilateral CVAT

Musculoskeletal FROM all extremities, joints without erythema/edema/enlargement/deformities

Neurological

Mental status: Disoriented to person, place, and time

Sensory: Intact to light touch, other assessments deferred

Cranial Nerves: CN II–XII intact; CN I deferred

Motor: Size equal bilaterally; tone firm and supple throughout; strength: unable to follow directions and assess; no involuntary movements

Cerebellar Function: Deferred—cannot follow directions

Reflexes:

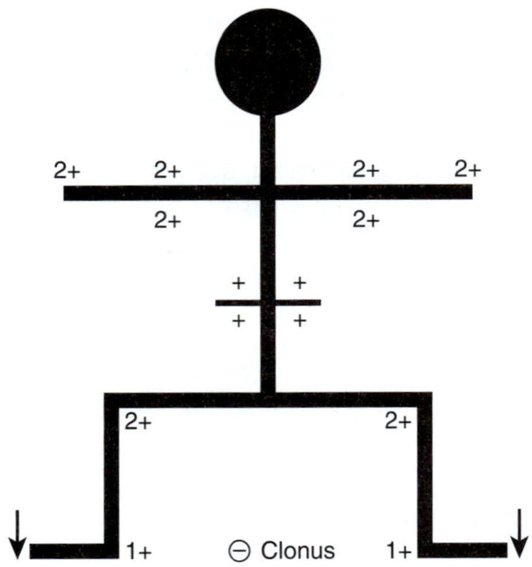

Scale = 4+

Genitalia and Rectum Scrotum without masses or lesions, no penile lesions, rectal examination deferred

LABORATORY RESULTS (selected)

Urine and Blood Cultures Sent to laboratory

Chest X-ray Bibasilar consolidation

Test	Client's Values	Normal Values
CBC		
WBC	15 k/mm^3	4.0–11.0 k/mm^3
RBC	3.1 M/mm^3	4.0–5.2 M/mm^3
Hgb	8.8 g/dL	12.0–16.0 g/dL
Hct	26.4%	37.0–47.0%
Platelet	350 k/mm^3	140–400 k/mm^3
Chemistry		
Sodium	130 mEq/L	135–145 mEq/L
Potassium	4.9 mEq/L	3.5–5.0 mEq/L
Chloride	101 mEq/L	100–108 mEq/L
Carbon Dioxide	20 mEq/L	24–30 mEq/L
BUN	33 mg/dL	8–25 mg/dL
Creatinine	1.7 mg/dL	0.6–1.5 mg/dL
Glucose	112 mg/dL	70–100 mg/dL
Calcium	8.7 g/dL	8.5–10.5 g/dL
Protein, total	5.9 g/dL	6.0–8.5 g/dL
Albumin	3.0 g/dL	3.5–5.0 g/dL
AST	42 units/L	0–40 units/L
ALT	59 units/L	0–55 units/L
Bilirubin, total	1.5 mg/dL	0.1–1.2 mg/dL
Alkaline phosphatase	87 units/L	25–150 units/L

CLINICAL JUDGMENT IN ACTION

1. What cues indicate that the client is having clinical distress?
2. What interventions have the highest priority?
3. What assessment findings indicate clinical improvement or decline in this client?

Review Questions

1. A 76-year-old client is confused after arriving for a physical examination. What is the first assessment that should be performed?
   a. Obtain a history from the client, family, or caregivers
   b. Complete a mental status examination
   c. Nothing, this is normal
   d. Obtain a complete blood cell count

2. Which of the following actions is appropriate to assess a client's functional abilities?
   a. Calling the client's adult children and asking them how the client is doing at home
   b. Performing a functional assessment using a valid and reliable tool with the client
   c. Arranging for a home health nurse to assess the client in the home environment
   d. Inviting a social worker to spend a few hours with the client to monitor the client's actions

3. Which of the following functional assessment tools is most appropriately used with a client who lives independently to assess safety in the home environment?
   a. PAINAD assessment
   b. Mini-Mental State assessment
   c. Falls Risk assessment
   d. Lawton IADL assessment

4. Most older adults live in which of the following setting?
   a. A nursing home
   b. Assisted living community
   c. In their children's home
   d. In their own home

5. You are caring for a hospitalized 93-year-old client who is alert and oriented. The client lives alone in an apartment. The client is hard of hearing and left the hearing aids at home. How can you best communicate with the client?
   a. Speak loudly so that the client can better hear you.
   b. Write out notes to the client with instructions.
   c. Call the client's family and speak with them.
   d. Place the ear pieces of a stethoscope in the client's ears and speak into the diaphragm of the stethoscope.

6. 73-year-old Felix is brought to the hospital by a neighborhood friend, Diego. Diego went to Felix's house to pick him up for their prearranged lunch. Diego reports that Felix seemed fine yesterday but today was distracted and did not recognize him. Felix's speech was rambling and incoherent. Diego reported that Felix was having a conversation with his deceased wife. Felix is coughing and has a temperature of 100.4°F (38°C). Which of the following does the nurse conclude is most likely happening with Felix?
   a. Felix is depressed and has delusions.
   b. Felix has dementia as evidenced by an inappropriate affect.
   c. Felix is experiencing delirium.
   d. Felix has a speech disorder.

7. The nurse conducts a mood assessment on 88-year-old Marta. Which of the following responses indicates that Marta may be depressed? Select all that apply.
   a. Martha admits to being bored.
   b. Martha feels helpless.
   c. Marta prefers staying at home rather than going out to a movie with a friend.
   d. Marta feels full of energy.
   e. Marta believes most people are better off than she is.

8. Which of the following describes some of the physiological changes in the older adult's lungs and thorax? Select all that apply.
   a. The cough reflex decreases.
   b. The diaphragm flattens out.
   c. A barrel chest develops.
   d. Forced vital capacity increases.
   e. Total lung capacity decreases.

9. Which of the following changes occur in the eyes of an older adult? Select all that apply.
   a. The pupils increase in size.
   b. The lens cortex becomes denser.
   c. Peripheral vision is decreased.
   d. Red and pink colors are more difficult to discern.
   e. Presbyopia develops.

10. The nurse assists an 84-year-old bed-bound client with a bath. The nurse conducts a physical examination while assisting the client. Which of the following physical examination findings is normal for an older adult? Select all that apply.
    a. Reduced muscle mass
    b. Decreased chest wall expansion
    c. Increased fat in the abdomen
    d. An elongated scrotal sac
    e. Irregular, flat, and deeply pigmented areas on sun-exposed areas

UNIT

V Putting It All Together

Chapter 27 The Complete Health History and Physical Examination, 928

CHAPTER 27

The Complete Health History and Physical Examination

Rather, ten times, die in the surf, heralding the way to a new world, than stand idly on the shore.

Florence Nightingale

Learning Objectives

1. Identify legal and ethical considerations for the health history and physical examination.
2. Discuss how the use of technology has altered access to and delivery of health care.
3. Conduct a comprehensive health history and physical examination.
4. Discuss the components of a preparticipation sports physical examination and how it differs from a nonpreparticipation sports physical examination.
5. Explain how to use the objectives of *Healthy People 2030* in clinical practice.

Performing a complete health history and physical examination is a skill that takes time and practice to develop. You must concentrate on perfecting interviewing techniques and examination skills. You must be able to accurately recognize normal findings in order to appreciate abnormal and pathological findings. Practicing in an academic laboratory setting or on a volunteer client is a crucial step leading to skill mastery. Learning the examination techniques system by system, as described in this text, allows you to gradually build on previously developed skills.

Keep in mind that, as you perfect your examination skills, the amount of time it takes to perform them will decrease. Plan on spending between 30 and 90 minutes conducting the complete health history and physical examination. If the client's chief complaint is not of an urgent or critical nature, the client's first visit to the health-care facility is the ideal time to perform a comprehensive assessment. Interval or follow-up visits frequently require partial assessments that document changes from the initial database; these visits require substantially less time.

It is important to develop a routine that is comfortable so that steps in the assessment process will not be overlooked. The client's physical, emotional, or mental state may necessitate a change in the usual progression of the examination. Clinical judgment and experience will dictate when specific steps should be omitted, deferred, or repeated.

Once the content of Chapters 9 to 23 is learned and you are comfortable performing each skill, it is time to integrate the entire health assessment and physical examination. This chapter provides a step-by-step approach to guide you through the entire process for an adult client. With time, you will develop a personal rhythm.

Advanced techniques are normally inserted in the assessment process at different phases, depending on the techniques to be performed and the client's condition. Experience will guide you in determining when these advanced techniques are warranted. They are omitted from the following examination sequence, which illustrates a "typical" head-to-toe examination.

Legal Considerations

The increasingly litigious nature of society has not bypassed the nursing profession. More and more nurses are being named as codefendants in lawsuits. Legally, nurses are expected to conduct themselves in a reasonably prudent manner at all times. Some specific guidelines are:

- Document all client interactions (e.g., face-to-face, teleconference, telehealth visit, FaceTime, media platforms [i.e., ZOOM], telephone, letters, faxes).
- Respect the client's confidentiality. Do not discuss any client's case in a public area or with colleagues who are not on that client's care team; keep discussions at a strictly professional level.
- Report any disease that is considered a public health concern (according to local, state, and federal regulations).
- Respect a client's right to privacy.
- Respect a client's right to refuse treatment or examinations (document thoroughly).
- When appropriate, ask the client for permission to perform various examinations, especially those that may be uncomfortable (breast, genitalia, rectal). If the client denies permission, explain the importance of the examination and repeat the request. If the client still denies permission, omit the examination and document the client's refusal.
- Know your institution's policies and standards of practice, and practice within those guidelines.
- Know your state's Nurse Practice Act and practice within that scope.
- Consult with your nurse manager, risk manager, supervisor, or institutional/practice attorney when indicated.

These guidelines are neither foolproof nor comprehensive. When in doubt, use your professional judgment.

Ethical Considerations

It is helpful to keep in mind the following ethical principles to guide your critical thinking within an ethical framework:

- **Autonomy**: a client's right to self-determination; the duty to respect a client's thoughts and actions as to what the client thinks is best for themself
- **Beneficence**: to do what is "good" for the client
- **Nonmaleficence**: to do no harm to the client
- **Justice**: to be fair and impartial to the client
- **Fidelity**: the duty to be faithful to the client
- **Veracity**: to be truthful to the client
- **Utilitarianism**: the duty to perform the greatest good for the greatest number of people

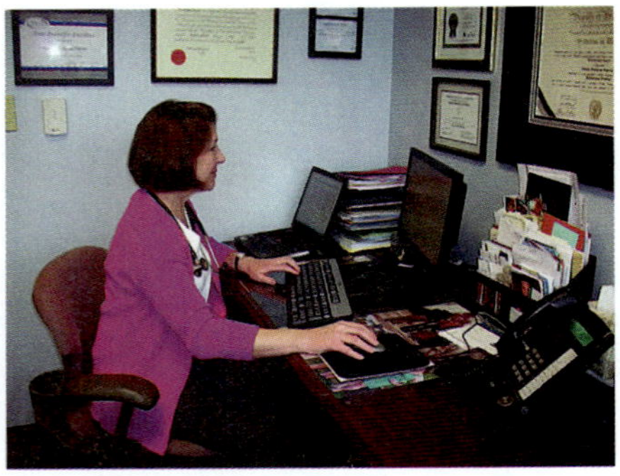

Figure 27-1 Computers are used in most health-care settings for client documentation and communication.

These principles may create challenges for you and the client when an ethical dilemma arises in the clinical setting. The principles are not foolproof, nor are they always easy to practice. Nevertheless, having an awareness of them helps to guard the rights of the client, which is ultimately one of the key roles of the nurse.

Many institutions have a multidisciplinary ethics committee. Some institutions employ an ethicist. Many professional nursing organizations issue ethics statements, both general and specific in nature, to help guide nursing actions. For example, in 2025 the ANA published a code of ethics to guide nurses' actions as they face unprecedented challenges with the evolving role of nurses in the 21st century. Use these or whatever resources are available to you when presented with ethical dilemmas or questions.

Electronic Health Records

Electronic health records (EHRs) or electronic medical records (EMRs) create a paperless system that reduces charting/documentation time once the clinician is familiar with the system (Fig. 27-1). EHRs enable the nurse to use voice recognition, narrative writing, and/or check boxes with drop-down menus to record clients' histories and examination findings. Other advantages of EHRs are their legibility, easy accessibility, ability to be accessed by multiple users simultaneously at different workstations in different areas in real time, and capability of accessing real-time laboratory and diagnostic studies.

Some systems interface with clients' monitors and automatically transfer vital signs from the client to the EHR. Integrated systems can enhance coordination of client care as all providers network with one another to share information. Nurses need to be comfortable with these technologies if they are to remain leaders in the health-care environment.

> **NURSING TIP**
> **Personal Health Record**
> Another example of client-centered technology is the personal health record (PHR), which is used to assist in accurately relaying client information. The PHR is a digital medical record of a client that is secured on a Web page. The PHR contains basic client information, current clinical diagnoses, medications, test results, and progress notes. The client frequently wears a bracelet or necklace that provides the Web address of the PHR with the password so that the record can be accessed in an emergency situation.

Advances in Technology

Technology is constantly evolving in the health-care system. Computers are used at the hospital bedside to document every facet of client care. Most all other clinical settings use computer-based systems to document client care. Health-care providers use computers to link directly to pharmacies when prescribing medications, even controlled substances. Clients too are active participants in their health care via technology. Clients can access special Internet portals to view or record their health information, schedule appointments, obtain test results, and query their health-care providers. With advances in technology members of the health-care team as well as clients can access electronic health records via smartphones. Current technology allows easy access to protected client information from just about anywhere in the world. Unfortunately, hacking of health-care systems has become an all-too-frequent situation, in which client health data is compromised. The privacy and legal issues inherent in health-care technology use are complex and evolving.

Technology has allowed unmanned aerial vehicles, or drones, to be used successfully in rural areas in the United States and around the world for health care. Drones can play a key role in delivering critical supplies in disaster relief areas. Drones have delivered medications, medical equipment, blood products, human organs, and food/water. In August 2015 nurse practitioners from The Health Wagon saw the potential in drone technology to assist their clients in a rural and underserved area of Appalachia in Southwest Virginia. They engineered the first U.S.-approved drone medication delivery in history! This historic event revolutionized client access to health-care supplies (The Health Wagon, 2016). The Health Wagon's drones delivered insulin when roads were impassable due to large snowfalls and delivered critical supplies during the COVID-19 pandemic!

Artificial Intelligence

Artificial intelligence (AI) in health care has been used for many years. AI is used in research, especially the development of new medications. Robots are used in hospitals for surgical assistance, for disinfection of clinical areas, for medication and supply deliveries, and for assistance in client care tasks. Simulation labs in schools of nursing also use AI to educate and train students in real-life medical scenarios. With the advent of ChatGPT in November of 2022, a whole new dimension of AI has evolved and impacted many aspects of health care and medicine. AI tools gather large and diverse data, process it, and devise an outcome based on developed algorithms. The goal is to improve diagnosis and treatment with improved clinical outcomes. AI can also predict adverse complications. AI is used in almost every clinical area of medicine. For instance, AI is used in dermatology to diagnose skin lesions more accurately; AI is used in gastroenterology to diagnose the results of endoscopies and colonoscopies more precisely; AI is used in radiology to interpret radiological imaging, including mammograms, and the list goes on and on. Ultimately, the hope of AI is to decrease health-care costs, decrease medical errors, and decrease workload, while providing improved client care and outcomes. However, there are negative aspects of AI, both ethical and legal. Inherent bias may be written in the diagnostic algorithm whether that was the intent of the developer or not. A diagnostic algorithm may not be accurate for every client. A nurse's clinical judgment and experience need to partner with AI. AI cannot measure the value of the nurse-client relationship and human elements such as touch, empathy, and caring. Nurses cannot become subservient to an AI algorithm. New standards need to be devised to protect confidential client data used in AI. The client has the right to retain autonomy with AI's use. Nurses and all health-care personnel have a professional responsibility to use AI ethically and legally. The AI revolution will continue to evolve, and nurses must be partners in the development of AI use and ultimately incorporate it into their practice.

NURSING TIP
Fostering Client Cooperation

The success of any health history and physical examination depends, in part, on obtaining and maintaining the client's cooperation. Guidelines to assist you in this endeavor include:

- Have the client wait as little as possible before the examination; explain any delays that occur.
- Greet the client first, shake hands, and put the client at ease (Fig. 27-2).
- Proceed in an efficient and organized manner.
- Encourage the client to actively participate in the process (e.g., provide information and ask questions).
- Use terms the client will understand.
- Ask the client to repeat home-care or self-examination instructions and to demonstrate learned skills when appropriate to verify client understanding.
- Be honest; do not offer false reassurance or jump to conclusions.
- Discuss findings first without diagnosing; validate findings when indicated.
- Arrange for the presence of a third party if requested.

NURSING TIP
Tips for a Successful Encounter

- Ensure that the examination table is at a comfortable height for you and the client, with easy access on all sides.
- Respect the client's modesty.
- Have the client make as few position changes as possible.
- Ensure that all of the equipment is accessible and arranged in a logical manner.
- Keep interruptions to a minimum.
- Teach self-assessment while the client is gowned or during specific system examinations.
- Advise the client before procedures about potential discomfort or sensations.
- Ask the client about pain or other sensations during certain examinations.
- Offer cleaning wipes or tissues to the client following certain examinations (e.g., the pelvic and rectal examinations).
- Provide the client with privacy for redressing.

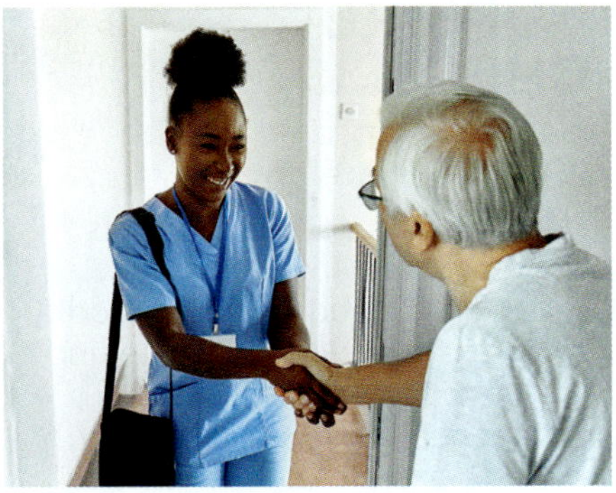

Figure 27-2 A friendly greeting will help to get the examination off to a successful start.

NURSING TIP
Merging the Health History and Public Health Issues

It is the professional responsibility of every nurse to remain clinically competent and stay abreast of emerging health-care issues. Remaining clinically relevant takes many forms and includes an awareness of public health conditions. A recent example was the September 2024 catastrophic flooding from the Category 4 hurricane Helene in Florida, Georgia, Tennessee, Virginia, and the Carolinas. Catastrophic flooding and tornadoes led to many injuries and fatalities. In situations such as hurricanes and tornadoes, injury and death can result not only from contaminated flood waters, but also from drowning, flying debris, downed power lines and loss of power for people who depend on electricity to run their medical equipment, heat exhaustion, and carbon monoxide poisoning from gas generators that were inadequately ventilated. A thorough health history of possible work environment, hobbies and leisure activities, travel history, and review of symptoms might elicit information valuable in analyzing a client's health status in a specific situation. In other words, whether a person is exposed to harmful bacteria in flood zones, parasites from food in a developing area, airborne dust from devastating earthquakes, or other atypical conditions, the nurse must maintain an awareness of events/occurrences in the immediate region as well as in the world to better understand the forces that affect a person's health.

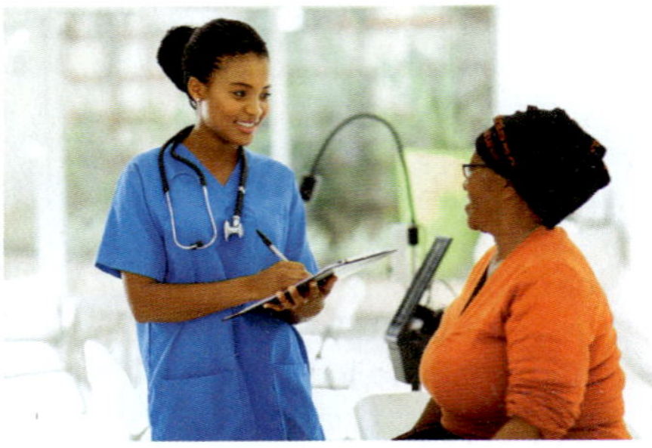

Figure 27-3 The nurse and client review health history information during the initial interview.

Health History

Conduct the health history (Fig. 27-3). Depending on the client's reason for the visit, this can be the complete, episodic, interval (follow-up), or emergency health history. The client can be dressed in street clothes for this interview.

Components of the developmental, cultural, and spiritual assessments are continually evaluated during the course of the client interaction. Thorough assessments of any or all of these special areas can be completed if dictated by the client's situation. The inspection component of the nutrition assessment is noted during the health history. Refer to Chapters 4 through 7.

Physical Examination

This text has provided a head-to-toe examination format in order to discuss body systems in their entirety. However, in practice, a head-to-toe examination combines systems when assessing most body parts. For example, when examining the hands and wrists, components of the skin, musculoskeletal, peripheral vasculature, and neurological examinations are employed. The sample case study at the end of this chapter documents a standard format of the head-to-toe physical examination.

NURSING CHECKLIST
General Approach to the Physical Examination

- Develop an approach that is logical but allows flexibility.
- Use clinical judgment to modify the examination sequence and adapt it to circumstances.
- Allow time at the conclusion of the examination to discuss relevant findings and to allow the client to ask questions.
- Assist older clients or clients with a differing ability to focus on how well they can meet the demands of daily life rather than on their limitations.
- Remember that a physical examination can be tiring, both for you and for the client.

NURSING TIP
Empowering Clients

In 2002, The Joint Commission launched the Speak Up™ campaign. The aim of this program was to empower clients and make them active participants in their own health care to prevent health-care errors and promote client safety. It was updated in 2018 after extensive market research and input from clients and their families. The Speak Up™ initiatives include:

- **S**peak up
- **P**ay attention
- **E**ducate yourself
- **A**dvocates (family members and friends) can help
- **K**now about your new medicine
- **U**se a quality health-care organization
- **P**articipate in all decisions about your care

Print and video resources are available on the Joint Commission's website. Retrieved December 13, 2025, from *https://www.jointcommission.org/en-us/knowledge-library/for-patients/speak-ups/about-your-care*.

General Survey

The client's general appearance is assessed during the health history (Fig. 27-4). Incorporate the following into this assessment:

1. Physical Presence
   Age: stated age versus apparent age
   General appearance
   Body fat
   Stature: posture, proportion of body limbs to trunk
   Motor activity: gait, speed, and effort of movement; weight-bearing; absence or presence of movement in different body areas
   Body and breath odors
2. Psychological Presence
   Dress, grooming, and personal hygiene
   Mood and manner
   Speech
   Facial expressions
3. Distress
   Physical
   Psychological
   Emotional
4. Pain

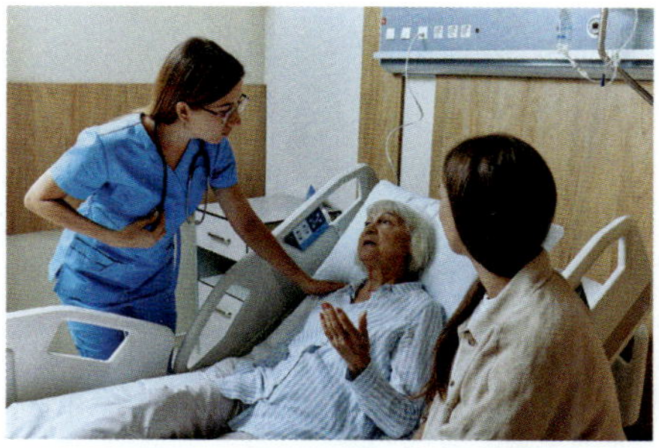

Figure 27-4 Observe the client's overall appearance and demeanor during the interview.

> **NURSING TIP**
> **Assessment of Assistive Devices**
> During inspection, remember to incorporate assessment of the client's assistive devices into your physical examination. Record these data as you would the physical examination findings.

> **NURSING CHECKLIST**
> **General Examination Reminders**
> - Understand illness in human terms, not just scientific terms.
> - Approach the client from a holistic viewpoint and try to understand the client's perspective.
> - Remember that nursing is both art and science.
> - Follow your judgment; critical thinking incorporates the consideration of objective and subjective data. Always ask yourself, "Why?"
> - Act unhurried.
> - Act in a professional manner at all times; remember that the client is simultaneously examining you (e.g., mannerisms, facial expressions, hesitations in speech).
> - Recognize both the client's potential stressors as well as your own (e.g., work, home environment, schedules) and try to account for them.
> - Acknowledge emotional reactions to illness (e.g., anger, fear, anxiety, disbelief, confusion, guilt, shame, blame, hurt, and betrayal).
> - Embrace sensitivity to cultural and spiritual issues.
> - Show respect for clients and their circumstances.
> - Maintain a sense of self-awareness to guide your actions.

> **NURSING TIP**
> **Verifying Assessment Data**
> Always verify assessment data that are extreme. For instance, if you obtain a blood pressure reading of 300/100 mm Hg, double-check it. If in doubt, ask a colleague to assess the parameter in question. Do not be embarrassed to get a second opinion; it is the hallmark of a professional to consult with a colleague when in doubt. Ultimately, the client will benefit from this consult.

Measurements

Record the client's:

1. Height
2. Weight
3. Temperature
4. Pulse (radial is the preferred site in adults) (Fig. 27-5)
5. Respirations
6. Blood pressure (both arms)
7. Anthropometric measurements (if indicated)

Neurological System

1. Assess mental status: facial expression, affect, level of consciousness, fund of information, attention span, memory, judgment,

insight, spatial perception, calculations, abstract reasoning, thought processes, and content.

After the mental status examination, ask the client to undress (Fig. 27-6) and don an examination gown; underwear may be worn. Ask the client to empty the bladder before commencing the examination process. The urine may be collected for a specimen if indicated. Ask the client to sit on the examination table with the legs hanging over the front. A second drape or sheet can be provided to cover the lap and legs. Stand in front of the client.

Skin

Throughout the entire head-to-toe examination, inspect the skin for the following characteristics (Fig. 27-7):

1. Color
2. Bleeding
3. Ecchymosis
4. Vascularity
5. Lesions

Throughout the entire head-to-toe examination, palpate the skin for:

1. Moisture
2. Temperature
3. Texture
4. Turgor
5. Edema

Head and Face

1. Inspect the shape of the head.
2. Inspect and palpate the head and scalp.
3. Inspect the color and distribution of the hair. Note any infestations; palpate the hair.
4. Inspect the face for expression, shape, symmetry (cranial nerve [CN] VII), and symmetry of eyes, eyebrows, ears, nose, and mouth.
5. Instruct the client to raise the eyebrows, frown, smile, wrinkle the forehead, show the teeth, purse the lips, puff the cheeks, and whistle (CN VII).
6. Palpate the temporal pulses. Palpate the temporalis muscles (CN V).
7. Palpate and auscultate the temporomandibular joints.
8. Palpate the masseter muscles (CN V).

Eyes

1. Test distance vision (Fig. 27-8A) and near vision (CN II).
2. Test color vision (Fig. 27-8B).

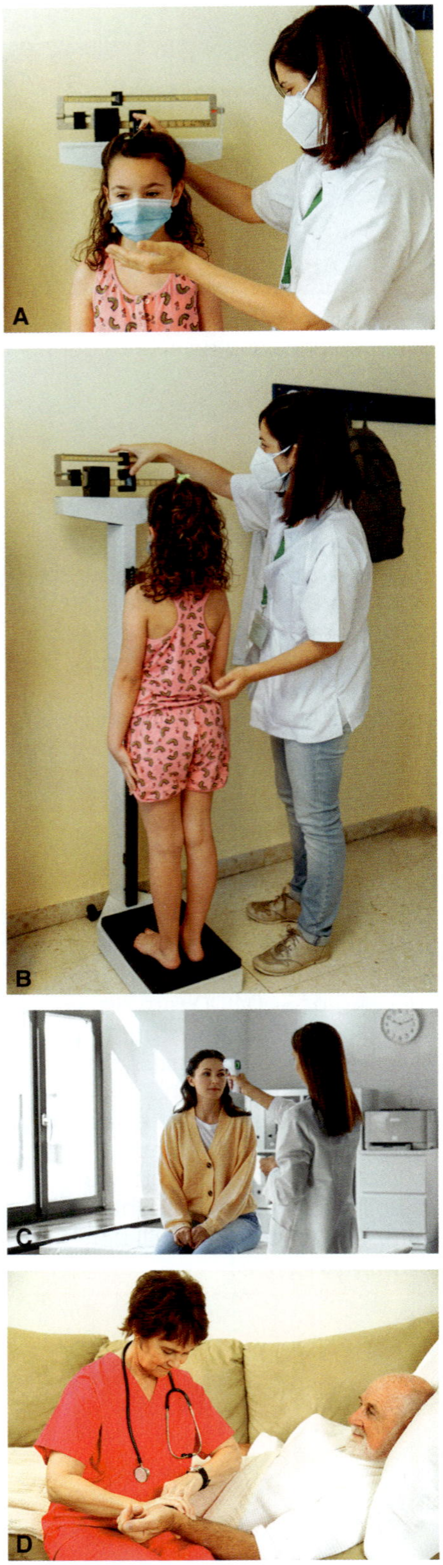

Figure 27-5 General measurements. **A.** Height. **B.** Weight. **C.** Temperature. **D.** Pulse.

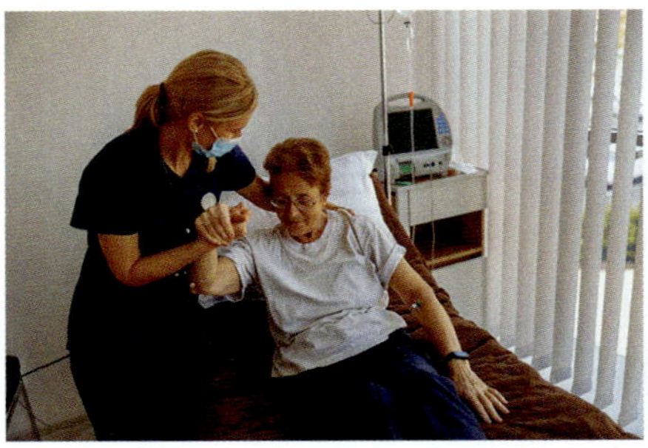

Figure 27-6 It may be necessary to assist the client with certain tasks, such as moving onto the examination table or donning an examination gown.

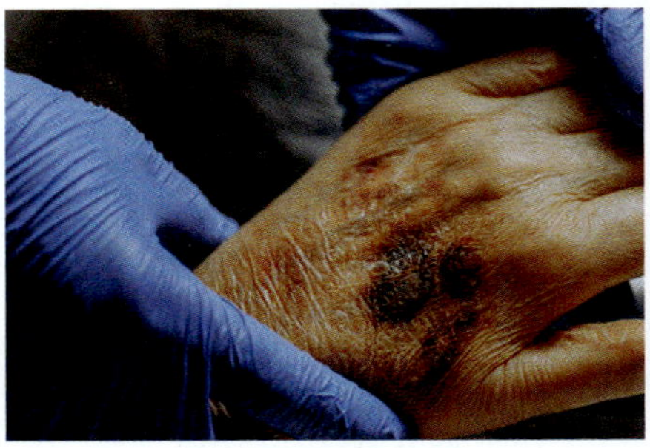

Figure 27-7 Inspect the characteristics of the skin.

3. Test visual fields via confrontation (CN II).
4. Assess extraocular muscle mobility: cover/uncover test, corneal light reflex, and six cardinal fields of gaze (CNs III, IV, VI).
5. Assess direct and consensual light reflexes and accommodation (CN III).
6. Inspect the eyelids, eyebrows, palpebral fissures, and position of eyes.
7. Inspect and palpate the lacrimal apparatus.
8. Inspect the conjunctiva, sclera, cornea, iris, pupils, and lenses.
9. Assess the corneal reflex.
10. Conduct funduscopic examination: retinal structures, macula.

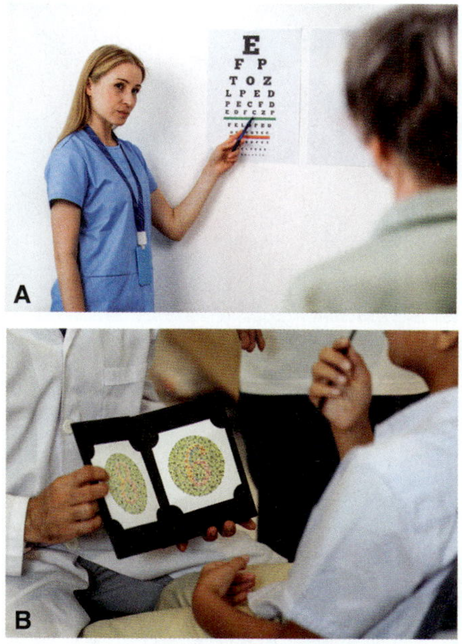

Figure 27-8 Vision assessment. **A.** Assessing distance vision with the Snellen chart. **B.** Assessing color vision.

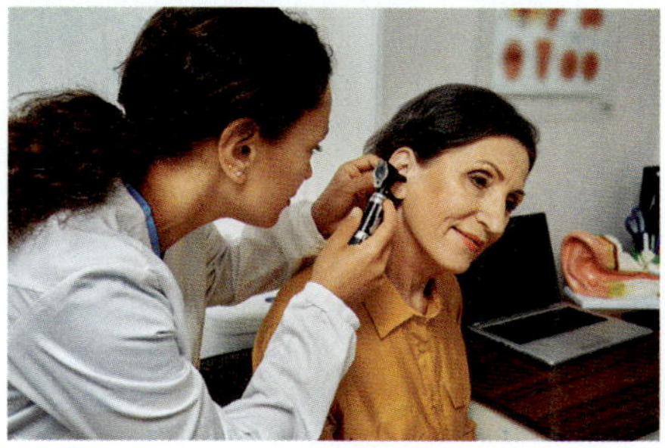

Figure 27-9 The otoscopic examination.

Ears

1. Test gross hearing: voice-whisper test or watch-tick test (CN VIII).
2. Assess ear alignment.
3. Inspect and palpate the external ear.
4. Conduct otoscopic examination: external auditory canal and tympanic membrane (Fig. 27-9).
5. Perform Weber and Rinne tests.

Nose and Sinuses

1. Inspect the external surface of the nose.
2. Assess nostril patency bilaterally.
3. Test olfactory sense (CN I).
4. Conduct internal examination with nasal speculum: mucosa, turbinates, and septum.
5. Inspect, percuss, and palpate frontal and maxillary sinuses.

Mouth and Throat

1. Note breath odor.
2. Inspect the lips, buccal mucosa, gums, and hard and soft palates.
3. Inspect the teeth; count the teeth.
4. Inspect the tongue; ask the client to stick out the tongue (CN XII).
5. Inspect the uvula; note movement when the client says "ah" (CNs IX, X).
6. Inspect the tonsils; note grade.
7. Inspect the oropharynx.
8. Test gag reflex (CNs IX, X).
9. Test taste (CN VII).
10. Palpate the lips and mouth if indicated.

Neck

1. Inspect the musculature of the neck.
2. Inspect range of motion, shoulder shrug, and strength of sternocleidomastoid and trapezius muscles (CN XI).
3. Palpate the musculature of the neck.
4. Inspect and palpate the trachea.
5. Palpate the carotid arteries (one at a time).
6. Inspect the jugular veins for distention; estimate jugular venous pressure if indicated.
7. Inspect and palpate the thyroid (use only one approach, either anterior or posterior).
8. Auscultate the thyroid and carotid arteries.
9. Inspect and palpate the lymph nodes: preauricular, postauricular, occipital, submental, submandibular, tonsillar, anterior cervical chain, posterior cervical chain, supraclavicular, and infraclavicular.

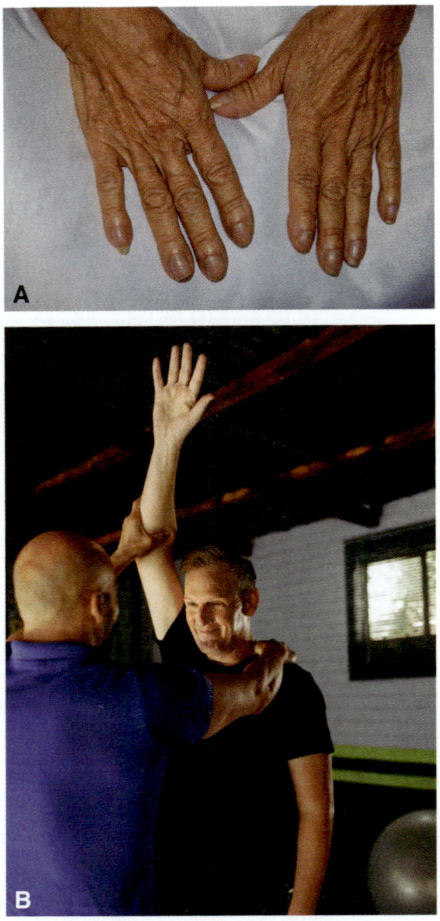

Figure 27-10 Upper extremity assessment. **A.** Inspecting the hands. Note the nail clubbing. **B.** Assessing range of motion of the shoulders.

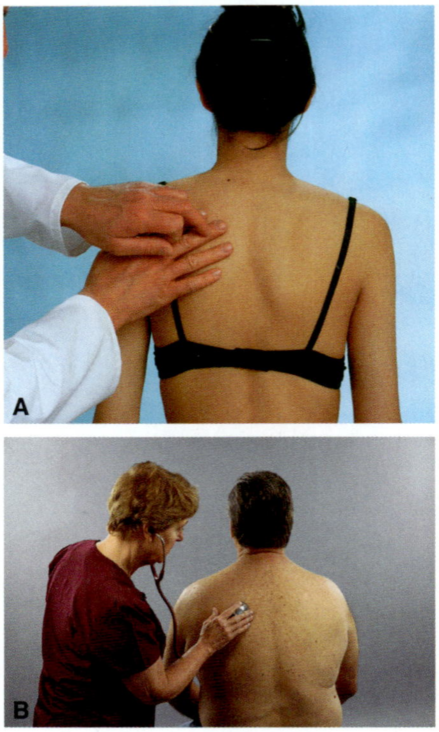

Figure 27-11 Posterior thorax assessment. **A.** Percussion. **B.** Auscultation.

Upper Extremities

1. Inspect nailbed color, shape, and configuration (Fig. 27-10A); palpate nailbed texture.
2. Assess capillary refill on nailbed.
3. Inspect muscle size and palpate muscle tone of hands, arms, and shoulders.
4. Palpate the joints of fingers, wrists, elbows, and shoulders.
5. Assess range of motion and strength of fingers, wrists, elbows, and shoulders (Fig. 27-10B).
6. Test position sense of the fingers.
7. Palpate radial and brachial pulses.
8. Palpate the epitrochlear node.
9. Move behind the client. Untie the gown so that the entire back is exposed. The gown should cover the shoulders and the anterior chest.

Back, Posterior and Lateral Thoraxes

1. Palpate the thyroid (posterior approach).
2. Inspect and palpate the spinous processes; inspect range of motion of the cervical spine.
3. Note thoracic configuration, symmetry of shoulders, and position of scapula.
4. Palpate the posterior thorax and lateral thorax.
5. Perform posterior thoracic expansion.
6. Perform tactile fremitus on the posterior thorax and lateral thorax.
7. Percuss the posterior thorax (Fig. 27-11A) and lateral thorax.
8. Perform diaphragmatic excursion.
9. Palpate the costovertebral angle; percuss the costovertebral angle with your fist.
10. Auscultate the posterior thorax (Fig. 27-11B) and lateral thorax; perform voice sounds if indicated.

Move in front of the client. Drape the client's gown at waist level (females may cover their breasts).

Anterior Thorax

1. Inspect shape of the thorax, symmetry of the chest wall, presence of superficial veins, costal angle, angle of ribs, intercostal spaces, muscles of respiration, respirations, and sputum (Fig. 27-12).
2. Palpate the anterior thorax.
3. Perform anterior thoracic expansion.
4. Perform tactile fremitus.
5. Percuss the anterior thorax.
6. Auscultate the anterior thorax; perform voice sounds if indicated.

Heart

1. Auscultate the cardiac landmarks: aortic, pulmonic, mitral, and tricuspid areas and Erb point (Fig. 27-13).

Female Breasts

Ask the female client to uncover their breasts.

1. Inspect the breasts for color, vascularity, thickening and edema, size, symmetry, contour, lesions and masses, and discharge with

the client in these positions: arms at side (Fig. 27-14), arms raised over the head, hands pressed into hips, hands in front, and client leaning forward.

2. Palpate the breasts with the client's arms first at the sides and then raised over the head.
3. Palpate the brachial, central axillary, pectoral, and subscapular lymph nodes.
4. Teach breast self-examination.

Male Breasts

1. Repeat the sequence used for female breasts. Having the client lean forward is usually unnecessary unless gynecomastia is present.

Assist the client into a supine position with the chest uncovered. Drape the abdomen and legs. Stand on the right side of the client.

Jugular Veins

As the client changes from a sitting to a supine position for the remainder of the breast examination, observe the jugular veins when the client is at a 45° angle. Examine again when the client is supine.

1. Inspect the jugular veins for distention; estimate jugular venous pressure if indicated.

Female and Male Breasts

1. Palpate each breast. The arm on the same side as the examined breast should be raised over the head.
2. Compress the nipple to express any discharge.

Heart

1. Inspect the cardiac landmarks for pulsations.
2. Palpate the cardiac landmarks for pulsations, thrills, and heaves.
3. Palpate the apical impulse.
4. With the diaphragm of the stethoscope, auscultate the cardiac landmarks; count the apical pulse.
5. With the bell of the stethoscope, auscultate the cardiac landmarks.
6. Turn the client on the left side and repeat auscultation of the cardiac landmarks.
7. Return the client to a supine position. Cover the client's anterior thorax with the gown. Uncover the abdomen from the symphysis pubis to the costal margin.

Abdomen

1. Inspect contour, symmetry, pigmentation, and color (Fig. 27-15A).
2. Note scars, striae, visible peristalsis, masses, and pulsations.
3. Inspect the rectus abdominis muscles (supine and with head raised) and respiratory movement of the abdomen.
4. Inspect the umbilicus.
5. Auscultate bowel sounds.
6. Auscultate for bruits, venous hum, and friction rub.
7. Percuss all four quadrants.
8. Percuss liver span and liver descent; percuss liver with fist if indicated.
9. Percuss the spleen, stomach, and bladder.
10. Lightly palpate all four quadrants.
11. Note any muscle guarding.

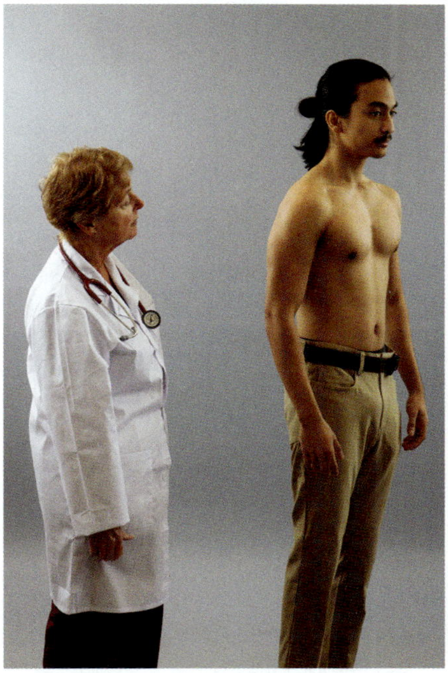

Figure 27-12 Inspect the thorax for shape and symmetry.

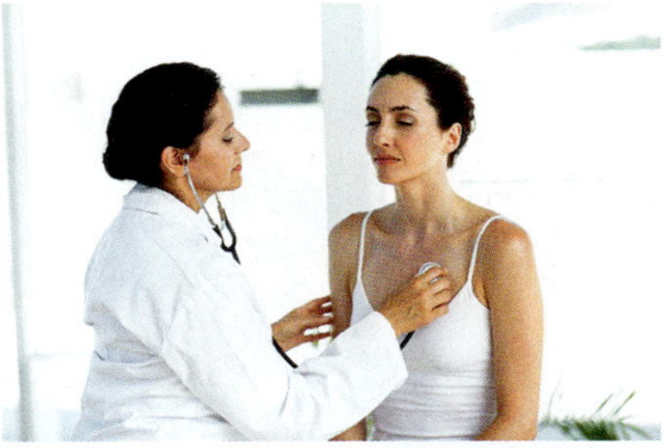

Figure 27-13 Auscultate the heart.

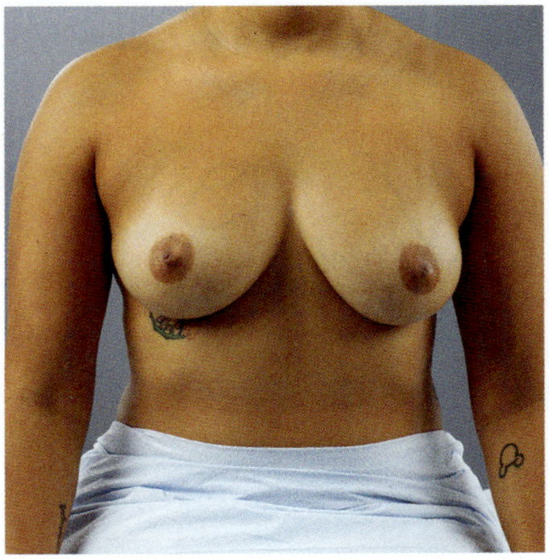

Figure 27-14 Inspect the breasts with the client in a sitting position.

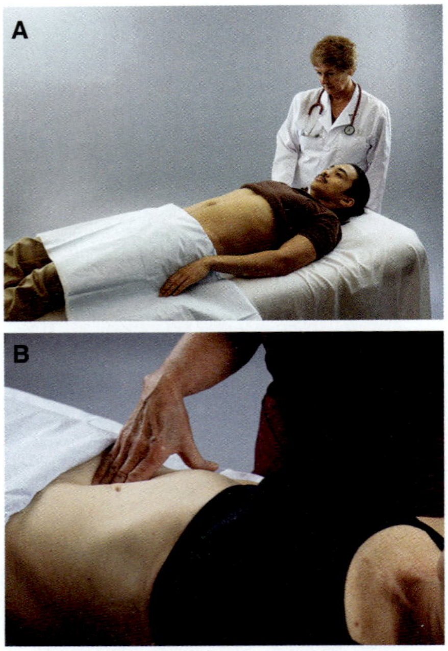

Figure 27-15 Abdominal assessment. **A.** Inspection. **B.** Palpation.

12. Deeply palpate all four quadrants (Fig. 27-15B).
13. Palpate the liver, spleen, kidney, aorta, and bladder.
14. Assess superficial abdominal reflexes.
15. Perform hepatojugular reflux if indicated.

Inguinal Area

1. Inspect and palpate the inguinal lymph nodes.
2. Inspect for inguinal hernias.
3. Palpate the femoral pulses.
4. Auscultate the femoral pulses for bruits.

Cover the exposed abdomen with the gown. Lift the drape from the bottom to expose the lower extremities.

Lower Extremities

1. Inspect for color, capillary refill, edema, ulcerations, hair distribution, and varicose veins.
2. Palpate for temperature, edema, and texture.
3. Palpate the popliteal, dorsalis pedis, and posterior tibial pulses.
4. Inspect muscle size and palpate muscle tone of the legs and feet.
5. Palpate the joints of the hips, knees, ankles, and feet.
6. Assess range of motion and strength of the hips, knees, ankles (Fig. 27-16), and feet.
7. Test position sense of the toes.
8. Assess for clonus.

Drape the lower extremities. Assist the client to a sitting position and note the ease with which the client sits up. Have the client dangle the legs over the edge of the examination table.

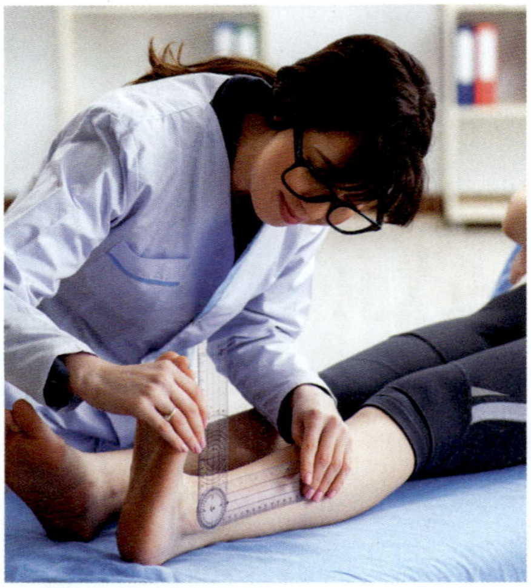

Figure 27-16 Assessing range of motion of the ankle.

Neurological System

1. Assess light touch: face (CN V), hands, lower arms, abdomen, feet, and legs.
2. Assess superficial pain (sharp and dull): face (CN V), hands, lower arms, abdomen, feet, and legs.
3. Assess two-point discrimination: tongue, lips, fingers, dorsum of hand, torso, and feet.
4. Assess vibration sense: fingers and toes.
5. Assess stereognosis, graphesthesia, and extinction.
6. Assess cerebellar function: finger to nose, rapid alternating hand movements, touching thumb to each finger, running heel down shin, and foot tapping.
7. Assess deep tendon reflexes: biceps, triceps, brachioradialis, patellar, and Achilles.
8. Assess plantar reflex.

Ask the client to stand barefoot on the floor. If the client is unsteady, use caution when performing the next few tests. Remain physically close to the client at all times.

NURSING TIP

Assessing the Comatose Client

For the comatose client, the family and prior health-care records can provide valuable information for the health history. Do not let the client's condition deter you from conducting a thorough physical examination. Omit components of the examination that require volition and client cooperation; complete the remainder of the examination as indicated.

Remember to assess neurological status thoroughly. Consider assessing doll's eyes phenomenon, corneal reflex, Babinski reflex, and pain responses.

Musculoskeletal System

1. Assess mobility: casual walk, heel walk, toe walk, tandem walk, backward walk, stepping to the right and left, and deep knee bends (one knee at a time). Note any indications of discomfort. Stand behind the client.
2. Assess range of motion of the spine.
   Open the client's gown to expose the back. Ask the client to bend forward at the waist.
3. Inspect the spine for scoliosis.
   Close the client's gown. Stand in front of the client.

Neurological System

1. Perform the Romberg test; assess pronator drift.
2. Assess the ability to hop on one foot, run heel down shin, and draw a figure 8 with foot.

Female Genitalia, Anus, and Rectum

Assist the client back to the examination table. Ask the client to assume the lithotomy position. Drape the client (Fig. 27-17). Sit on a stool in front of the client's legs.

1. Inspect pubic hair and skin color and condition: mons pubis, vulva, clitoris, urethral meatus, vaginal introitus, sacrococcygeal area, perineum, and anal mucosa.
2. Palpate the labia, urethral meatus, Skene glands, vaginal introitus, and perineum.
3. Insert the vaginal speculum.
4. Inspect the cervix: color, position, size, surface characteristics, discharge, and shape of cervical os; inspect the vagina.
5. Collect specimens for cytological smears and cultures.
   Stand in front of the client's legs.
6. Perform bimanual examination of the vagina, cervix, fornices, uterus, and adnexa.
7. Perform rectovaginal examination.
8. Palpate the anus and rectum.
9. If stool is on the glove, test for occult blood.

Assist the client to a sitting position. Offer tissues to wipe the perineal area. Ask the client to redress. Questions can be answered when the client is dressed.

Male Genitalia

Ask the male client to stand. Sit on a stool in front of the client. Have the client lift the gown to expose the genitalia.

1. Inspect hair distribution, penis, scrotum, and urethral meatus.
2. Palpate the penis, urethral meatus, and scrotum.
3. Palpate the inguinal area for hernias.
4. Auscultate the scrotum if indicated.
5. Teach testicular self-examination.

Ask the client to bend over the examination table (Fig. 27-18). If the client is bedridden, the knee-chest or left lateral position may be used. Expose the buttocks. Stand behind the client.

Male Anus, Rectum, and Prostate

1. Inspect the perineum, sacrococcygeal area, and anal mucosa.
2. Palpate the anus and rectum.
3. Palpate the prostate.
4. If stool is on the glove, test for occult blood.

NURSING TIP
Communicating Bad News

Be sensitive when communicating bad or unexpected news to the client, significant other(s), or caregiver. Talk to the client in a quiet, private room. Be specific and straightforward. Speak in terms that will be understood. Give the client time to process the information, alone if desired. Convey the same high level of respect that you have shown throughout the interview and examination process. Finally, allow time for questions.

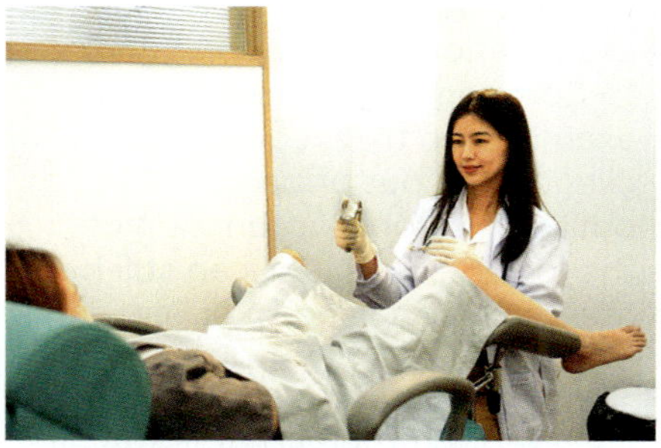

Figure 27-17 Assist the female client into the lithotomy position and drape the abdomen and legs for the genital examination.

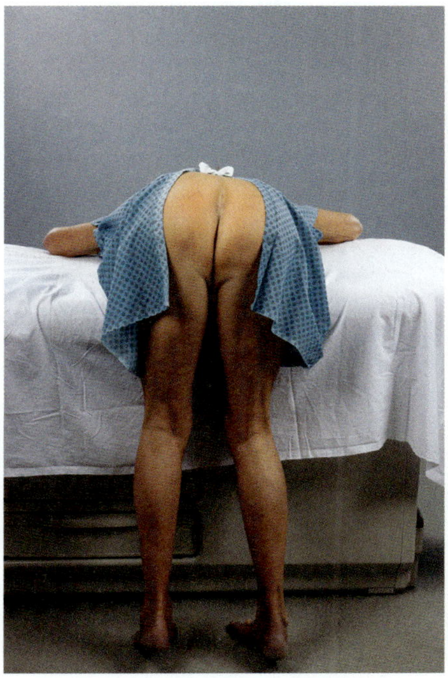

Figure 27-18 Ask the male client to bend over the examination table for the rectal examination.

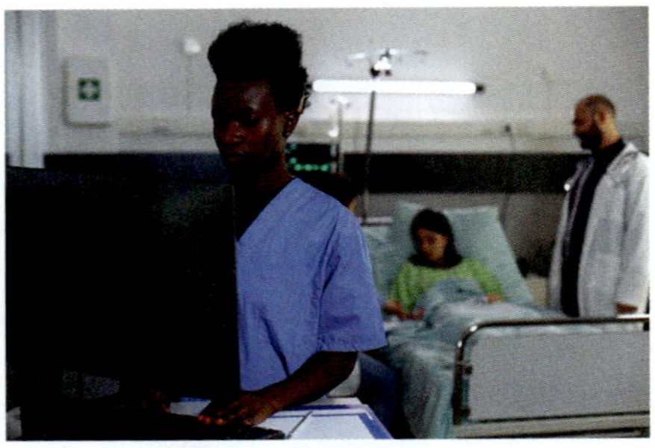

Figure 27-19 Be certain to carefully document all examination findings and client responses.

> **NURSING TIP**
> **Examining the Bedridden Client**
>
> The bedridden client may be capable of cooperating for the health history and physical examination.
>
> Components of the physical examination that require the client to be out of bed can be omitted. Cerebellar function of the lower extremities can still be assessed by having the client run the heel of each foot down each shin and draw a figure 8 with each foot on the bed or in the air.
>
> Frequently, examining the bedridden client requires the assistance of a second person to help hold the client in a side-lying position while the examination is conducted. If the client can tolerate a sitting position, the second person can help hold the client in this position while an assessment of the head, face, neck, and anterior thorax is conducted. Always use extra caution to protect the client against falls.

Cover the buttocks. Ask the client to stand up and redress. Offer tissues to wipe the rectal area. Questions can be answered when the client is dressed.

The client has the opportunity to think about questions about the examination while getting dressed. It is often difficult for clients to discuss future plans when wearing an examination gown. For this reason, give the client a few minutes to redress in private before you proceed. Always thank the client and explain what can be expected next.

When completing the examination, ensure that you return the client to the requested or required position. For example, for the bedridden client, ensure that the side rails are up (if appropriate) and that the call bell is readily accessible. Ask the client if there is anything else that can be done for comfort.

Now that you have all of this information, what do you do with it and how do you make sense of it? (Fig. 27-19). Refer back to Chapter 1, which discussed how to make the leap from gathering health assessment information and examination findings to using critical thinking to prioritize and plan evidence-based nursing care.

Laboratory and Diagnostic Data

The laboratory and diagnostic data that are obtained from the client vary according to presenting symptoms and clinical examination. Order only those tests that are necessary. Consider the risks, time, discomfort, cost, limitations, and contraindications of each test. Actively involve the client in preparing for each test and incorporate clinical teaching when appropriate. Remember that technology can never replace the art of listening to what your client is saying and the skill with which you perform physical examinations.

Problem List

The health history, physical examination, and laboratory and diagnostic data provide the data on which clinical action is based. As described in Chapter 1, similar signs, symptoms, and findings are clustered together in a meaningful way. These clusters are then named. Some nurses may use nursing diagnoses to name the clusters of meaningful information. Other nurses may use a medical model approach and formulate a problem list. The problem list is a provider-generated list of active and inactive health problems. Each problem is numbered and referred to in the client record by number. The onset date of each problem is noted, as is the date of problem resolution. Many electronic health records have a section where the problem list information is contained. The Problem Number may or may not be used. An example of a problem list is shown in the following table:

Onset Date	Problem Number	Active Problem	Inactive Problem
	1		Pneumonia
1984	2		Idiopathic thrombocytopenia purpura
2004	3	Bilateral ovarian cysts	
2009	4	Allergic rhinitis	
2010	5	Reactive airway disease	
2017	6	Left plantar fasciitis	
2020	7	Cystocele	

NURSING TIP

ISMP's List of Error-Prone Abbreviations

There are over 20,000 brand-name and generic prescription medications available in the United States. With such a large number of medications, not counting over-the-counter medications and home remedies, it is not surprising that adverse medication outcomes occur. It is estimated that 7,000 to 9,000 deaths occur annually from medication errors. Care for medication-associated errors costs the United States over $40 billion dollars each year (Tariq, Vashisht, Sinha, & Scherbak, 2021). Thus, medication errors pose a significant risk to the client and a burden to the economy. The Institute for Safe Medication Practices (ISMP) is a nonprofit organization whose mission is to prevent medication errors. Work by ISMP "has resulted in numerous necessary changes in clinical practice, public policy, and drug labeling and packaging." The ISMP has identified error-prone abbreviations and symbols that should be avoided and **never** used to prevent medication errors. By avoiding the use of the error-prone abbreviations, the risk of medication and clinical error decreases. The ISMP provides a list of error-prone abbreviations in the following categories:

- Abbreviations for dose/measurement units
- Abbreviations for route of administration
- Abbreviations frequency/instructions for use
- Miscellaneous abbreviations associated with medication use
- Drug name abbreviations
- Stemmed/coined drug names
- Dose designations and other information
- Symbols
- Apothecary or household abbreviations

Every health-care professional needs to be familiar with these abbreviations and symbols and they must be avoided in all verbal, electronic, and handwritten documentation/communication. Retrieved December 13, 2025, from *https://www.ismp.org/system/files/resources/2024-04/ISMP_ErrorProneAbbreviations_List.pdf*

From this problem list, a care plan is developed to address each active problem. The implementation and evaluation of the care plan then ensue. A SOAP note is one method that can be used to document this process.

Long COVID and Worldwide Pandemic

COVID-19 has caused a worldwide public health crisis since it was first identified in Wuhan, China, in late 2019. The COVID-19 pandemic has led to more than 778 million confirmed cases worldwide and over 7.1 million fatalities (WHO, 2025a,b). COVID-19 has impacted every body system as well as developmental, cultural, spiritual, and nutritional aspects of peoples' lives. Many individuals had and continue to have symptoms that linger after the acute phase of COVID-19. This cluster of symptoms has been called long COVID or post COVID-19 condition. The World Health Organization (WHO, 2025c) defines long COVID as a clinical condition that is "the continuation or development of new symptoms 3 months after the initial SARS-CoV-2 infection, with these symptoms lasting for at least 2 months with no other explanation." The National Academies of Sciences, Engineering, and Medicine (2024) defines long COVID as "an infection-associated chronic condition that occurs after SARS-CoV-2 infection and is present for at least 3 months as a continuous, relapsing and remitting, or progressive disease state that affects one or more organ systems." There are no diagnostic tests that diagnose or confirm long COVID.

The most common complaints of long COVID are fatigue, cough, shortness of breath, chest pain, and palpitations. Additional symptoms include decreased memory and concentration, "brain fog," depression, anxiety, headache, vomiting, diarrhea, altered sleep, joint pain, myalgias, and altered sense of taste and smell. According to WHO, approximately 6% of people who have the COVID-19 virus develop long COVID, though this number is lower than in the early stages of the pandemic (WHO, 2025c). Females, older adults, smokers, overweight/obese people and those with pre-existing chronic medical conditions have a higher risk of developing long COVID (WHO, 2025b). Long COVID can occur in children as well as adolescents. Individuals who had a mild case of COVID-19 can develop long COVID, as well as those who experienced severe illness. Long COVID can affect a person's functional ability and challenge those who have the condition. Long COVID can be considered a disability under the Americans with Disabilities Act (ADA), Section 504 and Section 1557 if substantial limitations impact one or more major life activities (HHS, 2021). Ultimately, treatment plans must be individualized for each person with long COVID to maintain health and improve quality of life.

On May 5, 2023, the WHO (2023) announced that COVID-19 no longer qualified as a global health emergency. Just a few days later, on May 11, 2023, the Centers for Disease Control and Prevention (CDC) ended the U.S. Federal COVID-19 Public Health Emergency. These organizations recognized that although COVID-19 remains an ongoing global infection of great concern, the death toll has greatly declined, hospitalizations from COVID-19 have decreased, and intensive care unit admissions due to COVID-19 have decreased. The availability of the original COVID-19 vaccines and the newer vaccines have led to a large number of people who have some immunity to COVID-19. Both the WHO and CDC are committed to ongoing research on COVID-19 as new variants emerge. It may be years or possibly decades to fully understand the devastation and effect the COVID-19 virus has brought to the world.

Preparticipation Athletic Evaluation

Nurses frequently evaluate school-age and adolescent children for their ability to participate in athletic activities. The purpose of the preparticipation sports physical examination is to establish the child's physical fitness, identify any health condition(s) that poses real or potential health risks, and determine whether the child can safely engage in the desired sport. If a child is unable to participate in the desired organized sport for health reasons, the nurse can suggest other activities that can safely provide a physical outlet. The evaluation encompasses both a thorough family and personal health history (especially cardiovascular and musculoskeletal) and a physical examination (also emphasizing cardiovascular and musculoskeletal health).

It is important to remember which conditions contraindicate participation in competitive aerobic sports: atlantoaxial instability, carditis, hypertrophic cardiomyopathy, uncontrolled severe hypertension, suspected coronary artery disease, specific electrocardiogram (ECG/EKG) abnormalities (e.g., long QT interval), absence of a paired organ, poorly controlled seizure disorder, Marfan syndrome, and hepatosplenomegaly. Many relative contraindications must be evaluated on a case-by-case basis, taking into consideration the child's history and the intended sport. Conditions such as history of concussions, cardiopulmonary conditions (e.g., asthma, heart valve pathology), dizziness/fainting, and family history of exercise-induced mortality should be evaluated more thoroughly to determine whether the child may safely participate in sports. There is no consensus on the necessity of every potential student athlete getting an EKG to assess for potential abnormalities. If indicated, an EKG and echocardiogram can be performed under the supervision of a pediatric cardiologist.

The American Academy of Pediatrics publishes an athletic evaluation form that can be used to conduct the preparticipation athletic evaluation (see References). Also, many school districts have developed their own forms to be completed by the person conducting the evaluation. Each state mandates the frequency with which the preparticipation athletic evaluation needs to be conducted.

Healthy People 2030

The U.S. government established measurable health goals for the population in the document *Healthy People 1990,* which was an outgrowth of *Healthy People: The Surgeon General's Report on Health Promotion and Disease Prevention* from 1979 (U. S. Department of Health and Human Services, 2021). The main goals of this document were to increase the population's lifespan by improving health, preventing disease, and enabling access to preventative care. Later initiatives included reducing health disparities among people living in the United States. The Healthy People public health program is revised every 10 years. The fifth version of this program launched in August 2020 and is entitled *Healthy People 2030. Healthy People 2030* identifies 355 objectives to improve health and well-being for the next 10 years. Objectives were identified based on their national importance, were evidence-based, and addressed health disparities and equity (Fig. 27-20). The newly revised format boasts easily accessed content with cross referencing information by:

- Health Conditions (e.g., addiction, dementia, osteoporosis)
- Health Behaviors (e.g., drug and alcohol use, injury prevention, sleep)
- Populations (e.g., infants, parents or caregivers, workforce)
- Settings and Systems (e.g., community, housing and homes, schools)
- Social Determinants of Health (e.g., economic stability, education access and quality, health-care access and quality)

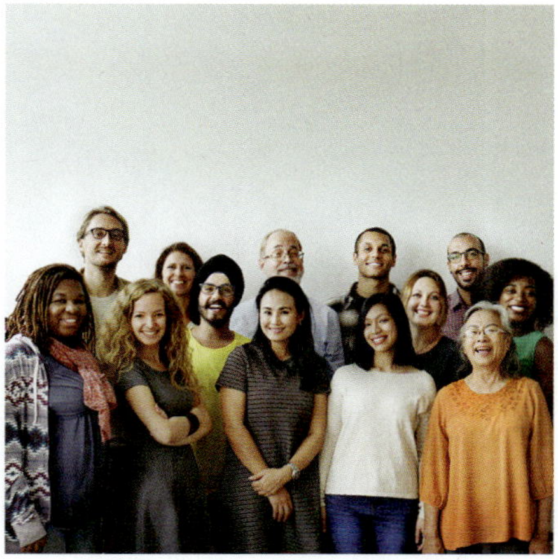

Figure 27-20 *Healthy People 2030* strives to eliminate health disparities for all people.

Leading Health Initiatives identify high-priority objectives from the 355 total objectives as being of vital importance to improving health. For the first time, personal and organizational Health Literacy is a component of *Heathy People* (U. S. Department of Health and Human Services, 2020).

It is vital that nurses be aware of this public health initiatives as it is a major force that contributes to health promotion and disease prevention. Whether a bedside nurse, school nurse, home health nurse, nurse practitioner, nurse anesthetist, or other advanced practice nurse, we all are responsible for improving the health of our clients and our community. *Healthy People 2030* provides a framework from which to start.

The Future of Nursing

After conducting a 2-year study, the Institute of Medicine (IOM) (2010), with funding from the Robert Wood Johnson Foundation (RWJF), published key messages on the future of the nursing profession:

- Nurses should practice to the full extent of their education and training.
- Nurses should achieve higher levels of education and training through an improved education system that promotes seamless academic progression.
- Nurses should be full partners, with physicians and other health-care professionals, in redesigning health care in the United States.
- Effective workplace planning and policy making require better data collection and information infrastructure.

The IOM report advocated for the removal of barriers so that nurses could practice to the fullest extent of their education, training, and the law. The IOM concluded that "nurses are well-positioned to lead change and advance health." The study validated what nurses have known for some time: that they are experts in advancing client health (Fig. 27-21). Possessing refined assessment and examination skills is the foundation of providing high-quality client care.

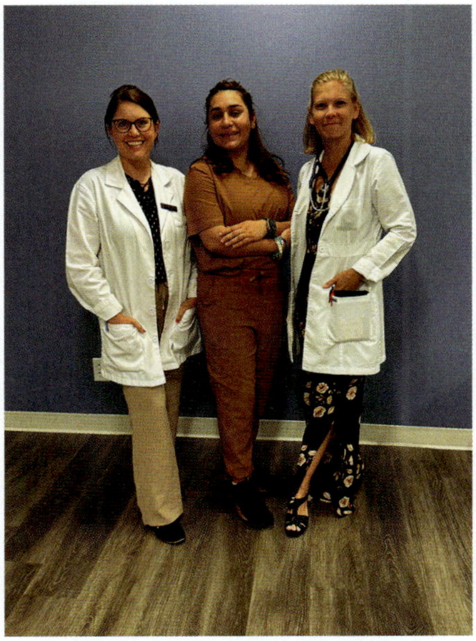

Figure 27-21 Nurses are experts in advancing client health and are well positioned to promote positive change in the health-care arena.

In May 2021 the National Academy of Medicine, with funding from the RWJF, launched a consensus study entitled, *The Future of Nursing 2020–2030, Charting a Path to Achieve Health Equity.* In addition to continuing to advocate for nurses to practice to the fullest extent of their education and training, the expert committee plans to address:

- "The role of nurses in improving the health of individuals, families, and communities by addressing social determinants of health and providing effective, efficient, equitable, and accessible care for all across the care continuum, as well as identifying the system facilitators and barriers to achieving this goal.
- The current and future deployment of all levels of nurses across the care continuum, including in collaborative practice models, to address the challenges of building a culture of health.
- System facilitators and barriers to achieving a workforce that is diverse, including gender, race, and ethnicity, across all levels of nursing education.
- The role of the nursing profession in assuring that the voice of individuals, families and communities are incorporated into design and operations of clinical and community health systems.
- The training and competency-development needed to prepare nurses, including advanced practice nurses, to work outside of acute care settings and to lead efforts to build a culture of health and health equity, and the extent to which current curriculum meets these needs.
- The ability of nurses to serve as change agents in creating systems that bridge the delivery of health care and social needs care in the community.
- The research needed to identify or develop effective nursing practices for eliminating gaps and disparities in health care.
- The importance of nurse well-being and resilience in ensuring the delivery of high quality care and improving community health.
- The role of nurses in response to emergencies that arise due to natural and man-made disasters and the impact on health equity." (National Academy of Medicine, 2021)

Only time will tell what the nursing profession and the U.S. health-care system will look like in 2030. Nurses need to become active in the nursing profession at the local, state, and national levels. We need to continue to be change agents to facilitate a health-care system where respect and dignity are afforded to all clients as we deliver high-quality, evidenced-based, cost-effective care.

Conclusion

Today's nurse is a sophisticated professional prepared to meet the demands of the health-care system. Hospitalized clients have a greater acuity and are being discharged at a faster rate to the home environment. The home health nurse is therefore seeing a greater variety of clients who are sicker. Nurses in advanced practice settings are providing care to clients who are positioned at different points on the health-illness continuum. Because the entire plan of care is based on client assessment, all nurses must possess expert examination skills. This text has supplied the information to assist both the novice and the experienced nurse in acquiring, refining, and perfecting health history and physical examination skills. The pathophysiological basis for the physical examination findings empowers the nurse to fully understand the client's clinical state and make appropriate clinical decisions. Ultimately, the clients are the benefactors of your knowledge, wisdom, and experience.

CASE STUDY
The Client With Multisystem Problems

Every nurse is a unique individual, and this is reflected in health-care documentation. There is no "right" or "wrong" way to document client data as long as one documents accurately and in legally advisable terms.

This case study illustrates the application and objective documentation of a head-to-toe physical examination. Carmen is anxious because she is scheduled to leave tomorrow for a weeklong trip to Iceland. It has been a lifelong dream to see the Aurora Borealis. This trip has been planned for over 1 year, and she does not want to miss it. Carmen has experienced increasingly painful urination the past 2 days. She presents to an urgent care clinic for an evaluation and treatment.

HEALTH HISTORY

TODAY'S DATE

March 15, 2026

BIOGRAPHICAL DATA

Client Name Carmen Monzon
Home Address 5022 Sydney Court, Unit 975
San Diego, CA 92122
Home Phone Number (858) 654-0000
Cell Phone Number (858) 654-1000
Date of Birth February 28, 1971
Birthplace San Diego, CA
Social Security Number xxx-xx-1234
Occupation Travel agent
Work Address 4400 Eastgate Mall
San Diego, CA 92121
Work Phone Number (877) 414- 4678
Insurance Information United Health Care
Usual Source of Health Care San Diego Internal Medicine
Source of Referral Self
Emergency Contact Bonita Pereira (friend)
Preferred Language English or Spanish
Source and Reliability of Information Client, good historian
Advance Medical Directive No; not aware of what this is

CLIENT PROFILE

Age 55
Sex Female
Gender Identity Woman
Preferred Name Cami
Sexual Orientation Asexual
Race Hispanic
Marital Status Single

CHIEF COMPLAINT

"It hurts when I pee."

HISTORY OF PRESENT ILLNESS

Client was in her usual state of good health until 2 days ago. At that time painful urination started and the urine appeared cloudy with an odor. There was no hematuria. Client increased water intake but that did not help the symptoms. Client reports urinating every hour and it feels like the bladder is never completely empty. There is some lower abdominal discomfort (4/10 intensity). The past two nights reports getting up to urinate every 4 hours. Self-administered OTC phenazopyridine hydrochloride 95 mg twice daily yesterday with little relief (2/10). Client denies low back pain, flank pain, urinary incontinence, vaginal discharge, change in bowel habits, and fever. No sexual activity in over 10 years. Client has never had a UTI and has no history of kidney stones.

PAST HEALTH HISTORY

Medical History

- Allergic rhinitis since age 13; allergy tested showed reaction to mold, pollen, grasses; controls with OTC medications
- Reactive airway disease since age 13; stable with medication use

Surgical History

- Appendectomy age 20 without sequelae; no adverse reaction to general anesthesia
- Wisdom teeth extraction age 18 under local anesthesia without sequelae

Allergies

Sulfa: rash

Denies allergies to: foods, latex, insect bites/bee stings

Medications

Fluticasone propionate/salmeterol 100 mcg/50 mcg—one inhalation daily, rinses after

Albuterol 90 mcg/inhalation HFA—1 to 2 inhalations every 4 to 6 hours as needed, last used 2 months ago

Loratadine 10 mg daily

Triamcinolone acetonide 55 mcg per nasal spray—2 sprays each nostril daily

Multivitamin daily

Vitamin D 2,000 IU daily

Communicable Diseases Denies recent STI; acknowledges history of past STIs (client declines providing more information); denies hepatitis, HIV

Injuries and Accidents Cut self with kitchen knife 3 years ago on left index finger, urgent care clinic cleaned wound, applied steri-strips, no sutures or antibiotics were required

Differing Abilities Denies

Blood Transfusions Denies

Childhood Illnesses Recalls chickenpox as a child and frequent ear infections

Immunizations Client reports being up to date, gets annual flu vaccine, last tetanus 3 years ago when she cut herself with a knife; no immunizations for travel the past 10 years

FAMILY HEALTH HISTORY

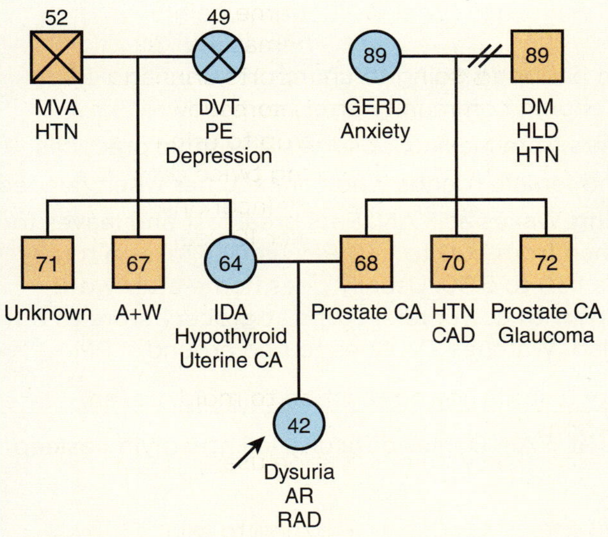

Denies family history of stroke, migraines, gout, emphysema, obesity, drug addiction, violence, suicide attempts/completions

Legend

- Living female
- Living male
- Deceased female
- Deceased male
- Points to client
- Couple in a relationship*
- Divorced/No relationship

*The line connecting clients can denote a union, whether that be a marriage or other type of relationship

A+W	Alive and well
AR	Allergic rhinitis
CA	Cancer
CAD	Coronary artery disease
DM	Diabetes mellitus
DVT	Deep vein thrombosis
GERD	Gastroesophageal reflux disease
HLD	Hyperlipidemia
HTN	Hypertension
IDA	Iron deficiency anemia
MVA	Motor vehicle accident
PE	Pulmonary embolus
RAD	Reactive airway disease

SOCIAL HISTORY

Alcohol Use One beer after work each night and 2 beers over the weekend (Friday, Saturday, Sunday)

Tobacco Use Denies use of tobacco in all forms

Recreational Drug Use Used marijuana every weekend junior and senior years of high school, not since. Denies use of injectable illicit substance; denies snorting any substance and use of any illicit substance

Domestic and Intimate Partner Violence Denies

Sexual Practice No sexual activity in over 10 years. Client provided no further elaboration.

Travel History Has been to all 7 continents. Never developed any illness with travel

Work Environment Works as a travel agent in an office in the city. Office was built 5 years ago. The work environment does not bother client's reactive airway disease or allergies.

Home Environment Lives in apartment building that is 10 years old. Contains all modern appliances including air conditioning. Has smoke detectors and carbon monoxide detectors. Changes the batteries every year on her birthday

Hobbies and Leisure Activities Enjoys going to the beach on the weekends with friends. Every Thursday is Happy Hour with coworkers after work. Watches TV most nights

Stress "I've been planning this trip to Iceland for a long time with my travel agent friends. I can't miss it!"

Education High school graduate

Economic Status Can pay the bills

Military Service Denies

Religion Nondenominational Christian. Stopped going to church 15 years ago. Is thinking about getting involved in a church community after her trip

Ethnic Background Great-grandparents from Mexico, observes no ethnic practices

Roles and Relationships Has male and female friends who can help her when needed

Characteristic Patterns of Daily Living Wakes at 7 AM. Eats breakfast and leaves for work by 8:30 AM. Works 9-1. Eats lunch from 1:00 to 1:30 PM, usually takes a turkey sandwich or salad from home. Works 1:30 to 5:30. Usually goes home after work except on Thursday Happy Hour night with coworkers. Stops at grocery store to buy a rotisserie chicken and premade salad. Watches TV. Goes to bed around 11 PM

HEALTH MAINTENANCE ACTIVITIES

Sleep Goes to bed at 11 PM and wakes at 7 AM Denies difficulty falling/staying asleep until 2 days ago.

Diet Regular

Exercise No regular exercise, will walk on the beach on weekends

Stress Management Watching TV

Use of Safety Devices Wears seat belt

Health Checkups

- Usually sees internist when a refill is needed for prescription medications—usually once a year, is overdue for check up
- Dentist annually
- Gynecological examination—believes about 5 years ago
- Mammogram more than 3 yrs ago
- Eye examination—over 10 years ago

REVIEW OF SYSTEMS

General Denies: fatigue, fever, chills, night sweats

Skin Lives near the beach. Uses sunscreen only if in the sun for more than 4 hr. Has history of severe sunburns since her teens. Denies change in size, shape or color of moles, moles not itchy, none have bled spontaneously. Denies: skin cancer, warts, psoriasis, eczema, rashes, odors, sweating, acne

Hair Denies: alopecia, scalp lesions, dandruff, hirsutism

Nails Denies: change in texture, splitting, breaking, onychomycosis

Eyes Has never worn glasses or contacts. Can get itchy eyes with grass exposure. Denies: diplopia, eye pain, halos around objects, photophobia, glaucoma, cataracts

Ears Gets itchy ears with grass exposure. Denies: discharge, vertigo, otalgia, tinnitus, phonophobia, hearing aid, hearing problems

Nose and Sinuses Gets clear rhinorrhea with grass exposure and occasional sneezing. Denies: epistaxis, change in sense of smell, sinusitis

Mouth Brushes teeth three times a day and flosses after meals. Uses no dental appliance. Denies: halitosis, toothache, tooth abscess, bleeding/swollen gums, difficulty chewing, change in taste

Throat and Neck Denies: hoarseness, dysphagia, goiter, change in voice

Breasts and Axilla Last mammogram was at least 5 years ago, it was normal. Does not perform breast self-examination.

Denies: pain, tenderness, discharge, lumps, dimpling

Respiratory Can increase fluticasone propionate/salmeterol 100 mcg/50 mcg to one inhalation twice daily if shortness of breath occurs (usually occurs with URI once a year). Has not needed to do this since last year. Does not do peak flow measurements at home.

Denies: pneumonia, frequent bronchitis, pulmonary emboli, hemoptysis, tuberculosis

Cardiac Denies: arrhythmia, heart murmur, congestive heart failure, myocardial infarction, valvular disease, chest pain, orthopnea, palpitations

Peripheral Vasculature Denies: feet/ankle edema, cyanosis, syncope, cold or discolored hands/feet, leg cramps, deep vein thrombosis, thrombophlebitis, varicose veins, intermittent claudication

Gastrointestinal

Stools are brown and soft every 2 to 3 days. Had explosive diarrhea a week ago that resolved after 24 hrs

Never had a colonoscopy

Denies: change in appetite, hemorrhoids, hematochezia, nausea, vomiting, diarrhea, constipation, reflux, abdominal pain, hepatitis, inflammatory bowel disease, diverticulitis, cholecystitis

Urinary Client takes nightly bubble baths

Musculoskeletal Denies: arthralgia, myalgia, decreased range of motion of limbs, low back pain, sprains, fractures, gout

Neurological Denies: headaches, change in balance or coordination, loss of movement, paresthesia, change in speech, syncope, tremors, seizures, head injury, tremor, tic

Psychological Denies: mood changes/swings, anxiety, depression, sadness, difficulty concentrating, eating disorders

Female Reproductive All past Pap smears have been negative. Last menstrual period was 7 days ago. Denies: vaginal pain, vaginal discharge and odor. Has never been pregnant

Nutrition Weighs 182 lbs (82.7 kg) today, usual weight 190 lbs (86.4 kg); tried to lose weight before the Iceland trip, is happy with current weight. Started to gain weight at age 30. Likes and eats most foods

Endocrine Denies: fatigue, heat/cold intolerance, polydipsia, polyphagia, increased sweating; swelling in anterior neck, diabetes

Lymph Nodes Denies: enlargement, tenderness

Hematological Blood type unknown

Denies: easy bruising/bleeding

PHYSICAL EXAMINATION

General Survey and Vital Signs Well-developed, well-nourished Hispanic woman in no acute distress who appears her stated age

No obvious deformity

Height: 5′7″ (170 cm)

Weight: 182 lbs (82.7 kg)

Temperature: 98.6°F (37°C)

Pulse: 96

Respiratory Rate: 18

Blood Pressure:

136/70 mm Hg (left arm sitting)

134/72 mm Hg (left arm supine)

132/74 mm Hg (right arm sitting)

Skin, Hair, and Nails Dark, tanned skin throughout; left posterior leg with 7 mm elevated brownish-tan lesion with irregular borders; no rash, ecchymoses, bleeding; warm to touch without diaphoresis; smooth texture hair shiny black without infestations, evenly distributed; nailbeds pink, firm, without clubbing; 3 second capillary refill

Head Normocephalic without lesions, masses, depressions, or tenderness; face symmetrical without involuntary movement or swelling; scalp shiny and intact without lesions or masses; temporomandibular joint articulates smoothly without clicking or crepitus

Eyes Acuity by Snellen chart: right eye: 20/20, left eye 20/20; has no difficulty reading magazine at 14 inches; color vision intact, visual fields by confrontation intact, eyebrows full and symmetrical, eyelashes evenly distributed and without inflammation, no ptosis or lid lag; lacrimal apparatus without inflammation or discharge, corneal light reflex symmetrical without strabismus, cover-uncover test without deviation, extraocular muscle movements intact, no nystagmus, conjunctiva pink, no foreign bodies, no tearing, sclera white without exudate, pupils equally round, reactive to light and accommodation at 3 mm

Funduscopic: positive red reflex, discs flat with sharp margins, background uniformly pink without hemorrhages or exudate; arterial-to-venous width ratio of 2:3

Ears Gross hearing intact by watch-tick test; pinna without masses, lesions, nodules, inflammation, or tenderness; external auditory canal clear without inflammation; tympanic membranes dull, landmarks visible, with small amount fluid, air bubbles lower left quadrants; no bulging or perforation

Weber—midline; Rinne—air conduction greater than bone conduction

Nose and Sinuses No: deformities, bleeding, lesions, masses, swelling; nares patent, nontender; septum midline without perforation; mucosa pale with clear discharge, turbinates enlarged 50%; sinuses nontender, resonant

Mouth and Throat Lips pink without swelling or lesions; gums and mucosa pink and moist; teeth in good repair; tongue midline, well papillated, and without fasciculations, lesions, swelling, or bleeding; hard and soft palates intact without lesions or masses; pharynx mildly erythematous; uvula midline and rises with phonation; no tonsillar enlargement or erythema; positive gag reflex

Neck Supple without masses or spasms, neck symmetrical without masses or tenderness, no lymphadenopathy, trachea midline, thyroid nontender with 1.5 cm solitary nodule in the right lobe, no thyroid bruit, no jugular venous distention at 90°, 45°, and supine

Breasts No: thickening, edema, vascularity, erosion, fissures, lesions, masses, retraction, discharge; areola and nipples dark in pigmentation; nonpalpable lymph nodes

Thorax and Lungs Anteroposterior to transverse chest diameter 1:2, chest wall symmetrical without dilated superficial veins, costal angle less than 90°, angle of the ribs with sternum is 45°, no bulging of intercostal spaces or retractions, no use of accessory muscles, inspirations regular; no sputum; thorax nontender without pulsations, masses, or crepitus; thoracic expansion 4 cm anterior and 4 cm posterior, tactile fremitus is decreased bilaterally; trachea midline; lungs resonant, diaphragmatic excursion 4 cm bilaterally with inspiration at 10th thoracic vertebrae, clear breath sounds; sonorous wheeze in right lower lobe posterior thorax and clears with coughing, muffled voice sounds all lobes; pulse oximetry 99%

Heart Precordium without pulsations/heaves/thrills, apical pulse 96, apical impulse 1 cm at left 5th intercostal space 1 cm to left of midclavicular line, S_1 and S_2 present, without murmur/ gallop/ rub, no S_3 or S_4

	Carotid	Brachial	Radial	Femoral	Popliteal	Dorsalis Pedis	Posterior Tibial
R	2+	2+	2+	2+	2+	2+	2+
L	2+	2+	2+	2+	2+	2+	2+

Scale: 0–4+

Peripheral Vasculature and Lymphatic System No pedal edema; no ulcerations, negative Homan sign, pulses regular and strong, no pulsus paradoxus, no bruits; no epitrochlear/inguinal/popliteal lymphadenopathy

Abdomen Rounded, no: dilated veins, pulsations, hernias, striae, incisions; rectus abdominis muscle intact; positive bowel sounds in 4 quadrants, no: bruits, venous hum, friction rub; tympanic, abdomen soft, mildly tender lower quadrants with light/deep palpation, no masses; kidneys/bladder nonpalpable; liver span 6 cm in right midclavicular line; no hepatosplenomegaly, no muscle guarding, negative costovertebral angle tenderness

Musculoskeletal Gait within normal limits; spine without scoliosis/lordosis; muscles without atrophy, equal in size bilaterally with adequate tone; no involuntary movements, extremities with full range of motion, 5/5 strength upper/lower extremities; joints without erythema/swelling/nodules/warmth

Neurological Mental Status: appropriate affect, mood, and behavior; cooperative; awake, alert, and oriented to person, place, and time; thought processes and memory intact

CNs II–XII intact, CN I deferred

Sensory: light touch, pain, position/vibration senses intact; stereognosis, graphesthesia, and 2-point discrimination intact

Motor: negative pronator drift

Cerebellar: tandem walk steady, draws figure 8 with each foot, finger-to-nose and rapid alternating hand movements intact without tremor

Reflexes:

Deep tendon reflexes

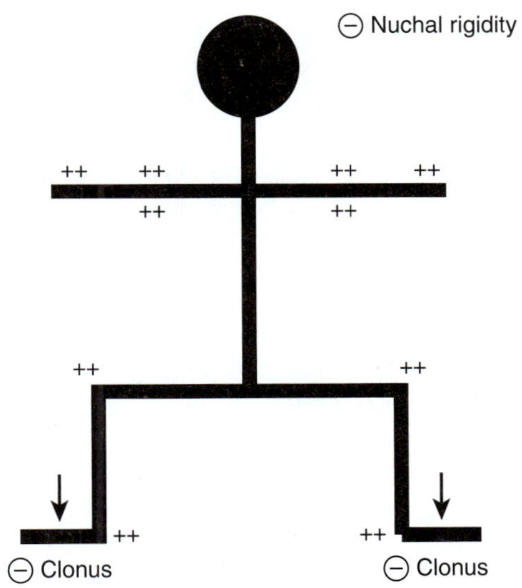

Scale = 4+

Genitalia and Rectum Client declined

Urinalysis Positive white blood cells and nitrites, microscopic hematuria; specimen sent to laboratory for culture & sensitivity

PROBLEM LIST

Onset Date	Problem Number	Active Problem	Inactive Problem
1994	1	Allergic rhinitis	
1994	2	Reactive airway disease	
1999	3		Wisdom teeth extraction
2001	4		Appendectomy
2011	5	Overweight	
2020	6		Injury to left index finger

CLINICAL JUDGMENT IN ACTION

1. What cues indicate that the client is having multiple clinical issues?
2. What interventions have the highest priority?
3. What assessment findings indicate clinical improvement?

Review Questions

Questions 1-2 refer to the following scenario: Sunitha is 55 years old and in good health. She presents today for a preoperative appointment to discuss having a colonoscopy. Sunitha's parents both died from colon cancer in their 60s.

1. The nurse answers the client's questions concerning colonoscopy preparation. At the end of the visit Sunitha states that she has decided not to have the colonoscopy for fear of colon perforation. The nurse recognizes that Sunitha has a right to self-determination in her health-care decisions. Though the nurse disagrees with Sunitha the nurse respects the client's action. Which ethical principle does this illustrate?
   a. Autonomy
   b. Beneficence
   c. Justice
   d. Veracity

2. The nurse communicates the client's decision to the gastroenterologist. Which of the following statements reflects legally advisable actions? Select all that apply.
   a. Respecting Sunitha's right to refuse the colonoscopy.
   b. Informing the gastroenterologist that the client was told that a colon perforation would never happen because the physician is so skilled.
   c. Documenting the discussion the nurse had with Sunitha.
   d. Calling Sunitha at home to insist on a change in the decision.
   e. Announcing over the intercom system that Sunitha refused a colonoscopy and the name needs to be removed from the colonoscopy schedule.

3. Which ethical principle is the duty to perform the greatest good for the greatest number of people?
   a. Nonmaleficence
   b. Fidelity
   c. Professional duty
   d. Utilitarianism

4. What are the goals of *Healthy People*? Select all that apply.
   a. Increase the U.S. population's lifespan
   b. Prevent disease
   c. Enable access to preventative care
   d. Reduce health disparities
   e. Address health literacy

5. The Speak Up™ campaign includes which of the following components? Select all that apply.
   a. Educate yourself
   b. Advocate for self and others
   c. Know what insurance covers
   d. Participate in care decisions
   e. Pay your health-care bill promptly

Questions 6-9 refer to the following situation: Natasha is a 17-year-old high school junior. Natasha's school requires an athletic preparticipation athletic evaluation before the softball season begins. Natasha has never played a high school sport and never had an athletic preparticipation athletic evaluation.

6. What is the purpose of the preparticipation athletic evaluation? Select all that apply.
   a. Establish a child's physical fitness
   b. Renew prescription medication
   c. Identify any health conditions
   d. Order laboratory tests
   e. Recommend a physical therapist

7. Which of the following body systems are most heavily evaluated in the preparticipation physical examination?
   a. Respiratory and mental health
   b. Eyes and neurological
   c. Skin and abdomen
   d. Musculoskeletal and cardiovascular

8. Which of the following conditions is an absolute contraindication for Natasha and would prevent her from playing softball?
   a. Prehypertension
   b. Controlled seizure disorder
   c. Hepatosplenomegaly
   d. Eczema

9. Which of the following sequences best describes the order in which Natasha's head-to-toe physical examination would proceed?
   a. Eyes, ears, mouth
   b. Neck, abdomen, throat
   c. Anterior thorax, upper extremities, vital signs
   d. Heart, thyroid, face

10. Which of the following statements are true about technology in health care? Select all that apply.
    a. Electronic health records provide easy accessibility.
    b. Nursing school simulation labs provide real-life experiential learning.
    c. Electronic medical records are used primarily by physicians.
    d. Hacking of electronic records is not a concern for nurses.
    e. Robots can be used to disinfect client rooms and assist in certain aspects of client care.

Appendix A

Functional Assessments: Instrumental Activities of Daily Living (IADLs) and Physical Self-Maintenance Activities

I. Instrumental Activities of Daily Living

A. Ability to use telephone
1. Operates telephone independently—looks up and dials numbers
2. Dials a few well-known numbers
3. Answers phone but does not dial or use touch-tone
4. Does not use telephone at all

B. Housekeeping
1. Maintains house independently or with occasional assistance for "heavy work"
2. Performs light tasks such as bedmaking and dishwashing
3. Performs light daily tasks but cannot maintain adequate level of cleanliness
4. Needs assistance with all home maintenance tasks
5. Does not participate in any tasks

C. Laundry
1. Does personal laundry completely
2. Launders small items such as socks and stockings
3. All laundry must be done by others

D. Mode of transportation
1. Independently drives own car or uses public transportation
2. Arranges own travel via taxi or special transportation services, but does not use public transportation and does not drive
3. Travels on public transportation when assisted or with others
4. Travel limited to taxi or auto with assistance
5. Does not travel at all

E. Responsibility for medications
1. Takes medication in correct dosages at correct time independently
2. Takes medication if medication is prepared in advance in separate doses
3. Not capable of dispensing own medications

F. Ability to handle finances
1. Independently manages finances—writes checks, pays bills, keeps track of income
2. Manages own finances with assistance
3. Not capable of managing own finances

G. Shopping
1. Does all the shopping independently
2. Shops for small purchases independently
3. Not able to go shopping without assistance
4. Unable to shop for any purchase

H. Food preparation
1. Able to prepare and serve food without assistance
2. Prepares adequate meals if supplied with food
3. Able to heat and serve prepared meals
4. Unable to prepare and serve meals

Adapted from *"Assessment of Older People: Self-Maintaining and Instrumental Activities of Daily Living"* by M. Lawton and E. Brody, 1969, The Gerontologist, 9, pp. 179–186.

II. Physical Self-Maintenance Activities

A. Feeding
   1. Eats without assistance
   2. Eats with minor assistance at meal times and helps in cleaning up
   3. Feeds self with moderate assistance
   4. Requires extensive assistance—all meals
   5. Does not feed self at all and resists efforts of others to feed them

B. Toilet
   1. Cares for self completely; no incontinence
   2. Needs to be reminded or needs help in cleaning self
   3. Soils the bed while asleep—more than once a week
   4. Soils clothing while awake—more than once a week
   5. No control of bladder or bowel

C. Grooming (hair, nails, hands, face)
   1. Able to care for self
   2. Occasional minor assistance needed (e.g., with shaving)
   3. Moderate and regular assistance needed
   4. Needs total grooming care, but accepts some
   5. Actively negates efforts of others to maintain grooming

D. Bathing
   1. Bathes self without help
   2. Bathes self with help into and out of tub or shower
   3. Can wash face and hands only
   4. Does not wash self but is cooperative
   5. Does not try to wash self and resists efforts of others to help

E. Dressing
   1. Dresses, undresses, and selects clothes from wardrobe
   2. Dresses and undresses with minor assistance
   3. Needs moderate assistance in dressing or selection of clothes
   4. Needs major assistance
   5. Completely unable to dress self and resists efforts of others to help

F. Ambulation
   1. Ambulates about grounds or city without assistance
   2. Ambulates within residence or nearby
   3. Ambulates with assistance of
      a. another person
      b. a railing
      c. cane
      d. walker
      e. wheelchair
   4. Sits unsupported in chair or wheelchair but cannot propel self
   5. Bedridden more than half the time

Appendix B

Abbreviations

A, A, & O × 3	awake, alert, and oriented times three (to person, place, and time)
AAA	abdominal aortic aneurysm
ABD/abd	abdomen/abdominal
AC	air conduction
ACL	anterior cruciate ligament
ACS	American Cancer Society
ADHD	attention-deficit/hyperactivity disorder
ADL	activities of daily living
AF; A fib	atrial fibrillation
AGA	appropriate for gestational age
AHA	American Heart Association
ALS	amyotrophic lateral sclerosis
ANA	American Nurses Association
AOM	acute otitis media
AP	apical pulse; anteroposterior
A&P	anterior and posterior; auscultation and percussion; anatomy and physiology
AROM	active range of motion; artificial rupture of membranes
AS	aortic stenosis
ASA	acetylsalicylic acid (aspirin)
ASD	atrial septal defect
AV	arteriovenous
A-V	atrioventricular
A&W	alive and well
BC	bone conduction
BCC	basal cell carcinoma
BCG	Bacille Calmette-Guérin vaccine
BCP	birth control pills
BMI	body mass index
BP	blood pressure
BPH	benign prostatic hypertrophy
BPM	beats per minute
BS	bowel sounds; breath sounds
BSE	breast self-examination
BX/bx	biopsy
°C	degrees Celsius/degrees centigrade
C section	Cesarean section
CA	cancer
CABG	coronary artery bypass graft
CAD	coronary artery disease
CC/cc	chief complaint/cubic centimeters
CCD	congenital cardiovascular defect
CDC	Centers for Disease Control and Prevention
CHD	childhood diseases; congenital heart disease
CHF	congestive heart failure
CHI	closed head injury; creatinine height index
CKD	chronic kidney disease
cm	centimeter
CMT	cervical motion tenderness

CMV	cytomegalovirus
CN I–XII	cranial nerves I–XII
CN II-XII	cranial nerves II-XII
CNS	central nervous system
C/O; c/o	complaining of/complaints of
CO	carbon monoxide; cardiac output
CO_2	carbon dioxide
COA	coarctation of the aorta
COPD	chronic obstructive pulmonary disease
CP	chest pain; cerebral palsy
CPAP	continuous positive airway pressure
CPD	cephalopelvic disproportion
CT	computerized tomography
CV	cardiovascular
CVA	costovertebral angle; cerebrovascular accident (stroke)
CVAT	costovertebral angle tenderness
CVP	central venous pressure
CX/cx	cervix
CX-ray	chest X-ray
DBP	diastolic blood pressure
D&C	dilation and curettage
DDH	developmental dislocation of the hip
DDST II	Denver Developmental Screening Test II
DES	diethylstilbestrol
DJD	degenerative joint disease
DM	diabetes mellitus
D/O; d/o	disorder
DOB	date of birth
DOE	dyspnea on exertion
DTR	deep tendon reflex
DUB	dysfunctional uterine bleeding
DVT	deep vein thrombosis
DX/dx	diagnosis
DZ/dz	disease
EAC	external auditory canal
ECG/EKG	electrocardiogram
ED	emergency department; erectile dysfunction
EDC	expected date of confinement (delivery date)
EDD	estimated date of delivery
EENT	eyes, ears, nose, and throat
EHR	electronic health record
EMR	electronic medical record
ENAP	examination, normal findings, abnormal findings, pathophysiology
ENT	ears, nose, and throat
EOM	extraocular muscle movements
EOMI	extraocular muscle movements intact
ER	emergency room
ETOH	ethyl alcohol
°F	degrees Fahrenheit
FHH	family health history
FHR	fetal heart rate
FHT	fetal heart tone
FM	fetal movement
FOB	father of baby
FOBT	fecal occult blood test
FROM	full range of motion
FSH	follicle-stimulating hormone
FTT	failure to thrive
FX/fx	fracture; function
GC	gonorrhea and chlamydia
GCS	Glasgow Coma Scale
GDM	gestational diabetes mellitus
GERD	gastroesophageal reflux disease

GI	gastrointestinal
GSW	gunshot wound
GU	genitourinary
GYN	gynecology, gynecological
H/A; HA	headache
HbA1c	glycosylated hemoglobin
HCG	human chorionic gonadotropin
HDL	high-density lipoprotein
HDP	hypertensive disorders of pregnancy
HELLP	hemolysis, elevated liver enzymes, low platelets syndrome
HF	heart failure
HIV	human immunodeficiency virus
HL/hl	health
HLD	hyperlipidemia
HMA	Health Maintenance Activities
H/O; h/o	history of
HPI	history of present illness
HPV	human papillomavirus
HR	heart rate; hour(s)
HRT	hormone replacement therapy
HSM	hepatosplenomegaly
HSV	herpes simplex virus
HT/ht	height
HTN	hypertension
HX/hx	history
IADL	instrumental activities of daily living
IBS	irritable bowel syndrome
IBW	ideal body weight
ICP	intracranial pressure
ICS	intercostal space
IDA	iron deficiency anemia
IHD	ischemic heart disease
IOP	intraocular pressure
IPPA	inspection, palpation, percussion, auscultation; inspection, percussion, palpation, auscultation
IPV	intimate partner violence
ITP	idiopathic thrombocytopenia purpura
IUD	intrauterine device
IUGR	intrauterine growth retardation
IUP	intrauterine pregnancy
IV	intravenous
JVD	jugular venous distension
JVP	jugular venous pressure
KUB	kidneys, ureters, bladder
L	liter
LA	left atrium; left arm
LAD	left anterior descending (coronary artery)
LBP	low back pain
LBS/lbs	pounds
LCL	lateral collateral ligament
LCM	left costal margin
LDL	low-density lipoprotein
LE	lower extremity
LGA	large for gestational age
LGBTQIA+	lesbian, gay, bisexual, transgender, queer, intersex, asexual, and other sexual and gender minorities
LH	luteinizing hormone
LLE	left lower extremity
LLL	left lower lobe (of lung)
LLQ	left lower quadrant (of abdomen)
LLSB	left lower sternal border
LMP	last menstrual period
LOC	level of consciousness/loss of consciousness

LPM/lpm	liters per minute (of oxygen)
LSB	left sternal border
LUE	left upper extremity
LUL	left upper lobe (of lung)
LUQ	left upper quadrant (of abdomen)
LV	left ventricle
LVH	left ventricular hypertrophy
MAC	mid-arm circumference
MAL	midaxillary line
MAMC	mid-arm muscle circumference
MCL	midclavicular line; medial collateral ligament
MD	muscular dystrophy; medical doctor
MGR	murmur, gallop, rub
MI	myocardial infarction
mL	milliliter
mm Hg	millimeters of mercury
MMR	measles, mumps, rubella
MMSE	Mini-Mental State Examination
MRI	magnetic resonance imaging
MS	multiple sclerosis; musculoskeletal
MSAFP	maternal serum alpha fetal protein
MVA	motor vehicle accident
MVI	multivitamin
MVP	mitral valve prolapse
N/A	not applicable
NAD	no acute distress/no apparent distress
NCHD	normal childhood diseases
NKA	no known allergies
NKDA	no known diagnosed allergies/no known drug allergies
NP	nurse practitioner
NPO	nothing by mouth
NSAID	nonsteroidal anti-inflammatory drug
NSR	normal sinus rhythm
NSVD	normal spontaneous vaginal delivery
N&V	nausea and vomiting
NVD	nausea, vomiting, diarrhea
NVDC	nausea, vomiting, diarrhea, constipation
O_2	oxygen
OA	osteoarthritis
OAB	overactive bladder
OB	obstetrics
OC	oral contraceptive
OCP	oral contraceptive pills
OD	overdose
OM	otitis media
OME	otitis media with effusion
ORIF	open reduction and internal fixation
OSA	obstructive sleep apnea
OTC	over the counter (medications)
PAD	peripheral artery disease
Pap	Papanicolaou test
PAR	perennial allergic rhinitis
PCL	posterior cruciate ligament
PCN	penicillin
PCP	primary care provider
PDA	patent ductus arteriosus
PE	pulmonary embolus; physical examination
PERRLA	pupils equally round, reactive to light and accommodation
pH	potential of hydrogen
PH	present health
PHH	past health history
PID	pelvic inflammatory disease
PMH	past medical history

PMI	point of maximal intensity/point of maximal impulse
PMS	premenstrual syndrome
PNA	pneumonia
PND	paroxysmal nocturnal dyspnea; postnasal drip
PPD	packs per day (smoking); purified protein derivative (skin test for TB)
PRN/prn	as necessary
PROM	passive range of motion; premature rupture of membranes
PS	pulmonic stenosis
PSA	prostate-specific antigen
PT	physical therapy
PTA	prior to admission/prior to arrival
PTSD	post-traumatic stress disorder
PUD	peptic ulcer disease
PVC	premature ventricular complex/premature ventricular contraction
PVD	peripheral vascular disease
RA	rheumatoid arthritis; right arm; right atrium
RCA	right coronary artery
RCM	right costal margin
RHD	rheumatic heart disease
RLE	right lower extremity
RLL	right lower lobe (of lung)
RLQ	right lower quadrant (of abdomen)
RLS	restless legs syndrome
RML	right middle lobe (of lung)
RN	registered nurse
ROM	range of motion
ROS	review of systems
RR	respiratory rate; red reflex
RSB	right sternal border
RSV	respiratory syncytial virus
RT	radiation therapy
RUE	right upper extremity
RUL	right upper lobe (of lung)
RUQ	right upper quadrant (of abdomen)
RV	right ventricle
Rx	prescription; prescription medication
SAR	seasonal allergic rhinitis
SBE	subacute bacterial endocarditis
SBP	systolic blood pressure
SCA	sickle cell anemia
SCC	squamous cell carcinoma
SCM	sternocleidomastoid
SDH	subdural hematoma
SEM	systolic ejection murmur
SGA	small for gestational age
SH	social history
SIDS	sudden infant death syndrome
SLE	systemic lupus erythematosus
SOB	shortness of breath
S/P	status post
SROM	spontaneous rupture of membranes
S/S	signs and symptoms
SSCP	substernal chest pain
ST	sore throat
STD	sexually transmitted disease
STI	sexually transmitted infection
SUID	sudden unexpected infant death
SX/sx	symptom
SZ/sz	seizure
T&A	tonsillectomy and adenoidectomy
TAH	total abdominal hysterectomy
TB	tuberculosis
TBI	traumatic brain injury

TIBC	total iron-binding capacity
THA	total hip arthroplasty
THR	total hip replacement; target heart rate
TIBC	total iron-binding capacity
TKR	total knee replacement
TM	tympanic membrane
TMJ	temporomandibular joint
TORCH	toxoplasmosis, rubella, cytomegalovirus, herpes
TPAL	number of: term infants, preterm infants, abortion (spontaneous or induced), living children
TPR	temperature, pulse, respirations
TSE	testicular self-examination
TSF	triceps skinfold
TVH	total vaginal hysterectomy
T1DM	type 1 diabetes mellitus
T2DM	type 2 diabetes mellitus
TX/tx	treatment
U/A	urinalysis
UC	uterine contraction; ulcerative colitis
UCHD	usual childhood diseases
UE	upper extremity
URI	upper respiratory infection
UTD	up-to-date
UTI	urinary tract infection
VBAC	vaginal birth after cesarean
VE	vaginal examination
VS	vital signs
VSD	ventricular septal defect
VSS	vital signs stable
VTX/vtx	vertex
WNL	within normal limits
WT/wt	weight
YO/yo	year old (age)
YR/yr(s)	year(s)

Glossary

A

Accommodation Visual focusing from a far to a near point as pupils constrict and eyes converge.

Acculturation Informal process of adaptation through which the beliefs, values, norms, and practices of a dominant culture are learned by a new member born into a different culture.

Acini *See* **Alveoli (of the Breast)**.

Acrocyanosis Normal phenomenon in light-skinned newborns whereby the hands and feet are blue and the rest of the body is pink.

Acromegaly Abnormal enlargement of the skull, bony facial structures, and bones of the extremities, caused by excessive secretion of growth hormone.

Action Response Attempt to stimulate clients to make some change in their thinking and behavior.

Active Listening Act of perceiving what is said both verbally and nonverbally.

Adnexa Uterine (fallopian) tubes, ovaries, and their supporting ligaments.

Advance Medical Directive A legal document that a client completes expressing what care should be provided if the client is unable to communicate these wishes due to illness or incapacity.

Adventitious Breath Sound Added breath sound that is superimposed on normal breath sounds.

Afterload Initial resistance that the ventricles must overcome in opening the semilunar valves to propel the blood into both the systemic and the pulmonary circulation.

Ages and Stages Developmental Theory Belief that individuals experience similar sequential physical, cognitive, socioemotional, and moral changes during the same age periods, each of which is termed a developmental stage.

Ageusia Loss of the sense of taste.

Aggravating Factors Events that worsen the severity of the client's chief complaint.

Agnosia Inability to recognize the form and nature of objects or persons.

Agnostic Person who is unsure if God exists.

Agonal Respirations Irregular respirations that signal impending death.

Agraphia Loss of the ability to write.

Air Trapping Abnormal respiratory pattern with rapid, shallow respirations and forced expirations; the lungs have insufficient time to fully exhale and air becomes trapped, leading to overexpansion of the lungs.

Albinism A generalized whiteness of the skin, hair, and eyebrows, caused by a congenital inability to form melanin.

Albumin Protein that transports nutrients, blood, and hormones and helps maintain osmotic pressure.

Alexia Loss of the ability to grasp the meaning of written words and sentences; also known as word blindness.

Allen Test Test used to assess for patency of the radial and ulnar arteries.

Alleviating Factors Events that decrease the severity of the client's chief complaint.

Ally A person who actively supports the rights of a marginalized community even though that person is not a member of that community; for example, a heterosexual person who campaigns for the rights of gay people.

Alopecia Partial or complete loss of hair.

Alveoli (of the Breast) Milk-producing glands located in the lobules; also called acini.

Alveoli (of the Lung) Smallest functional unit of the respiratory system; where gas exchange occurs.

Amblyopia Permanent loss of visual acuity resulting from certain uncorrected medical conditions.

Amenorrhea Absence of menses.

Anal Canal Terminal 1¼ to 1⅝ inches (3 to 4 cm) of the large intestine.

Anal Columns Longitudinal folds of mucosa in the superior portion of the anal canal.

Anal Fissure Linear tear in the epidermis of the anal canal.

Anal Incontinence Involuntary release of rectal contents.

Anal Orifice Exit to the gastrointestinal tract; located at the seam of the gluteal folds.

Anal Sinuses Pockets in the anal canal that lie superior to the anal valves; secrete mucus when compressed by feces.

Anal Valves Folds in the anal canal that are formed by joining anal columns.

Analgesia Absence of normal sense of pain.
Anemia Decreased number of circulating red blood cells or decreased hemoglobin.
Anencephaly Condition in which the cerebral cortex or cranium does not develop.
Anergy Diminished reaction to antigens.
Aneroid Manometer Blood pressure measurement equipment with a calibrated dial and indicator that points to numbers representing blood pressure.
Anesthesia Partial or complete absence of touch sensation with or without loss of consciousness.
Angina Myocardial ischemia that manifests as chest, neck, or arm pain.
Angle of Louis (Manubriosternal Junction, Sternal Angle) Junction of the manubrium and the sternum.
Animism Belief that all things in nature have souls or that spirits inhabit natural objects and creatures.
Anisocoria Difference in pupil sizes.
Anoderm Epithelial tissue that lies in the lower ¾ inches (2 cm) of the anal canal.
Anorectal Abscess Undrained collection of perianal pus in the tissue spaces in and adjacent to the anorectum.
Anorectal Fistula Hollow, fibrous tract lined by granulation tissue and filled with purulent or serosanguineous discharge; has an opening inside the anal canal or rectum, and one or more orifices in the perianal skin.
Anorectum Area where the anal canal fuses with the rectum.
Anosmia Loss of the sense of smell.
Anterior Axillary Line Vertical line drawn from the origin of the anterior axillary fold along the anterolateral aspect of the thorax.
Anterior Chamber Space anterior to the pupil and iris.
Anterior Triangle Area of the neck formed by the mandible, the trachea, and the sternocleidomastoid muscle; contains the anterior cervical lymph nodes, the trachea, and the thyroid gland.
Anthropometric Measurements Measurements of the human body, including height, weight, and body proportions.
Anticipatory Guidance Approach covering health promotion and education; designed to inform at-risk individuals of physical, cognitive, psychological, and social changes that may occur and help them explore their needs.
Antigen Skin Testing Test of immune function.
Apex (of the Heart) Inferior aspect of the heart.
Apex (of the Lung) Superior aspect of the lung.
Apgar Score A system for evaluating the newborn at 1 and 5 minutes of age, giving 0 to 2 points for heart rate, respiratory effort, muscle tone, reflex irritability, and color.
Aphasia Impairment or absence of language function.
Aphonia Total loss of voice.
Apnea Lack of spontaneous respirations for 10 or more seconds.
Apneustic Respirations Prolonged gasping during inspiration followed by a very short, inefficient pause that can last 30 to 60 seconds.
Apocrine Glands Sweat glands that are associated with hair follicles.
Appendicular Skeleton Peripheral skeleton including the limbs, pelvis, scapula, and clavicle.
Apraxia Inability to convert intended speech into the motor act of speech; inability to perform purposeful acts or to manipulate objects.
Arcus Senilis Hazy, gray ring about 2 mm in size and located just inside the limbus; most commonly found in older individuals.
Areola Pigmented area, approximately 1 to 4 inches (2.5 to 10 cm) in diameter, that surrounds the nipple.
Arrector Pili Muscle Muscle that causes contraction of the skin and hair, resulting in "goose bumps."
Arrhythmia A malfunction of the electrical conduction system of the heart leading to an irregular heart rhythm; also known as a dysrhythmia.
Ascites Excess accumulation of fluid in the abdominal cavity.
Asexual Describes a person who experiences little or no sexual attraction to others. Asexual people may still engage in sexual activity.
Associated Manifestations Signs and symptoms that accompany a client's chief complaint.
Astereognosis Inability to recognize the nature of objects by touch.
Asystole Absence of cardiac activity; no pulse, flat line on electrocardiogram.
Ataxic Respirations *See* **Biot Respirations**.
Atheist Person who does not believe in any god.
Atherosclerosis Development of lipid plaques in arteries that can lead to arterial occlusion.
Atlas First cervical vertebra.
Atrial Kick Final phase of ventricular diastole, when the atria contract to complete the final 20% to 30% of ventricular filling.
Atrioventricular Node One of the heart's pacemakers that delays the impulse from the atria before it goes to the ventricles; inherent rate is 40 to 60 beats per minute.
Atrioventricular Valves Valves that prevent blood from entering the ventricles until diastole and prevent retrograde blood flow during systole; composed of the tricuspid and mitral valves.

Atrophy Reduction in muscle size.
Auricle External flap of the ear; also called the pinna.
Auscultation Process of active listening to sounds within the body to gather information on a client's health status.
Auscultatory Gap A silent interval that may be heard between the systolic and diastolic blood pressures that can occur in hypertensive clients; this can lead to a falsely elevated high diastolic or falsely low systolic blood pressure measurement.
Autonomy A client's right to self-determination; the duty to respect a client's thoughts and actions as to what they thinks is best for themself.
Axial Skeleton Central skeleton, including the facial bones, skull, auditory ossicles, hyoid bone, ribs, sternum, and vertebrae.
Axillary Nodes Lymph nodes composed of four groups: brachial (lateral), central axillary (midaxillary), pectoral (anterior), and subscapular (posterior).
Axis Second cervical vertebra.

B

Ballottement Palpation technique that displaces excess fluid in the knee or abdominal cavity; used to identify an organ or mass.
Baroreceptors Receptors located in the walls of most of the great arteries that sense hypotension and initiate reflex vasoconstriction and tachycardia to bring the blood pressure back to normal.
Barrel Chest Abnormal thorax configuration where the ratio of the anteroposterior diameter to the transverse diameter of the chest is approximately 1:1.
Bartholin Glands (Greater Vestibular Glands) Glands located in the cleft between the labia minora and the hymenal ring; secrete a clear, viscid, odorless, alkaline mucus that improves the viability and motility of sperm along the female reproductive tract.
Base (of the Heart) Superior aspect of the heart.
Base (of the Lung) Inferior aspect of the lung.
Bell Palsy Idiopathic facial palsy of cranial nerve VII resulting in asymmetry of the palpebral fissures, nasolabial folds, mouth, and facial expression on the affected side.
Beneficence Doing what is "good" for the client.
Biases Social stereotypes that can be conscious or unconscious, whereby, nurses may generalize about clients based upon appearance (e.g., tattoos, piercings, obesity, levels of education, place of employment, and place of residence). These biases, which are socially constructed, are generalizations that may influence decisions in interactions and care.
Biot (Ataxic) Respirations Irregularly irregular respiratory pattern caused by damage to the medulla.
Bisexual A sexual orientation that describes a person who is emotionally and physically attracted to women/females and men/males. Some people define bisexuality as attraction to all genders.
Blepharitis Inflamed, scaly, red-rimmed eyelids, sometimes with loss of the eyelashes.
Blood Pressure Vital sign collected to assess cardiac output and vascular resistance; it measures the force exerted by the flow of blood pumped into the large arteries.
Body Mass Index (BMI) Measurement that indicates body composition based on a person's height and weight; an increased BMI indicates obesity and a decreased BMI indicates possible malnutrition.
Bohn Nodules Small, white cysts that may appear on the gums of a newborn.
Borborygmi Loud, audible, gurgling bowel sounds.
Bouchard Node Bony enlargement of the proximal interphalangeal joint of the finger.
Bow Legs *See* **Genu Varum**.
Bradycardia Pulse rate under 60 beats per minute in a resting adult.
Bradypnea Respiratory rate under 12 breaths per minute in a resting adult.
Braxton Hicks Contractions A pattern of intermittent, painless uterine contractions that occurs more frequently at the end of pregnancy (every 10–20 minutes or even more frequently). These are not true labor pains.
Breasts Pair of mammary glands located on the anterior chest wall and extending vertically from the second to the sixth rib and laterally from the sternal border to the axillae.
Bregma Junction of the coronal and sagittal sutures.
Bronchophony Use of a voice sound, where the client says the words "ninety-nine" or "one, two, three," to determine if the lung is filled with air or fluid, or is solid.
Bruit Adventitious blowing sound that can be auscultated when blood flow becomes turbulent as it rushes past a partial obstruction.
Brushfield Spots Small, white flecks located around the perimeter of the iris, associated with Down syndrome.
Bulbar Conjunctiva Covering of the anterior surface of the sclera.
Bulbourethral Glands Pea-sized glands located below the prostate; secretions are emptied from here at the time of ejaculation.
Bursae Sacs filled with fluids.

C

Cachexia Extreme malnutrition in which the client exhibits wasting.

Callus Thickening of the skin due to prolonged pressure.

Calorie *See* **Kilocalorie**.

Canthus Nasal or temporal angle where the eyelids meet.

Caput Medusae Venous pattern of congested veins around the umbilicus; attributed to obstruction of the portal vein and seen in liver dysfunction.

Caput Succedaneum Swelling over the occipitoparietal region of the skull that occurs during delivery of the newborn.

Carbohydrate Major source of energy for various functions of the body; supplies fiber and assists in the utilization of fat.

Cardiomegaly Enlargement of the heart.

Carotenemia Orange-yellow coloration of palmar and plantar surfaces caused by elevated levels of serum carotene.

Caruncle Round, red structure in the inner canthus; contains sebaceous glands.

Castration Anxiety Young boys' fear of having the penis cut off or mutilated.

Cataract Opacity in the lens of the eye that gives the pupil a pearly gray appearance.

Cephalohematoma Localized subcutaneous swelling over one cranial bone that occurs during delivery of the newborn.

Cephalocaudal Head to toe.

Cerumen Waxlike substance produced in the ear canal.

Cervix Inferior aspect of the uterus that protrudes into the vagina.

Chadwick Sign A blue, soft cervix, normally during pregnancy.

Chalazion Chronic inflammation of the meibomian gland in the upper or lower eyelid.

Chancre Reddish, round ulcer or small papular lesion with a depressed center and raised, indurated edges.

Chancroid Tender, ulcerated, exudative, papular lesion with an erythematous halo, surrounding edema, and a friable base.

Chandelier Sign Cervical motion tenderness on palpation.

Characteristic Patterns of Daily Living Client's normal daily routines/timetable; includes meal, work, and sleeping schedules and patterns of social interactions.

Chemosis Swelling of the palpebral conjunctiva.

Cherry Angioma Bright red, circumscribed area that may be flat or raised and that darkens with age.

Cheyne-Stokes Respirations Crescendo or decrescendo respiratory pattern interspersed between periods of apnea.

Chief Complaint Sign, symptom, or problem that causes the client to seek health care.

Chloasma *See* **Melasma**.

Cholesterol Lipid found only in animal products; it is transported in the body by high-density lipoproteins and low-density lipoproteins.

Choroid Vascular tissue of the posterior uveal tract lining the inner surface of the globe of the eye, beneath the retina; provides nutrition to the retina and helps absorb excess light.

Ciliary Body Extension of the uveal tract that produces aqueous humor.

Circadian Rhythm Normal fluctuation of body temperature, pulse, and blood pressure during a 24-hour period.

Cisgender Refers to a person whose gender identity corresponds to the sex assigned at birth.

Click Extrasystolic heart sound that is high-pitched and can radiate in the chest wall.

Client Profile Demographics that may be linked to health status.

Clinical Reasoning A disciplined, creative, and reflective approach used with critical thinking to establish potential strategies for clients to reach their health goals.

Clitoris Cylindrical erectile body located at the superior aspect of the vulva, between the labia minora; contains erectile tissue and has a significant supply of nerve endings.

Clonus Rhythmic oscillation of involuntary muscle contraction.

Clubfoot *See* **Talipes Equinovarus**.

Cochlea Snail-shaped structure in the bony labyrinth of the inner ear.

Colloquialism Word or phrase particular to a community and used in informal conversation and writing.

Coloboma Defect of the choroid and retina resulting when development in utero is interrupted.

Colostrum A thin, milky secretion expressed by the breast during pregnancy and for a few days after parturition; it is rich in antibodies.

Complete Health History Comprehensive history of the client's past and present health status; includes physical, emotional, psychological, developmental, cultural, and spiritual data.

Concha *See* **Turbinate**.

Condyloma Acuminatum Genital wart.

Cone Retinal structure in the macula that is responsible for color vision.

Confabulation Fabrication of answers, experiences, or situations unrelated to facts.

Congenital Dermal Melanocytosis Various irregularly sized areas of deep bluish pigmentation on the upper back, shoulders, buttocks, and lumbosacral area of newborns of African, Latino, and Asian descent (formerly known as Mongolian spots).
Conservation The understanding that altering the physical state of an object does not change the basic properties of that object.
Constructional Apraxia Inability to reproduce figures on paper.
Cooper Ligaments Ligaments that extend vertically from the deep fascia through the breast to the inner layer of the skin; provide support for the breast tissue.
Corn Conical area of thickened skin.
Cornea Transparent covering of the iris.
Costal Angle Angle formed by the intersection of the costal margins at the sternum.
Costal Margin Medial border created by the articulation of the false ribs.
Cradle Cap Seborrheic dermatitis manifesting as greasy-appearing scales on an infant's scalp.
Craniosynostosis Abnormal shape of the skull due to premature ossification of one or more suture lines before brain growth is complete.
Craniotabes Softening of the skull.
Creatinine Substance found in muscle and excreted in the urine.
Crepitus Subcutaneous emphysema; beads of air escape from the lungs and create a crackling sound when palpated. A grating or crackling sound that can be felt/heard with joint movement.
Crescendo Heart murmur configuration that proceeds from soft to loud.
Critical Thinking A purposeful, goal-directed thinking process that strives to problem solve client care issues through clinical reasoning.
Cryptorchidism Condition in which a testicle has not descended into the scrotum.
Cullen Sign Bluish discoloration encircling the umbilicus and indicative of blood in the peritoneal cavity.
Cult A small, created religious organization often headed by a single charismatic leader and viewed as spiritually innovative or heretical in nature.
Cultural Awareness The process of critical self-reflection of one's own biases toward other cultures and exploration of one's own cultural background.
Cultural Competence The process by which the nurse demonstrates culturally congruent practice.
Cultural Diversity Different combinations of cultural and subcultural minorities (e.g., ethnic, racial, national, religious, generational, marital status, socioeconomic, occupational, health status, and preference in life partner orientations) coexisting in a given location.
Cultural Humility An awareness of personal bias. It encompasses a life-long approach to working with diversity and the recognition of the role of power in health-care interactions. Cultural humility enables the nurse to develop respectful partnerships with clients to achieve equity in the delivery of health care.
Cultural Norms Often unwritten but generally understood prescriptions for acceptable behavior by members of a cultural group.
Cultural Relativity Belief that no culture is either inferior or superior to another; that behavior must be evaluated in relation to the cultural context in which it occurs; and that respect, equality, and justice are basic rights for all racial, ethnic, subcultural, and cultural groups.
Cultural Rituals Highly structured and prescribed patterns of behavior used by a cultural group to respond to or in anticipation of specific life events such as birth, death, illness, healing, marriage, and worship.
Cultural Values Fundamental, often unshakable and unchanging, set of principles on which the cultural beliefs, behaviors, and customs of all members of the culture are based.
Culturally Congruent Care The application of evidence-based nursing practice that aligns with the client/consumer's cultural values, beliefs, and worldview, and practices.
Culture Learned and socially transmitted orientation and way of life specific to a group of people, with similar lifeways.
Cutaneous Hypersensitivity Stimulus detecting specific zones of peritoneal irritation.
Cyanosis Blue coloration of the skin or nails that occurs when more than 5 g/dL of hemoglobin is deoxygenated in the blood.
Cystocele Bulging of the anterior vaginal wall.
Cystourethrocele Bulging of the anterior vaginal wall, bladder, and urethra into the vaginal introitus.

D

Dacryoadenitis Acute inflammation of the lacrimal gland.
Dacryocystitis Inflammation of the lacrimal duct.
Decerebrate Rigidity Involuntary rigidity and sustained contraction of extensor muscles that occur in severe brain damage.
Decorticate Rigidity Involuntary hyperflexion of the arms, hyperextension and internal rotation of the legs, and plantar flexion that occur in severe brain damage.
Decrescendo Heart murmur configuration that proceeds from loud to soft.

Deep Palpation Palpating the body's internal structures to a depth of 1⅝ to 2 inches (4 to 5 cm) to elicit information on organs and masses, including position, size, shape, mobility, consistency, and areas of discomfort.
Defecation Expulsion of feces from the rectum.
Dehydration Lack of fluid in the body's tissues.
Dermatome Skin area innervated by afferent spinal nerves from a specific nerve root.
Dermis Corium, or the second layer of the skin.
Desquamation Shedding of old skin cells as new cells are pushed up from the lower layers of the epidermis.
Development Patterned and predictable increases in the physical, cognitive, socioemotional, and moral capacities of individuals that enable them to successfully adapt to their environments.
Developmental Dislocation of the Hip Dislocated hip found in newborns and young infants; related to familial factors, maternal hormones, firstborn children, oligohydramnios, and breech presentations.
Developmental Stage One of multiple sequential age periods during which individuals experience similar physical, cognitive, socioemotional, and moral changes.
Developmental Task Specific physical or psychosocial skill that must be achieved during a developmental stage.
Diaphragmatic Excursion Technique used to assess the client's depth of ventilation.
Diaphragmatic Hernia Protrusion of intestines into the thoracic cavity.
Diaphysis Central shaft of a long bone.
Diastasis Recti Separation of the rectus muscle of the abdominal wall.
Diastole Phase in the cardiac cycle when the heart is at rest.
Dietary Guidelines for Americans An evidence-based publication by the Dietary Guidelines Advisory Committee that seeks to promote health and reduce the morbidity and mortality of diseases through diet and physical activity.
Dietary Reference Intakes Nutrient reference values developed by the Institute of Medicine that are used to assess a person's diet; comprised of four components: Adequate Intake, Estimated Average Requirement, Tolerable Upper Intake Level, and Recommended Dietary Allowances.
Diopter A unit of refractive measurement.
Direct (Immediate) Auscultation Active listening to body sounds via the unaided ear.
Direct Fist Percussion Using the ulnar aspect of a closed fist to strike the client's body to elicit tenderness over specific body areas.
Direct Inguinal Hernia Protrusion of the bowel and/or omentum directly through the external inguinal ring.
Direct (Immediate) Percussion Striking of an area of the body directly with the index or middle finger pad or fist to elicit sound.
Discrimination Overt or covert actions that limit opportunities based upon cultural/racial biases.
Dislocation Complete dislodgement of a bone from its joint cavity.
Distress Negative stress that is harmful and unpleasant.
Down Syndrome Congenital chromosomal aberration marked by slanted eyes with inner epicanthal folds; a short, flat nose; a protruding, thick tongue; and intellectual limitations.
Ductus (Vas) Deferens Tube that permits sperm to exit from the epididymis and pass from the scrotal sac upward into the abdominal cavity.
Dullness Descriptor for a percussible sound that is moderate in intensity, moderate in duration, of high pitch, thudlike, and normally located over organs.
Duration (of Percussion) Time period over which a sound is heard.
Dysarthria Disturbance in muscular control of speech.
Dyscalculia Inability to perform calculations.
Dysdiadochokinesia Inability to perform rapid alternating movements.
Dysesthesia Abnormal interpretation of a stimulus such as burning or tingling from a stimulus such as touch or superficial pain.
Dysmenorrhea Pain or cramping during menses.
Dysmetria Impairment of judgment of distance, range, speed, and force of movement.
Dyspareunia Painful sexual intercourse.
Dysphagia Difficulty swallowing.
Dysphonia Difficulty in making laryngeal speech sounds.
Dyspnea Subjective feeling of shortness of breath.
Dysrhythmia *See* **Arrhythmia**.
Dyssynergy Lack of coordinated action of the muscle groups.

E

Ecchymosis A red-purple discoloration of varying size caused by extravasation of blood into the skin; a black-and-blue mark.
Eccrine Glands Sweat glands that are not associated with hair follicles.
Echolalia Involuntary repetition of a word or sentence that was uttered by another person.
Eclampsia Life-threatening complication of hypertensive disorder of pregnancy that can cause a seizure.

Ecomap A diagram depicting a person's relationship with their family and with significant friends, peers, neighbors, and work associates.
Ectodermal Galactic Band *See* **Milk Line**.
Ectopic Pregnancy A pregnancy other than intrauterine; nonviable and often requires surgical intervention.
Ectropion (Eversion, of the Cervix) A red, inflamed appearance of the cervix as the columnar epithelium extends from the os past the normal squamocolumnar junction.
Ectropion (of the Eye) Turning outward or eversion of the eyelid, usually the lower.
Edema Accumulation of fluid in the intercellular spaces, leading to swelling of any part of the body, usually the feet and hands.
Ego Personality component that is conscious, rational, emerges during the first year of life, and seeks realistic and acceptable ways to meet needs.
Egocentrism Viewing the world in terms of the self only and interpreting one's own actions and all other events in terms of the consequences they have for self.
Egophony Use of a voice sound, where the client says the sound "ee," to determine if the lungs are filled with air or fluid, or are solid.
Ejaculatory Ducts Ducts located posterior to the urinary bladder; they eject sperm into the prostatic urethra prior to ejaculation.
Electra Complex Young girls' sexual attraction toward their fathers and rivalry with their mothers for their fathers' attention.
Electrocardiogram Record of the electrical activity of the heart.
Emergency Health History History taken from the client or other sources when the client is experiencing a life-threatening state.
Enculturation The process of adapting to the dominant cultural patterns of one's society.
Entropion Turning inward or inversion of the eyelid, usually the lower.
Epidermis Multilayered outer covering of the skin, consisting of four layers throughout the body, except for the palms of the hands and soles of the feet, where there are five layers.
Epididymis Comma-shaped organ that lies along the posterior border of each testis; consists of a tightly coiled tube where sperm maturation occurs.
Epimysium Connective tissue sheath covering the muscle belly.
Epiphysis Rounded end of a long bone.
Episodic Health History History taken from the client for a specific problem or need.
Epispadias Congenital abnormality in which the urethral meatus lies on the dorsal surface of the penis.
Epstein Pearls Small, hard, white cysts found on a newborn's hard palate and gum margins.
Eructation Belching.
Escutcheon Characteristic triangular pattern of coarse, curly hair that develops over the mons pubis at puberty.
Esophoria Latent misalignment of the eye; nasal, or inward, drift.
Esotropia Inward deviation of the eye.
Ethnic Identity A subjective self-identification with an ethnic group.
Ethnocentrism Condition that occurs when individuals or groups of people perceive their own cultural group and cultural values, beliefs, norms, and customs to be superior to all others and have disdain for the expression of any way of life but their own.
Eupnea Normal breathing; respirations are 12 to 20 per minute for the resting adult.
Eustachian Tube Auditory tube that serves as an air channel connecting the middle ear to the nasopharynx to allow equalization between the air pressure in the ear and in the atmosphere.
Eustress Positive stress that challenges, provides motivation, and prevents stagnation.
Eversion (of the Cervix) *See* **Ectropion**.
Evidence-Based Practice Uses the outcomes of well-designed and executed scientific studies to guide clinical decision making and clinical care.
Exophoria Latent misalignment of the eye; temporal, or outward, drift.
Exophthalmos Abnormal protrusion of the globe of the eye.
Exotropia Outward deviation of the eye.

F

Faith Orientation to a belief structure.
Fallopian Tubes *See* **Uterine Tubes.**
False Ribs Rib pairs 8 to 10.
Fat-Soluble Vitamin Vitamin stored in dietary fat and absorbed in the fat portions of the body's cells.
Fats Substances that supply essential fatty acids, which form a part of the structure of all cells.
Femoral Hernia Protrusion of the omentum or bowel through the femoral wall.
Fetoscope Special stethoscope for hearing fetal heart tones.
Fidelity The duty to be faithful to the client.
Fissure Groove separating the different lobes of the lungs.
Flatfoot *See* **Pes Planus**.

Flatness Descriptor for a percussible sound that is soft in intensity, short in duration, of high pitch, and normally located over muscle or bone.

Flatulence Passage of excess gas via the rectum.

Floating Ribs Rib pairs 11 and 12; they do not articulate at their anterior ends.

Fluid Wave Physical examination finding in a client with ascites; the lateral aspect of the abdomen is delivered a blow and the examiner's hand feels for the wave on the contralateral side.

Folk Illness Illness believed to be caused by disharmony, an imbalance, or as punishment.

Folk Practitioner Healer or other individual who is not part of the scientific care system but is believed to have special knowledge or power to prevent, treat, or provide resources needed to heal folk illnesses.

Follow-Up Health History *See* **Interval Health History**.

Fornices Pouchlike recesses around the cervix.

Fourchette Transverse fold of skin of the posterior aspect of the labia minora; also known as a frenulum.

Fovea Centralis Center of the macula; the area of sharpest vision.

Frenulum (of the Mouth) Tissue that connects the tongue to the floor of the mouth and the upper lip to the gums.

Friability Susceptibility to bleeding from the cervix.

Frontal bossing Prominent protruding forehead that may occur with protruding eyebrow ridges.

Functional Health Assessment Documents a person's ability to perform instrumental activities of daily living and physical self-maintenance activities.

Fundus Superior aspect of the uterus.

G

Gallop Extra heart sound; an S_3 is a ventricular gallop, whereas an S_4 is an atrial gallop.

Ganglion Cyst Benign, cystic growth.

Gay A sexual orientation describing people who are primarily emotionally and physically attracted to people of the same sex and/or gender as themselves. Commonly used to describe men who are primarily attracted to men but can also describe women attracted to women.

Gender Identity How a person manifests or expresses their gender, including male, female, or nonbinary.

Genogram Pictorial representation of a client's family health history.

Genomics Study of the genetic makeup of the human cell.

Genu Valgum Inward deviation toward the midline at the level of the knees; also known as knock-knees.

Genu Varum Outward deviation away from the midline at the level of the knees; also known as bow legs.

Glans Penis Bulbous end of the penis.

Glasgow Coma Scale International scale used in grading neurological response.

Glaucoma Disease of the eye in which intraocular pressure is elevated leading to optic nerve atrophy and possible blindness.

Glycosuria Glucose in the urine.

Goiter Enlargement of the thyroid gland.

Goniometer Device used to measure the angle of the skeletal joint during range of motion; a protractor with two movable arms.

Granulation Tissue Inflamed tissue, new vessels, and white blood cells at the base of a wound in the process of healing.

Graphanesthesia Inability to identify numbers, letters, or shapes drawn on the skin.

Graphesthesia Ability to identify numbers, letters, or shapes drawn on the skin.

Greater Vestibular Glands *See* **Bartholin Glands**.

Gynecomastia Enlargement of male breast tissue; may occur normally in adolescent and older adult males.

H

Hallux Valgus Lateral deviation of the big toe and medial deviation of the first metatarsal with enlargement and inflammation of the metatarsophalangeal joint; also known as a bunion.

Hammertoe Flexion of the proximal interphalangeal joint and hyperextension of the distal metatarsophalangeal joint.

Harlequin Color Change Condition in which one-half of a newborn's body is red or ruddy and the other half appears pale.

Health Maintenance Activities Practices that a person incorporates into a lifestyle to promote healthy living.

Healthy People 2030 A public health initiative, by the US Department of Health and Human Services, that strives to increase each American's quality of life and number of years of healthy life, and to eliminate disparities in health.

Heave Lifting of the cardiac area secondary to an increased workload and force of left ventricular contraction; also known as a lift.

Heberden Node Bony enlargement of the distal interphalangeal joint of the finger.

HELLP Syndrome Complication of hypertensive disorder of pregnancy: the acronym represents hemolysis, elevated liver enzymes, and low platelets syndrome.

Hematemesis Vomiting of blood.
Hematocrit Measurement to determine the percentage of red blood cells to the volume of whole blood.
Hemiparesis Unilateral weakness or paralysis; also known as hemiplegia.
Hemiplegia *See* **Hemiparesis**.
Hemoglobin The iron component that transports oxygen in the blood.
Hemorrhoids Dilated hemorrhoidal veins in the anorectum.
High-Density Lipoprotein Substance that carries cholesterol away from the heart and arteries and toward the liver.
Hirsutism Excessive body hair.
History of the Present Illness Chronological account of the client's chief complaint and the events surrounding it.
Holosystolic Murmur that is heard throughout all of systole; also known as pansystolic.
Homan Sign Pain in the calf when the foot is dorsiflexed; can be a sign of venous thrombosis of the deep veins of the calf.
Hordeolum Infection of a sebaceous gland in the eyelid; often called a stye.
Hydrocele Fluid collection within the tunica vaginalis of the testis.
Hydrocephalus Enlargement of the head without enlargement of the facial structures; due to increased accumulation of cerebrospinal fluid within the ventricles of the brain.
Hymen Avascular, thin fold of connective tissue surrounding the vaginal introitus; may be annular or crescentic in shape.
Hypalgesia Diminished sensitivity to pain.
Hyperalgesia Increased sensitivity to pain.
Hyperemesis Gravidarum Excessive nausea and vomiting during pregnancy.
Hyperesthesia Abnormal acuteness to the sensitivity of touch.
Hyperglycemia Increase in serum glucose.
Hyperkinetic Increased movement.
Hyperopia Farsightedness.
Hyperphoria Latent misalignment of the eye; an upward turning of the eye.
Hyperpnea Breath that is greater in volume than the resting tidal volume.
Hyperresonance Descriptor for a percussible sound that is very loud in intensity, long in duration, of very low pitch, boomlike, and normally not found in the healthy adult.
Hypertelorism Abnormal width between the eyes.
Hypertension A systolic blood pressure of 130 to 139 mm Hg or diastolic blood pressure of 80 to 89 mm Hg as defined be the 2025 ACC/AHA high blood pressure guidelines in an adult. Refer to Chapter 9 for pediatric parameters.
Hyperthermia Generalized or localized excessive warming of the skin; body temperature that exceeds 101.5°F or 38.5°C.
Hypertrophy Increase in muscle size due to an increase in the bulk of muscle fibers.
Hypesthesia Diminished sense of touch; also called hypoesthesia.
Hyphema Condition in which there is blood in the anterior chamber of the eye.
Hypoesthesia *See* **Hypesthesia**.
Hypogeusia Diminution of taste.
Hypoglycemia Decrease in serum glucose.
Hypokinetic Decreased movement.
Hypophoria Latent misalignment of the eye; a downward turning of the eye.
Hypospadias Congenital abnormality in which the urethral meatus lies on the ventral surface of the penis.
Hypotension Blood pressure that is lower than what is needed to maintain adequate tissue perfusion and oxygenation.
Hypothermia Generalized or localized cooling of the skin; body temperature that is below 95.2°F or 35°C.
Hypotonicity Decrease in normal muscle tone (flaccidity).

I

Id Personality component that is inborn, unconscious, and driven by biological instincts and urges to seek immediate gratification of needs such as hunger, thirst, and physical comfort.
Immediate Auscultation *See* **Direct Auscultation**.
Immediate Percussion *See* **Direct Percussion**.
Indirect Fist Percussion Using the closed ulnar aspect of the fist of the dominant hand to strike the nondominant hand to elicit tenderness over specific body areas on the client.
Indirect Inguinal Hernia Portions of the bowel or omentum that enter the inguinal canal through the internal inguinal ring and exit at the external inguinal ring.
Indirect (Mediate) Auscultation Active listening to body sounds via some amplification or mechanical device, such as a stethoscope or Doppler transducer.
Indirect (Mediate) Percussion Using the plexor to strike the pleximeter to elicit sound.
Infarction (Myocardial) Necrosis of cardiac muscle due to decreased blood supply.

Inferior Angle of Scapula Thoracic landmark located at the inferior border of the scapula; this level corresponds to the seventh rib or intercostal space.

Injection Redness around the cornea.

Inspection Use of one's senses to consciously observe the client; in physical examination, vision, hearing, smell, and touch are used.

Insufficiency *See* **Regurgitation**.

Integument Skin, or cutaneous tissue.

Intensity (of Percussion) Relative loudness or softness of sound; amplitude.

Intercostal Space Area between the ribs.

Intermediary Individual who assists with communication between the client and another individual, usually a member of the health-care team.

Interpleural Space *See* **Mediastinum**.

Intersex Describes a group of congenital conditions in which the reproductive organs, genitals, and/or other sexual anatomy do not develop according to traditional expectations for females or males. Intersex can also be used as an identity term for someone with one of these conditions. The medical community sometimes uses the term differences of sex development to describe intersex conditions; however, the term intersex is recommended by several intersex community members and groups.

Interval (Follow-Up) Health History History that builds on the client's last health-care visit and documents resolution or nonresolution of a problem or health-care need.

Intussusception Formation of a sausage-shaped mass in the upper abdomen that results when the ileocecal region of the intestine telescopes into the ileum.

Iris Most anterior portion of the uveal tract; provides a distinctive color for the eye.

Ischemia (Myocardial) Local and temporary lack of blood supply to the heart; may progress to an infarction if left untreated.

Isoelectric Line Electrical resting period after the T wave on the electrocardiogram.

Isthmus (of the Thyroid) Narrow portion of the thyroid gland that connects the two lobes and lies over the tracheal rings.

Isthmus (of the Uterus) Constricted area between the body of the uterus and the cervix.

J

Jaundice Yellow-green to orange cast or coloration of skin, sclera, or mucous membranes; caused by an elevated bilirubin level.

Joining Stage Introduction or first stage of the interview process, during which the nurse and client establish rapport.

Joint Union between two bones.

Justice To be fair and impartial to the client..

K

Kilocalorie Amount of heat required to raise 1 gram of water 1 degree centigrade; also called calorie.

Knock-Knees *See* **Genu Valgum**.

Korotkoff Sounds Sounds generated when the flow of blood through an artery is altered by the inflation of a blood pressure cuff around an extremity.

Kussmaul Respirations Respirations characterized by extreme increased rate and depth, as in diabetic ketoacidosis.

Kwashiorkor Severe protein malnutrition usually seen in children in developing countries.

Kyphosis Excessive convexity of the thoracic spine; known as "humpback."

L

Labia Majora Two longitudinal folds of adipose and connective tissue that extend from the clitoris anteriorly and gradually narrow to merge and form the commissure of the perineum posteriorly.

Labia Minora Two thin folds of skin that enclose the vulval vestibule and extend to form the prepuce, or hood, of the clitoris anteriorly and a transverse fold of skin that forms the fourchette posteriorly.

Labyrinth Bony and membranous system of interconnecting tubes in the inner ear; essential for hearing and equilibrium.

Lacrimal Apparatus Lacrimal gland and ducts.

Lactiferous Ducts Openings at the nipple through which milk and colostrum are excreted.

Lagophthalmos Condition in which the client is unable to completely close the eyelid.

Lanugo Fine, downy hair present during gestational life, which gradually disappears toward the end of pregnancy; it remains in smaller quantities over the temples, back, shoulders, and upper arms after birth.

Lens Crystalline structure of the eye that changes shape to refract light from various focusing distances.

Lesbian A sexual orientation that describes a woman who is primarily emotionally and physically attracted to other women.

Lesion Circumscribed, pathological change in tissue.

Lichenification Localized thickening, hardening, and roughness of the skin; can be a result of chronic pruritus.
Life-Event or Transitional Developmental Theory Belief that development occurs in response to specific events, such as new roles (e.g., parenthood), and life transitions (e.g., career changes).
Lift *See* **Heave**.
Ligament Strong, fibrous, connective tissue that connects bones to each other at a joint.
Light Palpation Superficial palpation; depressing the skin ⅜ inch (1 cm) to elicit information on skin texture and moisture, masses, fluid, muscle guarding, and superficial tenderness.
Lightening Descent of the presenting fetal part into the pelvis.
Limbus Junction of the sclera and cornea.
Linea Alba Tendinous tissue that extends from the sternum to the symphysis pubis in the middle of the abdomen.
Linea Nigra Darkening of the abdominal linea alba during pregnancy.
Linear Raphe Linear ridge in the middle of the hard palate.
Lipoma Nonmobile, fatty mass with a smooth, circular edge.
List Leaning of the spine.
Listening Response Attempt made by the nurse to accurately receive, process, and respond to the client's messages.
Lobes (of the Breast) Glandular breast tissue arranged radially in the form of 12 to 20 spokes.
Lobules (of the Breast) Grapelike bunches that are clustered around several lactiferous ducts; each lobe is composed of 20 to 40 lobules that contain milk-producing glands called alveoli or acini.
Lordosis Excessive concavity of the lumbar spine.
Low-Density Lipoprotein Substance that carries cholesterol toward the heart.
Lunula White, crescent-shaped area at the proximal end of each nail.
Lymph Node (Lymph Gland) Bean-shaped structures of the immune system that are located throughout the body that filter lymphatic fluid, protect the body from pathogens and recognize and remove abnormal cells.
Lymphatic Drainage Yellow, alkaline drainage originating in the lymph vessels and composed primarily of lymphocytes.
Lymphedema A condition in which the lymphatic system is obstructed and localized swelling occurs.
Lymphocyte White blood cell that plays a key role in the body's immune system.

M

Macromineral Major mineral needed by the body in large amounts.
Macrosomia Newborn weighing more than 4,000 grams.
Macula Tiny, darker area in the temporal area of the retina. It is responsible for central vision.
Manubriosternal Junction *See* **Angle of Louis**.
Manubrium Upper bone of the sternum; articulates with the clavicles and the first pair of ribs.
Marasmus Extreme protein calorie malnutrition in which the body has little fat and muscle stores primarily seen in children in developing countries.
Mast Cells Body's major source of tissue histamine, which triggers the body's reaction to invasive allergens.
Mastectomy Excision, or surgical removal, of the breast.
Matrix Undifferentiated epithelial tissue from which keratinized cells arise to form the nail plate.
McBurney Point Anatomic location that is approximately at the normal location of the appendix in the right lower quadrant; point of increased tenderness in appendicitis.
Meconium Dark-green, sticky, stool-like material excreted from the rectum of the newborn within the first 24 hours after birth.
Mediastinum (Interpleural Space) Area between the lungs.
Mediate Auscultation *See* **Indirect Auscultation**.
Mediate Percussion *See* **Indirect Percussion**.
Medullary Cavity Interior of the diaphysis; contains the bone marrow.
Melanocytes Cells that produce pigmented substances that provide color to the hair, skin, and choroid of the eye.
Melasma Irregular pigmentation on the face due to pregnancy; also known as chloasma.
Melena Black, tarry stool.
Menarche Onset of menstruation.
Menopause Cessation of menstruation.
Menorrhagia Heavy menses.
Metabolic Syndrome Cluster of conditions that if present, cumulatively increase the risk of an adult developing cardiovascular disease and diabetes.
Metatarsus Varus Medial forefoot misalignment.
Microcephaly Small brain with a resultant small head.
Micromineral Trace mineral needed by the body in small amounts.
Microphallus Small penis for developmental stage.
Mid-Arm Circumference Anthropometric measurement that provides information on skeletal muscle mass and adipose tissue.

Mid-Arm Muscle Circumference Anthropometric measurement derived from mid-arm circumference; provides information on skeletal muscle mass and adipose tissue.

Midaxillary Line Vertical line drawn from the apex of the axilla; lies midway between the anterior and the posterior axillary lines.

Midclavicular Line Vertical line drawn from the midpoint of the clavicle.

Midspinal (Vertebral) Line Vertical line drawn from the midpoint of the spinous processes.

Midsternal Line Vertical line drawn from the midpoint of the sternum.

Milia Plugged sebaceous glands manifesting as small, white papules and appearing on the infant's head, especially on the cheeks and nose.

Milk Line Ectodermal galactic band that develops from the axilla to the groin during the fifth week of fetal development.

Mineral Inorganic element that regulates body processes and builds body tissue; classified into macrominerals and microminerals.

Miotic Describes a pupil that constricts to less than 2 mm in diameter.

Molding Condition in which the newborn's parietal bone overrides the frontal bone as a result of increased pressure during delivery.

Monotheism Belief in one all-powerful, omnipresent, and omnipotent God.

Monounsaturated Fats Fatty acids that contain one double bond between carbon atoms.

Mons Pubis Pad of subcutaneous fatty tissue lying over the anterior symphysis pubis.

Montgomery Tubercles Sebaceous glands present on the surface of the areola.

Multicultural Identity Unique combination of cultural influences that results from membership in a variety of subcultures within the primary culture.

Mydriatic Describes a pupil that dilates to more than 6 mm in diameter.

Myopia Nearsightedness.

N

Nabothian Cysts Small, round, yellow cystic lesions on the cervical surface.

Nail Plate Tissue that covers and protects the distal portion of the fingers and toes.

Nail Root Nail portion that is posterior to the cuticle and attached to the matrix.

Nailbed Vascular bed located beneath the nail plate.

Naturalistic Illness Illness believed to be caused by an imbalance or disequilibrium between essentially impersonal factors (e.g., hot and cold).

Neologism Word coined by a client that is meaningful only to the client.

Neuropathic Pain Pain that results from lesions in the central nervous system or the peripheral nervous system.

Nevi Pigmented moles that may be flat or elevated.

Nipple A round, hairless, pigmented protrusion of erectile tissue approximately ¼ to ⅝ inches (0.5 to 1.5 cm) in diameter located in the center of the breast.

Nitrogen Component of amino acids and proteins.

Nociception A multistep process that involves the nervous system and other body systems in perceiving pain.

Nociceptive Pain Pain that arises from somatic or visceral stimulation.

Nociceptors Receptive neurons of pain sensation that are located in the skin and various viscera.

Nociplastic Pain Pain that "arises from altered nociception despite no clear evidence of actual or threatened tissue damage causing the activation of peripheral nociceptors or evidence for disease or lesion of the somatosensory system causing the pain" (IASP, 2017).

Nocturia Excessive urination at night.

Nonbinary Individuals who do not identify with one specific gender, instead view themselves as somewhere on the spectrum and may also identify as gender-fluid, whereby, gender identity may change across the life span of the individual.

Nonmaleficence To do no harm to the client.

Nonverbal Communication Communicating a message without using words.

Nulliparous Descriptor for a woman who has not given birth.

Numeric Rating Scale Pain assessment tool that uses a numeric scale to rate pain.

Nutrient Substance found in food that is nourishing and/or useful to the body.

Nutrition Processes of the human body that metabolize and utilize nutrients.

Nystagmus Involuntary oscillation of the eye.

O

Obesity Having a body mass index of 30 gm/m^2 or higher.

Object Permanence Ability to form a mental image of an object and to recognize that, although removed from view, the object still exists.

Objective Data Data that are tangible or visible and can be corroborated by others; unbiased data not based on opinion or feeling.

Obturator Sign Differential technique for assessing appendicitis; indicative of an irritated obturator internus muscle.

Oedipus Complex Boys' sexual attraction toward their mothers and feelings of rivalry toward their fathers.

Oogenesis Development and formation of an ovum.

Optic Disc Round area on the nasal side of the retina, where retinal fibers join to form the optic nerve.

Orchitis Acute onset of testicular swelling.

Orthopnea Difficulty breathing except in an upright position.

Orthostatic Hypotension Hypotension that occurs when changing positions such as from a supine to an upright position.

Ossicles Three tiny bones in the middle ear that play a crucial role in the transmission of sound: the malleus, the incus, and the stapes.

Osteoporosis Disease characterized by reduced bone density and mass leading to weak, fragile bones.

Otitis Media Inflammation or infection of the middle ear.

Ovaries Pair of almond-shaped glands, approximately 1¼ to 1⅝ inches (3 to 4 cm) in length, in the upper pelvic cavity; oogenesis and hormonal production are the ovaries' principal functions.

P

Pack/Year History Term used to describe the quantity of cigarettes smoked over a period of time.

Paganism A nonmonotheistic religion or belief system whose principles reflect an animistic, and usually polytheistic, spirit-filled orientation.

Pain An "unpleasant sensory or emotional experience associated with actual or potential tissue damage, or described in terms of such damage" (IASP, 1979).

Pallor Lack of color.

Palpation Touching the client in a diagnostic manner to elicit specific information.

Palpebral Conjunctiva Mucous membrane covering the interior surface of the eyelid.

Palpebral Fissure Opening between the eyelids.

Palpitation Irregular and rapid heartbeat, or sensation of fluttering of the heart.

Pansystolic *See* **Holosystolic**.

Pantheism A religion in which God is believed to be in everything that exists; that God is the world and the world is God.

Papilla Small projection on the dorsal surface of the tongue that contains openings to taste buds.

Papillary Layer Upper layer of the dermis; composed primarily of loose connective tissue, small elastic fibers, and an extensive network of capillaries that serve to nourish the epidermis.

Paranasal Sinuses Air-filled cavities in the cranial bones that are lined with mucous membranes.

Paraphimosis Condition in which the retracted foreskin develops a fixed constriction proximal to the glans penis.

Paraurethral Glands *See* **Skene Glands**.

Paresthesia An abnormal sensation such as numbness, pricking, or tingling.

Parietal Pericardium Pericardial layer that lies close to the fibrous tissues.

Parietal Pleura Lining of the chest wall and the superior surface of the lungs.

Parous Descriptor for a woman who has given birth to one or more neonates.

Past Health History History that covers the client's health from birth to the present.

Pastoral Care Care and response needed when a person is in spiritual crisis.

Peau d'Orange Thickening or edema of the breast tissue or nipple; may present as enlarged skin pores that give the appearance of an orange rind.

Pectus Carinatum Abnormal thorax configuration in which there is a marked protrusion of the sternum; known as "pigeon chest."

Pectus Excavatum Abnormal thorax configuration in which there is a depression in the lower body of the sternum; known as "funnel chest."

Penis Cylindrical male organ of copulation and urination.

Penis Envy Young girls' desire to have a penis.

Percussion Striking one object against another to cause vibrations that produce sound used to evaluate underlying structures.

Pericarditis Inflammation of the pericardium.

Perineum External surface located between the fourchette and the anus.

Peripheral Vasculature Resistance Opposing force against which the left ventricle must contract to pump blood into the aorta; also known as systemic vascular resistance or afterload.

Periungual Tissue Tissue that surrounds the nail plate and the free edge of the nail.

Personalistic Illness Illness that is believed to occur either because an individual committed some offense and is being punished, or because of acts of aggression (sometimes unintentional) by other individuals.

Pertinent Negatives Manifestations that might be expected to be present in the client with a suspected pathology but that are denied by the client or are absent.

Pes Cavus Foot with an exaggerated height to the arch.

Pes Planus Foot with a low, longitudinal arch; also known as flatfoot.
Pes Valgus Foot that is turned laterally away from the midline.
Pes Varus Foot that is turned inward toward the midline.
Petechiae Reddish-purple skin discoloration that is less than ¼ inch (0.5 cm) in diameter and does not blanch.
Peyer's Patches Clusters of lymphatic nodules that line the ileum of the small intestine.
Phimosis Constriction of the distal penile foreskin that prevents normal retraction over the glans.
Phoria Latent misalignment of an eye.
Physiologic Cup Pale, central area of the optic disc.
Physiological Weight Loss Tendency of a neonate to lose approximately 10% of birth weight within a few days after birth and to regain it by 2 weeks of age.
Pica Craving for substances other than food (e.g., dirt, clay, starch, ice cubes).
Pinguecula Yellow nodule on the nasal, or temporal, side of the bulbar conjunctiva.
Pinna External flap of the ear; also called the auricle.
Pitch (of Percussion) Highness or lowness of a sound.
Plagiocephaly A unilateral flattened head or back of the head caused by placing the infant in the same position over a prolonged period of time.
Pleura Serous sac that encases the lung.
Pleural Friction Fremitus Palpable grating that feels more pronounced on inspiration when there is an inflammatory process between the pleura.
Pleximeter Stationary finger of the nondominant hand used in indirect percussion.
Plexor Middle finger of the dominant hand used to strike the pleximeter to elicit sound in indirect percussion.
Polycythemia Elevated number of red blood cells.
Polydactyly Extra digits on the hand or foot.
Polypharmacy The simultaneous use of numerous medications to treat medical conditions.
Polytheism Belief in many gods of different levels of power and status.
Posterior Axillary Line Vertical line drawn from the posterior axillary fold.
Posterior Chamber Space immediately posterior to the iris.
Posterior Triangle Area of the neck between the sternocleidomastoid and the trapezius muscles, with the clavicle at the base; contains the posterior cervical lymph nodes.
Prealbumin The transport protein for thyroxine and retinol-binding protein; also called thyroxine-binding prealbumin.
Precordium Anterior area of the body that lies over the heart, its great vessels, the pericardium, and some pulmonary tissue.
Prediabetes A clinical state of hyperglycemia that places the individual at risk for developing diabetes and heart disease, but the blood glucose levels are not yet high enough to classify as diabetes.
Prejudice Negative, harmful preconceived attitudes, beliefs directed toward an individual, group, culture, gender, or behavior, which limits accurate perceptions. Examples of prejudice include homophobia, Islamophobia, and antisemitism.
Preload Resting force on the myocardium as determined by the pressure in the ventricles at the end of diastole.
Prepuce Foreskin covering the glans penis.
Presbycusis Hearing loss commonly found in older individuals.
Presbyopia Impaired near vision occurring in middle-aged or older individuals.
Priapism Abnormal prolonged penile erection unrelated to sexual desire.
Prognathism A protruding upper jaw, lower jaw, or both.
Proprioception Position sense.
Prostate Glandular organ that lies anterior to the wall of the rectum and encircles the urethra; an accessory male sex organ.
Protein Group of complex nitrogenous compounds, each containing amino acids.
Proteinuria Presence of protein in the urine.
Prurigo Itchy skin eruptions of unknown cause.
Pruritus Severe itching.
Pterygium Triangular, yellow thickening of the bulbar conjunctiva, extending from the nasal side of the cornea to the pupil.
Ptosis Drooping of the eyelid.
Ptyalism Excessive secretion of saliva.
Puddle Sign Percussion technique that identifies an ascitic abdomen.
Pulse Palpable expansion of an artery in response to cardiac functioning; used to determine heart rate, rhythm, and estimated volume of blood being pumped by the heart.
Pulse Deficit Apical pulse rate greater than the radial pulse rate; occurs when some heart contractions are too weak to produce a palpable pulse at the radial site.
Pulse Pressure Difference between systolic and diastolic blood pressures.
Pulsus Paradoxus Pathological decrease in systolic blood pressure by 10 mm Hg or more on inspiration.
Puncta Opening at the inner canthus of the eye through which tears drain.

Pupil Opening in the center of the iris; regulates the amount of light entering the eye.
Purpura Condition characterized by the presence of confluent petechiae or confluent ecchymosis over any part of the body.

Q

Quality (of Percussion) Timbre; how a sound is perceived musically.
Queer An umbrella term describing people who think of their sexual orientation or gender identity as outside of societal norms. Some people view the term *queer* as more fluid and inclusive than traditional categories for sexual orientation and gender identity. Although queer was historically used as a slur, it has been reclaimed by many as a term of empowerment. Nonetheless, some still find the term offensive.
Questioning Describes a person who is unsure about or is exploring their sexual orientation and/or gender identity.
Quickening First fetal movements felt by a pregnant woman.

R

Race Classification of individuals based on shared biological traits and physical characteristics such as skin color, physical features, and hair texture genetically inherited from biological ancestors, as a result of climate and diet.
Rash Cutaneous skin eruption that may be localized or generalized.
Reason for Seeking Health Care Problem or health-care need that brought the client to seek health care.
Rebound Tenderness Pain elicited during deep palpation, frequently associated with peritoneal inflammation or appendicitis.
Recommended Dietary Allowances Recommended amount of nutrients to be eaten daily; recommendations differ according to sex, age, and pregnancy or lactation status.
Rectal Prolapse Protrusion of the rectum through the anal orifice.
Rectocele Bulging of the posterior vaginal wall with a portion of the rectum.
Rectouterine Pouch Deep recess formed by the outer layer of the peritoneum; the lowest point in the pelvic cavity, encompassing the lower posterior wall of the uterus, the upper portion of the vagina, and the intestinal surface of the rectum.
Rectum Lower portion of the large intestine; passes downward in front of the sacrum.
Red Reflex Light reflection elicited from the retina in the ophthalmoscopic examination of the eye.
Reepithelialization Reformation of epithelium over denuded skin.
Regurgitation Backward flow of blood through a diseased heart valve; also known as insufficiency.
Resonance Descriptor for a percussible sound that is loud in intensity, moderate to long in duration, low in pitch, hollow, and normally located in healthy lungs.
Respiration Act of breathing that supplies oxygen to the body and occurs in response to changes in the concentration of oxygen, carbon dioxide, and hydrogen in the arterial blood.
Reticular Layer Lower layer of the dermis that is formed by a dense bed of vascular connective tissue; it also includes nerves and lymphatic tissue.
Retina Innermost layer of the eye (an extension of the optic nerve).
Retromammary Adipose Tissue Tissue that composes the bulk of the breast.
Reversibility The understanding that an action need not be experienced or performed before one can anticipate the results or consequences of the action.
Review of Systems The client's subjective responses to a series of body system–related questions; serves as a double-check that vital information is not overlooked.
Rhonchal Fremitus Coarse, palpable vibration produced by the passage of air through thick exudate in the large bronchi or the trachea.
Rinne Test Method of evaluating hearing loss by comparing air and bone conduction with tuning fork vibrations.
Rod Retinal structure responsible for peripheral vision and dark or light discrimination.
Rovsing Sign Technique to elicit referred pain indicative of peritoneal inflammation.

S

Saturated Fats Lipids derived primarily from animal and other (e.g., butters, shortening, coconut oil) sources. Saturated fats are solid when at room temperature.
Scapular Line Vertical line drawn from the inferior angle of the scapula.
Scientific Illness Illness in which the presence of pathology is the defining characteristic.
Sclera Opaque covering of the eye; appears white.
Scoliosis Lateral curvature of the spine.
Scrotum Pouchlike supporting structure of the testes.
Sebaceous Glands Sebum-producing glands that are found almost everywhere in the dermis except the palmar and plantar surfaces.
Seborrhea Dandruff.
Sebum Oily secretion that is thought to retard evaporation and water loss from the epidermal surface.

Seizure Transient disturbance of cerebral function caused by an excessive discharge of neurons.

Semicircular Canals Anterior, posterior, and lateral canals in the bony labyrinth of the inner ear that provide balance and equilibrium.

Seminal Vesicles Paired pouches located posteriorly to and at the base of the bladder; fluid from here forms 60% of the volume of semen.

Septum (of the Heart) Wall that divides the left side of the heart from the right side.

Sequelae Aftermath.

Shifting Dullness Abnormal clinical finding elicited during abdominal percussion that detects ascites.

Sighing Normal respiration interrupted by a deep inspiration and followed by a deep expiration.

Sign Objective finding.

Sinoatrial Node Normal pacemaker of the heart; intrinsic adult rate is approximately 60 beats per minute.

Skene Glands (Paraurethral Glands) Glands that open in a posterolateral position to the urethral meatus and provide lubrication to protect the skin.

Skinfold Thickness Anthropometric measurement used to determine body fat stores and nutritional status.

Smegma White, cottage-cheeselike substance sometimes found under the female labia minora or the male foreskin.

Snap High-pitched sound that is heard in early diastole; usually occurs in mitral stenosis.

Snellen Chart Chart used for testing distance vision; contains letters of various sizes with standardized visual acuity numbers at the end of each line of letters.

Social Determinants of Heath Economic and social conditions that influence the health status of individuals and groups, e.g., achieved education, immigration status, employment/income, housing, access to health care, and the lived environment.

Social History Information related to the client's lifestyle that can impact health.

Spasticity Increase in muscle tension on passive stretching, especially rapid or forced stretching of a muscle.

Spermatic Cord Connective tissue sheath made up of arteries, nerves, veins, lymphatic vessels, and the cremaster muscle.

Spermatocele Well-defined cystic mass on the superior testes.

Spermatogenesis Production of sperm.

Sphygmomanometer Gauge used to measure blood pressure; consists of a blood pressure cuff with an inflatable bladder, connecting tubes, bulb air pump, and a manometer.

Spider Angioma Bright-red, star-shaped vascular marking that often has a central pulsation; it blanches in the extensions when pressure is applied.

Spinnbarkeit Elasticity of cervical mucus during ovulation.

Spirituality A private and personal form of religion, divorced from the rites, rituals, and codified beliefs of organized religion, usually concerned with the meaning and purpose of life.

Sputum Substance that is produced by the respiratory tract and can be expectorated or swallowed; composed of mucus, blood, purulent material, microorganisms, cellular debris, and, occasionally, foreign objects.

Squamocolumnar Junction Cervical area between the squamous epithelial surface and the columnar epithelial surface.

Standard Precautions Practices that health-care providers use to prevent the exchange of blood and body fluids when coming into contact with a client; outlined by the Centers for Disease Control and Prevention (CDC).

Steatorrhea Pale yellow, greasy, fatty stool.

Stenosis Narrowing or constriction (e.g., diseased heart valve).

Stensen Ducts Openings from the parotid glands; located just opposite the upper second molars.

Stereognosis Ability to identify objects by manipulating and touching them.

Stereotyping Classifying individuals/groups based upon culture/race with rigid, characteristics, while failing to recognize individual/group variations.

Sternal Angle *See* **Angle of Louis**.

Strabismus Deviation of gaze due to extraocular muscle dysfunction; the eyes do not align when looking at an object.

Stratum Corneum Horny layer; outer layer of the epidermis.

Stratum Germinativum Basal cell layer; deepest layer of the epidermis.

Stratum Granulosum Epidermal layer where skin cell death occurs; overlays the stratum spinosum.

Stratum Lucidum Additional skin layer found exclusively on the palmar and plantar surfaces.

Stratum Spinosum Epidermal layer that overlays the stratum germinativum and consists of layers of polyhedral cells.

Stress Physiologically defined response to changes that disrupt the resting equilibrium of an individual.

Striae Atrophic lines or scars commonly found on the abdomen, breasts, thighs, or buttocks.

Striae Gravidarum Stretch marks that occur in pregnancy.

Subculture Group of people whose values and experiences differ from those in the dominant culture, with whom they identify.

Subcutaneous Tissue Superficial fascia composed of loose areolar connective tissue or adipose tissue, depending on its location in the body; lies below the dermis.
Subjective Data Information perceived by the client to be real; such data cannot always be verified by an independent observer.
Subluxation Partial dislodgement of a bone from its place in the joint cavity.
Sulcus Terminalis Midline depression separating the anterior two-thirds from the posterior one-third of the tongue.
Superego Personality component that represents the internalization of the moral values formed as children interact with their parents and significant others.
Supernumerary Nipples Extra nipples or breast tissue along the milk line resulting from incomplete atrophy of the galactic band.
Suprasternal Notch Visible and palpable depression in the midsternal line superior to the manubrium.
Sutures Immovable joints connecting the cranial bones.
Sweat Glands Glands that produce perspiration; composed of two types: eccrine and apocrine glands.
Symptom Subjective finding.
Syncope Fainting; transient loss of consciousness due to decreased oxygen or glucose supply to the brain.
Syndactyly Fusion between two or more digits on the hand or foot.
Synovial Effusion Excessive synovial joint fluid.
Systemic Vascular Resistance *See* **Peripheral Vasculature Resistance**.
Systole Phase in the cardiac cycle during which the myocardial fibers contract and tighten to eject blood from the ventricles; correlates with the first Korotkoff sound.

T

Tachycardia Pulse rate greater than 100 beats per minute in an adult.
Tachypnea Respiratory rate greater than 20 breaths per minute in an adult.
Tactile (Vocal) Fremitus Palpable vibration of the chest wall that is produced by the spoken word.
Tail of Spence Upper outer quadrant of the breast that extends into the axilla.
Talipes Equinovarus (Clubfoot) Medially adducted and inverted toes and forefoot.
Tangential Lighting Light that is shone at an angle on the client to accentuate shadows and highlight subtle findings.
Tarsal Plates Connective tissue that gives shape to the upper eyelid.
Telehealth Telehealth is the delivery of health-care services remotely through the use of telecommunication technology. It can include both audio and audiovisual components.
Telenursing Telenursing is the use of telehealth to deliver health care.
Temperature Vital sign collected to assess core body heat.
Tendons Epimysium ends that attach a muscle to a bone.
Terminal Hair Coarse body hair in the axillary and pubic areas as well as the eyebrows, eyelashes, scalp, and, in men, the chest and face.
Termination Stage Last segment of the interview process, during which information is summarized and validated.
Testes Pair of ovoid glands located in the scrotum.
Thelarche The beginning of breast development in puberty.
Thenar Eminence Rounded prominence at the base of the thumb.
Thoracic Expansion The extent and symmetry of chest wall expansion.
Thrill Vibration related to turbulent blood flow that feels similar to what one feels when a hand is placed on a purring cat.
Tilts Set of blood pressure values taken in supine, sitting, and standing positions.
Torticollis Lateral deviation of the neck; intermittent or sustained dystonic contraction of the muscles on one side of the neck.
Total Iron-Binding Capacity Amount of iron with which transferrin can bind.
Transferrin Protein that regulates iron absorption.
Transgender Describes a person whose gender identity and assigned sex do not correspond based on traditional expectations; for example, a person assigned female sex who identifies as a man; or a person assigned male sex who identifies as a woman. Transgender can also include people with gender identities outside the girl/woman and boy/man gender binary structure, for example, people who are gender fluid or nonbinary.
Transitional Developmental Theory *See* **Life-Event**.
Transmission-Based Precautions Infection control practices involving contact, droplet, and airborne transmission of microorganisms that are known to exist in a client or are suspected in a client. They are practiced in conjunction with Standard Precautions.
Triceps Skinfold Anthropometric measurement used to determine body fat stores and nutritional status.
Triglyceride Substance that accounts for most of the fat stored in the body's tissues.
True Ribs *See* **Vertebrosternal Ribs**.

Turbinate (Concha) Projection from the lateral wall of the nose that is covered with mucous membranes that greatly increase the surface area within the nose.

Turgor Elasticity of the skin; reflects the skin's state of hydration.

Tussive Fremitus Palpable vibration produced by coughing.

Twelfth Rib Posterior thoracic landmark.

Tympany Descriptor for a percussible sound that is loud in intensity, long in duration, of high pitch, drumlike, and normally located over a gastric air bubble.

U

Urethra Duct from the urinary bladder to the urethral meatus; carries urine and, in the male, semen.

Uterine (Fallopian) Tubes Female reproductive organs that extend from the cornu of the uterus to the ovaries and are supported by the broad ligaments. The site of egg fertilization.

Uterus Inverted, pear-shaped, hollow, muscular organ in which the impregnated ovum develops into a fetus.

Utilitarianism The duty to perform the greatest good for the greatest number of people.

Uvula Fingerlike projection hanging down from the center of the soft palate.

V

Vagina Pink, hollow, muscular tube extending from the cervix to the vulva, located posterior to the bladder and anterior to the rectum.

Vaginal Introitus Entrance to the vagina, situated at the inferior aspect of the vulval vestibule.

Value Orientation Patterned principles (time, human nature, activity, relations, and people-to-nature) that provide order and give direction to an individual's thoughts and behaviors related to the solution of commonly occurring human problems.

Varicocele Bluish mass resulting from abnormal dilation of the veins of the pampiniform plexus of the spermatic cord.

Vas Deferens *See* **Ductus (Vas) Deferens**.

Vellus Hair Fine, faint hair that covers most of the body.

Venous Hum Continuous, medium-pitched sound originating in the inferior vena cava and associated with obstructed portal circulation.

Venous Star Linear or irregularly shaped, blue vascular pattern on the skin; does not blanch when pressure is applied.

Veracity To be truthful to the client.

Vernix Caseosa Protective integumentary mechanism of the newborn; consists of sebum and shed epithelial cells.

Vertebra Prominens The long spinous process of the seventh cervical vertebra.

Vertebral Line *See* **Midspinal Line**.

Vertebrosternal (True) Ribs Rib pairs 1 to 7; articulate via the costal cartilage to the sternum.

Vertigo Dizziness or lightheadedness.

Vestibule Boat-shaped area between the labia minora and containing the urethral meatus, the openings of Skene glands, the hymen, the openings of Bartholin glands, and the vaginal introitus.

Vestibule (of the Ear) Part of the inner ear located between the cochlea and the semicircular canals.

Visceral Pericardium Pericardial layer that lies against the heart muscle.

Visceral Pleura Lining of the external surface of the lungs.

Vital Signs Measurements, including temperature, pulse, respirations, and blood pressure, that provide an index of a client's physiological status.

Vitamin Organic substance needed to maintain the function of the body.

Vitiligo Patchy, symmetrical areas of white on the skin.

Vitreous Humor Gelatinous material that fills the center cavity of the eye; helps maintain the shape of the eye and the position of the internal structures.

Vocal Fremitus *See* **Tactile Fremitus**.

Voice Sounds An examination skill used to assess whether the lungs are filled with air or fluid, or are solid.

W

Water-Soluble Vitamin Vitamin soluble in water; is not stored in the body but is excreted in the urine.

Weber Test Tuning fork test to evaluate hearing loss and determine whether the loss is conductive or sensorineural.

Wharton Ducts Openings from the submaxillary glands; located on either side of the frenulum.

Whispered Pectoriloquy Use of a voice sound, where the client whispers the words "ninety-nine" or "one, two, or three," to determine if the lungs are filled with air or fluid, or are solid.

Working Stage That segment of the interview process during which most data are collected.

X

Xanthelasma Creamy, yellow plaque on or around the eyelid caused by hypercholesterolemia.

Xerosis Excessive dryness of the skin.

Xiphoid Process Cartilaginous process at the base of the sternum; does not articulate with the ribs.

Y

Yang Traditional Chinese medicine term for "hot" forces.
Yin Traditional Chinese medicine term for "cold" forces.

+ The + sign refers to people who feel that none of the usual sexual-orientation categories, such as lesbian, gay, bisexual, transgender, etc., correctly identify their sexual or gender identity.

Index

A-V junction, 469
A-V nicking, 346
A-V node, 468, 469, 469f
A-V valve, 464–465
a wave, 513, 515
AAA. *See* Abdominal aortic aneurysm (AAA)
Abbreviations, 941b
ABCDE mnemonic, 279b
Abdomen, 533–572
- abdominal cavity, 533
- anatomical regions, 537f
- anatomy and physiology, 533–539
- assistive devices, 551b
- bladder, 539, 556, 558, 565
- bladder cancer, 556b
- case study (pancreatitis), 568–571
- colorectal cancer, 545b, 560b, 567b
- differentiating abdominal pain, 544t
- esophageal cancer, 548b
- four-quadrant anatomical map, 535t
- gallbladder, 539
- health history, 540–544
- hepatitis, 554–555b
- kidneys, 539, 558, 558f, 562, 562f, 563b
- large intestine, 537–538
- liver, 538–539, 560–561, 561f
- liver cancer, 560b
- musculature, 534f
- older adult client, 895, 915
- pancreas, 539
- pancreatic cancer, 556b
- pediatric client, 834, 868–870
- peritoneum, 533–534
- physical examination. *See* Abdominal examination
- pregnant client, 788, 805–806
- quadrants, 535f, 535t, 536–537t
- renal cancer, 562b
- small intestine, 535, 537
- spleen, 539, 556, 561
- stomach, 535, 556
- stomach cancer, 555b
- USPSTF recommendations, 567b
- vasculature, 534, 535f, 552f
- vermiform appendix, 539

Abdominal anatomical regions, 537f
Abdominal aortic aneurysm (AAA), 510t, 527b, 567b
Abdominal assistive devices, 551b
Abdominal ballottement, 565b, 565f
Abdominal cavity, 533
Abdominal cavity drain, 551b
Abdominal contours, 547, 547f
Abdominal distention, 547b
Abdominal examination
- abdominal distention, 547b
- abdominal inflammation, 563b, 563f
- abdominal mass, 565b, 565f
- abdominal muscle guarding, 559
- aorta, 562–563
- appendicitis, 563b, 564b
- ascites, 557f, 557t, 558b, 558f
- auscultation, 550–552
- ballottement, 565b, 565f
- bladder, 556, 558, 565, 565f
- bowel sounds, 550, 552
- cancer. *See* Abdomen
- cholecystitis, 561b
- contour, 547, 547f
- cutaneous hypersensitivity, 564b, 564f
- equipment, 547
- examination landmarks, 537f
- friction rubs, 552
- general approach, 546b
- inspection, 547–550
- kidneys, 558, 558f, 562, 562f, 563b
- liver, 560–561, 561f
- liver border, 554, 554f
- liver descent, 553–554
- liver span, 553, 553f
- masses and nodules, 549
- overview, 546
- palpation, 559–565
- pelvic abscess, 564b, 564f
- percussion, 552–559
- peristalsis, 549
- pigmentation and color, 548
- pulsation, 549
- rebound tenderness, 563b, 563f
- rectus abdominis muscles, 548
- respiratory movement, 549
- scars, 548–549, 548f
- spleen, 556, 556f, 561, 561f
- stomach, 556
- striae, 549, 549f
- symmetry, 547–548
- umbilicus, 550
- urinary incontinence, 565, 565–566b, 566f
- urinary tract infection (UTI), 566–567b
- vascular sounds, 552
- venous hum, 552

Abdominal examination landmarks, 537f
Abdominal inflammation, 563b, 563f
Abdominal mass, 565b, 565f
Abdominal muscle guarding, 559
Abdominal musculature, 534f
Abdominal pain, 541
Abdominal quadrants, 535f, 535t, 536–537t
Abdominal reflexes, 684, 684f
Abdominal scars, 548–549, 548f
Abdominal striae, 549, 549f
Abdominal vasculature, 534, 535f, 552f
Abducens nerve, 644t, 675
Abduction, 576t
ABI. *See* Ankle-brachial index (ABI)
Abstract reasoning, 663
Abuse. *See also* Sexual assault
- elder abuse and neglect, 916b
- pregnant client, 791b
- rectal, 774b
- sexual, 715b
- shaken baby syndrome, 858
- signs of, 265b

Acanthosis nigricans, 265, 265f
Accommodation, 341
Acculturation, 122
ACE. *See* Adverse childhood experiences (ACE)
Acetone (fruity) breath, 377
Achilles reflex, 683, 683f, 917
Achilles tendon rupture, 626b, 626f
Acini, 394
ACL. *See* Anterior cruciate ligament (ACL)
Acne papules and nodules, 273, 273f
Acne rosacea, 273, 273f
Acne scarring, 273, 273f
Acne vulgaris, 273
Acoustic nerve, 644t, 677
Acoustic stethoscope, 215, 215f
Acral lentiginous melanoma, 289
Acrochordon, 278
Acrocyanosis, 848, 848f
Acromegaly, 305, 305f, 585
Acromioclavicular joint separation, 601
ACS. *See* Acute coronary syndrome (ACS)
Actinic keratosis, 279, 279f, 910–911, 911f
Action responses
- collaborating, 31
- confronting, 31
- exploring, 30
- focusing, 30
- informing, 31
- limit setting, 31–32
- normalizing, 32
- presenting reality, 30–31

Action tremor, 590t
Active listening, 25
Acute arterial occlusion, 510t
Acute bacterial prostatitis, 776b
Acute confusion, 664t
Acute coronary syndrome (ACS), 474t, 482t
Acute otitis externa, 371, 372t

Acute otitis media (AOM), 371, 372*b*, 372*t*
Acute pain, 244, 248
ADA. *See* Americans with Disabilities Act (ADA)
Adams forward bend test, 629*b*
Adduction, 576*t*
Adie's pupil, 342*t*
Adnexa, 699, 728–729
Adolescents, 107–108. *See also* Pediatric client
  AAP blood pressure categories, 238, 238*t*
  alternative alcohol consumption, 878*b*
  calorie needs, 159*t*
  childhood fears, 831*b*
  developmental assessment tools, 113*t*, 114*t*
  developmental tasks, 108
  growth spurts, 222
  HEEADSSS 3.0 assessment, 840*b*
  immunization schedule, 839*t*
  inguinal hernia, 881
  milestones, 108*t*
  nutrition, 170–171, 170*b*, 171*f*
  physical growth, 824
  pulse rate, 228*t*
  respiratory rate, 226*t*
  STI education, 879*b*
Adoption, 850*b*
Adulthood
  developmental assessment tools, 113*t*, 114*t*, 115*t*
  late. *See* Older adult client
  middle. *See* Early middle adulthood; Late middle adulthood
  young. *See* Young adults
Advance medical directive, 48
Advance medical directives, 904
Advanced techniques, 929
Adventitious breath sounds, 449, 450*t*, 455*t*
Adverse childhood experiences (ACE), 101
Aerobic exercise, 72–73
AF. *See* Atrial fibrillation (AF)
Affect, 654
Affirmative care, 127
AFI. *See* Amniotic fluid index (AFI)
Afterload, 494
Age
  blood pressure, 238, 238*t*
  body temperature, 230
  ensuring accurate chronological age, 48*b*
  pain, 244
  pulse rate, 228*t*
  respiratory rate, 226*t*
  stated age vs. apparent age, 220–221
Ages and stages developmental theories, 92, 94–95*t*
Ages and Stages Questionnaire, 112*t*
Ageusia, 677
Aggravating factors, 51
Agnosia, 661
Agonal respirations, 434, 434*f*
Agoraphobia, 665*t*
Agraphia, 655
AI. *See* Artificial intelligence (AI)
Air conduction, 365, 366, 366*f*
Air trapping, 434*f*, 435
Airborne Precautions, 204*f*
Airborne transmission, 203
Ala nasi, 356, 358*f*
Albinism, 264, 264*f*
Albumin, 188
Alcohol assessment tools, 61
Alcohol use/abuse. *See also* Drug use/abuse
  alternative alcohol consumption, 878*b*
  grade B recommendations, 80*b*
  social history, 61, 62*b*
Alcohol Use Disorders Identification Test (AUDIT-C), 61, 62*b*, 114*t*, 118
Alexia, 655
Allen test, 523–524*b*, 524*f*
Allergic conjunctivitis, 337
Allergic contact dermatitis, 275, 275*f*
Allergic facies, 307, 307*f*
Allergic rhinitis, 307, 859
Allergic shiners, 307
Alleviating factors, 51, 51*b*
Ally, 38
Alopecia, 287, 709, 743
Alopecia areata, 287, 287*f*
Alopecia totalis, 288
Alphatocopherol, 161*t*
Alternative alcohol consumption, 878*b*
Alveoli, 394, 418*f*, 421
Amblyopia, 327
Amenorrhea, 704
American Nurses Association (ANA), 123
American Sign Language interpreter, 39
Americans with Disabilities Act (ADA)
  deafness, 39
  speech impairment, 40
  visual impairment, 39
Amniocentesis, 814*t*
Amniotic fluid index (AFI), 814*t*
Amphiarthroses, 577*t*
Amsler grid, 348*b*, 349*f*
ANA. *See* American Nurses Association (ANA)
ANA code of ethics, 930
ANA Standards of Professional Nursing Practice
  assessment, 6–8, 6*t*
  diagnosis, 6*t*, 8–9
  evaluation, 12–13
  implementation, 12
  outcomes identification, 6*t*, 10
  overview, 6*t*
  planning, 6*t*, 10–12
  respectful and equitable practice, 123–124
Anal canal, 763, 764*f*
Anal columns, 764, 764*f*
Anal culture, 726
Anal fissure, 771, 771*f*
Anal glands, 771
Anal incontinence, 766, 771
Anal orifice, 697, 763–764
Anal Pap, 772*b*
Anal psychosexual stage, 94*t*, 97
Anal reflex, 685
Anal sinuses, 764, 764*f*
Anal skin tags, 770
Anal sphincter, 764, 764*f*
Anal stenosis, 774*t*
Anal valves, 764, 764*f*
Anal wink, 685
Analgesia, 669
Analog stethoscope, 215
Anatomical snuff box, 605
Androgenetic alopecia, 287*f*
Anencephaly, 854*b*
Anergy, 187
Anesthesia, 669
Aneurysm, 510*t*
Angel kiss, 849
Angina, 465
Angioedema, 287*f*, 287*t*
Angle-closure glaucoma, 339
Angle of Louis, 420*b*
Angle of the ribs, 430–431, 431*f*, 453*t*
Angular cheilosis, 378, 378*f*
Animals in health-care setting, 203
Animism, 142
Anisocoria, 341, 342*t*
Ankle-brachial index (ABI), 524–525*b*
Ankle sprain
  anterior drawer test, 623*b*, 623*f*
  talar tilt test, 623*b*, 624*f*
Ankles and feet, 620–626
  anatomy, 621*f*
  ankle sprain, 623*b*, 623*f*, 624*f*
  callus, 623, 623*f*
  case study (numbness in hands and feet), 689–693
  corn, 622, 622*f*
  distal limbs and digits, 625*b*
  hallux valgus (bunion), 622, 622*f*
  hammertoe, 622, 622*f*
  ligaments of the ankle, 624*f*
  pes planus (flat feet), 622
  physical examination, 620–623
  ruptured Achilles tendon, 626*b*, 626*f*
  toe abnormalities, 622, 622*f*
Ankyloglossia, 380, 381*f*
Ankylosing spondylitis, 585
Annular lesions, 269*f*
Annuloaortic ectasia, 474*t*
Annulus, 355, 355*f*
Anoderm, 764
Anomic aphasia, 656*t*
Anorectal abscess, 771
Anorectal cancer, 775, 775*b*
Anorectal examination, 769–778. *See also* Anus, rectum, and prostate
  anal mucosa, 770–773
  anal Pap, 772*b*
  client positions, 769*b*, 769*f*
  documenting anal abnormalities, 771*b*
  equipment, 768
  general approach, 769*b*
  hemorrhoids, 770, 770*f*, 774, 774*f*, 778–781
  index finger, 773, 773*f*, 774*f*
  inspection, 769–773
  palpation, 773–777
  perineum and sacrococcygeal area, 769–770
  rectal abuse, 774*b*
  rectal bleeding, 774*b*
  stools, 774*t*
Anorectal fistula, 771, 771*f*, 775
Anorectum, 763
Anorexia nervosa, 170, 174
Anosmia, 672
ANS. *See* Autonomic nervous system (ANS)
Antalgic gait, 588*t*
Anteflexed uterus, 698*f*
Anterior axillary line, 420*b*
Anterior cerebral artery, 642*f*, 642*t*
Anterior chamber, 322, 339–340, 340*f*, 912
Anterior corticospinal tract, 641, 641*f*
Anterior cruciate ligament (ACL), 619*b*
Anterior drawer test, 618*b*, 618*f*, 623*b*, 623*f*

Anterior spinothalamic tract, 641, 642*f*
Anterior triangle, 299, 299*f*
Anteverted uterus, 698, 698*f*
Anthropometric measurements, 179–185
 body mass index (BMI), 182–183
 height, 181
 interpreting, 182*b*
 malnutrition, 184, 184*b*
 midarm and midarm muscle circumferences, 183–184
 skinfold thickness, 185, 185*f*
 standardized charts, 179
 uses, 179
 waist circumference/waist-to-hip ratio, 183
 weight, 181–182
Antibacterial stations, 199*b*, 201*f*
Anticipatory guidance, 167
Antiembolic stockings, 521*b*
Antigen skin testing, 187
Anus, rectum, and prostate, 763–782
 acute bacterial prostatitis, 776*b*
 anatomy and physiology, 763–765
 anorectal cancer, 775, 775*b*
 anus, 696*f*, 697*f*, 763–765, 771*b*
 benign prostatic hypertrophy (BPH), 776, 777*f*
 case study (enlarged prostate and hemorrhoid), 778–781
 head-to-toe examination, 939–940, 940*f*
 health history, 765–768
 older adult client, 898, 918
 pediatric client, 881–882
 physical examination. *See* Anorectal examination
 prostate, 764*f*, 765
 prostate cancer, 775*b*, 777, 777*b*, 777*f*
 PSA, 776*b*, 777*b*
 rectum, 763, 764*f*
 USPSTF recommendations, 778*b*
Anxiety disorders, 665–666*t*, 688*b*
Anxious or angry client, 41
AOM. *See* Acute otitis media (AOM)
Aorta, 534, 562–563
Aortic area, 483, 483*f*
 auscultation, 489
 inspection, 484
 palpation, 486
Aortic dissection, 482*t*, 510*t*
Aortic ejection click, 490*f*
Aortic regurgitation or insufficiency, 474*t*, 495*t*
Aortic stenosis (AS), 474*t*, 476*t*, 489, 495*t*
Apgar score, 847–848, 848*t*
Aphasia, 655, 656*t*
Aphonia, 655
Aphthous ulcer, 380, 380*f*, 382
Apical impulse, 486*b*, 487, 487*f*, 864
Apical pulse, 227, 228, 228*f*
Apley grinding sign, 617*b*, 617*f*
Apnea, 226, 433, 434*f*
Apneustic respirations, 433, 434*f*
Apocrine glands, 253*f*, 254
Appendicitis, 563*b*, 564*b*
Appendicular skeleton, 574, 574*f*
Appendix, 506*f*, 534*f*
Apraxia, 655, 662
Apraxic gait, 588*t*
Arachnoid mater, 638, 638*f*
Arachnoid villi, 638, 638*f*
Arcus senilis, 339, 339*f*
Areola, 393, 393*f*
Argyll Robertson pupil, 342*t*
Arrector pili muscle, 253*f*, 254
Arrhythmia, 229, 469, 474*t*
Arterial hypertension, 489
Arterial insufficiency, 520*b*, 521*t*
Arterial pulse examination, 516–518
Arterial ulceration, 519, 519*f*
Arteries, 503, 504*f*
Arterioles, 502–503
Arteriosclerosis, 239
Arteriovenous (A-V) nicking, 346
Arthritis, 222
Artifacts, 129
Artificial cardiac pacemaker, 495–496*b*
Artificial intelligence (AI), 931
Ascites, 557*f*, 557*t*, 558*b*, 558*f*
Ascorbic acid, 163*t*
ASD. *See* Atrial septal defect (ASD)
Asexual, 38
Asian clients, 61*b*
Assessment
 advanced techniques, 929
 ANA Standard, 6–8
 assistive devices, 933*b*
 cultural, 134, 135*t*
 growth and development. *See* Developmental assessment
 nutrition. *See* Nutritional assessment
 overview, 6*t*
 putting it all together. *See* Complete health history and physical examination
 religion. *See* Spiritual assessment
 verifying assessment data, 933*b*
Assistive devices, 77
Associated manifestations, 51
Asterixis, 590*t*
Asthma, 453–455*t*, 456*f*
Asymptomatic bacteriuria, 806
Asystole, 228, 229
Ataxic respirations, 433
Atelectasis, 446, 453–455*t*, 456*f*
Atherosclerosis, 171, 474*t*
Athetosis, 590*t*
Athlete's foot, 272
Athletic evaluation, 942–943. *See also* Sports
Atlas, 299, 299*f*
Atopic dermatitis, 275, 849, 849*f*
Atrial fibrillation (AF), 469*b*
Atrial kick, 468
Atrial septal defect (ASD), 478*t*
Atrial systole, 467*f*, 468
Atrioventricular canal defect, 479*t*
Atrioventricular (A-V) node, 468
Atrioventricular septal defect, 479*t*
Atrioventricular (A-V) valve, 464–465
Atrophic testicle, 743, 752
Atrophic vaginitis, 726
Atrophy, 271*f*, 589, 589*f*
Attention, 659–660
AUDIT-C, 61, 62*b*, 114*t*, 118
Augmentation mammoplasty, 411
Auricle, 354, 355*f*
Auricular tophi, 367, 367*f*
Auscultation, 215–216
Auscultatory gap, 240*t*
Autism, 224
Autoerotic experience, 66*b*
Autonomic nervous system (ANS), 643, 645
Autonomy, 929
Autonomy vs. shame and doubt stage, 94*t*, 98
Awake tummy time, 831*b*
Awareness, 656
Axial skeleton, 574, 574*f*
Axillary thermometer, 231*t*, 233, 233*f*, 844

B cells, 506, 507*f*
Babinski reflex, 686, 875, 876*f*
Baby Boomers, 889
Bachmann bundle, 468, 469*f*
Bacterial sinusitis, 374
Bacterial vaginosis (BV), 713, 713*t*, 725
Bad breath, 223
Bad news, 939*b*
Bag of worms, 739, 752
BAI. *See* Beck Anxiety Inventory (BAI)
Baker cyst, 616*b*, 617*f*
Balanitis, 744, 744*f*
Ball and socket joint, 577*t*
Ballism, 590*t*
Ballottement
 abdominal examination, 565*b*, 565*f*
 patellar, 616–617*b*, 617*f*
Barlow maneuver, 872, 873
Baroreceptors, 235, 519*b*
Barrel chest, 428, 428*f*
Bartholin glands, 697
Bartholinitis, 715*f*
Basal cell carcinoma (BCC)
 generally, 279, 279*f*
 older adult client, 911, 911*f*
 physical examination, 378, 379*f*
 risk factors, 280*b*
Basal ganglia, 638
Basilar artery, 642*f*, 642*t*
Battle's sign, 367
BCC. *See* Basal cell carcinoma (BCC)
BDI. *See* Beck Depression Inventory (BDI)
BE FAST, 657*b*
Beau lines, 291, 292*f*
Beck Anxiety Inventory (BAI), 114*t*
Beck Depression Inventory (BDI), 113*t*
Bedridden client, 940*b*
Bell palsy, 306, 306*f*, 676, 676*f*
Beneficence, 929
Benign prostatic hypertrophy (BPH), 776, 777*f*
Bethesda system, 723
Biases, 123
Biceps reflex, 682–683, 682*f*
Biceps tendinitis, 601
Bicuspid aortic valve, 477*t*
Bicuspid valve, 465
Bigeminal pulse, 517*f*
Bilateral cataract, 343
Bilateral hypertrophy, 589
Bile, 539
Bilevel positive airway pressure (BiPAP), 438*b*
Biliary drain, 551*b*
Bimanual method of deep palpation, 559, 559*f*
Bimanual method of liver palpation, 560, 561*f*
Binge eating, 170
Biophysical profile, 814*t*
Biot respirations, 433, 434*f*

Biotin, 163*t*
Bipolar disorder, 667*t*
Birth. *See* Pregnant client
Birth defects, 840*b*
Bisexual, 38
Blackhead, 273
Bladder, 534*f*
  older adult client, 897
  physical examination, 556, 558, 565, 565*f*
  urine, 539
Bladder cancer, 566*b*
Blepharitis, 332, 332*f*
Blepharospasm, 332
Blindness vs. legal blindness, 331*b*
Blocking, 663
Blood pressure, 234–241
  AAP blood pressure categories, 238, 238*t*
  ACC/AHA guidelines, 238–239, 239*t*
  age, 238, 238*t*
  auscultatory gap, 240*t*
  automatic blood pressure measurement, 237–238, 238*f*
  baroreceptors, 235
  documenting BP, 237*b*
  equipment, 236, 236*f*
  errors in BP measurement, 240*t*
  example BP readings, 237*b*
  home monitoring devices, 235*b*
  hypertension. *See* Hypertension
  hypotension, 240
  Korotkoff sounds, 235
  manual blood pressure measurement, 236–237, 237*f*
  mean arterial pressure (MAP), 235
  measurement sites, 236
  older adult client, 891, 909–910
  palpation method, 238*b*
  pediatric client, 844*b*
  pregnant client, 787
  pulse pressure, 235, 239
  systolic/diastolic pressure, 235, 240*t*
Blood supply, 641, 642*t*
Bloody vomitus, 540
BMI. *See* Body mass index (BMI)
BMI calculator, 182–183
BNBAS. *See* Brazelton Neonatal Behavioral Assessment Scale (BNBAS)
Body and breath odors, 222–223
Body fat, 221–222
Body fat distribution, 183
Body mass index (BMI), 171, 182–183
Body Mass Index for Age growth chart, 824, 828*f*
Body Mass Index for Age Percentiles growth chart, 824, 829*f*
Body movements, 222
Body piercings, 262*b*, 263*f*
Body temperature. *See* Temperature
Bohn nodules, 861
Boil, 273, 273*f*
Bone conduction, 365, 366, 366*f*
Bone density scan, 191
Bones, 574
Bony labyrinth, 355
Bottled water, 166*f*
Bouchard node, 607, 607*f*
Bounding pulses, 229, 517*f*
Boutonnière deformity, 607, 607*f*
Bow legs (genu varum), 616, 616*b*, 616*f*, 872
Bowel sounds, 550, 552
BPH. *See* Benign prostatic hypertrophy (BPH)
Brace, 631*b*
Brachial-femoral lag, 868
Brachioradialis reflex, 682, 682*f*
Bradycardia, 228
Bradypnea, 226, 433, 434*f*
Brain, 638–639, 639*f*, 642*f*, 642*t*, 896
Brain death, 659*t*
Brainstem, 639, 639*f*
Braxton Hicks contractions, 790
Brazelton Neonatal Behavioral Assessment Scale (BNBAS), 112*t*
Breast asymmetry, 403, 403*f*. *See also* Breasts
Breast augmentation, 411
Breast cancer
  hereditary breast cancer syndromes, 397*t*
  incidence rates, 392
  long-term survival rates, 392
  males, 411, 412
  mastectomy, 409–410, 409*f*, 409*t*
  reconstruction techniques, 410
  risk factors, 397*t*
  screening, 400*t*, 412*b*
  types, 402*t*
  USPSTF recommendations, 400*t*, 412*b*
Breast discharge, 398, 404–405
Breast examination, 401–411. *See also* Breasts
  breast augmentation clients, 411
  breast self-examination (BSE), 410*b*, 410*f*
  chief complaint (health history), 398
  clinical breast examination (CBE), 405*b*
  color, 401–402
  consistency, 406
  contour, 403
  discharge, 398, 404–405
  general approach, 400*b*
  inspection, 401–405
  males, 412
  masses/lesions. *See* Breast mass
  mastectomy clients, 409–410, 409*f*, 409*t*
  palpation, generally, 405
  palpation, sitting position, 406, 406*f*
  palpation, supine position, 407–408, 408*f*
  positioning of client for inspection, 401, 401*f*, 402*f*
  pregnant and breastfeeding client, 408*b*
  size and symmetry, 403, 403*f*
  thickening/edema, 402
  vascularity, 402
Breast hypertrophy, 403, 403*f*
Breast mass
  case study, 412–414
  chief complaint (health history), 398
  common pathologies, 404*t*
  documenting breast mass characteristics, 409*b*
  generally, 403–404
Breast milk jaundice, 849
Breast reconstruction, 410
Breast self-examination (BSE), 410*b*, 410*f*
Breast tenderness, 398
Breasts, 392–416
  anatomy and physiology, 393–395
  benign breast disease, 405*b*
  breast development throughout life span, 395
  cancer. *See* Breast cancer
  case study (breast mass), 412–414
  examination. *See* Breast examination
  female, 392–414
  function of female breast, 394
  head-to-toe examination, 936–937, 937*f*
  health history, 396–399
  male, 395*b*, 411–412
  masses/lesions. *See* Breast mass
  older adult client, 894, 914
  pediatric client, 833
  pregnant client, 408*b*, 786, 786*b*, 804–805, 804*b*, 804*f*
  quadrants, 393–395
  sexual maturity rating (SMR), 395, 396*t*
  Tanner staging, 395, 396*t*
  transgender men, 395*b*
Breath sounds, 448–451, 455*t*, 863–864
Breech presentation, 810*f*, 812
Bregma, 298
Brief Pain Inventory, 248
Bristol Stool Form Scale, 538*b*, 538*f*
Broca aphasia, 656*t*
Broca area, 639*f*
Bronchi, 418*f*, 421
Bronchial breath sound, 448, 449*f*, 449*t*
Bronchiectasis, 453–455*t*, 456*f*
Bronchitis, 453–455*t*, 456*f*
Bronchophony, 452
Bronchovesicular breath sounds, 448, 449*f*, 449*t*, 863
Brudzinski sign, 688*b*
Bruit, 516, 518
Brushfield spots, 857
BSE. *See* Breast self-examination (BSE)
Buccal mucosa, 358, 381–382
Bulbar conjunctiva, 319, 336–337
Bulbocavernosus reflex, 685
Bulbourethral glands, 736, 736*f*
Bulge sign, 616*b*, 616*f*
Bulimia, 170
Bullae, 270*f*
Bundle branch system, 469
Bundle of His, 469, 469*f*
Bunion, 622, 622*f*
Burns, 283, 284*f*
Bursae, 575
BV. *See* Bacterial vaginosis (BV)

c wave, 513
Cachexia, 182, 182*f*, 307
Café au lait spots, 265, 265*f*, 281, 548
CAGE-AID assessment tool, 114*t*
CAGE assessment tool, 114*t*
Calcium (Ca), 164*t*, 624*b*
Calcium carbonate, 173*b*
Calcium citrate, 173*b*
Calcium supplements, 173*b*
Calgary Family Assessment and Intervention Model (CFAM/CFIM), 115*t*
Callus, 623, 623*f*
Calorie, 159
CAM. *See* Confusion Assessment Method (CAM)
Candida, 748
Candida albicans, 770
Candida vaginitis, 713, 713*t*
Candidiasis, 270, 271*f*, 379, 380*f*
Cane, 630–631*b*

Canines, 359, 359*f*
Canker sore, 380, 380*f*
Cannabis, 63*b*, 447*b*, 650*t*
Canthus, 319
Cao gio, 132
Capillaries, 503
Caput medusae, 548
Caput succedaneum, 853, 853*f*
Carbohydrates, 159–160
Cardiac assistive devices, 495–496*b*
Cardiac cycle, 467–468, 467*f*
Cardiac disorders, 474–475*t*
Cardiac ischemia, 482*t*
Cardiac landmarks, 483–484, 483*f*
Cardiac muscle, 574
Cardiac tamponade, 474*t*, 496–499
Cardiac thrill, 210
Cardinal fields of gaze, 335–336, 335*f*
Cardiogenic shock, 474*t*
Cardiomegaly, 471
Cardiomyopathy, 474*t*
Carina, 418*f*, 421
Carotenemia, 263
Carpal tunnel syndrome
  anatomy and nerve distribution
  Phalen sign, 610*b*, 610*f*
  Tinel sign, 609*b*, 610*f*
Cartilage, 574–575
Caruncle, 320*f*, 321
Case study
  acute shoulder pain, 632–635
  atrophic vaginitis, 731–733
  breast mass, 412–414
  cardiac tamponade, 496–499
  COVID-19 and pneumonia, 458–461
  divorce, ineffective coping, 116–119
  dysmenorrhea, 135–137
  ear pain and hydrocele, 883–887
  enlarged prostate and hemorrhoid, 778–781
  examples of health histories. *See* Health history — examples
  eyes, 349–352
  ill client, 84–88
  lip lesion, 293–296
  multisystem problems, 945–951
  numbness in hands and feet, 689–693
  older adult, 920–924
  pancreatitis, 568–571
  pediatric client, 883–887
  penile lump and Peyronie disease, 759–761
  peripheral vasculature and lymphatic systems, 508–510
  pneumonia and altered mental status, 920–924
  pregnant client, 818–821
  spiritual assessment, 153–155
  streptococcal pharyngitis, 387–390
  thyroid nodule, 315–317
  underweight client, 192–195
  well client, 80–84
Cast, 631*b*
Castration anxiety, 97
Cataract, 341, 341*f*, 343, 344*b*
Catholics, 142, 151
Cauda equina, 640*f*, 643, 669
Cauliflower ear, 366, 367*f*
Cavities, 384
CBE. *See* Clinical breast examination (CBE)
CC. *See* Chief complaint (CC)
Cecum, 534*f*, 538
Cellulitis, 263*f*, 273, 273*f*
Celsius temperature scale, 230, 230*f*
Central nervous system (CNS), 638–641
Central sleep apnea, 433
Cephalohematoma, 853, 853*f*
Cerebellar arteries, 642*f*, 642*t*
Cerebellar ataxia gait, 588*t*
Cerebellar function, 653*t*, 679–681
Cerebellum, 639, 639*f*
Cerebral cortex, 638, 638*f*
Cerebral lobes, 638, 639*f*
Cerebral palsy (CP), 871
Cerebrovascular accident (CVA), 510*t*, 657*b*
Cerebrum, 638, 639*f*
Cerumen, 354, 366, 369*b*
Cervical cancer, 695, 719, 720, 720*b*, 723*t*
Cervical candidiasis, 719, 719*f*
Cervical nerves, 640*f*, 643
Cervical os, 720, 722*f*
Cervical polyp, 719, 719*f*
Cervical smear, 724, 724*f*
Cervical spine, 597–599
Cervical venous distention (CVD), 515, 515*f*
Cervical venous pressure (CVP), 514–515
Cervix, 697*f*, 698, 699*f*, 717–720
  bimanual examination, 727–728
  cervical cancer, 695, 719, 720, 720*b*, 723*t*
  cervical candidiasis, 719, 719*f*
  cervical os, 720, 722*f*
  cervical polyp, 719, 719*f*
  color, 718
  discharge, 719
  nabothian cysts, 719, 719*f*
  physical examination, 717–718
  position, 718
  size, 719
  strawberry, 718, 718*f*
  surface characteristics, 719
CFAM/CFIM. *See* Calgary Family Assessment and Intervention Model (CFAM/CFIM)
CGM. *See* Continuous glucose monitor (CGM)
Chadwick sign, 718, 790*t*
Chalazion, 333, 333*f*
Chancre, 378, 378*f*
  females, 710, 710*f*
  males, 744, 745*f*
Chancroid
  females, 715, 715*f*, 726*f*
  males, 745, 745*f*
  perineal, 715, 715*f*, 773, 773*f*
Chandelier sign, 727
Characteristic patterns of daily living, 71
Checklist of Non-Verbal Pain Indicators (CNPI), 903
Cherry angioma, 266, 267*f*
Chest pain, 470, 482*t*
Chest tubes, 496*b*
Chestfeeding, 167
Cheyne-Stokes respirations, 433, 434*f*
CHF. *See* Congestive heart failure (CHF)
CHI. *See* Creatinine height index (CHI)
Chickenpox, 275, 275*f*
Chief complaint (CC)
  aggravating factors, 51
  alleviating factors, 51, 51*b*
  associated manifestations, 51
  location, 50
  meaning and impact, 52
  mnemonics to remember characteristics of CC, 50*b*
  negative findings, 51
  positive findings, 51
  quality, 50
  quantity, 50–51
  radiation, 50
  setting, 51–52
  timing, 52
Chilblains, 264
Childhood fears, 830–831*b*
Childhood obesity, 169*b*, 169*f*
Children. *See* Pediatric client
Chlamydia, 719, 719*f*
Chlamydia culture specimen, 724
Chloride (Cl), 164*t*
Choking, 168*b*
"Choking game," 66*b*
Cholecalciferol, 161*t*
Cholecystitis, 561*b*
Cholesteatoma, 371, 371*f*
Cholesterol, 160, 186
Chorea, 590*t*
Chorionic villi sampling (CVS), 814*t*
Choroid, 321*f*, 322
Christian population, 141*f*
Christian Scientists, 143
Chromium (Cr), 165*t*
Chromosome studies, 814*t*
Chronic malignant/nonmalignant pain, 244, 248
Church of Christ, Scientist, 143
Chvostek sign, 597*b*, 597*f*
Chyme, 535
Cialis, 758*b*
Cigarette smoking, 62–63, 62*b*
Ciliary body, 321*f*, 322
Circadian rhythm, 230
Circle of Willis, 641, 642*f*
Circumcision, 744*b*, 880*b*
Circumduction, 576*t*
Cleft lip, 860, 860*f*
Cleft palate, 860, 860*f*
Client
  bedridden, 940*b*
  child. *See* Pediatric client
  comatose, 938*b*
  "difficult." *See* Client with differing abilities
  elderly. *See* Older adult client
  empowering, 932*b*
  fostering cooperation, 931*b*
  interviewing. *See* Client interview
  pregnancy. *See* Pregnant client
Client interview, 20–45
  approach, 22
  client's role, 21
  communication pointers. *See* Communication
  conclusion of interview, 77
  confidentiality, 23
  "difficult" clients. *See* Client with differing abilities
  environment, 22–23
  eye contact, 43

general principles of effective interviewing, 43–44
HIPAA, 23
humor, 30*b*
motivational interviewing, 21–22
multitasking, 43
note taking, 23–24
nurse's role, 21
older adult client, 898–900
personal questions asked by client, 32*b*
preparation, 22*b*
problematic interviewing techniques, 35–37
role of client, 21
self-awareness, 24
sensitive topics, 64*b*
stages of interview process, 24
time, length, duration, 24
touch, 26*b*, 39
Client outcomes, 10
Client profile, 49
Client with differing abilities
anxious or angry, 41
crying, 41
deafness of hard-of-hearing, 39
eliciting birthplace information from reluctant client, 48*b*
hostile client, 42
illiteracy, 40
impairment by alcohol or drugs, 42
interpreters, 40, 41*b*
low level of understanding, 41
non-English speaking, 40–41
sexually aggressive client, 42
speech impairment or aphasia, 39–40
very-ill client, 42–43
visual impairment, 39
Clinical breast examination (CBE), 405*b*. *See also* Breast examination
Clinical judgment, 3, 6
Clinical reasoning, 3
Clitoris, 696, 697*f*, 712, 712*f*
Clonus, 684, 686
Closed questions, 27
Clubbing, 291, 291*f*, 293
Clubfoot (talipes equinovarus), 872, 872*f*
Clue cells, 725, 725*f*
CNPI. *See* Checklist of Non-Verbal Pain Indicators (CNPI)
CNS. *See* Central nervous system (CNS)
CNS stimulants, 650*t*
Coarctation of the aorta, (COA), 476–477*t*, 867*b*, 868
Coarse crackle, 450*t*
Cobalamin, 162*t*
Coccygeal nerves, 640*f*
Cochlea, 355*f*, 356
Cognitive function, 659–665
abstract reasoning, 663
acute confusion, 664*t*
assessment tools, 660*b*
attention, 659–660
calculation, 662
COVID-19 pandemic, 660
delirium, 664*t*
dementia, 664*t*
insight, 661
judgment, 660–661
memory, 660
older adult client, 907
Piaget's theory of cognitive development, 93, 94–95*t*, 96
spatial perception, 661–662
suicide/suicidal ideation, 665, 665*b*
thought process and content, 663–664
Cold (frio)/hot (caliente), 131, 131*t*, 132
Cold sores, 378
Collaborative interventions, 11
Collapsing pulse, 517*f*
Collateral blood flow murmur, 868
Collateral family kinship patterns, 133–134
Collateral family structure, 133
Coloboma, 347
Color return (CR), 523*b*
Color Vision Testing Made Easy tool, 856
Colorectal cancer, 545*b*, 560*b*, 567*b*
Colostomy, 551*b*
Colostrum, 394, 786
Columns of Morgagni, 764
Coma, 659*t*
Comatose client, 938*b*
Comedones, 273, 273*f*
Communication
action responses, 30–32
bad news, 939*b*
closed questions, 27
distance, 25
facilitating, 27
ineffective techniques, 32–37. *See also* Nontherapeutic communication techniques
listening, 25
listening responses, 27–30
mental status assessment, 654–655, 656*t*
nonverbal cues, 25
open-ended questions, 26
personal space, 26
problematic interviewing techniques, 35–37
silence, 27
Communication board, 42–43
Communication failures, 17
Communion, 142*f*
Compartment syndrome, 625*b*
Complete health history, 48–77. *See also* Health history
biographical data, 48–49
case studies, 80–84, 84–88
chief complaint, 49, 50–52, 50*b*
client profile, 49
family health history, 59–61
health maintenance activities, 71–74
history of the present illness (HPI), 49–52
past health history. *See* Past health history
reason for seeking health care, 49
review of systems (ROS), 74–76
social history, 61–71. *See also* Social history
source and reliability of information, 49, 49*b*
today's date, 48
what is it?, 47
Complete health history and physical examination, 928–953
advanced techniques, 929
case study (client with multisystem problems), 945–951
EHR/PHR, 930, 931*b*
ethical considerations, 929–930
general approach to physical examination. *See* Physical examination
head-to-toe examination. *See* Head-to-toe examination
health history, 932, 932*b*. *See also* Health history
legal considerations, 929
time commitment, 928
Compression bandage, 522*b*, 522*f*
Concentric circles breast palpation, 408*f*
Conchae, 356
Concrete operational stage, 94*t*, 96
Conduction aphasia, 656*t*
Conductive hearing loss, 365, 913
Condyloid joint, 577*t*
Condyloma acuminatum, 710, 745, 746*f*, 750, 750*f*, 772
Condyloma latum, 710, 710*f*
Cones, 322
Confabulation, 663
Confidentiality, 23
Confluent lesions, 269*f*
Confrontation, 329, 330*f*
Confronting, 31
Confusion, 656*b*, 659*t*, 664*t*
Confusion Assessment Method (CAM), 907
Congenital dermal melanocytosis, 848, 848*f*
Congenital heart defects, 476–481*t*
Congestive heart failure (CHF), 453–455*t*, 456*f*, 474*t*, 865, 865*f*
Conjunctiva, 320*f*, 336–338
Conjunctivitis, 337, 337*f*
Conservation, 96
Constipation, 538*f*, 541, 766–767
Constructional apraxia, 662, 662*f*
Contact Precautions, 204*f*
Continuous glucose monitor (CGM), 188*b*
Continuous murmur, 868
Contraction stress test (CST), 814*t*
Convex abdomen, 547
Cooper's ligaments, 393, 393*f*
Coordination, 680–681
Corn, 622, 622*f*
Cornea, 321, 321*f*, 338–339
Corneal laceration, 339, 339*f*
Corneal light reflex, 334
Corneal reflex, 674, 675*f*
Corneal scar, 339, 339*f*
Corneal ulceration, 338, 339*f*
Cornu, 699*f*
Coronary arteries and veins, 466*f*
Coronary artery disease, 474*t*
Coronary circulation, 465–467
Corpus callosum, 638
Corpus cavernosum, 736*f*, 737
Corpus spongiosum, 736*f*, 737
Cortical sensation, 671–672
Corticospinal tract, 641, 641*f*
Costal angle, 420*b*, 430, 431*f*
Costovertebral angle tenderness, 806
Cotton wool spots, 347, 347*f*
Cough, 424
Cover/uncover test, 334, 335*f*, 855
"Cover Your Cough" poster, 201, 202*f*
COVID-19 pandemic, 941–942
ageusia/hypogeusia, 677
antibacterial stations, 199*b*
attention span, 660
"Cover Your Cough" poster, 201, 202*f*

discrimination, 129
growth and development, 116
long COVID, 941–942
memory difficulties, 660
pediatric client, 882
pertussis, 436*b*
pneumonia, 452, 458–461
pulmonary condition, 452
religious and spiritual beliefs, 143
spiritual assessment, 152–153
telehealth, 43
vaccine, 57
COVID brain fog, 660
Cowper glands, 736, 736*f*
Coxa plana, 871
CP. *See* Cerebral palsy (CP)
CR. *See* Color return (CR)
Crackle, 450*t*
Cradle cap, 851, 852*f*
CRAFFT, 113*t*
Cranial nerves, 308*b*, 672–679
abducens nerve, 644*t*, 675
acoustic nerve, 644*t*, 677
examination skill, 653*t*
facial nerve, 644*t*, 675–677
glossopharyngeal nerve, 644*t*, 677–678
hypoglossal nerve, 644*t*, 679
mnemonics, 644*b*
oculomotor nerve, 644*t*, 673
olfactory nerve, 644*t*, 672–673, 672*b*
optic nerve, 644*t*, 673
pediatric client, 876–877
spinal accessory nerve, 644*t*, 678
trigeminal nerve, 644*t*, 673–675
trochlear nerve, 644*t*, 673
vagus nerve, 644*t*, 677–678
Craniosynostosis, 305, 852
Craniotabes, 305
Creatinine, 189
Creatinine height index (CHI), 189
Cremasteric reflex, 685, 685*f*
Crepitus, 267, 308, 309, 441, 592–593, 594
Crescendo-decrescendo murmur, 493, 493*f*
Crescendo murmur, 493, 493*f*
CRIES tool, 248
Critical thinking
defined, 3
evaluation, 4
explanation, 4
inference, 4
interpretations of situations, 3–4
self-regulation, 4
UIS. *See* Universal Intellectual Standards (UIS)
Crohn disease, 773
Crust, 271*f*
Crutches, 630*b*
Crying client, 41
Cryptic tonsil, 385
Cryptorchidism, 753*f*, 754, 881
CST. *See* Contraction stress test (CST)
Cullen sign, 548
Cult, 142
Cultural assessment
assessment tools, 134, 135*f*
basic principles (general approach), 134*b*
case study (Vietnamese au pair with dysmenorrhea), 135–137
cultural identity. *See* Cultural identity
nurse's role, 123
older adult client, 901
Cultural awareness, 123–125
Cultural beliefs, 130
Cultural care accommodation or negotiation, 132
Cultural care preservation or maintenance, 132
Cultural care repatterning or restructuring, 132
Cultural competence, 124–125
Cultural congruence, 123–124
Cultural diversity, 122
Cultural health beliefs, 130, 130*t*
Cultural humility, 123
Cultural identity, 125–134. *See also* Cultural assessment
artifacts, 129
communication patterns, 128
communication variables, 128
cultural health beliefs, 130, 130*t*
cultural meaning of symptoms, 133
cultural norms, 128
cultural rituals, 133
cultural values, 128, 130*t*
ethnic customs, 133
ethnicity, 126
family and kinship relations, 133–134
folk illnesses, 131
folk medicine remedies, 132
gender identity, 127
hot (caliente)/cold (frio), 131, 131*t*, 132
language, 127
potential for harm associated with cultural beliefs, 132
prejudice, discrimination, stereotyping, 129
race, 125–126
self-care practices, 132
sexual orientation, 126–127
subculture, 125–127
symbols, 129
value orientations, 129–130, 130*t*
Cultural norms, 128
Cultural relativity, 122
Cultural rituals, 133
Cultural values, 128, 130*t*
Culture, 121
Cushing syndrome, 221, 307, 308*f*
Customs, 133
Cutaneous horn, 279, 279*f*
Cutaneous hypersensitivity, 564*b*, 564*f*
Cutaneous pain, 243
Cuticle, 255, 255*f*
CVA. *See* Cerebrovascular accident (CVA)
CVD. *See* Cervical venous distention (CVD)
CVP. *See* Cervical venous pressure (CVP)
CVS. *See* Chorionic villi sampling (CVS)
Cyanosis, 262–263, 848
Cyanotic defects, 479–481*t*
Cyclothymia, 667*t*
Cyst, 270*f*
Cystocele, 714, 714*f*
Cystourethrocele, 714, 714*f*
Cytobrush, 722

Dacryocystitis, 333, 333*f*, 856
Dandruff, 288
Dangerous abbreviations, acronyms, and symbols, 78
Dangerous sexual practices, 66*b*
DASH diet, 173*b*
DCIS. *See* Ductal carcinoma in situ (DCIS)
DDH. *See* Developmental distortion of the hip (DDH)
DDST. *See* Denver II (DDST)
De Quervain tenosynovitis, 610*b*, 610*f*
Deaf client, 39
Decerebrate rigidity, 679, 679*f*
Decibel scale, 356*f*
Decorticate rigidity, 679, 679*f*
Decrescendo murmur, 493, 493*f*
Deep palpation, 211–212, 211*f*
Deep tendon reflexes, 682–684
Deep vein thrombosis (DVT), 511*t*, 522*b*
Defecation, 764
Deformity, 579–580
Dehydration, 166*f*, 286
Delirium, 664*t*, 907, 908*t*
Delusions, 650*t*
Dementia, 664*t*, 907, 908*t*
Dennie-Morgan lines, 307
Dental caries, 384, 384*f*
Dental disease, older adults, 894, 894*f*
Denver II (DDST), 112*t*, 840, 841*f*
Dependent edema, 287*t*
Depression
acronym (IN SAD CAGES), 663*b*
assessment tool (GDS-15), 115*t*, 907, 909*t*
joint range of motion, 576*t*
major depressive disorder, 666*t*
norepinephrine, 896
older adult client, 907, 908*t*
overview, 664*t*, 908*t*
perinatal, 813*b*
USPSTF recommendation, 688*b*
Dermatofibroma, 278
Dermatomes, 643, 643*f*
Dermis, 253–254, 253*f*
DES. *See* Diethylstilbestrol (DES)
Development, 92
Developmental assessment, 92–120
adolescents, 107–108, 113*t*, 114*t*
adverse childhood experiences (ACE), 101
ages and stages developmental theories, 92, 94–95*t*
assessment tools, 112, 112–115*t*
basic principles (general approach), 112*b*
case study (ineffective coping after divorce), 116–119
COVID-19, 116
early middle adulthood, 109–110
Erikson's epigenetic theory of personality, 94–95*t*, 98–99
Freud's psychoanalytic theory, 94*t*, 96–98
general approach, 100
growth charts, 824, 825–829*f*
infants, 102–104
internalized racism, 101–102
Kohlberg's theory of moral development, 94–95*t*, 99–100
late adulthood, 111
late middle adulthood, 110–111
older adult client, 113*t*, 114*t*, 115*t*, 900–901
pediatric client, 840, 841*f*
Piaget's theory of cognitive development, 93, 94–95*t*, 96
preschoolers, 105–106

school-age children, 106–107
social determinants of health (SDOH), 101
structural racism, 101
toddlers, 104–105
young adults, 108–109
Developmental assessment tools, 112, 112–115*t*
Developmental distortion of the hip (DDH), 872, 873
Developmental stage, 92
Developmental tasks, 92
adolescents, 108
early middle adulthood, 110
infants, 104
late adulthood, 111
late middle adulthood, 110–111
preschoolers, 106
school-age children, 107
toddlers, 105
young adults, 109
Deviated nasal septum, 374, 374*f*
DEXA scan, 191, 613*b*
Dextrocardia, 488*b*, 488*f*
DHT. *See* Dihydrotestosterone (DHT)
Diabetes, 171, 188
Diabetic peripheral neuropathy, 687*b*, 687*f*
Diabetic retinopathy, 346, 347, 347*f*
Diagnosis, 6*t*, 8–9
Diagnostic algorithm, 931
Diagnostic and laboratory data, 8
Diaper dermatitis, 850, 850*f*
Diaphragm, 418*f*, 422
Diaphragmatic hernia, 869
Diaphysis, 574
DIAPPERS, 565–566*b*
Diarrhea, 538*f*, 541, 767
Diarthroses, 577, 577*t*
Diascopy, 267*b*
Diastasis, 467*f*, 468
Diastasis recti, 788
Diastole, 467, 467*f*, 517*f*
Diastolic murmur, 493, 495*t*, 868
Diastolic pressure, 235, 240*t*
Diencephalon, 638–639, 639*f*
Diet, 72. *See also* Nutrition
Diet history, 179*t*
Dietary Guidelines for America, 158, 166
Dietary reference intakes (DRIs), 158
Diethylstilbestrol (DES), 719, 720*b*, 720*f*, 743
Differences of sex development (DSD), 38
"Difficult" clients. *See* Client with differing abilities
Digit hypoperfusion, 625*b*
Digital stethoscope, 216*b*, 217*f*
Dihydrotestosterone (DHT), 765
Diopter, 343
Direct fist percussion, 214, 214*f*, 558*f*
Direct inguinal hernia, 756, 756*f*, 757*t*
Direct percussion, 213, 213*f*
Disappearing penis phenomenon, 880
Discrete lesions, 269*f*
Discrimination, 129
Disinfectant stations, 199*b*
Dislocation, 591
Distal limb, 625*b*
Distress, 69, 69*f*, 224–225
DNA, 60
DNR. *See* Do Not Resuscitate (DNR)
Do no harm (fundamental value), 132
Do Not Resuscitate (DNR), 904
Documentation, 77–79, 940*f*
anal abnormalities, 771*b*
blood pressure, 237*b*
breast masses, 409*b*
dangerous abbreviations, acronyms, and symbols, 78
examination-specific documentation guidelines, 78–79
frequently used documentation methods, 18
general documentation guidelines, 77–78
handwritten client records, 78
progress note, 18
pulses, 229*b*, 229*f*
SOAP notes, 18
Dogma, 141
Doll's eye phenomenon, 673*b*
Dominant-hemisphere lesions, 655*b*
Donovanosis, 748. *See also* Granuloma inguinale
Doppler ultrasonic stethoscope, 216, 216*f*
Dorsal horn, 640, 642*f*, 645*f*
Dorsal recumbent position, 208*f*
Dorsalis pedis pulse, 516*f*
Dorsiflexion, 576*t*
Dot hemorrhage, 346
Down syndrome, 306, 306*f*
Drawer test, 618*b*, 618*f*
Dress, grooming, and personal hygiene, 223
DRIs. *See* Dietary reference intakes (DRIs)
Driving, older adult client, 904*b*
Drones, 930–931
Drop arm test, 601*b*, 601*f*
Droplet Precautions, 204*f*
Drug use/abuse. *See also* Alcohol use/abuse
cannabis, 63*b*, 447*b*, 650*t*
chest pain, 482*t*
CNS stimulants, 650*t*
drug overdose, 249–250
drug safety categories in pregnancy, 794*b*
grade B recommendations, 80*b*
hallucinogens, 650*t*
marijuana, 63*b*, 447*b*, 650*t*
marijuana poisoning, 878*b*
narcotics, 650*t*
neurological signs of drug ingestion, 650*t*
sedative-hypnotics, 650*t*
Drusen, 347, 347*f*
Dual-energy x-ray absorptiometry (DEXA) scan, 191, 613*b*
Duchenne muscular dystrophy (MD), 871
Ductal carcinoma in situ (DCIS), 402*t*
Ductus deferens, 736
Duke Activity Status Index, 473
Dullness, 213*t*, 444
Duodenum, 534*f*, 535
Dupuytren contracture, 607, 608*f*
Dura mater, 637, 638*f*
Durable power of attorney, 904
DVT. *See* Deep vein thrombosis (DVT)
Dwarfism, 585
Dysarthria, 655
Dyscalculia, 662
Dysdiadochokinesia, 681
Dysesthesia, 669
Dysmenorrhea, 704
Dysmetria, 681
Dysphagia, 175, 655*b*, 893
Dysphonia, 655, 655*b*
Dyspnea, 424
Dysrhythmia, 229, 469
Dyssynergy, 681
Dysthymia, 667*t*
Dystonia, 590*t*
Dysuria, 542, 806

E-cigarettes, 447*b*
EAC. *See* External auditory canal (EAC)
Ear. *See also* Ears, nose, mouth, and throat
anatomy, 354–356
AOM, OME, and otitis externa, 371, 371*f*, 372*t*
auditory screening, 364–375
case study (ear pain and hydrocele), 883–887
chief complaint (health history), 360–361
clearing EAC of cerumen, 369*b*
decibel scale, 356*f*
EAC foreign body, 369, 369*b*
examination, 364–372
external, 354, 355*f*, 366–368
head-to-toe examination, 935, 935*f*
hearing aids, 386*b*
inner, 355–356, 355*f*
middle, 355, 355*f*
observing client with decreased hearing, 365*b*
older adult client, 893, 913–914
otalgia, 360
otorrhea, 361
otoscopic examination, 368–372
pediatric client, 858–859, 859*b*
Rinne test, 366, 366*f*
risk factors, 372*b*
tinnitus, 360–361
tuning fork tests, 365
voice-whisper test, 364–365
Weber test, 365, 365*f*
Early diastolic murmur, 868
Early Language Milestones Scale (PEDS), 112*t*
Early middle adulthood, 109–110
calorie needs, 159*t*
developmental assessment tools, 113*t*, 114*t*
developmental tasks, 110
nutrition, 171–172
Early systole, 468
Ears, nose, mouth, and throat, 354–391
anatomy and physiology, 354–359
assistive devices, 386–387*b*
case study (streptococcal pharyngitis), 387–390
ear. *See* Ear
examination, 363*b*, 364–386
health history, 360–363
mouth. *See* Mouth
nose. *See* Nose
sinuses. *See* Sinuses
teeth, 359, 359*f*, 383–384
throat. *See* Throat
Eating disorders, 170, 171*f*, 222
EBP. *See* Evidence-based practice (EBP)
Ebstein anomaly, 477*t*
Ecchymosis, 265, 265*b*, 266*f*
Eccrine glands, 253*f*, 254
ECG. *See* Electrocardiogram (ECG or EKG)

ECG monitoring, 496*b*
Echolalia, 663
Eclampsia, 789, 802*t*
Ecomap, 134
Ectodermal galactic band, 393, 394*f*
Ectopic pregnancy, 807*b*
Ectropion, 332, 332*f*, 719, 807
Eczema, 274, 274*f*, 275, 849
EDD. *See* Estimated date of delivery (EDD)
Edema, 286, 286*b*, 287*f*, 287*t*, 518*f*, 803
Edinburg Postnatal Depression Scale (EDPS), 114*t*
EDPS. *See* Edinburg Postnatal Depression Scale (EDPS)
Eggshell nails, 291
Ego, 96
Ego integrity vs. despair stage, 95*t*, 99
Egocentrism, 96
Egophony, 452
EHR. *See* Electronic health record (EHR)
Eisenmenger complex or syndrome, 479*t*
Ejaculatory duct, 736, 736*f*
Ejection click, 489, 490*f*, 491*f*
Ejection murmur, 866
EKG. *See* Electrocardiogram (ECG or EKG)
Elastic cartilage, 575
Elbows, 602–604
Elder abuse and neglect, 916*b*
Elderly persons. *See* Older adult client
Elderspeak, 898
Electra complex, 97
Electrocardiogram (ECG or EKG), 468
Electromechanical dissociation, 229
Electronic cigarettes, 447*b*
Electronic health record (EHR), 47, 930
Electronic thermometer, 232*f*, 233
Elevation, 576*t*
Emergency health history, 47
Emergency response system (electronic device), 903*b*
Emotional distress, 224–225
Emphysema, 453–455*t*, 456*f*
Enculturation, 122
Endemic goiter, 310
Endocardial cushion defect, 479*t*
Endocarditis, 474*t*
Endocervical smear, 722–723, 722*f*
Endolymph, 356
Endometrial cancer, 720–721*b*
Endometrium, 697*f*, 698, 699*f*
Endotracheal tube, 439*b*
Enteral tubes, 551*b*
Entropion, 331, 332*f*
Epicondylitis, 603
Epidermis, 252–253, 253*f*
Epididymis, 736, 736*f*, 752, 752*f*
Epididymitis, 753, 753*f*
Epimysium, 574
Epiphora, 333
Epiphysis, 574
Episodic health history, 47
Epispadias, 749, 749*f*
Epitrochlear lymph nodes, 506*f*, 525, 525*f*
Eponychium, 255, 255*f*
Epstein's pearls, 861
Epworth Sleepiness Scale, 71, 902
Equilibratory coordination, 680
Erb's point, 483, 483*f*
Erectile dysfunction, 738*b*, 740, 758*b*
Erikson's epigenetic theory of personality, 98–99
  autonomy vs. shame and doubt stage, 94*t*, 98
  ego integrity vs. despair stage, 95*t*, 99
  generativity vs stagnation stage, 95*t*, 99
  identity vs. role confusion stage, 94*t*, 99
  industry vs. inferiority stage, 94*t*, 98–99
  initiative vs. guilt stage, 94*t*, 98
  intimacy vs. isolation stage, 95*t*, 99
  overview, 94–95*t*
  trust vs. mistrust stage, 94*t*, 98
Erosion, 271*f*
Error-prone abbreviations, 941*b*
Erysipelas, 272–273, 272*f*
Erythema, 264, 264*f*
Erythema infectiosum, 277, 277*f*
Erythema migrans, 277, 278*f*
Erythema toxicum, 849
Escutcheon, 696
Esophageal cancer, 548*b*
Esophageal rupture, 482*t*
Esophoria, 335, 335*f*
Esotropia, 334, 334*f*, 855, 855*f*
Essential hypertension, 239
Estimated date of delivery (EDD), 795*f*, 795*t*
Ethical considerations, 929–930
Ethmoid sinus, 357*f*
Ethnic customs, 133
Ethnic discrimination, 129
Ethnic group, 126
Ethnic identity, 126
Ethnicity, 126
Ethnocentrism, 124
Eupnea, 432, 434*f*
Eustachian tube, 355, 355*f*, 831–832
Eustress, 69
Evaluation, 12–13
Eversion, 576*t*, 719, 807
Evidence-based practice (EBP), 2, 12
Evil eye, 131, 131*f*
Examination of thorax and lungs, 428–457
  adventitious breath sounds, 449, 450*t*, 455*t*
  angle of the ribs, 430–431, 431*f*, 453*t*
  assessing oxygenation, 430*b*
  assessing thoracic skin, 440*b*
  auscultation, 446–452, 455*t*
  breath sounds, 448–451, 455*t*
  comparison of selected respiratory conditions, 453–455*t*, 456–457*f*
  costal angle, 430, 431*f*
  crepitus, 441
  general approach, 426–427*b*
  inspection, 428–440, 453*t*
  intercostal space (ICS), 431–432
  masses, 440–441
  overview, 426–427*b*
  palpation, 440–444, 454*t*
  percussion, 444–446, 454*t*
  pulsations, 440
  respirations, 432–437
  respiratory assistive devices, 438–439*b*
  respiratory patterns, 433–434, 434*f*, 435
  respiratory rate, 432–433, 432*b*, 453*t*
  shape of thorax, 428–429, 453*t*
  sputum, 424, 437–438, 438*t*
  superficial veins, 429–430
  symmetry of chest wall, 429
  tactile fremitus, 442–443, 442*f*, 443*f*, 454*t*
  thoracic expansion, 441–442, 441*f*, 454*t*
  thoracic tenderness, 441
  tracheal position, 443–444, 443*f*, 454*t*
  voice sounds, 451–452, 455*t*
Examples. *See* Case study; Health history — examples
Exanthem subitum, 276
Exanthematous drug eruption, 278*f*
Excoriation, 271*f*
Exercise, 72–73, 72*f*, 73*b*
Exhalation, 225
Exome gene sequencing, 60
Exophoria, 335, 335*f*
Exophthalmos, 307, 307*f*, 331
Exostoses, 370, 370*f*
Exotropia, 334, 334*f*, 855
Expiration (exhalation), 225, 422*f*, 423
Expired medications, 53*b*
Extension, 576*t*
External anal sphincter, 764, 764*f*
External auditory canal (EAC), 354, 355*f*, 369*b*
External ear, 354, 355*f*, 366–368, 913
External inguinal ring, 737
External os, 699, 699*f*
External respiration, 423
External rotation, 576*t*
Exteroceptive sensation, 668–670
Extinction, 672
Extraocular muscles, 321, 334, 334*b*, 334*f*
Extrapyramidal rigidity, 679
Extrapyramidal tract, 641
Extreme talkativeness, 36
Extremity pain, 508–509
Eye, 319–353
  anatomy and physiology, 319–323. *See also* Eye examination
  blindness vs. legal blindness, 331*b*
  case study (stye, conjunctivitis, diabetic retinopathy), 349–352
  cataract, 341, 341*f*, 343, 344*b*
  color vision, 854–855
  diabetic retinopathy, 346, 347, 347*f*
  extraocular muscles, 321, 334, 334*b*, 334*f*
  glaucoma, 340*b*
  head-to-toe examination, 934–935, 935*f*
  health history, 323–325
  hygiene tips, 336*b*
  inner layer, 321*f*, 322
  lacrimal apparatus, 320–321, 333
  macular degeneration, 347*b*, 348*b*, 349*t*
  middle layer, 321*f*, 322
  older adult client, 893, 912–913, 913*b*
  outer layer, 321–322, 321*f*
  pediatric client, 853–858
  physical examination. *See* Eye examination
  posterior segment structures, 343
  visual pathway, 322, 323*f*
Eye contact, 43, 64*b*
Eye examination, 326–348. *See also* Eye
  anterior chamber, 339–340, 340*f*
  cardinal fields of gaze, 335–336, 335*f*
  color vision, 328–329
  comprehensive examination, 344*b*
  conjunctiva, 336–338
  cornea, 338–339
  corneal light reflex, 334
  cover/uncover test, 334, 335*f*
  diseases/disorders. *See* Eye

distance vision, 327–328
equipment, 326, 343, 343*f*, 344*t*
extraocular muscles, 334, 334*b*, 334*f*
eye refraction, 329*f*
eyes, eyelids, eyebrows, and eyelashes, 330–333
general approach, 327*b*
Hirschberg test, 334
iris, 340
lacrimal apparatus, 333
lens. *See* Lens
macula, 347–348, 348*f*
near vision, 328
ophthalmoscope, 343, 343*f*, 344*t*
overview, 326
pupil. *See* Pupil
retinal structures, 344–347, 344*f*
sclera, 338
visual acuity, 326–329
visual fields, 329, 330*f*
Eye refraction, 329*f*
Eyebrows, 319, 320*f*
Eyelashes, 319, 320*f*
Eyelids, 320*f*, 856

Face, 298, 299*f*, 306–307
FACES Pain Rating Scale, 248, 248*f*, 840
Facial asymmetry, 306, 306*f*
Facial expression, 654
Facial expressions, 224
Facial nerve, 644*t*, 675–677
Fad diets/exercise regimens, 171
Fahrenheit temperature scale, 230, 230*f*
Faith, 141
Falls, 902–903
False reassurances, 33–34
False ribs, 418
Family and kinship relations, 133–134
Family health history, 59–61
FAQ. *See* Functional Activities Questionnaire (FAQ)
Fasciculation, 590*t*
FASE. *See* Functional Assessment Screening in the Elderly (FASE)
FAST, 657*b*
Fat intake in young children, 877*b*
Fat-soluble vitamins, 161, 161*t*
Fats, 160–161
Fecal incontinence, 770, 898
Fecal odor, 223
Feet. *See* Ankles and feet
Female athlete triad, 619*b*
Female genitalia, 695–734. *See also* Females
Female genitalia examination, 706–730. *See also* Females
adnexa, 728–729
anal culture, 726
anus, 714–715
bimanual examination, 727–728
cancer, 720–721*b*
cervical smear, 724, 724*f*
cervix, 717–720. *See also* Cervix
chlamydia culture specimen, 724
client positioning, 709, 709*f*
clitoris, 712, 712*f*
endocervical smear, 722–723, 722*f*
equipment, 707–708
external genitalia, 708–715, 715–717
fishy odor, 713*t*, 725
five percent acetic acid wash, 725–726
fornices, 728
general approach, 706*b*
genital self-examination, 717*b*
gonococcal culture specimen, 725
hysterectomy, 729*b*
internal genitalia (speculum examination), 717–720
KOH prep, 725
labia, 715
milking the urethra, 716, 716*f*
mons pubis, 710–711
overview, 707
Pap smear, 721–724
perineum, 714–715, 717
preparing for gynecological examination, 708*b*
pubic hair, 709
rectovaginal examination, 729–730, 729*f*
saline mount ("wet prep"), 725
self-collection for HPV and STI testing, 726*b*
skene glands, 716
skin color and condition, 710–711
urethral meatus, 712, 712*f*, 716
USPSTF recommendations, 723*t*, 730*b*
uterine leiomyoma, 728*b*
uterus, 728
vagina, 727
vaginal introitus, 713–714, 715
vaginal wall, 726
vulva, 710–711
Females. *See also* Gender differences
anatomy and physiology, 695–699
breastfeeding, 167, 167*f*
case study (atrophic vaginitis), 731–733
cervical cancer, 695, 719, 720, 720*b*, 723*t*
client education, 699*b*
diethylstilbestrol (DES), 720*b*, 720*f*
endometrial cancer, 720–721*b*
external genitalia, 695–697, 708–715
gynecological examination. *See* Female genitalia examination
head-to-toe examination, 939
health history (female genitalia), 702–704
hernias, 717*b*
HPV vaccination, 724*b*
internal genitalia, 697–699
long COVID, 941–942
maintaining gynecological health, 707*b*
menarche (onset of menstruation), 700, 702*b*
menopause - hormone replacement therapy, 717*b*
menopause - maintaining sexual function, 730*b*
menstrual cycle, 700, 700*f*
older adult client, 897, 917–918
ovarian cancer, 721*b*
ovarian cycle, 699–700, 700*f*
pain tolerance, 244
pear-shaped appearance, 183
pediatric client, 834, 877–879
pregnant client, 789–790, 807, 809
progesterone and body temperature, 230
puberty, 700–701
pubic hair, 701*t*, 709
reproductive cycle, 699–701
transgender male client, 730*b*
vaginal cancer, 721*b*
vaginal discharge, 713*t*
vaginal infections, 713*b*
vulvar cancer, 721*b*
Femoral hernia, 756, 757*f*, 757*t*
Festinating gait, 588*t*
Fetal heart rate (FHR), 811*b*
Fetal heart tone (FHT), 809–810, 810*f*, 811, 811*b*
Fetal movement count, 814*t*, 817*b*
Fetor hepaticus, 223, 377
Fetoscope, 798
Fetus. *See* Pregnant client
FEV. *See* Forced expiratory volume (FEV)
Fever blister, 378, 378*f*
FHR. *See* Fetal heart rate (FHR)
FHT. *See* Fetal heart tone (FHT)
Fibrillation, 590*t*
Fibroadenoma, 404*f*
Fibrocartilage, 575
Fibroids, 728*b*
Fibroma, 384, 385*f*
Fibromyalgia, 592, 592*f*
FICA spiritual assessment tool, 146, 154–155
Fidelity, 929
Fifth disease, 277
Figure 8, 681*f*
Fimbriae, 699, 699*f*
Fine crackle, 450*t*
Fine motor skills
adolescents, 108*t*
infancy, 102–103*t*
school-age children, 107*t*
toddlers, 104–105*t*
Finger anomalies, 607, 607*f*
Fingerprints, 254
Fingertip-to-nose touch, 680*f*
Finkelstein test, 610, 610*f*
First-degree burn, 283, 284*f*
Fish, 160*b*
Fishy odor, 713*t*, 725
Fissure, 271*f*
Fissured tongue, 380, 381*f*
Fist percussion
kidney, 214–215, 214*f*, 215*f*, 558, 558*f*
liver, 558–559, 559*f*
FIT acronym, 73*b*
Five percent acetic acid wash, 725–726
FLACC Behavioral Pain Assessment Scale, 248
Flat bones, 574
Flat feet, 622
Flatness, 213*t*
Flatulence, 537, 541–542
Flexion, 576*t*
Flight of ideas, 663
Floating ribs, 418
Flu vaccines, 427*b*
Fluid wave, 557*b*, 558*f*
Fluoride (F), 165*t*
Folacin, 163*t*
Folic acid, 163*t*, 190
Folk illness, 130, 131
Folk medicine remedies, 132
Folk practitioner, 130
Folliculitis, 281, 281*f*
Follow-up health history, 47
Folstein Mini-Mental State Examination (MMSE), 115*t*, 907
Fontanel, 852

Food. *See* Nutrition
Food diary, 177
Food intake history, 177, 179*t*
Foot drop gait, 588*t*
Forced expiratory volume (FEV), 455*b*
Fordyce spots, 381, 382*f*
Foreskin (prepuce), 736*f*, 737
Formal operational stage, 94–95*t*, 96
Fornix (fornices), 697, 699*f*, 728
Fossa, 356
Foster care, 850*b*
4 + tonsils, 386, 386*f*
Fourchette, 696, 696*f*
Fourth-degree burn, 283, 284*f*
Fovea centralis, 322
Fragility fracture, 587
Frenulum, 358, 359*f*, 696
Freud's psychoanalytic theory, 96–98
  anal psychosexual stage, 94*t*, 97
  castration anxiety, 97
  genital psychosexual stage, 94*t*, 98
  id, ego, superego, 96
  latency psychosexual stage, 94*t*, 97
  Oedipus/Electra complexes, 97
  oral psychosexual stage, 94*t*, 97
  overview, 94*t*
  penis envy, 97
  personality, 96
  phallic psychosexual stage, 94*t*, 97
Friability, 790, 807
Friction rubs, 552
Frontal lobe, 639*f*
Frontal sinus, 357*f*, 358
Frozen shoulder, 600–601
Fruity (acetone) breath, 377
Functional Activities Questionnaire (FAQ), 114*t*
Functional Assessment Screening in the Elderly (FASE), 115*t*
Functional health assessment, 71
Functional incontinence, 566*b*
Functional scoliosis, 628
Fundal height, 809
Fundus of uterus, 698, 699*f*
Funduscopic examination, 344*f*
Funnel chest, 429
Furuncle, 273, 273*f*
Furunculosis, 370
Future of Nursing 2020-2030, 123, 944

Gag reflex, 385*b*
Gait, 222, 586–587, 588*t*, 647–648
Galant reflex, 876, 876*f*
Galeazzi's sign, 873
Gallbladder, 534*f*, 539
Gallop, 492, 492*f*
Ganglion cyst, 607, 607*f*
Gangrene, 267, 267*f*
Gardasil 9, 724*b*
Gas gangrene, 267, 267*f*
Gastrostomy, 551*b*
Gay, 38
GCS. *See* Glasgow coma scale (GCS)
GDS-15. *See* Geriatric Depression Scale-15 (GDS-15)
Gender differences. *See also* Females; Males
  calorie needs, 159*t*
  dysthymia, 667*t*
  growth spurts, 824
  major depressive disorder, 665*t*
  panic disorder, 665*t*
  schizophrenia, 667*t*
  serum iron, 186
  thyroid cartilage (Adam's apple), 310
Gender identity, 127
General survey, 219–225, 933
  body and breath odors, 222–223
  body fat, 221–222
  distress, 224–225
  dress, grooming, and personal hygiene, 223
  environmental cues, 220*b*
  equipment, 220
  facial expressions, 224
  general appearance, 221
  mood and manner, 223
  motor activity, 222
  overview, 220
  physical presence, 220–223
  psychological presence, 223–224
  speech, 224
  stated age vs. apparent age, 220–221
  stature, 222
Generalized anxiety disorder, 665*t*
Generalized lesions, 269*f*
Generativity vs stagnation stage, 95*t*, 99
Genetic testing, 814*t*
Genetics Information Nondiscrimination Act (GINA), 61
Genetics testing, 60–61, 61*b*
Genital herpes simplex, 711*f*
Genital psychosexual stage, 94*t*, 98
Genital self-examination, 717*b*
Genital warts, 726, 745, 746*f*
Genogram, 59*f*
Genomics, 60
Genu valgum (knock knees), 615, 615*f*, 616*b*, 872
Genu varum (bow legs), 616, 616*b*, 616*f*, 872
Geographic tongue, 380, 381*f*
Geriatric Depression Scale-15 (GDS-15), 115*t*, 907, 909*t*
Geriatric syndromes, 901–902. *See also* Older adult client
German measles, 277
Gestation calculation wheel, 795*f*
Gestational age at birth, 797, 797*b*
Gestational hypertension, 801*t*
Get Up and Go test, 906
GINA. *See* Genetics Information Nondiscrimination Act (GINA)
Gingival hyperplasia, 383, 383*f*
Gingival recession, 383, 383*f*
Gingivitis, 383, 383*f*
Glabellar reflex, 686
Glans penis, 736*f*, 737
Glasgow coma scale (GCS), 657–658, 658*f*, 659*t*
Glaucoma, 339, 340*b*
Glaucomatous cupping, 346, 346*f*
Gliding, 576*t*
Gliding joint, 577*t*
Global aphasia, 656*t*
Glossopharyngeal nerve, 644*t*, 677–678
Gloves
  genitalia, 711*f*, 745*f*
  latex allergies, 201*b*
  PPE, 200*f*
  toxins/caustic substances, 261*b*
GLP-1 medications, 183*b*
Glucose, 188, 188*b*, 188*f*
Glycosuria, 789
Glycosylated hemoglobin (HbA1c), 188–189
Goiter, 310, 310*f*
Golden rules of physical examination, 216–217
Golfer's elbow, 604–605
Goniometer, 583, 595, 595*f*
Gonococcal culture specimen, 725
Gonococcal proctitis, 773
Gonococcal vaginal discharge, 713*t*
Gonorrhea, 713, 719, 752*f*
Goodell sign, 727, 790*t*
Goose bumps, 254
Gout, 591*f*, 593, 593*f*, 594
Gout tophus, 593, 593*f*
Gower's sign, 871
Graafian follicle, 699, 700
Grade A recommendations, 79
  anus, rectum, and prostate, 778*b*
  bladder cancer, 567*b*
  blood pressure, 527
  female genitalia, 730*b*
  HIV, 80*b*
  hypertension, 250*b*
  male genitalia, 758*b*
  older adults, 918*b*
  pediatric client, 882*b*
  pregnant client, 191*b*, 817*b*
  tobacco use, 80*b*, 458*b*
Grade B recommendations, 79
  abdominal aortic aneurysm (AAA), 527*b*, 567*b*
  alcohol use/abuse, 80*b*
  anus, rectum, and prostate, 778*b*
  anxiety disorders, 688*b*
  breasts, 412*b*
  cardiac disease risk factors, 496*b*, 527*b*
  colorectal cancer, 567*b*
  depression, 688*b*
  drug use/abuse, 80*b*
  female genitalia, 730*b*
  intimate partner violence (IPV), 80*b*
  latent tuberculosis infection (LBTI), 458*b*
  lung cancer with low-dose computed tomography (LDCT), 458*b*
  male genitalia, 758*b*
  nutrition/nutritional assessment, 191*b*
  older adults, 919*b*
  osteoporosis, 632*b*
  pediatric client, 883*b*
  pregnant client, 817*b*
  skin cancer, 293*b*
  statins, 496*b*, 527*b*
Grade C recommendations, 79
Grade D recommendations, 79
Grade E recommendations, 79
Granulation tissue, 256*b*
Granuloma annulare, 281, 281*f*
Granuloma inguinale
  females, 711, 711*f*
  males, 748, 748*f*
Graphanesthesia, 671
Graphesthesia, 671, 671*f*
Graves disease, 307, 311
Graves speculum, 707, 707*f*
Gravida/para (TPAL), 795*b*
Greater vestibular glands, 697

Grip strength, 608*b*, 608*f*
Gross cyst, 404*f*
Gross motor skills
  adolescents, 108
  infancy, 102–103*t*
  school-age children, 106*t*
  toddlers, 104–105*t*
Grouped lesions, 269*f*
Growth and development, 92. *See also* Developmental assessment
Growth charts, 824, 825–829*f*
Gulf War Illness, 70
Gums, 359, 382–383
Gynecological examination. *See* Female genitalia examination
Gynecomastia, 411, 411*f*

Habit tick deformity, 292, 293*f*
Hair. *See also* Skin, hair, and nails
  anatomy/physiology, 256
  color, 287
  distribution, 287–288
  function, 256
  health history questions (hair care habits), 260*b*
  inspection, 286–288
  lesions, 288
  older adult client, 892, 910–911, 910*b*, 912*b*
  palpation, 288–289
  signs of physical abuse, 265*b*
  texture, 288–289
Halitosis, 361–362, 377, 386
Hallucinations, 650*t*
Hallucinogens, 650*t*
Hallux valgus (bunion), 622, 622*f*
Hammertoe, 622, 622*f*
Hand, 210, 210–211*f*. *See also* Wrists and hands
Hand-foot-mouth disease, 850, 850*f*
Hand hygiene, 199, 200*f*, 201*f*
Hand-off, 16–17
Handedness, 655*b*
Handwritten client records, 78
Hard exudates, 347, 347*f*
HARK screening tool, 66*b*
Harlequin color change, 849
HAV. *See* Hepatitis A virus (HAV)
Hawkins impingement sign, 602*b*, 602*f*
HbA1c. *See* Glycosylated hemoglobin (HbA1c)
HBV. *See* Hepatitis B virus (HBV)
HCG. *See* Human chorionic gonadotropin (HCG)
HCV. *See* Hepatitis C virus (HCV)
HDL, High-density lipoproteins (HDL)
HDL cholesterol, 186
HDV. *See* Hepatitis D virus (HDV)
Head, neck, and lymph nodes, 298–318
  anatomy and physiology, 298–300
  blood supply, 300
  case study (thyroid nodule), 315–317
  cranial nerves, 308*b*
  equipment, 304
  face, 298, 299*f*, 306–307
  general approach to physical examination, 304*b*
  head, palpation of, 305
  head, shape of, 304–305
  health history, 300–303
  lymph nodes, 300, 300*f*, 313–315
  mandible, 299*f*, 307–308
  neck, 299, 299*f*, 300*f*, 308–309, 309*b*
  older adult client, 892, 911–912
  parathyroid disease, 312*t*
  pediatric client, 831, 832*f*, 851–854
  scalp, 305–306
  skull, 298, 299*f*
  thyroid. *See* Thyroid gland
Head circumference, 826*f*, 846–847, 846*f*
Head lice, 288, 289*f*
Head-to-toe examination, 933–951. *See also* individual body systems/parts
  abdomen, 937–938, 938*f*
  anterior thorax, 936, 937*f*
  back, posterior and lateral thoraxes, 936, 936*f*
  breasts, 936–937, 937*f*
  ears, 935, 935*f*
  eyes, 934–935, 935*f*
  female anus and rectum, 939
  female breasts, 936–937, 937*f*
  female genitalia, 939
  general approach to physical examination, 932*b*. *See also* Physical examination
  general survey, 933
  head and face, 934
  heart, 936, 937*f*, 938
  inguinal area, 938
  laboratory and diagnostic data, 940
  lower extremities, 938, 938*f*
  male anus, rectum, and prostate, 939–940, 940*f*
  male breasts, 937
  male genitalia, 939
  measurements, 933, 934*f*
  mouth and throat, 935
  musculoskeletal system, 939
  neck, 935
  neurological system, 933–934, 938, 939
  nose and sinuses, 935
  problem list, 940–941
  skin, 934, 934*f*
  upper extremities, 936, 936*f*
Headache, 303*t*, 304*b*
Headpiece mnemonic, 215*b*
Health checkup information, 74
Health history, 46–90, 931
  basic principles (general approach), 48*b*
  breasts and regional lymph nodes, 396–399
  complete. *See* Complete health history
  computerization (EHR), 47–48
  conclusion of interview, 77
  examples. *See* Health history — examples
  family, 59–61
  merging health history and public health issues, 932*b*
  preparing for, 47
  subjective data, 7
  system-specific, 76–77
  types, 47
Health history — examples
  abdomen, 540–544
  anus, rectum, and prostate, 765–768
  case studies. *See* Case study
  ears, nose, mouth, and throat, 360–363
  eyes, 323–325
  female genitalia, 702–704
  female reproductive history, 705*t*
  head, neck, and regional lymph nodes, 300–303
  heart, 470–473
  ill client, 84–88
  male genitalia, 739–742
  musculoskeletal system, 578–581
  neurological system, 646–650
  nutritional assessment, 174–176
  pain, 245–247
  pediatric client, 834–839
  peripheral vascular and lymphatic systems, 508–510
  pregnant client, 791–794
  skin, hair, and nails, 257–260, 260*b*
  thorax and lungs, 423–426
  well client, 80–84
Health Insurance Portability and Accountability Act (HIPAA), 23
Health maintenance activities, 71–74
  diet, 72
  exercise, 72–73, 72*f*, 73*b*
  health checkups, 74
  safety devices, 73
  sleep, 71–72
  stress management, 73, 73*f*
Health promotion diagnosis, 9
Healthy People: The Surgeon General's Report, 943
Healthy People 2030, 157, 943
Hearing aids, 386*b*
Hearing/hearing loss. *See* Ear
Heart, 463–501
  anatomy and physiology, 463–469
  cardiac assistive devices, 495–496*b*
  cardiac cycle, 467–468, 467*f*
  cardiac disorders, 474–475*t*
  cardiac landmarks, 483–484, 483*f*
  case study (cardiac tamponade), 496–499
  chambers, 464, 465*f*
  chest pain, 470, 482*t*
  conduction system, 468–469, 469*f*
  congenital heart defects, 476–481*t*
  coronary arteries and veins, 466*f*
  coronary circulation, 465–467
  dextrocardia, 488*b*, 488*f*
  ECG, 468
  exercise (physical activity), 468*b*, 473
  head-to-toe examination, 936, 937*f*, 938
  health history, 470–473
  mechanical circulatory support devices, 486*b*
  NYHA classification, 473
  older adult client, 895, 915
  palpitations, 470–471
  pediatric client, 864–868
  pericardium, 463–464, 464*f*
  physical examination. *See* Heart examination
  pregnant client, 786–787, 805
  prosthetic heart valves, 494–495
  risk factors for cardiac disease, 484*b*
  sounds. *See* Heart sounds
  target heart rate (THR) zone, 468*b*
  USPSTF recommendations, 496*b*
  valves, 464–465, 494–495
Heart chambers, 464, 465*f*
Heart examination, 482–495
  aortic area. *See* Aortic area

apical impulse, 486*b*, 487, 487*f*
auscultation, 488*b*, 489–495
cardiac assistive devices, 495–496*b*
cardiac landmarks, 483–484, 483*f*
equipment, 482
general approach, 483*b*
heart sounds. *See* Heart sounds
heaves, 486, 487
inspection, 484–486
midprecordial area. *See* Midprecordial area
mitral area. *See* Mitral area
murmurs, 493–494, 493*f*, 494*t*, 495*t*
overview, 483
palpation, 486–488
pericardial friction rub, 494, 494*b*, 495*t*
precordium, 482–484
pulmonic area. *See* Pulmonic area
pulsations, 486, 486*f*, 487
thrills, 486, 486*f*, 487
tricuspid area. *See* Tricuspid area
Heart murmurs, 866–868
Heart palpitations, 470–471
Heart pulsations, 486, 486*f*, 487
Heart rate, 226–227
Heart sounds, 866–868
S_1, 468, 489, 490, 490–492*f*, 491, 866
S_2, 468, 489, 490–492*f*, 866
S_3, 492, 492*b*, 492*f*, 866
S_4, 492, 492*f*, 493*b*, 866
Heart valves, 464–465, 494–495
Heaves, 486, 487, 865
Heberden node, 607, 607*f*
HEEADSS 3.0, 113*t*
HEEADSSS 3.0 assessment, 840*b*
Heel slide, 680*f*
Hegar sign, 790*t*
Height, 181, 910
HELLP syndrome, 802*t*
Hemangioma, 380, 381*f*
Hematemesis, 540
Hematocrit, 185
Hematoma, 265, 266, 266*f*
Hemiparesis, 596
Hemiplegia, 596
Hemodynamic monitoring, 496*b*, 521*b*
Hemoglobin, 185
Hemorrhoids, 715, 770, 770*f*
case study, 778–781
internal, 774, 774*f*
pregnant client, 800*t*
Hemotympanum, 370, 370*f*
Hendrich Fall Risk Assessment, 903
Hepatitis A virus (HAV), 554*b*
Hepatitis B virus (HBV), 554*b*
Hepatitis C virus (HCV), 555*b*
Hepatitis D virus (HDV), 555*b*
Hepatitis E virus (HEV), 555*b*
Hepatojugular reflux, 515–516, 516*f*
Hepatomegaly, 870
Herbal products, 55*b*
Hernia
diaphragmatic, 869
direct inguinal, 756, 756*f*, 757*t*
females, 717*b*
femoral, 756, 757*f*, 757*t*
indirect inguinal, 756, 756*f*, 757*t*
inguinal, 756, 756*f*, 757*t*, 881
umbilical, 550, 550*f*, 869, 869*f*
ventral, 550, 550*f*
Herniated disc
Milgram test, 630*b*
straight leg raising test, 629–630*b*, 630*f*
Herpes simplex virus, 275, 275*f*, 276
Herpes zoster, 276, 276*f*
Herpes zoster ophthalmicus, 276, 276*f*
Heterograft valve, 495
HEV. *See* Hepatitis E virus (HEV)
High-Fowler's position, 208*f*
Hing joint, 577*t*
HIPAA. *See* Health Insurance Portability and Accountability Act (HIPAA)
Hippus phenomenon, 341
Hips, 610–614
Hirschberg test, 334, 855
Hirsutism, 288, 288*f*
History of the present illness (HPI), 49–52
HITS screening tool, 66*b*
HIV/AIDS
grade A recommendations, 80*b*
risk factors, 746*b*
screening guidelines for men having sex with men (MSM), 747*b*
Hives, 278, 278*f*
Hoarseness, 541
Hobbies and leisure activities, 69
Holosystolic murmur, 491, 493, 866, 868
Homan sign, 522*b*
Home safety, 581*b*
Homeless persons, 69*b*
Homograft valve, 495
Hook method of liver palpation, 561, 561*f*
HOPE tool, 146
Hordeolum, 332, 332*f*
Horizontal recumbent position, 208*f*
Horner's syndrome, 342*t*
Horny layer, 253
Hospital chaplain, 151
Hostile client, 42
Hot (caliente)/cold (frio), 131, 131*t*, 132
Household Pulse Survey, 126
HPV. See Human papillomavirus
Human chorionic gonadotropin (HCG), 700
Human Genome Project, 60
Human papillomavirus (HPV)
anal carcinoma, 775
anal region, 772*f*
cervix, 726
condylomata acuminata, 772
females (vaccination), 724*b*
males (vaccination), 746*b*
penile, 747*f*
Human trafficking, 65*b*, 66*f*
Humor, 30*b*
Humpback, 429
Hutchinson's incisors, 384, 384*f*
Hutchinson's sign, 289
Hyaline cartilage, 574–575
Hydration, 166*f*
Hydrocele, 750, 750*f*, 881, 883–887
Hydrocephalus, 305, 847, 854*b*
Hymen, 696*f*, 697
Hypalgesia, 669
Hyperactive deep tendon reflexes, 684
Hyperalgesia, 669
Hyperemesis gravidarum, 804
Hyperesthesia, 669
Hyperextension, 576*t*
Hyperglycemia, 188
Hyperkinetic pulsations, 486, 517*f*
Hyperkinetic states, 222, 229
Hypernea, 434*f*, 435
Hyperopia, 328, 329*f*
Hyperparathyroidism, 312*t*
Hyperphoria, 335
Hyperresonance, 213*t*, 444
Hypertelorism, 307
Hypertension, 511*t*. *See also* Blood pressure
AAP guidelines, 238*t*
ACC/AHA guidelines, 239*t*
DASH diet, 173*b*
essential, 239
pregnant client, 799, 799*b*, 801–802*t*
secondary, 239
stage 1/stage 2, 238*t*, 239*t*
USPSTF recommendation, 250*b*
Hyperthermia, 234, 284
Hyperthyroidism, 224, 311*t*
Hypertrophia, 855
Hypertrophy, 589, 589*f*, 591*b*
Hyperventilation, 433, 434*f*
Hyphae, 725, 725*f*
Hyphemia, 340
Hypoesthesia, 669
Hypogeusia, 677
Hypoglossal nerve, 644*t*, 679
Hypoglycemia, 188
Hypogonadism, 752
Hypokinetic pulsations, 485, 517*f*
Hypoparathyroidism, 312*t*
Hypophoria, 335
Hypopigmentation, 264
Hypoplastic left heart syndrome, 481*t*
Hypospadias, 749, 749*f*, 880
Hypotension, 240
Hypothalamus, 639
Hypothermia, 234, 284, 285
Hypothyroidism, 284, 307, 311*t*
Hypotonicity, 592
Hypoventilation, 435
Hypovitaminosis D, 190
Hysterectomy, 729*b*

IADL. *See* Instrumental activities of daily living (IADL); Lawton Instrumental Activities of Daily Living Scale (IADL)
IBC. *See* Inflammatory breast cancer (IBC)
Ichthyosis vulgaris, 284, 284*f*
ICS. *See* Intercostal space (ICS)
Id, 96
IDC. *See* Infiltrating ductal carcinoma (IDC)
Identity vs. role confusion stage, 94*t*, 99
IJ veins. *See* Internal jugular (IJ) veins
ILC. *See* Infiltrating lobular carcinoma (ILC)
Ileal conduit, 551*b*
Ileostomy, 551*b*
Ileum, 534*f*, 537
Iliopsoas muscle test, 564*b*, 564*f*
Illiterate client, 40
Immediate auscultation, 215
Immediate percussion, 213
Immobilizer, 631*b*
Immunization schedule, 839*t*
Immunization schedules, 57*b*, 58*t*
Impaired client (drugs/alcohol), 42
Impella, 486*b*
Impetigo, 272, 272*f*
Impingement syndrome, 602*b*, 602*f*

Implementation, 12
IN SAD CAGES, 663*b*
Incisors, 359, 359*f*
Incongruency, 31
Incus, 355, 355*f*
Independent nursing interventions, 11
Indirect auscultation, 215–216
Indirect fist percussion, 214–215, 215*f*, 558*f*, 559*f*
Indirect inguinal hernia, 756, 756*f*, 757*t*
Indirect percussion, 213–214, 214*f*
Individualism, instrumental purpose, and exchange stage, 94*t*, 100
Individualistic kinship patterns, 133
Industry vs. inferiority stage, 94*t*, 98–99
Indwelling catheter, 551*b*
Infants, 102–104. *See also* Pediatric client
  awake tummy time, 831*b*
  breast milk jaundice, 849
  chest circumference, 847, 847*f*
  chest configuration, 833, 833*f*
  childhood fears, 830*b*
  choking, 168*b*
  cleft palate, 860, 860*f*
  congestive heart failure, 865, 865*f*
  cranial nerve function, 877
  developmental assessment tools, 112*t*
  developmental distortion of the hip (DDH), 872, 873
  developmental tasks, 104
  esotropia, 855, 855*f*
  fontanel, 852
  genu varum (bowleg), 872
  head control, 851–852
  heart, 833
  immunization schedule, 839*t*
  inguinal hernia, 881
  iris, 857
  milestones, 102–103*t*
  myelomeningocele, 850, 850*f*
  nutrition, 167–168, 168*b*
  physical growth, 824
  pseudostrabismus, 855*b*
  pulse rate, 228*t*
  reflexes, 874–876
  respiratory rate, 226*t*
  SIDS, 831*b*
  sleep position, 831*b*
  strabismus screening, 855
  suture lines, 852
  talipes equinovarus (clubfoot), 872, 872*f*
  teeth, 832, 832*f*
  thrush, 860*f*
  transillumination of skull, 854*b*
  vernix caseosa, 851, 851*f*
  weight, 845, 845*f*
  wheezing, 864
Infarction, 465
Inferior angle of scapula, 420*b*
Infiltrating ductal carcinoma (IDC), 402*t*
Infiltrating lobular carcinoma (ILC), 402*t*
Inflammatory breast cancer (IBC), 402*t*
Influenza vaccine, 427*b*
Infundibulum, 699, 699*f*
Ingrown hair, 281
Ingrown nail, 291, 292*f*
Inguinal area, 751, 755–756, 938
Inguinal canal, 737
Inguinal hernia, 756, 756*f*, 757*t*, 881
Inguinal ligament, 737
Inguinal lymph nodes, 506*f*, 526, 526*f*
Initial Pain Assessment Inventory, 248
Initiative vs. guilt stage, 94*t*, 98
Inner ear, 355–356, 355*f*
Innocent heart murmurs, 866, 867*t*
Insight, 661
Inspection, 209
Inspiration (inhalation), 225, 422–423, 422*f*
Instrumental activities of daily living (IADL), 71
Insufficiency, 494
Insulin resistance syndrome, 171, 475*t*
Integumentary system, 252. *See also* Skin
Intellectual disability, client with, 41
Intention tremor, 590*t*
Intercostal space (ICS), 419, 419*b*, 419*f*, 431–432
Intermittent pneumatic compression pump, 522*b*
Internal anal sphincter, 764, 764*f*
Internal hemorrhoids, 774, 774*f*. *See also* Hemorrhoids
Internal jugular (IJ) veins, 513
Internal os, 699, 699*f*
Internal respiration, 423
Internal rotation, 576*t*
Internalized racism, 101–102
Internet gaming disorder, 69*b*
Interpleural space, 421
Interpreter, 39, 40, 41*b*
Interrupting the client, 35–36
Intersex, 38
Interstitial cells of Leydig, 737
Interval health history, 47
Interventions, 11
Interviewing the client. *See* Client interview
Intestinal diversions, 551*b*
Intestinal tubes, 551*b*
Intimacy vs. isolation stage, 95*t*, 99
Intimate distance, 25
Intimate partner violence (IPV)
  grade B recommendations, 80*b*
  IPV screening tools, 65, 66*b*
  social history, 64–65
Intra-aortic balloon pump, 486*b*
Intraductal papilloma, 408
Intravenous (IV) catheter, 521*b*
Introitus mucosa, 713
Intuition, 2
Inversion, 576*t*
Involuntary muscle movements, 590*t*
Iodine (I), 165*t*
IPV. *See* Intimate partner violence (IPV)
Iris, 321*f*, 322, 340, 857
Iron (Fe), 165*t*
Iron deficiency, 163
Irregular bones, 574
Irregular pulse, 227
Ischemia, 465
Ishihara color test, 856
ISMP's list of error-prone abbreviations, 941*b*
Isoelectric line, 468
Isthmus, 299, 299*f*, 698–699, 699*f*
IV catheter. *See* Intravenous (IV) catheter

Jargon, medical, 36
Jaundice, 263, 264*f*, 548, 848*f*, 849
Jehovah's Witnesses, 143
Jejunum, 534*f*, 535, 537
Joining stage, 24
Joints
  defined, 576
  grading of joint swelling, 594*t*
  older adult client, 916
  physical examination, 589–591, 593–594, 594*t*
  range of motion (ROM), 576*t*
  skeletal, 577, 577*t*
  synovial, 577, 577*f*, 577*t*
Judaism, 141–142
Judgment, 660–661
Jugular venous pressure (JVP), 513–515
Justice, 929
JVP. *See* Jugular venous pressure (JVP)

Kaposi sarcoma, 274, 274*f*
Katz Index of Independence in Activities of Daily Living (Katz ADL), 114*t*, 906
Kawaski disease, 849
Keloid, 271*f*, 276, 276*f*
Keratoconus, 339, 339*f*
Kernig sign, 687*b*
Ketonuria, 806
Kidneys, 539, 558, 558*f*, 562, 562*f*, 563*b*
Kiesselbach's plexus, 356, 375, 375*f*
Kilocalories (kcal), 159
Kinship relations, 133–134
Klinefelter syndrome, 181
Klippel-Feil syndrome, 599
Knee-chest position, 208*f*
Knees, 614–620
  ACL, 619*b*
  Baker cyst, 616*b*, 617*f*
  cruciate ligaments, 618*b*, 618*f*
  genu valgum, 615, 615*f*, 616*b*, 872
  genu varum, 616, 616*b*, 616*f*, 872
  large effusions (patellar ballottement), 616–617*b*, 617*f*
  LCL, 620*b*, 620*f*
  MCL, 620*b*, 620*f*
  meniscal tears, 617–618*b*, 617*b*, 617*f*
  physical examination, 614–616
  small effusions (bulge sign), 616*b*, 616*f*
Knock knees (genu valgum), 615, 615*f*, 616*b*, 872
Koenig, Harold, 143
KOH prep, 725
Kohlberg's theory of moral development, 99–100
  conventional level, 94*t*, 100
  individualism, instrumental purpose, and exchange stage, 94*t*, 100
  morality stage, 94*t*, 100
  mutual expectations, relationships, and conformity to moral norms stage, 94*t*, 100
  overview, 94–95*t*
  postconventional level, 95*t*, 100
  preconventional level, 94*t*, 100
  social contract or utility, and individual rights stage, 95*t*, 100
  social system and conscience stage, 94*t*, 100
  universal ethical principles stage, 95*t*, 100
Koilonychia, 291
Koplik spots, 276, 277*f*
Korotkoff sounds, 235

Kussmaul respirations, 434*f*, 435
Kwashiorkor, 184, 184*f*
Kyphosis, 429, 585*f*, 628, 628*f*, 629*f*

Labia majora, 696, 696*f*, 697*f*
Labia minora, 696, 696*f*, 697*f*
Labial commissure, 358, 358*f*
Labial tubercle, 358, 358*f*
Labium (labia), 715
Laboratory data, 185–190
 albumin, 188
 antigen skin testing, 187
 cholesterol, 186
 creatinine height index (CHI), 189
 folic acid, 190
 glucose, 188, 188*b*, 188*f*
 glycosylated hemoglobin (HbA1c), 188–189
 hematocrit and hemoglobin, 185
 lipids, 185–186
 nitrogen balance, 189
 prealbumin, 187–188
 total lymphocyte count (TLC), 187
 transferrin, TIBC, and iron, 186–187
 vitamin B_{12}, 190
 vitamin D, 189–190
Labyrinth, 355
Lacrimal apparatus, 320–321, 333, 856
Lacrimal gland, 320*f*
Lacrimal punctum, 320*f*
Lactose intolerance, 168*b*
LAD. *See* Left anterior descending (LAD)
Ladin sign, 790*t*
Lagophthalmos, 331
Landau reflex, 876
Language skills
 adolescents, 108
 infancy, 102–103*t*
 school-age children, 106*t*
 toddlers, 104–105*t*
Lanugo, 831
Large intestine, 537–538
Lasègue test, 629–630*b*
Late adulthood. *See* Older adult client
Late middle adulthood, 110–111
 calorie needs, 159*t*
 developmental assessment tools, 113*t*, 114*t*
 developmental tasks, 110–111
 midlife crisis, 110
 nutrition, 171–172
Late systole, 468
Latency psychosexual stage, 94*t*, 97
Latent tuberculosis infection (LBTI), 458*b*
Lateral collateral ligament (LCL), 620*b*, 620*f*
Lateral epicondylitis, 603
Lateral spinothalamic tract, 641, 642*f*
Latex allergies, 201*b*
Lawton Instrumental Activities of Daily Living Scale (IADL), 115*t*, 906
LBB. *See* Left bundle branch (LBB)
LBTI. *See* Latent tuberculosis infection (LBTI)
LCL. *See* Lateral collateral ligament (LCL)
LCX. *See* Left circumflex (LCX)
LDCT. *See* Lung cancer with low-dose computed tomography (LDCT)
LDL. *See* Low-density lipoproteins (LDL)
LDL cholesterol, 186
Leading questions, 35
Left anterior descending (LAD), 465, 466
Left bundle branch (LBB), 469
Left circumflex (LCX), 466
Left lower quadrant (LLQ), 535*f*, 535*t*, 536–537*t*
Left upper quadrant (LUQ), 535*f*, 535*t*, 536*t*
Left ventricular hypertrophy, 487
Leg claudication, 527–530
Legal considerations, 929
Legg-Calvé disease, 871
Leininger, Madeline, 132
Leiomyomas, 728*b*
Lens
 generally, 321*f*, 322
 older adult, 912
 pediatric client, 857
 physical examination, 341, 341*b*, 343
Lentigines, 910
Lentigo, 270, 271*f*
Leopold maneuver, 811–812, 812*f*
LEP. *See* Limited English proficient (LEP) individuals
Lesbian, 38
Lesions
 breasts, 403
 cauda equina, 669
 dominant-hemisphere, 655*b*
 hair, 288
 lip, 293–296
 mouth and throat, 362
 penis, 740
 peripheral nerve, 669
 skin. *See* Skin lesions
 spatial perception, 661–662
 trigeminal nerve, 675
 upper/lower motor neuron, 686*t*
Lethargy, 659*t*
Leukocoria, 345, 345*f*
Leukonychia, 289, 289*f*
Leukonychia totalis, 289, 289*f*
Leukoplakia, 378, 379*f*, 380, 380*f*, 381, 382*f*, 726
Leukorrhea, 807
Level of consciousness (LOC), 656–658, 659*t*
Levitra, 758*b*
LGBTQIA+ individuals
 biases/disparities, 126
 health disparities, 743*b*
 mistrust and fear of health-care system, 127
 National LGBTQIA+ Health Education Center, 37
 nonbinary individuals, 127
 terminology, 37, 38
 transgender persons. *See* Transgender individuals
Lichen plenus, 382, 382*f*, 748, 748*f*
Lichen sclerosus, 711, 711*f*
Lichenification, 271*f*
Lid lag, 331
Life-event theories, 93
Ligaments, 575
Light palpation, 211, 211*f*
Light reflex, 345
Light touch, 668, 668*f*, 674, 674*f*
Lightening, 790
Limb circumference, 591*b*, 591*f*
Limb length, 613*b*, 613*f*
Limbic lobe, 638
Limbus, 319, 320*f*
Limit setting, 31–32
Limited English proficient (LEP) individuals, 40–41, 127
Lindsey's nails, 290
Linea alba, 533
Linea nigra, 785, 785*f*
Linear alopecia, 287*f*, 288
Linear family, 133
Linear lesions, 269*f*
Linear raphe, 358, 359*f*
Lip blister, 859, 859*f*
Lip lesion, 293–296
Lipids, 185–186
Lipoma, 306
Lips, 377–379, 859–860
Liraglutide, 183*b*
List, 628, 628*f*, 629
Listening, 25
Listening responses, 27–30
 clarifying, 28–29
 encouraging comparisons, 29
 interpreting, 29
 making observations, 28
 reflecting, 28
 restating, 28
 sequencing, 29
 summarizing, 29
Lithotomy position, 208*f*
Liver, 534*f*, 538–539, 560–561, 561*f*, 870
Liver border, 554, 554*f*
Liver cancer, 560*b*
Liver descent, 553–554
Liver scratch test, 554, 554*f*
Liver span, 553, 553*f*
Liver spots, 910
Lives Daily Hassles Scale (LIVES-DHS), 114*t*
Living will, 904
LLQ. *See* Left lower quadrant (LLQ)
Lobules, 735, 736*f*
LOC. *See* Level of consciousness (LOC)
Locked-in syndrome, 659*t*
Long COVID, 941–942
Long-term memory, 660
Longitudinal fissure, 638
Longitudinal melanonychia, 289, 290*f*
Longitudinal ridging, 291
Lordosis, 628, 628*f*
 pediatric client, 871
 pregnant client, 789, 789*f*
Loud S_1, 491, 491*f*
Low-density lipoproteins (LDL), 160
Lower abdominal reflex, 684
Lower motor neuron lesions, 686*t*
Lower motor neurons, 641, 641*f*
Lower respiratory tract, 417
Lumbar nerves, 640*f*
Lung cancer, 437–438*b*, 458*b*
Lung cancer with low-dose computed tomography (LDCT), 458*b*
Lung fissures, 419, 421*f*
Lungs, 418*f*, 419, 420*f*, 421*f*. *See also* Thorax and lungs
Lunula, 255, 255*f*
LUQ. *See* Left upper quadrant (LUQ)
LV. *See* Lymphogranuloma venereum (V)
Lyme disease, 278*f*, 306*f*, 687*b*
Lymph, 504

Lymph nodes, 506
  anatomy, 507*f*
  epitrochlear, 506*f*, 525, 525*f*
  head and neck, 300, 300*f*, 313–315
  inguinal, 506*f*, 526, 526*f*
  location, 506*f*
  palpation, axillary node region, 406–407
  palpation, head and neck, 313–315
  palpation, supraclavicular and infraclavicular, 405–406
  pediatric client, 862
  popliteal, 506*f*, 526, 526*f*
  regional, 394, 395*f*
Lymphadenitis, 512*t*
Lymphadenopathy, 313*f*, 509, 512*t*, 756
Lymphatic system. *See also* Peripheral vasculature and lymphatic systems
  anatomy and physiology, 503–507
  inspection and palpation, 525–526, 525*b*
  lymph nodes. *See* Lymph nodes
  lymphatic drainage, 505
  lymphatic organs, 506, 506*f*
  lymphatic vessels, 504–505
Lymphedema, 287*t*, 507, 511*t*, 512*f*, 522*b*, 522*f*
Lymphocytes, 503
Lymphogranuloma venereum (V), 756
Lymphoma, 511*t*, 525*b*

M-CHAT-R/F. *See* Modified Checklist for Autism Toddlers (M-CHAT-R/F)
Macewen's sign, 853
Macrominerals, 163
Macrosomia, 809
Macula, 322, 347–348, 348*f*
Macular degeneration, 347*b*, 348*b*, 349*t*, 912
Macule, 270*f*
Magnesium (Mg), 164*t*
Magnification, 267*b*
Major depressive disorder, 666*t*. *See also* Depression
Major minerals, 163, 164*t*
Male genitalia, 735–762. *See also* Males
  head-to-toe examination, 939
  older adult client, 897, 918
Male genitalia examination, 742–758. *See also* Males
  epididymis/epididymitis, 752, 752*f*, 753, 753*f*
  equipment, 742
  general approach, 742*b*
  hair distribution, 743
  inguinal area, 751, 755–756
  overview, 742
  penis. *See* Penis
  scrotum. *See* Scrotum
  sexual maturity rating (SMR), 738*t*, 743
  STIs, 752*b*
  testicular mass, 752, 752*f*
  testicular self-examination (TSE), 754*b*, 755*f*
  testicular torsion, 753, 753*b*, 753*f*
  transillumination of scrotum, 755*b*, 755*f*
  urethral meatus, 750–751, 751–752
  USPSTF recommendations, 758*b*
Male sexual assault (MSA), 747*b*
Males. *See also* Gender differences
  anatomy and physiology, 735–738
  apple-shaped appearance, 183
  balding, 287
  breasts/breast cancer, 411–412
  case study (penile lump and Peyronie disease), 759–761
  ducts, 736–737
  erectile dysfunction, 738*b*, 758*b*
  health history, 739–742
  HIV, 746*b*, 747*b*
  male sexual assault (MSA), 747*b*
  men having sex with men (MSM), 747*b*
  pediatric client, 879–882
  physical examination. *See* Male genitalia examination
  sexual act, 738
  sexual development, 737, 738*t*
  sexual history, 739*b*
  spermatogenesis, 737
  terminal facial and chest hair, 287
  testicular cancer, 754*b*
  transgender men, 395*b*, 730*b*
  unique health issues, 737*b*
Malignant melanoma, 280–281, 280*f*
Malleus, 355, 355*f*
Malnutrition, 184, 184*b*, 191*f*
MALT. *See* Mucosal-associated lymphoid tissue (MALT)
Mammary duct ectasia, 406
Mandible, 299*f*, 307–308, 359*f*
Manganese (Mn), 165*t*
Manicure, 261*b*
Manual compression tests, 522*b*
Manubriosternal junction, 420*b*
Manubrium, 355, 417
MAP. *See* Mean arterial pressure (MAP)
Marasmic kwashiorkor, 184
Marasmus, 184, 184*f*
Marcus Gunn pupil, 341
Marfan syndrome, 181, 222, 474*t*, 585
Marijuana, 63*b*, 447*b*, 650*t*
Marijuana poisoning, 878*b*
Maslow's hierarchy of needs, 10–11, 11*f*
Masseter muscle, 674, 674*f*
Mastectomy, 409–410, 409*f*, 409*t*
Mastitis, 406
Maxillary sinus, 357*f*, 358
McCaffrey Initial Pain Assessment Tool, 248
McDonald sign, 790*t*
McGill Pain Questionnaire, 248
MCL. *See* Medial collateral ligament (MCL)
McMurray sign, 617–618*b*, 617*f*
Mean arterial pressure (MAP), 235
Measles, 276, 277
Mechanical circulatory support devices, 486*b*
Mechanical ventilation, 439*b*
Medial collateral ligament (MCL), 620*b*, 620*f*
Medial epicondylitis, 604
Median sulcus, 765
Mediastinum, 418*f*, 421
Mediate auscultation, 215
Mediate percussion, 213
Medical history, 53
Medical jargon, 36
Medications
  error-prone abbreviations, 941*b*
  expired, 53*b*
  general medication questions, 55
  GLP-1, 183*b*
  herbal products, 55*b*
  hirsutism, 288, 288*f*
  obtaining accurate medication history, 54*b*
  over-the-counter, 54
  pain, 249
  prescription, 54
  vitamin B_{12} deficiency, 190
Medulla oblongata, 639, 639*f*
Medullary cavity, 574
Mees bands, 289
Meibomian glands, 320*f*
Melanin, 253
Melanoma, 280–281, 280*b*, 280*f*, 290*f*
Melanonychia, 289
Melasma, 785, 785*f*
Melena, 774*t*
Memory, 660
Memory centers, 660
Memory disorders, 648
Men. *See* Males
Men having sex with men (MSM), 747*b*
Menarche, 700, 702*b*
Ménière disease, 677
Meninges, 637–638, 638*f*
Meningitis, 687–688*b*
Meningococcal B meningitis vaccine, 688*b*
Meningococcal meningitis, 688*b*
Meningococcal (A, C, W, Y) vaccine, 688*b*
Meniscal tears
  Apley grinding sign, 617*b*, 617*f*
  McMurray sign, 617–618*b*, 617*f*
Menopause, 717*b*, 730*b*
Menorrhagia, 704
Menstrual cycle, 700, 700*f*
Mental status and neurological system, 637–694
  anatomy and physiology, 637–646
  arteries of the brain, 642*f*, 642*t*
  autonomic nervous system (ANS), 643, 645
  blood supply, 641, 642*t*
  brainstem, 639, 639*f*
  case study (numbness in hands and feet), 689–693
  central nervous system (CNS), 638–641
  cerebellum, 639, 639*f*
  cerebral lobes, 638, 639*f*
  cerebrovascular accident (CVA), 657*b*
  cerebrum, 638, 639*f*
  cranial nerves, 643, 644*f*, 644*t*
  diabetic peripheral neuropathy, 687*b*, 687*f*
  diencephalon, 638–639, 639*f*
  examination of neurological system. *See* Neurological examination
  extrapyramidal tract, 641
  health history, 646–650
  Lyme disease, 687*b*
  meninges, 637–638, 638*f*
  meningitis, 687–688*b*
  meningococcal meningitis, 688*b*
  mental status assessment. *See* Mental status assessment
  older adult client, 896, 916–917, 920–924
  parasympathetic nervous system, 645, 645*t*
  pediatric client, 873–877
  peripheral nervous system, 642–643
  posterior column, 641
  pregnant client, 789*b*, 807
  preventing traumatic injuries, 645*b*
  pyramidal tract, 641
  reflexes. *See* Reflexes
  scalp/skull, 637

spinal cord, 639–640, 639*f*
spinal nerves, 640*f*, 643
spinothalamic tracts, 641, 642*f*
stroke, 657*b*
sympathetic nervous system, 645, 645*t*
traumatic brain injury (TBI), 662*b*
USPSTF recommendations, 688*b*
Mental status assessment, 652–667. *See also* Mental status and neurological system
abstract reasoning, 663
affect, 654
anxiety disorders, 665–666*t*, 688*b*
application of painful stimuli, 657*b*
attention, 659–660
calculation, 662
client history, 654*t*
cognitive abilities and mentation, 659–665
communication, 654–655, 656*t*
confusion, 656*b*, 664*t*
delirium, 664*t*
dementia, 664*t*
depression, 663*b*, 664*t*, 666*t*, 688*b*
dress, grooming and personal hygiene, 653–654
examination skills, 653*t*
facial expression, 654
Glasgow coma scale (GCS), 657–658, 658*f*, 659*t*
insight, 661
judgment, 660–661
level of consciousness (LOC), 656–658, 659*t*
memory, 660
mood disorders, 666–667*t*
physical appearance and behavior, 652–654
posture and movements, 652
schizophrenia, 667*t*
spatial perception, 661–662
suicide/suicidal ideation, 665, 665*b*, 668*b*
thought process and content, 663–664
when specific assessment to be made?, 652*b*
Mercury thermometer, 230*b*
Metabolic syndrome, 171–172, 475*t*
Metamorphopsia, 348*b*
Metatarsus varus, 872
Meth mouth, 384, 384*f*
Microaneurysms, 346, 347*f*
Microcephaly, 847
Microminerals, 163
Microphallus, 743, 880
Microtia, 366, 367*f*
Mid-diastole, 468
Midarm and midarm muscle circumferences, 183–184
Midaxillary line, 419, 420*f*, 421*f*
Midbrain, 639, 639*f*
Midclavicular line, 419, 420*f*, 421*f*
Middiastolic murmur, 868
Middle-aged adults. *See* Early middle adulthood; Late middle adulthood
Middle cerebral artery, 642*f*, 642*t*
Middle ear, 355, 355*f*
Midlife crisis, 110
Midprecordial area, 483, 483*f*
auscultation, 490
inspection, 485
palpation, 487
Midspinal line, 420*b*
Midsternal line, 420*b*, 420*f*, 421*f*
Migraine headache, 304*b*
Milia, 851, 851*f*
Military service
health history, 70
traumatic brain injury (TBI), 662*b*
Milk line, 393
Milking the urethra, 716, 716*f*
Minerals, 163, 164*t*, 165*t*
Mini-Cog, 652, 907
Mini-Mental State Examination (MMSE), 115*t*, 660*b*, 907
Mini-Nutritional Assessment (MNA), 902
Mini-stroke. *See* Transient ischemic attack (TIA)
Minimum Data Set (MDS 3.0), 115*t*
Miotic pupil, 341
Mitral area, 483*f*, 484
auscultation, 491, 492
inspection, 485
palpation, 487
Mitral regurgitation or insufficiency, 475*t*, 487, 491–492, 495*t*
Mitral stenosis, 475*t*, 487, 495*t*
Mitral valve, 465
MMSE. *See* Folstein Mini-Mental State Examination (MMSE)
MNA. *See* Mini-Nutritional Assessment (MNA)
MoCA. *See* Montreal Cognitive Assessment (MoCA)
Modified Checklist for Autism Toddlers (M-CHAT-R/F), 112*t*
Modified radical mastectomy, 409*t*
Molars, 359, 359*f*
Molding, 853, 853*f*
Molluscum contagiosum, 278, 278*f*
females, 711, 711*f*
males, 748, 748*f*
Molybdenum (Mo), 165*t*
Mongolian spots, 848, 848*f*
Moniliasis, 270
Monk Skin Tone (MST) scale, 256*b*, 256*f*
Mononucleosis, 861
Monosynaptic reflex, 645*f*, 646
Monotheistic religions, 142
Monounsaturated fats, 160
Mons pubis, 696, 696*f*, 710–711
Montgomery's tubercles, 393
Montreal Cognitive Assessment (MoCA), 660*b*
Mood and manner, 223
Mood disorders, 666–667*t*
Moon face, 307, 308*f*
Morality stage, 94*t*, 100
Moralizing, 34
Moro reflex, 876, 876*f*
Motivational interviewing, 21–22
Motor system, 653*t*, 679
Motorized scooter, 631*b*
Mouth. *See also* Ears, nose, mouth, and throat
anatomy, 358–359, 358*f*, 359*f*
breath, 377
buccal mucosa, 381–382
cancer, 381*b*
chief complaint (health history), 361–362
examination, 377–379
gums, 359, 382–383
lips, 377–379
older adult client, 893–894, 914
oral appliances, 387*b*
palate, 384–385
teeth, 359, 359*f*, 383–384
tongue, 358, 379–380
MSA. *See* Male sexual assault (MSA)
MSM. *See* Men having sex with men (MSM)
MST scale. *See* Monk Skin Tone (MST) scale
McBurney point, 563*b*
Mucocele, 378, 379*f*
Mucosal-associated lymphoid tissue (MALT), 507
Multicultural identity, 125
Multitasking, 43
Mumps, 307, 308*f*, 861, 861*f*
Murmurs, 866–868
Murphy sign, 561*b*
Muscle cramps, 789*b*
Muscle stretch reflexes, 684
Muscles
classification, 574
involuntary muscle movements, 590*t*
major muscles of body, 575*f*
size and shape, 587, 589
spasm, 592, 599
strength, 595–596, 595*t*
tone, 591–593
Muscles of respiration, 422, 422*f*
Musculoskeletal examination, 582–629. *See also* Musculoskeletal system
ankles and feet, 620–626. *See also* Ankles and feet
carpal tunnel syndrome, 609*b*, 609*f*, 610*b*, 610*f*
cervical spine, 597–599
comprehensive, 604*b*
De Quervain tenosynovitis, 610*b*, 610*f*
DEXA screening, 613*b*
digit hypoperfusion, 625*b*
distal limbs, 625*b*
elbows, 602–604
finger anomalies, 607, 607*f*
gait and mobility, 586–587, 588*t*
grip strength, 608*b*, 608*f*
herniated disc, 629–630*b*, 630*f*
hips, 610–614
impingement syndrome, 602*b*, 602*f*
inspection, 587–591
joints, 589–591, 593–594
knees, 614–620. *See also* Knees
limb circumference, 591*b*, 591*f*
limb length, 613*b*, 613*f*
muscle size and shape, 587, 589
muscle strength, 595–596, 595*t*
muscle tone, 591–593
neuroexcitability, 597*b*, 597*f*, 604*b*
osteoarthritis, 630*b*
osteoporosis, 612*b*
overall appearance, 585–588
overview, 582
palpation, 591–596
posture, 586
range of motion (ROM), 594–595
relative energy deficiency in sport (RED-S), 619–620*b*
rotator cuff damage, 601*b*, 601*f*, 602*b*, 602*f*
scoliosis, 629, 629*b*, 629*f*
shoulders, 599–602, 632–635

spine, 626–630. *See also* Spine
sports injuries, 604*b*
temporomandibular joint, 596, 596*f*, 597*f*
toe abnormalities, 622, 622*f*
wrists and hands, 605–610. *See also* Wrists and hands
Musculoskeletal system, 573–636
anatomy and physiology, 573–577
assistive devices, 630–631*b*
axial/appendicular skeleton, 574, 574*f*
bones, 574
bursae, 575
cartilage, 574–575
case study (acute shoulder pain), 632–635
head-to-toe examination, 939
health history, 578–581
involuntary muscle movements, 590*t*
joints. *See* Joints
ligaments, 575
muscles, 574, 575*f*
older adult client, 896, 915–916
pediatric client, 870–873
physical examination. *See* Musculoskeletal examination
pregnant client, 788–789, 807
tendons, 574
USPSTF recommendations, 632*b*
Muslims, 144, 144*f*, 149
Mutual expectations, relationships, and conformity to moral norms stage, 94*t*, 100
Mydriatic pupil, 341
Myelomeningocele, 850, 850*f*
Myocardial infarction, 475*t*
Myocarditis, 475*t*
Myocardium, 465
Myoclonus, 590*t*
Myocutaneous flap breast reconstruction, 410
Myometrium, 697*f*, 698, 699*f*
Myopia, 327, 329*f*
MyPlate Food Guide, 158, 158*f*
MyPyramid Food Guide, 158
Myringosclerosis, 370, 370*f*
Myxedema, 307

Nabothian cysts, 719, 719*f*
Naegele rule, 795*t*
Nail pitting, 292, 293*f*
Nails. *See also* Skin, hair, and nails
anatomy/physiology, 256, 256*f*
angle of the nail base, 290, 290*f*, 291
clubbing, 291, 291*f*, 293
color, 289–290
function, 256
health history questions (nail care habits), 260*b*
inspection, 289–292
manicure/pedicure, 261*b*
older adult client, 892, 910–911, 910*b*, 912*b*
palpation, 293
shape and configuration, 290–292
texture, 293
NANDA-I nursing diagnoses, 8
Narcotics, 650*t*
Nares, 356, 358*f*
NAS. *See* Neonatal abstinence syndrome (NAS)
Nasal polyps, 374, 375*f*
Nasal rinse devices, 387*b*
Nasal salute, 307, 308*f*
Nasogastric suction tubes, 551*b*
Nasolacrimal duct, 320*f*
National Human Trafficking Center, 65*b*
National LGBTQIA+ Health Education Center, 37
Naturalistic illnesses, 131
Nausea, 540
NCJMM. *See* Nursing Clinical Judgment Measurement Model (NCJMM)
Neck, 299, 299*f*, 300*f*, 308–309, 309*b*
Necrosis, 267, 267*f*
Neer impingement sign, 602*b*, 602*f*
Neologism, 663
Neonatal abstinence syndrome (NAS), 873*b*
Neonates. *See* Newborns
Neovascularization, 346, 347
Neuroexcitability
Chvostek sign, 597*b*, 597*f*
Trousseau sign, 604*b*
Neurofibroma, 281
Neurofibromatosis, 549*f*
Neurofibromatosis type I, 281
Neurological examination, 652–686
cerebellar function, 653*t*, 679–681
coordination, 680–681
cranial nerves. *See* Cranial nerves
equipment, 652
examination skills, 653*t*
head-to-toe examination, 933–934, 938, 939
mental status. *See* Mental status assessment
motor system, 653*t*, 679
neurological flow sheet, 658*f*
overview, 651, 653*t*
reflexes, 682–686. *See also* Reflexes
sensation. *See* Sensory examination
station, 681
Neurological flow sheet, 658*f*
Neurological system. *See* Mental status and neurological system
Neuropathic pain, 243
Neurovascular deterioration, 625*b*
Nevus flammeus, 266, 267*f*
Nevus vascularis, 266
New Age movements, 142
Newborns. *See also* Pediatric client
acrocyanosis, 848, 848*f*
Apgar score, 847–848, 848*t*
apnea, 226
birth defects, 840*b*
BNBAS, 112*t*
caput succedaneum, 853, 853*f*
cephalohematoma, 853, 853*f*
chest, 833
circumcision, 880*b*
cleft lip, 860, 860*f*
cyanosis, 848
gestational age at birth, 797, 797*b*
jaundice, 848*f*, 849
lanugo, 831
lip blister, 859, 859*f*
milia, 851, 851*f*
molding, 853, 853*f*
neonatal abstinence syndrome (NAS), 873*b*
optical blink reflex, 857
pulse rate, 228*t*
respiratory rate, 226*t*
sclera, 857
tears, 831
thrush, 860
visual acuity, 831
weight, 845
Niacin B_3, 162*t*
NIC. *See* Nursing interventions classification (NIC)
Nicotinic acid, 162*t*
9-valent HPV vaccine, 746*b*
Nipple, 393, 393*f*
Nipple inversion, 403
Nitrites, 806
Nitrogen, 189
Nitrogen balance, 189
NOC outcomes, 10
Nociception, 242, 242*f*
Nociceptive pain, 242–243, 242*f*
Nociplastic pain, 243
Nocturia, 542, 789
Nodule, 270*f*
Non-English speaking client, 40–41, 127
Nonbinary individuals, 127. *See also* LGBTQIA+ individuals
Noncontact infrared thermometer, 232*t*, 234, 234*f*
Noninflammatory edema, 287*t*
Nonmaleficence, 929
Nonpitting edema, 287*t*
Nonstress test (NST), 814*t*
Nontherapeutic communication techniques, 32–37
advising, 35
defending, 34–35
giving approval or disapproval, 34
offering false reassurance, 33–34
probing, 33
problematic interviewing techniques, 35–37
requesting an explanation, 32–33
Nontoxic diffuse goiter, 310, 311
Nonverbal communication, 25, 41
Normalizing, 32, 64*b*, 65
Nose. *See also* Ears, nose, mouth, and throat
anatomy, 356–357
chief complaint (health history), 361
examination, 373–375
head-to-toe examination, 935
nasal rinse devices, 387*b*
older adult client, 893, 914
pediatric client, 859
sinuses. *See* Sinuses
Nostrils, 356
NST. *See* Nonstress test (NST)
Nuchal rigidity, 687*b*
Nuclear family, 133, 134, 134*f*
Numeric Rating Scale, 51, 247
Nurse. *See also* Nursing
client interview, 21
cultural assessment, 123
first, do no harm, 132
professional intuition, 2
SANE, 64*b*
spiritual assessment, 144
Nursing. *See also* Nurse; Nursing process
assistive devices, 933*b*
clinical judgment. *See* Nursing Clinical Judgment Measurement Model (NCJMM)

communicating bad news, 939*b*
culturally competent practice, 124
empowering clients, 932
ethical considerations, 929–930
fostering client cooperation, 931*b*
future of, 943–944
hand-off, 16–17
Healthy People 2030, 943
interviewing the client. *See* Client interview
legal considerations, 929
medication-associated errors, 941*b*. *See also* Medications
merging health history and public health issues, 932*b*
putting it all together. *See* Complete health history and physical examination
Scope and Standards of Practice, 5–6, 6*t*
technological advances, 930–931
tips for successful encounter, 931*b*
verifying assessment data, 933*b*
Nursing: Scope and Standards of Practice, 6*t*, 123
Nursing Clinical Judgment Measurement Model (NCJMM)
analyze cues, 13–14
evaluate outcomes, 16
generate solutions, 15
nursing process, compared, 7*t*
prioritize hypotheses, 14–15
recognize cues, 13
take action, 15–16
what is it?, 6
Nursing diagnosis, 8–9
Nursing interventions, 11
Nursing interventions classification (NIC), 11
Nursing outcomes classification (NOC), 10
Nursing process
dynamic process, 6
NCJMM, compared, 7*t*
six steps, 6. *See also* ANA Standards of Professional Nursing Practice
Nutrition. *See also* Nutritional assessment
adolescents, 170–171, 170*b*, 171*f*
calcium supplements, 173*b*
calorie needs, 159*t*
carbohydrates, 159–160
cholesterol, 160, 186
cultural differences, 174
DASH diet, 173*b*
dietary guidelines, 158
eating disorders, 170, 171*f*
fad diets/exercise regimens, 171
fats, 160–161
healthy eating/safe food handling objectives, 157
infants, 167–168, 168*b*
metabolic syndrome, 171–172
minerals, 163, 164*t*, 165*t*
MyPlate Food Guide, 158, 158*f*
nutrients, 158–166
obesity. *See* Obesity
older adult client, 173, 173*b*, 902
pregnant and lactating clients, 172, 172*b*, 172*f*
preschoolers, 169, 170*b*
protein, 160
psychosocial implications of food, 174*b*
school-age children, 169, 170*b*
toddlers, 168, 170*b*
vitamins, 161, 161*t*, 162–163*t*
water, 166, 166*b*
young and middle-aged adults, 171–172
Nutritional assessment, 157–196. *See also* Nutrition
anthropometric measurements. *See* Anthropometric measurements
basic principles (general approach), 179*b*
case study (underweight client), 192–195
comprehensive assessment, 178*t*
DEXA scan, 191
diet history, 179*t*
equipment, 177, 179*b*
food intake history, 179*t*
laboratory data. *See* Laboratory data
malnutrition, 184, 184*b*
nutritional health history, 174–176, 177, 179*t*
overview, 177
radiographic studies, 191
signs and symptoms of poor nutritional status, 180*t*
USPSTF recommendations, 191*b*
Nystagmus, 336

Obesity
back pain, 585
body fat, 221
body mass index (BMI), 171
children, 169*b*, 169*f*
defined, 171
tactile fremitus, 443
tidal volume, 435
type 2 diabetes, 171
yo-yo dieting/weight cycling, 171
Objective data, 7
Obsessive-compulsive disorder, 666*t*
Obstruction defects, 476–477*t*
Obstructive sleep apnea, 386, 433
Obturator muscle test, 564*b*, 564*f*
Occipital lobe, 639*f*
Oculocephalic reflex, 673*b*, 673*f*
Oculomotor nerve, 644*t*, 673
Oedipus complex, 97
OLD CARTS, 50*b*
Older adult client, 111
abdomen, 895, 915
advance medical directives, 904
anus, rectum, and prostate, 898, 918
bladder, 897
breasts, 894, 914
calorie needs, 159*t*
case study (pneumonia and altered mental status), 920–924
client interview, 898–900
cognitive assessment, 907
cultural assessment, 901
dental disease, 894, 894*f*
developmental assessment, 113*t*, 114*t*, 115*t*, 900–901
developmental tasks, 111
DNR, 904
driving, 904*b*
ears, 893, 913–914
elder abuse and neglect, 916*b*
elderspeak, 898
emergency response system (electronic device), 903*b*
epidemiology, 889–890
eyes, 893, 912–913, 913*b*
falls assessment, 902–903
female genitalia, 897, 917–918
functional assessment, 906
geriatric syndromes, 901–902
head and neck, 892, 911–912
heart, 895, 915
height and weight, 910
male genitalia, 897, 918
mental status and neurological system, 896, 916–917, 920–924
mouth and throat, 893–894, 914
musculoskeletal system, 896, 915–916
nose, 893, 914
nutrition, 173, 173*b*, 902
pain assessment, 903
palliative care, 904
peripheral vasculature, 895, 915
physical examination, 904–905*b*
quick screen, 906*t*
self-determination assessment, 903–904
skin, hair, and nails, 892, 910–911, 910*b*, 912*b*
sleep assessment, 902
spiritual assessment, 901
STIs, 917*t*
thorax and lungs, 894–895, 915
urinary system, 896–897
USPSTF recommendations, 918–919*b*
variations in presentation, 890–891
vital signs, 891, 907–910
Older adult quick screen, 906*t*
Olecranon bursitis, 604, 604*f*
Olfactory nerve, 644*t*, 672–673, 672*b*
Olfactory sense (smell), 209
OME. *See* Otitis media with effusion (OME)
Omega-3-fatty acids, 160*b*
One-handed method of deep palpation, 559, 559*f*
Onychatrophia, 291
Onychauxis, 291, 292*f*
Onychocryptosis, 291, 292*f*
Onycholysis, 291, 292*f*
Onychomycosis, 290, 290*f*
Onychophagy, 292, 292*f*
Onychorrhexis, 292, 292*f*
Onychoschizia, 292, 293*f*
Oogenesis, 699
Open-ended questions, 26
Open Invite, 146
Opening snap, 491, 492*f*
Operation Desert Storm, 70
Ophthalmoplegia, 336
Ophthalmoscope, 343, 343*f*, 344*t*
Opioid crisis, 249–250
Opposition, 576*t*
Optic disc, 322, 345*f*
Optic nerve, 321*f*, 644*t*, 673
Optical blink reflex, 857
Oral appliances, 387*b*
Oral hairy leukoplakia, 380, 381*f*
Oral psychosexual stage, 94*t*, 97
Oral temperature, 231*t*, 232, 232*f*
Orchitis, 754
Orientation, 656
Oropharynx, 861
Orthodox Christians, 142, 149, 151
Orthopnea, 437
Orthostatic hypotension, 519*b*
Ortolani maneuver, 872, 872*f*, 873

Ossicles, 355
Osteoarthritis, 309, 607, 630*b*
Osteogenesis imperfecta, 338
Osteonecrosis of the jaw, 596
Osteoporosis, 172, 172*f*, 191, 585, 612*b*, 632*b*
Otalgia, 360
Otitis externa, 371, 372*t*
Otitis media, 371, 372*b*, 372*t*, 859*b*
Otitis media with effusion (OME), 369, 370*f*, 371, 371*f*
Otorrhea, 361
Oucher Pain Assessment Tool, 248, 248*f*, 840
Outcomes identification, 6*t*, 10
Outflow valves, 465
Ovarian cancer, 721*b*
Ovarian cycle, 699–700, 700*f*
Ovary, 699, 699*f*
Overflow incontinence, 566*b*
Overload, 494
Oxygen, as respiratory assistance, 438*b*
Oxygen-poor/oxygen-rich blood, 503*f*

Pack/year history, 62
Packs per day (PPD), 63
PAD. *See* Peripheral artery disease (PAD)
Paganism, 142
Paget disease, 402*t*
Pain, 241–249
  acute, 244, 248
  age, 244
  assessment tools, 247–248, 247*f*, 248*f*
  chronic malignant/nonmalignant, 244, 248
  culture, 244–245
  cutaneous, 243
  defined, 241
  effects of pain on body, 247
  females, 244
  fifth vital sign, 242
  health history, 245–247
  key points, 241
  medications, 249
  neuropathic, 243
  no cure (decreasing severity of pain symptoms), 249
  nociceptive, 242–243, 242*f*
  nociplastic, 243
  nonpharmacological treatments, 249
  older adult client, 903
  pediatric client, 840, 842
  perception of, 244
  physiological responses, 247
  physiology of pain perception, 242*f*
  referred, 243
  somatic, 243
  visceral, 243
PAINAD tool, 248, 903
Palate, 384–385
Palatine arches and pillars, 359
Palatine perforation, 385, 385*f*
Palatine tonsils, 357*f*, 359, 359*f*
Palliative care, 904
Palliative shunt murmur, 868
Pallor, 523*b*
Palmar grasp reflex, 874, 874*f*
Palpation, 209–212
Palpebral conjunctiva, 319, 337, 337*f*
Palpebral fissure, 319, 320*f*
Pancreas, 534*f*, 539
Pancreatic cancer, 556*b*
Pancreatitis, 568–571
Panic attack, 665*t*
Panic disorder, 665*t*
Pansystolic murmur, 491, 493, 868
Pantheism, 142
Pantothenic acid, 163*t*
Pap smear, 721–724
Papillae, 358
Papillary layer, 254
Papilledema, 346, 346*f*
Papule, 270*f*
Parallel lines breast palpation method, 408*f*
Paranasal sinuses, 357, 357*f*
Paraphimosis, 748, 749*f*
Parasympathetic nervous system, 645, 645*t*
Parathyroid disease, 312*t*
Paraurethral glands, 696
Paresthesia, 647, 669
Parietal lobe, 639*f*
Parietal pain, 544*t*
Parietal pericardium, 464, 464*f*
Parietal peritoneum, 534
Parietal pleura, 420
Parkinson disease, 307, 307*f*
Paronychia, 291, 292*f*
Parotitis, 382, 382*f*, 861, 861*f*
Pars flaccida, 355, 355*f*
Pars tensa, 355, 355*f*
Past health history, 52–58
  allergies, 53, 53*b*
  blood transfusions, 56
  childhood illnesses, 56–57
  communicable diseases, 55
  differing abilities, 56
  immunizations, 57, 57*b*, 58*t*
  injuries and accidents, 56
  medical history, 53
  medications, 53*b*, 54–55, 54*b*
  surgical history, 53
Pastoral care, 151
Patch, 270*f*
Patellar ballottement, 616–617*b*, 617*f*
Patellar reflex, 683, 683*f*
Patent ductus arteriosus (PDA), 481*t*
Pathological jaundice of the newborn, 849
Pathological reflexes, 685–686
Patient. *See* Client
Patient Health Questionnaire, 2 items (PHQ-2), 113*t*
Patient Health Questionnaire, 9 items (PHQ-9), 113*t*
PDA. *See* Patent ductus arteriosus (PDA)
PDE 5 inhibitors. *See* Phosphodiesterase type 5 (PDE 5) inhibitors
PE tubes. *See* Pressure equalization (PE) tubes
Peau d'orange, 402, 402*t*
Pectus carinatum, 428, 429, 429*f*
Pectus excavatum, 429, 429*f*
Pederson speculum, 707, 707*f*
Pediatric client, 823–888
  abdomen, 834, 868–870
  adolescence. *See* Adolescents
  adoption, 850*b*
  alternative alcohol consumption, 878*b*
  Apgar score, 847–848, 848*t*
  blood pressure, 844*b*
  breasts, 833
  case study (ear pain and hydrocele), 883–887
  choking, 861*b*
  client cooperativeness, 844*b*
  COVID-19 pandemic, 882
  developmental assessment, 840, 841*f*
  eustachian tube, 831–832
  eyes, ears, nose, mouth, and throat, 831–832, 859–861
  fat intake in young children, 877*b*
  female genitalia, 834, 877–879
  foster care, 850*b*
  growth charts, 824, 825–829*f*
  head, 831, 832*f*, 846–847, 846*f*, 851–854
  health history, 834–839
  heart, 833, 864–868
  height, 846, 846*f*
  immunization schedule, 839*t*
  infant. *See* Infants
  male genitalia, 834, 879–882
  marijuana poisoning, 878*b*
  musculoskeletal system, 834, 870–873
  neurological system, 834, 873–877
  order of examination procedures, 212*b*
  pain assessment, 840, 842
  penis, 880
  peripheral vasculature, 833, 868
  physical examination. *See* Pediatric physical examination
  physical growth, 823–829
  preschooler. *See* Preschoolers
  salmonellosis, 833*b*
  school-age children. *See* School-age children
  sexual abuse, 881*b*
  sinuses, 831–832, 832*f*
  skin and hair, 831, 848–851
  stridor, 863*b*
  teeth, 832, 832*f*, 860
  thorax and lungs, 833, 862–864
  toddler. *See* Toddlers
  urinary system, 834
  USPSTF recommendations, 882–883*b*
  vital signs, 830, 844–845
  weight, 845–846, 845*f*
Pediatric physical examination. *See also* Pediatric client
  abdomen, 868–870
  anus, 881–882
  Apgar score, 847–848, 848*t*
  apical impulse, 864
  breasts, 862
  breath sounds, 863–864
  chest circumference, 847, 847*f*
  coarctation of the aorta, 867*b*, 868
  color vision, 854–855
  cranial nerve function, 876–877
  ears, 858–859, 859*b*
  equipment, 843
  eyelids, 856
  eyes, 853–858
  feet, 872
  female genitalia, 877–879
  fontanel, 852
  general approach, 842*b*
  hair, 850
  head, 851–854
  head circumference, 826*f*, 846–847, 846*f*
  heart, 864–868
  heart sounds, 866–868
  height, 846, 846*f*
  hip and femur, 872–873

inguinal hernia, 881
joints, 871, 872
lacrimal apparatus, 856
length or height, 846, 846*f*
lens, 857
lips, 859–860
liver, 870
lymph nodes, 862
male genitalia, 879–882
mouth and throat, 859–861
murmurs, 866–868
muscle strength, 870*b*
musculoskeletal system, 870–873
neck, 861–862
neurological system, 873–877
nose, 859
oropharynx, 861
overview, 843
penis, 880
peripheral vasculature, 868
red reflex, 857
respiratory distress, 863
respiratory rate, 845
retina, 858
scrotum, 881
skin, 848–851
tactile fremitus, 863
teeth, 860
temperature, 844–845
thorax and lungs, 862–864
thrills, 865
thyroid, 862
tibiofemoral bones, 872
vision screening, 854, 854*f*
vital signs, 844–845
weight, 845–846, 845*f*
Pediatric Symptom Checklist (PSC), 113*t*
Pediculosis capitis, 288
Pediculosis pubis, 709
Pedicure, 261*b*
PEDS. *See* Early Language Milestones Scale (PEDS)
Pelvic abscess, 564*b*, 564*f*
Pelvic pain, 703
Penile cancer, 745, 745*b*, 746*f*
Penile carcinoma, 745, 746*f*
Penile lesion, 740
Penis, 737
body piercing, 744*b*
cancer, 745, 745*b*, 746*f*
disappearing penis phenomenon, 880
inspection, 743–749
palpation, 751, 751*f*
pediatric client, 880
penile lump and Peyronie disease, 759–761
uncircumcised, 744*b*
Penis envy, 97
PEP. *See* Polymorphic eruptions in pregnancy (PEP)
Percussion, 212–215
Percussion pitch, 212*f*
Percussion sounds, 212, 213*t*
Percussion strike, 214*f*
Perforated eardrum, 371, 372*f*
Pericardial friction rub, 494, 494*b*, 495*t*
Pericarditis, 475*t*, 482*t*
Pericardium, 463–464, 464*f*
Perichondrial hematoma, 366, 367*f*
Perichondritis, 367, 367*f*
Perifollicular papules, 281
Perilymph, 356
Perimetrium, 699*f*
Perinatal depression, 813*b*
Perineal chancroid, 715, 715*f*, 773, 773*f*
Perineum, 696*f*, 697, 714–715, 717, 769–770
Periodontitis, 383
Peripheral artery disease (PAD), 511*t*, 520*b*
Peripheral edema, 508
Peripheral nerve lesions, 669
Peripheral nervous system, 642–643
Peripheral neuropathy, 687*b*, 687*f*
Peripheral perfusion, 518–520
Peripheral pulmonary arterial stenosis, 867*t*
Peripheral pulse rates, 227*f*
Peripheral vasculature and lymphatic systems, 502–532
anatomy and physiology, 502–507
ankle-brachial index (ABI), 524–525*b*
arterial insufficiency vs. venous insufficiency, 520*b*, 521*t*
arterial pulse examination, 516–518
arterial system anatomy, 504*f*
arterial ulceration, 519, 519*f*
assessing arterial system, 523–524*b*
assessing venous system, 522–523*b*
assistive devices, 521–522*b*
case study (leg claudication), 527–530
cervical venous distention (CVD), 515, 515*f*
cervical venous pressure (CVP), 514–515
disorders/diseases, 510–512*t*
equipment, 512
health history, 508–510
hepatojugular reflux, 515–516, 516*f*
jugular venous pressure (JVP), 513–515
lymphatic system. *See* Lymphatic system
older adult client, 895, 915
orthostatic hypotension examination, 519*b*
oxygen-poor/oxygen-rich blood, 503*f*
pediatric client, 833, 868
peripheral artery disease (PAD), 520*b*
peripheral perfusion, 518–520
physical examination, 512–526, 513*b*
pregnant client, 787, 805
pulsus paradoxus, 517*f*, 518*b*
Raynaud phenomenon, 519, 520*f*
systemic and pulmonary circuits, 503*f*
TIA (mini-stroke), 512*b*
USPSTF recommendations, 527*b*
varicose veins, 522*b*, 522*f*, 523*b*
venous system anatomy, 505*f*
venous ulceration, 520, 520*f*
Peristalsis, 549
Peritoneal cavity, 534
Peritoneal dialysis catheter, 551*b*
Peritoneum, 533–534, 697*f*, 698
Peritonsillar abscess, 386
Periungual tissue, 255, 255*f*
Permanent vegetative state, 659*t*
Personal distance, 25
Personal health record (PHR), 930*b*
Personal hygiene, 653–654
Personal protective equipment (PPE), 199, 200*f*, 202*f*
Personal space, 26
Personalistic illnesses, 131
Pertinent negatives, 51
Pertussis, 436*b*
Pes cavus, 622
Pes planus (flat feet), 622
Pes valgus, 622
Pes varus, 622
Petechiae, 265, 266*f*
Peyer's patches, 506*f*, 507
Peyronie disease, 749, 749*f*, 759–761
Phalen sign, 610*b*, 610*f*
Phallic psychosexual stage, 94*t*, 97
Pharmacogenetic testing, 61*b*
Pharyngeal tonsil, 507
Philtrum, 358, 358*f*
Phimosis, 748, 749*f*, 880, 880*f*
Phobias, 665*t*
Phoria, 334, 335
Phosphodiesterase type 5 (PDE 5) inhibitors, 758*b*
Phosphorus (P), 164*t*, 624*b*
PHQ-2. *See* Patient Health Questionnaire, 2 items (PHQ-2)
PHQ-9. *See* Patient Health Questionnaire, 9 items (PHQ-9)
PHR. *See* Personal health record (PHR)
Physical activity (exercise), 72–73, 72*f*, 73*b*
Physical appearance and behavior, 652–654
Physical examination, 198–218. *See also* Head-to-toe examination
appropriate client placement, 201, 208*f*
auscultation, 215–216
ending the visit, 207
equipment, 203, 205, 206*f*
general approach, 206–207, 932*b*
general examination reminders, 933*b*
golden rules, 216–217
hand hygiene, 199, 200*f*, 201*f*
head-to-toe approach, 7–8
inspection, 209
legal considerations, 216
nurse's role, 199
objective data, 7
olfactory sense (smell), 209
order of examination procedures, 212*b*
palpation, 209–212
percussion, 212–215
personal protective equipment (PPE), 199, 200*f*, 202*f*
positioning and draping techniques, 207, 208*f*
practicing physical examination techniques, 209*b*
preparing for, 205
purposes, 198
safe injection practices, 203
Standard Precautions, 199, 200*f*
stethoscope, 215–216, 215*f*, 216*b*, 216*f*
Transmission-Based Precautions, 203, 204*f*
visual inspection, 209
Physiological cup, 322, 345, 345*f*, 346
Physiological hyperplasia, 310
Pia mater, 638, 638*f*
Piaget's theory of cognitive development, 93–96
concrete operational stage, 94*t*, 96
conservation, 96
egocentrism, 96
formal operational stage, 94–95*t*, 96
overview, 94–95*t*
preoperational stage, 94*t*, 96
reversibility, 96
sensorimotor stage, 94*t*, 95

Pigeon chest, 428
Pilonidal cyst, 769, 769*f*
Pilonidal disease, 769
Pinguecula, 337, 337*f*
Pink nevus simplex, 849, 849*f*
Pinna, 354, 355*f*
Pitting edema, 286, 286*f*, 287*t*
Pityriasis rosea, 272, 272*f*
Pivot joint, 577*t*
Placing reflex, 876, 877*f*
Plagiocephaly, 831*b*
Planning, 6*t*, 10–12
Plantar flexion, 576*t*
Plantar grasp reflex, 875, 875*f*
Plantar reflex, 684, 684*f*
Plantar wart, 278*f*
Plaque, 270*f*
Plaques of pregnancy (PUPP), 803
Plateau murmur, 493, 493*f*
Pleura, 418*f*, 420–421
Pleural effusion, 443, 446, 453–455*t*, 456*f*
Pleural friction fremitus, 443
Pleural friction rub, 450*t*, 494*b*
Pleximeter, 213
Plexor, 213
PLLR. *See* Pregnancy/lactation labeling rule (PLLR)
PMI. *See* Point of maximal impulse (PMI)
Pneumatic compression stockings, 522*b*
Pneumonia
  case study, 458–461, 920–924
  chest pain, 482*t*
  older adult, 920–924
  risk factors, 457*b*
  selected respiratory conditions, compared, 453–455*t*, 457*f*
Pneumothorax, 453–455*t*, 457*f*, 482*t*
Point of maximal impulse (PMI), 485, 486*b*
Polycyclic lesions, 269*f*
Polycythemia, 262, 264
Polydactyly, 871
  fingers, 607, 607*f*
  toes, 622, 622*f*
Polymorphic eruptions in pregnancy (PEP), 803
Polymyalgia rheumatica, 592
Polypharmacy, 907
Polyps, 545*b*
Polysynaptic reflex, 645*f*, 646
Polytheistic religions, 142
Pons, 639, 639*f*
Popliteal lymph nodes, 506*f*, 526, 526*f*
Port-wine stain, 266
Positioning and draping techniques, 207, 208*f*
Posterior axillary line, 420*b*
Posterior cerebral artery, 642*f*, 642*t*
Posterior chamber, 322
Posterior column, 641
Posterior drawer test, 618*b*, 618*f*
Posterior thorax percussion, 214*f*, 445
Posterior triangle, 299, 299*f*
Posttraumatic stress disorder (PTSD), 666*t*
Posture, 586, 652
Potassium (K), 164*t*
Potassium hydroxide (KOH), 725
Potbelly, 869
Pouch of Douglas, 698
Poupart ligament, 737
PPD. *See* Packs per day (PPD)
PPE. *See* Personal protective equipment (PPE)
PRESTO, 50*b*
Prayer, 146, 146*f*
Prealbumin, 187–188
Precordium, 482–484
Preeclampsia, 801–802*t*
Prediabetes, 188
Pregnancy/lactation labeling rule (PLLR), 794*b*
Pregnant client, 784–822
  abdomen, 788, 805–806
  abuse, identifying, 791*b*
  adolescents (pregnant teens), 816
  anatomy and physiology, 784–791
  antepartum tests and evaluations, 814*t*
  anus and rectum, 791, 813
  blood pressure, 787
  Braxton Hicks contractions, 790
  breasts, 408*b*, 786, 786*b*, 804–805, 804*b*, 804*f*
  breech presentation, 810*f*, 812
  case study, 818–821
  center of balance, 789*b*
  client education, 816–817*b*
  common complaints, 800–801*t*
  danger signs, 815*t*
  drug safety categories, 794*b*
  ectopic pregnancy, 807*b*
  endocrine system, 791, 813
  estimated date of delivery (EDD), 795*f*, 795*t*
  eyes, ears, nose, and throat, 804
  female genitalia, 789–790, 807, 809
  fetal heart tone (FHT), 809–810, 810*f*, 811, 811*b*
  friability, 790, 807
  fundal height, 809
  gastrointestinal health, 788*b*
  general assessment, 798–799
  gestational age at birth, 797, 797*b*
  gravida/para (TPAL), 795*b*
  hair treatments, 785*b*
  head and neck, 785–786, 804
  health history, 791–794
  heart, 786–787, 805
  high-risk factors, 796–797*t*
  hypertensive disorders, 799, 799*b*, 801–802*t*
  laboratory tests, 808*t*
  Leopold maneuver, 811–812, 812*f*
  lightening, 790
  lordosis, 789, 789*f*
  muscle cramps, 789*b*
  musculoskeletal system, 788–789, 807
  neurological system, 789*b*, 807
  nutrition, 172, 172*b*, 172*f*
  nutritional assessment, 172*b*
  pelvic organs, 790*t*
  perinatal depression, 813*b*
  peripheral vasculature, 787, 805
  physical examination, 797*b*
  prenatal visits, 798, 816
  prenatal vitamins, 172
  psychosocial assessment and learning needs, 813–816
  quickening, 816*b*
  signs and symptoms of pregnancy, 799*b*
  skin and hair, 785, 803–804
  supine hypotension and lower extremity edema, 787, 787*b*, 787*f*
  thorax and lungs, 786, 805
  urinary system, 788, 788*b*, 806–807
  USPSTF recommendations, 817*b*
  uterine and abdominal enlargement, 789*f*, 809
  vertex presentation, 810*f*, 812
  waddle of pregnancy, 789
Pregnant teens, 816
Prehn sign, 753*b*
Prejudices, 129
Preload, 494
Premature ventricular complex (PVC), 227
Premolars, 359, 359*f*
Prenatal visits, 798, 816
Prenatal vitamins, 172
Preoperational stage, 94*t*, 96
Preparticipation athletic evaluation, 942–943
Prepuce (foreskin), 736*f*, 737
Presbycusis, 893
Presbyopia, 328, 893
Preschoolers, 105–106. *See also* Pediatric client
  calorie needs, 159*t*
  childhood fears, 830*b*
  cranial nerve function, 877
  developmental tasks, 106
  heart, 833
  immunization schedule, 839*t*
  inguinal hernia, 881
  milestones, 106*t*
  nutrition, 169, 170*b*
  physical growth, 824
  potbelly, 869
  readiness for school, 106
  weight, 845, 845*f*
Pressure equalization (PE) tubes, 369, 369*f*
Pressure injuries, 282*b*, 283*b*, 283*f*
Presystolic murmur, 868
Priapism, 748–749
Prince Albert piercing, 744*b*
Prioritization, 10–11
Problem-focused diagnosis, 9
Problem list, 940–941
Problematic interviewing techniques, 35–37
  authoritativeness, 36–37
  hidden agendas, 37
  interrupting the client, 35–36
  leading questions, 35
  medical jargon, 36
  multiple questions, 36
  neglecting to ask pertinent questions, 36
  talkativeness, 36
Professional intuition, 2
Progress note, 18
Prolapse of urethral mucosa, 712, 712*f*
Pronation, 576*t*
Pronator drift, 679
Prone position, 208*f*
Proprioceptive sensation, 670–671
Proptosis, 331, 331*f*
Prostate, 764*f*, 765. *See also* Anus, rectum, and prostate
Prostate cancer, 775*b*, 777, 777*b*, 777*f*
Prostate-specific antigen (PSA), 776*b*, 777*b*
Prostatitis, 776*b*
Prosthetic eye, 331, 331*f*
Prosthetic heart valves, 494–495
Protein, 160
Proteinuria, 789, 807
Protraction, 576*t*

Protuberant abdomen, 547, 547*f*
Pruritic urticarial papules, 803
Pruritus, 257, 767, 770, 892
Pruritus ani, 770–771
PS. *See* Pulmonary stenosis (PS)
PSA. *See* Prostate-specific antigen (PSA)
PSC. *See* Pediatric Symptom Checklist (PSC)
Pseudofolliculitis barbae, 281
Pseudostrabismus, 855*b*
Psoriasis, 274, 274*f*
Psychedelics, 63*b*
Psychological presence, 223–224
Pterygium, 292, 338, 338*f*
Ptosis, 331, 331*f*
PTSD. *See* Posttraumatic stress disorder (PTSD)
Ptyalism, 786
Puberty, 700–701. *See also* Sexual maturity rating (SMR)
Pubic hair
 females, 701*t*, 709
 males, 738*t*, 743
Pubic lice, 709, 709*f*
Public distance, 25
Puddle sign, 557*b*, 557*f*
Pulmonary atresia, 480*t*
Pulmonary edema, 453–455*t*, 457*f*
Pulmonary embolus, 482*t*
Pulmonary flow murmur, 867*t*
Pulmonary regurgitation or insufficiency, 475*t*, 495*t*
Pulmonary stenosis (PS), 475*t*, 476*t*
Pulmonic area, 483, 483*f*
 auscultation, 489–490
 inspection, 484–485
 palpation, 487
Pulmonic ejection click, 491*f*
Pulmonic regurgitation or insufficiency, 475*t*, 495*t*
Pulmonic stenosis, 495*t*
Pulse, 226–229
 apical, 227, 228, 228*f*
 asystole, 228, 229
 bradycardia, 228
 charting peripheral pulses, 229*b*, 229*f*
 deficit, 228, 229
 dysrhythmias/arrhythmias, 229
 older adult client, 891, 909
 peripheral pulse sites, 227*f*
 radial, 228, 228*f*
 rate, 226–227, 228, 228*t*
 rhythm, 227, 229
 site, 227, 227*f*
 tachycardia, 228
 volume, 227, 227*t*, 229
Pulse deficit, 228, 229
Pulse oximeter, 439*b*, 439*f*
Pulse pressure, 235, 239
Pulse rate, 226–227, 228, 228*t*
Pulseless electrical activity, 229
Pulsus alternans, 517*f*
Pulsus bisferiens, 517*f*
Pulsus paradoxus, 517*f*, 518*b*
Punctum (puncta), 320, 320*f*
Pupil
 abnormalities, 342–343*t*
 generally, 321*f*, 322
 older adult client, 912–913
 physical examination, 340–341, 341*f*
PUPP. *See* Plaques of pregnancy (PUPP)
Purkinje fibers, 469, 469*f*
Purpura, 265, 266*f*
Pursed-lip breathing, 437, 437*f*
Pustular psoriasis, 274, 274*f*
Pustule, 270*f*
PVC. *See* Premature ventricular complex (PVC)
Pyramidal tract, 641
Pyridoxine, 162*t*

Queer, 38
Questioning, 38
Quickening, 816*b*

R-PDQ. *See* Revised Prescreening Developmental Questionnaire (R-PDQ)
Race, 125–126
Racial prejudice, 129
Racism, 101–102
Radial pulse, 228, 228*f*
Radical mastectomy, 409*t*
R.A.L.E. Respiratory, 452*b*
Range of motion (ROM), 594–595
RAS. *See* Reticular activating system (RAS)
Rash, 257–258
Raynaud phenomenon, 292, 511*t*, 519, 520*f*
RBB. *See* Right bundle branch (RBB)
RCA. *See* Right coronary artery (RCA)
RDA. *See* Recommended dietary allowances (RDA)
Rebound tenderness, 563*b*, 563*f*
Recommended dietary allowances (RDA), 158
Recreational drug use, 63, 63*b*
Rectal abuse, 774*b*
Rectal bleeding, 766, 774*b*
Rectal pain, 766
Rectal polyps, 775*f*
Rectal prolapse, 771, 772*f*, 775, 898
Rectal temperature, 231*t*, 232–233, 844–845
Rectocele, 714, 714*f*
Rectouterine pouch, 697*f*, 698
Rectovaginal examination, 729–730, 729*f*
Rectovaginal septum, 697*f*
Rectum, 763, 764*f*. *See also* Anus, rectum, and prostate
Rectus abdominis muscles, 548
Red marrow, 574
Red pulp, 507
Red reflex, 344, 344*f*, 345, 857
RED-S. *See* Relative energy deficiency in sport (RED-S)
Reepithelialization, 256*b*
Referred pain, 243, 544*t*, 545*f*
Reflexes, 682–686
 abdominal, 684, 684*f*
 Achilles, 683, 683*f*
 anal, 685
 Babinski, 686
 biceps, 682–683, 682*f*
 brachioradialis, 682, 682*f*
 bulbocavernosus, 685
 clonus, 686
 corneal, 674, 675*f*
 cremasteric, 685, 685*f*
 deep tendon, 682–684
 examination skill, 653*t*
 glabellar, 686
 monosynaptic/polysynaptic, 645*f*, 646
 muscle stretch, 684
 oculocephalic, 673*b*, 673*f*
 patellar, 683, 683*f*
 pathological, 685–686
 plantar, 684, 684*f*
 reflex action, defined, 645
 superficial, 684–685
 triceps, 683, 683*f*
Regional lymph nodes, 394, 395*f*. *See also* Lymph nodes
Regular pulse, 227
Regurgitation or insufficiency, 494
Relative energy deficiency in sport (RED-S), 619–620*b*
Religion, 70, 141. *See also* Spiritual assessment
Renal cancer, 562*b*
Resonance, 213*t*
Respirations
 audibility, 436
 client position, 436–437, 437*f*
 depth, 434–435
 mode of breathing, 437, 437*f*
 older adult client, 891
 pattern, 433–434, 434*f*, 435
 rate, 432–433, 432*b*, 453*t*
 symmetry, 435–436
Respiratory assistive devices, 438–439*b*
Respiratory cycle, 432
Respiratory distress, 225, 225*f*, 863
Respiratory patterns, 433–434, 434*f*, 435
Respiratory rate, 226*t*, 432–433, 432*b*, 453*t*, 845
Respiratory tract, 417, 418*f*. *See also* Thorax and lungs
Reticular activating system (RAS), 639, 656
Reticular formation, 639
Reticular layer, 254
Retina, 321*f*, 322
Retinal structures, 344–347, 344*f*
Retinitis pigmentosa, 346*f*
Retinoblastoma, 857
Retinol, 161*t*
Retraction, 576*t*
Retroflexed uterus, 698*f*
Retrograde filling, 523*b*
Retroperitoneal organs, 534
Retroverted uterus, 698*f*
Reversibility, 96
Review of systems (ROS), 74–76
Revised-Denver II, 840, 841*f*
Revised Prescreening Developmental Questionnaire (R-PDQ), 112*t*
Rheumatoid arthritis, 593, 607
Rhinitis, 374
Rhonchal fremitus, 443
Rib cage angles, 430–431, 431*f*, 453*t*
Riboflavin, 162*t*
Ribs, 418, 419*f*
Rickets, 191, 191*f*, 429
Right bundle branch (RBB), 469
Right coronary artery (RCA), 466–467
Right lower quadrant (RLQ), 535*f*, 535*t*, 536–537*t*
Right upper quadrant (RUQ), 535*f*, 535*t*, 536*t*
Right ventricular failure, 489
Ringworm, 288
Rinne test, 366, 366*f*
Risk nursing diagnosis, 9

Rituals, 141
RLQ. *See* Right lower quadrant (RLQ)
Road Wide Driver Course, 904*b*
Rocky Mountain spotted fever, 277, 278*f*
Rods, 322
ROM. *See* Range of motion (ROM)
Romberg test, 681*b*
Roofing reflex, 874, 874*f*
ROS. *See* Review of systems (ROS)
Rosacea rhinophyma, 274, 274*f*
Rosenbaum Pocket Vision Screener, 329
Roseola, 276, 276*f*
Rotator cuff damage, 601*b*, 601*f*, 602*b*, 602*f*
Roth spots, 346
Rounded abdomen, 547*f*
Rounded bones, 574
Rovsing sign, 563*b*
Rubella, 277, 277*f*
Rubeola, 276, 277*f*
Ruptured Achilles tendon, 626*b*, 626*f*
RUQ. *See* Right upper quadrant (RUQ)

S_1, 468, 489, 490, 490–492*f*, 491, 866
S_2, 468, 489, 490–492*f*, 866
S_3, 492, 492*b*, 492*f*, 866
S_4, 492, 492*f*, 493*b*, 866
S-A (sinoatrial) node, 226, 468, 469*f*
Sacral nerves, 640*f*
Sacrament of the Anointing of the Sick, 144, 144*f*, 151
Saddle joint, 577*t*
Saddle pattern of sensation loss, 669
Safe home environment, 581*b*
Safe injection practices, 203
Saline mount ("wet prep"), 725
Salmon patch, 849
Salmonellosis, 833*b*
SANE nurse, 64*b*
SARS-CoV2, 201. *See also* COVID-19 pandemic
SASQ. *See* Single Alcohol Screening Question (SASQ)
Saturated fats, 160
SBAR, 17, 17*t*
Scab formation, 256*b*
Scabies, 275, 275*f*
Scales, 271*f*
Scalp, 305–306, 637, 638*f*
Scaphoid abdomen, 547, 547*f*
Scapular line, 420*b*
Scapular winging, 600
Scar, 271*f*
Scar formation, 256*b*
Scarification, 262*b*, 263*f*
Scarlet fever, 277, 277*f*
SCC. *See* Squamous cell carcinoma (SCC)
Schizophrenia, 667*t*
School-age children, 106–107. *See also* Pediatric client
  calorie needs, 159*t*
  childhood fears, 831*b*
  developmental assessment tools, 112*t*, 113*t*
  developmental tasks, 107
  immunization schedule, 839*t*
  inguinal hernia, 881
  milestones, 107*t*
  nutrition, 169, 170*b*
  physical growth, 824
  pulse rate, 228*t*
  respiratory rate, 226*t*
  weight, 845
Scientific illness, 130
Scissors gait, 588*t*
Sclera, 321, 321*f*, 322, 338, 857
Scleral icterus, 338, 338*f*
Scleroderma, 307, 307*f*
Scoliometer, 629*b*, 629*f*
Scoliosis, 429, 626, 628, 628*f*, 629, 629*b*, 629*f*
Scooter, motorized, 631*b*
Scope and Standards of Practice, 5–6, 6*t*, 123–124. *See also* ANA Standards of Professional Nursing Practice
Scotomata, 348*b*
Scrotal edema, 754, 754*f*
Scrotal tongue, 380, 381*f*
Scrotum, 736*f*, 737
  auscultation, 757
  condylomatous lesions, 750*f*
  inspection, 749–750
  pain, 740
  palpation, 752–754
  pediatric client, 881
  scrotal edema, 754, 754*f*
  transillumination, 755*b*, 755*f*
Scurvy, 191
SDOH. *See* Social determinants of health (SDOH)
Sebaceous cyst, 750
Sebaceous glands, 253*f*, 254
Sebaceous hyperplasia, 910
Sebaceous keratosis, 910, 911*b*
Seborrhea, 288
Seborrheic dermatitis, 288, 289*f*, 851, 852*f*
Sebum, 254
Second-degree burn, 283, 284*f*
Secondary hypertension, 239
Sedative-hypnotics, 650*t*
See High-density lipoproteins (HDL), 160
Seizure, 646–647
Selenium (Se), 165*t*
Self-care practices, 132
Self-determination, 903–904
Self-harm/self-mutilation, 281, 281*f*
Semaglutide, 183*b*
Semi-Fowler's position, 208*f*
Semicircular canals, 355*f*, 356
Semilunar valves, 465, 468
Seminal vesicles, 736, 736*f*
Seminiferous tubules, 735, 736*f*
Senile cataract, 341
Senile lentigo, 910, 910*f*
Senile pruritus, 892
Senile purpura, 910
Sensation. *See* Sensory examination
Sense of Coherence Scale (SOC) Scale, 113*t*
Sensorimotor stage, 94*t*, 95
Sensory ataxia gait, 588*t*
Sensory examination
  cortical sensation, 671–672
  examination skill, 653*t*
  exteroceptive sensation, 668–670
  extinction, 672
  general approach, 667*b*
  graphesthesia, 671, 671*f*
  light touch, 668, 668*f*
  motion and position, 670
  proprioceptive sensation, 670–671
  stereognosis, 671, 671*f*
  superficial pain, 668–669
  temperature, 669
  two-point discrimination, 671–672, 671*f*
  vibration sense, 670–671, 670*f*
Sensory skills
  adolescents, 108
  infancy, 102–103*t*
  school-age children, 106*t*
  toddlers, 104–105*t*
Separated shoulder, 601
Septa, 464
Septal defects, 478–479*t*
Serial 3s, 660
Serial 7s, 660, 662
Serous otitis media, 372*f*
Serpiginous lesions, 269*f*
Serum iron, 186, 187
Sesamoid bones, 574
Sexual assault. *See also* Abuse
  females, 715*b*
  male sexual assault (MSA), 747*b*
  SANE nurse, 64*b*
  sexual abuse in children, 881*b*
Sexual assault nurse examiner (SANE) nurse, 64*b*
Sexual maturity rating (SMR)
  female breast development, 395, 396*t*
  female pubic hair, 701, 701*t*
  male genitalia, 738*t*, 743
Sexual orientation, 126–127. *See also* LGBTQIA+ individuals
Sexual practice, 65–66, 66*b*
Sexually abused client, 715*b*
Sexually aggressive client, 42
Sexually transmitted infections (STIs), 752*b*, 879*b*, 917*b*
Shahada, 149
Shaken baby syndrome, 858
Shifting dullness, 557*b*, 557*f*
Shingles, 276, 276*f*
Short bones, 574
Short leg gait, 588*t*
Shoulders, 599–602, 632–635
Sibilant wheeze, 450*t*
Side lying position, 208*f*
SIDS. *See* Sudden infant death syndrome (SIDS)
Sighing, 434*f*, 435
Sildenafil (Viagra), 758*b*
Silence, 27
Simple mastectomy, 409*t*
Sims' position, 208*f*
Single Alcohol Screening Question (SASQ), 61, 62*b*, 114*t*
Single-sided dual-frequency acoustic stethoscope, 215*f*
Sinoatrial (S-A) node, 226, 468, 469*f*
Sinuses. *See also* Ears, nose, mouth, and throat
  anatomy, 357–358, 357*f*
  examination, 375–376
  transillumination, 376*b*, 377*f*
Sinuses of Valsalva, 465
Sitting position, 208*f*
Situs inversus, 488*b*
Situs solitus, 488*b*
6-Minute Walk Test, 452*b*
Skeletal joints, 577, 577*t*

Skeletal muscle, 574
Skene glands, 696, 696*f*, 716
Skin, 261–286
anatomy and physiology, 252–254
avoiding integumentary damage, 912*b*
bleeding, ecchymosis, and vascularity, 265–266
burns, 283, 284*f*
case study (lip lesion), 293–296
color, 262–265
dermis, 253–254, 253*f*
edema, 286, 286*b*, 287*f*, 287*t*
enhancement techniques, 267*b*
epidermis, 252–253, 253*f*
female genitalia, 710–711
function, 256
general approach to physical examination, 261*b*
head-to-toe examination, 934, 934*f*
health history questions (skin care habits), 260*b*
inspection, 261–282
lesions. *See* Skin lesions
moisture, 283–284
Monk Skin Tone (MST) scale, 256*b*, 256*f*
older adult client, 892, 910–911, 910*b*, 912*b*
palpation, 283–286
pediatric client, 848–851
pressure injuries, 282*b*, 283*b*, 283*f*
reducing exposure to integumentary irritants, 261*b*
sebaceous glands, 254
self-examination, 281*b*, 282*f*
signs of abuse, 265*b*
subcutaneous tissue, 254
sunscreen/other protection tips, 281*b*
sweat glands, 254
tattoos, body piercings, scarification, 262*b*, 263*f*
temperature, 284–285
tenderness, 285
texture, 285
turgor, 285–286, 285*f*
USPSTF recommendation, 293*b*
wound evaluation, 262*b*
wound healing and scar formation, 256*b*
Skin, hair, and nails, 252–297
anatomy and physiology, 252–256
case study (lip lesion), 293–296
general approach to physical examination, 261*b*
hair. *See* Hair
health history, 257–260, 260*b*
nails. *See* Nails
older adult client, 892, 910–911, 910*b*, 912*b*
skin. *See* Skin
Skin cancer, 293*b*
Skin lesions, 268–281
ABCDE mnemonic, 279*b*
anatomical locations, 268*t*
arrangement of lesions, 269*f*
basal and squamous cell carcinoma, 280*b*
cancerous lesions, 280*b*
melanoma, 280–281, 280*b*, 280*f*
morphology, 270*f*, 271*f*
risk factors, 280*b*
sunscreen/other protection tips, 281*b*
Skin self-examination, 281*b*, 282*f*
Skin tags, 278, 278*f*
Skin turgor, 285–286, 285*f*
Skinfold thickness, 185, 185*f*
Skull, 298, 299*f*, 637
Sleep, 71–72, 902
Sleep apnea, 433
Slipped capital femoral epiphysis, 871
Small intestine, 535, 537
Smart stethoscope, 216*b*
Smegma, 744
Smell (olfactory sense), 209
Smoking cessation, 62*b*
Smooth muscle, 574
SMR. *See* Sexual maturity rating (SMR)
Snap, 491
Snellen chart, 326, 328*f*, 854
SOAP notes, 18, 941
SOC (Sense of Coherence Scale) Scale, 113*t*
Social contract or utility, and individual rights stage, 95*t*, 100
Social determinants of health (SDOH), 101, 125
Social distance, 25
Social history, 61–71
alcohol use, 61, 62*b*
characteristic patterns of daily living, 71
economic status, 70
education, 70
ethnic background, 71
functional health assessment, 71
hobbies and leisure activities, 69
home environment, 67–69
intimate partner violence (IPV), 64–65
military service, 70
recreational drug use, 63, 63*b*
religion, 70
roles and relationships, 71
sensitive topics, 64*b*
sexual practice, 65–66, 66*b*
stress, 69–70
tobacco use, 62–63, 62*b*
travel history, 67, 67*b*, 67*f*
Social phobia, 665*t*
Social system and conscience stage, 94*t*, 100
Sodium (Na), 164*t*
Soft palate, 357*f*, 359, 359*f*
Soft S_1, 491, 492*f*
Solar keratosis, 910–911
Solar lentigo, 910
Solitary thyroid nodule, 311, 312*f*
Somatic afferent fibers, 641
Somatic pain, 243
Sonorous wheeze, 450*t*
Spasm, 590*t*, 592
Spastic hemiplegia gait, 588*t*
Spasticity, 592
Spatial perception, 661–662
Speak Up campaign, 932*b*
Spector, Rachel, 134, 135*f*
Speculum, 707, 707*f*, 717*f*, 718*f*
Speech, 39–40, 224
Spermatic cord, 736*f*, 737
Spermatocele, 750, 750*f*
Spermatogenesis, 737
Sphenoid sinus, 357*f*
Spider angioma, 266, 266*f*
Spinal accessory nerve, 644*t*, 678
Spinal cord, 639–640, 639*f*
Spinal nerves, 640*f*, 643
Spinal shock, 684
Spine, 626–630
cervical, 597–599
herniated disc, 629–630*b*, 630*f*
kyphosis, 628, 628*f*, 629*f*
list, 628, 628*f*, 629
lordosis, 628, 628*f*
normal, 626
scoliosis, 626, 628, 628*f*, 629, 629*b*
Spinnbarkeit test, 699*b*
Spinothalamic tracts, 641, 642*f*
Spiritual assessment, 140–156, 901
actions to avoid, 151–152, 152*t*
assessment tools, 146
basic principles (general approach), 145, 146*b*
case study, 153–155
client history as source of information, 145
clues to client's spirituality, 147*b*
COVID-19, 152–153
cult, 142
definitions, 141
discussing religious/spiritual beliefs, 147*b*
dogma, 141
FICA tool, 146, 154–155
God, 142
harmful outcomes, 143–144
health effects of religion and spirituality, 143–144
hospital chaplain, 151
mobilizing client's spiritual resources, 150–151
monotheistic/polytheistic religions, 142
New Age movements, 142
nurse's role, 144
nursing interventions, 150*t*, 151–152
ongoing therapeutic relationship, 147
prayer, 146, 146*f*
praying with client, 149–150, 149*f*
purpose, 145
religion and spirituality in U.S., 140–141, 141*f*
religion/spirituality, distinguished, 142
resistance to, 147, 150*t*
showing respect/allowing clients to practice their religion, 148–149
signs of decrease in client's spiritual distress, 152
"Why Me?" question, 152*b*
Spleen, 506*f*, 507, 534*f*, 539, 556, 561
Splint, 631*b*
Splinter hemorrhage, 290, 290*f*
Sports
female athlete triad, 619*b*
injuries, 604*b*
preparticipation athletic evaluation, 942–943
relative energy deficiency in sport (RED-S), 619–620*b*
traumatic brain injury (TBI), 662*b*
Sputum, 424, 437–438, 438*t*
Squamocolumnar junction, 699
Squamous cell carcinoma (SCC)
generally, 279, 279*f*
older adult client, 911, 911*f*
physical examination, 378, 378*f*
right neck mass, 308*f*
risk factors, 280*b*

Standard Precautions, 199, 200*f*
Standing position, 208*f*
Stapedius, 355
Stapes, 355, 355*f*
Startle reflex, 876
Station, 681
Stature, 222
Staxyn, 758*b*
STEADI. *See* Stopping Elderly Accidents, Deaths & Injuries (STEADI)
Steatorrhea, 774*t*
Stenosis, 494
Stensen's ducts, 359, 359*f*, 381, 382
Steppage gait, 588*t*
Stepping reflex, 875, 875*f*
Stereognosis, 671, 671*f*
Stereophonic stethoscope, 216
Stereotyping, 129
Sternal angle, 420*b*
Sternocleidomastoid muscle, 299, 299*f*, 678, 678*f*
Sternum, 417–418
Stethophone, 216*b*
Stethoscope, 215–216, 215*f*, 216*b*, 216*f*
Stevens-Johnson syndrome, 276, 276*f*
Stiffness, 579
Stills, 867*t*
STIs. *See* Sexually transmitted infections (STIs)
Stomach, 534*f*, 535, 556
Stomach cancer, 555*b*
Stool types, 538*b*, 538*f*, 774*t*
Stopping Elderly Accidents, Deaths & Injuries (STEADI), 903
Stork bites, 849
Strabismus, 334, 334*f*
Strabismus screening, 855
Straight leg raising test, 629–630*b*, 630*f*
Stratum corneum, 253, 253*f*
Stratum germinativum, 252–253, 253*f*
Stratum granulosum, 253, 253*f*
Stratum lucidum, 253, 253*f*
Stratum spinosum, 253, 253*f*
Strawberry cervix, 718, 718*f*
Strawberry hemangioma, 266, 267*f*
Strawberry spots, 719
Streptococcal pharyngitis, 314, 386, 386*f*, 387–390
Stress, 69–70
Stress incontinence, 566*b*
Stress management, 73, 73*f*
Striae, 402, 549, 549*f*
Striae gravidarum, 785, 785*f*
Stridor, 450*t*, 863*b*
Stroke, 657*b*
Structural racism, 101
Structural scoliosis, 626, 628, 629*b*
Stupor, 659*t*
Stye, 332
Subacromial bursitis, 601
Subaortic stenosis, 477*t*
Subconjunctival hemorrhage, 338, 338*f*
Subculture, 125–127
Subcutaneous emphysema, 441
Subcutaneous mastectomy, 409*t*
Subcutaneous tissue, 254
Subdural space, 637, 638*f*
Subjective data, 7
Sublingual glands, 359, 359*f*
Subluxation, 591
Submaxillary glands, 359
Substance abuse. *See* Drug use/abuse
Subungual hematoma, 291, 292*f*
Sucking reflex, 874, 874*f*
Sudden infant death syndrome (SIDS), 831*b*
Suicide/suicidal ideation, 665, 665*b*, 668*b*
Sulcus terminalis, 359
Sulfur (S), 164*t*
Summation gallop, 492, 492*f*
Sunburn, 264
Sunscreen/other skin protection tips, 281*b*
Superego, 96
Superficial pain, 668–669
Superficial reflexes, 684–685
Supernumerary digits, 871
Supernumerary nipple, 393, 394*f*, 403
Supination, 576*t*
Supine hypotension, 787, 787*b*, 787*f*
Supine position, 208*f*
Supranuclear facial palsy, 676
Suprasternal notch, 420*b*
Surgical history, 53
Suture lines, 852
Sutures, 298
Swallowing problems, 648, 893
Swan neck deformity, 607, 607*f*
Sweat glands, 254
Symbols, 129, 129*f*
Sympathetic nervous system, 645, 645*t*
Synarthroses, 577*t*
Syncope, 508, 647
Syndactyly, 871
  fingers, 607, 607*f*
  toes, 622, 622*f*
Synovial joints, 577, 577*f*, 577*t*
Synthetic opioids, 249
Syphilitic chancre
  females, 710, 710*f*
  males, 745, 745*f*
Syphilitic glossitis, 380
System-specific health history, 76–77
Systemic lupus erythematosus, 274, 274*f*
Systole, 467, 467*f*, 478, 517*f*
Systolic ejection murmur, 866
Systolic murmur, 493, 495*t*
Systolic pressure, 235, 240*t*

T cells, 506, 507*f*
Tachycardia, 228, 491
Tachypnea, 226, 432, 434*f*
Tactile fremitus, 210, 442–443, 442*f*, 443*f*, 454*t*, 863
Tadalafil (Cialis), 758*b*
Tail of Spence, 393
Talar tilt test, 623*b*, 624*f*
Talipes equinovarus (clubfoot), 872, 872*f*
Talkativeness, extreme, 36
TandemHeart ventricular assist device, 486*b*
Tangential lighting, 209
Tanner staging. *See* Sexual maturity rating (SMR)
Tanner's Clinical Judgment Model, 6
Target heart rate (THR) zone, 468*b*
Tarsal plate, 320, 320*f*
Laryngotracheobronchitis, 863*b*
Tattoos, 262*b*, 263*f*
TB. *See* Tuberculosis (TB)
TBI. *See* Traumatic brain injury (TBI)
Teal Wand, 726*b*
Technology addiction, 69*b*
Teeth
  deciduous and permanent, 359*f*, 832, 832*f*
  dental caries, 384
  generally, 383–384, 860
  Hutchinson's incisors, 384, 384*f*
  incisors, 359, 359*f*
  meth mouth, 384, 384*f*
  molars, 359, 359*f*
  tooth numbering system, 359*b*, 359*f*
TEF. *See* Tracheoesophageal fistula (TEF)
Telangiectasia, 266, 266*f*
Telehealth, 43
Telenursing, 43
Temperature, 230–234
  axillary method, 231*t*, 233, 233*f*
  circadian rhythm, 230
  electronic thermometer method, 233
  Fahrenheit/Celsius scale, 230, 230*f*
  hyperthermia/hypothermia, 234
  measurement routes, 230–234
  mercury thermometers, 230*b*
  noncontact infrared method, 232*t*, 234, 234*f*
  normal range, 231–232*t*
  older adult client, 891, 909
  oral method, 231*t*, 232, 232*f*
  pediatric client, 844–845
  rectal method, 231*t*, 232–233
  sensory examination, 669
  temporal artery method, 232*t*, 233–234, 233*f*
  tympanic artery method, 232*t*, 233, 233*f*
  variables affecting body temperature, 230
Temporal arteritis, 305
Temporal artery thermometer, 232*t*, 233–234, 233*f*
Temporal lobe, 639*f*
Temporalis muscle, 674, 674*f*
Temporomandibular joint, 596, 596*f*, 597*f*
Tendons, 574
Tennis elbow, 603
Tensor tympani, 355
Terminal hair, 255, 287
Termination stage, 24
Testes, 735
Testicles, 735, 736*f*
Testicular cancer, 752, 754*b*
Testicular mass, 752, 752*f*
Testicular self-examination (TSE), 754*b*, 755*f*
Testicular torsion, 753, 753*b*, 753*f*
Testosterone, 737, 897
Tetanus, 675
Tetany, 590*t*
Tetrahydrocannabinol (THC), 878*b*
Tetralogy of Fallot, 479*t*
THC. *See* Tetrahydrocannabinol (THC)
The Health Wagon, 930–931
The Lawton Instrumental Activities of Daily Living Scale (IADL), 115*t*
Thenar eminence, 605
Therapeutic touch, 73*f*
Thermometer, 230–234. *See also* Temperature
Thiamine, 162*t*
Third-degree burn, 283, 284*f*
Thomas test, 614

Thompson squeeze test, 626*b*, 626*f*
Thoracic aneurysm, 510*t*
Thoracic dissection, 482*t*
Thoracic expansion, 441–442, 441*f*, 454*t*
Thoracic landmarks, 420*b*
Thoracic nerves, 640*f*
Thoracic tenderness, 441
Thoracolumbar system, 645
Thorax and lungs, 417–462
 alveoli, 421
 anatomy, 417–422
 breath sounds, 448–451, 455*t*
 bronchi, 421
 case study (COVID-19 and pneumonia), 458–461
 control of breathing, 423
 diaphragm, 422
 disorders/diseases. *See* Examination of thorax and lungs
 equipment, 428
 external respiration, 423
 forced expiratory volume (FEV), 455*b*
 health history, 423–426
 imaginary thoracic lines, 421*f*
 intercostal space (ICS), 419, 419*b*, 419*f*, 431–432
 internal respiration, 423
 landmarks, 420*b*
 lung auscultation practice, 452*b*
 lungs, 418*f*, 419, 420*f*, 421*f*
 maintaining respiratory health, 430*b*
 mediastinum, 421
 muscles of respiration, 422, 422*f*
 older adult client, 894–895, 915
 pediatric client, 833, 862–864
 physical examination. *See* Examination of thorax and lungs
 physiology, 422–423
 pleura, 420–421
 pregnant client, 786, 805
 preventing aspiration, 448–451, 455*t*
 respiratory assistive devices, 438–439*b*
 rib cage angles, 430–431, 431*f*, 453*t*
 ribs, 418, 419*f*
 risk factors of lung cancer, 437–438*b*
 sternum, 417–418
 USPSTF recommendations, 458*b*
 ventilation, 422–423
 voice sounds, 451–452, 455*t*
Thought process and content, 663–664
THR zone. *See* Target heart rate (THR) zone
3 + tonsils, 386, 386*f*
Thrills, 486, 486*f*, 487, 865
Throat. *See also* Ears, nose, mouth, and throat
 anatomy, 359
 cancer, 381*b*
 case study (streptococcal pharyngitis), 387–390
 chief complaint (health history), 362
 inspection, 385–386
 older adult client, 893–894, 914
Thrombophlebitis, 511*t*
Thrombus/embolus, 511*t*
Thrush, 379, 380*f*, 860, 860*f*
Thymus gland, 506, 506*f*
Thyroid adenoma, 311
Thyroid cancer, 312*b*
Thyroid disease, 311*t*
Thyroid gland
 anatomy, 299, 299*f*
 anterior approach to examination, 310–311, 310*f*
 auscultation, 312
 case study (thyroid nodule), 315–317
 hypothyroidism/hyperthyroidism, 311*t*
 inspection, 309–310
 palpation, 310–311, 310*f*
 posterior approach to examination, 310, 310*f*
 solitary thyroid nodule, 311, 312*f*
 thyroid cancer, 312*b*
Thyroid nodule, 315–317
TIA. *See* Transient ischemic attack (TIA)
TIBC. *See* Total iron-binding capacity (TIBC)
Tibiofemoral bones, 872
Tic, 590*t*
Tic douloureux, 675
Tinea barbae, 281, 281*f*
Tinea capitis, 288, 288*f*
Tinea corporis, 272, 272*f*
Tinea cruris, 748, 750
Tinea pedis, 272, 272*f*
Tinea versicolor, 271, 271*f*
Tinel sign, 609*b*, 610*f*
Tinnitus, 360–361
Tirzepatide, 183*b*
TLC. *See* Total lymphocyte count (TLC)
Tobacco use, 62–63, 62*b*, 80*b*
Toddlers, 104–105. *See also* Pediatric client
 calorie needs, 159*t*
 childhood fears, 830*b*
 cranial nerve function, 877
 developmental assessment tools, 112*t*
 developmental tasks, 105
 fontanel, 852
 genu valgum (knock-knee), 872
 heart, 833
 immunization schedule, 839*t*
 milestones, 104–105*t*
 nutrition, 168, 170*b*
 physical growth, 824
 pulse rate, 228*t*
 respiratory rate, 226*t*
 teeth, 832, 832*f*
 weight, 845
Toe abnormalities, 622, 622*f*
Tongue, 358, 379–380
Tonic neck reflex, 875, 875*f*
Tonic pupil, 342*t*
Tonsil stone, 386
Tonsillitis, 386, 386*f*, 387–390
Tonsils, 506*f*, 507
Tophus (tophi), 367, 367*f*, 593, 593*f*, 594, 594*f*
Torticollis, 309, 309*f*, 861
Torus mandibularis, 381, 382*f*
Torus palatinus, 384, 384*f*
Total anomalous pulmonary venous connection, 481*t*
Total iron-binding capacity (TIBC), 186
Total lymphocyte count (TLC), 187
Touching the client, 26*b*, 39
TPAL, 795*b*
Trace minerals, 163, 165*t*
Trachea, 418*f*, 421, 444
Tracheoesophageal fistula (TEF), 861
Tracheostomy, 437, 437*f*
Tracheostomy tube, 439*b*
Traditional nuclear family, 133, 134, 134*f*
Transcortical motor aphasia, 656*t*
Transcortical sensory aphasia, 656*t*
Transferrin, 186–187
Transgender individuals
 prostate cancer, 775
 transgender, defined, 38
 transgender men, 395*b*, 730*b*
 transgender women, 757*b*
Transient ischemic attack (TIA), 511*t*, 512*b*
Transillumination
 scrotum, 755*b*, 755*f*
 sinuses, 376*b*, 377*f*
 skull, 854*b*
Transitional developmental theories, 93
Transitional Impact Scale, 114*t*
Transmission-Based Precautions, 203, 204*f*
Transposition of the great arteries, 480*t*
Trapezius (trapezii), 299, 299*f*, 678, 678*f*
Traumatic brain injury (TBI), 662*b*
Travel history, 67, 67*b*, 67*f*
Travel medicine clinics, 67
Tremor, 590*t*, 647
Trench mouth, 383
Trendelenburg gait, 588*t*
Trendelenburg test, 523*b*, 612*b*
Triceps reflex, 683, 683*f*
Triceps skinfold (TSF), 184, 185, 185*f*
Trichomonas vaginitis, 713, 713*t*, 720*f*
Trichomoniasis, 725
Trichotillomania, 288, 288*f*
Tricuspid area, 483, 483*f*
 auscultation, 490–491, 492
 inspection, 485
 palpation, 487
Tricuspid atresia, 480*t*
Tricuspid regurgitation or insufficiency, 475*t*, 495*t*
Tricuspid stenosis, 475*t*, 495*t*
Tricuspid valve, 464–465
Trigeminal nerve, 644*t*, 673–675
Trigeminal neuralgia, 675
Triglycerides, 160, 186
Tripod position, 437, 437*f*
Trochlear nerve, 644*t*, 673
Trousseau sign, 604*b*
True ribs, 418
Truncus arteriosus, 481*t*
Trust vs. mistrust stage, 94*t*, 98
TSE. *See* Testicular self-examination (TSE)
TSF. *See* Triceps skinfold (TSF)
Tuberculosis (TB), 439–440*b*
Tumbling E vision chart, 328*f*, 854, 854*f*
Tumor, 270*f*
Tunica adventitia, 502
Tunica albuginea, 735, 736*f*
Tunica externa, 502
Tunica intima, 502
Tunica media, 502
Tunica vaginalis, 735, 736*f*
Tuning fork tests, 365
Turbinates, 356
Turner syndrome, 861
Tussive fremitus, 443
24-hr recall, 177
Two-parent households, 134
Two-point discrimination, 671–672, 671*f*
Tympanic membrane, 355, 355*f*, 369, 369*b*

Tympanic membrane perforation, 372*f*
Tympanic thermometer, 232*t*, 233, 233*f*
Tympanosclerosis, 370
Tympanostomy tubes, 369
Tympany, 213*t*
Tyndall effect, 253
Type 2 diabetes, 171
Tzanck test, 747

UIS. *See* Universal Intellectual Standards (UIS)
Ulcer, 271*f*
Ultraviolet light, 267*b*
Umami, 358, 359
Umbilical hernia, 550, 550*f*, 869, 869*f*
Umbilicus, 550
Underweight client, 192–195
Undescended testis, 753, 753*f*, 754
Unilateral anosmia, 672
Unilateral cataract, 341
United States
  cultural diversity, 122
  ethnic groups, 126
  LGBTQIA+ community, 126
  races, 126
  religion and spirituality, 140–141, 141*f*
  two-parent households, 134
Universal ethical principles stage, 95*t*, 100
Universal Intellectual Standards (UIS)
  accuracy, 4
  breadth, 5
  clarity, 4
  depth, 5
  fairness, 5
  logic, 5
  precision, 5
  relevance, 5
  significance, 5
Upper abdominal reflex, 684
Upper motor neuron lesions, 686*t*
Upper motor neurons, 641, 641*f*
Upper respiratory tract, 417
Uremic frost, 221
Ureter, 539
Ureteral stents, 551*b*
Urethra
  females, 697*f*
  males, 736–737, 736*f*
Urethral caruncle, 712, 712*f*
Urethral discharge, 739
Urethral meatus
  females, 696*f*, 712, 712*f*, 716
  males, 750–751, 751–752
Urge incontinence, 566*b*
Urinary bladder. *See* Bladder
Urinary diversions, 551*b*
Urinary incontinence, 542, 565, 565–566*b*, 566*t*
Urinary system
  older adult client, 896–897
  pediatric client, 834
  pregnant client, 788, 788*b*, 806–807
Urinary tract infection (UTI), 566–567*b*, 712
Urticaria, 278, 279*f*
Urticarial rash, 278, 278*f*
U.S. Preventive Services Task Force (USPSTF)
  breasts/breast screening, 400*t*, 412*b*
  cervical cancer screening, 723*t*
  developmental assessment tools, 114*t*
  grade A recommendations, 79. *See also* Grade A recommendations
  grade B recommendations, 79. *See also* Grade B recommendations
  grade C recommendations, 79
  grade D recommendations, 79
  grade E recommendations, 79
  IPV screening tools, 65
  preventive service guidelines, 79
USPSTF. *See* U.S. Preventive Services Task Force (USPSTF)
Uterine bleeding, 702
Uterine leiomyoma, 728*b*
Uterine prolapse, 716, 716*f*, 718
Uterine tube, 699, 699*f*
Uterus, 698, 728
UTI. *See* Urinary tract infection (UTI)
Utilitarianism, 929
Uvula, 359

V-A ECMO. *See* Veno-arterial extracorporeal membrane oxygenator (V-A ECMO)
v wave, 513, 515
Vagina, 697, 697*f*, 727
Vaginal adenosis, 719
Vaginal cancer, 721*b*
Vaginal discharge, 703, 713*t*
Vaginal infections, 713*b*
Vaginal introitus, 696*f*, 697, 713–714, 715
Vaginal speculum, 707, 707*f*, 717*f*, 718*f*
Vaginal wall, 726
Vagus nerve, 644*t*, 677–678
Valgus stress test, 620*b*, 620*f*
Value orientations, 129–130, 130*t*
Values, 128
Vaping, 447*b*
Vardenafil (Levitra), 758*b*
Vardenafil HCl (Staxyn), 758*b*
Varicella, 275, 275*f*
Varicocele, 750, 750*f*
Varicose veins, 522*b*, 522*f*, 523*b*, 711
Varus stress test, 620*b*, 620*f*
VAS. *See* Visual Analog Scale (VAS)
Vas deferens, 736, 736*f*
Vasculitis, 511*t*
Veins, 503, 505*f*
Vellus hair, 255, 287
Veno-arterial extracorporeal membrane oxygenator (V-A ECMO), 486*b*
Venous filling time (VFT), 523*b*
Venous hum, 552, 867*t*
Venous insufficiency, 521*t*
Venous star, 266, 267*f*
Venous ulceration, 520, 520*f*
Ventral hernia, 550, 550*f*
Ventral horn, 640, 645*f*
Ventricular aneurysm, 475*t*
Ventricular bigeminy, 227
Ventricular septal defect (VSD), 478*t*
Venules, 503
Veracity, 929
Vermiform appendix, 539
Vermilion zone, 358, 358*f*
Vermis, 639
Vernix caseosa, 831, 851, 851*f*
Verruca vulgaris, 278, 278*f*
Vertebra prominens, 299, 420*b*
Vertebrosternal ribs, 418
Vertex presentation, 810*f*, 812
Vertical septa, 464
Vertigo, 648, 677
Vesicle, 270*f*
Vesicular breath sound, 448, 449*f*, 449*t*
Vestibule, 355*f*, 356, 696, 696*f*
VFT. *See* Venous filling time (VFT)
Viagra, 758*b*
Vibration sense, 670–671, 670*f*
Vincent stomatitis, 383
Virchow node, 314
Virchow triad, 522*b*
Visceral afferent fibers, 641
Visceral pain, 243, 544*t*
Visceral pericardium, 464, 464*f*
Visceral peritoneum, 534
Visceral pleura, 420
Vision. *See* Eye
Visual acuity, 326–329
Visual Analog Scale (VAS), 247, 247*f*
Visual field defects, 330*f*
Visual fields, 329, 330*f*
Visual inspection, 209
Visual pathway, 322, 323*f*
Visually impaired client, 39
Vital signs, 225–241, 830, 844–845. *See also* individual elements
  blood pressure, 234–241
  general approach to vital sign assessment, 225*b*
  older adult client, 891, 907–910
  pulse, 226–229
  respiration, 225–226, 226*b*
  temperature, 230–234
Vitamin A, 161*t*
Vitamin B_1, 162*t*
Vitamin B_2, 162*t*
Vitamin B_6, 162*t*
Vitamin B_{12}, 162*t*, 190
Vitamin C, 163*t*
Vitamin D, 161*t*, 189–190, 624*b*
Vitamin D 25-OH, 190
Vitamin D deficiency, 190
Vitamin E, 161*t*
Vitamin K, 162*t*
Vitamins, 161, 161*t*, 162–163*t*
Vitiligo, 264, 265*f*
Vitreous humor, 322
Voice sounds, 451–452, 455*t*
Voice-whisper test, 364–365
Vomiting, 540–541
von Recklinghausen disease, 281, 281*f*
VSD. *See* Ventricular septal defect (VSD)
Vulva, 710–711
Vulvar cancer, 721*b*

Waddle of pregnancy, 789
Waist circumference, 183
Waist-to-hip ratio, 183
Walker, 631*b*, 632*f*
Wart, 278, 278*f*
Water, 166, 166*b*
Water-hammer pulse, 517*f*
Water-soluble vitamins, 161, 161*t*
WE CAN!, 169*b*
Weak pulse, 517*f*
Weber test, 365, 365*f*
Wedge breast palpation, 408*f*

Weight
  anthropometric measurements, 181–182
  BMI, 171, 182–183
  case study (underweight client), 192–195
  eating disorders, 170, 171*f*
  gain/loss, 175
  obesity. *See* Obesity
  older adult client, 910
Weight-bearing status, 584*b*
Weight cycling, 171
Wernicke aphasia, 656*t*
Wernicke area, 639*f*
Wet prep (saline mount), 725
Wharton's ducts, 359, 359*f*
Wheal, 270*f*
Wheelchair, 631*b*
Wheeze, 450*t*
Wheezing, 864
Whiff test, 725
Whispered pectoriloquy, 452
White pulp, 507
White reflex, 345
Whole genome sequencing, 60
Whooping cough video, 436
"Why Me?" question, 152*b*
Wickham's striae, 382
Witchcraft, 131
Women. *See* Females
Wong-Baker FACES Pain Rating Scale, 248, 248*f*, 840
Wood's lamp, 267*b*
Working stage, 24
Wound evaluation, 262*b*
Wound healing and scar formation, 256*b*
Wrinkling, 892
Wrists and hands, 605–610
  carpal tunnel syndrome, 609*b*, 610*b*, 610*f*
  case study (numbness in hands and feet), 689–693
  De Quervain tenosynovitis, 610, 610*f*
  finger anomalies, 607, 607*f*
  grip strength, 608*b*, 608*f*
  physical examination, 605–609

x descent, 513
Xanthelasma, 333, 333*f*
Xanthoma striata palmaris, 263
Xerosis, 284
Xerostomia, 382
Xiphoid process, 418

y descent, 514
Yellow marrow, 574
Yin and yang, 131
Yo-yo dieting, 171
Young adults, 108–109
  calorie needs, 159*t*
  developmental assessment tools, 113*t*, 114*t*
  developmental tasks, 109
  nutrition, 171–172
  socializing (hookah/Arabic tea), 133*f*

Zinc (Zn), 165*t*
Zonules, 322
Zosteriform lesions, 269*f*